Primary Care of Women: A Guide for Midwives and Women's Health Providers

Barbara Hackley, MS, CNM
Assistant Professor
Yale University School of Nursing
New Haven, Connecticut
Assistant Director of Women's Health
South Bronx Health Center for Children and Families
Montefiore Medical Center, Albert Einstein College of Medicine
Bronx, New York

Jan M. Kriebs, CNM, MSN, FACNM
Assistant Professor
Department of Obstetrics, Gynecology, and Reproductive Sciences
Director of Midwifery
University of Maryland
Baltimore, Maryland

Mary Ellen Rousseau, MS, CNM, FACNM
Clinical Professor and Director
Yale University School of Nursing
Midwifery Specialty
New Haven, Connecticut

JONES AND BARTLETT PUBLISHERS
Sudbury, Massachusetts
BOSTON   TORONTO   LONDON   SINGAPORE

World Headquarters

Jones and Bartlett Publishers	Jones and Bartlett Publishers Canada	Jones and Bartlett Publishers International
40 Tall Pine Drive	6339 Ormindale Way	Barb House, Barb Mews
Sudbury, MA 01776	Mississauga, Ontario L5V 1J2	London W6 7PA
978-443-5000	CANADA	UK
info@jbpub.com		
www.jbpub.com		

Jones and Bartlett's books and products are available through most bookstores and online booksellers. To contact Jones and Bartlett Publishers directly, call 800-832-0034, fax 978-443-8000, or visit our website, www. jbpub.com. Substantial discounts on bulk quantities of Jones and Bartlett's publications are available to corporations, professional associations, and other qualified organizations. For details and specific discount information, contact the special sales department at Jones and Bartlett via the above contact information or send an email to special sales@jbpub.com.

The authors, editor, and publisher have made every effort to provide accurate information. However, they are not responsible for errors, omissions, or for any outcomes related to the use of the contents of this book and take no responsibility for the use of the products described. Treatments and side effects described in this book may not be applicable to all patients; likewise, some patients may require a dose or experience a side effect that is not described herein. The reader should confer with his or her own physician regarding specific treatments and side effects. Drugs and medical devices are discussed that may have limited availability controlled by the Food and Drug Administration (FDA) for use only in a research study or clinical trial. The drug information presented has been derived from reference sources, recently published data, and pharmaceutical research data. Research, clinical practice, and government regulations often change the accepted standard in this field. When consideration is being given to use of any drug in the clinical setting, the healthcare provider or reader is responsible for determining FDA status of the drug, reading the package insert, reviewing prescribing information for the most up-to-date recommendations on dose, precautions, and contraindications, and determining the appropriate usage for the product. This is especially important in the case of drugs that are new or seldom used.

Library of Congress Cataloging-in-Publication Data
Hackley, Barbara.
   Primary care of women : a guide for midwives and women's health
providers / Barbara Hackley, Jan M. Kriebs, Mary Ellen Rousseau.
     p. ; cm.
   Includes bibliographical references and index.
   ISBN 0-7637-1650-2 (pbk.)
   1. Midwives. 2. Primary care (Medicine) 3. Women's health ser-
vices.   I. Kriebs, Jan M. II. Rousseau, Mary Ellen. III. Title.
   [DNLM: 1. Primary Health Care. 2. Midwifery. 3. Women's Health.
W 84.6 H122p 2006]
RG950.H33 2006
618.2′0233—dc22

2005023402

6048

Production Credits
Acquisitions Editor: Kevin Sullivan
Associate Editor: Amy Sibley
Production Director: Amy Rose
Associate Production Editor: Kate Hennessy
Senior Marketing and Project Manager: Emily Ekle
Composition: Auburn Associates, Inc.
Manufacturing and Inventory Coordinator: Amy Bacus
Cover Design: Timothy Dziewit
Printing and Binding: Malloy, Inc.
Cover Printing: Malloy, Inc

Printed in the United States of America
10 09 08 07 06   10 9 8 7 6 5 4 3 2 1

Contents

Chapter 18: The Abdomen: Kidney, Bladder, and Reproductive Problems 679

By Diane Hodgman, Edie McConaughey, and Diane Angelini

Chapter 19: Breast Health and Disease 719

By Mary Ellen Rousseau

Contributors

Todd Ambrosia, PhD, MSN, CRNP
Family Nurse Practitioner, Assistant Professor, and
    Director
Division of Family Primary Care
School of Nursing
University of Maryland
Baltimore, Maryland

Diane Angelini, EdD, CNM, FACNM, FAAN
Clinical Associate Professor
Department of OB-Gyn
Brown University
Director, Nurse Midwifery
Women and Infants' Hospital
Providence, Rhode Island

Melissa D. Avery, CNM, PhD, FACNM
Associate Professor and Director
Nurse-Midwifery Program
School of Nursing
University of Minnesota
Minneapolis, Minnesota

Karyn D. Baum, MD, FACP
Assistant Professor of Medicine
School of Medicine
University of Minnesota
Minneapolis, Minnesota

Margaret W. Beal, PhD, CNM
Associate Professor and Director
Graduate Entry Prespecialty in Nursing
Yale University School of Nursing
New Haven, Connecticut

Diane Berry, PhD, CANP
Assistant Professor
School of Nursing
The University of North Carolina at Chapel Hill
Chapel Hill, North Carolina

Mary Ellen Bouchard, CNM, MS
Midwife Consultant
Arlington, Virginia

Barbara Hackley, MS, CNM
Assistant Professor
Yale University School of Nursing
New Haven, Connecticut
Assistant Director of Women's Health
South Bronx Health Center for Children and
    Families
Montefiore Medical Center, Albert Einstein
    College of Medicine
Bronx, New York

Diane Hodgman, MS, CNM
Nurse Midwife
Clinical Teaching Associate
Brown University School of Medicine
Providence, Rhode Island

Ruth E. Johnson, MSN, MPA, CNM, CS
Private Practice in Psychotherapy and
    Psychopharmacology
Wellesley, Massachusetts

Deborah Karsnitz, MSN, CNM
Course Coordinator
Frontier School of Midwifery and Family
    Nursing
Lexington, Kentucky

Thomas J. Kidder, LCSW, MSW, ACSW, SAP
Associate Professor
Western Connecticut State University
Danbury, Connecticut
Director of the HIV/AIDS Division
Hill Health Corporation
New Haven, Connecticut

Jan M. Kriebs, CNM, MSN, FACNM
Assistant Professor
Department of Obstetrics, Gynecology, and
    Reproductive Sciences
Director of Midwifery
University of Maryland
Baltimore, Maryland

Julie Marfell, ND, BC, FNP
Chairperson, Department of Family Nursing
Frontier School of Midwifery and Family
    Nursing
Lexington, Kentucky

Edie McConaughey, CNM, MSN
Nurse Midwife
Department of Nurse Midwifery
Women and Infants' Hospital
Providence, Rhode Island

Patricia A. Paluzzi, CNM, DrPH
President and Chief Executive Officer
Healthy Teen Network
Washington, DC

Molly Fey Persinger, FNP-C, MSN
East Hartford Community Health Center
East Hartford, Connecticut

Valerie A. Roe, CNM, MS
Assistant Professor
Midwifery Education Program
SUNY Downstate Medical Center
Brooklyn, New York

Mary Ellen Rousseau, MS, CNM, FACNM
Clinical Professor and Director
Yale University School of Nursing
Midwifery Specialty
New Haven, Connecticut

Karen A. Stemler, MS, APRN, FNP-BC
Family Nurse Practitioner
Yale University School of Nursing
New Haven, Connecticut

Kimberly Updegrove, CNM, MSN, MPH
Clinical Coordinator
Mother's Milk Bank at Austin
Austin, Texas

Diane C. Viens, DNSc, CFNP, FAANP
Associate Professor of Nursing
Yale University School of Nursing
New Haven, Connecticut

Donna Vivio, MS, MPH, CNM, FACNM
Director
Maternal & Child Health Center of Excellence
JHPIEGO
Baltimore, Maryland

Kimberly Whitfill, MS, CNM
New York, New York

Eileen Barrett Wyner, MS, APRN, BC
Newton Wellesley Hospital
Adjunct Faculty, Boston University
School of Public Health Maternal Child Health
  Program
Newton, Massachusetts

Preface

In recognition of the pivotal role that midwives have in the provision of comprehensive, integrated, and holistic care to women, the American College of Nurse Midwives released its first statement designating nurse–midwives as primary care providers in 1997. Over the intervening years, it has become increasingly clear that textbooks currently available in primary care were insufficient to meet the needs of the profession. And as educators, we were frustrated by having to use texts that did not reflect midwifery practice and were not designed to meet the needs of our students. This text, *Primary Care of Women: A Guide for Midwives and Women's Health Providers*, is an important addition to the field. It is the first textbook to specifically address primary care in midwifery practice and will be useful to midwives already in practice, who desire an up-to-date compilation of primary care content, and midwifery students, who also need guidance in understanding how to incorporate primary care fits into practice. Women's health providers, who practice primarily in obstetrics and gynecology, also experience many of these same frustrations and will find this text useful.

The most essential element of *Primary Care of Women* is that it presents primary care material in a manner that matches midwifery scope of practice and will provide midwives the background they need in order to meet the health care needs of their clients. Meeting the primary health care needs of women requires knowledge about health promotion, screenings, immunizations, and environmental health, as well as lifestyle changes needed to prevent long-term health problems. It also requires being able to manage a wide range of infections and mild presentations of chronic conditions, and an understanding of when, where, and to whom to refer women with more complicated clinical presentations.

Users of this text should find the organization particularly helpful. Each chapter begins with a discussion of common symptoms and suggestions on how to evaluate various clinical presentations and concludes with a discussion of the management of specific conditions. Each chapter also discusses how management of these conditions is affected by pregnancy. Easy-to-use tables summarize diagnostic possibilities, treatment recommendations, and other key points, and are found throughout each chapter, making information easy to retrieve.

Because many midwives and women's health providers care predominantly for younger reproductive-aged women, they have the unique opportunity to help women adopt healthier lifestyle behaviors early enough to prevent chronic conditions, such as cardiovascular disease, diabetes, and cancer, which are leading causes of death and disability in women. They also have the skills and ability to help women, with already established health conditions, better manage their care. Our hope is that this text will help us, as a profession, more effectively "be with women across the lifespan."

Acknowledgments

While it is impossible to thank everyone whose support has made the "birth" of this text possible, we would be remiss if we did not extend special thanks to at least some of those whose help and encouragement were most critical to the completion of these text.

A special loving thank you to my husband, Tom Baker, whose universal good cheer and positive energy gave me encouragement when I most needed it, to my older daughter Kai, whose artistic eye recognized the diversity of women cared for by midwives and captured this diversity in pictures which grace sections of this text, and to my younger daughter Emma who, with a maturity and generosity of spirit beyond her years, gave me the time I needed to write and edit.

I also want to acknowledge with great gratitude my fellow faculty of Yale University School of Nursing, in particular Heather Reynolds, Sara Gottlieb, Terri Clark, and Saras Vedum, who graciously covered many of my academic responsibilities while I was working on this text, and in particular my co-authors, Jan Kriebs and Mary Ellen Rousseau, for their vision, flexibility, and willingness to "roll with the punches"—without them, this text would not be possible.

Lastly I would like to thank all of my students whose quest for excellence was the impetus for this text.

- Barbara Hackley

This work is my thank you to all the women who have trusted their health to me over the years, believing that I will care as much about their general well-being as I do their reproductive health. It could not have been completed without the support of my department, and particularly the midwifery division—Jenifer Fahey, Jennifer Kaye, Rachel Lovett, Courtney Marshall, and Kathy O'Brien. And finally, thank you, David, for understanding how important this is to me.

- Jan M. Kriebs

I would like to acknowledge the loving support and encouragement, for working on this project, as well as many others, from my family—Tom, my husband, and my children, Aaron, Shannon, Patrick, and Kate—who understand what it means to be a midwife. Additionally, I would like to thank my fellow faculty and my patients—from whom I have learned and continue to learn so much.

- Mary Ellen Rousseau

Chapter 1

Defining Primary Care

Jan M. Kriebs

Healthy women may be well served by having as their primary contact with the health system a midwife focused on health maintenance, age-appropriate screening, and patient education.[1]

Primary care has been described in many ways: by provider type, by specialty, and by care provided. The most comprehensive definition was developed by the Institute of Medicine's (IOM) Committee on the Future of Primary Care in 1994:

"Primary care is the provision of integrated, accessible health care services by clinicians who are accountable for addressing a large majority of personal health care needs, developing a sustained partnership with patients, and practicing in the context of family and community."[2]

In explicating this definition, the IOM avoided specifying the type of provider or location of service required to provide primary care. Instead, the statement emphasized characteristics of clinicians and systems, such as the ability to provide care that addresses health and social needs as well as illness management, cultural competence, and ability to work in the context of an individual's social network. Structural aspects of care such as the provision or coordination of care for most of an individual's needs, acting as a point of entry to the health care system, and persistence of relationships over time were also emphasized.[2]

The importance of identifying oneself, or one's profession, as able to offer primary care services can easily be seen in the economic consequences of direct patient access as opposed to requirements for referral or restrictions on authority to treat. For clinicians such as midwives and other women's health practitioners, the recognized ability to treat an expanded range of conditions affects state and institutional scope of practice, prescriptive authority, third party reimbursement, and a host of other pragmatic business survival factors. A small study published in 2002 indicated that midwives identified lack of reimbursement, institutional policies, state laws, and public perception of scope of care as barriers to their providing primary care.[3]

Midwives as Primary Care Providers

Regardless of the credentialing or financial benefits that might accrue from identification as primary care clinicians, the traditional scope of midwifery (maternity cycle care) did not meet the definition. Whether midwives could reasonably act in this role was addressed by the American College of Nurse-Midwives (ACNM) in the position statement entitled, "Certified Nurse Midwives and Certified Midwives as Primary Care Providers/Case Managers" as early as 1992.[4] Appropriate populations for midwifery primary care were identified as healthy women and newborns, and the focus on health maintenance was emphasized. The Core Competencies for the Practice of Midwifery,[5] the document defining the scope of basic midwifery education, was revised in 1997 to include the knowledge and skills required to assess, diagnose, and treat conditions beyond the maternity cycle and well-women's gynecologic concerns.

Clinicians whose focus is on women's health care are often de facto primary care providers. Many healthy women choose to see their gynecologic provider for primary care on a regular basis, where the routine of an annual breast and pelvic examination establishes an ongoing relationship. Midwives already provide health screening, preventive health recommendations, and counseling about lifestyle changes to women. In addition, during pregnancy, many clinicians defer to the obstetric provider for the management of many health concerns probably because the "extra patient" complicates choices of therapy or medication. For essentially healthy women—the core group of patients who see midwives—conditions such as infections, mild or stable presentations of chronic conditions, immunizations, and symptomatic visits are among issues within the scope of independent midwifery practice to be addressed when the midwife is the primary provider. Women with significant medical diagnoses may still seek out a women's health provider for gynecologic care in addition to their primary care provider. For midwives, the ability to recognize medical problems, determine whether the plan of care is being followed and is effective, and make appropriate referrals within an integrated system of care remains a key function.

Midwives and the Provision of Primary Care

A key component of primary care is health maintenance. This is accomplished in several ways: through counseling and education to decrease lifestyle risks and promote health, disease prevention, and regular general health care examinations. Murphy[6] reported that for gynecologic patients seen by midwives, blood pressure evaluation and assessment of medication use were common; cholesterol assessment and determination of rubella immunity were provided by more than half of the clinicians. Those services provided to the fewest women included other immunizations. About half of the midwives asked women about other sources of primary care. Midwives identified lifestyle and psychosocial issues as counseling issues commonly addressed in their practice. The counseling services least often reported as provided included injury prevention, seat belt use, and work-related risks.[6]

A 1993 survey by Scupholme and Carr identified obesity, anemia, and upper respiratory and gastrointestinal infections as primary care diagnoses managed by more than 80% of midwives.[7] **Figure** 1-1 is a more comprehensive summary of practice in this sample.

Midwives surveyed by Stuart and Oshio[3] most commonly reported that their formal education included material related to acute respiratory, gastrointestinal, and genitourinary problems; and hematologic and metabolic conditions. Knowledge of behavioral, psychosocial, and sexual conditions was also reported by a large majority of the respondents. In each case, a somewhat smaller percentage managed these conditions independently.

Task analysis surveys, performed by the ACNM Certification Council to sample the current clinical content of midwifery practice, have been used to identify trends in practice. This information is included as the professional certifying examination is revised to reflect current practice. The results of the most recent task analysis, published in 2002,[8] surveyed midwives certified since 1995. Midwives in this group were the first for whom primary care was considered "basic practice." Aspects of primary care identified in prior analyses as frequently performed tasks within the maternity cycle and now identified as independently managed in primary care were: anemia, backache, constipation, and urinary tract infection. Other primary care tasks frequently managed independently according to the 2002 survey included ear infections, fungal infections (tinea), indigestion, insomnia, and oral herpes. As can be seen, midwives have brought forward knowledge that has been used to manage health problems during

Figure 1-1 Percentage of midwives who identify and manage selected health care problems.

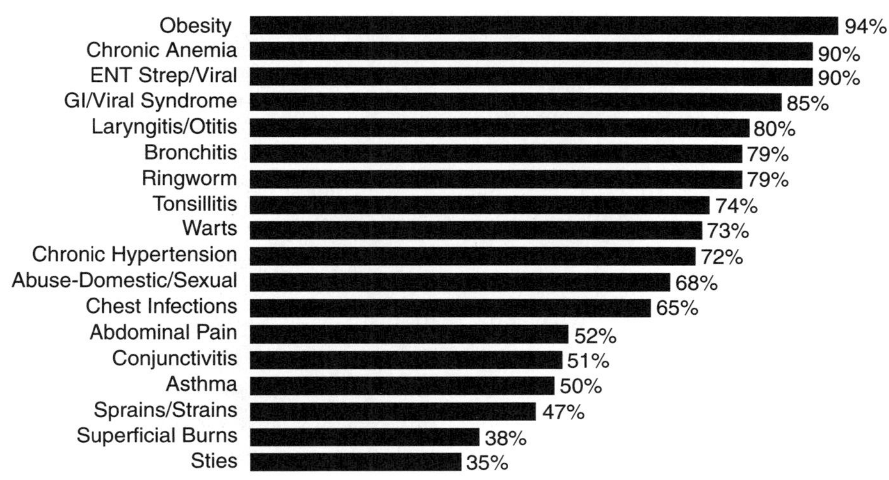

Source: Scupholme A, Carr KC. CNMs and primary care: Practice models and types of services. *Quickening* 1993;24(6):14. Reprinted by permission of the American College of Nurse-Midwives.

pregnancy to support the provision of primary care in their practices.

Common Health Problems in Primary Care

Reviewing the commonly identified problems, screening tests, and counseling during primary care visits helps to establish a basis for deciding when and to whom midwives can offer primary care services. Approximately 3004 office visits per 1000 persons occur every year.[9] Women are seen more frequently than men, whites than blacks, and elderly women than young women (excluding pregnancy).[10] On average, women see a primary care clinician 4.6 times per year.[9] Approximately 40% of visits by women are for acute care, 30% for management of a chronic condition, and 23% for preventive care.[11]

The federal government regularly reports on common diagnoses seen in ambulatory care. The National Ambulatory Medical Care Survey reports comprehensive access and diagnosis data every five years as well as yearly summaries.[10] These reports help identify the "substantial majority" of health problems a primary care clinician should be able to identify and manage or refer appropriately. **Table 1-1** shows common diagnoses reported for visits by women.

Among the services provided during office visits, blood pressure evaluation is by far the most common. Other tests ordered with some frequency include urinalysis, complete blood count, Papanicolau (Pap) smears, pregnancy testing, and cholesterol.[9] **Table 1-2** lists the most common topics for counseling. Virtually all of these are topics that midwives regularly encounter.

Finally, medications frequently prescribed or advised during office visits can be grouped for

Table 1-1 COMMON REASONS FOR VISITS TO AMBULATORY MEDICAL OFFICES BY WOMEN IN 2002

Primary Diagnosis	Percentage of All Visits
Essential hypertension	5.4
Normal pregnancy	3.3
Acute upper respiratory infection	3.1
Arthropathies, related disorders	2.8
General medical examination	2.5
Diabetes mellitus	2.3
Spinal disorders	2.3
Gynecologic examination	2.2
Rheumatism, other than back	1.9
Otitis media and Eustachian tube disorders	1.6
Chronic sinusitis	1.6
Allergic rhinitis	1.7
Malignant neoplasms	1.5
Asthma	1.5
Other heart disease	1.2
Acute pharyngitis	1.1
Lipid metabolism disorder	1.1
Ischemic heart disease	0.8

Source: Adapted from Cherry DK, Woodwell DA. National ambulatory medical care survey: 2002 survey. *Advance data from vital and health statistics,* No. 328. Hyattsville, MD: National Center for Health Statistics; June 5, 2002.

identification. Vaccines and antisera are the most commonly prescribed, followed by nonsteroidal analgesics, antihistamines, antihypertensives, and anti-asthma medications.[10] Data including only women show non-narcotic analgesics, antidepressants, and hormones to be the leading prescriptions.[9]

While the preceding data identify a number of conditions that preclude the midwife or other

Table 1-2 OFFICE-BASED PATIENT COUNSELING

Topic	Frequency (% of visits)
Diet	15.3
Exercise	11.1
Breast self exam	4.2
Stress	2.9
Mental health	2.8
Family planning	2.8
Tobacco	2.7
Injury prevention	1.8
Skin cancer	1.7
HIV/STD	1.3

women's health clinicians from acting as the primary source of medical care (e.g., insulin dependent diabetics need endocrinologist supervision), these women can be identified on history and physical examination, and then referred as necessary. Far more women need health education, preventive services and screening, and general examinations that fall well within the midwife's scope of practice.

Disparities in Health Care

Having looked at common components of primary care visits, midwives must also consider how disparities in health and access to health care can affect practice. Disparities in services sought and provided can be found across ethnic groups, age groups, rural versus urban locations, and economic strata. The 2002 report from the IOM, *Unequal Treatment: Confronting Racial and Ethnic Disparities in Health Care,*[11] documents the significant disparities across racial lines in the United States. One difficulty in studying the disparities found between racial and cultural groups is that U.S. studies tend to use race as a marker for class or socioeconomic status.[12] Within racially and ethnically defined groups, those with less education, lower incomes, and working class jobs fare more poorly.

The first National Healthcare Disparities Report noted that, "there are complicated interrelationships between race, ethnicity, and socioeconomic status that may result in healthcare disparities"[13, (p.8)]. As an initial evaluation of the state of health care disparities, they offered seven key findings to their targeted audience of policy, clinical, and community leaders:

1. Inequality in quality persists.
2. Disparities come at a personal and societal price.
3. Differential access may lead to disparities in quality.
4. Opportunities to provide preventive care are frequently missed.
5. Knowledge of why disparities exist is limited.
6. Improvement is possible.
7. Data limitations hinder targeted improvements.

Anyone who is interested in improving health care equity should consider these steps in evaluating their own clinical practice and ask questions such as: Have I asked all of my patients about substance abuse? About violence? About immunizations? How can I make my practice more accessible to women in the community? Am I treating my patients with as much respect as I would want to be treated?

Although the public perception of midwives is closely tied to birth and to care of normal women, since the earliest days of Frontier Nursing Service, American midwives have cared for women at risk from poor nutrition, poverty, and other socioeconomic problems. A 1998 survey reported that midwives continue to care for a population that is disproportionately adolescent, of color, immigrant, and poor.[14] As midwives continue to provide care to underserved women, it is important to be aware that the midwife is, and can be, the primary health care provider for many women. Because midwives are skilled at being "with women," they can evaluate the needs of women under their care, provide high quality services, and refer women requiring more in-depth care to the appropriate consultants.

Seventy percent of U.S. mortality is the result of chronic diseases. Monitoring for causes of death from chronic diseases uses indicators linked to cancer, cardiovascular disease, diabetes, asthma, renal disease, and osteoporosis. Lifestyle factors including nutrition, exercise, tobacco and alcohol use, oral health, and the "overarching" factors of poverty, education, and insurance status are also followed for their contribution to the development of diseases.[15]

Causes of death can be viewed in two ways, and most people are used to the report of disease states (**Table 1-3**). However, another way to consider the burden of disease is to show the contribution of factors that promote disease. The information on actual causes of death is based on lifestyle and environmental factors that precipitate disease or are directly responsible for death. **Table 1-4** includes all adults of either gender and any racial group.

One example of educational needs to prevent long-term morbidity and mortality can be found in heart disease, which is the cause of 29% of deaths among American women. Women are both under-diagnosed and under-treated for heart disease. Studies have found that women regularly underestimate the risk of heart disease as opposed to the risk of breast cancer as a health problem.[19]

In addition to the mortality from chronic disease, ongoing morbidity must be considered. According to the Centers for Disease Control and Prevention (CDC), more than 10% of all Americans live with a chronic, disabling health condition. While life expectancies for women are higher than for men, elderly women are more likely to be disabled.[20] Heart disease, diabetes, and breast cancer all are more common among women of color than among whites.[21]

The REACH 2010 Risk Factor Study for 2001–2002 found that although more minorities (African American, Hispanic, Asian Pacific Islander, and Native American) reported poor health than whites, they did not access health care because of cost.[22] Both educational levels and income were lower for minorities than for the average of the area being surveyed. However, the health risk factors and access to care varied both between populations and between communities. Outreach and intervention strategies need to be tailored to each community, just as health care interventions are targeted to the individual to be most effective.

Cultural Competence in Practice

Simply knowing about disparities in health access and health care is not enough to make one an effective provider. Awareness of and respect for the diversity among women can help remove a common barrier to care. Culture has been defined as "a socially transmitted design for living which includes traditional values, beliefs, rituals, and behaviors."[23] Within groups there is diversity and change over time; cultures are not

Table 1-3 LEADING CAUSES OF DEATH AND ACTUAL CAUSES OF DEATH IN THE UNITED STATES, 2000[16,17]

Leading cause of death*	Percentage (of all deaths) (%)	Actual cause(s) of death[†]	Percentage (of all deaths) (%)
Heart disease	30	Tobacco	18.1
Cancer	23	Poor diet, physical inactivity	16.6
Stroke	7	Alcohol consumption	3.5
Chronic lower-respiratory disease	5	Microbial agents (e.g., influenza, pneumonia)	3.1
Unintentional injuries	4	Toxic agents (e.g., pollutants, asbestos)	2.3
Diabetes	3	Motor vehicles	1.8
Pneumonia/influenza	3	Firearms	1.2
Alzheimer's disease	2	Sexual behavior	0.8
Kidney disease	2	Illicit drug use	0.7

Sources: *Miniño AM, Arias E, Kochanek KD, Murphy SL, Smith BL. Deaths: final data for 2000. *National Vital Statistics Reports.* 2002;50(15):1–120.
[†]Mokdad AH, Marks JS, Stroup DF, Gerberding JL. Actual causes of death in the United States, 2000. *JAMA.* 2004;291 (10):1238–1246.

monolithic. Dunn[24] describes the characteristics of any culture as dynamic, shared, learned, and integrated. Other authors have suggested that health care providers form a culture based on a common set of knowledge and behaviors, including a use of language that is not common in the community,[25] and that medicine sees itself as culture-free, while identifying anyone with a different perspective as being "cultural."[26]

Cultural competence is the skill of learning and appreciating cultural differences and similarities between groups, and being able to act on that understanding. Nunez[27] suggested that the term *cross-cultural efficacy* is more appropriate than *cultural competence*, because it represents an understanding of equalities between cultures. Whether one uses efficacy or competence as a goal, the first barrier for many health care providers is recognizing that persons from different communities have different practices and belief systems, and that their reality, their truth, is based in those practices and beliefs. Lack of understanding on the part of the clinician is a barrier to care, both because it decreases the chance that data are collected, and because the patients can identify this as bias against their cultural or racial identity.

It has been demonstrated that race, education, source of care (defined as having a regular provider), and other variables all play a role in the patient's perception of bias from his or her providers, and that racial identity is a more powerful factor when asking about system bias. Regardless of education or financial status, nonwhite groups tended to perceive system bias

Table 1-4 LEADING CAUSES OF DEATH, WOMEN ONLY[18]

All Races, Females	Percent*
1. Diseases of the heart (heart disease)	29.9
2. Malignant neoplasms (cancer)	21.8
3. Cerebrovascular diseases (stroke)	8.4
4. Chronic lower-respiratory diseases	5.1
5. Diabetes mellitus (diabetes)	3.1
6. Influenza and pneumonia	3.0
7. Alzheimer's disease	2.9
8. Accidents (unintentional injuries)	2.8
9. Nephritis, nephrotic syndrome, and nephrosis (kidney disease)	1.6
10. Septicemia	1.4

*Percent of total deaths due to the cause indicated.

Source: CDC Office of Women's Health. Available at: http://www.cdc.gov/od/spotlight/nwhw/lcod/00all.htm. Accessed April 22, 2004.

based on cultural identity and use of English.[28] Among the specific factors suggesting a lack of cultural sensitivity to patients were a failure to provide ethnically sensitive office materials, such as illustrations or reading materials, and office staff behavior.[29] In this study, the language barrier was more important to Latinos, while environmental factors that suggested respect for African-American culture were more important to African Americans.

Other factors that primary care patients have identified as indicators of culturally sensitive care include people skills and effective communications, individualized treatment plans, and technical skill. Positive characteristics used to describe physician behavior in one study included listening, demonstrating concern, and good communication skills.[29] Beck's review of the literature on patient-provider relations identified more than 20 nonverbal and verbal behaviors that had positive associations.[30] Among these were friendliness, courtesy, and empathy, which are behaviors that suggest acceptance of the person.

In medicine, providers also need to be respectful of the traditions and "folk illnesses" of their patients.[25] These issues may cause women to delay coming for care, utilize parallel care (medical plus traditional healers), or cause behaviors that the provider interprets as noncompliance when in fact the patient is following his or her own script for healing. Some illnesses do not fit a Western biomedical model, but are deeply rooted in cultural beliefs. Awareness and responsiveness to different cultural expectations can help to identify instances of parallel treatment, practices, and therapies that may be harmful, and improve communication.

Conclusion

Primary care is a complex construct. It requires that care be available and that a clinician take the responsibility for paying attention to the whole person, not only one organ system or disease. It is best provided when the clinician can see across the divides of race, education, culture, and financial status, working to understand the individual and community network to provide care that works for the woman.

Many women rely on their midwife or other gynecologic caregiver to recognize and address all of their health care needs. When considering the focus on education, empowerment for shared decision making, psychosocial interventions, and lifestyle changes to improve health that are components of primary care, it is not surprising that midwives can be considered primary care providers. Fulfilling that expectation—and triaging those who are not appropriate for midwifery primary care to a different clinician—requires knowledge. The basics of that knowledge are in the following chapters.

References

1. Kriebs JM. Primary care and midwifery. In: Varney H, Kriebs JM, Gegor CL, editors. *Varney's Midwifery.* Sudbury, MA: Jones and Bartlett Publishers; 2004. p. 135.

2. Donaldson MS, Yordy KD, Lohr KN, Vanselow NA, editors. *Primary Care: America's Health in a New Era.* Washington, DC: National Academy Press; 1996.

3. Stuart D, Oshio S. Primary care in midwifery practice: A national survey. *J Midwifery Women's Health.* 2002;47(2):104–109.

4. American College of Nurse-Midwives. *Certified Nurse Midwives and Certified Midwives as Primary Care Providers/Case Managers.* Washington, DC: ACNM; 1992, revised 1997.

5. American College of Nurse-Midwives. *Core Competencies for the Practice of Midwifery.* Washington, DC: ACNM; 2002.

6. Murphy PA. Primary care for women: Health assessment, health promotion, and disease prevention services. *J Nurse-Midwifery.* 1996;41(2):83–91.

7. Scupholme A, Carr KC. CNMs and primary care: Practice models and types of services. *Quickening.* 1993;24(6):14.

8. Oshio S, Johnson P, Fullerton J. The 1999–2000 task Analysis of American nurse-midwifery/midwifery practice. *J Midwifery Women's Health.* 2002;47(1): 35–41.

9. National Center for Health Statistics. *Health Care in America: Trends in Utilization 2004.* Hyattsville, MD: National Center for Health Statistics; 2004.

10. Woodwell DA, Cherry DK. National ambulatory medical care survey: 2002 survey. *Advance Data from Vital and Health Statistics*, No. 346. Hyattsville, MD: National Center for Health Statistics; August 26, 2004.

11. Smedley BD, Stith AY, Nelson AR, editors. *Unequal Treatment: Confronting Racial and Ethnic Disparities in Health Care.* Washington, DC: National Academy Press; 2003.

12. Navarro V. Race or class versus race and class: Mortality differentials in the United States. In: Lee PR, Carroll LE, editors. *The Nation's Health.* 5th ed. Sudbury, MA: Jones and Bartlett Publishers; 1997. pp. 32–36.

13. Agency for Healthcare Quality and Research. *The National Healthcare Disparities Report.* Rockville, MD: United States Department of Health and Human Services; 2003.

14. Declerq ER, Williams DR, Koontz AM, Paine LL, Streit EL, McKloskey L. Serving women in need: Nurse-midwifery practice in the United States. *J Midwifery Women's Health.* 2001;46(1):11–16.

15. Centers for Disease Control and Prevention. Indicators for chronic disease surveillance. *MMWR.* 2004;53 (No.RR-11).

16. Miniño AM, Arias E, Kochanek KD, Murphy SL, Smith BL. Deaths: Final data for 2000. *Natl Vital Stat Rep.* 2002;50(15):1–120.

17. Mokdad AH, Marks JS, Stroup DF, Gerberding JL. Actual causes of death in the United States, 2000. *JAMA.* 2004;291(10):1238–1246.

18. CDC Office of Women's Health. Leading causes of death, all females, United States – 2000. [database on the Internet]. Atlanta (GA): Centers for Disease Control [cited 2004 April 22]. Available from: http://www.cdc.gov/od/spotlight/nwhw/lcod/00all.htm.

19. Mosca L, Jones WK, King KB, Ouyang P, Redberg RF, Hill MN, for the American Heart Association Women's Heart Disease and Stroke Campaign Task Force. Awareness, perception, and knowledge of heart disease risk and prevention among women in the United States. *Arch Fam Med.* 2000;9:506–515.

20. Centers for Disease Control and Prevention. Chronic Disease Overview. [cited 2005 February 13] Available from: http://cdc.gov/nccdphp/overview.htm.

21. Liao Y, Tucker P, Okoro CA, Giles WH, Mokdad AH, Harris VB. *REACH 2010 Surveillance for Health Status in Minority Communities—United States, 2001–2002.* Atlanta, GA: Division of Adult and Community Health, National Center for Chronic Disease Prevention and Health Promotion, Centers for Disease Control and Prevention (CDC); 2002.

22. Adler NE, Boyce WT, Chesney MA, Folkman S, Syme SL. Socioeconomic inequalities in health: No easy solution. In: Lee PR, Carroll LE, editors. *The Nation's Health.* 5th ed. Sudbury, MA: Jones and Bartlett Publishers; 1997. pp. 18–31.

23. Lenberg CB, Lipson JG, Demi AL, Blaney DR, Stem PN, Schultz PR, et al. Promoting cultural competence in and through nursing education: A critical review

and plan for action. Washington, DC: American Academy of Nursing; 1995. Quoted in Dunn AM. Cultural competence and the primary care provider. *J Pediatr Health Care.* 2002;16:105–111.

24. Dunn AM. Cultural competence and the primary care provider. *J Pediatr Health Care.* 2002;16:105–111.

25. Pachter LM. Culture and clinical care: Folk illness beliefs and their implications for health care delivery. *JAMA.* 1994;271:690–694.

26. Taylor JS. Confronting "culture" in medicine's "culture of no culture." *Acad Med.* 2003;78:555–559.

27. Nunez AE. Transforming cultural competence into cross cultural efficacy in women's health education. *Acad Med.* 2000;75:1071–1080.

28. Johnson RL, Saha S, Arbelaz JJ, Beach MC, Cooper LA. Racial and ethnic differences in patient perceptions of bias and cultural competence in health care. *J Gen Intern Med.* 2004;19:101–110.

29. Tucker CM, Herman KC, Pedersen TR, Higley B, Montrichard M, Ivery P. Cultural sensitivity in physician-patient relationships. *Med Care.* 2003;41:859–870.

30. Beck RS, Daughtridge R, Sloane PD. Physician-patient communication in the primary care office: A systematic review. *J Am Board Fam Pract.* 2002;15:25–38.

Recommended Resources

Smedley BD, Stith AY, Nelson AR, editors. *Unequal Treatment: Confronting Racial and Ethnic Disparities in Healthcare.* Washington, DC: National Academy Press; 2003.

Agency for Healthcare Quality and Research. *The National Healthcare Disparities Report.* Rockville, MD: United States Department of Health and Human Services; 2003.

Chapter 2

Immunizations

Barbara Hackley

Immunizations are widely acknowledged to be one of the most effective health interventions. In the pre-vaccine era, over one million Americans became infected with a vaccine-preventable illness every year.[1] After widespread implementation of vaccination, rates of reported vaccine-preventable illnesses have declined by 93% for pertussis, by more than 98% for diphtheria, tetanus, measles, mumps, and rubella, and by 100% for polio and smallpox.[1] More recently, the introduction of a varicella vaccine has led to significant declines in the incidence of varicella. In 2003, the Centers for Disease Control and Prevention (CDC) estimated that the incidence of varicella declined as much as 67% to 82% in selected states since 1990.[2]

Immune Response

Vaccines provide either active or passive immunity.[3] Active immunity is long-lasting because it triggers the immune system to develop antibodies. The protection afforded by passive immunization wanes as the antibodies provided by the vaccine die off; the immune system is not stimulated to produce antibodies with passive immunization. Examples of vaccines providing active immunity include measles, mumps, and rubella vaccines; those providing passive immunity include vaccines containing immunoglobulin. Passive transmission of antibodies can also occur via transplacental transport from mother to fetus and by receipt of some blood products.

Active vaccines work by exposing the immune system to a substance that triggers a similar immune response to that which occurs upon exposure to wild infection.[3] Vaccines use a modified live antigen, such as a virus or bacterium, or a manufactured one with a structure very similar to the wild form. The essential qualities of a wild virus or bacterium are mimicked so that the immune system will create antibodies to these antigens without allowing an active infection to develop.

Exposure to a vaccine triggers both humoral and cellular immunity and creates immunological memory.[3,4] These basic mechanisms of the immune response create pathways that allow the body to inactivate free virus and eliminate infected cells. Cellular immunity is a result of the activity of T cells, which are produced in the thymus. The two major types of T cells, killer T cells (also known as cytotoxic T lymphocytes) and helper T cells, each play a different role. Killer T cells directly attack the infected cells and are particularly aggressive in eliminating cells infected with viruses and malignant cells. Helper T cells are essential in coordinating the overall immune response and stimulate other cells, such as B cells, needed for the body to mount an effective immune response. Humoral immunity is responsible for long-term protection; its primary mechanism is to trigger the development of antibodies produced by B cells, which combat viruses and bacteria on entry to the body and so prevent infection. Antibodies prevent infection from developing and modify the course of infection once it is established by using several different mechanisms. Antibodies directed to surface antigens can cause viruses to aggregate, making them easier to clear out of the body by the immune system. Other kinds of antibodies change the structure of antigens, rendering them noninfectious. Others neutralize antigens, not by changing their structure, but by not allowing viruses to attach to human cells. Antibodies work synergistically and by doing so effectively attack viruses and bacteria. Both systems—cellular and humoral—work in concert to prevent and eliminate infection.[3,4] Once infection is eradicated, levels of antibodies wane. However, following re-exposure to an antigen, memory B cells (which circulate in the blood and are also present in bone marrow), recognize the antigen and rapidly reproduce antibodies to levels high enough to prevent infection. This immunologic memory can last for years, sometimes for a lifetime, and provides long-term protection from infection.[3,4]

Types of Vaccinations

There are two basic types of immunizations: attenuated-live and inactivated vaccines.[3] *Attenuated live vaccines* use weakened viruses and bac-

teria to induce low-level replication in the individual receiving the vaccine. The immune response from exposure to the low levels of viruses and bacteria induced by attenuated live vaccines is almost identical to that produced by wild infection. Occasionally receipt of attenuated live vaccines results in clinical infection, but often these infections are much milder than wild infections and cause few problems. Because they are so effective, attenuated live vaccines can usually achieve an effective immune response with only one dose. In contrast, *inactivated vaccines* are less effective, may require multiple doses to induce an adequate immune response, and need additional boosters to maintain adequate antibody levels. Inactivated vaccines are developed by modifying live viruses and bacteria so that they cannot reproduce and then using various portions of these inactivated viruses or bacteria to stimulate an immune response. *Whole cell inactivated vaccines*, such as polio and pertussis, use the entire bacteria or virus; other *fractional vaccines* use viral subunits, polysaccharide components of bacterial cell walls, or toxins produced by a bacterium, to stimulate the immune system. *Recombinant vaccines* are "manufactured" vaccines using genetic engineering technology and are the newest class of inactivated immunizations. **Table 2-1** explains the vaccine types.

Vaccine Safety

As with all medications, the use of vaccines may result in unwanted effects. Up to 50% of all vaccinations may be associated with mild local reactions.[5] Systemic symptoms such as fever and malaise are less common. More serious reactions can occur but are rare, and are commonly referred to as *vaccine adverse events (VAE)*. VAEs can result from a reaction to any of the additives or

Table 2-1 TYPES OF VACCINES[3]

Types	Examples	Mechanism of Action	Problems
Attenuated Live Vaccines			
Viral	Measles, mumps, rubella, varicella, yellow fever	Viral or bacterial replication induces subclinical infection	Ineffective if vaccine damaged by light or heat. Rendered ineffective by circulating antibodies if recent receipt of immunoglobulins or blood products
Bacterial	BCG, oral typhoid		
Inactivated Vaccines			
Whole Cell			
Viral	Polio, hepatitis A	Exposure to whole virus, made incapable of reproducing, induces immune response	Less effective than attenuated live viral vaccine. Requires multiple doses. Immunity wanes over time if no boosters given
Fractional			
Subunit	Hepatitis B, influenza	Exposure to viral or bacterial components induces immune response	Same as whole cell
Toxoid	Tetanus, diphtheria	Same as subunit	Same as whole cell
Polysaccharide	Pneumococcal, meningococcal	T cell independent	Ineffective in children <2 years of age due to their immature immune system. Less effective than other inactivated vaccines, which are protein based and induce stronger and longer lasting immune responses, because polysaccharide

(continues)

Table 2-1 TYPES OF VACCINES *(continued)*

Types	Examples	Mechanism of Action	Problems
Polysaccharide (continued)			vaccines trigger predominantly IgM, not IgG, antibody
Conjugated polysaccharide	Hib Pneumococcal	T cell dependent	Conjugation fixes many of the problems found in polysaccharide vaccines, making them more effective in young children and capable of being "boosted" with multiple doses
Recombinant Vaccines Viral	Hepatitis B, Typhoid, Nasally administered influenza vaccine	Exposure to highly purified viral subunits induces immunity.	Requires multiple boosters

immunologic components of the vaccine; from medication errors, such as reconstituting a vaccine with the wrong dilutant or using poor technique during administration; or from errors made during the manufacturing process. VAEs also may be coincidental and unrelated to vaccine receipt.[5]

Trying to determine whether a reaction is truly a result of vaccine exposure or co-incidental can be difficult depending on the presentation. More severe and more immediate effects are most likely to be identified as possible vaccine-related reactions.[6] Subtle or later developing reactions are more easily missed. Concern has been expressed in a few communities that receipt of some vaccines is related to the development of multiple sclerosis, autism, and other autoimmune disorders.[7] Others have suggested that receipt of pertussis vaccine is as-sociated with the development of severe neurological damage in children.[8] These concerns prompted the Institute of Medicine to convene an expert panel to examine the safety of vaccines, initially in 1991,[9] and then again in response to more recent concerns in 2001.[10] This expert panel, also known as the Immunization Safety Review Committee, has published a series of reports on the safety of individual vaccines, evaluating possible relationships between the receipt of measles-mumps-rubella (MMR) vaccine and autism, thimerosal-containing vaccines and neurodevelopmental disorders, childhood vaccines and sudden infant death syndrome (SIDS) as well as other possible VAEs. The Immunization Safety Review Committee uses the same methodology in all of its reports. The committee evaluates whether the relationships between various vaccines and VAEs are biologically plausible and also analyzes the available research to determine whether the evidence is of sufficient quality and quantity to determine if a causal relationship exists. In many cases, the Immunization Safety Review Committee found that the evidence was insufficient to draw clear conclusions. **Table 2-2** is a synopsis of the findings of these reports.[10]

The evaluation of vaccine safety is based on pre-licensure research and post-licensure surveillance. In order to receive Food and Drug Administration (FDA) approval for use, a vaccine must be evaluated by a series of pre-licensure research studies consisting of Phase 1, Phase 2, and Phase 3 clinical trials.[18] Phase 1 trials have few participants and are designed to determine whether an intervention passes minimal safety standards. Phase 2 trials are larger and designed to evaluate effectiveness, determine dosage, and identify the more frequent minor and major side effects. Phase 3 trials are the largest, often comprising over 1000 participants, and help to further refine the dosage needed to maximize benefits and minimize risks, and provide better data on the safety profiles of vaccines. However, because serious reactions are rare, VAEs may not be picked up in pre-licensure trials, making post-licensure surveillance essential.

Post-licensure surveillance is conducted through several different avenues. One is by Phase 4 clinical trials.[18] To be approved for licensure, the FDA, in addition to requiring Phase 1, 2, and 3 trials, sometimes also requires the manufacturer to conduct a Phase 4 trial, which is a continuation of the Phase 3 trial using a much larger cohort, sometimes as large as 10,000 individuals. While this large sample size helps identify other previously unrecognized reactions or subpopulations at increased

risk of developing VAEs, it is not sufficiently large enough to pick up rare events.[19] For example, the relationship between the rotavirus vaccine and bowel obstruction was not suspected to be a problem in pre-licensure trials of over 17,000 individuals.[20,21] This relationship became evident only after 1.5 million doses were distributed and led to a recall of this vaccine.[22]

To improve vaccine safety monitoring, the Vaccine Adverse Events Reporting System (VAERS), a national passive reporting system, was established in 1990.[18,23] VAERS is jointly administered by the CDC and the FDA. Health care providers are mandated to report all suspected vaccine-related adverse events, but reports submitted by the general public are also accepted. These case reports are reviewed to determine if a suspected link exists between a vaccine and a specific adverse event, if problems are occurring in certain manufacturer lots, or if rates of adverse events are increasing. If potential problems are identified, further research is needed. Because the VAERS is a collection of case reports, it cannot prove causality; rather, VAERS data are used to generate hypotheses better evaluated by other research modalities.

Two systems that can evaluate hypotheses generated by VAERS data are large linked data sets (LLDS), such as the Vaccine Safety Datalink, and the Clinical Immunization Safety Assessment (CISA) Network.[18] These systems complement each other and can be used to answer different kinds of research questions.

LLDS are computerized data sets of health care information generated from health maintenance organizations or large insurance systems such as Medicaid that make it possible to link information about the health status of individuals receiving vaccination to the receipt of specific vaccines.[18,23] Consequently, this system

Table 2-2 SUMMARY OF FINDINGS OF VACCINE SAFETY REVIEW REPORTS

Possible Vaccine-Related Event	Year of Publication	Findings
MMR and Autism[11]	2001	• Evidence favors rejection of a relationship. • Evidence does not exclude the possibility that a relationship exists for a small subset of exposed individuals. The epidemiological evidence is not precise enough to assess rare occurrences.
Thimerosal-Containing Vaccines and Neuro-development Disorders[12]	2001	• Biologically plausible. • Evidence insufficient to accept or reject a causal relationship. • Recommended removing thimerosal in vaccines administered to infants, children, and pregnant women in the United States. • Further research recommended.
Multiple Vaccine Receipt and Immune Dysfunction[13]	2002	• Evidence favors rejection of a causal relationship between multiple immunizations and an increased risk of type 1 diabetes or the development of heterologous infections. • Evidence inadequate to evaluate the relationship between multiple immunizations and allergic disease including asthma. • Evidence for proposed biological mechanisms for a relationship between multiple vaccinations and type 1 diabetes and autoimmune disease ranges from theoretical to weak. • Proposed biological mechanism for a relationship with multiple vaccines and heterologous infections is strong. • Further research recommended.
Hepatitis B Vaccine and Demyelinating Disorders[14]	2002	• Evidence favors no relationship between hepatitis B vaccine and the development or relapse of multiple sclerosis. • Evidence is inadequate to determine a relationship between hepatitis B vaccine and optic neuritis, brachial neuritis, Guillian-Barré syndrome (GBS), and transverse myelitis.
Vaccines and SIDS[15]	2002	• Evidence favors acceptance of relationship between DTwP and death due to anaphylaxis. • Evidence favors no relationship between DTwP and SIDS. • Evidence favors no relationship between receipt of multiple vaccines and SIDs.

Table 2-2 SUMMARY OF FINDINGS OF VACCINE SAFETY REVIEW REPORTS *(continued)*

Possible Vaccine-Related Event	Year of Publication	Findings
Influenza Vaccine and Neurological Disorders[16]	2003	• Inadequate evidence exists to determine if a relationship exists between receipt of individual vaccines and SIDS. • Evidence favors acceptance of a relationship between 1976 swine flu vaccine and GBS. • Insufficient evidence to evaluate if a relationship between receipt of other influenza vaccines and GBS exists. • Evidence favors no relationship between influenza vaccine and exacerbation of multiple sclerosis.
Vaccines and Autism[17]	2004	• Evidence favors no causal relationship between autism and receipt of MMR or thimerosal-containing vaccines.

can better answer questions about the incidence of specific vaccine-related adverse events, the normal background incidence of these reactions in patients who have not recently received a vaccine, and subgroups at higher risks of vaccine-related complications. However, health data entered in these LLDS may not be completely accurate as information is being collected, not for research purposes, but as part of routine health care.[23] Errors may occur in coding.[24] Reactions too minor to warrant medical attention will be lost to analysis. Nor are these data sets likely to include a sufficient number of unvaccinated individuals who can serve as controls.[23] Because over 95% of the U.S. population has received recommended childhood vaccinations,[25] relatively few unvaccinated controls are available. In addition, these individuals may be significantly different in their genetic makeup, lifestyle, or environmental exposures from the general public. Therefore, LLDS are best at identifying problems with new vaccines or with changes in recommendations on the initiation or use of older ones.[23] Because of the lack of a vaccine-naïve control group, LLDS cannot easily answer lingering questions regarding the safety of older vaccines already in widespread use, about the risks of cumulative vaccine exposure, or about the relationship between vaccine receipt and the future development of autoimmune disorders. However, despite these limitations, LLDS are a significant improvement that allows a more sophisticated analysis of vaccine safety than was previously available.

The CISA Network is designed to serve several purposes. First, it allows individuals who experience a VAE to receive expert advice and monitoring. The CISA Network consists of designated referral centers where information, such as how to properly investigate a suspected VAE as well as how best to care for the individual experiencing one, can be obtained.[18] Second, because support for both providers and patients can be standardized, data collected through the CISA Network can aid in the development and promotion of uniform guidelines for the management of specific

VAEs.[18] Finally, because of the standardized scrutiny each case reported to the CISA network receives, the CISA network may be able to identify differences in the genetic make-up, environmental exposures, or physiology of individuals that may predispose them to the development of vaccine-related reactions. Identifying idiosyncratic differences that predispose individuals to VAEs may be particularly useful in the future development of safer vaccines.

For post-surveillance to be most effective, all providers who order or administer vaccines need to report potential adverse reactions, whether they are major or minor, to VAERS and seek further advice from the CISA Network if needed.[18,26] Because the background incidence of many reactions attributed to vaccines, such as Guillian-Barré syndrome, autism, or multiple sclerosis, is unknown, it is very difficult or impossible to quantify the relationship between vaccine receipt and these events. Consequently, VAERS data are often quoted as a surrogate measure of prevalence. For example, the rate of serious VAEs associated with hepatitis A vaccine has been reported to be 1.4 VAEs per 100,000 distributed doses.[27] This statistic does not describe a causal relationship, only an association. However, it is useful in counseling patients to have some understanding of how rare VAEs are thought to be. The use of VAERs data in this fashion can only be accurate if all suspected reactions are reported. **Table 2-3** lists the Web sites where VAERS reporting forms and other vaccine safety-related information can be obtained.

Communicating Vaccine Risk

Unlike medications used to treat already established disease, vaccines are given to healthy individuals to prevent an infection that might occur with future exposure to a pathogen. Of course, this future exposure may not occur, making vaccine receipt unnecessary. Consequently, vaccines must adhere to the highest level of safety. Even rare reactions may make some individuals reluctant to accept vaccination.[28–31] If enough individuals refuse to participate in community innoculation, the ability of vaccines to protect the general public will decline. Not only do vaccines provide individual protection, but they also induce herd immunity if enough individuals are protected. *Herd immunity* protects unvaccinated individuals by disrupting transmission. If a vaccine-preventable illness enters a community with high levels of immunity, only a few isolated cases, if any, will develop. Transmission does not occur, and the infection dies out. However, if infection enters a community with uneven or no vaccination coverage, infection can be transmitted to unvaccinated individuals and lead to widespread illness. The level of community acceptance needed to induce herd immunity varies depending on the inherent effectiveness of the vaccine, the prevalence and virulence of infection, and the mode of transmission.[32] For example, it is thought that approximately 70% of the population needs to be vaccinated against diphtheria[33] in order to induce herd immunity compared to more than 93% for measles.[34] Therefore, while the decision to accept vaccination is made by the individual, the individual's decision to accept or reject vaccination affects the health of the entire community. In areas where vaccination levels have fallen, such as in Japan and parts of the former Soviet Union, vaccine-preventable illnesses have risen, in some cases to epidemic levels.[28,35,36]

The perception of the risks and benefits related to vaccination differs depending on whether they are viewed from the individual or societal perspective.[37] From the individual

Table 2-3 WEB RESOURCES

Organization	Information Available	Web site
National Academy Press	Full text, online books, and reports sponsored by the Institute of Medicine	http://books.nap,edu/books/ 0309074479/html/related.html
Immunization Safety Review	Minutes and full text reports of the committee	http://www.iom.edu/project. asp?id=4705
VAERS	VAERS report forms	http://www.fda.gov/cber/vaers/ vaers.htm
National Immunization Program	General information, adult and childhood vaccine schedules, links to most recent ACIP recommendations	http://www.cdc.gov/nip/
World Health Organization	Information on vaccines and vaccine preventable diseases worldwide	http://www.who.int/vaccines/
VARIVAX Pregnancy Registry	Site where reports of pregnant women immunized inadvertently with varicella vaccine should be reported	http://www.merckpregnancy registries.com/varivax.html
National Vaccine Information Center	Alternative views on vaccinations; links to state by state school immunization requirements	http://www.nvic.org/state-site/ state-exemptions.htm
National Center for Infectious Diseases Travelers Health	Recommended vaccinations and prophylactic medications according to travel destination	http://www.cdc.gov/travel/ destinat.htm
National Network for Immunization Information	Searchable link for state school immunization requirements	http://www.immunizationinfo.org/ vaccineInfo/index.cfm#state

perspective, vaccines provide protection but also are associated with minor side effects and some very rare but serious risks. From the societal perspective, vaccines carry no risk. They promote the general health of the community because large-scale acceptance leads to herd immunity, which protects those individuals who cannot afford or do not have access to immunizations, those whose immunity has unknowingly waned, and those who forgo immunization because of underlying medical conditions that place them at higher risk of vaccine-related complications. However, because the risks of vaccination are borne by the individual, some may decide against immunization and rely on chance or on the protection afforded by herd immunity.[38] Others may decide to be vaccinated for their own individual protection, as well as for the public good. Others do not actively evaluate their choices and simply follow the example of the majority of individuals around them. Individuals accept or reject vaccinations because of differences in their underlying beliefs about the importance of individual rights versus the public good, their understanding and preference for various types and degrees of risk, and their interpretation of the statistics used to describe the risks and benefits of vaccination.[38]

Understanding the underlying values affecting decision making and the ways that individuals evaluate risk is essential in order to provide the level of counseling needed to help women decide whether they want to receive, or have their family members receive, vaccinations.[39] In general, individuals contemplating a choice among "risky" options will be more likely to choose an intervention where the associated risks are familiar, voluntary, and natural.[38,40] Risks that are human-made, that is, they result from an imposed choice or are unknown and unquantified, are less acceptable. Individuals are also more likely to accept vaccination if it provides protection against catastrophic events, such as death or severe disability, even if these events are rare.

Other values affect vaccine decision making. Individuals will have different preferences for risks associated with omission or commission.[37,38] Does a woman prefer to expose her child to the potential risk of a serious reaction associated with receipt of a vaccine or does she prefer the risks associated with contracting a vaccine-preventable illness? To a certain extent, the preference for risks associated with omission or commission is partially based on a woman's understanding of the frequency that these risks might occur as well as her perception about the likelihood that her child could contract a vaccine-preventable illness.[40] Individuals differ in their perception of the meaning of statistics used to describe these events.[40] In addition, health providers have their own set of values and

ways of interpreting the data used to describe the benefits and risks of vaccines, which can color their discussion of these issues with their clients.[40]

After weighing all the pros and cons, some women will decide against immunization either for themselves or their families. These women often experience pressure from other health professionals and from institutions such as schools, workplaces, and childcare centers to accept vaccination. Women need to be counseled in an accepting manner about the risks associated with various infections, the likelihood that infection with a vaccine preventable infection will occur, and the type and frequency of vaccine-related side effects. **Table 2-4** lists vaccine-preventable diseases and **Table 2-5** contains some commonly used adult vaccines.

Women who decide to forgo immunizations should be informed that herd immunity provides limited protection from vaccine-preventable illnesses. Several studies have shown that un-immunized children are more likely to contract pertussis and measles than immunized children, and they can spread infection to already immunized children whose immunity has lapsed due to primary vaccine failure or waning antibody levels. In studies of school-aged children, exemptors were 22[66] to 35 times[67] more likely to develop measles and 6 times more likely to develop pertussis.[66] In addition, Feikin[66] found that 11% of vaccinated children who developed measles acquired their infection through exposure to an un-immunized child. However, the overall incidence of infection remained low. The annual incidence of measles in unvaccinated children was 32 cases per 100,000 compared to 1.4 cases per 100,000 for vaccinated children; the incidence of pertussis was 80 cases per 100,000 for unvaccinated children

Table 2-4 VACCINE-PREVENTABLE DISEASES

Infection	Incubation	Presentation	Complications
Diphtheria[41]	2–5 days	Commonly infects tonsils and pharynx. Begins with malaise, sore throat, low grade fever, progressing to development of blue-white membrane covering tonsils and soft palate. Covering turns to grey-green to black in color. If larnynx is involved, membrane can cause airway obstruction. Skin infections are rare and more common in tropics.	Prostration, coma, myocarditis, neuritis. Case fatality rate: 5%–10%.
Hepatitis A[42]	28 days, range 15-50 days	Abrupt onset of malaise, headache, abdominal pain, nausea, anorexia, dark urine, and jaundice. 30% of adults can be asymptomatic. Usually resolves within two weeks.	Hospitalization rates: 11%–22%; Rare: fulminant hepatitis A; Case fatality rate: 0.3%.
Hepatitis B[43,44]	Average 120 days, range 6 weeks to 6 months	50% are asymptomatic. If symptomatic, initial presentation consists of malaise, anorexia, nausea, right upper quadrant pain, skin rashes, arthalgias, and dark urine. Icteric phase (jaundice, light or gray stools, hepatomegaly, and hepatic tenderness) lasts from one to three weeks. Malaise and fatigue can last for several months.	Fulminant hepatitis 1% to 2%; 6% to 10% of adults will become chronic carriers (more frequent in infants and children)[44]; 25% of chronic carriers develop chronic active hepatitis B, which increases risk of cirrhosis, liver failure, and cancer.

(continues)

Table 2-4 Vaccine-Preventable Diseases *(continued)*

Infection	Incubation	Presentation	Complications
Influenza[45]	2 days, range 1–4 days	Abrupt onset of fever, malaise, myalgia, cough, and sore throat.	Secondary bacterial infections; myocarditis; worsening of asthma or chronic bronchitis. Deaths 0.5–1 per 1000 cases, primarily in the elderly.
Meningitis[46]	3–4 days, range 2–10 days	Sudden onset of headache, fever and stiff neck. Other symptoms such as photophobia, nausea, vomiting, and altered mental status common.	Case fatality rates 9% to 12%. Up to 20% of survivors have permanent disability.
Measles[47–49]	10–12 days to prodrome, 14 days to rash	Prodrome of fever, cough, runny nose progressing to rash on mucous membranes (Kopliks spots) to rash. Rash is maculopapular, begins on face and progresses downward and outward to feet. Rash initially blanches under pressure, but by 3–4 days does not blanch when pressed. Rash fades in same order in which it appears.	Otitis media 7% Pneumonia 6% Encephalitis 0.1% Seizures 0.6% Thrombocytopenia 1 out of 3000 cases. Subacute sclerosing panencephalitis (rare) 25% of survivors with CNS dysfunction have permanent disability. Case fatality rate 1–2 deaths per 1000 reported cases.[47]
Mumps[50]	14–18 days	Prodrome is nonspecific. Parotitis occurs in 30%–40%. Up to 20% of cases are asymptomatic.	Orchitis in 50% of postpubertal males, sterility is rare. Oophoritis occurs in 5% of postpubertal females, fertility unaffected. Deafness in 1 per 20,000 cases.

Table 2-4 **VACCINE-PREVENTABLE DISEASES** *(continued)*

Infection	Incubation	Presentation	Complications
Rubella[51]	Average 14 days, range 12–23 days	Symptoms can be mild. Up to 50% are subclinical. Nonspecifc prodrome progresses to rash beginning on day 2–6 after onset of symptoms. Rash is fainter than in measles, but has similar head to toe progression. Rash lasts about 3 days. Lymphadenopathy common.	Encephalitis 2 out of 100,000 cases, one case reported per year between 1980 and 1999. Arthritis/arthralgia in 70% women, rare in children and men. Encephalitis occurs in 1 out of 6000 cases, more common in women. Thrombocytopenia in 1 out of 3000 cases, more common in children.
Pneumococcal[52]	1–3 days	Abrupt onset of fever, chills, and rigor. Also can present with pleuritic chest pain, productive cough, dyspnea, tachypnea, hypoxia, tachycardia, malaise, and weakness.	Bacteremia in 25%–30%. Bacterial meningitis.
Tetanus[53]	3–21 days	80% of cases are generalized tetanus, which presents with lockjaw, stiff neck, difficulty swallowing, laryngospasm, muscle spasms, and fever. Recovery usually complete in 4–6 weeks. Infection does not confer immunity.	Fractures from severe muscle spasms. Aspiration pneumonia. 11% case fatality rate, highest in elderly.

(continues)

Table 2-4 **VACCINE-PREVENTABLE DISEASES** *(continued)*

Infection	Incubation	Presentation	Complications
Varicella[54]	14–15 days from exposure, range 10–21 days	Prodrome of malaise and fever for one to days before rash. Rash usually starts on head, progresses to trunk, and then to extremities with lesions concentrated on trunk. Rash evolves from macules to papules to vesicles to crusting. All stages of lesions can be present at the same time. Lesions also present on mouth, vagina, and mucous membranes.	Complications much more common in adults than children. Secondary bacterial skin infection. Pneumonia. Encephalitis in 1.6 per 10,000 cases. Herpes zoster. Case fatality in children 1 per 100,000 cases. Case fatality in adults older than 30 is 25.2 per 100,000.

and 13 cases per 100,000 for vaccinated children.[66]

Women who choose not to vaccinate their children can request a school waiver so that their children do not have to comply with state immunization requirements in order to attend school. Each state has established specific regulations governing eligibility, what vaccines are covered, and the exact steps an individual must follow in order to be deemed exempt from vaccine requirements. All states grant medical exemptions; 48 grant exemptions for religious beliefs, but only 18 grant exemptions based on personal values (Table 2-3).[68]

Principles of Vaccination

Proper administration of vaccines is critical. Using improper technique, spacing vaccine boosters incorrectly, or administering vaccines simultaneously with antibody-containing products can all undermine the effectiveness of vaccines. Following a few essential principles can ensure that vaccines will provide long-lived immunity.

Give Vaccines Simultaneously Where Possible

The simultaneous administration of vaccines (e.g., giving MMR, varicella, and tetanus all at the same visit) will not impair the immune response to any of the vaccines generally used in adult practice.[5] The immune response to vaccines administered simultaneously is robust and confers long-lasting protection. Nor does the safety profile of vaccines seem to change with simultaneous administration. Because patients and providers are often pressed for time, simultaneous administration

Table 2-5 COMMONLY USED ADULT VACCINES

Vaccine	Type and Schedule	Efficacy	Indications	Contra-indications	Precautions	Use in Pregnant and HIV Positive Women	Vaccine-Associated Side Effects
Hepatitis A[27,42]	Inactivated: Two doses separated by 6 months.[42]	After first dose, protective levels of antibody develop in 94%–100%. After second dose, 100% protective.[42] Duration of protection is unknown. Current data estimate that protection may last 20 years or more.[42]	High-risk groups: Travelers to countries with intermediate (former Soviet Union) or high disease endemicity (Central and South America, Africa, Asia); individuals engaging in anal intercourse in nonmonogamous relationships; IV drug users; persons with clotting-factor disorders or chronic liver disease; persons who work with HAV-infected primates or in research laboratory settings with exposure to HAV.[42]	Allergy to alum, to the preservative 2-phenoxyethanol, or other vaccine component.	Moderate-to-severe illness.	Pregnancy: no data. Theoretically safe because vaccine is inactivated. HIV+: safe.	Soreness at injection site (20%–50%).[42] Malaise, fever <10%.[42] No serious vaccine-related adverse reactions have been causally attributed to hepatitis A vaccine use. Rate of serious events temporally related to vaccine use is 1.4/100,000 adult recipients and includes reports of neurological events, autoimmune disorders, and hematological problems.[27]

(continues)

Table 2-5 COMMONLY USED ADULT VACCINES *(continued)*

Vaccine	Type and Schedule	Efficacy	Indications	Contra-indications	Precautions	Use in Pregnant and HIV Positive Women	Vaccine-Associated Side Effects
Hepatitis B[43,48,54–56]	Recombinant vaccine: 3 doses, second dose 1–2 months after the first, third dose 4–6 months after the first.[43] Alternative regimen available to adolescents age 11–15 years: 2 dose series.[55]	Vaccine response declines with age. After 3 dose series, 90% of adults age 40 will respond, but by 60 years only 75% of recipients will develop immunity. Overall efficacy is 80%–100%. Immunity lasts for at least 15 years.[43]	Persons at risk of exposure to blood. Clients and staff in institutions for the developmentally disabled.[43] Household contacts and sex partners of those with chronic HBV infection. Injecting drug users. Men who have sex with men (MSM). Individuals with multiple sex partners or recent STD. Inmates of long-term correctional institutions. Hemodialysis patients.	Anaphylactic allergy to yeast, alum, or other vaccine component.[43]	Moderate-to-severe illness.[43]	Pregnancy: no data; theoretically safe as the vaccine does not contain live viral particles.[43] HIV+: safe, but response may be suboptimal depending on the severity of immunosuppression. Vaccine doses may need to be doubled or special formulation used.[43]	Pain at injection site 13%–29%.[43] Fatigue, headache, and irritability in 11%–17%.[43] Fever in 1%.[43] Possible association with alopecia and vaccine receipt.[56] Serious adverse events have rarely been reported. Unlike with plasma-derived vaccines, no association has been found between Guillain-Barre Syndrome (GBS) and receipt of recombinant hepatitis B vaccine.[57] Anaphylaxis is rare. Based on VAERS data anaphylaxis is estimated to

			Travelers to areas with epidemic levels of HBV. Family members of adoptive children who are HBV+.[43]				occur once per 600,000 vaccine-distributed doses.[48] Conflicting evidence regarding the relationship between vaccine receipt and multiple sclerosis.[14,50]
Influenza[45,58]	TIV Inactivated virus generally containing two A and one B subtypes as either whole or split cell vaccine.	TIV With a good match between the vaccine and the strains of influenza in circulation, the influenza vac-	TIV Can be used in anyone older than 6 months. Specific target groups: Adults ≥ 50 years. Nursing home residents.	TIV and LAIV Anaphylactic allergy to eggs or other vaccine component.[45]	TIV and LAIV Moderate-to-severe illness.[45] History of a GBS episode within 6 weeks of vaccine receipt.[45]	TIV Pregnancy: Recommended for routine use after 14 weeks of gestation in all pregnant women, due to	TIV Pain, redness, and induration at the injection site in 15%–20% of recipients.[45]

(continues)

Table 2-5 COMMONLY USED ADULT VACCINES *(continued)*

Vaccine	Type and Schedule	Efficacy	Indications	Contra-indications	Precautions	Use in Pregnant and HIV Positive Women	Vaccine-Associated Side Effects
	Given annually.[59] Live-attenuated influenza vaccine (LAIV) administered via nasal spray. Given annually.[59]	cine will prevent illness in 90% of adults and 30% to 40% of the frail elderly. Vaccine use among the elderly reduces the risk of hospitalization by 50%-60% and of death by 80%. Immunity lasts less than one year.[45] LAIV Same efficacy.[45]	Persons with chronic cardiac or pulmonary conditions including asthma. Women in their 2nd or 3rd trimester of pregnancy during the flu season. Individuals on long-term aspirin therapy. Individuals who can infect high-risk persons. Anyone desiring to reduce the risk of acquiring influenza.[45] LAIV Only given to healthy individuals between ages of 5 and 49.[45]			the increased rate of complications from influenza infection in pregnancy. Pregnant women with high-risk medical conditions should be vaccinated before the start of the flu season even if vaccination occurs in the first trimester of pregnancy.[45] HIV+: Recommended for use regardless of the level of immunosuppression. Response may be suboptimal. LAIV contraindicated for use in pregnant or HIV+ individuals.	Fever, malaise, myalgias, and chills have been reported in <1%.[45] Rare allergic reactions.[45] Little if any increased risk of GBS with current vaccine. Worse case scenario estimates one additional case of GBS per million vaccinated individuals.[59] LAIV Cough, runny nose, nasal congestion, sore throat, chills in 10%–40%.[45]

Meningitis[46,60]	Purified bacterial capsular polysaccharide vaccine (MPSV4).[52]	Clinical effectiveness >85% for serogroups A and C. Efficacy assumed but not documented for Y and W-135 subgroups. Clinical protection lasts a minimum of 3 years.[60]	Control of serogroup C meningococcal outbreaks.[52] Research, industrial, or clinical laboratory personnel exposed to *N. meningitides*.[52] Travel where infection is epidemic (parts of sub-Saharan Africa).[52] Those with asplenia.[52]	Allergy to vaccine components.[52]	Moderate-to-severe illness.[52]	Safe if indicated.[52] HIV+: safe if indicated.[52]	Pain and redness at injection site 5% to 10%.[52] Headache and malaise 5%–10%. Transient fever 3%.[52] Allergic reaction (urticaria, wheezing, rash) 0.0–0.1 per 100,000 vaccine doses.[60] Anaphylaxis <0.1 per 100,000 vaccine doses.[60] Rarely seizures, paresthesias.[60]
	Quadrivalent conjugate vaccine (MCV 4).[61]	Clinical effectiveness thought to be similar to polysaccharide vaccine.[61]	Routine use in pre-adolescents, college freshman living in dormitories, and those in high-risk categories.[61]	Same as in polysaccharide vaccine.[61]	Same as in polysaccharide vaccine.[61]	Pregnancy: use in pregnancy to be avoided unless necessary since safety data are not yet available. Safe for use in HIV+ individuals.[61]	Pain, redness, induration at injection site 10%–17%. Arthralgia 17%–19%, Malaise 21%. Fever 1.5%–5%.[63]
Measles[47,48,50,62]	Live virus vaccine available as single agent measles (M) measles-rubella (MR) or measles-mumps-rubella (MMR); MMR is preferred. At least one dose after the first birthday.	Efficacy: 95% after one dose, 99% after two. Duration is lifelong.[47]	Adults born after 1956 without written documentation of immunization on or after the first birthday. Travelers to foreign countries. College students.[47]	Severe immunosuppression or on immunosuppressive therapy.[62] Anaphylactic allergy to neomycin, gelatin, or other vaccine component.[62] Active untreated TB.[62]	Moderate-to-severe illness. Recent receipt of Immunoglobulin or blood product.[62] Egg allergy is no longer considered a contraindication, consultation suggested.[47]	Pregnancy: contraindicated.[47] Recommended for all asymptomatic HIV infected persons.[47] Contraindicated in severely immunosuppressed HIV+ persons.[47]	Fever 5%–15% and rash in 5% of recipients, usually seen seven to ten days after vaccination.[48] Thrombocytopenia 1:30,000 doses.[48]

(continues)

Table 2-5 COMMONLY USED ADULT VACCINES *(continued)*

Vaccine	Type and Schedule	Efficacy	Indications	Contra-indications	Precautions	Use in Pregnant and HIV Positive Women	Vaccine-Associated Side Effects
Measles (continued)	Two doses, separated by a minimum of one month, are required for health care workers, travelers to foreign countries, and college students.[47]				Use with caution in persons with a prior history of thrombocytopenia or thrombocytopenia purpura.[62]		Encephalopathy >1/1,000,000 doses.[50] Anaphylaxis >1/1,000,000 doses.[64] Death from vaccine-induced infection (5 deaths in <200 million doses of administered vaccine) has occurred only in severely immunocompromised individuals.[48] (See rubella and mumps sections below if giving MMR.)
Mumps (*See notes under measles.*)[50]	Single agent vaccine available or combined with measles and/or rubella; MMR preferred. One dose.	Efficacy: 95%. Duration: >25 years, probably lifelong.	(See under measles.)	(See under measles.)	(See under measles.)	(See under measles.)	Usually given as MMR. Most reactions to MMR are attributed to either measles or rubella component. Parotitis (rare), CNS dysfunction, deafness, and allergic reac-

							tions have occurred after receipt of mumps component.
Rubella *(See notes under measles.)*[51]	(See under measles.) Vaccine in current use in U.S. is RA 27/3. Single agent vaccine available or combined with mumps/measles.	Efficacy: 95% Duration is lifelong.	(See under measles.) Specific to rubella component, target susceptible adolescents and adults, particularly women of reproductive age.	(See under measles.)	(See under measles.)	(See under measles.)	Commonly given as MMR. Most reactions thought to be due to measles component (see measles). Rubella component thought to cause fever, lymphadenopathy, and arthralgia. 25% of susceptible women develop arthralgias, 10% develop acute arthritis.[51]
Pneumococcal PPV[52]	Polysaccharide vaccine; one dose. Second dose repeated 5 years after the first, only for those at highest risk of severe pneumococcal infection.	PPV is 60% to 70% effective in preventing invasive disease. Response may be suboptimal in the elderly and those with some chronic conditions or immunodeficiency.	All adults ≥65 years. Younger adults with serious chronic cardiac or pulmonary conditions (such as DM, CHF, COPD, emphysema, renal failure, organ transplant, splenic dysfunction, immunosuppression).	Allergy to vaccine component(s).	Moderate-to-severe illness.	Pregnancy: safety is unknown. Women at high risk for pneumococcal infection should be vaccinated before pregnancy. HIV+: recommended for use even with severe immunosuppression.	Local reactions occur in 30%–50% of recipients. Fever, myalgias, and other moderate systemic reactions occur in <1% of recipients. Serious adverse events are rare.

(continues)

Table 2-5 COMMONLY USED ADULT VACCINES (continued)

Vaccine	Type and Schedule	Efficacy	Indications	Contra-indications	Precautions	Use in Pregnant and HIV Positive Women	Vaccine-Associated Side Effects
Tetanus[5,41,53,62]	Toxoid (TT) Single agent tetanus; tetanus-diphtheria (Td) preferred. Dose: 2 doses 4–8 weeks apart; 3rd dose 6–12 months after the 2nd. Booster after 10 years.	Tetanus toxoid has a clinical efficacy approaching 100%.[53] Diphtheria toxoid has a clinical efficacy of 95%. Duration of protection 10 years or less.[41]	All adults.[41]	Severe allergic reaction to prior dose.[41]	Moderate-to-severe illness.[62] Recent GBS episode (within last 6 weeks).[62] Any unstable evolving neurologic condition.[62] Seizure or shock-like state.[62]	Pregnancy: safe.[50] HIV+: safe.[5]	Local reactions such as erythema, induration, pain common. Arthritis-like reactions: (extensive painful swelling 2–8 hours after injection). Most common in those with very high antitoxin levels from frequent immunization. People with arthritis-like reactions should not receive boosters ≤ every 10 years. Severe: Very rarely, brachial neuritis (1/2 to 1 case per 100,000 recipients of tetanus toxoid) and possibly GBS in susceptible individuals.[48]

Varicella[54,62,65]	Attenuated live virus vaccine. For persons aged ≥13 years: two doses separated by 4–8 weeks.[55]	Vaccine efficacy of 80%–90%. Duration of protection unknown, estimated to be as long as 7 to 10 years, may be lifelong.[54]	Susceptible adults, particularly high-risk groups such as: employees at risk of exposure (i.e., health care workers, child care providers, teachers, residents and staff of institutional settings) individuals, mothers, and other family members of young children; family and health care workers with contact with immunosuppressed individuals.[54] Individuals with a history of varicella can be assumed to be immune and do not need vaccination. Those who do not know may be screened serologically to determine vaccine need.[54]	Anaphylactic allergy to gelatin, neomycin, or other vaccine component.[54,62] Untreated active tuberculosis (TB).[62] Immunosuppression due to leukemia, lymphoma, generalized malignancy, immune deficiency disease, or high dose immunosuppressive therapy.[54] Symptomatic or immunosuppressed HIV+.[62]	Moderate-to-severe illness.[54] Recent receipt of immunoglobulin or blood products.[54]	Pregnancy: contraindicated. If woman is inadvertently exposed, enroll case in Varicella Vaccine Pregnancy Registry [1 (800) 986-8999].[54] Asymptomatic HIV+.[54]	Local reactions (soreness, redness, or swelling) in 24% and varicella-like rash occurs in 4%–6% of adult recipients after first dose. Local reactions occur in 33% and varicella-like rash in 1% of recipients after second dose.[54] Varicella-like rash occurs at the site of injection in 1% of adults.[54] Fever within 42 days of receipt occurs in 10% of adults.[54] Secondary transmission is rare and most likely to occur if the recipient is immunocompromised and has a rash.[65]

(continues)

Table 2-5 COMMONLY USED ADULT VACCINES *(continued)*

Vaccine	Type and Schedule	Efficacy	Indications	Contra-indications	Precautions	Use in Pregnant and HIV Positive Women	Vaccine-Associated Side Effects
Varicella (continued)							Post-vaccine zoster thought to occur less frequently after vaccine receipt than after wild infection.[65] Less than 1% of vaccine recipients will experience vaccine failure and contract infection. Breakthrough infections are mild.[54]

is often recommended because it is more practical. Compared to having the patient return for repeated vaccinations of single products, simultaneous administration is more likely to result in the timely completion of any needed immunization series.

However, when immunizations are not given simultaneously, correct spacing becomes important. Incorrect spacing may interfere with the immune response, leaving the patient vulnerable to vaccine-preventable diseases. Inactivated vaccines are not affected by non-simultaneous administration, but live viral vaccines are. If two live parenteral viral vaccines, such as the MMR and varicella vaccines, are not given simultaneously, then they should be administered a minimum of four weeks apart.[5] Giving parenteral live viral vaccines too close together will inhibit the immune response of the second vaccine. In this case, the second vaccine should be repeated or the patient should have serologic confirmation that immunity developed. Only parenteral vaccines need to follow these guidelines. Oral live vaccines, such as oral poliovirus vaccine, are not affected by non-simultaneous administration and may be given as needed.

Space Boosters Correctly

The immune response also can be inhibited by too early administration or by too close spacing of boosters.[5] Both live and inactivated vaccines can be affected by these errors. Recommendations for what age to start a vaccine series, the number of doses needed in the primary series, and the need for subsequent boosters are based on such considerations as when exposure is expected to occur, the physiology of the immune response, and the maturity of the immune system. Childhood vaccine series start as early as birth and as late as 15 months. Beginning at an earlier age than recommended will result in inadequate antibody levels because the immune system is too immature to mount a permanent response. If multiple doses are required, adherence to the recommended time intervals between doses is also important. Giving vaccines too close together will not "boost" the immune system because too early administration will not be recognized as a separate event. Immunologic memory is induced only by repeated separate exposures to an antigen. However, boosters given at longer intervals than recommended will still induce an adequate immune response.

Because the types of vaccines and the number of vaccines needed to complete a primary series is different for adults than children, the management of adults whose records indicate that vaccines were given incorrectly is different than if these errors occur with children. For example, a primary series of tetanus vaccine for children consists of a total of five doses, whereas the adult primary series consists of only three. Therefore adults who did not receive a primary series of tetanus vaccine in childhood do not need to "make up" missed doses and need to receive only three doses to complete their primary series.

Recommendations regarding the management of spacing errors are the same for children and adults. Vaccines requiring multiple doses should not be given at shorter time intervals than recommended.[5] If this occurs, the dose given too early should not be counted as part of the series and should be repeated at the correct time. Boosters given at longer intervals than recommended still induce an appropriate response and may be counted as part of the series. In this case, the vaccine series does not need to be restarted no matter how much time has elapsed between doses.

Table 2-6 shows an adult immunization schedule and describes the types and timing of vaccines recommended for general use in adults. Adults who will be traveling to areas of the world where vaccine-preventable illnesses not commonly seen in the United States occur should consult resources on the Internet (Table 2-3) for current travel recommendations. These recommendations change frequently, so midwives should refer these clients to local or state health departments and/or the National Center for Infectious Diseases Travelers Health Web site for up-to-date information.

Use Proper Technique

Correct administration of vaccine products requires that proper technique be used.[70] Some vaccines should be administered intramuscularly and others subcutaneously to work effectively.[70] Some vaccines, such as measles, require that their distribution and administration follow "cold chain" principles. Other vaccines require that they be stored only at room temperature. Failure to keep vaccines at the proper temperature during each step of the distribution process, from the manufacturer to the patient, can result in loss of vaccine potency.[70] Consequently, practices that provide immunizations to their clients need to follow all manufacturers' instructions on the correct handling and storage for each specific vaccine.

Vaccines should not be co-administered with products that can inhibit the immune response. Passive acquisition of antibodies through receipt of immunoglobulins, whole blood, or other blood products can reduce the effectiveness of some vaccines if the vaccines and antibody-containing products are administered simultaneously.[5] Inactivated vaccines are not affected; however, the immune response of live antigen vaccines can be compromised if they are given too close to the receipt of antibody-containing products. If the vaccine is given first, then two or more weeks should elapse before an antibody-containing product is given.[5] If an antibody-containing product is given first, then three or more months should elapse before receipt of a live antigen vaccine.[5] Allowing a minimum interval between receipt of an antibody-containing product and a live antigen vaccine will permit levels of passively acquired antibodies to decline to low enough levels so that the development of a permanent immune response will not be affected. The recommended window of time needed to elapse before immunizing with a live antigen vaccine differs according to which type of antibody-containing product was given (Table 2-7).[70]

In obstetrical practice, one time that a woman might need both a live viral vaccine and an antibody-containing product would be the Rh negative woman who needs both rubella vaccine and an Rh immune globulin (RhoGAM) injection postpartum. However, the levels of antibodies found in RhoGAM are so low that they are not thought to interfere with the development of an effective immune response to the rubella vaccine in most cases.[5] Even in cases where a postpartum blood transfusion is needed, the CDC recommends vaccinating rubella-susceptible women.[5] Postpartum immunization with the rubella vaccine is a critical strategy used to reduce the incidence of infection and congenital rubella syndrome. Serologic confirmation of immunity is suggested by the Advisory Committee on Immunization Practices (ACIP) when a woman receives RhoGAM or other antibody-containing product after her delivery.[5] The timing of serologic confirmation varies according to which antibody-

Table 2-6 RECOMMENDED ADULT IMMUNIZATION SCHEDULE BY VACCINE AND AGE GROUP UNITED STATES OCTOBER 2004–SEPTEMBER 2005[69]

Age Group Vaccine	19–49	50–64	≥65	Comments*
Tetanus Diphtheria (Td)	1 dose booster every 10 years			
Influenza		1 dose annually	1 dose annually	Priority groups and age recommendations may vary each year according to vaccine availability
Pneumococcal (polysaccharide)		1 dose	1 dose	Generally one lifetime dose. May repeat once five years after first dose for those at highest risk.*
Hepatitis B	3 doses (0, 1–2, 4–6 months)			
Hepatitis A	2 doses (0, 6–12 months)			
Measles, Mumps, Rubella (MMR)	1 or 2 doses			
Varicella	2 doses (0, 4–8 weeks)			
Meningococcal (polysaccharide)	1 dose			

◇ For all persons in this group
◇ For persons at risk (medical/exposure indications)
◈ For persons lacking documentation of vaccination or evidence of disease
◆ Contraindicated
* See text for further details

Table 2-6A RECOMMENDED ADULT IMMUNIZATION SCHEDULE BY VACCINE AND MEDICAL CONDITIONS AND WORK STATUS UNITED STATES OCTOBER 2004–SEPTEMBER 2005[69]*

Vaccine	Pregnancy	Diabetes, heart disease, chronic pulmonary disease, chronic liver disease (including chronic alcoholism)	Congenital immunodeficiency, leukemia, lymphoma, generalized malignancy, large amounts of corticosteroids	HIV	Health Care Workers
Tetanus Diphtheria (Td)					
Influenza		Asthma is an indication			
Pneumococcal (polysaccharide)		Asthma is NOT an indication			
Hepatitis B					
Hepatitis A					No data to support a recommendation
Measles, Mumps, Rubella (MMR)				Withhold if evidence of severe immunosuppression	
Varicella					

◇ For all persons in this group

◈ For persons lacking documentation of vaccination or evidence of disease

◈ For persons at risk (medical/exposure indications)

◆ Contraindicated

* See specific recommendations by the ACIP for individuals with cochlear implants, renal failure/end stage renal disease, recipients of hemodialysis or clotting factor concentrates, asplenia, elective splenectomy, terminal complement component deficiencies, therapy with alkylating agents, antimetabolites, CSF leaks, or radiation.

Table 2-7 SPACING OF LIVE ANTIGEN VACCINES AFTER RECEIPT OF ANTIBODY-CONTAINING PRODUCTS[70]

Antibody-Containing Products	Months Needed to Elapse Before Vaccinating with Live Vaccine
Varicella immunoglobulin	5
Hepatitis B immunoglobulin	3
Packed red blood cells	6
Whole blood	6
Plasma/platelet products	7

containing product a woman received. If RhoGAM was given, serology should be obtained at three or more months postpartum (Table 2-7).[70]

Screen for Contraindications to Vaccine Receipt

Very few true contraindications exist for vaccine receipt. Vaccines have been inappropriately withheld for many reasons. These "missed opportunities" are one of the most common reasons why individuals may not be adequately immunized (**Table 2-8**). According to the CDC, there are only two absolute permanent contraindications: anaphylactic reaction to a vaccine or vaccine component and the development of encephalopathy within seven days of receiving pertussis vaccine.[5] The most common concern is an egg allergy. Individuals who experience severe allergy symptoms, such as generalized hives, itching of the mouth or throat, shortness of breath, hypotension, or shock, after ingesting eggs should not receive the yellow fever or influenza vaccine.[5] Historically, egg allergy has been thought to be responsible for allergic reactions after the receipt of the MMR vaccine, since the MMR vaccine utilizes egg embryos in its manufacturing process. However, in 1998, the ACIP removed anaphylactic allergy to eggs from the list of contraindications to receive the MMR vaccine. Further research suggests that gelatin is the most likely agent causing allergic reactions to the MMR vaccine.[5] The section on the MMR vaccine has further details on the recommendations governing administration to individuals with a history of allergies to eggs.

Other allergies can also be problematic, in particular, allergies to neomycin, yeast, alum, or gelatin. Most individuals with allergies to these substances develop contact dermatitis, not anaphylaxis, after exposure. Those who experience only contact dermatitis may receive vaccines without concern; however, those who have had an anaphylactic reaction should not receive vaccines that contain the offending substance(s).[62] **Table 2-9** shows vaccines and allergies, and the clinician should carefully read the package inserts that come with vaccine products for details.

Latex allergies are also of concern. Latex and latex derivatives (natural rubber latex and dry natural rubber) are used in the manufacture of medical gloves, IV tubing, vaccine vials, and syringes. Other materials, such as vinyl, can be used in the manufacture of these products and do not contain the substances found in latex and latex derivatives, making these products safe for use by those with allergies to latex. Those who

Table 2-8 CONDITIONS AFFECTING THE DECISION TO ORDER VACCINATIONS[5]

Appropriate Reasons to Withhold Some Vaccines	Inappropriate Reasons for Withholding Vaccination
<ul><li>Pregnancy for some but not all vaccines*</li><li>Moderate or severe illness</li><li>Anaphylactic reaction to vaccine or vaccine components</li><li>Anaphylactic reaction to eggs, neomycin, or other vaccine component</li><li>Household members with immunosuppression may be a contra-indication for some but not all vaccines*</li><li>Immunosuppression for some but not all vaccines*</li></ul>	<ul><li>Mild illness</li><li>Antibiotic use</li><li>Pregnancy in the household</li><li>Breastfeeding</li><li>Premature birth</li><li>Need for multiple vaccines</li><li>Non-specific allergies</li><li>Family history of SIDS or seizures</li><li>Nonanaphylactic allergies to vaccine components</li></ul>

*See section on pregnancy and immunosuppression for further details.

experience anaphylactic reactions from exposure to latex should not receive vaccines supplied in vials or syringes that contain natural rubber of any type.[70] Those who report contact dermatitis with use of latex gloves may be vaccinated with products that contain dry natural rubber or natural rubber latex.[70] Synthetic rubber and synthetic latex products may be used in all allergic individuals.[5]

Other situations may occur that are labeled "Precautionary." Vaccines may be given in these cases if the chance of acquiring a vaccine preventable illness is high, but withholding the vaccine until the precautionary condition or situation resolves is preferable. The following are precautions listed by the CDC[5]:

- A condition that increases the likelihood that a VAE may occur or could increase the severity of a VAE (Table 2-5)
- A condition or situation that may inhibit the immune response to a vaccine
- Precautions that apply specifically to the pertussis vaccine include any of the

following reactions occurring within 48 hours of receiving a prior dose of pertussis vaccine: temperature >105°F, hypotonic hyporesponsive episode, or inconsolate crying lasting more than three hours; or a seizure occurring within three days of receiving a dose of pertussis vaccine

Individuals with moderate-to-severe illness should wait to receive vaccinations until the illness has resolved. These individuals do not seem to be at higher risk of impaired immunity or vaccine reactions; rather, the underlying illness may make the recognition of a VAE, particularly fever, more difficult to ascertain.

Before administering vaccines, the clinician should ask a few screening questions regarding conditions that would make vaccine receipt problematic. Patients should be queried about allergies, particularly food allergies; whether they and/or anyone living in their household have problems with their immune system; if they ever had any reaction to the receipt of any

Table 2-9 VACCINES AND ALLERGIES[62]

Anaphylactic Allergy	Vaccines to Avoid
A specific vaccine	That vaccine
Alum	Hepatitis A
Gelatin	MMR, varicella
Neomycin	MMR, varicella
Yeast	Hepatitis B
Egg	Influenza

other vaccines; their current state of health; and the likelihood they could be pregnant.[5] Table 2-8 summarizes the conditions that impact the decision to administer vaccines.

When a Vaccine History Is Unknown

Three different approaches are acceptable for women whose immunization status is unknown.[70] The midwife can determine immunity by obtaining serologic titers and administer vaccine(s) if low titers indicate a vaccine is needed. Testing for titers is expensive but will avoid unnecessary vaccine administration. However, giving a vaccine without documenting immunity is also acceptable if no contraindications are present. This approach may be less expensive and easier to implement than obtaining titers. The third approach is to obtain immunization records from school and medical records, analyze these records to determine what vaccinations are needed, and immunize accordingly. This approach will avoid unneeded vaccination, but will be more difficult and time-consuming to implement. Midwives should discuss these options with their clients and suggest the one that best meets the needs of the client and the system in which care is provided.

Immunization in Special Populations

Pregnancy and Lactation

All inactivated vaccines are considered safe to give in pregnancy. However, live viral vaccines should be avoided. Live viral vaccines induce low-level replication similar to that seen in wild infection and could theoretically cause infection in the fetus. Rubella is the vaccine of most concern because wild infection in the mother can lead to fetal infection and the development of congenital rubella syndrome in a significant percentage of infected fetuses.[64] Between 1971 and 1989, the CDC followed 324 women who received the rubella vaccine between three months before conception and the third month of pregnancy.[64] None of the infants born to these women had congenital rubella syndrome, and only five had serologic evidence of subclinical infection. Therefore, women who inadvertently receive the vaccine during pregnancy should be informed of these theoretical risks but do not need to be advised to terminate their pregnancy.[64] Pre-vaccination pregnancy tests are also not recommended, but women should be advised to avoid pregnancy for one month after receiving the vaccine.[64]

Exposure to other live viral vaccines during pregnancy is of less concern because it is unlikely that exposure to these vaccines will lead to adverse fetal effects. No cases of adverse fetal effects have been documented after receipt of mumps, measles, or varicella vaccines.[64,71] Infections targeted by these vaccines are not thought to lead to significant increases in birth defects, although depending on the causative agent, maternal infection in pregnancy has been reported to increase the risk of preterm delivery, spontaneous abortion, and intrauterine growth restriction.[72] Maternal infection with varicella during pregnancy can lead to congenital varicella syndrome in exposed fetuses, which can present with skin lesions, limb hypoplasia, cataracts, microophthalmia, and other malformations.[72] However, the incidence of congenital varicella syndrome is low and has been estimated to occur in 0.6% of infants born to mothers infected in the first trimester.[72] Because the virulence of the attenuated strain used in the varicella vaccine is much less than that of wild virus, fetuses exposed to the vaccine are unlikely to be affected. Women should be advised to avoid pregnancy for one month after receipt of the vaccine, but those who inadvertently received the vaccine one month before conception or in pregnancy do not need to be advised to terminate their pregnancy.[71] Women who are exposed to the varicella vaccine in the month before pregnancy and/or early pregnancy should be reported to the VARIVAX Pregnancy Registry, so that more accurate information regarding the safety of the varicella vaccine is available in the future (Table 2-3).

All vaccines can safely be given during lactation. While live viral vaccines replicate in the mother's body, there is little evidence that vaccine-virus other than rubella is excreted in the breast milk. There are only a few reports in the literature linking the presence of virus in breast milk to infection in the infant, and the resulting infections have been well tolerated. Therefore, the ACIP recommends that breastfeeding mothers and their infants follow the routine adult and childhood immunization schedule.[70]

Pregnancy provides an ideal opportunity to "catch-up" on needed vaccines. It is a time when many women, including those who would otherwise not seek health care, are seen repeatedly over a relatively short time span in the same institution or practice. Many vaccines needed by adults require boosters, and most are safe to administer in pregnancy or in the early postpartum period. The vaccines of particular concern for women during this time period are tetanus, hepatitis B, rubella, and varicella.

HIV and Other Immunosuppressive Conditions

Severe immunosuppression can be caused by cancer, chemotherapy, human immunodeficiency virus (HIV) infection, or high-dose corticosteroid use, and less commonly can be found in some congenital disorders. Inactivated, recombinant, subunit, polysaccharide, conjugate, and toxoid vaccines can safely be given to all immunocompromised individuals, although response to vaccination may be suboptimal.[70]

Live viral vaccines can be problematic for immunosuppressed individuals.[5] Uncontrolled replication has led to fatal cases of polio and measles infection in immunocompromised HIV-positive individuals after vaccine administration. Live viral vaccines are contraindicated in those with severe immunosuppression.[5] However, those with milder immunosuppression can receive live vaccines and may need their protection. Recommendations vary by vaccine and by level of immunosuppression (**Table 2-10**). Ensuring that asymptomatic HIV-positive individuals and others receive vaccines at a time when the immune system is healthy enough to mount an effective response may protect these individuals from serious infection later when their immune system begins to fail.

Table 2-10 LIVE VACCINES AND IMMUNOSUPPRESSION

Product	Vaccinate	Hold Vaccination	Household Contact
Varicella vaccine[5,65]	• Asymptomatic HIV positive individuals[5] • Mildly immunosuppressed HIV positive children (defined as age specific CD4+ T-lymphocyte% ≥ 25%) • Low dose corticosteroid use (aerosols, topicals, short course, alternative day)	• Cellular immunodeficiency[65] • High dose corticosteroid use (≥20 mg/day) • Symptomatic HIV+ individuals	Vaccinate
MMR[5,64]	• Low dose corticosteroid use (aerosols, topicals, short course, alternative day)[5] • Asymptomatic HIV+ individuals[5] • Mildly immunosuppressed HIV+ individuals (defined in those ≥13 years of age as ≥200 µ/L total CD4+ T-lymphocyte **OR** ≥14% CD4+ T-lymphocytes as % of total lymphocytes)[64]	• High dose corticosteroid use (≥20 mg/day)[5] • Symptomatic or severely immunosuppressed HIV+ individuals[5]	Vaccinate[64]

Commonly Used Adult Vaccines

The specific vaccines recommended for general use in adults vary according to age, exposure potential, vaccine history, and the presence of underlying medical conditions (Tables 2-5, 2-6, and 2-6A).

Tetanus/Diphtheria Vaccine

Tetanus is caused by toxins released by *Clostridium tetani*. The infection can lead to paralysis, laryngospasm, hypertension, and fractures.[53] Infection occurs when the organism, commonly found in soil, enters the body usually but not always through non-intact skin. Adults are the most at risk. While immune levels remain high for as long as 10 to 20 years after vaccination, many adults do not receive booster shots and their immune levels wane over time. Between 1998 and 2000, over 80% of all cases of tetanus occurred in adults over 30 years of age.[73] Others at higher risk include diabetics (12% of cases) and IV drug users (15% of cases).[73] The majority of deaths occurred in individuals over 60 years of age.[73]

Many pregnant women are not protected from tetanus. In a survey of over 200 pregnant women, Kalaca found that 35% of subjects were not immune.[74] Despite inadequate levels of maternal immunity in some individuals, neonatal infection is rare in the United States; only two cases of neonatal tetanus have been reported in the United States since 1989. One occurred in a child born to a Mexican woman who had resided in the United States for several years, received prenatal care and delivered in a U.S. hospital, yet never received the tetanus vaccine.[75] Many countries primarily target pregnant women, whereas in the United States adults have generally received a complete series in childhood. Midwives need to be aware of the immunization practices of the countries of origin for the women in their care. Areas of the world with high prevalence rates of neonatal tetanus include China, India, Pakistan, Nepal, Brazil, and parts of Africa and Southeast Asia.[76] The other case of neonatal tetanus occurred in an infant born to an American woman who had never received the vaccine due to personal beliefs.[77] Exposure was thought to occur via inappropriate cord care, which led to subsequent infection. Both of these cases point out the importance of ensuring that pregnant women are protected from tetanus and, if vaccination is not acceptable to a client, that mothers receive instruction on appropriate ways to clean and wrap the umbilical cord for infants after birth.

The tetanus vaccine is usually combined with diphtheria vaccine and given to adults and adolescents as Td.[53] Other formulations, such as the DT, DPT, and DTaP vaccines, are available but are given only to young children. A new formulation (Tdap) containing pertussis have just recently been approved for use in adolescents and adults. In June 2005, the ACIP voted to recommend that Tdap replace the Td booster previously recommended for adolescents aged 11 to 12. They also recommended that adolescents ages 13 to 18 years of age who missed the Td booster at age 11 to 12 be vaccinated with Tdap and to consider use of this new vaccine in adolescents between 11 and 18 who already received Td in order to protect them from pertussis infection. As of June 2005, the ACIP has not released recommendations regarding the use of this product in adults.[78] Currently, the recommended adult primary series consists of three doses of Td with boosters every ten years. Patients do not require more frequent doses except in special circumstances. **Table 2-11** describes when a tetanus vaccination is needed in the event of an injury.[53]

Diphtheria is much more common than tetanus and is easily spread via person-to-person contact from infected respiratory secretions. Diphtheria can be mild and mimic the common cold, but more severe infection can lead to tonsillar and laryngeal disease.[41] Epidemics have occurred, such as in Eastern Europe in the 1990s when immunization levels fell in the aftermath of the dissolution of the Soviet Union.[36] Immunizing with a combined tetanus-diphtheria vaccine is recommended by the ACIP as an effective approach to keeping diphtheria under control.[41]

MMR Vaccine

Measles infection is one of the leading causes of death and disability worldwide. Over 50% of all childhood deaths from vaccine preventable illnesses worldwide are estimated to be due to complications from measles.[79] Measles is highly infectious; the highest rates of complications occur in individuals less than 5 years of age or older than 20 years.[47] Infection can lead to diarrhea, otitis media, and pneumonia.

Table 2-11 TETANUS IMMUNIZATION AND WOUND MANAGEMENT[53]

Vaccine History	Clean Minor Wound	Other More Severe Wounds
Unknown or incomplete primary series	Vaccinate	Vaccinate
Complete series	Vaccination not needed unless has not received booster in last 10 years	Vaccinate if <5 years since last booster

Other less common complications include encephalitis, seizures, and subacute sclerosing panencephalitis (SSP).[47] SSP, while rare, can be devastating. It is a degenerative disease of the central nervous system (CNS) that slowly progresses from intellectual and behavioral impairment to ataxia, myoclonic seizures, and ultimately death.

In 1990, the World Summit for Children set a goal to immunize 90% of the world's children by 2000.[80] Measles has many of the attributes that make it amenable to eradication: 1) the only reservoir is humans; 2) a highly effective and affordable vaccine has been developed; 3) subclinical infections are rare, making diagnosis easier; and 4) serological tests are available that can confirm infection and/or immunity, making it possible to monitor success and pinpoint geographical areas or at-risk populations that may require further vaccine coverage.[81,82] Significant progress toward worldwide eradication has been made, particularly in the Americas. Between 1999 and 2001, 68% of the 41 countries in the region, including the United States, Canada, Cuba, the English-speaking Carribean countries, and most of Central and South America, were free of endemic measles.[83] Most of the cases of measles that did occur were a result of importation from Europe, Asia, or Africa. Thanks to implementation of "catch-up" campaigns targeting children younger than age 5, indigenous spread of wild infection has been eliminated in the Western hemisphere since 2002.[83] However, importation of measles from other parts of the world remains a constant threat.[34] Maintaining high vaccine coverage rates in the Americas is an essential part of the World Health Organization (WHO) strategy for eliminating measles worldwide.

The mumps vaccine is commonly given as a combined product containing the measles and rubella vaccines. Mumps is caused by a paramyxovirus. Its initial presentation is nonspecific and similar to that seen in upper respiratory infections.[50] Up to 40% of infected individuals will develop parotitis. More serious complications are rare but can include orchitis, oophoitis, pancreatitis, and hearing loss. Serious side effects associated with use of the mumps vaccine are rare. It is estimated that CNS dysfunction after receipt of mumps vaccine occurs in one out of one million administered doses.[50]

Rubella is rare in the United States but remains of major concern because of the devastating consequences for the fetus from maternal infection during pregnancy. Maternal infection in pregnancy is associated with major congenital defects such as deafness, cardiac anomalies, microcephaly, mental retardation, cataracts, glaucoma, and other problems. The probability that infection will lead to congenital defects varies by stage of pregnancy. Up to 85% of fetuses will be affected if infection occurs during the first trimester.[51]

While vaccine coverage is high in the United States, rubella vaccine use is more sporadic in other parts of the world and over 40% of other countries do not include it as part of their recommended vaccine schedule.[84] Therefore, importation into the United States is possible, particularly into immigrant communities with lower immunity levels. In recent years, most cases in the United States have occurred in Hispanic adults who have immigrated from parts of the world where rubella vaccine is not commonly given.[51]

Vaccines against measles, mumps, and rubella are available as single agent or combined products. The ACIP recommends the MMR vaccine as the preferred product, since it can protect against several diseases.[51] Because these vaccines are attenuated live viral vaccines, they are highly effective and in general need only one dose to achieve long-lasting immunity, although the ACIP recommends that individuals living or working in high-risk settings such as schools receive two doses. As with all live vaccines, these vaccines are contraindicated for use in pregnancy and in some circumstances for immunosuppressed individuals, discussed earlier in this chapter. Side effects and adverse reactions can result from exposure to vaccine components, but also from viral replication, which very rarely can lead to clinical disease (Table 2-4).

Varicella Vaccine

Historically, varicella has been endemic in the United States with over 85% of the population infected by age 15.[54] However, since varicella vaccine became available in 1995, the incidence of infection has plummeted. Between 1995 and 2001, the numbers of reported cases fell by 76%.[54] Because vaccine campaigns to date have focused on children, a subset of adults remains at risk, particularly those between 20 and 30 years of age who were less likely to have been exposed as children to endemic infection and too old to have been offered varicella vaccine as part of routine childhood immunizations. Adults are much more likely to experience significant complications from varicella infection than children. Consequently, all adults should be screened and offered varicella vaccine as appropriate.

The decision on whether immunization is needed is based on patient history; serological testing is generally not needed. Unlike other vaccine-preventable illnesses, varicella causes few subclinical infections and has a distinctive rash, making it easy to diagnose. Serological studies have confirmed that relying on patient history is a cost-effective approach. In one study, over 97% of those who gave a history of having had varicella had seropositive titers indicating immunity. Even those with a negative history were likely to be immune: 71% to 93% of these individuals were seropositive.[71] Therefore, if a patient has a history of varicella, neither serological confirmation of immunity or vaccination is needed. Those who do not know or don't think they had varicella earlier in life should be screened via serological testing and immunized if needed.

The varicella vaccine is a live viral vaccine, making it contraindicated for use in pregnancy and in some immunosuppressed individuals (detailed earlier in this chapter). Serious adverse events are thought to be rare with use of this vaccine, but ongoing monitoring is essential given that it is a relatively new addition to the childhood and adult immunization schedule. Suspected reactions should be reported to VAERS. Pregnant women exposed to the vaccine in early pregnancy or in the month prior to conception should be reported to the VARIVAX Pregnancy Registry.

In addition to causing chickenpox, the varicella-zoster virus also can cause herpes zoster. After the primary infection resolves, the *Varicella-virus* lies dormant in the dorsal root ganglia. If the virus becomes reactivated, it travels down the nerves to the skin resulting in a painful vesicular rash. This rash typically presents in a classic pattern, following the distribution of the affected dermatome. Not all individuals infected with varicella develop zoster. The likelihood seems to be increased in those who were infected at a young age (in utero or less than 18 months of age) and in immunocompromised individuals.[71] Herpes zoster is rare in childhood (if infection occurs after 18 months) and increases with age.[71] The incidence has been reported to be 2.5 per 1000 in people 20 to 50 years of age, rising to 7.8 cases per 1000 in individuals older than 60 years.[85] Post-herpetic neuralgia or pain that resolves slowly (sometimes as long as one year) after resolution of the rash is an uncommon, but debilitating, complication. It also occurs more often in older adults, increasing from 3% to 4% in individuals aged 30 to 49 years to 21% in those between 60 and 70 years of age to 34% in those more than 80 years.[85]

One of the concerns expressed in the medical community when the varicella vaccine was added to the routine childhood schedule was whether use of the vaccine would shift the prevalence of disease upward and increase the incidence of infection in older individuals.[86–88] Complications are 6 to 15 times higher and deaths 24 times higher in adults than children.[85] In addition, there is epidemiological evidence that naturally circulating wild infection may also play a role in providing "natural boost-

ing" and by doing so maintain immunity to chickenpox and prevent herpes zoster.[89] To date, preliminary evidence seems to indicate that use of the varicella vaccine may be protective against the development of herpes zoster. The incidence of herpes zoster in vaccinated children from VAERS reports is 2.6 cases per 100,000 distributed doses compared to 68 cases in healthy children younger than 20 years of age per 100,000 person-years after natural infection.[65] However, since rates of herpes zoster tend to increase with age, it is too early to tell whether the cohort of children currently receiving varicella vaccine will experience continued lower rates of herpes zoster as they age. Consequently, it is possible that vaccine use could increase morbidity and mortality associated with the varicella virus, at least in the short run, if infections increase in older individuals and if natural boosting does play a role in maintaining protective levels of antibodies.

An analysis of the impact of vaccine use on the epidemiology and health consequences of varicella infection using various estimates of vaccine effectiveness, vaccine coverage rates, and disease-related complications was published in 2003.[89] This model predicts that routine infant immunization with 90% coverage would reduce inpatient hospital stays by approximately half a day from complications related to varicella but increase inpatient hospital stay by one day due to complications secondary to herpes zoster.[89] However, after 65 years of vaccine use, it is predicted that widespread universal use of the varicella vaccine would lead to decreased morbidity. Midwives should check for periodic updates regarding the use of varicella vaccine because the recommendations governing the timing of administration, number of doses, and need for boosters may change as these issues become clarified.

Hepatitis B Vaccine

Since 1991, the CDC has recommended a multifaceted approach to eliminating hepatitis B infection in the United States. These include: universal screening of pregnant women; immunoprophylaxis of exposed newborns; routine vaccination of all infants; catch-up vaccination of adolescents; and vaccination of high risk adults. These efforts have resulted in significant declines in the number of cases reported to the CDC. Between 1990 and 2002, rates of acute hepatitis B infection have declined by 89% in children and adolescents ages 0 to 19 years,[90] by 67% in adults aged between 20 and 39 years, and by 39% in adults aged over 40 years.[91] However, while the overall incidence has been declining, certain subgroups, such as men 20 years or older and women 40 years or older, have experienced increasing rates of infection in the last few years.[91] Individuals who engage in such high risk behaviors as having multiple partners, men who have sex with men (MSM), and IV drug users are at particular risk. The CDC recommends continued emphasis on screening and immunizing adults who engage in these behaviors.[91]

Screening and immunizing adults as needed may help prevent morbidity and mortality associated with hepatitis B infection. While adults are significantly less likely to become chronic carriers than infants or children after infection, many more of them become infected. Therefore, over 70% of all chronic infections in the United States are estimated to be due to infections acquired in adulthood.[44] Not only can adults transmit infection to their sexual partner(s), but pregnant women who become acutely infected during pregnancy are much more likely to transmit infection perinatally than chronic carriers. As many as 90% to 95%

of infants born to mothers infected in the last three months of pregnancy develop chronic infection compared to 10% to 85% of infants born to chronic carriers.[57,92] (Note: Use of hepatitis B immune globulin prophylaxis after birth significantly lowers these risks.) Pregnant women should be counseled about high risk behaviors and offered immunization if their lifestyle poses potential maternal or fetal risks.

Over 40% of the population of the world lives in areas where hepatitis B is endemic.[43] High prevalence areas are defined as locations where more than 8% of the population is HBsAG positive; moderate prevalence is between 2% and 7%, and low prevalence is below 2%.[43] In areas of the world with high prevalence, more than 60% of the population becomes acutely infected,[43] often in infancy or during childhood, and 8% develop chronic infection.[14] In areas of low prevalence, less than 20% become acutely infected, most often in adulthood, and chronic infection is present in less than 1% of the population.[43]

In 1992, WHO set a goal to have all countries integrate hepatitis B vaccination into their routine childhood immunization schedule by 1997.[93] As of 2001, 66% of WHO member countries had adopted universal infant or childhood vaccination with hepatitis B.[93] Many of those countries not providing universal vaccination programs are in areas where hepatitis B is endemic. Women from areas such as China, South East Asia, the Middle East, Africa, and the Pacific Islands[43] are unlikely to have received hepatitis B vaccination in their native country, and need to be screened for evidence of active or past infection and immunized as appropriate.

Serologic markers that can help indicate whether a woman needs to be immunized are hepatitis B core antibody (HBcAb), hepatitis B surface antibody (HBsAb), and hepatitis B antigen (HBAg).[43] Individuals who are immune will test positive for one or both of the antibodies (HBcAb, HBsAb) and negative for the antigen (HBAg). Those who acquired immunity via vaccination usually test positive for HBsAb, whereas those who acquired immunity from resolved infection usually test positive for HBcAb. Individuals who are chronically infected test negative for antibodies (HBcAb, HBsAb) and positive for antigen (HBAg). **Table 2-12** shows commonly used markers to evaluate hepatitis B immunity.

Hepatitis B vaccines have been available since 1981. The vaccine in current use is a recombinant vaccine, which is formed by inserting the hepatitis B antigen into Baker yeast cells.[43] These yeast cells produce HBAg, which is then harvested, purified, and used as a basis for the vaccine. The final product contains no infectious components and is incapable of causing active infection. Usually the hepatitis B vaccine is given as a single agent in a three-dose series. However, a combined product containing both hepatitis A and hepatitis B vaccine components has been available since 2001.[43] The combined product is available for use in individuals older than 18 years of age and is recommended for individuals with chronic liver disease, those who have clotting factor conditions requiring receipt of therapeutic blood products, IV drug users, and MSM.[94] Effectiveness and side effects are similar to those seen in

Table 2-12 MARKERS USED IN EVALUATING HEPATITIS B IMMUNITY[43]

Status	Serologic Markers	Notes
Susceptible	HBsAb Negative HBcAb Negative HBAg Negative	Vaccinate
Immune from Infection	HBsAb Negative HBcAb Positive HBAg Negative	Vaccination not necessary
Immune from Vaccine	HBsAb Positive HBcAb Negative HBAg Negative	Vaccination not necessary
Four possibilities 1) Recovering from acute infection 2) Distantly immune with very low levels of HBsAb 3) Susceptible with false positive HBcAb 4) Chronically infected with undetectable HBAg	HBsAb Negative HBcAb Positive HBAg Negative	Repeat serologic markers to rule out false positive results. Screen with IGM HBcAb, which is positive early in the course of acute infection. Screening with liver function tests can help uncover low level chronic infections.

single product hepatitis A and hepatitis B vaccines.[94]

Reactions are rare after hepatitis B vaccine receipt. Pain at the injection site is the most commonly reported side effect; less than 1% of recipients report fever.[43]

One potential VAE that has been investigated is whether the hepatitis B vaccine triggers the development of multiple sclerosis or relapse in those who already have the disease. Multiple sclerosis is more common in women and is frequently diagnosed between 20 and 40 years of age.[14] The cause is unknown, but environment exposure and genetics are thought to be involved in the etiology. Case reports of women developing multiple sclerosis in France in the mid-1990s after receiving the vaccine prompted widespread public concern and resulted in routine hepatitis B vaccination being dropped from school health clinics despite assertions from WHO that the vaccine was safe.[95–97] After an intensive review of the available research, the Immunization Safety Review Committee released a report in 2002 agreeing with this assessment.[14] Two of the strongest studies weighed heavily in their evaluation.[98,99] Ascherio evaluated 192 cases and 645 matched controls to determine whether vaccination could trigger the development of multiple sclerosis. Immunization history was initially obtained by self-report and those who indicated receipt of hepatitis B vaccination had their vaccination history confirmed by employee health care records. Timing of symptom onset and disease diagnosis was assessed by patient and physician surveys. The results indicated no association between vaccination and the development of multiple sclerosis (confidence interval [CI] 0.5–1.6).[98] Confavreux found no association with receipt of the hepatitis B vaccination and relapse in 643 women with established disease.[99] However, newer research contradicts these findings. A nested case control study of 163 cases and over 1600 controls found that the odds ratio of developing multiple sclerosis within three years after immunization with the hepatitis B vaccine was 3.1 (CI 1.5–6.3).[58] No increased risk was found after tetanus or influenza vaccination. This study used rigorous definitions of important study variables. It used the date of symptom onset consistent with multiple sclerosis, not the date of diagnosis, as the measure of concern and confirmed symptom onset, date of diagnosis, and vaccine history by review of the paper medical record and computerized vaccine history. This discrepancy between an authoritative evaluation of the literature and more recent research points out the importance of staying abreast of the newest updates on vaccine safety. While consensus opinion does not change on the basis of one study, a well-designed study contradicting established thought warrants careful consideration.

Another safety issue of concern in the late 1990s was whether incorporating hepatitis B vaccines into the infant immunization schedule would raise infants' exposure to mercury to unsafe levels. Many vaccines, including the hepatitis B vaccine, have historically used thimerosal, which contains mercury as a preservative. It was commonly added to multidose vials to prevent contamination and until 1999 was present in 30 vaccines licensed and marketed in the United States.[14] Until 1991, the only vaccine given to infants that contained thimerosal was DTP. In 1991, hepatitis B and HIB vaccines, both of which contained thimerosal, were recommended for routine use in infants less than one year of age.[14] This expanded immunization schedule was estimated by the FDA to increase the exposure of infants younger than 6 months to mercury levels that exceeded Environmental Protection Agency (EPA) body-weight recommendations.[14] The FDA recommended that vaccine manufacturers remove mercury from vaccines or justify why its continued use was necessary. In 1999, the American Academy of Pediatrics and the Public Health Service released a statement recommending that thimerosal-containing vaccines be used in infants and children only until thimerosal-free alternatives became available.[100] Since mid-2001, vaccines administered to children are either thimerosal-free or contain only trace amounts.[70] The Immunization Safety Review Committee also recommends the use of thimerosal-free vaccines in infants and children as well as in pregnant women.[12] Thimerosal is present in some adult vaccines (Td, DT, one of two adult hepatitis B vaccines, and influenza vaccine).[70]

Hepatitis A Vaccine

Hepatitis A is spread through contact or ingestion of contaminated food or water via fecal-oral routes. The source of infection is unknown in many cases. Over 40% of cases occur in individuals with no known risk factors; 14% occur after exposure to an infected individual, 10% occur in MSM, and 8% occur in IV drug users.[42] Symptoms include fever, malaise, abdominal pain, dark urine, and jaundice and vary by age. Over 70% of children less than age 6 are asymptomatic, whereas over 70% of older children and adults report symptoms.[42] Most infections resolve within two months.

The hepatitis A vaccine was licensed for use in 1995 in children age two or older.[42] It is recommended for use only in selected situations, such as for those who live in communities with high prevalence and those whose lifestyle places

them at higher risk of exposure. Prevalence is much higher in children who live in the Western United States. Between 1987 and 1997, over 50% of the cases occurred in Arizona, Arkansas, California, Oregon, Oklahoma, New Mexico, North Dakota, Utah, and Washington.[42] In 1999, the ACIP recommended that children older than age 2 living in higher prevalence communities receive hepatitis A vaccine as part of the routine childhood immunization schedule. Individuals living in communities with double the normal background incidence of hepatitis A (20 cases per 100,000) should be offered the vaccine; those living in above-average prevalence communities (10 to 20 cases per 100,000) should be informed of the availability of the vaccine and vaccinated as appropriate.[42] Other high-risk individuals such as IV drug users, MSM, those at occupational risk, or those with underlying liver disease should also be offered the vaccine.[42] Child care workers, those who work in sanitation-related jobs, and food handlers are not considered to be at higher risk and do not need routine vaccination.[42]

The hepatitis A vaccine is an inactivated vaccine and requires two doses separated by six months.[42] Side effects are minimal (Table 2-5). Hepatitis A vaccine is also available as a combined product containing hepatitis B vaccine.

Influenza Vaccine

The influenza virus has three subtypes: A, B, and C.[45] Influenza A infects humans and animals and causes moderate to severe illness. Influenza B also infects humans but generally causes milder disease. Influenza C rarely infects humans; when infection occurs, it tends to be subclinical. Influenza viruses constantly evolve. Minor changes in subtypes are called antigenic drift; major changes are called antigenic shifts.

Both changes can lead to epidemics, but antigenic shifts, which generally result from genetic recombinations between influenza A viruses that infect humans and birds, can lead to pandemics. Pandemics (disease that infects a region, country, or that is global) spread along travel routes and have high attack rates in all age groups. While disease severity tends to remain unchanged, because so many more individuals are infected during pandemics, mortality can be high.

Each year, the influenza vaccine is reformulated to match the subtypes expected to be circulating during the flu season. The ideal time to vaccinate is in October and November, before the start of the flu season that typically runs from November to March. If a good match exists between the current vaccine and circulating subtypes, vaccine efficacy is high (90%) in healthy young adults.[45] Influenza vaccine is less effective, even with a good match, in the frail elderly, but can mitigate the severity of infection. Use of the influenza vaccine in the elderly is estimated to prevent infection in only 30% to 40% of recipients, but is 50% to 60% effective in preventing hospitalization and 80% effective in preventing death.[45]

The influenza vaccine comes in two formulations: trivalent-inactivated influenza vaccine (TIV) and live-attenuated influenza vaccine (LAIV).[45] The TIV vaccine, which is administered intramuscularly, has been available since the 1940s. The newest influenza vaccine, approved for use in 2003, is the LAIV vaccine administered as a nasal spray. Both vaccines contain the same subtypes: type A (H1N1), type A (H3N2), and type B.[45] Some versions of the TIV vaccine use thimerosal as a preservative; others use only reduced amounts or are preservative-free.[59] The LAIV vaccine is thimerosal-free.[59]

Both vaccines are grown in chicken eggs and contain trace amounts of egg protein. Therefore, patients should not receive either vaccine if they have developed hives, swelling of the lips or tongue, acute respiratory distress, or collapse after ingesting eggs.[59] Individuals with milder reactions to egg exposure may also be at increased risk for allergic reactions. Those at high risk of complications from influenza may either receive prophylactic antiviral medication or be desensitized before receiving the vaccine. Consultation with a vaccine expert is recommended for egg-allergic individuals before being immunized with an influenza vaccine.[58]

While the efficacy is similar for both vaccines, recommendations on who should receive them differ significantly. Viral shedding has occurred for two to three days after receipt of the LAIV vaccine but not after receipt of the TIV vaccine.[59] Therefore, the LAIV has the potential to cause clinical illness in the recipient and to be spread to close contacts, but studies to date indicate that this rarely occurs. In a study of transmissibility of the LAIV in a childcare setting, the probability of acquiring vaccine virus after close contact with a vaccinated child was only 0.58% to 2.4%.[59] Complaints of runny nose, headaches, and sore throat are more common in LAIV recipients than in the placebo group but clinical infection is rare.[59] Because of the remote possibility that clinical illness and/or transmission may occur with LAIV, the ACIP recommends that the use of LAIV be limited to healthy individuals between ages 5 and 49.[59] In contrast, TIV is approved for use in individuals aged 6 months or older and in those with underlying medical conditions, HIV infected individuals, and pregnant women. Both vaccines may be given to family members and close personal contacts of individuals with mild-to-moderate immunosuppression; those in contact with individuals with severe immunosuppression should receive the TIV vaccine.[59]

Pneumococcal Vaccine

Infection with *Streptococcus pneumoniae* causes between 13% and 19% of all cases of bacterial meningitis and 36% of all cases of community-acquired pneumonia in adults.[52] Invasive pneumococcal disease is most common in children under 2 years of age and in adults 65 years or older. The ACIP recommends routinely vaccinating individuals in these age groups as well as all individuals regardless of age who have underlying chronic illness or immunosuppression.[52]

Two vaccines are available.[52] Conjugate vaccine is available for use in children. The pneumococcal polysaccharide vaccine is recommended for use in adults. The current adult vaccine contains antigen from 23 types of pneumococcal bacteria and the childhood vaccine contains seven.[52] The antibody response to the polysaccharide vaccine is poor in children under 2 years of age, but robust after receipt of the conjugate vaccine. Therefore, the conjugate vaccine is preferred for use with children. Antibody response to the polysaccharide vaccine is also reduced in some older adults and in some adults with underlying medical conditions, particularly immunosuppression. Even though some adult recipients may have a suboptimal antibody response to vaccination, the ACIP recommends that influenza vaccine be administered even to those unlikely to mount a full and sustained antibody response because most recipients are afforded some level of protection from infection.[52]

Immunity wears off over time. Antibody levels decline over five to ten years and can decline faster in those individuals whose initial response was poor. Because boosters do not seem to improve protection, revaccination is not recommended except for those at the highest risk of complications from infection. High-risk individuals who are candidates for revaccination are those with asplenia, transplants, chronic renal failure, nephritic syndrome, or immunosuppression.[52] These individuals should receive a one-time booster five or more years after receipt of their original pneumococcal vaccine.[52]

Serious reactions to the pneumococcal vaccine are rare. While 30% to 50% of recipients can develop pain and soreness at the injection site, less than 1% develop fever and malaise.[52]

Meningitis

Neisseria meningitidis is the most common cause of bacterial meningitis in the United States.[46] Case fatality rates are high (9%–12%) even with appropriate antibiotic coverage. Up to 20% of survivors have neurological damage, hearing loss, or other permanent disability.[46] Infection is uncommon but varies with age. Incidence rates are highest in infants less than one year of age, decline during childhood, rise again in adolescence and early adulthood, and fall in older adults.[46] One subgroup at slightly higher risk is college students living in dormitories. However, because the risk is only slightly increased, the ACIP has not historically recommended requiring vaccination for college students in general, college freshmen, or students living in dormitories; rather, they had recommended counseling all students, particularly freshmen who will be living in dormitories and their parents, about meningitis, the availability of the vaccine, and making vaccination available for those who want it.[101] However, in February 2005 a new vaccine (Menactra™) was approved by the FDA for the prevention of invasive meningococcoccal disease caused by the Neisseria meningitides serogroups A, C, Y, W-135. The ACIP released a new statement in March 2005 recommending that it be incorporated into the routine immunization schedule at the pre-adolescent pediatric visit at ages 11 to 12 years and be made a requirement for high school entry. They also recommend its routine use in college freshman living in dormitories and for others at higher risk of exposure or disease complications.[102] Routine use for adults aged 20 to 55 is not recommended as rates of disease are low in this age group.

Until February 2005, the only vaccine recommended for use in adults was a polysaccharide vaccine. It was recommended for use in college freshmen as outlined above, but has also been used in the control of outbreaks, for travelers to areas of the world where *Neisseria meningitides* is endemic, in individuals at higher risk of exposure (such as laboratory technicians), and in those at higher risk of complications (such as those with asplenia).[52] The meningococcal polysaccharide vaccine requires only one dose and confers protection in over 90% of recipients. Protection begins to wane two to three years after receipt; therefore revaccination may be recommended in selected cases for some high-risk individuals.[52] The newest vaccine (Menactra™) is a quadrivalent conjugate vaccine. Pre-licensure studies indicate that it has equivalent efficacy to the polysaccharide vaccine, but it is hoped that it may induce longer and more durable immunity.

Conjugation changes the immunologic pathway induced by vaccination from a T cell independent to a T cell dependent one, which results in a more robust initial response and stronger anamnestic response upon reexposure. It also seems to reduce nasopharygeal carriage of bacteria and may therefore protect unvaccinated individuals by improving herd immunity.[61] Local reactions appear to occur slightly more frequently with the use of conjugate than polysaccharide vaccine, but serious reactions to date have been rare.[61]

Vaccines: The Future

The numbers of vaccines commonly used has increased from 9 in 1985 to 15 in 2000, and is projected to increase to 35 in 2020. Some of these new vaccines as well as some older ones may be recommended for use in pregnant women to better protect the newborn from pertussis, *Streptococcus pneumoniae*, *Haemophilus influenzae* type B, and Group B streptococcal infections. Other vaccines currently under development against herpes simplex, HIV, human papillomavirus, and cytomeglovirus would directly impact the health of women and infants. New non-injection based technologies are under development. Immunizations may eventually play a role, not just in the prevention of infection, but in the treatment of cancer or autoimmune disorders. Therefore, midwives need to stay abreast of the constantly evolving changes in the vaccine field and be able to evaluate the clinical utility of proposed new vaccines, incorporate changes regarding use of older vaccines into their clinical practice, monitor for vaccine safety, and provide the level of counseling needed by the women considering vaccination.

References

1. CDC. Appendix A: Impact of vaccines in the 20th century. In: Atkinson W, Hamborski J, Wolfe C, editors. *Epidemiology and Prevention of Vaccine-Preventable Diseases: The Pink Book.* 8th ed. Waldorf, MD: Public Health Foundation; 2004. p. A24.

2. CDC. Decline in annual incidence of varicella-selected states, 1990–2001. *MMWR.* 2003;52(37): 884–885.

3. CDC. Principles of vaccination. In: Atkinson W, Hamborski J, Wolfe C, editors. *Epidemiology and Prevention of Vaccine-Preventable Diseases: The Pink Book.* 8th ed. Waldorf, MD: Public Health Foundation; 2004.

4. Murphy B, Chanock R. Immunizations against viral disease. In: Knipe D, Howley P, Griffin D, Lamb R, Martin M, Roizman B, et al., editors. *Fields Virology.* 4th ed. Baltimore: Lippincott Williams & Wilkins; 2001. pp. 435–460.

5. CDC. General recommendations on immunizations. In: Atkinson W, Hamborski J, Wolfe C, editors. *Epidemiology and Prevention of Vaccine-Preventable Diseases: The Pink Book.* 8th ed. Waldorf, MD: Public Health Foundation; 2004.

6. Ward B. Vaccine adverse events in the new millennium: Is there reason for concern? *Bull WHO.* 2000;782:205–216.

7. Poland G, Jacobson R. Understanding those who do not understand: A brief review of the anti-vaccine movement. *Vaccine.* 2001;19(17–19):2440–2445.

8. Rock A. The lethal dangers of the billion-dollar vaccine business. *Money.* 1996:148–164.

9. Institute of Medicine (IOM). *Adverse Effects of Pertussis and Rubella Vaccines.* Washington, DC: National Academy Press; 1991.

10. IOM. Immunization Safety Review [monograph on the Internet]. Washington, DC: National Academy Press [cited 2004 Aug 29]. Available from: http://www.iom.edu/project.asp?id=4705.

11. Immunization Safety Review Committee. *Immunization Safety Review: Measles-Mumps-Rubella Vaccine and Autism.* Washington, DC: Institute of Medicine, Board on Health Promotion and Disease Prevention, National Academy Press; 2001.

12. Immunization Safety Review Committee. *Immunization Safety Review: Thimerosal–Containing Vaccines and Neurodevelopmental Disorders.* Washington, DC:

Institute of Medicine, Board on Health Promotion and Disease Prevention, National Academy Press; 2001.

13. Immunization Safety Review Committee. *Immunization Safety Review: Multiple Immunizations and Immune Dysfunction.* Washington, DC: Institute of Medicine, Board on Health Promotion and Disease Prevention, National Academy Press; 2002.

14. Immunization Safety Review Committee. *Immunization Safety Review: Hepatitis B Vaccine and Demyelinating Neurological Disorders.* Washington, DC: Institute of Medicine, Board on Health Promotion and Disease Prevention, National Academy Press; 2002.

15. Immunization Safety Review Committee. *Immunization Safety Review: Vaccinations and Sudden Unexpected Death in Infancy.* Washington, DC: Institute of Medicine, Board on Health Promotion and Disease Prevention, National Academy Press; 2003.

16. Immunization Safety Review Committee. *Immunization Safety Review: Influenza Vaccines and Neurological Complications.* Washington, DC: Institute of Medicine, Board on Health Promotion and Disease Prevention, National Academy Press; 2004.

17. Immunization Safety Review Committee. *Immunization Safety Review: Vaccines and Autism.* Washington, DC: Institute of Medicine, Board on Health Promotion and Disease Prevention, National Academy Press; 2004.

18. CDC. Vaccine safety. In: Atkinson W, Hamborski J, Wolfe C, editors. *Epidemiology and Prevention of Vaccine-Preventable Diseases: The Pink Book.* 8th ed. Waldorf, MD: Public Health Foundation; 2004.

19. Jacobson R, Adeqbenro A, Pankratz S, Poland G. Adverse events and vaccination-the lack of power and predictability of infrequent events in pre-licensure study. *Vaccine.* 2001;19(17–19):2428–2433.

20. ACIP. Rotavirus vaccine for the prevention of rotavirus gastroenteritis among children, recommendations of the Advisory Committee on Immunization Practices (ACIP). *MMWR Recomm Rep.* 1999; 48(RR-s):1–23.

21. Anonymous. Intussusception among recipients of rotavirus vaccine–United States, 1998–1999. *MMWR.* 1999;48(27):577–581.

22. Anonymous. Withdrawal of rotavirus vaccine. *MMWR.* 1999;48(43):1007.

23. Chen R, DeStefano F, Davis R, Jackson L, Thompson R, Mullooly J, et al. The Vaccine Safety Datalink: Immunization research in health maintenance organizations in the USA. *Bull WHO.* 2000; 78(2):186–194.

24. Mullooly J, Drew L, DeStefano F, Maher J, Bohlke K, Immanuel V, et al. Quality assessments of HMO diagnosis databases used to monitor childhood vaccine safety. *Methods Inf Med.* 2004;43(2):163–170.

25. CDC. National, state, and urban area vaccination coverage among children aged 19–35 months, United States, 2003. *MMWR.* 2004;53(29):658–661.

26. Committee to Study New Research on Vaccines. Research strategies for assessing adverse events associated with vaccines: A workshop summary. In: Stratton K, Howe C, Johnston R, editors. *Research Strategies for Assessing Adverse Events Associated with Vaccines.* Washington, DC: National Academy Press; 1994. pp. 1–24.

27. ACIP. Prevention of hepatitis A through active or passive immunization. *MMWR.* 1999;48(RR 12):1–37.

28. Gangarosa EJ, Galazka AM, Wolfe CR, Phillips LM, Gangarosa RE, Miller E, et al. Impact of anti-vaccine movements on pertussis control: The untold story. *Lancet.* 1998;351(9099):356–361.

29. Reagan L. Show us the science: An exclusive mothering report on the Second International Public Conference of the National Vaccine Information Center. *Mothering.* 2001;March/April:38–55.

30. Wechsler P. *Shot in the Dark.* New York; 1996. pp. 39–45.

31. Fisher BL. Shots in the dark: Attempts at eradicating infectious diseases are putting our children at risk. *Next City.* 1999(Summer):33–55.

32. De Jong M, Bouma A. Herd immunity after vaccination: How to quantify it and how to use it to halt disease. *Vaccine.* 2001;19(17–19):2722–2728.

33. Dadswell J. Susceptibility to diphtheria. *Lancet.* 1978;1(8061):428–430.

34. Meissner H, Strebel P, Orenstein W. Measles vaccines and the potential for worldwide eradication of measles. *Pediatrics.* 2004;114(4):1065–1069.

35. Galazka A, Robertson S, Oblapenko G. Resurgence of diphtheria. *Eur J Epidemiol.* 1995;11(1):95–105.

36. Galazka A, Robertson S. Diphtheria: Changing patterns in the developing world and the industrialized world. *Eur J Epidemiol.* 1995;11(1):107–117.

37. Fine P, Clarkson J. Individual versus public priorities in the determination of optimal vaccination policies. *Am J Epidemiol.* 1986;124:1012–1020.

38. Institute of Medicine. Risk communication and vaccination: Summary of a workshop. In: Evans G, Bostrom A, Johnston R, Fisher B, Stoto M, editors. *Risk Communication and Vaccination.* Washington, DC: National Academy Press; 1997. pp. 1–35.

39. Chen R, Hibbs B. Vaccine safety: Current and future challenges. *Pediatr Ann.* 1998;27(7):445–455.

40. Ball L, Evans G, Bostrom A. Risky business: Challenges in vaccine risk communication. *Pediatrics.* 1998;101(3):453–458.

41. CDC. Diphtheria. In: Atkinson W, Hamborski J, Wolfe C, editors. *Epidemiology and Prevention of Vaccine-Preventable Diseases: The Pink Book.* 8th ed. Waldorf, MD: Public Health Foundation; 2004. pp. 55–54.

42. CDC. Hepatitis A. In: Atkinson W, Hamborski J, Wolfe C, editors. *Epidemiology and Prevention of Vaccine-Preventable Diseases: The Pink Book.* 8th ed. Waldorf, MD: Public Health Foundation; 2004. pp. 177–189.

43. CDC. Hepatitis B. In: Atkinson W, Hamborski J, Wolfe C, editors. *Epidemiology and Prevention of Vaccine-Preventable Diseases: The Pink Book.* 8th ed. Waldorf, MD: Public Health Foundation; 2004. pp. 191–212.

44. Meheus A. Risk of hepatitis B in adolescence and young adulthood. *Vaccine.* 1995;13(Suppl 1): S31–S34.

45. CDC. Influenza. In: Atkinson W, Hamborski J, Wolfe C, editors. *Epidemiology and Prevention of Vaccine-Preventable Diseases: The Pink Book.* 8th ed. Waldorf, MD: Public Health Foundation; 2004. pp. 213–231.

46. CDC. Meningococcal disease. In: Atkinson W, Hamborski J, Wolfe C, editors. *Epidemiology and Prevention of Vaccine-Preventable Diseases: The Pink Book.* 8th ed. Waldorf, MD: Public Health Foundation; 2004. pp. 247–255.

47. CDC. Measles. In: Atkinson W, Hamborski J, Wolfe C, editors. *Epidemiology and Prevention of Vaccine-Preventable Diseases: The Pink Book.* 8th ed. Waldorf, MD: Public Health Foundation; 2004. pp. 115–133.

48. ACIP. Update: Vaccine side effects, adverse reactions, contraindications, and precautions. Recommendations of the Advisory Committee on Immunization Practices (ACIP). *MMWR Recomm Rep.* 1996;45(RR-12):1–35.

49. Gershon A. Measles (Rubeola). In: Fauci A, Braunwald E, Isselbacher K, Wilson J, Maring J, Kasper D, et al., editors. *Harrison's Principles of Internal Medicine.* 14th ed. New York: McGraw-Hill; 1998. pp. 1123–1125.

50. CDC. Mumps. In: Atkinson W, Hamborski J, Wolfe C, editors. *Epidemiology and Prevention of Vaccine-*

Preventable Diseases: The Pink Book. 8th ed. Waldorf, MD: Public Health Foundation; 2004. pp. 135–143.

51. CDC. Rubella. In: Atkinson W, Hamborski J, Wolfe C, editors. *Epidemiology and Prevention of Vaccine-Preventable Diseases: The Pink Book.* 8th ed. Waldorf, MD: Public Health Foundation; 2004. pp. 145–158.

52. CDC. Pneumococcal disease. In: Atkinson W, Hamborski J, Wolfe C, editors. *Epidemiology and Prevention of Vaccine-Preventable Diseases: The Pink Book.* 8th ed. Waldorf, MD: Public Health Foundation; 2004. pp. 233–245.

53. CDC. Tetanus. In: Atkinson W, Hamborski J, Wolfe C, editors. *Epidemiology and Prevention of Vaccine-Preventable Diseases: The Pink Book.* 8th ed. Waldorf, MD: Public Health Foundation; 2004. pp. 65–73.

54. CDC. Varicella. In: Atkinson W, Hamborski J, Wolfe C, editors. *Epidemiology and Prevention of Vaccine-Preventable Diseases: The Pink Book.* 8th ed. Waldorf, MD: Public Health Foundation; 2004. pp. 159–175.

55. Anonymous. Notice to readers: Alternative two-dose hepatitis B vaccination schedule for adolescents aged 11–15 years. *MMWR.* 2000;49(12):261.

56. Sepkowitz S. Hair loss after immunization. *JAMA.* 1998;279(2):117–118.

57. ACIP. Hepatitis B virus: A comprehensive strategy for eliminating transmission in the United States through universal childhood vaccination: Recommendations of the Immunization Practices Advisory Committee (ACIP). *MMWR Recomm Rep.* 1991; 40(RR 13):1–19.

58. Hernan M, Jick S, Olek M, Jick H. Recombinant hepatitis B vaccine and the risk of multiple sclerosis: A prospective study. *Neurology.* 2004;63(5): 838–842.

59. ACIP. Prevention and control of influenza: Recommendations of the Advisory Committee on Immunization Practices (ACIP). *MMWR Recomm Rep.* 2004; 53(RR06):1–40.

60. ACIP. Control and prevention of meningococcal disease: Recommendations of the Advisory Committee on Immunization Practices (ACIP). *MMWR Recomm Rep.* 2000;49(RR07):1–10.

61. CDC Prevention and Control of Meningococcal Disease Recommendations of the Advisory Committee on Immunization Practices (ACIP). *MMWR.* 2005;54 (RR-7):1–17.

62. CDC. Appendix A: Contraindications and precautions tables. In: Atkinson W, Hamborski J, Wolfe C, editors. *Epidemiology and Prevention of Vaccine-Preventable Diseases: The Pink Book.* 8th ed. Waldorf, MD: Public Health Foundation; 2004.

63. Prescribing Information: Meningococcal (Groups A, C, Y and W-135) Polysaccharide Diphtheria Toxoid Conjugate Vaccine Menactra. Accessed September 2005 at http://www.vaccineshoppe.com/US_PDF/MENACTRA_LE4714-15_Jan19.pdf.

64. ACIP. Measles, mumps, and rubella–vaccine use and strategies for elimination of measles, rubella, and congenital rubella syndrome and control of mumps: recommendations of the Advisory Committee on Immunization Practices. *MMWR Recomm Rep.* 1998; 47(RR-8):1–57.

65. ACIP. Prevention of varicella: Updated recommendations of the Advisory Committee on Immunization Practices (ACIP). *MMWR.* 1999;48(RR06):1–5.

66. Feikin D, Lezotte D, Hamman R, Salmon D, Chen R, Hoffman R. Individual and community risks of measles and pertussis associated with personal exemptions to immunization. *JAMA.* 2000;284(24): 3145–3150.

67. Salmon D, Haber M, Gangarosa E, Phillips L, Smith N, Chen R. Health consequences of religious and philosophical exemptions from immunization laws: Individual and societal risk of measles. *JAMA.* 1999;282(1):47–53.

68. National Vaccine Information Center 2004. Legal Exemptions to Vaccination [monograph on the Internet]. Vienna, VA [cited 2005 Aug 29]. Available from: http://www.909shot.com/state-site/legal-exemptions.htm.

69. ACIP. Recommended adult immunization schedule, October 2004 to September 2005. *MMWR.* 2004; 53(45):Q1–Q4.

70. ACIP. General Recommendations on Immunization Recommendations of the Advisory Committee on Immunization Practices (ACIP) and the American Academy of Family Physicians (AAFP). *MMWR.* 2002;51(RR 2):1–34.

71. ACIP. Prevention of varicella: Recommendations of the Advisory Committee on Immunization Practices (ACIP). *MMWR Recomm Rep.* 1996; 45(RR-11):1–25.

72. Alger L. Common viral infections. In: Cohen W, editor. *Cherry & Merkatz's Complications of Pregnancy.* 5th ed. Lippincott Williams & Wilkins; 2000. pp. 709–743.

73. Pascual B, McGinley E, Zanardi L, Cortese M, Murphy T. Tetanus surveillance–United States, 1998–2000. *MMWR.* 2003;52(SS03):1–8.

74. Kalaca S. Missed opportunities for tetanus vaccination in pregnant women, and factors associated with seropositivity. *Public Health.* 2004;118(5):377–382.

75. Craig A, Reed G, Mohon R, Quick M, Swarner O, Moore W, et al. Neonatal tetanus in the United States: A sentinel event in the foreign born. *Pediatr Infect Dis J.* 1997;16(10):955–959.

76. WHO. Progress towards the global elimination of neonatal tetanus, 1990–1998. *Wkly Epidemiol Rec.* 1999;74(10):74–80.

77. Anonymous. Neonatal Tetanus–Montana, 1998. *MMWR.* 1998;47(43):928–930.

78. ACIP. ACIP Recommends Adolescent Vaccination for Tetanus, Diphtheria and Pertussis Vaccine, June 30, 2005. Accessed September 9, 2005, http://www.cdc.gov/nip/pr/pr_tdap_jun2005.htm.

79. Strebel P, Cochi S, Grabowsky M, Bilous J, Hersh B, Okwo-Bele J, et al. The unfinished measles immunization agenda. *J Infect Dis.* 2003;187(Suppl 1): S1–S7.

80. Anonymous. Update: Global Measles Control and Mortality Reduction–Worldwide, 1991–2001. *MMWR.* 2003;52(20);471–475.

81. Losos J. Report of the Workgroup on Viral Diseases. *MMWR Supplements.* 1999;48(SU01):126–137.

82. Fenner F. Candidate viral diseases for elimination or eradication. MMWR Supplements. 1999;48(SU01): 86–90.

83. de Quadros C, Izurieta H, Venczel L, Carrasco P. Measles eradication in the Americas: Progress to date. *J Infect Dis.* 2004;189(Suppl 1):S227–S235.

84. Robertson S, Featherstone D, Gacic-Dobo M, Hersh B. Rubella and congenital rubella syndrome: Global update. *Rev Panam Salud Publica/Pan Am J Public Health.* 2003;14(5):306–314.

85. Arvin A. Varicella-zoster virus. In: Knipe D, Howley P, Griffin D, Lamb R, Martin M, Roizman B, et al., editors. *Fields Virology.* 4th ed. Baltimore: Lippincott Williams & Wilkins; 2001. pp. 2746–2749.

86. Lallier C. Questions about varicella vaccine. *Pediatrics.* 1996;98(6):1226.

87. Spingarn R, Benjamin J. Universal vaccination against varicella. *N Engl J Med.* 1998;338(10): 683–684.

88. Macfarlane L, Sanders M, Carek P. Concerns regarding universal varicella immunization: Time will tell. *Arch Fam Med.* 1997;6(6):537–541.

89. Brisson M, Edmunds W, Gay N. Varicella vaccination: Impact of vaccine efficacy on the epidemiology of VZV. *J Med Virol.* 2003;70(Suppl 1):S31–S37.

90. Anonymous. Acute hepatitis B among children and adolescents–United States, 1990–2002. *MMWR.* 2004;53(43):1015–1018.

91. Anonymous. Incidence of Acute Hepatitis B–United States, 1990–2002. *MMWR.* 2004; 52(51):1252–1254.

92. Esteban R. Risk of Hepatitis B in infancy and childhood. *Vaccine.* 1995;13(Suppl 1):S35–S36.

93. CDC. Global progress toward universal childhood hepatitis B vaccination. *MMWR.* 2003;52(36): 868–870.

94. Anonymous. Notice to readers: FDA approval for a combined hepatitis A and B vaccine. *MMWR.* 2001;50(37):806–807.

95. WHO. Press Release WHO/67: No scientific justification to suspend hepatitis B immunization [monograph on the Internet]. Geneva, Switzerland; Oct 2, 1998. Available from: http://www.who.int/inf-pr-1998/en/pr98-67.html.

96. Marshall E. A shadow falls on hepatitis B vaccination effort. *Science.* 1998;281(5377):630–631.

97. Halsey N. Limiting infant exposure to thimerosal in vaccines and other sources of mercury. *JAMA.* 1999;282(18):1763–1766.

98. Ascherio A, Zhang S, Hernan M, Olek M, Coplan P, Brodovicz K, et al. Hepatitis B vaccination and the risk of multiple sclerosis. *N Engl J Med.* 2001; 344(5):327–332.

99. Confavreux C, Suissa S, Saddier P, Bourdes V, Vukusic S. Vaccinations and the risk of relapse in multiple sclerosis. *N Engl J Med.* 2001;344:319–326.

100. Anonymous. Thimerosal in vaccines: A joint statement of the American Academy of Pediatrics and the Public Health Service. *MMWR.* 1999;48(26): 563–565.

101. ACIP. Meningococcal disease and college students: Recommendations of the Advisory Committee on Immunization Practices (ACIP). *MMWR Recomm Rep.* 2000;49(RR07):11–20.

102. CDC. Meningococcal Conjugate Vaccine Meningococcal (Groups A, C, Y and W-135) Conjugate Vaccine (MCV-4) ACIP Recommends Meningococcal Vaccine for Adolescents and College Freshmen. National Immunization Program, March 9, 2005. Accessed September 9, 2005:http://www.cdc.gov/nip/vaccine/mening/mcv4/mcv4_acip.htm.

Chapter 3

Health Screenings

Barbara Hackley

Because of widespread acceptance of vaccination and improved access to clean water and sanitation services in the United States, deaths due to infectious diseases have plummeted over the last century, and the percentage of morbidity and mortality associated with chronic diseases has proportionately grown. With the control of infectious diseases, screening for the early detection and treatment of chronic disease is the next area where significant improvements in the health and well-being of the general public can be made. For example, countries that have adopted Pap smear screening programs have reduced deaths from cervical cancer by 20% to 60%[1]; those countries with the most extensive coverage and organized follow-up have been able to reduce the incidence of cervical cancer by 80%.[2] Similar benefits have been found in studies evaluating the impact of screening and treatment for hypertension and hyperlipidemia. Survival rates have improved most dramatically for those with more severe disease. Studies have reported that appropriate treatment of malignant hypertension increases five-year survival rates from 0% to 75%. Controlling less severe presentations has been estimated to reduce mortality by 16% to 20%.[3] Drug treatment for hyperlipidemia, which affects approximately 20% of women older than 20 years of age, has been estimated to reduce the incidence of coronary heart disease events by 30%.[4] The use of effective screening tests can save lives by identifying preclinical stages of disease, which offers the opportunity to intervene early enough in the course of the disease to avert death and disability.

However, screening is expensive and has limited effectiveness unless certain criteria are met. Screening programs generally target those who are most at risk. Which groups to target, with what specific tests, and how frequently to screen these groups are controversial issues. Different professional groups, such as the American Cancer Society (ACS) and the American College of Obstetricians and Gynecologists (ACOG), and national authorities, such as the United States Preventive Services Task Force (USPSTF), issue recommendations depending on their risk-benefit analyses of the efficacy and cost of screening as well as the prevalence, morbidity, and mortality associated with the disease in question. Each authority also issues periodic updates as newer information becomes available. Therefore, this chapter is not meant to provide clinicians with the most current recommendations issued by various authorities; rather, it presents the background needed to be able to evaluate screening recommendations and an understanding of the diversity of opinion held by various authorities. **Table 3-1** lists Internet resources where the most current guidelines can be found.

Principles of Screening

Criteria for Successful Screening Programs

For a screening program to significantly reduce the negative health consequences of a specific disease, the condition being considered must meet several criteria. First, the disease in question must cause substantial morbidity or mortality in a significant percentage of the population. Second, prevention or treatment options that can effectively reduce the likelihood of disease progression must be available. Third, a screening test must be available that is inexpensive, reliable, effective, and acceptable to patients. Use of the screening test must identify illness when the disease is asymptomatic. Early intervention during these preclinical stages must result in improved outcomes compared to care begun when the disease is clinically obvious (**Table 3-2**).

Screening programs that do not meet these criteria will be less effective and, in some cases,

Table 3-1 RESOURCES ON THE INTERNET

Agency	Resources	Web Site
Agency for Healthcare Research and Quality	Links to flow sheets that can be inserted into a patient's chart and used to track preventive counseling, screening, and immunizations	http://www.ahrq.gov/clinic/ppipix.htm
	Materials available to help integrate preventive services into a clinical practice setting	
News releases in preventive services (from the United States Preventive Services Task Force [USPSTF])	Newest updates to the USPSTF *Guide to Clinical Preventive Services*, 3rd ed., 2000-2004	http://www.ahrq.gov/clinic/prevnew.htm
USPSTF home page	Recommendations released by the USPSTF, past and present	http://www.ahrq.gov/clinic/uspstfix.htm
National Guideline Clearinghouse	Searchable collection of guidelines issued by different authorities	http://www.guideline.gov
Canadian Task Force on Preventive Health Care	Links to most recent recommendations	http://www.ctfphc.org/index2.htm

---

Table 3-2 CRITERIA FOR AN EFFECTIVE SCREENING TEST

Condition	Screening Test
• Common • Associated with significant morbidity and/or mortality • Intervention in preclinical stage of illness can prevent disease progression and sequelae • Early intervention leads to improved outcomes compared to those achieved with treatment started later in the course of the disease	• Available • Inexpensive • Accurate • Reliable • Acceptable to patients • Able to pick up disease earlier than routine clinical care

---

worthless. Screening can also be potentially harmful if the further evaluation of abnormal results requires the use of invasive tests. For example, lung cancer is one of the leading causes of cancer-related mortality. It is usually asymptomatic and commonly clinically detected late in the course of the disease. While lung cancer meets some of the criteria necessary for effective screening programs, it does not meet all of them. Screening tests are minimally effective at detecting preclinical stages of lung cancer. Follow-up of abnormal chest x-rays may require the use of bronchoscopy or biopsies, which pose risks for some patients. Treatment outcomes are poor and the five-year survival rate is estimated to be only 14%.[5] Therefore, no authorities currently recommend screening for lung cancer in asymptomatic individuals, even if risk factors such as smoking are present.[6] Other conditions, such as colorectal cancer, do meet all of the necessary criteria, but may be detected using screening tests (serial fecal occult blood testing, sigmoidoscopy, and colonoscopy) that are less acceptable to patients. In studies of community-based screening programs, only 15% to 30% of patients complied with recommendations to obtain serial fecal occult testing, and compliance rates for sigmoidoscopy were even lower.[7]

Currently, only 35% of the population aged 50 or older are estimated to have obtained a fecal occult test within the last two years and only 37% have ever received a sigmoidoscopy, far short of the 2010 Healthy People goal of 50%.[8] Failure to convince enough at-risk individuals to obtain screening tests will lower the effectiveness of a screening program.

Accuracy of Screening Tests

The accuracy of screening tests is determined by their sensitivity, specificity, positive predictive value, and negative predictive value. Sensitivity and specificity answer these two questions: "If the disease is present, will the test be positive?" or "If the disease is absent, will the test be negative?" *Sensitivity* refers to the likelihood that the screening test will be positive if an individual has the disease. *Specificity* is the opposite; it describes the likelihood that the test will be negative if the individual is healthy. However, sensitivity and specificity are of less clinical value to providers than positive or negative predictive values. From a provider's perspective, the more important questions are, "If the test is positive,

Table 3-3 SCREENING TEST RESULTS: A 2 × 2 TABLE

Test	Disease Present	Disease Absent
Positive	A = True Positive	B = False Positive
Negative	C = False Negative	D = True Negative

does the patient have the disease?" (positive predictive value) and "If the test is negative, is the patient disease-free?" (negative predictive value). **Table 3-3** describes the criteria used in **Table 3-4**, which defines the values used to describe the accuracy of a screening test.

In addition to having high sensitivity and specificity, a good screening test must be reliable. Values should be consistent across time so that differences are assumed to be because of the presence or absence of disease, and are not related to factors such as normal diurnal fluctuations, changes in diet or activity level, variations in laboratory techniques or personnel, or other external factors.

Impact of Disease Prevalence

Disease prevalence has a direct and powerful impact on the success of screening programs. Prevalence is more important than the quality of the screening test, the seriousness of the disease, or the effectiveness of treatment. Disease conditions that are more prevalent can be more readily identified by screening tests and will have higher positive and negative predictive values, even if the screening test used has relatively poor sensitivity and specificity. For example, the positive predictive value of a screening test is 95%

Table 3-4 DEFINITIONS: VALUES USED TO DESCRIBE THE ACCURACY OF SCREENING TESTS

Value	Definition	Formula
Sensitivity	If the **disease** is present, will the test be positive?	A/ A&C or True Positive/Disease Present
Specificity	If the **disease** is absent, will the test be negative?	D/ B & D or True Negative/ Disease Absent
Positive Predictive Value	If the **test** is positive, will the disease be present?	A/ A & B or True Positive/ All Positive Tests
Negative Predictive Value	If the **test** is negative, will the disease be absent?	D/ C & D or True Negative/ All Negative Tests

Table 3-5 IMPACT OF PREVALENCE ON POSITIVE PREDICTIVE VALUE[9]

Prevalence (%)	Sensitivity 90% Specificity 90%	Sensitivity 95% Specificity 95%	Sensitivity 99% Specificity 99%
0.1	0.9	1.9	9.0
1	8.3	16.1	50
2	15.5	27.9	66.9
5	32.1	50	83.9
50	90	95	99

Source: Reprinted with permission from Lippincott Williams & Wilkins.

for a condition that occurs in 50% of the population and the screening test used has a sensitivity and specificity of 95%. However, if prevalence is lower and affects only 5% of the population, this same excellent screening test can only detect 50% of individuals with the disease (**Table 3-5**).

Prevalence also affects whether any interventions implemented as a result of screening are likely to improve health outcomes. Less effective interventions targeting more prevalent diseases improve health at the population level better than more effective interventions for less common diseases (**Table 3-6**). Therefore, authorities such as the USPSTF whose recommendations are based on population rather than individual health considerations do not recommend screening for rare diseases even if highly effective treatment is available.

Prevalence has such strong influence on the effectiveness of screening programs that many authorities recommend directing screening efforts to subpopulations at higher risk of a particular health problem rather than to the general population. Guidelines commonly recommend that particular screening strategies be directed to subgroups based on their age, lifestyle, or risk profile.

Biases in Screening Tests

Screening tests are subject to biases, such as lead time and length time biases, which make screening tests appear to be effective in improving health outcomes when, in fact, they

Table 3-6 EFFECTIVENESS OF MORTALITY RATE ON TOTAL DEATHS PREVENTED[10]

Reduction in Mortality with Intervention	Deaths per Year from Target Population	Total Deaths Prevented with Intervention
50%	10	5
1%	100,000	1,000

are not. *Lead time bias* occurs when a screening test identifies a disease earlier than usual clinical care, but treatment begun earlier does not improve outcomes. Screening tests for cancer, for example, may falsely appear to improve survival rates by allowing earlier detection, thereby increasing the length of time from detection to death but not truly increase survival (**Figure 3-1**).

Length time bias is also problematic. This bias is present if screening identifies only slowly progressing or more benign forms of a condition, which are more likely to have better outcomes, and miss more aggressive forms. Treatment for indolent forms of the disease may appear to, but will not actually improve outcomes, if most of the deaths occur with more aggressive disease. For example, controversy over the effectiveness

Figure 3-1 Algorithm showing lead time bias. (A) Effective screening test. (B) Lead time bias. (C) Natural course of disease with care starting at the symptomatic stage.

A. Effective Screening Test

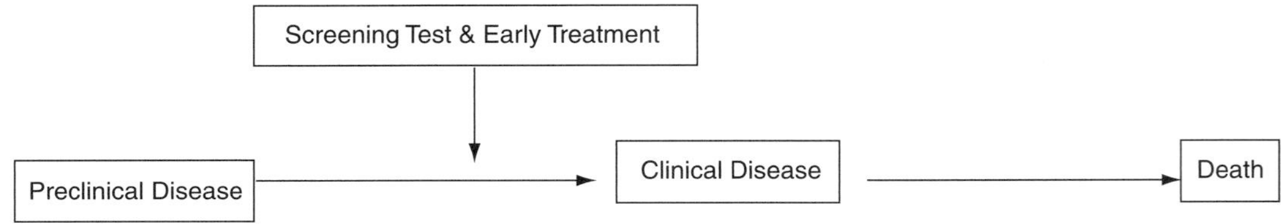

B. Lead Time Bias

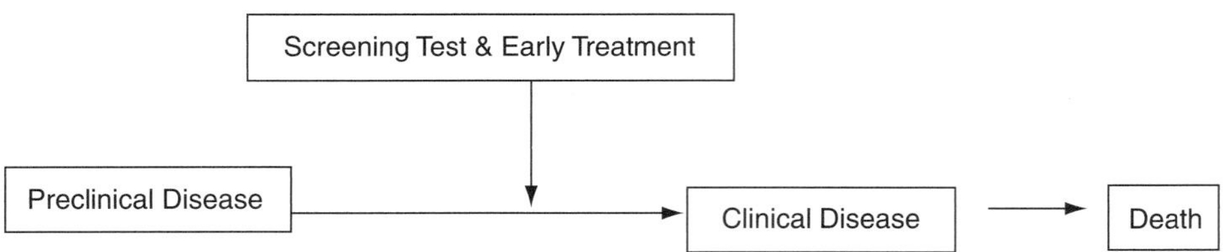

C. Natural Course of Disease with Care Starting at Symptomatic Stage

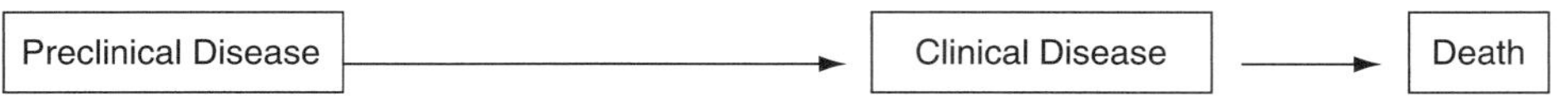

of prostate cancer screening is due to differences in interpretations of the effect of length time bias on the success of prostate cancer screening (**Figure 3-2**).

Recommendations of Various Organizations

Many professional and national organizations issue screening guidelines. These guidelines differ in many ways, including what conditions should be screened; what tests should be used; which groups should be targeted; when screening tests should be initiated; and how often (if at all) they should be repeated. These differences reflect an organization's cost-effectiveness analysis as well as its underlying interest. Determining the incidence and health impact of disease, the accuracy of a particular screening test, or the effectiveness of early treatment in preventing death and disability is not an exact science. Using more conservative or more liberal estimates of these numbers can dramatically change the cost-benefit equation. In addition, only limited resources are available for health care in general and screening in particular. It may be that health care dollars and provider and patient time devoted to marginally effective screening programs are better used in other ways.

Differences exist in the way organizations evaluate these competing demands. For example, the USPSTF makes recommendations based on population benefit, whereas others, such as the ACS and the National Osteoporosis Foundation, are concerned about the impact of one condition. In general, therefore, the USPSTF tends to issue more conservative screening recommendations, while condition-specific organizations tend to be more aggressive in their

Figure 3-2 Algorithm showing length time bias. With length time bias, the screening test is more likely to detect more indolent forms of the cancer that tend to have better prognosis, giving the false impression of improved survival. More aggressive forms of cancer rapidly lead to death and are missed with screening.

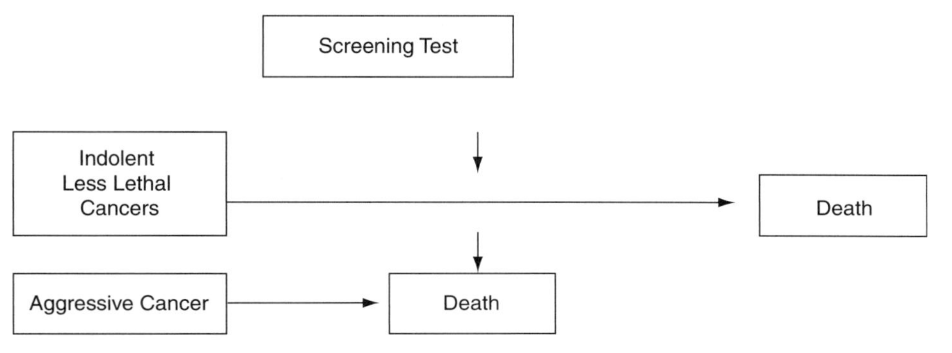

recommendations. **Table 3-7** compares some of the recommendations issued by different authorities.

Conclusion

All clinicians must exercise clinical judgment when offering screening tests to their clients. Screening can save lives. However, women who are considered at low risk may incur additional expense, discomfort, and worry during the evaluation of false-positive tests that can result from overzealous screening. In midwifery and women's health, striking the correct balance depends on understanding the prevalence and sequelae of the common health problems found in the communities in which a provider practices, an ability to evaluate the risk status of individual clients, and a willingness to devote time during a health care visit to these issues. Providers who do this will successfully improve the health of women while minimizing the risks and expense associated with screening.

Table 3-7 COMPARISON OF SCREENING RECOMMENDATIONS FROM VARIOUS ORGANIZATIONS

Condition	More Conservative				More Aggressive
Obesity	Organization	CTFPHC[11]	USPSTF[12]	ACOG[13]	ACPM[14]
	Year	1999	2003	2000	2001
	Screening Test	BMI	BMI preferred, waist circumference alternative.	Weight	BMI & Counseling for all irrespective of BMI on diet and exercise.
	Recommendation	Insufficient evidence to recommend for or against BMI measurement in the periodic health examination for general public; fair evidence to support use of BMI for obese individuals with obesity-related disease.	Screen all adults.	Screen all women.	Screen all adults.
	Frequency	Unspecified	Unspecified	At time of periodic assessment, timing unspecified.	At time of periodic exam, timing unspecified.
Lipids	Organization	USPSTF[4]	ACOG[15]	NCEP[16]	AHA[17]
	Year	2001	2002	2002	2002
	Screening Test	Total cholesterol, HDL. Can be fasting or non-fasting.	Cholesterol for low-risk women, lipid profile for high-risk women.	Fasting lipoprotein profile (total cholesterol, LDL cholesterol, HDL cholesterol, and triglyceride) or if nonfasting total cholesterol and HDL.	Fasting serum lipoprotein profile (or total and HDL if fasting is unavailable).

(continues)

Table 3-7 COMPARISON OF SCREENING RECOMMENDATIONS FROM VARIOUS ORGANIZATIONS *(continued)*

Condition	More Conservative	←		→ More Aggressive
Recommendation	Screen all women aged ≥45. Screen earlier in higher risk individuals aged 20–45 yr: diabetes; family history of cardiovascular (CV) disease before age 60 in female relatives; family history suggestive of hyperlipidemia; multiple CV disease risk factors.	Screen low-risk women aged ≥45 yr. Screen earlier if high risk: women with elevated cholesterol level; history of parent or sibling with cholesterol level of 240 mg/dL; first degree relative with disease (<55 years of age for men, <65 years for women); personal history of coronary heart disease; diabetes, or smoker.	Screen all adults aged ≥20 yr.	Screen all adults aged ≥20 yr.
Frequency	Optimal frequency uncertain. Reasonable to repeat every 5 yr, sooner if results borderline, longer intervals if repeatedly normal.	For low-risk women, begin at age 45, repeat every 5 yr. For high-risk women, timing unspecified; can be earlier or more frequent.	A fasting lipoprotein (or if nonfasting a total cholesterol and HDL) should be obtained once every 5 yr. If the sample is nonfasting, only total cholesterol and HDL cholesterol will be usable. In such a case, if total cholesterol is >200 mg/dL or HDL is <40 mg/dL, a follow-up lipoprotein profile is needed for appropriate management based on LDL.	Beginning at age 20, should be measured according to patient's risk for hyperlipidemia at least every 5 yr; if risk factors are present, every 2 yr.

Hypertension	Organization	CTFPHC[17]	USPSTF[19]	ACOG[13]	AHA[17]
	Year	1994	2003	2000	2002
	Screening Test	BP	BP	BP	BP
	Recommendation	Good evidence to include BP as part of periodic exam for adults ages 21–64 yr.	Screen all adults aged 18 years or older.	Screen all women.	Screen all adults beginning at age 20.
	Frequency	Unspecified.	Unspecified.	At time of periodic assessment, timing unspecified.	Every 2 yr for low risk adults.
Tuberculosis	Organization	CTFPHC[20]	USPSTF[21]	ACOG[15]	CDC[22]
	Year	1994	1996	2002	2000
	Screening Test	PPD	PPD	PPD	PPD
	Recommendation	Screen high-risk individuals only.	Screen high-risk individuals only.	Screen high-risk women only. Defined as: HIV+, close contact with someone known or suspected to have infection, personal medical risk factors that increase risk of disease if infected, born in country with high TB prevalence, low income, medically underserved, IVDU, alcoholism, resident of long-term care facility, health care professional working in high-risk facility.	Screen high-risk individuals only. Defined as: those at high risk of disease based on exposure (immigrants from areas of the world where disease is endemic and in U.S. for less than 5 yr, residents or employees of high risk congregated at institutions such as homeless shelters), or those at risk for disease progression because of underlying medical condition (HIV+, IVDU, organ transplants, etc.).

(continues)

Table 3-7 COMPARISON OF SCREENING RECOMMENDATIONS FROM VARIOUS ORGANIZATIONS *(continued)*

Condition	More Conservative			More Aggressive
	Frequency	Unspecified.	Unspecified.	At time of periodic assessment, timing unspecified.	Unspecified.
Skin Cancer	Organization	USPSTF[23,24]	CTFPHC[25]	ACOG[13,15]	ACS[39]
	Year	2001, 2003	1994	2000, 2002	2004
	Screening Test	Physical exam & counseling	Total skin examination (TSE) & self exam (SE) & counseling	Physical exam & counseling	General physical exam & counseling
	Recommendation	Insufficient evidence for or against including skin exam or to include counseling on prevention in periodic visit for general public.	Poor evidence to include TSE for general public, fair evidence to include for high-risk individuals with family history of malignant melanoma. Poor evidence to include SE or use of sunscreen for general public. Fair evidence to advise use of protective clothing and avoidance of sun exposure.	Evaluate and counsel all women on skin exposure to ultraviolet rays. Screen high-risk women only: Work or play a lot outdoors, family or personal history of skin cancer, have precancerous lesions.	Screen all adults.
	Frequency	NA.	Unspecified.	At time of periodic assessment, timing unspecified.	Begin at age 20, frequency unspecified, to be done at the time of a general periodic health exam.
Thyroid	Organization	CTFPHC[26]	USPSTF[27,28]	ACOG[15]	ATA[29]
	Year	1994	2004, 1996	2002	2000
	Screening Test	NA	NA	TSH	TSH
	Recommendation	Poor evidence exists to include or exclude	Insufficient evidence to recommend for or		Screen all asymptomatic adults

		screening of post-menopausal women using clinical examination or TSH. Recommended maintaining a high level of suspicion in perimenopausal women since incidence of disease higher in this group.	against routine screening for thyroid dysfunction or cancer in asymptomatic adults		
	Frequency	NA	NA	Unspecified	Start age 35 and screen every 5 yr
Diabetes	Organization	CTFPHC[30]	USPSTF[31]	ACOG[15]	AHA[17]
	Year	2005	2003	2002	2002
	Screening Test	Fasting blood glucose	Evaluated various options	Fasting glucose & urinalysis	Fasting blood glucose
	Recommendation	Fair evidence to recommend screening for diabetes in individuals with hypertension or hyperlipidemia.	Evidence is insufficient to recommend for or against routinely screening asymptomatic adults for type 2 diabetes, impaired glucose tolerance, or impaired fasting glucose.	Screen low-risk women age 45 or older. Screen high-risk women, timing and frequency at provider discretion: obesity, first-degree relative with diabetes, member of high-risk ethnic group (African American, Hispanic, Native American, Asian, Pacific Islander), delivered a baby 9 pounds or more, history of gestational diabetes, hypertensive, low HDL levels, high triglyceride levels of more than 250mg/dl, history of impaired glucose tolerance.	Screen all women beginning at age 20.

(continues)

Table 3-7 Comparison of Screening Recommendations from Various Organizations *(continued)*

Condition		More Conservative			More Aggressive
	Frequency	Unspecified	Unspecified	Low-risk women: Begin at age 45, repeat fasting blood glucose every 3 yr. Beginning at age 65, obtain a yearly urinalysis to check for glycosuria. High-risk women: Timing and frequency unspecified.	Varies according to risk status. Minimum every 5 yr; if risk factors are present, every 2 yr.
Vision and Glaucoma	Organization	CTFPHC[32]	USPSTF[33,34]	ACOG[13]	Department of Veterans Affairs[35]
	Year	1994	1996, 2005	2000	2000
	Screening Test	Varies	Varies	Evaluation and counseling for visual acuity and glaucoma.	Physical exam, intraocular pressure, other techniques to evaluate presence of glaucoma.
	Recommendation	Fair evidence to include screening for visual acuity in people 65 years of age and older in periodic health exam. Fair evidence to include screening for diabetic retinopathy, using fundoscopy or retinal photography for	Insufficient evidence for or against screening for glaucoma. Good evidence that treatment of elevated intraocular pressure reduces visual field defects and progression of disease, but also found that early treatment is associated with a number of po-	Screen women age 65 and older.	Screen individuals age 40 or more.

		persons aged 65+ with diabetes in periodic health exam. Insufficient evidence to include or exclude screening for age-related macular degeneration aged 65+ in periodic health exam. Insufficient evidence to include or exclude screening for glaucoma using fundoscopy, tonometry, or automated perimetry in periodic health exam. Patients at high risk for age-related macular degeneration or glaucoma may better be evaluated by an eye specialist.	tential harms. Concludes that evidence is insufficient to determine if screening provides enough benefit to offset these risks. Recommends screening for visual acuity in the elderly.		
	Frequency	Unspecified.	Unspecified.	Unspecified.	Every 1 to 2 yr, depending on risk status.
Oral Cancer	Organization	CTFPHC[36,37]	USPSTF[38]	ACOG[13]	ACS[39]
	Year	1995, 1999	2004	2000	2004
	Recommendation	Evidence insufficient to recommend for or against screening for oral cancer in general population. Good evidence to include smoking cessation counseling for all adults in the periodic health visit as a way to reduce oral cancer.	Evidence insufficient to recommend for or against routine screening for oral cancer in adults.	Include counseling on smoking cessation in periodic visit. Screen for oral cancer via visual inspection for women beginning at age 40.	Inspect oral cavity at time of periodic exam for oral cancer screening for all adults. Counsel regarding risk factors for oral cancer.

(*continues*)

Table 3-7 **Comparison of Screening Recommendations from Various Organizations** (*continued*)

Condition	More Conservative	←		→ More Aggressive
	Frequency	At time of periodic visit. Those at high risk (smokers, excessive alcohol users) could consider annual screening by physician or dentist.	NA	Counsel at time of periodic assessment, timing unspecified for all women. Begin inspection of oral cavity at age 40 at time of periodic assessment, frequency unspecified.	Begin at age 20, frequency unspecified.
Breast Cancer Clinical Breast Exam (CBE)*	Organization	CTFPHC[40]	USPSTF[41]	ACOG[42]	ACS[43]
	Year	1994, wording updated 1998	2002	2003	2003
	Screening Test	CBE done in combination with mammogram	NA	CBE	CBE alone for women <40 years of age, and prior to mammogram for women aged ≥40.
	Recommendation	Screen women aged 50–69 yr.	Evidence is insufficient to recommend for or against routine CBE alone to screen for breast cancer.	Screen all women	Screen all women aged ≥40.
	Frequency	Every 1 to 2 yr	NA	Annually as part of the physical examination	CBE every 3 years as part of periodic health examination from 20–40 years, and annually thereafter.
Breast Cancer Breast Self Exam (BSE)*	Organization	CTFPHC[44]	USPSTF[41]	ACOG[42]	ACS[43]
	Year	2001	2002	2003	2003
	Recommendation	Because there is fair evidence of no benefit and good evidence of harm, CTFPHC recommends	Evidence is insufficient to recommend for or against teaching or	Despite a lack of evidence for or against BSE, BSE has the potential to detect pal-	Should be told about the benefits and limitations of BSE. If a woman chooses to do

		CTFPHC[40,44,45]	USPSTF[41]	ACOG[42]	ACS[43]
		against including BSE in the periodic health visit for women between the ages of 40 and 70 years. There is not sufficient evidence for or against SBE for younger or older women.	performing routine BSE.	pable breast cancer and can be recommended.	BSE, she should be instructed on proper technique and be observed to make sure her technique is correct.
	Target Group	NA	NA	All women.	Women in their 20s and older.
	Frequency	NA	NA	Unspecified.	Unspecified. Acceptable to do BSE irregularly or not at all.
Breast Cancer Mammogram*	Organization	CTFPHC[40,44,45]	USPSTF[41]	ACOG[42]	ACS[43]
	Year	2001, 1994	2002	2003	2003
	Screening Test	Mammogram.	Mammogram +/− clinical breast exam.	Mammogram.	Mammogram for women of average risk, other screening modalities can be considered for women of higher risk.*
	Recommendation	Evidence does not support including or excluding screening mammogram for women aged 40–49. Recommends screening beginning at age 50.	Recommends screening mammography, with or without clinical breast examination beginning at age 40.	Screen all woman age ≥40.	Screen all women aged ≥40 of average risk; can consider earlier or more frequent screening if at above-average risk.
	Frequency	Every 1 to 2 yr between ages 50 and 69.	For women aged ≥40 screen every 1 to 2 yr.	Every 1 to 2 yr between 40 and 49 years; annually aged 50 or older.	Annually, no specified end point as long as woman is in good health.

(continues)

Table 3-7 COMPARISON OF SCREENING RECOMMENDATIONS FROM VARIOUS ORGANIZATIONS *(continued)*

Condition	More Conservative	←			→ More Aggressive
Colorectal Cancer**	Organization	CTFPHC[46]	USPSTF[47]	ACOG[15]	ACS[48]
	Year	2001	2002	2002 (book)	2001
	Screening Test	Several options (see frequency) Recommended options vary by risk status.	Insufficient evidence to recommend one strategy over another (see frequency).	Several options (see frequency).	Several options (see frequency).
	Recommendation	Screen all individuals aged ≥50.	Strongly recommends that clinicians screen men and women ≥50 yr. Earlier screening may be considered for those at higher risk (those with a first-degree relative diagnosed with colorectal cancer before age 60 yr). Expert guidelines have been established for those at highest risk.*	Screen low risk women age ≥50 yr. Suggests following ACS recommendations for high-risk women.	Screen low-risk women age ≥50 yr.
	Frequency	Normal risk individuals: 1) fecal occult blood test (FOBT): Good evidence to include	1) FOBT 2) Flexible sigmoidoscopy alone 3) FOBT & flexible sigmoidoscopy	1) Annual FOBT 2) Flexible sigmoidoscopy every 5 yr	1) Annual FOBT; best technique is to collect two samples from three consecu-

		CTFPHC[49]	USPSTF[50–52]	ACOG[13]	CDC[53]
		every 1 to 2 yr as part of periodic exam 2) Flexible sigmoidoscopy: fair evidence to include as part of periodic exam 3) FOBT & flexible sigmoidoscopy: insufficient evidence to recommend one test over another or a combination of tests 4) Colonoscopy: Insufficient evidence to include or exclude as initial screening test in average risk individuals Above average risk individuals 1) Genetic testing and colonoscopy for individuals with a family history of familial adenomatous polyposis or hereditary nonpolyposis colon cancer 2) Colonoscopy if first degree relative with polyps or colorectal cancer	4) Double contrast barium enema 5) Colonoscopy Reviews risks and effectiveness of various approaches. Makes no specific recommendations on which test(s) to use or how frequently they should be repeated	3) Annual FOBT & flexible sigmoidoscopy every 5 yr 4) Double-contrast barium enema every 5–10 yr 5) Colonoscopy every 10 yr	tive specimens at home. 2) Flexible sigmoidoscopy every 5 yr 3) Annual FOBT plus flexible sigmoidoscopy every 5 yr (combined approach preferred over FOBT alone or flexible sigmoidoscopy alone) 4) Double-contrast barium enema every 5 yr 5) Colonoscopy every 10 yr
Sexually Transmitted Disease (STD)	Organization	CTFPHC[49]	USPSTF[50–52]	ACOG[13]	CDC[53]
	Year	1996	2001, 1996	2000	2002
	Screening Test	Only addresses chlamydia	Chlamydia, gonorrhea, and HIV	Chlamydia, gonorrhea, and HIV	Chlamydia, gonorrhea, and HIV

(continues)

Table 3-7 COMPARISON OF SCREENING RECOMMENDATIONS FROM VARIOUS ORGANIZATIONS *(continued)*

Condition	More Conservative			More Aggressive
	Recommendation	Screen all pregnant women in first trimester of pregnancy without regard to risk. Screen high-risk, nonpregnant women annually. High risk defined as: sexually active women ≤25 years of age; women with new sexual partners; women or men with multiple sexual partners during the previous year; women who use nonbarrier contraceptive methods; and women who have symptoms of chlamydia infection (cervical friability, mucopurulent cervical discharge or intermenstrual bleeding). Fair evidence to reject screening low-risk general population.	Gonorrhea and chlamydia: Strongly recommend that clinicians routinely screen all sexually active women aged ≤25 yr, and other asymptomatic older women at increased risk for infection. Also recommends screening high-risk pregnant women aged ≤25 years. High risk defined as: has new or multiple sexual partners; those in settings where chlamydial or gonorrhea infection is common; and those with a past STD). Makes no recommendation for or against routinely screening asymptomatic low-risk pregnant and low-risk non-pregnant women in the general population for chlamydial or gonorrhea infection. *HIV* Screen everyone for risk factors. Test only those at high risk: those seeking treatment for STDs, men who have had sex with men after	Gonorrhea and chlamydia: Screen high risk only (history of multiple partners or partner with multiple contacts; sexual contacts with persons with STD; history of repeated episodes of STDs). Routine screening for chlamydia and gonorrhea infection in all sexually active adolescents as well as older asymptomatic women at high risk. *HIV* Screen high risk only: Treated for STD, IVDU, history of prostitution, partner with HIV or who injects drugs or is bisexual, long-term resident or birth in area with high prevalence, history of transfusion from 1978 to 1985, invasive cervical cancer, pregnancy, offer to all women seeking preconception care	Pregnant women: All pregnant women should be offered HIV, gonorrhea, chlamydia, syphilis, and hepatitis B screening at the first prenatal visit. Women at higher risk should be rescreened in the third trimester for hepatitis B and HIV (women who use illicit drugs; have STDs during pregnancy; have multiple sex partners during pregnancy; or have HIV-infected partners), for Chlamydia (same risk factors as HIV, additionally age less than 25), or gonorrhea (same risk factors as for HIV, additionally living in higher prevalence communities). *Chlamydia* All sexually active adolescent women screened at least annually, even if symptoms are not present. Annual screening of all sexually active women aged 20–25 years is also recommended, as is screening of older

		CTFPHC[54]	USPSTF[55]	ACOG[56]	ACS[57]
			1975, past or present injection drug users, persons who exchange sex for money or drugs and their sex partners, women and men whose past or present sex partners were HIV-infected, bisexual, or injection drug users and persons with a history of transfusion between 1978 and 1985). Test pregnant women who are high risk or live in communities with high prevalence of infection.		women with risk factors (e.g., those who have a new sex partner and those with multiple sex partners). More frequent screening is appropriate for some women. *Gonorrhea* Screen all women at risk for STDs. *HIV* Screen all women at risk or currently being treated for STD(s).
	Frequency	Annually for high-risk individuals	Unspecified	At time of periodic assessment, timing unspecified	
Cervical Cancer[+]	Organization	CTFPHC[54]	USPSTF[55]	ACOG[56]	ACS[57]
	Year	1994	2003	2003	2002
	Screening Test	Cytology	Cytology	Cytology	
	Recommendation	Annual screening is made following initiation of sexual activity or age 18 (whichever is first); after 2 normal smears, screen every 3 years to age 69. Consider increasing	Strongly recommends screening for cervical cancer in women who have been sexually active and have a cervix. Recommends against routinely screening women >65 yr for cervical cancer if they have had adequate recent screening with normal PAP smears	Screen within 3 yr of onset of sexual activity or age 21, and then annually until age 30. Women older than 30 may be screened every 2–3 yr if have had 3 consecutive negative smears. Women with HIV infection, immunosuppression or who were exposed to	Screen within 3 yr of onset of sexual activity or age 21. Annually with slide-based or every 2 yr with liquid-based cytology tests until age 30, then every 2 to 3 yr if had 3 consecutive normal and technically adequate samples until

(continues)

Table 3-7 COMPARISON OF SCREENING RECOMMENDATIONS FROM VARIOUS ORGANIZATIONS *(continued)*

Condition	More Conservative	←		→	More Aggressive
		frequency for women with risk factors: age of first sexual intercourse <18 yr; many sexual partners or consort with many partners; smoking; or low socioeconomic status.	and are not at high risk for cervical cancer. Recommends against screening women who had a total hysterectomy for benign disease. Evidence is insufficient to recommend for or against the routine use of *human papillomavirus* (HPV) testing as a primary screening test for cervical cancer.	diethylstilbestrol in utero are at higher risk and may benefit from more frequent screening. HIV+ women should be screened twice in the first year after diagnosis and then annually. Those with a history of CIN2, CIN3, or cancer should be screened annually. If follow-up smears negative x 3 for those with a history of CIN 2 or 3, can reduce frequency of pap smear screening. Upper age range of when to stop screening is uncertain.	age 70 yr. After age 70 yr women with an intact cervix can cease if had 3 normal adequate tests and no abnormal smears within the last 10 yr. (Note that pending FDA approval, 2002 guidelines preliminarily recommended liquid-based cytology with HPV serotyping be performed every 3 yr for women aged 30 or older.)
Ovarian Cancer	Organization Year Recommendation	CTFPHC[58] 1994 Fair evidence to exclude screening for ovarian cancer by all modalities from the periodic health examination of asymptomatic pre- and post-menopausal women. Insufficient evidence to recommend for or against screening in	USPSTF[59] 2004 Recommends against screening for ovarian cancer.	ACOG[60] 2000 No screening tests have been proven effective. CA 125 and ultrasound screening ineffective for population-based screening.	ACS[39] 2004 General cancer screening done at periodic visit via physical exam.

		individuals with one or more first-degree relatives with ovarian cancer. Expert opinion currently suggests that higher risk individuals be referred to an academic research center for regular combination screening with pelvic examination, ultrasonography, and CA 125 levels.			
	Frequency	NA	NA	NA	Start at age 20, frequency unspecified, to be done at the time of a "general periodic health exam"
Osteoporosis	Organization	ACOG[13]	USPSTF[61]	CTFPHC[62]	NOF[63]
	Year	2000	2002	2004	2003
	Screening Test	Counsel regarding calcium intake and exercise, No specific recommendations on bone density testing in the 2000 report. ACOG participated as one of the panel members developing the 2003 NOF guidelines.	Bone density measurements	Bone density measurements	Bone density measurements
	Recommendation	All women	Recommends that women aged ≥65 yr be screened routinely for osteoporosis. Begin at age 60 if at increased risk for	Screen all postmenopausal women for presence of high risk criteria: 1) history of previous fracture;	Counsel all women regarding calcium/vitamin D intake, exercise, fall prevention, and lifestyle for

(continues)

Table 3-7 Comparison of Screening Recommendations from Various Organizations *(continued)*

Condition	More Conservative				More Aggressive
			osteoporotic fractures (no agreement on risk factors of enough concern, other than weight, that would prompt screening). Makes no recommendations for or against routine screening in women <60 yr of age or those between 60 and 65 who are low-risk	2) age ≥ 65 yr; 3) ORAI score of 9 or 4) SCORE score of 6. Screen is considered positive if woman meets any one of these criteria. See Table 3-8. In women without documented osteoporosis, there is fair evidence to recommend calcium and vitamin D. There is fair evidence that HRT prevents total fractures in this population; however, risks may outweigh benefits. Insufficient evidence to recommend for or against exercise, raloxifene, bisphosphonates, calcitonin, parathyroid hormone, fluoride, or combination therapy to prevent osteoporotic fractures in women without osteoporosis.	prevention of osteoporosis. Bone density measurements for all women aged 65 or older. Screen younger women if two or more risk factors (other than being white, postmenopausal) are present: *Major risks* personal history of fracture, bone fragility in first degree relative, weight less than 127 pounds, current smoking, use of oral corticosteroids for more than 3 months. *Minor risks* impaired vision, estrogen deficiency at less than 45 years of age, poor health/fragility, recent fall, lifelong low calcium intake, low physical activity, >2 drinks a day.
Frequency	Unspecified	Unspecified		At time of periodic assessment, timing unspecified	If negative on screening criteria, assess lifestyle and reevaluate in 1–2 yr. Counsel to increase calcium intake to 1000–1500 mg/d and

Vitamin D to 400–800 IU/d; exercise 3 times a week for 20–30 minutes, decrease caffeine intake to less than 4 cups a day; and to stop smoking.

If positive on any criteria, then do DEXA screening. If DEXA screening is normal, repeat in 2 yr and provide lifestyle counseling. If osteopenia is found, consider medication, counsel on lifestyle, and repeat DEXA in 1 to 2 yr. If woman has osteoporosis, provide treatment, lifestyle counseling, and repeat DEXA in 1 to 2 yr.

Abbreviations are: CTFPHC, Canadian Task Force on Preventive Health Care; USPSTF, United States Preventive Services Task Force; ACOG, American College of Obstetricians & Gynecologists; ACPM, American College of Preventive Medicine; NCEP, National Cholesterol Education Program; National Heart, Lung, and Blood Institute, National Institutes of Health; AHA, American Heart Association; ACS, American Cancer Society; NOF, National Osteoporosis Foundation; yr, year(s); BMI, body mass index; BSE, breast self exam; CBE, clinical breast exam; CV, cardiovascular (disease); FOBT, fecal occult blood test; HDL, high-density lipoprotein; HIV, human immunodeficiency virus; IVDU, intravenous drug user; LDL, low-density lipoprotein; NA, not applicable; ORAI, Osteoporosis Risk Assessment Instrument; PPD, purified protein derivative of tuberculin; SCORE®, Simple Calculation for Osteoporosis Risk Evaluation; SE, self exam; STD, sexually transmitted disease; TB, tuberculosis; TSE, total skin examination; TSH, thyroid stimulating hormone.

* ACS 2003 Breast Cancer Screening for those at Higher Risk.[43] Evidence is insufficient, but you can consider offering more aggressive screening using MRI and/or ultrasound in addition to mammogram for those at higher risk of developing breast cancer. Individuals at higher risk include those who test positive for *BRAC-1* and *BRAC-2* mutations or have a family history suggestive of increased genetic risk (i.e., 2 or more relatives with breast or ovarian cancer; breast cancer occurring before age 50 in affected relative; relatives with both breast and ovarian cancer; 1 or more relatives with two cancers [breast and ovarian cancer or two independent breast cancers; family history of breast or ovarian cancer and Ashkenazi Jewish heritage]; family history of male breast cancer. ACS recommends considering the following screening options: 1) earlier initiation of mammography at age 30 years, rarely sooner; 2) more frequent screening via mammography every 6 months; or 3) use of MRI and ultrasound, frequency is unspecified.

** ACS 2001 Colorectal Cancer Screening for those at Higher Risk.[48] Those at higher risk need more aggressive screening. Screening test and frequency vary according to high-risk conditions. High-risk conditions are defined as: a personal history of adenomatous polyps or colorectal cancer; family history of either colorectal cancer or colorectal adenomas diagnosed in a first-degree relative before age 60 years or in 2 first-degree relatives of any age; history of inflammatory bowel disease, Crohn's disease, or chronic ulcerative colitis; family history of or genetic testing indicating the presence of familial adenomatous polyposis or hereditary non-polyposis colon cancer.

(continues)

Table 3-7 Comparison of Screening Recommendations from Various Organizations *(continued)*

+ ACS 2002 Cervical Cancer Screening in Special Circumstances.[57] 1) Total hysterectomy done for benign reasons: no need for further screening. 2) Subtotal hysterectomy: Follow usual screening recommendations. 3) Hysterectomy with a history of CIN1/2: Follow until 3 consecutive negative adequate samples over 10 years with no abnormal smears. 4) Hysterectomy with a history of cervical cancer or in utero exposure to DES: continue screening as long as the woman is in reasonable health.

§Screening in Those at Higher Risk of Ovarian Cancer, 2004 Recommendations.[64] Higher risk profile is the same as that for those at higher risk of breast cancer. Screening recommendations are controversial, but some authorities suggest more aggressive surveillance via clinical pelvic exams every six months and transvaginal ultrasound and CA 125 levels beginning at age 25 to 35 years and repeated every 6 to 12 months.

Table 3-8 Methods Used to Determine if Bone Density Test Needed

ORAI Scoring[65]:

Variable	Score
Age, years	
75 or older	15
64–74	9
55–64	6
45–54	0
Weight	
<60 kg (≤132 lbs)	
60–69 kg (132–152 lbs)	9
≥70 kg (≥154 lbs)	3
Current Estrogen Use	0
Yes	2
No	0
Score	≥ 9 needs bone density screening

Score Questionnaire[66]:

Question	Answer	Score
1) Are you Caucasian or Asian?	If yes, add 5 points. If no, add 0 points.	+ _______
2) Do you take estrogen?	If yes, add 0 points. If no, add 1 point.	+ _______
3) Do you have rheumatoid arthritis?	If yes, add 4 points. If no, add 0 points.	+ _______
4) Do you have a fractured wrist, hip, or spine from a minor fall or accident?	If yes, add 4 points. If no, add 0 points.	+ _______
5) Take the first number of your age and multiply by 3. (Example: Age 60 = 6 × 3 = 18)	Calculate your score (Example, add 18)	+ _______
6) Take your weight and divide by 10. Round off to the nearest whole number. (Example: Weight 120 lbs = 120 ÷ 10 = 12)	Subtract your score (Example, subtract 12)	− _______
Total Score		≥6 needs **DEXA** screening

References

1. United States Preventive Services Task Force (USP-STF). Screening for cervical cancer. In: *Guide to Clinical Preventive Services.* 2nd ed. Baltimore: Williams & Wilkins; 1996. pp. 105–118.

2. Sankaranarayanan R, Budukh AM, Rajkumar R. Effective screening programmes for cervical cancer in low- and middle-income developing countries. *Bull WHO.* 2001;79(10):954–962.

3. USPSTF. Screening for hypertension. In: *Guide to Clinical Preventive Services.* 2nd ed. Baltimore: Williams & Wilkins; 1996. pp. 39–52.

4. USPSTF. Screening adults for lipid disorders: Recommendations and rationale. *Am J Prev Med.* 2001; 20(3S):73–76.

5. Reich J. Improved survival and higher mortality: The conundrum of lung cancer screening. *Chest.* 2002; 122(1):329–337.

6. USPSTF. *Lung Cancer Screening: Recommendation Statement.* Rockville, MD: Agency for Healthcare Research and Quality; 2004.

7. USPSTF. Screening for colorectal cancer. In: *Guide to Clinical Preventive Services.* 2nd ed. Baltimore: Williams & Wilkins; 1996. pp. 89–104.

8. Centers for Disease Control and Prevention & National Institutes of Health. Healthy People Progress Report. Cancer. [monograph on the Internet] Atlanta and Bethesda, 2004. Available from: http://www.healthy people.gov/document/html/volume1/03cancer.htm.

9. Selection and interpretation of diagnostic tests. In: Goroll A, May L, Mulley A, editors. *Primary Care Medicine.* 4th ed. Philadelphia: Lippincott Williams & Wilkins; 2000.

10. USPSTF. Introduction: Methodology Table 4. In: *Guide to Clinical Preventive Services.* Baltimore: Williams & Wilkins; 1996.

11. Douketis J, Feightner J, Attia J, Feldman W. Periodic health examination, 1999 update: 1. Detection, prevention and treatment of obesity. Canadian Task Force on Preventive Health Care. *CMAJ.* 1999;160(4): 513–525.

12. USPSTF. *Screening for Obesity in Adults: Recommendations and Rationale.* Rockville, MD: Agency for Healthcare Research and Quality; 2003.

13. ACOG Committee on Gynecologic Practice. Committee Opinion Number 246. *Primary and Preventive Care: Periodic Assessment.* Washington, DC: American College of Obstetricians and Gynecologists; 2000.

14. Nawaz H, Katz D. American College of Preventive Medicine medical practice policy statement: Weight management counseling for overweight adults. *Am J Prev Med.* 2001;21(1):73–78.

15. *Guidelines for Women's Health Care.* 2nd ed. Washington, DC: American College of Obstetricians and Gynecologists; 2002.

16. National Cholesterol Education Program Detection, National Heart, Blood and Lung Institute. *Third Report of the National Cholesterol Education Program (NCEP) Expert Panel on Detection, Evaluation, and Treatment of High Blood Cholesterol Adult Treatment Panel III.* NIH publication 02-5215. Bethesda: National Institutes of Health; 2002.

17. Pearson T, Blair S, Daniels S, et al. AHA guidelines for primary prevention of cardiovascular disease and stroke: 2002 update. *Circulation.* 2002;106(3):388–391.

18. Logan A. Screening for hypertension in young and middle-aged adults. In: Examination. Canadian Task Force on the Periodic Health Examination, editor. *Canadian Guide to Clinical Preventive Health Care.* Ottawa: Health Canada; 1994. pp. 636–648.

19. USPSTF. *Screening for High Blood Pressure: Recommendations and Rationale.* Rockville, MD: Agency for Healthcare Research and Quality; 2003.

20. Walmsley S. Screening and isoniazid prophylactic therapy for tuberculosis. In: Examination Canadian Task Force on the Periodic Health Examination, editor. *Canadian Guide to Clinical Preventive Health Care.* Ottawa: Health Canada; 1994. pp. 754–765.

21. USPSTF. Screening for tuberculosis infection. In: *Guide to Clinical Preventive Services.* 2nd ed. Baltimore: Williams & Wilkins; 1996. pp. 277–286.

22. ATS/CDC statement committee on latent tuberculosis infection membership list. Targeted tuberculin testing and treatment of latent tuberculosis infection. *MMWR Recomm Rep.* 2000;49(RR06):1–54.

23. UPSTF. Screening for skin cancer: Recommendations and rationale. *Am J Prev Med.* 2001;20(3 Suppl):44–46.

24. USPSTF. Counseling to prevent skin cancer: Recommendations and rationale. Rockville, MD: Agency for Healthcare Research and Quality; 2003.

25. Feightner J. Prevention of skin cancer. In: Examination Canadian Task Force on the Periodic Health

Examination, editor. *Canadian Guide to Clinical Preventive Health Care.* Ottawa: Health Canada; 1994. pp. 850–859.

26. Beaulieu M. Screening for thyroid disorders and thyroid cancer in asymptomatic adults. In: Examination Canadian Task Force on the Periodic Health Examination, editor. *Canadian Guide to Clinical Preventive Health Care.* Ottawa: Health Canada; 1994. pp. 612–618.

27. USPSTF. *Screening Thyroid Disease: Recommendation Statement.* Rockville, MD: Agency for Healthcare Research and Quality; 2004.

28. USPSTF. Screening for thyroid cancer. In: *Guide to Clinical Preventive Services.* 2nd ed. Baltimore: Williams & Wilkins; 1996.

29. Ladenson P, Singer P, Ain K, et al. American Thyroid Association guidelines for detection of thyroid dysfunction. *Arch Intern Med.* 2000;160(11):1573–1575.

30. Feig D, Palda V, Lipscombe L with the Canadian Task Force on Preventive Health Care. Screening for type 2 diabetes mellitus to prevent vascular complications: Updated recommendations from the Canadian Task Force on Preventive Health Care. *CMAJ.* 2005; 172(2):177–180.

31. USPSTF. Screening for type 2 diabetes mellitus in adults: Recommendations and rationale. In: Agency for Healthcare Research and Quality. Rockville, MD: USPSTF; 2003.

32. Canadian Task Force on the Periodic Health Examination. Periodic health examination, 1995 update: 3. Screening for visual problems among elderly patients. *CMAJ.* 1995;152(8):1211–1222.

33. USPSTF. Screening for visual impairment. In: *Guide to Clinical Preventive Services.* 2nd ed. Baltimore: Williams & Wilkins; 1996. pp. 373–382.

34. USPSTF. Screening for Glaucoma: Recommendation Statement. AHRQ Publication No. 04-0548-A, March 2005. Agency for Healthcare Research and Quality, Rockville, MD. http://www.ahrq.gov/clinic/uspstf05/glaucoma/glaucrs.htm.

35. Department of Veterans Affairs (U.S.). Screening for glaucoma in the primary care setting. [monograph on the Internet] Washington, DC: Office of Quality and Performance; 2000. Available from: http://www.oqp.med.va.gov/cpg/Glaucoma/GLA_GOL.htm.

36. Lewis D, Ismail A. Canadian Task Force on the Periodic Health Examination Periodic Health Examination, 1995 update: 2. Prevention of dental caries. *CMAJ.* 1995;152(6):836–846.

37. Hawkins R, Wang E, Leake J. Preventive health care, 1999 update: Prevention of oral cancer mortality. The Canadian Task Force on Preventive Health Care. *J Can Dent Assoc.* 1999;65(11):617.

38. USPSTF. Screening for oral cancer: Recommendation statement. In: *Agency for Healthcare Research and Quality.* Rockville, MD: USPST; 2004.

39. Smith R, Cokkinides V, Eyre H. American Cancer Society AC. American Cancer Society guidelines for the early detection of cancer, 2004. *CA Cancer J Clin.* 2004;54(1):41–52.

40. Morrison B. Screening for breast cancer (revised by the Canadian Task Force on the Periodic Health Examination 1998). Canadian Task Force on the Periodic Health Examination, editor. *Canadian Guide to Clinical Preventive Health Care.* Ottawa: Health Canada; 1994. pp. 788–795.

41. USPSTF. *Screening for Breast Cancer: Recommendations and Rationale.* Rockville, MD: Agency for Healthcare Research and Quality; 2002.

42. ACOG Committee on Practice Bulletins. *ACOG Practice Bulletin Clinical Management Guidelines for Obstetrician-Gynecologists Breast Cancer Screening.* Number 42, April 2003. Washington, DC: American College of Obstetricians and Gynecologists; 2003.

43. Smith R, Saslow D, Sawyer K, Burke W, Costanza M, Evans W, et al. American Cancer Society Guidelines for Breast Cancer Screening Update 2003. *CA Cancer J Clin.* 2003;53(3):141–169.

44. Baxter N, Care Canadian Task Force on the Periodic Health Examination. Preventive health care, 2001 update: Should women be routinely taught breast self-examination to screen for breast cancer? *CAMJ.* 2001;164(13):1837–1846.

45. Ringash J, Canadian Task Force on Preventive Health Care. Preventive health care, 2001 update: Screening mammography among women aged 40-49 years at average risk of breast cancer. *CMAJ.* 2001;164(4): 469–476.

46. Canadian Task Force on Preventive Health Care. Colorectal cancer screening: Recommendation statement from the Canadian Task Force on Preventive Health Care. *CMAJ.* 2001;165(2):206–208.

47. USPSTF. *Screening for Colorectal Cancer: Recommendations and Rationale.* Rockville, MD: Agency for Healthcare Research and Quality; 2002.

48. Smith R, von Eschenbach A, Wender R, Levin B, Byers T, Rothenberger D, et al. American Cancer Society guidelines for the early detection of cancer:

Update of early detection guidelines for prostate, colorectal, and endometrial cancers. *CA Cancer J Clin.* 2001;51(1):38–75.

49. Davies H, Wang E, Canadian Task Force on the Periodic Health Examination. Periodic health examination, 1996 update: Screening for chlamydial infections. *CMAJ.* 1996;154(1):1631–1644.

50. USPSTF. Screening for chlamydial infection: Recommendations and rationale. *Am J Prev Med.* 2001; 20(3S):90–94.

51. USPSTF. Screening for gonorrhea. In: *Guide to Clinical Preventive Services.* 2nd ed. Baltimore: Williams & Wilkins; 1996. pp. 293–302.

52. USPSTF. Screening for human immunodeficiency virus infection. In: *Guide to Clinical Preventive Services.* 2nd ed. Baltimore: Williams & Wilkins; 1996. pp. 303–323.

53. CDC. Sexually transmitted diseases treatment guidelines: 2002. *MMWR Recomm Rep.* 2002;51(RR 6): 1–77.

54. Morrison B, Canadian Task Force on the Periodic Health Examination. Screening for cervical cancer. In: *Canadian Guide to Clinical Preventive Health Care.* Ottawa: Health Canada; 1994. pp. 870–881.

55. USPSTF. Screening for cervical cancer: Recommendations and rationale. In: AHRQ Publication No. 03-515A. Rockville, MD: Agency for Healthcare Research and Quality; 2003.

56. ACOG Committee on Practice Bulletins. ACOG Practice Bulletin: Clinical management guidelines for obstetrician-gynecologists. Number 45, August 2003. Cervical cytology screening (replaces committee opinion 152, March 1995). *Obstet Gynecol.* 2003;102(2):417–427.

57. Saslow D, Runowicz C, Solomon D, Moscicki A, Smith R, Eyre H, et al. American Cancer Society guideline for the early detection of cervical neoplasia and cancer. *CA Cancer J Clin.* 2002;52(6): 342–362.

58. Gladstone C, Canadian Task Force on the Periodic Health Examination. Screening for ovarian cancer. In: *Canadian Guide to Clinical Preventive Health Care.* Ottawa: Health Canada; 1994. pp. 870–881.

59. USPSTF. *Screening for Ovarian Cancer: Recommendation Statement.* Rockville, MD: Agency for Healthcare Research and Quality; 2004.

60. ACOG Committee on Gynecologic Practice. *ACOG Committee Opinion Routine Cancer Screening # 247.* Washington, DC: American College of Obstetricians and Gynecologists; 2000.

61. USPSTF. *Screening for Osteoporosis in Postmenopausal Women: Recommendations and Rationale.* Rockville, MD: Agency for Healthcare Research and Quality; 2002.

62. Cheung A, Feig D, Kapra lM, Diaz-Granados N, Dodin S, Canadian Task Force on Preventive Health Care. Prevention of osteoporosis and osteoporotic fractures in postmenopausal women: Recommendation statement from the Canadian Task Force on Preventive Health Care. *CMAJ.* 2004;170(11):1665–1667.

63. National Osteoporosis Foundation. Physician's guide to prevention and treatment of osteoporosis. [monograph on the Internet] Washington, DC: National Osteoporosis Foundation; 2003. Available from: http://www.nof.org/physguide/.

64. Sifri R, Gangadharappa S, Acheson L. Identifying and testing for hereditary susceptibility to common cancers. *CA Cancer J Clin.* 2004;54(6):309–326.

65. Cadarette S, Jaglal S, Kreiger N, McIssac W, Darlington G, Tu J. Development and validation of the Osteoporosis Risk Assessment Instrument to facilitate selection of women for bone densiometry. *CMAJ.* 2000;162(9):1289–1294.

66. Lydick E, Cook K, Turpin J, Melton M, Stine R, Byrnes C. Development and validation of a simple questionnaire to facilitate identification of women likely to have low bone density. *Am J Manag Care.* 1998;4(1):37–48.

Chapter 4

Environmental Health

Donna Vivio

The history of environmental health as a competency area in midwifery in the United States is simultaneously very recent and, in some ways, quite established. Midwives and others who care for women of childbearing age are well aware of the potential exogenous and environmental risks to women and their unborn children before, during, and after pregnancy. In addition to counseling women about radiologic exposures, medications (e.g., thalidomide, rubella vaccine), the need for folic acid, and the hazards of smoking, midwives have asked women questions about their occupation and household conditions. However, the midwifery community continues to be in need of additional information on environmental health issues and on the related responsibilities of the profession to the women that it serves. The purpose of this chapter is to introduce environmental health into the clinician's consciousness and offer a guide to appropriate resources to improve care.

Why Midwives?

According to Dr. Kenneth Olden, Director of the National Institute of Environmental Health Sciences and the National Toxicology Program, the term *environment* includes industrial and agricultural chemicals, foods and nutrients, and physical and biological agents.[1] Environmental exposures can occur anywhere—at home, in the workplace, in schools, in health care settings—and are often influenced by social, economic, and cultural factors (e.g., income, housing, and food sources and preparation). Exposures to environmental hazards can be chronic, such as indoor air quality, or acute, such as an industrial accident.[2] As the public and the health care community are becoming increasingly aware of the hazards of exposure to environmental toxins, increasing emphasis is being placed on identifying risk factors, developing prevention strategies, and translating knowledge into practice to prevent human illness.

Environmental hazards are among the top health concerns of parents for their children.[3] One example of this is media coverage, including the local press coverage of past and current arsenic and mercury exposures to citizens.[4] Many environmental hazards can have an adverse effect on the health of pregnant women, the developing fetus, and children. Exposure to these hazards can result in diseases such as asthma, lead poisoning, childhood cancer, and developmental disorders. Additionally, recent research has demonstrated a relationship between fetal deaths and air pollution.[5]

It is the responsibility of health care providers, including midwives, to be current in their knowledge of environmental health and to use this knowledge in their practices. Because health care providers generally have strong credibility with the public, they have both the opportunity and the responsibility to aid in the prevention of problems occurring from exposure to environmental toxins. Additionally, because midwives have multiple visits with women during pregnancy and provide continuity of care before, between, and after pregnancies, they are in a prime position to have a positive effect on the health of women and children. Careful history taking and physical evaluation, laboratory screening, and anticipatory guidance are all tools to identify and treat problems.

In addition to answering their patients' questions, clinicians need to assess the risk within the home, at work, and in the community. Midwives need to respond to the expanding research showing adverse effects of detrimental environmental events such as air pollution (including indoor air pollution) and pesticide use, and to address the questions of their patients regarding pertinent and sensitive issues such as breast cancer and safety of breastfeeding.

The Clinical Setting

In developed countries, the major causes of morbidity and mortality are not easily treated or cured, making prevention a more attractive avenue for management of chronic diseases.[1] Indeed, most chronic diseases arise from a complex array of factors including intrinsic genetic susceptibility, environmental exposures, behavior, age, and stage of development. Examples of diseases whose development can be attributed to environmental factors are lung disease (air pollutants), impaired intelligence (lead exposure), breast cancer (steroidal estrogens), and cardiovascular disease (air pollutants).[2,6]

The midwife's role in the clinical setting, relative to environmental health, is to understand and apply the related knowledge and risks. Assessment of risk and prevention of illness are two of the ways that this application is manifested in practice. Anticipatory guidance, counseling, and referral are ways that environmental health practice is implemented.

Assessment of Risk

Assessment of risk, which includes a health history of the patient, should be made at initial health care visits and updated at subsequent visits as indicated (**Table 4-1**). Although it is difficult to include time for additional information gathering in an already busy patient care visit, questions about a woman's environment are basic to the health history. This is particularly true if there are signs and symptoms that are not easily accounted for, and/or if the primary care visit is for pre-conception counseling. For a woman planning pregnancy or for any woman who is of childbearing age, discussion about the environment is crucial because the effects of exposure to environmental toxins vary depending on the developmental stage of the fetus.[3]

Environmental exposures can trigger illnesses or cause exacerbations of underlying medical conditions. For example, in respiratory illnesses such as asthma and other airway diseases, tobacco smoke is the most commonly associated

Table 4-1 CONTENTS OF HEALTH CARE VISITS RELATIVE TO ENVIRONMENTAL HEALTH

Visit Type	Environmental History	Focused Environmental History	Anticipatory Guidance	Focused Physical Exam	Appropriate Laboratory and Testing	Appropriate Consultation or Referral
Preconception	▒		▒		▒	▒
Initial Prenatal	▒					
Prenatal		▒	▒			
Inter-conceptional		▒	▒	▒	▒	▒
Post-childbearing		▒	▒	▒	▒	▒
Sick visit		▒	▒	▒	▒	▒

Shaded boxes indicate that these visits should include the particular action.

Includes appropriate screenings for cancer dependent on age, history, family history, and other factors, such as breast examination and mammogram.

environmental toxin. Lead poisoning may present with recurrent abdominal pain, seizures, irritability, constipation, developmental delays, or unexplained coma.[3] Most often, because there are not symptoms that immediately suggest an environmental cause, it is important to actively consider environment when presented with a case that has atypical symptoms or that is unresponsive to treatment. Some questions to ask are similar to those used to evaluate pain:

- Are the symptoms present or worse in certain locations (e.g., the workplace)?
- What is the timing of the symptoms (e.g., every day, only during the week, only on weekends)?
- Is there something else associated with the symptoms (e.g., a particular activity)?
- Does anyone else that you know have the same symptom(s)?
- If yes, who are they or how are they associated with you?

History

To elicit basic information on environmental risks or concerns at a routine health visit, participants at the 2002 annual meeting of the American College of Nurse-Midwives (ACNM) reviewed a sample environmental health history questionnaire developed from *Nursing, Health and the Environment* (**Table 4-2**).[7] The goal was

---

Table 4-2 POTENTIAL ENVIRONMENTAL HAZARD ASSESSMENT TOOL[7]

How to use this tool:

Complete this form, focusing particularly on potential problem areas. If the answer to a question is yes, ask for more details and use appropriate resources to evaluate the problem. Explore relationships and think about reasonable options for your patient.

1. Has anyone in your home or workplace been diagnosed with or suspected to have a health problem or birth defect that could be attributed to environmental exposure (e.g., mold, damp house, lead paint chips, chemicals in the workplace)?
2. Do you have trouble breathing, or do you cough or wheeze in your home or workplace?
3. Do you live or work in the immediate vicinity of a refinery, smelter, factory, industrial plant, hazardous waste site, landfill, or other potential pollution source? (If yes, determine dosage/exposure level.)
4. Do you live, work, or regularly visit a building that is undergoing renovation, has peeling or chipped lead paint, new carpeting, or is being painted?
5. Do you smoke cigarettes, cigars, pipes, or chew tobacco? Do you have regular exposure to secondhand smoke[a]?
6. Are you exposed to pesticides, mothballs, hobby glues or paints, or chemicals of any nature in your home or workplace? Are you aware of any chemical odors or strong fumes in your environment?
7. Is there evidence of mold in your home or workplace?
8. What ventilation systems are used in your workplace?
9. Which of the following do you use in your home?
   - Air conditioner or air purifier
   - Electric, wood, or gas stove
   - Humidifier
   - Wood fireplace or gas fireplace
   - Unvented kerosene heater or gas heater
10. What is your source of drinking water?
    - Community water system
    - Private well
    - Bottled water
11. If you eat fish or seafood, what types and how often?
12. How do you spend most of your day?
13. If you have headaches… (explore relationships.)
14. Are you aware of hazards in the environment that may hurt you, your baby, and/or your family?
15. Are you exposed to anything in your home or your work that you are concerned about?
16. Where does your partner work?

---

[a]Secondhand smoke is also called "passive smoke" or "environmental tobacco smoke."

to create an environmental history tool that is both relevant to midwifery and also quick and easy to use. Any warning signs or red flags identified need further investigation and may require consultation or referral. It should be used as any health history tool is used. Complete the tool, focusing particularly on potential problem areas. If the answer to a question is yes, ask for more details, and focus the remainder of the patient encounter (physical exam, testing, etc.) on the most likely exposure.

To sensitize midwives to potential environmental hazards and to their need to consider environmental exposures during client visits, workshop attendees were asked to identify possible environmental hazards in the home, community, workplace, and school. **Table 4-3** is a list of possible environmental hazards identified by the participants that can be used in conjunction with a basic history to pinpoint potential exposures of concern for an individual woman.

Physical Examination

The physical examination should proceed as usual, with additional attention focused on areas of interest flagged in the history. For example, a thorough skin exam is important with those exposures that could lead to contact dermatitis and a neurologic exam for those that affect the brain. Areas of concern may require laboratory testing, consultation, or referral for evaluation by an expert in environmental health. Consultation with a physician and/or appropriate referral should be pursued as indicated.

Laboratory

Further laboratory testing is dependent on the history and the findings on physical examination. Specific laboratory tests that can be used to identify excessive exposures are not available for many suspected toxins. There are some exceptions, including tests for lead and mercury levels, although normal blood levels do not exclude mercury poisoning. Even if such tests were readily available, few, if any, treatments exist that can effectively eliminate toxins from the body or mitigate their short- or long-term effects. Therefore, laboratory testing is of limited value in environmental health, particularly in the primary health care setting.[3]

Diagnosis, Treatment, and Referral

A diagnosis of a problem secondary to environmental exposures could warrant additional testing, consultation, and/or referral to a physician. Although environmental health is emerging in the consciousness of all clinicians, only a few of those clinicians can be classified as "experts" in this realm. Therefore, discussion with the midwife or practitioner's consultant is the first step in referral. Additionally, contact with the local or state Health Department may be another way to locate appropriate consultants or to gain information on particular environmental hazards to which the midwife's patient may have been exposed (thus aiding in diagnosis). As in any diagnosis, a plan should be developed that includes further testing, consultation, referral, and other interventions, as appropriate.

Anticipatory Guidance

Many of the toxins that may be causing problems or concerns do not have known treatments other than prevention of further exposure. Therefore, anticipatory guidance is the key intervention in clinical practice. The guidance given depends on the reason for the

Table 4-3 POSSIBLE ENVIRONMENTAL HAZARDS FOR PATIENTS

Home	Community	Workplace	School
• Well water	• Global warming	• Computers	• Immunizations
• Radon	• Landfills	• Asbestos	• Art supplies
• Cleaning supplies	• Urban sprawl	• Air conditioning	• Asbestos
• Lead paint/pipes	• Carbon monoxide	• Hazardous waste	• Cleaning supplies
• Pesticides	• Smog	• Hospitals	• Radon
• Non-organic garden	• Waste incineration	• Radioactive materials	• Water
• Hair spray	• Farms (odors, runoff,	• Microorganisms	• Food
• Car oil	salmonella)	• Bottled water	• Infectious diseases
• Gasoline	• Petting zoos	• People exposure	• Carpet
• Antifreeze	• Lead paint/pipes	• Secondhand smoke	• Bad Air
• Freon	• Pressure-treated wood	• Water	• Drugs
• Mercury	• Chlorine	• Food	• Lead
• Carpet/fabric gas	• Drug byproducts in	• Cleaning supplies	• Pesticides
• Gas or wood stove	water system	• Carpet	• Vectors
• Furnace	• Water	• Toxic waste	• Cockroaches
• Pet supplies	• Infectious diseases	• Chemical exposure	
• Suntan lotions	• Pesticides	• Bad air	
• Deodorant	• Sewage and water	• Blood	
• Prescription meds and	treatment	• Noise	
vitamins	• Hot tubs/pools/	• Fuels	
• Food	saunas	• Solvents	
• Asbestos	• Vectors	• Gases	
• Air pollution	• Toxic waste		
• Mold	• Bad air/pollution		
• Animal/litter box	• Mercury in water		
• Iron	• Electrical wires		
	• Ultraviolet light		

health care visit and individual characteristics such as the patient's childbearing status. Is the primary focus mainly on prevention? For example, a preconception visit would focus on past and present environmental risks such as chemical exposures and smoking that the woman should avoid or minimize. In this example, the woman could be counseled on the risks to the fetus associated with smoking, and a smoking cessation program could be offered. To address the realities of a busy practice as well as the enormity of discussion or intervention for possible environmental exposures, **Table 4-4** was developed by midwives during the 2002 ACNM Workshop. It lists information and interventions for specific hazards that midwives felt were relatively easy to fit into each visit, as well as such information that was important to give to women. While the information in this table is not exhaustive,

Table 4-4 INFORMATION AND INTERVENTIONS TO GIVE TO WOMEN TO PREVENT EXPOSURES TO ENVIRONMENTAL TOXINS

Important to Give	Easy to Give	Intervention
• Fish consumption limits • Smoking cessation • Pesticides • Household chemicals • Fresh air • Lead • Nutrition • Resource kit • Hand washing	• Fish consumption limits • Smoking cessation • Fresh air • Lead • Hand washing	• Breast milk better (dioxin issue) • Humidifier cleaning (filter, vinegar) • Ventilation • Less toxic paints • Iron and calcium supplements to offset lead • Smoking cessation

it will help to "triage" the crucial information for women.

Environmental and Patient Care Issues and Foundation

Two key issues provide the foundation and main justification for health care providers' responsibilities vis-à-vis environmental health: the precautionary principle and the issue of environmental justice.

The *precautionary principle* is the basis on which much of the environmental health movement works. It states that the first priority is protection of health. It calls for seeking out the safest ways to accomplish human activities while recognizing the limits of scientific knowledge. In other words, even though there may be no "proof" that a particular substance is dangerous to human health, in order to protect health it is best to be cautious about increasing exposure to that substance. Thus, the precautionary principle is at the heart of many environmental policies based on clean production and pollution prevention.[8,9] One definition of the precautionary principle, developed at the Wingspread Conference in 1998, states:

> *When an activity raises threats of harm to human health or the environment, precautionary measures should be taken even if some cause and effect relationships are not fully established scientifically. In this context the proponent of an activity, rather than the public, should bear the burden of proof. The process of applying the precautionary principle must be open, informed and democratic and must include potentially affected parties. It must also involve an examination of the full range of alternatives, including no action.*[8]

The precautionary principle is incorporated into many international environmental agreements and European environmental policies. One such example is the Rio Declaration, which is an international agreement signed by the United States at the 1992 United Nations Conference on Environment and Development in Rio de Janeiro.

The concept of environmental justice has emerged because much of the exposure to and many of the effects from environmental pollutants in the United States disproportionately affect lower socioeconomic groups. *Environmental justice* is achieved when everyone enjoys the same degree of protection from environmental health hazards and has equal access to the decision-making process to have a healthy environment in which to live, learn, and work.[10]

Midwives have an opportunity to move this environmental justice and environmental health agenda forward by continuing to provide services to and advocate for vulnerable populations. Approximately 70% of the women and newborns seen by midwives are considered vulnerable by virtue of age, socioeconomic status, education, ethnicity, or place of residence. As of 2002, nearly 60% of the population served by midwives in the United States received public sources of insurance coverage indicating near or at poverty level. Such populations often have the least access to information that can help them to make informed decisions about their health care. These same populations also share many of the same characteristics as the communities served by environmental justice grants made by the federal government.[11]

Two issues are particularly relevant to midwifery practice and to midwives' patients: breastfeeding and breast cancer. In addition to a discussion of these two issues, the next section reviews a few of the more common toxins that are particularly hazardous to women, fetuses, and children. A focus that includes children is appropriate for discussion because it is the woman and her major concerns (which often center on her children) that are the reasons for the primary care visit. Thus, some of the information provided here about specific toxins fo-cuses on effects on children because they are disproportionately affected by these toxins, for example, by their developmental stages and behaviors (e.g., hand-to-mouth activity).

Breastfeeding

The goodness of breast milk—and indeed a mother's very ability to produce it—is now being compromised by the presence of toxic chemicals in the human food chain.... The question is not whether we should feed our babies chemically contaminated, yet clearly superior, breast milk or chemically uncontaminated, yet clearly inferior, formula. The question is, what do we need to do to get chemical contaminants out of clearly superior breast milk?[12]

There is increasing evidence that some of the most persistent pollutants in the environment are expressed in human breast milk. What are the implications of this evidence for the prospective mother? What are the risks and benefits of breastfeeding in light of this evidence? Are the same contaminants present in cow's milk, soy products, and/or infant formula?

In 2001, the popular press presented news about environmental pollutants that were being measured in human breast milk.[13] Although the environmental health research community has been aware of the presence of persistent pollutants in breast milk, this was new information to the midwifery community. As strong advocates for breastfeeding, it is imperative that midwives understand the possible health implications of the contaminants as they relate to the many benefits that breastfeeding affords both the baby and the mother.

The contaminants being measured included, but were not limited to, heavy metals, chlorinated pesticides (including DDT), halogenated hydrocarbons and biphenyls, various industrial chemicals, fungicides, furans, and other pesticides. Many of these chemicals are persistent in the environment and bio-accumulate as they move up the food chain. Humans, at the top of the food chain, receive the highest magnitude of these chemicals. Many of these same chemicals are lipophylic, meaning they are easily stored in body fat for years due to their lengthy half-lives. When a woman breastfeeds, these chemicals are released from fat cells into her breast milk. Contaminants have been found in breast milk of women from countries from around the world as diverse as Vietnam, the United States, Korea, Canada, the Netherlands, Kazakhstan, and Croatia.

Studies have examined trends in the composition and concentrations of these chemicals in human milk. Other studies have looked at the daily intakes and body burdens of various chemicals in infants, and the adverse effects that these chemicals may pose to the infant in utero and postnatally. Rogan and colleagues reported problems with exposure to polychlorinated biphenyls (PCBs) and dioxins in utero (such as lower developmental and intelligence scores, including lower psychomotor scores from newborn through 2 years), and hyporeflexia and hypertonia in infants.[14] Their studies did not find conclusive evidence of the adverse effects on breastfeeding infants and, therefore, there was insufficient evidence to warrant a recommendation to not breastfeed. However, other studies found effects associated with breastfeeding and exposure to pollutants. Some of these studies have found that postnatal pesticides and dioxins (from breast milk) have an effect on infant mental and psychomotor development.[15]

Breast milk substitutes may not be safe from environmental contaminants either. Concerns have been raised that cow's milk-based infant formulas may contain chemical and hormone residues, antibiotics, and bovine growth hormone. Milk and soy-based formulas are also subject to industrial poisoning accidents as well as preparation errors, including over- and under-concentration of the product. In addition to the occasions when these formulas are watered down or underconcentrated in an attempt to save on the cost of the formula (which can lead to malnutrition in the infant and possible growth and development problems), another concern about breast milk substitutes is that the product may be reconstituted with water that is contaminated with diarrhea-causing bacteria, pesticides, or heavy metals. These issues are particularly relevant for the developing world.

In addition, many infant formulas are delivered in plastic feeding bottles that may contain phthalates and nonphenols, which are hormone-disrupting chemicals (see "Sources of Exposure"). In Midwestern states that have a high agricultural production, many bottle-fed infants may be exposed to the pesticide atrazine when formula is reconstituted with contaminated tap water. Infant hair manganese levels are also high in formula-fed infants because of the high content of this element in infant formulas, especially soy-based formulas. Elevated levels of manganese may be associated with various attention problems in children. Soy-based formulas also have problems, because they may be made from genetically altered soy, the effects of which are unknown. Additionally, infant soy products have high levels of phytoestrogens.[16]

It has been widely demonstrated that the benefits of breastfeeding are substantial for both the infant and the mother. The American Academy of Pediatrics contends that breastfed infants are less likely to develop many illnesses such as pneumonia, diarrhea, ear infections, bacterial meningitis, bacteremia, urinary infections, and bacterial infections of the intestines.[17] Other clearly demonstrated benefits include maternal health improvements such as reduction in postpartum bleeding, earlier return to prepregnancy weight, reduced risk of premenopausal breast cancer, and reduced risk of osteoporosis.

Most researchers as well as national and international public health organizations currently agree that the benefits of breastfeeding far outweigh the possible risks that may or may not be associated with contaminants in human breast milk. In 1998, the World Health Organization working group concluded that the current evidence does not warrant altering the current recommendation to breastfeed, and that efforts should focus on controlling the sources of environmental pollutants. The U.S. Environmental Protection Agency (EPA) acknowledges infant exposure to pesticides from breast milk contamination, they also state that the potential risks of this exposure are offset by the known benefits of breastfeeding.[18]

ACNM POLICY STATEMENT: ENVIRONMENTAL POLLUTANTS IN BREAST MILK

The ACNM issued a policy statement on environmental pollutants in breast milk in 2003.

The American College of Nurse-Midwives believes that it is imperative that the public, especially women and families faced with infant feeding choices, be given comprehensive and accurate information, and be given the support they need to breastfeed. ACNM feels that despite environmental pollutants, breastfeeding is still the preferred method. We support funding for training programs and resource materials that provide health care professionals, women, and the community assistance in understanding the benefits and potential negatives of breastfeeding and formula feeding as it relates to the existence of environmental pollutants. ACNM also supports local, state, national, and international efforts to decrease environmental pollutants that enter and impact the human body, including breast milk. This may include measures to decrease mercury contamination, fuel, power plant, and incinerator emissions.[19]

Breast Cancer

Once primarily a disease of women beyond childbearing age, breast cancer increasingly is seen in women who are in their 20s and 30s. In the 1940s, a woman's lifetime risk of breast cancer was 1 in 22. Today, it is 1 in 7 and rising.[20] Known risk factors, including genetics and family history, account for only 50% of breast cancer cases. Some of the risk factors for breast cancer include:

- Earlier onset of menstruation (12 years or younger)
- Later menopause (55 years or older)
- Late first-term pregnancy (30 years or older)
- No children or no breastfeeding
- Early use of oral contraceptives
- More than 4 years' use of hormone replacement therapy
- Postmenopausal obesity
- Alcohol consumption
- Exposure to environmental tobacco smoke (ETS)
- Low physical activity
- Exposure to radiation

The other 50% of the cases remain unexplained. Evidence increasingly points to environmental exposures as potential triggers for the development of breast cancer.[20] Some of these exposures are related to the 85% of chemicals in use in the United States that have *not* been tested for safety in humans. Other sources of exposure to chemicals linked to breast cancer are from hormone-mimicking chemicals that are in cleaning products, pesticides, prescription drugs, and fuels. Seemingly innocuous sources include some cosmetics, plastic wrap on food (a source of phthalates), personal care items such as deodorant, and some fragrances. Pesticides, herbicides, fungicides, fuels, some prescription drugs, and other chemicals that mimic reproductive hormones have been strongly implicated in triggering breast cancer. In total, 150 chemicals, the majority of which are still in use today, have been found to cause mammary tumors in laboratory animals. The U.S. National Toxicology Program considers such evidence as being "reasonably anticipated to be carcinogenic to humans."[6]

Most of the toxins discussed here have been the subjects of government outreach to consumers and providers, and are known to the public. More extensive information on these and other toxins are available from a number of sources, most notably from the National Environmental Education and Training Foundation Web site, which contains the Pesticide Initiative Information Gateway.[21] Another important resource for midwives is a booklet published in 2002 by the ACNM and Health Care Without Harm. This booklet, entitled, *Green Birthdays*, provides important information for providers about environmental safety in the birthplace and offers practical ways to reduce exposure to toxins.[11]

Molds

SOURCES OF EXPOSURE

Molds can enter the home via doorways, windows, ventilation systems, and heating or air conditioning units. Mold thrives in damp areas such as unventilated bathrooms, flooded basements, and greenhouses and other areas where indoor plants are grown.

ROUTES OF CONTAMINATION

Exposure to molds is via inhalation and direct physical contact.

LEVELS OF EXPOSURE FOR CONCERN

Most of the effects of exposure to mold are in the mucous membranes of the respiratory system, eyes, nose, and throat. The clinical effects can be allergic (e.g., sneezing, eye irritation, rhinitis, coughing, and wheezing) or toxic. Toxic effects may be secondary to inhalation of mycotoxins, which are lipid-soluble and readily absorbed by the airways. In several cases, particularly with exposure to *Stachybotrys atra,* pulmonary hemorrhage in young infants was found to be associated with molds.[22,23]

WAYS TO MINIMIZE EXPOSURE

Water and all water-damaged items should be removed within 24 hours of a flood or leak as a preventive intervention. If some mold is already present, the affected area needs to be washed with soap and water, and then with a solution of 1 part bleach to 10 parts water. Protective gloves should be worn for any cleanup activities.

IMPACT ON PREGNANCY, LACTATION, AND THE FETUS

A review of the literature failed to uncover any evidence that there are specific additional impacts of molds on pregnant or lactating women or on the fetus.

Mercury

SOURCES OF EXPOSURE

Mercury is a neurotoxic heavy metal that is linked to numerous health effects in wildlife and people. It occurs in three forms: the metallic element, inorganic salts, and organic compounds (including methylmercury). When released into the environment, mercury is deposited onto land and water surfaces, where it remains indefinitely as either elemental mercury or as methylmercury. Microorganisms can convert elemental mercury to methylmercury, making it more biologically available, that is, more able to interact with and damage cells. Sources of mercury contamination include medical waste incineration and wastewater from hospitals. Health care facilities are among the largest sources of mercury released into the atmosphere.[24] Thermometers, sphygmomanometers, dilation and feeding tubes, batteries, and fluorescent lamps are all products that contain elemental mercury and are widely used in hospitals.

ROUTES OF CONTAMINATION

Methylmercury accumulates in the tissues of animals, especially fish and shellfish. Although nearly all fish and shellfish contain traces of methylmercury, larger fish that have lived longer have the highest levels. Fish that are higher on the food chain absorb the most mercury, and humans are contaminated after consuming these fish. Other routes of contamination are:

- Accidental mercury spills.
- Incinerators and facilities burning mercury-containing fuels (i.e., coal or other fossil fuels, mercury-containing wastes).

- In some cases, unborn children are exposed through the mother's blood, and infants may be exposed through breast milk.

LEVELS OF EXPOSURE FOR CONCERN

The National Academy of Sciences has determined that a reference dose for mercury is 0.1 mcg/kg per day.[3] A *reference dose* is an amount determined to be safe on the basis of available toxicity information and used to provide a basis for establishing safety standards and guidelines.

DIAGNOSIS

Diagnosis of mercury poisoning is made by history and physical examination. Some signs and symptoms are tremors, impaired vision and hearing, paralysis, insomnia, emotional instability, developmental deficits during fetal development, and attention deficit and developmental delays during childhood. Laboratory testing may demonstrate elevated blood mercury, although normal blood levels do *not* exclude mercury poisoning.[3]

TREATMENT

The treatment for exposure to mercury is to identify its source and eliminate it. Although chelating agents have been used for treatment of elemental and inorganic mercury poisoning, it is not clear whether this treatment helps. There is no chelating agent approved by the U.S. Food and Drug Administration (FDA) that is effective for organic (methylmercury) poisoning.

WAYS TO MINIMIZE EXPOSURE

Preventing mercury intake is the only way to prevent its effects. Due to potential neurotoxic risks to the fetus and child, fish consumption advisories for pregnant women, for women of childbearing age, and for children are in place in the United States. In 2001, the Centers for Disease Control and Prevention (CDC) estimated that 1 in 10 women have mercury levels high enough to cause neurological effects.[25] The FDA and the EPA advise women of childbearing age, pregnant and nursing women, and young children to avoid some types of fish and shellfish, even those lower in mercury. Their three recommendations are[26]:

1. Do not eat shark, swordfish, king mackerel, or tilefish.
2. Eat up to 12 ounces (2 average meals) a week of a variety of fish and shellfish that are lower in mercury. Examples of these are shrimp, canned light tuna, salmon, pollock, and catfish. Because albacore ("white") tuna has more mercury than canned light tuna, only up to 6 ounces of this tuna should be eaten per week.
3. Check local advisories about the safety of fish caught in local lakes, rivers, and coastal areas. If no advice is available, eat up to 6 ounces per week of fish caught from local waters, but do *not* consume any other fish during that week.

IMPACT ON HEALTH, INCLUDING PREGNANCY, LACTATION, AND THE FETUS

Mercury attacks the central nervous system, kidneys, and lungs. Ingested methylmercury (via fish consumption) crosses the placenta easily, and the critical effect on the infant from prenatal exposure is mental retardation. Even with minimal effects of maternal exposure, infants demonstrate nervous system damage.[27] Organic mercury, a powerful teratogen, causes disruption of the normal patterns of neuronal migration and nerve cell histology in the developing brain. Some of the gradually developing symptoms can include psychomotor retardation, blindness, deafness, and seizures.[3]

Polyvinyl Chloride Plastic, Phthalates, Dioxin

Polyvinyl chloride (PVC) plastic is a chlorinated plastic. PVC creates dioxin, a deadly carcinogen, when it is manufactured or burned. Thus, the use of PVC plastic leads to environmental contamination by two different toxins—dioxin and di-2-ethylhexyl phthalate (DEHP)—each of which has different toxic effects.

SOURCES OF EXPOSURE FOR DIOXIN AND DEHP (PHTHALATES)

Dioxin is created when materials that contain chlorine are burned. For example, when PVC plastic is burned in a medical or municipal waste incinerator, dioxin may be formed and emitted into the air. Dioxin first came to the attention of the U.S. public via Agent Orange, which was used as a defoliant during the Vietnam War. U.S. soldiers and Vietnamese exposed to dioxin now exhibit a number of different illnesses including chronic lymphocytic leukemia, soft tissue sarcoma, Hodgkin's disease, and chloracne. Although there has been controversy as to the cause of some illnesses, particularly chloracne, the National Academy of Sciences Report on Agent Orange states that there is sufficient evidence of an association between exposure to herbicides and these health outcomes.[28]

PVC plastic is made soft and flexible for most applications by the addition of DEHP. It is widely used by the food and construction industries, as well as the health care industry. Because the DEHP plasticizer is not chemically bound to PVC, it can leach into the environment. For example, medical devices containing PVC can release DEHP when in contact with fluids such as blood, plasma, and drug solutions, or it can be released and migrate when the device is heated. The rate of migration depends on the storage conditions (temperature of the fluid contacting the device, the amount of fluid, the contact time, the extent of shaking or flow rate of the fluid) and the lipophilicity of the fluid.[27] For an in-depth discussion of DEHP exposure from health care settings, please visit the Web site of Health Care Without Harm to read or order articles addressing this issue.[29]

PVC medical products are between 20%–80% DEHP by weight. Some common sources of dioxin and/or DEHP are:

- Building products (wall and floor coverings, carpet backing, piping).
- Personal care products (lotions, cosmetics, hair products, nail polish, perfume).
- Children's toys (teething rings, children's meal toy products).
- Food preparation and packaging (plastic wraps, plastic containers, vinyl gloves for food workers).
- Medical products such as IV bags and tubing, and other tubing related to medical procedures such as dialysis, cardiopulmonary bypass, and enteral and total parenteral nutrition.

ROUTES OF CONTAMINATION

Humans ingest dioxin in food after particles are distributed via incineration into the atmosphere by wind and rain. These particles become lodged in soil, lakes, and rivers, and settle on plants. In areas of the country where dioxin lev-

els are highest, animals eat and drink dioxin particles. When humans consume contaminated fish, meat, and dairy products, the bioaccumulative dioxin dose that the animal incurred over its lifespan and stored in its fatty tissue is also ingested. Additionally, the fats in breast milk can store dioxin. Some nursing infants may be exposed to dioxin levels at high concentrations. The intake of dioxin was found to be 50 times higher in two breastfed infants than in a formulafed infant.[30] However, the long-term impact of exposure to dioxin from breast milk seems to be minimal. While shorter term studies have shown an association between breast milk intake and adverse cognitive function from dioxin exposure, longer term studies do not.[31–33] Long-term studies following breast fed and formula fed infants ages 4 to 6 have found an association between pregnancy maternal body burden and poorer cognitive function, but no association between type of feeding and dioxin-related damage.[32,33] Therefore, there is NO recommendation to avoid breastfeeding infants due to dioxin exposure in the mother.[34] Rather the emphasis should be on reducing PCB body burden by minimizing exposure to these chemicals.

LEVELS OF EXPOSURE FOR CONCERN

Dioxin is a potent carcinogen at very low levels of exposure, and even daily exposures of dioxin measured in picograms or nanograms can cause toxic effects. The general population, through ordinary dietary exposures, carries a current body burden of dioxin that is near or above the levels that cause adverse effects in animal tests. Through food alone, Americans get 22 times the maximum daily dioxin exposure considered by the EPA to be without adverse effects. Daily human exposure to DEHP in the United States is significant, but occupational and clinical exposures from DEHP-plasticized medical devices (e.g., blood bags, hemodialysis tubing, nasogastric feeding tubes) further increase body burden levels. Prolonged exposures induce high levels of the gonadotropin luteinizing hormone and increase the serum concentrations of sex hormones, which could disrupt normal physiologic functioning in any body system containing estrogen receptors.[35]

Ways to Minimize Exposure to Dioxin and DEHP

To avoid exposure to PVC, dioxin, and phthalates, patients are counseled to:

- Choose products not made with vinyl for: children's toys, food containers, car seats, crib bumpers, wallpaper, wall coverings, and flooring.
- Avoid burning PVC (#3) plastic.
- Eat fewer fatty foods (e.g., cheese, red meats, whole milk).
- Avoid personal care products made with phthalates.[36] This requires some familiarity with chemical names or abbreviations.
- Additionally, health care workers can work to prevent the spread of DEHP by advocating that their health care facility use alternatives to those products manufactured with DEHP.

Impact on Pregnancy, Lactation, and the Fetus

There is no known way to lower body burdens of toxins generated by PVCs. Although breastfeeding lowers a mother's levels by approximately 20% for each 6 months of lactation, this suggests it would increase the risk to the baby. Thus far, the infant morbidity attributable to exposure to these compounds is believed to come from prenatal exposure to maternal body burden rather than from exposure through breast milk.[3] Some of these effects include lower developmental and intelligence scores, including lower psychomotor scores from newborns. However, breast milk is still considered to be the best food for infants (see "Breastfeeding" section above). Another impact of PVC exposure may be an increased cancer mortality overall, because studies have shown that prenatal exposure in rodents substantially increased their risk of breast cancer later in life.[34] Proven impacts include:

- Neonatal abnormalities: Decreases in the percentage of boys born; altered level of thyroid hormone.[37]
- Skin disorders: Chloracne.[28,37]
- Immune system: Change in immune system parameters/modulation.
- Endocrine system effects: Low levels of testosterone; increased glucose intolerance or diabetes; decreased estrogen and estrogen-receptor levels after fetal exposure in the newborn.

Based on its earlier safety assessment of DEHP, the FDA issued a public health notification in 2002, recommending that alternatives to DEHP-containing products be used when procedures that have a high risk of leaching DEHP into the body are performed on male newborns, pregnant women carrying male fetuses, and peripubertal males. Some of the highest risk procedures identified by the FDA are:

- Total parenteral nutrition in neonates (with lipids in PVC bags).
- Enteral nutrition in neonates and adults.
- Multiple procedures in sick neonates.

- Hemodialysis in peripubertal males or pregnant or lactating women.

Lead

Lead is a naturally occurring element. Blood levels are low in the absence of industrial activities or other sources indicated below.

SOURCES OF EXPOSURE

In the United States, the chief sources of lead exposure for children have been airborne (mainly from leaded gasoline combustion) and inhalation or ingestion of leaded chips or dust from lead-based paints. Lead levels in breast milk are low; lead has also been found in canned formula and evaporated milk.[16,38]

ROUTES OF CONTAMINATION

The most common way that lead poisoning occurs, particularly in children, is through the unintentional ingestion of lead-containing particles, such as lead dust from paint or soil, in water (including drinking "tap" water), or foreign bodies. Lead can also be inhaled as fumes and absorbed via the pulmonary tract.

LEVELS OF EXPOSURE FOR CONCERN

Actions are recommended for children whose blood lead levels are greater than or equal to 10 mcg/dL, although evidence exists showing adverse neurobehavioral effects at lower levels.[39,40] For adults, the only agency that has set an adult standard is the Occupational Safety and Health Association, which states ≤45 mcg/dL is the level of concern in workplace settings, although evidence of damage also exists for adults at far lower levels. The level of lead determines the recommended intervention, which ranges from environmental controls at lower levels to chela-

tion at higher levels.[3] The recognition that lead exposure can induce damage at levels lower than previously thought to be safe has prompted the CDC to convene a panel of experts to reconsider whether the lead level of concern for pregnant and lactating women should be lowered and if any changes should be made to recommended intervention strategies. The results of this workgroup are expected to be reported in 2007.[41]

WAYS TO MINIMIZE EXPOSURE

The public should know the lead level in their tap water source. This is especially important for infants who are being fed formula reconstituted with tap water. Additionally, prevention of ingestion or inhalation (lead-based paint chips and fuels) is important. Other possible sources of lead exposure are listed in **Table 4-5**. Encouraging women to consume adequate amounts of calcium and iron seems to minimize lead absorption from the environment and release of lead from bony body stores. Women should also be screened for pica behavior because cases of lead poisoning have been reported in women consuming lead-contaminated pottery and soil.[42,43] Pica also is associated with nutritional deficiencies.[44,45] Ensuring adequate intakes of vitamin C, iron, and calcium may be of even greater importance in these women because it may minimize further lead exposure from endogenous and exogenous sources.

IMPACT ON PREGNANCY, LACTATION, THE FETUS, AND CHILDREN

Lead levels in human milk are low. Due to laws enacted in the 1970s that banned lead in gasoline and paint, blood lead levels have declined substantially. Fatal lead encephalopathy has virtually disappeared. However, while lead

Table 4-5 SOURCES OF LEAD EXPOSURE[43]

Occupation Related	Hobbies and Other Activities	Folk Remedies
Lead abatement and home renovation/restoration	Making stained glass	Alkohl: black powder used as eye cosmetic and on umbilical stump (middle Eastern, African, Asian cultures)
Recycling operations	Copper enameling	Azarcon: bright orange powder used by Hispanic cultures for gastrointestinal upset and diarrhea
Manufacturing/installation of plumbing	Bronze casting	Bali Goli: a black bean dissolved in gripe water in Asian Indian cultures for stomach ache
Foundry work	Pottery with lead glaze and paint	Ghazard: brown powder used within Asian Indian cultures to aid digestion
Firing range work	Hunting and target shooting	Greta: yellow-orange powder used with Hispanic cultures to treat digestive problems
Production/use of chemicals	Jewelry making with lead solder	Pay-loo-ah: an orange red powder used within Southeast Asian cultures to treat rash or fever
Bridge, tunnel construction	Electronics with lead solder	Koo Sar: pills used by Cambodian women for the treatment of menstrual cramps
Auto repair shop	Glassblowing with leaded glass	Battery manufacture/repair
Printmaking and other fine arts	Manufacture of industrial machinery	Liquor distillation

Source: Reprinted with permission from: Hackley B, Katz-Jacobson A. Lead poisoning in pregnancy: A case study with implications for midwives. *Journal of Midwifery and Women's Health.* 2003; 48:30–38.

poisoning is less common, it still occurs, particularly in infants and children living in older substandard housing, in those who emigrated from parts of the world where lead exposures are high, and in pregnant women who engage in pica behavior (i.e., eating abnormal things like ash and chalk). In the human body, the main repository for lead is bone, where the turnover rate is approximately 25 to 30 years. Chronic lead exposure results in significant accumulation of lead in the skeleton. During pregnancy, lactation, and the perimenopausal transition, calcium turnover is greatly increased, which may trigger a release of lead stores from bone. The main effect on children is damage to the central nervous system. Evidence exists that low-level lead exposure may increase the risk of miscarriage, pre-eclampsia in pregnancy, and hypertension in non-pregnant women.[46–48]

Tobacco and Nicotine

SOURCES OF EXPOSURE

The main source of exposure is cigarette smoking. Exposure to ETS or passive smoke is a health risk.

ROUTES OF CONTAMINATION

Contamination occurs through inhalation (active or via secondhand smoke).

LEVELS OF EXPOSURE FOR CONCERN

All exposure to tobacco smoke is relevant. The causal relationship of smoking and lung cancer is well established.

WAYS TO MINIMIZE EXPOSURE

Exposure can be minimized by ceasing to smoke, not frequenting places where other people smoke, and banning smoking from the home and workplace.

IMPACT ON PREGNANCY, LACTATION, AND THE FETUS

Loss of ova from exposure to tobacco or tobacco smoke has resulted in decreased fertility.[3,49] Secondhand smoke has been linked to decreased birth weight, predisposition to persistent pulmonary hypertension in the newborn, and an increased risk of sudden infant death syndrome. Developing lungs are susceptible to secondhand smoke, and it has been strongly associated with asthma.

Conclusion

Environmental health is an enormous public health concern, and midwives can play a vital role in educating patients about the problem and its effect on a woman's health and that of her fetus and children. This education extends beyond the assessment and referral of patients for the possible ill effects of environmental hazards. Ideally, it includes anticipatory counseling to patients, which can minimize exposure.

The list of resources and bibliography in **Table 4-6** is the greater contribution of this chapter. These resources include Web sites, organizations, and books where the practicing midwife can find basic information and alternative tools such as history and data collection forms.

Table 4-6 FEDERAL AGENCIES AND OTHER RESOURCES FOR TOXICOLOGICAL INFORMATION

Resource	Explanation	Contact Information
American College of Nurse-Midwives	Green Birthdays[11]: Important information every health care provider should know about the environmental safety of the birthplace and practical steps to reduce their own and their patients' exposure to toxic chemicals. With Health Care Without Harm, 2001. Policy Statement on Environmental Pollutants in Breast Milk: ACNM supports local, state, national, and international efforts to decrease environmental pollutants that enter and impact the human body, including breast milk. This may include measures to decrease mercury contamination, fuel, power plant, and incinerator emissions.	http://www.midwife.org http://www.midwife.org/legis/pollutants-policystatement.cfm
Health Care Without Harm An international organization that campaigns for environmentally responsible health care.	HCWH has a wide array of publications and information as well as programs, on many of the health hazards encountered in the process of receiving health care. Some of these are listed here. Additionally, this organization has many opportunities for midwives and others in the health care industry to become involved in making health care safer for patients, families, and communities.[10,29,32,34]	http://www.noharm.org http://www.nottoopretty.org

(continues)

Table 4-6 FEDERAL AGENCIES AND OTHER RESOURCES FOR TOXICOLOGICAL INFORMATION *(continued)*

Resource	Explanation	Contact Information
U.S. Environmental Protection Agency	Excellent Web site and publications relevant to almost all aspects discussed in this chapter, including environmental justice, pregnancy and children's health, reproductive health, endocrine disruptor screening program.[28]	http://www.epa.gov/compliance/environmentaljustice Office of Children's Health Protection: 202-564-2188 http://yosemite.epa.gov/ochp/ochpweb.nst/homepage EPA Endocrine Disruptor Screening Program: http://www.epa.gov.scipoly/oscpend
National Institute of Environmental Health Sciences. National Institutes of Health	National Toxicology Program.[6] Center for the Evaluation of Risks to Human Reproduction: Information on the possible effects of chemical exposures on fertility, reproductive health, pregnancy, and child development. Also has links to related Web sites, expert panel reports, and monographs.	http://ntp-server.niehs.nih.gov http://cerhr.niehs.nih.gov/
American Academy of Pediatrics Committee on Environmental Health. Etzel RA, ed.[3]	Text that is geared toward the average pediatrician, although also very relevant to midwives. Extensive resource list at the end of the book, including lists of toxins. Very good discussion of communication of risk to patients as well as how to advocate for environmental policy.	http://www.aap.org
Agency for Toxic Substances and Disease Registry, U.S. Department of Health and Human Services	*Case Studies in Environmental Medicine: Taking an Exposure History.* Atlanta, GA: U.S. Department of Health and Human Services, Agency for Toxic Substances and Disease Registry: 2000. ATSDR Publication ATSDR-HE-CS-2001-0002. Toxicological Profiles	http://www.atsdr.cdc.gov/HEC/CSEM/exphistory/index.html Information Center Clearinghouse: 404-639-6360 Emergency Response Branch Phone: 404-639-0744 http://www.atsdr.cdc.gov/toxpr2.html

Table 4-6 FEDERAL AGENCIES AND OTHER RESOURCES FOR TOXICOLOGICAL INFORMATION *(continued)*

Resource	Explanation	Contact Information
National Academy of Sciences, Washington, DC	Nursing, Health and the Environment; Institute of Medicine report.[7] Report on Agent Orange.	http://books.nap.edu/books
Storey, Eileen, Kenneth Dangman, Paula Schenck, Robert L. DeBernardo, Chin S. Yang, Anne Bracker, Michael Hodgson, *Guidance for Clinicians on the Recognition and Management of Health Effects Related to Mold Exposure and Moisture Indoors.* Center for Indoor Environment and Health, University of Connecticut, Storrs, CT, September 2004[50]	A new publication that addresses mold-related illness. Title is self-explanatory.	University of Connecticut
Science and Environmental Health Network	Discussion of the Precautionary Principle.[8]	http://www.sehn.org/wing.html
National Environmental Education and Training Foundation	Several reports of interest to those midwives who are interested in public policy and in education of health care providers: National Strategies for Health Care Providers: Proceedings of a National Forum. June 2003. Nurses and Environmental Health: Success through Action, Illustrations from Across the Nation. September 2002.	202-833-2933 http://www.neetf.org

References

1. Olden K, editor. National strategies for health care providers' pesticides initiatives. In: *Proceedings of the National Forum of National Environmental Education and Training Foundation;* 2003 Jun 10–11; Washington, DC.

2. Evans N. State of the evidence: What is the connection between chemicals and breast cancer? *Breast Cancer Fund.* 1993;15(1):66–77.

3. Etzel RA, editor. *Pediatric Environmental Health.* 2nd ed. American Academy of Pediatrics Committee on Environmental Health. Elk Grove Village, IL: American Academy of Pediatrics; 2003.

4. Leonnig CD. Groundwater toxin near aqueduct: Army engineers faulted for inaction since 2003 finding. *The Washington Post.* 2004 Oct 27;Sect. B:1.

5. Pereira LA, Loomis D, Conceicao GM, Braga AL, Arcas RM, Kishi HS, et al. Association between air pollution and intrauterine mortality in Sao Paulo, Brazil. *Environ Health Perspect.* 1998;106:325–329.

6. *Report on Carcinogens,* 11th ed. U.S. Department of Health and Human Services, Public Health Service, National Toxicology Program. 2005. [Monograph on the Internet]. Available from: http://ntp.niehs.nih.gov/ntp/roc/eleventh/.

7. Pope AM, Snyder MA, Mood LH, editors. *Nursing, Health and the Environment.* Washington, D.C.: National Academy Press; 1995.

8. Science and Environmental Health Network. Wingspread Conference on the Precautionary Principle. [Monograph on the Internet]. Ames, IA, 1998 Jan 26 [cited 2004 Dec 20]; Available from: http://www.sehn.org/wing.html.

9. Bay Area Working Group. Bay Area Working Group on the Precautionary Principle [information sheet]. San Francisco, CA: Bay Area Working Group; Spring 2003.

10. Environmental Protection Agency. Environmental justice [monograph on the Internet]. Washington, DC [cited 2004 Dec 20; updated daily]. Available from: http://www.epa.gov/compliance/environmen taljustice.

11. Health Care Without Harm and American College of Nurse-Midwives. *Green birthdays: Important information every healthcare provider should know about the environmental safety of the birth place, and practical steps to reduce their own and their patients' exposure to toxic chemicals.* Washington, DC: Health Care Without Harm and American College of Nurse-Midwives; 2001.

12. Steingraber S. *Having Faith: An Ecologist's Journey to Motherhood.* Cambridge, MA: Perseus Publishing; 2001.

13. Tarkan L. Research is urged for healthier breast milk. *New York Times.* 2001;16 Oct. Late Edition - Final, Section F, Page 6, Column 1.

14. Rogan WJ, Blanton PJ, Portier CJ, Stallard E. Should the presence of carcinogens in breast milk discourage breastfeeding? *Regul Toxicol Pharmacol.*1991;13(3): 228–240.

15. Krauthacker B, Reiner E, Votava-Raic A, Tjesic-Drinkovic D, Batinic D. Organochlorine pesticides and PCBs in human milk collected from mothers nursing hospitalized children. *Chemosphere.* 1998; 37(1):27–32.

16. Walker M, editor. Summary of the hazards of infant formula, part two. *Proceedings of the International Lactation Consultants' Association.* 1998; Raleigh, NC: ILCA.

17. Anderson JW, Johnstone BM, Remely DT. Breastfeeding and cognitive development: A meta-analysis. *Am J Clin Nutr.* 1999;70(4):525–535.

18. Van Esterik, P. Rights, risks and regulation communicating about risks and infant feeding. [monograph on the Internet]. World Alliance for Breastfeeding Action. Available from: http://www.waba.org.my/RRR/penny1b.htm.

19. Moore J. Environmental pollutants in breast milk: ACNM policy statement [monograph on the Internet]. American College of Nurse-Midwives, Silver Spring, MD. 2003 Jan 25 [cited 2004 Dec 20]. Available from: http://www.midwife.org/legis/pollu tants-policystatement.cfm.

20. Breast Cancer Fund. Prevention starts here at the nexus of health and the environment. [Monograph on the Internet]. Breast Cancer Fund, San Francisco, CA. 2004 Nov 9 [cited 2004 Dec 20]; Available from: http://www.breastcancerfund.org/site/pp.asp?c=kwK XLdPaE&b=43969.

21. National Environmental Education and Training Foundation (NEETP). [Homepage on the Internet]. Washington, DC ©2001. Available from: http://www.neetf.org.

22. Centers for Disease Control and Prevention. Update: pulmonary hemorrhage/hemosiderosis among infants. *MMWR*. 2000;49:180–184.

23. Weiss A, Chidekel AS. Acute pulmonary hemorrhage in a Delaware infant after exposure to *Stachybotrys atra*. *Del Med J*. 2002;74:363–368.

24. United States Environmental Protection Agency. Mercury Report to Congress (1997) [Monograph on the Internet]. Washington, DC [updated daily]. Available from: http://www.epa.gov/mercury/report.htm.

25. Blood and hair mercury levels in young children and women of childbearing age—United States. *MMWR*. 1999;50(8):140.

26. United States Food and Drug Association and United States Environmental Protection Agency. What you need to know about mercury in fish and shellfish [pamphlet]. Washington, DC: United States Food and Drug Association and United States Environmental Protection Agency; 2004.

27. Health Care Without Harm. A summary of the expert panel report of the national toxicology program on DEHP and its risks to human reproduction. Washington, DC: Health Care Without Harm; 15 Oct 2001.

28. The National Academy Press: Veterans and Agent Orange: Update 2002. [Monograph on the Internet]. Board on Health Promotion and Disease Prevention and Institute of Medicine. 2003 [cited 2004 Dec 20]. Available from: http://books.nap.edu/books/030908 6167/html.

29. Health Care Without Harm. *Going Green: A Resource Kit for Pollution Prevention in Health Care*. [Materials on the Internet]. Available from: http://www.no harm.org.goingGreen.

30. Abraham K, Knoll A, Ende M, Papke O, Helge H. Intake, fecal excretion, and body burden of polychlorinated dibenzo-p-dioxins and dibenzofurans in breast-fed and formula-fed infants. *Pediat Res*. 40(5): 671-679.

31. Koopman-Esseboom C, Weisglas-Kuperus N, de Ridder MA, Van der Paauw CG, Tuinstra LG, Sauer PJ. Effects of polychlorinated biphenyl/dioxin exposure and feeding type on infants' mental and psychomotor development. *J Pediatr*. 1996;97(5): 700–706.

32. Patandin S, Lanting CI, Mulder PG, Boersma ER, Sauer PJ, Weisglas-Kuperus N. Effects of environmental exposure to polychlorinated biphenyls and dioxins on cognitive abilities in Dutch children at 42 months of age. *J Pediatr*. 1999;134: 33–41.

33. Boersma ER, Lanting CI. Environmental exposure to polychlorinated biphenyls (PCBs) and dioxins. Consequences for longterm neurological and cognitive development of the child lactation. *Adv Exp Med Biol*. 2000; 478:271–287.

34. Environmental Protection Agency. National Center for Environmental Assessment. Dioxin: Frequently asked questions. Published on the Internet by the Interagency Working Group on Dioxin. Available from:http://cfpub.epa.gov/ncea.

35. Akingbemi BT, Renshan G, Klinefelter GR, Zirkin BR, Hardy MP, editors. Phthalate-induced Leydig cell hyperplasia is associated with multiple endocrine disturbances. *Proc Natl Acad Sci*. 2004;101(3): 775–780. Epub 2004 Jan 8.

36. *Poisoned Cosmetics, Not Too Pretty*. [monograph on the Internet]. Women's Environmental Network, London, UK. 2004 [cited 2004 Dec 20]. Available from: http://www.nottoopretty.com/index.htm.

37. Mocarelli P, Gerthoux PM, Ferrari E, Petterson DG, Kieszak SM, Brambilla P, et al. Paternal concentrations of dioxin and sex ratio of offspring. *Lancet*. 2000;355:1858–1863.

38. Sinks T, Jackson R. International study finds breast milk free of significant lead contamination. *Environ Health Perspect*. 1999;107:A58–59.

39. Chiodo LM, Jacobson SW, Jacobson JL. Neurodevelopmental effects of postnatal lead exposure at very low levels. *Neurotoxicology & Teratology*. 2004; 26:359–371.

40. Canfield RL, Henderson CR Jr, Cory-Slechta DA, Cox C, Jusko TA, Lanphear BP. Intellectual impairment in children with blood lead concentrations below 10 microg per deciliter. *N Engl J Med*. 2003; 348: 1517–1526.

41. CDC. Advisory Committee On Childhood Lead Poisoning Prevention (ACCLPP) Work Groups. Accessed at http://www.cdc.gov/nceh/lead/ACCLPP/workGroups.htm.

42. Mycyk M, Leikin J. Combined Exchange Transfusion and Chelation Therapy for Neonatal Lead Poisoning. *Ann Pharmacotherap*. 2004:38(5):821–824.

43. Hackley B, Katz-Jacobson A. Lead poisoning in pregnancy: A case study with implications for midwives. *J Midwifery Women's Health*. 2003;48: 30–38.

44. Rainville AJ. Pica practices of pregnant women are associated with lower maternal hemoglobin level at delivery. *J Am Diet Assoc.* 1998;98:293–296.

45. Edwards CH, Johnson AA, Knight EM, Oyemade UJ, Cole OJ, Westney OE, Jones S, Laryea H, Westney LS. Pica in an urban environment. *J Nutr.* 1994;124(6 Suppl):954S–962S.

46. Borja-Aburto VH, Hertz-Picciotto I, Rojas Lopez M, Farias P, Rios C, Blanco J. Blood lead levels measured prospectively and risk of spontaneous abortion. *Am J Epidemiology.* 1999;150:590–597.

47. Nash D, Magder L, Lustberg M, Sherwin R, Rubin R, Kaufmann R, Silbergeld E. Blood lead, blood pressure, and hypertension in perimenopausal and postmenopausal women. *JAMA.* 2003;289:1523–1532.

48. Sowers M, Jannausch M, Scholl T, Li W, Kemp FW, Bogden JD. Blood lead concentrations and pregnancy outcomes. *Arch Environ Health.* 2002;57:489–495.

49. Munafo M, Murphy M, Whiteman D, Hey K. Does cigarette smoking increase time to conception? *J Biosoc Sci.* 2002:34:65–73.

50. Storey E, Dangman K, Schenck P, DeBernardo RL, Yang CS, Bracker A, et al. Guidance for clinicians on the recognition and management of health effects related to mold exposure and moisture indoors. Center for Indoor Environment and Health, University of Connecticut Health Center, Storrs, CT; 2004 Sept 30. Available for order at: http://oehc.uchc.edu/clinser/indoor.htm.

Chapter 5

Antibiotics

Valerie A. Roe

Antimicrobials are among the most widely prescribed medications in the primary health care setting. Responsible prescribing practices require understanding a significant body of scientific knowledge including microbiology; pharmacology; host factors that affect the infectious disease process, response to pharmacotherapy, and toxicity; as well as community and global patterns of resistance.

Further, the flora and fauna that normally inhabit the human body are in delicate balance. Initiation of antimicrobial therapy may upset that balance, offering the opportunity for superimposed infection. In addition, the primary care provider plays a significant role in combating the crisis of emerging antimicrobial resistance by adhering to appropriate prescribing practices, encouraging palliative therapy for viral infections, recommending immunizations when appropriate, and educating women and their families regarding the judicious use of antibiotics and simple infection control measures such as handwashing.

There may be additional health benefits associated with cautious prescribing habits and educating women regarding the appropriate use of antibiotics. For example, a case-control study, published in the *Journal of the American Medical Association* in February 2004, identified a relationship between antibiotic use and breast cancer. Researchers compared the computerized pharmacy records of 2266 women with primary, invasive breast cancer to the records of 7953 randomly selected women without breast cancer, and found that increasing antibiotic exposure was associated with an increase in the incidence of and mortality from breast cancer.[1] All participants were enrolled in the same health plan, and results were adjusted for age and length of enrollment. Two measures of antibiotic exposure were utilized based on data from the health plan pharmacy: cumulative number of days of antibiotic use and total number of antibiotic prescriptions. The relative risk of breast cancer increased in all categories of antibiotic use with each increment in days of use or number of prescriptions. Although this study does not demonstrate a causal relationship between antibiotic use and the risk of breast cancer, it does support prudent prescribing habits until additional research provides definitive answers.

The term *antimicrobial* refers to drugs used in the treatment of infections caused by bacteria, viruses, fungi, or protozoa. This chapter focuses on antibacterial therapy. It is designed to clarify the relationship between pathogen and antibacterial therapy, identify simple rules to follow before prescribing, and foster a level of confidence in initiating antibacterial therapy based on sound rationale. Specific pharmacotherapeutic guidelines for common health conditions encountered in the primary care setting as well as pharmacotherapy for viral, fungal, and protozoal infections are discussed in greater detail in other chapters.

Microbiology

A fundamental knowledge of microbiology is essential in understanding how antibacterials work. The most clinically useful antibacterials are selectively toxic chemicals that exploit the cellular and biochemical differences between pathogen and host in order to eradicate infection with the fewest host side effects. These differences in structure and function between bacterial cells and human cells provide a mechanism for antibacterials to interfere with the replication and growth of microorganisms (*bacteriostatic agents*) or kill invading pathogens (*bactericidal agents*). This distinction is important, because the bacteriostatic agents rely on an intact immune system for maximum therapeutic benefit.

Bacteria are *prokaryotes*, single cells or groups of cells without nuclei. DNA in the form of a single chromosome lies in the cytoplasm. The genetic material in human cells, *eukaryotes*, is contained within the cell nucleus, encased in the nuclear membrane. Unlike eukaryotes, the plasma cell membrane of bacteria is surrounded by a cell wall, composed primarily of *peptidoglycan*, a protein unique to bacteria. This bacterial cell wall is necessary to maintain the osmotic pressure of the cellular contents, es-

sentially preventing the cell from exploding. Interfering with cell wall synthesis is lethal to bacterial cells.

Differing biochemical functions within the host and bacterial invader also provide potential for interfering with the growth and development of pathogenic colonization. For example, both bacteria and human cells require folate in DNA synthesis. Although humans rely on dietary folate, bacteria must synthesize folate in order to reproduce. Hence, blocking bacterial folate synthesis effectively inhibits DNA replication.

Bacteria are classified as *Gram-positive* or *Gram-negative* depending on their color reaction to a staining technique developed by Hans Gram in 1884. The principal difference between Gram-positive and Gram-negative organisms is the composition of the cell wall. The cell wall of Gram-positive organisms is simple in structure. The complexity of the composition of the cell wall of Gram-negative organisms, in which the peptidoglycan layer is surrounded by lipopolysaccharides and encased in an outer lipid membrane, creates a more significant barrier to penetration by antibacterials.

The shape of individual bacteria may be spherical (*cocci*), rod-shaped (*bacilli*), or curved and spiral (*spirochetes*). Diplococci refer to cocci in pairs (e.g., *Neisseria gonorrhoeae*), streptococci refers to cocci in chains (e.g., *Streptococcus pyogenes*), and staphlyococci refers to clusters of cocci (e.g., *Staphylococcus aureus*). Bacteria are also classified as *aerobic* or *anaerobic* depending on their need for oxygen to grow and reproduce.

Some tiny Gram-negative bacteria, such as *Chlamydia* and *Mycoplasma*, do not share the common characteristics of other bacteria and were initially believed to be viruses. *Chlamydia*, the most primitive of bacteria, is an obligate intracellular parasite. Like viruses, *Chlamydia* depends on the host cell to perform essential metabolic processes; unlike viruses, these microbes contain both DNA and RNA. *Mycoplasmae* are the tiniest cellular microbes. Because they do not have a true cell wall, their shape is amorphous and they are resistant to antimicrobials that interfere with cell wall synthesis.

The integrity of the host immune system, including the presence of antibodies secondary to a previous exposure to a particular microorganism, affects the ability of the individual to actively fight infection. Other host factors may contribute to susceptibility to a particular infection. For example, *Chlamydia trachomatis* invades the columnar epithelium of the cervix. The adolescent is more likely than the adult woman to have a cervical ectropion, with columnar epithelium on the ectocervix. This makes the adolescent cervix more vulnerable to invasion by *Chlamydia*. The cervical ectropion associated with the use of combined hormonal contraceptives creates a similar situation, and a similarly increased risk.

Many bacterial infections are due to the overgrowth of bacteria that are part of the normal flora in a particular site. *Staphylococcus aureus* (*S. aureus*), for example, may be found on the skin of a healthy individual. These bacteria are opportunistic pathogens. In small numbers they are relatively harmless to the host; however, under certain host conditions, such as a break in the skin, *S. aureus* may proliferate, causing carbuncles, furuncles, mastitis, impetigo, or cellulitis. A viral or fungal infection may also provide the right conditions for opportunistic pathogens to multiply and cause a secondary infection. *Tinea pedis* causes breaks in the skin between the toes that may become secondarily infected with *S. aureus* or *Streptococcus pyogenes*,

another bacterium frequently found on the skin. The vesicles and ulcers of herpes simplex virus also provide these bacteria with a portal of entry into soft tissue.

Bacterial infections also occur as an organism migrates and proliferates from one anatomical site to another site that is not usually colonized by that organism. *Escherichia coli* (*E. coli*) is part of the flora of the colon. When transported to the urogenital tract, *E. coli* easily multiplies in the sterile environment of the bladder, causing cystitis.

Some bacterial infections are the result of exposure to microbes that are not part of the normal flora, such as *Bacillus anthracis* or *Chlamydia trachomatis*.

Tables 5-1, 5-2, and **5-3** summarize the characteristics, common anatomical sites of colonization, and primary care conditions associated with many common human pathogens.

Antibiotic Classifications

The term *antibiotic* actually refers to the earliest antibacterials that were produced by microorganisms, isolated, and harvested from culture. Newer drugs within a class are often semisynthetic derivatives of these antibiotics. Some drugs, like the quinolones, are entirely synthesized chemical compounds. Today the term antibiotic is commonly applied to all antibacterial agents regardless of origin.

Antibiotics may have a narrow spectrum of activity, effective against a select group of microbes, or a broad spectrum, effective against a number of different types of bacteria. Antibiotics are classified according to similarities in chemical structure, mechanism of action, and antibacterial activity. Drugs are also labeled by the Food and Drug Administration

Table 5-1 GRAM-POSITIVE AEROBIC BACTERIA

Organism	Common Anatomical Sites Where Organism May Colonize as Part of Flora	Common Infections Caused by Opportunistic Pathogenic Organisms
Cocci		
Streptococcus Group A	Respiratory	Strep pharyngitis, Scarlet fever, rheumatic fever
S. pyogenes	Skin	Impetigo, cellulitis, toxic shock syndrome
Streptococcus Group B *S. agalactiae*	Genitourinary	Neonatal sepsis
Streptococcus pneumoniae	Respiratory	Pneumonia, meningitis, sinusitis
Staphylococcus aureus	Skin and soft tissue Respiratory Gastrointestinal	Mastitis, carbuncles, furuncles, folliculitis, impetigo, cellulitis, sinusitis
Staphylococcus saprophyticus	Gastrointestinal tract	Urinary tract infection
Enterococcus	Gastrointestinal tract Genitourinary	Urinary tract infection Nosocomial infections
Rods		
Bacillis anthracis	Not part of normal flora: Spores enter through skin, respiratory, gastrointestinal routes.	Anthrax
Listeria	Not part of normal flora: ingested in contaminated food (cheese)	Listeriosis, meningitis, septicemia, abscess, encephalitis, septicemia
Corynebacterium *C. diphtheriae*	Genitourinary	Diptheria
Mobiluncus	Genitourinary	Bacterial vaginiosis
Lactobacillus	Genitourinary Gastrointestinal Skin	Nonpathogenic
Spirochetes		
Treponema pallidum	Not part of normal flora	Syphilis

(FDA) according to real and potential perinatal and neonatal effects when prescribed in pregnancy (**Table 5-4**).

Although the FDA pregnancy categories were created to simplify the selection of medications for pregnant women, they can be con-

Table 5-2 Gram-Negative Aerobic Bacteria

Organism	Common Anatomical Sites Where Organism May Colonize as Part of Flora	Common Infections Caused by Opportunistic Pathogenic Organisms
Cocci		
Neisseseria	Not part of normal flora: sexually transmitted	Gonorrhea of the urogenital tract, pharynx, arthritis
N. gonorrhoea		
N. meningitis	Respiratory	Meningitis
Rods		
E. coli	Gastrointestinal tract (colon)	Urinary tract infection
Klebsiella species	Gastrointestinal tract (colon)	Urinary tract infection Pneumonia
Proteus species	Gastrointestinal tract (colon)	Urinary tract infection
Moraxella		
M. catarrhalis	Respiratory	Pneumonia, sinusitis
Haemophilus influenzae	Respiratory	Meningitis, pneumonia Sinusitis, conjunctivitis, otitis media
Pseudomonas species *P. aeruginosa*	Skin	Otitis externa, skin and soft tissue infections
Helicobacter pylori	Gastrointestinal tract	Bacterial gastritis, duodenal ulcers
Primitive species		
Chlamydia	Not part of normal flora	Pneumonia
C. pneumoniae		Chlamydial cervicitis
C. trachomatis		Pelvic inflammatory disease Urethritis Newborn pneumonia Conjunctivitis/trachoma (neonatal and adult eye disease)
Mycoplasma pneumoniae	Respiratory	Atypical pneumonia

fusing and misleading when choosing pharmacotherapy, primarily because conducting randomized controlled trials in pregnant women is unethical. Limited data are available for most drugs. In general, the newer the drug, the less information is available. Pregnancy drug registries and meta-analyses of retrospective studies provide the most reliable information regarding drug use in pregnancy. A good example is the antiviral drug acyclovir (Zovirax). Acyclovir is FDA pregnancy category C. The acyclovir pregnancy registry[2] documents that in

Table 5-3 ANAEROBIC BACTERIA

Organism	Common Anatomical Sites Where Organism May Colonize as Part of Flora	Common Infections Caused by Opportunistic Pathogenic Organisms
Gram-Positive Anaerobic Rods		
Clostridium	Gastrointestinal tract Genitourinary	
C. difficile		Pseudomembranous colitis
C. tetani		Tetanus
Propionibacterium		
P. acnes	Skin (pilosebaceous glands)	Acne
Gram-Negative Anaerobic Rods		
Bacteroides	Gastrointestinal tract	Wound infection, peritonitis
Prevotella	Gastrointestinal tract, vagina	Abscesses
Fusobacterium	Gastrointestinal tract, respiratory	Oral and respiratory infections

over 25 years of clinical use, it has not been associated with an increased risk of birth defects or other adverse neonatal effects regardless of trimester of exposure. Valacyclovir, a newer antiviral and a prodrug of acyclovir, was given an FDA pregnancy category of B, essentially riding the coattails of the acyclovir registry. Why has acyclovir not been changed to FDA category B? It is costly to apply for a change in FDA category, and because acyclovir is now a generic drug, there is no monetary benefit to the pharmaceutical company in applying for a change in status.

Combined oral contraceptives are another example of how FDA labeling may cause confusion. Oral contraceptives are pregnancy category X not because they are associated with an increase in fetal abnormalities or evidence of fetal risk, but rather because there is no clear benefit in their use during pregnancy. The FDA has convened a committee to explore replacing FDA pregnancy categories with a narrative report that would be more helpful to clinicians in evaluating the risks and benefits of a particular drug during pregnancy.

Both the American Academy of Pediatrics (AAP) and the World Health Organization (WHO) publish recommendations regarding the use of medications during lactation. These organizations review the clinical literature to determine the amount of drug that is found in breast milk after maternal ingestion, serum levels of the drug in infants following exposure in breast milk as well as reported and possible adverse effects on the breastfeeding infant. AAP categories for breastfeeding are included here for each class of antibiotics.

There are numerous Internet resources that are helpful in selecting drug therapy, including indications, optimal route, dosage, adverse reactions, and precautions during pregnancy and lactation. Three of these resources are listed in

Table 5-4 FOOD AND DRUG ADMINISTRATION PREGNANCY CATEGORIES

FDA Category	Definition
A	Adequate studies in pregnant women have not demonstrated a risk to the fetus in first trimester of pregnancy, and there is no evidence of risk in later trimesters.
B	Animal studies have not demonstrated a risk to the fetus, but there are no adequate studies in pregnant women **OR** animal studies have shown an adverse effect, but adequate studies in pregnant women have not documented a risk to the fetus during the first trimester of pregnancy and there is no evidence of risk in later trimesters.
C	Animal studies have shown adverse effect to the fetus, but there are no adequate studies in humans **OR** there are no animal reproduction studies and no adequate studies in humans.
D	Evidence of human fetal risk. Potential benefits of use in pregnant women may be acceptable despite potential risk.
X	Studies in animals or humans demonstrate fetal abnormalities or adverse reactions; reports indicate evidence of fetal risk. Risk in pregnant women clearly outweighs any possible benefit.

Table 5-5. The adverse effects of particular classifications of drugs cited in this text are limited to those most commonly reported and those serious or toxic effects that are less common but associated with morbidity and mortality that warrant precaution. The Web sites noted in Table 5-5 provide a more detailed listing of infrequently encountered potential side effects.

The antibiotic classes and specific antibiotics discussed in detail are those most likely to be used in the primary care setting and include the following:

- Beta (β) Lactams
  - Penicillins
  - Cephalosporins
- Macrolides
  - Erythromycin
  - Azithromycin
  - Clarithromycin
- Lincosamides
  - Clindamycin
- Quinolones
  - Ciprofloxacin
  - Ofloxacin
  - Levofloxacin
- Tetracyclines
  - Tetracycline
  - Doxycycline
  - Minocycline
- Metronidazole
- Sulfonamides and Trimethoprim
- Aminoglycosides
  - Gentamycin
- Nitrofurantoin

Beta-Lactams (β-Lactams)

The β-lactams include the penicillins and cephalosporins that share a common core chemical structure: the four membered β-lactam ring. β-lactams are bactericidal agents that interfere with the synthesis of peptidoglycan, the principal component of the bacterial cell wall, resulting in

---

Table 5-5   WEB RESOURCES

www.perinatology.com/exposures/druglist2.htm: Provides an index to classification of drugs, FDA pregnancy category with a brief narrative, AAP recommendations and links to other Web sites and journal articles. Also provides a link to the WHO guidelines for prescribing during pregnancy and lactation.

www.medscape.com: Provides an extensive drug index including chemistry, indications, dosage, optimal route, and adverse effects.

www.AAP.org: American Academy of Pediatrics provides a detailed summary and chart regarding the transfer of drugs and other chemicals into human milk.

---

cell lysis. The β-lactams have little effect on the metabolic and biochemical functioning of human cells because human cells are *eukaryotes* and have no cell wall. As a result, there are few toxic effects associated with the β-lactams; however, the broad-spectrum drugs in this group may disturb the balance of microflora in the gut, causing gastrointestinal (GI) disturbance.

The most common adverse effects are nausea, vomiting, diarrhea, and headache. Urticaria and skin rash are less common as are true *hypersensitivity reactions*, which are characterized by life-threatening anaphylaxis and respiratory distress. Although rare, hypersensitivity reactions are the most serious sequelae of the use of β-lactams. When evaluating hypersensitivity reactions, the clinician should take a careful history to distinguish them from common adverse effects. Skin testing may be warranted in clinical situations when the β-lactams are the preferred therapeutic option in order to document a true allergic response. Cross hypersensitivity between the penicillins and cephalosporins may occur. When alternatives are viable, selection of another class of medications is prudent when there is a history of hypersensitivity to one or the other.

The natural penicillins were the first antimicrobial agents to be used in a wide variety of clinical situations. In 1928 Alexander Fleming discovered that a mold of the genus *Penicillium*, growing on a culture medium with staphylococci, produced an antibacterial substance. It was not until 1940 that Chain and Florey successfully harvested the first natural penicillins from cultures of *Penicillium notatum* and a year later demonstrated their effectiveness in combating bacterial infections in a human subject. Penicillin G became widely available by 1950 and continues to be an effective agent in the treatment of infections caused by many Gram-positive and Gram-negative cocci, anaerobes, and spirochetes such as *Treponema pallidum*. After more than 50 years of clinical use, penicillin remains the drug of choice for infections caused by group A and group B β hemolytic streptococcus as well as all stages of syphilis. Penicillin G is given parenterally because of its poor absorption from the GI tract. Penicillin VK is available as an oral preparation.

The effectiveness of the β-lactams depends on the presence of actively growing and dividing bacterial cells; therefore, when they are used in combination with bacteriostatic agents such as erythromycin or the tetracyclines, their effectiveness is compromised. The mechanism for resistance to this class of drugs is the evolution of β-lactamase–producing bacteria, particularly in Gram-positive organisms such as staphylococccus and *Neisseria gonorrhoeae,* as well as the Gram-negative enteric bacilli such as *E. coli, Klebsiella,* and *Proteus* species. Both of the β-lactamases, penicillinase and cephalosporinase, produced by resistant bacteria cleave the beta-lactam ring, inactivating the antimicrobial properties of the drug.

The emergence of β-lactamase–producing bacteria led to the development of penicillinase-resistant penicillins, semisynthetic compounds that include cloxacillin, dicloxacillin, oxacillin, methicillin, and nafcillin. These drugs have a narrow spectrum specific to the treatment of infections due to penicillinase-producing staphylococcus such as *S. aureus.* It should be noted that in the event of abscess formation, antibiotics are not a substitute for excision and drainage, because antibiotics do not penetrate pus.

The aminopenicillins, ampicillin (Omnipen) and amoxicillin (Amoxil), are also semisynthetic derivatives of natural penicillin that have a broader spectrum of activity than the natural penicillins, and provide better coverage of Gram-negative organisms including *E. coli, Haemophilus influenzae,* and *Proteus mirabilis.* Amoxicillin has higher bioavailability following oral administration, which allows for a less frequent dosing schedule (3 x/d) than ampicillin or penicillin VK (4 x/d). The half-life of the aminopenicillins and penicillin VK is one hour compared to the 30-minute half-life of penicillin G. Because it is better absorbed than ampicillin, amoxicillin is less likely to interfere with the balance of intestinal microflora and, therefore, is less likely to cause the watery diarrhea associated with pseudomembranous colitis.

β-lactamase inhibitors such as clavulanic acid and sulbactam have weak antibacterial activity alone, but when combined with the aminopenicillins extend the spectrum of activity of these drugs to include penicillinase-producing bacteria. Like all β-lactams, clavulanic acid and sulbactam contain a β-lactam ring that binds to β-lactamase, inactivating it. Augmentin is the combination of 125 milligrams (mg) of clavulanic acid with 250 mg, 500 mg, or 875 mg of amoxicillin. It should be noted that the dose of clavulanic acid is constant in all of these preparations; therefore, two 250-mg tablets may not be substituted for one 500-mg tablet. Ampicillin is combined with sulbactam to form the parenteral drug Unasyn.

The extended spectrum penicillins, ticarcillin (Ticar), mezlocillin (Mezlin), and piperacillin (Pipracil), are particularly useful in treating *Pseudomonas* infections. In combination with the β-lactamase inhibitors, they provide even broader coverage of β-lactamase–producing organisms.

The cephalosporins are defined in terms of generation. The first generation cephalosporins, the earliest developed, are rarely employed as first-line therapy, although there are a few exceptions. First generation cephalosporins are most active against Gram-positive aerobic cocci and are resistant to the β-lactamases produced by staphylococci. They are effective in treating skin and soft tissue infections caused by staphylococci and streptococci such as impetigo. Impetigo may manifest as a primary lesion or a secondary dermatological lesion. For example, the ulcers in a severe primary episode of herpes simplex virus may become *impetiginized,* that is, secondarily infected with Group A β-hemolytic streptococci.

The first generation parenteral cephalosporin, cefazolin (Ancef, Kefzol), is frequently employed as prophylactic therapy in surgical procedures. A Cochrane review of 51 trials showed that cefazolin and ampicillin were equally effective in preventing endometritis when prescribed as single agents during cesarean birth. Further, second or third generation cephalosporins or combination drug regimens offered no additional benefit.[3]

Moving from first to third generation, the cephalosporins exhibit greater Gram-negative coverage at the expense of Gram-positive coverage. Second generation cephalosporins, such as cefaclor (Ceclor) are effective in treating both otitis media and community acquired pneumonia, because of their activity against both Gram-positive streptococcus and Gram-negative *Moraxella* and *Haemophilus influenzae*. The third generation cephalosporins, parenteral ceftriaxone (Rocephin) and oral cefixime (Suprax), are effective single dose therapies for *Neisseria gonorrhoeae*. Ceftriaxone crosses the blood-brain barrier, making it an effective therapy for meningitis. In addition to renal excretion, ceftriaxone is 40% eliminated in bile and, therefore, unlike other cephalosporins, it does not require dose adjustment in individuals with renal impairment. Of the third generation cephalosporins, Ceftazidime (Fortaz, Tazidmime) offers the best coverage of *Pseudomonas*.

The β-lactams have variable absorption, depending on the specific drug and route of administration. All are widely distributed following oral or parenteral administration. With the exception of some of the third generation cephalosporins, they do not cross the blood-brain barrier. Elimination is primarily via the kidneys by tubular secretion. The β-lactams are pregnancy category B and are compatible with breastfeeding according to the AAP. **Table 5-6** lists the beta-lactams and their antibacterial activities.

Macrolides

The basic chemical structure of the macrolides, which include such antibiotics as erythromycin, clarithromycin, and azithromycin, is a lactone ring. Macrolides inhibit protein synthesis and are classified as bacteriostatic agents; however, in some concentrations and in some circumstances they may be bactericidal. Erythromycin, available in several different salts (erythromycin base, erythromycin estolate, erythromycin stearate, and erythromycin ethylsuccinate), has been in clinical use since the 1950s. Clarithromycin (Biaxin) and azithromycin (Zithromax), the newer macrolides, have longer serum half-lives than erythromycin, providing a more convenient oral dosing, schedule. Clarithromycin requires twice daily dosing and azithromycin is given once daily. Erythromycin is given four times daily. Azithromycin is also better absorbed than erythromycin, which may account for the fact that it has fewer GI side effects and can achieve and maintain high tissue levels for a longer period of time.

Macrolides are commonly used in clinical practice and are usually well tolerated. However, as with all drugs some side effects and adverse reactions can occur. Because these drugs are metabolized in the liver and are primarily eliminated in bile, they should be used with caution in patients with altered liver function. Macrolides are pregnancy category B and so may be prescribed during pregnancy and lactation, with the exception of erythromycin estolate, which is more likely to be associated with hepatotoxicity than the other formulations.

The most severe and frequent side effect of the macrolides is GI upset. Nausea, vomiting, diarrhea, abdominal cramping, and anorexia are

Table 5-6 BETA-LACTAMS BACTERICIDAL AGENTS

β-Lactam Agent	Antimicrobial Activity
Penicillins	
Natural penicillins	Narrow spectrum Gram-positive cocci Gram-negative cocci Some anaerobes Spirochetes

Penicillinase-resistant penicillins
    (cloxicillin, dicloxacillin, oxacillin,
    methicillin nafcillin)
	Penicillinase-producing staphylococcus

Aminopenicillins (ampicillin, amoxicillin)	Broad spectrum Gram-positive cocci Better Gram-negative cocci coverage Some anaerobes

Aminopenicillins + beta lactamase inhibitors
  Augmentin (amoxicillin + clavulanic acid)
  Unasyn (ampicillin + sulbactam)
  Extended spectrum penicillins
    (ticaricillin, mexlocillin, piperacillin)
	Extend the spectrum of the aminopenicillins to
	    include penicillinase-producing bacteria
	
	Pseudomonal infections

Cephlorosporins	
First Generation (cephalexin, cefazolin)	Antimicrobial Activity Similar to the penicillins

Second Generation
  (cefaclor)
	Moving from first to third generation, the
	  cephalosporins exhibit greater Gram-negative
	    coverage and less Gram-positive coverage

Third Generation (ceftrixone, cefixme, ceftazidime)	Ceftazidme covers *Pseudomonas aeruginosa*

common. Erythromycin interacts with many drugs and may be synergistic, causing increased blood levels and toxicity, as with theophylline and lovastatin, or may be antagonistic, such as when administered in conjunction with the penicillins. A thorough history of current medications should be obtained prior to the initiation of any antimicrobial therapy, because all of these agents have the potential to interact with other drugs.

In the primary care setting, the macrolides are most frequently prescribed for upper and lower respiratory tract infections from *Streptococcus pyogenes, Streptococcus pneumoniae, Haemophilus influenzae,* and *Mycoplasma pneumoniae.* Erythromycin base is one of the recommended treatments for *Chlamydia tracomatis* during pregnancy, with the caveat that frequent GI side effects may interfere with completing the course of therapy. Azithromax in a single one-gram dose is a Centers for Disease Control and Prevention (CDC) recommended treatment for *Chlamydia* in the nonpregnant woman, and although it is cited as an alternative therapy in pregnancy, the CDC states that clinical evidence supports its efficacy and safety during pregnancy.[4] In a single two-gram dose, azithromycin is also an effective treatment for *Neisseseria gonorrhoae*; however, it is not a first-line recommended therapy because of its potential for GI side effects and the cost of therapy. Ceftriaxone remains the "gold standard" for treatment of gonorrhea because of its low cost, few host side effects, and lack of reported cases of resistance. Erythomycin is frequently prescribed as an alternative in individuals who have a history of hypersensitivity to the beta-lactams, because it has a spectrum of activity similar to the penicillins. **Table 5-7** lists the macrolides and their antibacterial activity.

Lincosamides

Lincomycin, the first lincosamide, was first isolated from the mold *Streptomycin linconensis.* Clindamycin, a derivative of lincomycin, is formed by the replacement of a hydroxyl group with a chlorine atom. Because of its superior antibacterial activity and better oral bioavailability, clindamycin has essentially replaced lincomycin in clinical use.[5]

Like the macrolides, clindamycin is bacteriostatic and inhibits bacterial protein synthesis. It has a broad spectrum of activity that includes streptococci, staphylococci, and *Mycoplasma hominis.* Clindamycin does not cover Gram-positive enterococci or the aerobic Gram-negative bacilli such as *E. coli, Klebsiella, Proteus,* or *H. influenza.*

Clindamycin is often employed in treating mixed anaerobic infections, because it is effective against most anaerobes, with the exception of *Clostridium difficile (C. difficile).* Among the

Table 5-7 MACROLIDES BACTERIOSTATIC AGENTS

Macrolide	Antimicrobial Activity
First Generation	
erythromycin	Spectrum similar to the penicillins; many Gram-positive and Gram-negative aerobic bacteria; *Chlamydia trachomatis*
Second Generation	
azithromycin	Spectrum similar to the penicillins: Many Gram-positive and Gram-negative aerobic bacteria
clarithromycin	Azithromycin is active against both *Chlamydia* and gonorrhea

broad-spectrum antibiotics, clindamycin poses the most significant risk of pseudomembranous colitis. Because it effectively destroys competing flora, *C. difficile* proliferates, leading to profuse, watery diarrhea. Pseudomembranous colitis is a life-threatening condition and should be suspected when an individual presents with profuse watery diarrhea while taking any broad-spectrum antibiotic. Antibiotic therapy should be discontinued, fluid replacement initiated, and the individual observed for improvement of symptoms. Metronidazole and vancomycin (discussed below) are equally effective in treating *C. difficile*-associated diarrhea. However, metronidazole is the first-line therapy in order to reduce the risk of the development of vancomycin-resistant organisms.[6] A course of metronidazole is also less expensive than vancomycin.

Clindamycin is available in oral, topical, and parenteral preparations. Following oral or parenteral administration, clindamycin is rapidly distributed in tissue, including bone, which makes it particularly useful in treating staphylococcal infections of the bones and joints. The half-life of clindamycin is 21 hours; it is partially metabolized in the liver and excreted in urine and bile.

Like the macrolides, clindamycin is rated FDA pregnancy category B and is considered compatible with breastfeeding by the AAP. Topical clindamycin cream and oral clindamycin, in addition to metronidazole, are effective in the treatment of bacterial vaginosis. The CDC does not recommend the use of clindamycin cream during pregnancy.[4]

Fluoroquinolones

Fluoroquinolones are bactericidal. They impair synthesis and repair of bacterial DNA by inhibiting DNA gyrase. Like the cephalosporins, they can be categorized by generations. The first generation quinolone—nalidixic acid—was introduced in 1963 for the treatment of urinary tract infection. Because of rapid absorption and renal elimination following oral administration, this drug does not exhibit systemic effects. It is no longer used because of the prevalence of resistant organisms.

Second (ciprofloxacin, ofloxacin) and third generation (levofloxacin) fluoroquinolones are synthetic fluorinated analogs of nalidixic acid. Following oral administration, they are well absorbed from the gut with high bioavailabilty. Ciprofloxacin (Cipro) and ofloxacin (Floxin) are active against most Gram-negative aerobic rods, including drug-resistant *Pseudomonas* and *Enterobacter species*. They do not have effective anaerobic activity and have poor Gram-positive coverage with the exceptions of *Bacillus anthracis*, a Gram-positive aerobic rod, *Chlamydia*, and *Neisseria gonorrhoea*.

The third generation quinolone, Levofloxacin (Levaquin) has broad Gram-positive and Gram-negative coverage with better absorption, bioavailability (99%), and a longer half-life than the second generation drugs. It is given as a once daily dose and is excreted unchanged in urine. Levofloxacin is useful in treating upper and lower respiratory infections (sinusitis, pneumonia), infections of the skin and skin structures, and urinary tract infections. Due to its expense and the propensity for resistance to develop in the quinolones, it is best reserved for infections that are resistant to other drug therapies or when an agent with its broad spectrum of activity is clearly indicated. Levofloxacin is a good choice for highly resistant strains of *Streptococcus pneumoniae*.

Vancomycin (Vancocin), a glycopeptide in a class of its own, is another drug that is highly effective against resistant pneumococci. Vancomycin is bactericidal, inhibiting cell wall synthesis. Because of its efficacy against many resistant microbes, its use is reserved for circumstances in which there is no alternative therapy.[7] Given orally, vancomycin is not absorbed from the GI tract and is not useful in the primary care setting except as a therapeutic alternative to metronidazole in the treatment of pseudomembranous colitis. Vancomycin effectively covers *C. difficile* in the gut; however, it is not the first-line therapy because of cost and the potential to encourage resistance.

Like the tetracyclines, absorption of the quinolones is impaired in the presence of divalent or trivalent cations (magnesium, calcium, aluminum, and zinc), so antacids, vitamins, and dairy products containing these substances should be avoided for several hours before and after its administration. While ofloxacin is excreted almost entirely via the kidney, ciprofloxacin is metabolized in the liver and partially excreted via the biliary route.

The most common side effects of the quinolones include mild GI upset (nausea, vomiting, and diarrhea), dizziness, headache, rash, and photosensitivity. Studies in young animals have shown damage to growing cartilage, and children exposed to the fluoroquinolones have experienced transient arthralgias; therefore, they are not recommended in individuals younger than 18 years of age. For this reason also they are pregnancy category C and should be avoided in pregnancy because there are safer alternatives. The fluoroquinolones are considered compatible with breastfeeding by the AAP. **Table 5-8** lists the quinolones and their antibacterial activity.

Tetracyclines

Tetracyclines are broad-spectrum bacteriostatic agents that inhibit bacterial protein synthesis. Four fused cyclic rings form the common chemical structure of tetracycline, doxycycline, and minocycline. Doxycycline and minocycline have several advantages over tetracycline. The longer half-life of both doxycycline and minocycline allows for a less frequent dosing schedule and, unlike the other tetracyclines, food, milk, and antacids do not impair absorption. Unlike tetracycline, both doxycycline and monocycline are excreted in bile, and so are good choices for individuals with impaired renal function.

Table 5-8 QUINOLONES BACTERICIDAL AGENTS

Quinolones	Antimicrobial Activity
First Generation (nalidixic acid)	Gram-negative organisms associated with urinary tract infection
Second Generation (ciprofloxacin, ofloxacin)	Gram-negative aerobic rods Including *Pseudomonas* and *Enterobacter* species *Chlamydia trachomatis*, *Neisseria gonorrhoea*, and *Bacillus anthracis*
Third Generation (levofloxacin)	Gram-positive and Gram-negative aerobic bacteria

Common adverse effects include GI disturbance and photosensitivity. Minocycline has been associated with dizziness and vertigo. The tetracyclines are categorized as pregnancy category D because they chelate calcium ions and are deposited in deciduous teeth (causing discoloration) and bones (inhibiting bone growth and causing deformities). Because they are excreted in breast milk in low concentrations, and serum levels in breastfed infants exposed to these medications are undetectable, the tetracyclines are considered compatible with breastfeeding according to the AAP.

Tetracyclines were introduced in 1948. Their spectrum of activity includes many Gram-positive aerobes, including spirochetes, Gram-negative aerobes including *Mycoplasma* and *Chlamydia*, and some anaerobes such as *Bacteroides* species (**Table 5-9**). Increasing resistance and the availability of alternative drugs has undermined their clinical usefulness. They do remain an effective alternative for some conditions in individuals with penicillin allergy. Doxycycline is an alternative treatment for syphilis in nonpregnant penicillin-allergic individuals as well as a therapeutic option for chlamydial infections. Minocycline is an effective treatment for acne rosacea.

Nitroimidazoles

Metronidazole is the only drug in this class currently available in the United States (**Table 5-10**). The spectrum of activity includes most anaerobic bacteria, including *C. difficile*, and some protozoa, notably *Trichomonas*. Because it is the only effective therapeutic option for *Trichomonas* infection, individuals who are allergic to metronidazole must be desensitized prior to initiation of treatment. There have been reported cases of *Trichomonas* resistance to metronidaze, in which case consultation with an infectious disease specialist may be warranted.[8] Trichomoniasis is a multifocal infection that must be treated systemically, and sexual partners must be treated as well.

Oral, parenteral, topical, and vaginal preparations of metronidazole are available. Topical metronidazole is a treatment for rosacea (cystic acne). Oral metronidazole has almost 100% bioavailability. Metronidazole given either vaginally or orally is an effective treatment for the mixed anaerobic vaginal colonization of bacterial vaginosis.

Metronidazole is FDA category B. A meta-analysis of seven studies evaluating the use of metronidazole in pregnancy concluded that there was no increase in the incidence of mutagenic or teratogenic effects regardless of trimester exposure.[9] The AAP categorized metronidazole as a drug for which the effect on nursing infants is unknown but may be of concern. It further recommends that single dose therapy be given when possible during lactation, and that women

---

Table 5-9 **TETRACYCLINES BACTERIOSTATIC AGENS**

Tetracycline	Antimicrobial Activity
Tetracycline	Many Gram-positive aerobic bacteria including spirochetes
Doxycycline	Many Gram-negative aerobic bacteria including *Mycoplasma* and *Chlamydia*
Minocycline	Some anaerobes including *Bacteroide* species

Table 5-10 NITROIMIDAZOLES BACTERIOSTATIC AGENT

Nitroimidazole	Antimicrobial Activity
Metronidazole	Most anaerobic bacteria including *Clostridium*

---

should discontinue breastfeeding for 12 to 24 hours, pump their breasts, and discard the milk.

Metronidazole has no activity against aerobic bacteria,[5] a factor that increases its advantage in treating bacterial vaginosis. Hydrogen peroxide-producing lactobacillus, a Gram-positive rod, is largely responsible for maintaining the vaginal ecosystem, creating an acidic environment. Bacterial vaginosis occurs when colonization by lactobacilli is disrupted, the vaginal pH rises, and anaerobic bacteria thrive. Lactobacilli sparing treatment with metronidazole may allow for re-colonization and a return to the natural balance of flora in the genital tract.

Sulfonamides and Trimethoprim

The first antimicrobial agents found to be active in the treatment of bacterial infections were the sulfonamides. The sulfonamides, synthetic agents first formulated in 1932, are no longer employed as single agents because of the evolution of resistant microbes, the prevalence of hypersensitivity reactions, and the availability of alternative drugs with similar spectrum of activity and fewer potential side effects. When sulfamethoxazole is combined with trimethoprim (TMP-SMX), the resulting drug has enhanced Gram-positive and Gram-negative coverage and less risk of resistance than when either drug is used alone.

Sulfamethoxazole and trimethoprim are bacteriostatic agents alone and bactericidal in combination. Because each drug interferes with folate synthesis in a different metabolic step, their combination has a synergistic effect. Side effects of the sulfonamides include nausea, vomiting, headache, and allergic reactions. Hypersensitivity to the sulfonamides may be severe and life-threatening. Therapy should be discontinued with the onset of skin rash, sore throat, fever, cough, shortness of breath, or any signs of adverse reaction. Increasing fluid intake during the course of therapy is recommended to prevent crystalluria. The sulfonamides have been associated with hemolytic anemia in individuals with glucose-6-phosphate-dehydrogenase (G6PD) deficiency, including the term fetus.

TMP-SMX is rapidly absorbed following oral administration with peak blood levels at one to four hours. Elimination is primarily through the kidney. Because of the potential for this drug to interfere with folic acid metabolism, it should be avoided in individuals with folate deficiency (megaloblastic anemia). TMP-SMX is labeled pregnancy category C; however, near term it is category D. It should not be prescribed after 36 weeks' gestation because of the risk of hemolytic anemia in the newborn. TMP-SMX has low concentrations in breast milk and is considered compatible with breastfeeding by the AAP.

Aminoglycosides

Rarely employed in the primary care setting, the parenteral aminoglycosides gentamicin, amikacin, streptomycin, and tobramycin are reserved for severe systemic infections from Gram-negative aerobes resistant to other medications (**Table 5-11**). The high risk of ototoxicity and nephrotoxicity and a narrow therapeutic window require monitoring of blood levels. Toxicity is related to both serum levels and duration of therapy, so short courses of therapy are indicated. The aminoglycosides are bactericidal agents that inhibit bacterial protein synthesis. Gentamicin is frequently used in conjunction with penicillin or vancomycin, a combination that has a synergistic effect, increasing the efficacy of gentamicin. Elimination is via the kidney. The aminoglycosides are pregnancy category C, and because of their potential for toxicity they should not be prescribed in pregnancy except in severe infections with resistant organisms that have not responded to less toxic therapy. The aminoglycosides are considered compatible with breastfeeding by the AAP.

Oral preparations of neomycin and paromycin are poorly absorbed, so their use is limited to a few specific intestinal infections. Neomycin is used in conjunction with erythromycin to reduce bowel flora prior to elective colorectal surgery, and paromycin is effective against some intestinal protozoa.[5] Neomycin is also available as topical treatment for infections of the skin, eye, and ears (Neosporin, Cortisporin).

Nitrofurantoin

Nitrofurantoin, available as macrocrystals (Macrodantin) or monohydrate/macrocrystals (Macrobid), is a urinary antiseptic active against most organisms responsible for urinary tract infection with the exception of *Proteus* species. *Proteus* creates an alkaline urine that inhibits the activity of nitrofurantoin, a drug that works best in an acid environment. The absorption, metabolism, and renal excretion of nitrofurantoin are so efficient that there are no systemic antimicrobial effects and few host side effects, other than mild GI upset. Its mechanism of action is not known (**Table 5-12**).

As with the sufonamides, nitrofurantoin is associated with hemolytic anemia in individuals with G6PD deficiency, including neonates exposed in utero. Worldwide, an estimated 400 million individuals are affected by G6PD deficiency, the most common enzyme deficiency in humans. Hemolytic anemia and prolonged neonatal jaundice are the most serious, life-threatening conditions associated with G6PD deficiency. When alternative therapies are available, the sulfonamides and nitrofurantoin should be avoided after 36 weeks' gestation due to the potential risks. Nitrofurantoin is actively transported into breast milk, so it should be avoided in breastfeeding women with newborns affected by G6PD deficiency or who have prolonged, unexplained jaundice. Although nitrofurantoin is considered compatible with breastfeeding by the AAP, it is not the best choice for nursing mothers since alternative therapies are available.

Table 5-11 **AMINOGLYCOSIDES BACTERICIDAL AGENT**

Aminoglycoside	Antimicrobial Activity
Gentamicin	Penicillin/methicillin-resistant strains of staphy lococcus Gram-negative aerobic bacteria including *Enterobacter*, *E. coli*, *Klebsiella*, *Proteus*, and *Pseudomonas*

Table 5-12 NITROFURANTOIN URINARY ANTISEPTIC

Nitrofurantoin	Antimicrobial Activity
Macrocrystals (Macrodantin) Mohohydrate/macrocrystals (Macrobid)	Most organisms responsible for urinary tract infection except proteus species: *E. coli*, *Klebsiella*, *Enterococcus*, and *Enterobacter*

Antimicrobial Resistance

In response to WHO's identification of antimicrobial resistance as a global crisis,[10] many nations have implemented national programs to combat the threat of emerging microbes that are impervious to even the most powerful drugs. Since the advent of antibiotic use in the 1940s, bacteria have mutated to develop resistance and have acquired the capacity to genetically share that resistance with other microbes when they meet in the human GI tract.[11] Many factors contribute to antimicrobial resistance: incorrect prescribing practices by clinicians; misuse of antibiotics by consumers; and the use of antibiotics in animal husbandry, which has created a complex problem that requires multifaceted strategies.

The inappropriate use of antibiotics by providers and consumers is a primary factor in the emergence of resistant bacteria, prompting initiation of national campaigns designed to educate as well as change attitudes and behaviors of clinicians and the public. Upper respiratory infections and acute uncomplicated cystitis are two of the most common conditions for which individuals seek care in the ambulatory setting, and they both have the potential for errors in drug therapy.

Perhaps the most obvious error in prescribing practices is the use of antibiotics for viral infections. Several studies have documented that primary care providers may be swayed by patients to prescribe antibiotics even when they are not clinically indicated. A 1996 study involving 113 patients with respiratory infections concluded that 65% of these patients expected to receive antibiotics during the physician visit. Physicians in the study were more likely to prescribe antibiotics when they perceived that patients expected them even though most upper respiratory infections are viral in origin. More importantly, the study reported that patient satisfaction with the visit did not depend on a prescription, but rather the time the physician spent with them and their understanding of the disease when the visit was over.[12]

Selecting the wrong drug is another common error in the treatment of respiratory infections. A retrospective analysis for a 10-year period found that there were 6.7 million annual visits in the primary care setting by adults with sore throat in the United States. Although bacterial infections account for less than 20% of pharyngitis in adults, antibiotics were prescribed 73% of the time.[13] The Infectious Disease Society of America (IDSA) recommended treatment for Group A beta hemolytic streptococcal pharyngitis is penicillin, or erythromycin in the event of allergy to the beta-lactams, yet the researchers found an increase, over the 10-year period, in the use of such nonrecommended therapies as the extended-spectrum macrolides and fluoroquinolones.[13]

The first step in initiating antimicrobial therapy should be documentation of a bacterial infection and identification of the responsible pathogen. Identification of the suspected pathogenic organism is essential in that it directs prescription of an agent with a narrow spectrum of activity that targets that specific pathogen. The site of the infection, clinical symptoms, epidemiological data, and culture, when indicated and available, all contribute to identifying an organism or group of probable organisms for a particular infection.

Selecting a drug with a narrow spectrum reduces the risk of interfering with the host's normal microbial flora in addition to reducing the risk of encouraging resistance.

There are occasions when the clinician can make a diagnosis based on clinical symptoms alone. For example, when a client presents with dysuria, frequency of urination, and suprapubic pain, in the absence of evidence suggestive of complicated cystitis or pyelonephritis, there is ample clinical evidence to support the diagnosis of acute uncomplicated cystitis.[14] This diagnosis can be confirmed with a midstream urine dipstick positive for leukocyte esterase and nitrites.

Initiating empiric therapy requires knowledge about the most common pathogens for the identified infection as well as susceptibility and resistance patterns in the community. In the case of uncomplicated cystitis in women, *E. coli* is the most frequent uropathogen, accounting for more than 80% of infections; *S. saprophyticus* accounts for an additional 10% to 15%.[15] The emergence of *E. coli* strains that are resistant to the β-lactams has limited their usefulness in treating urinary tract infections. The aminopenicillins are no longer recommended for empiric treatment of uncomplicated cystitis because of the prevalence of resistant *E. coli*, which may be as high as 30%.

Prescribing patterns also suggest that health care professionals are affected by pharmaceutical marketing practices when selecting an antimicrobial agent. Although the IDSA recommends TMP/SMX (Bactrim) in a three-day course of therapy as a first-line empiric treatment for acute uncomplicated cystitis, a recently published study that reviewed the prescriptive histories in a cohort of over 13,000 individuals found that only 37% of physicians prescribed TMP/SMX for uncomplicated cystitis, and frequently it was prescribed for a longer duration than the recommended three-day course. Fluoroquinolones, heavily marketed by pharmaceutical companies for the treatment of cystitis and more expensive than Bactrim, were given in 32% of cases. Other drugs prescribed in the study included erythromycin, amoxicillin, azithromycin, and other β-lactams, none of which are appropriate therapies for cystitis. In their discussion, the researchers suggested that, "As fluoroquinolone resistance is increasing, it is likely that making the fluoroquinolones a first line treatment for acute, sporadic cystitis would accelerate resistance rates, and lead to more treatment failures and potentially less effective and safe alternatives."[16] Furthermore, they concluded that, "Steps should be taken to educate physicians and patients on the choice and dosage of antibiotics for cystitis to minimize emergence of antibiotic resistance."[16] The length of therapy is also significant, because shorter courses of therapy are often as effective as longer courses while offering less risk of contributing to the emergence of resistant organisms.

The IDSA recommendation regarding first-line therapy for cystitis comes with the caveat that regional *E. coli* resistance to Bactrim should be less than 20%. Emerging resistance to TMP/SMX is variable in the United States. A 1999 study revealed a wide range in *E. coli* regional resistance patterns, from 28.4% in the West-South-Central regions to 9.2% in the East-South-Central regions. The highest resistance was in Iowa (33%) and the lowest in Pennsylvania (7.4%).[17] This study underlines the significance of investigating community patterns of antimicrobial resistance before prescribing a therapeutic agent.

There are other instances when empiric therapy is warranted, such as when delaying treatment may cause serious morbidity or even death, or when there is a significant risk of transmitting the infection to others. When the invading microbe has not been identified, broad-spectrum antimicrobials or combinations of drugs may be employed to cover the greatest number of possible microorganisms. The clinician should switch to an agent with a narrower spectrum when supported by the results of culture and sensitivity.

The role of antibacterial soaps and cleaning agents in the proliferation of resistant microbes is not yet clear. Concern about the widespread use of these products has been raised in the scientific community.[18] It would seem prudent to limit the use of these products until their effect on antimicrobial resistance is documented. The American Medical Association advocates regulation by the FDA for antibacterials in home products with a potential link to antibiotic resistance and the removal of products that demonstrate a mechanism of antibiotic resistance.[18]

Primary care providers can minimize the development of antibiotic resistance by following appropriate prescribing practices. **Table 5-13** identifies simple rules to follow when initiating antimicrobial therapy in order to have the best

therapeutic effect and to reduce the risk of encouraging the emergence of resistant organisms.

There is a growing debate about the relationship between the use of antibiotics in animals, therapeutically, prophylactically, and as growth promoters, and the emergence of antibiotic resistance in humans.[19] Antibiotic-resistant organisms can be passed from animals to humans via the food chain. WHO recognizes the relationship between antibiotic use in animals as a contributory factor in global antibiotic resistance in humans. In response, the European Union has banned certain antibiotic growth promoters in animals.

Summary

The core of primary health care is health promotion and disease prevention. The holistic philosophy, inherent in the midwifery model of care, engages women as participants in their own health and wellness. Prescribing healthy lifestyle choices that boost the immune system such as good nutrition, exercise, smoking cessation, and stress reduction are important infection prevention techniques. Midwives traditionally have functioned under the Hippocratic tenet of, "First, do no harm." It is essential to adhere to this cautious approach to intervention, utilizing pharmacological therapy only when indicated and carefully choosing an evidenced-based course of therapy.

Clinicians can promote their patients' participation in this aspect of care by educating women about the natural history of their infection in addition to the rationale, risks, and benefits of drug therapy. Other teaching topics included in the plan of care are the importance of completing a course of medication and avoiding sharing or self-initiating drug therapy. Both pharmacological and non-pharmacological palliative therapies should be included in the plan.

Table 5-13 **INITIATING ANTIBACTERIAL THERAPY**[1,2,3]

Simple Rules	Rationale
Document a bacterial infection and identify a pathogen based on the site of infection, clinical evidence, epidemiological patterns, and culture when indicated.	Antibiotics are not effective in treating viral infections. Targeting a specific microbe is less likely to disturb the balance of microbial flora, thus reducing the risk of superimposed infection. Therapy directed at a specific organism reduces the risk of encouraging resistance.
Identify host factors that may influence pharmacodynamics and pharmacokinetics: age, weight, health, allergies, integrity of the immune system, impaired liver or kidney function, medications, pregnancy, and lactation.	Absorption, distribution, and elimination of drugs is host-dependent. Side effects and adverse reactions can be minimized when therapy is tailored to the individual.
Review patterns of antimicrobial resistance in the community and select an agent with the narrowest spectrum and best efficacy against the suspected pathogen.	Selecting an agent with a narrow spectrum reduces the risk of encouraging drug resistance in the individual and the community.
Carefully consider route, dosing schedule, and duration of therapy.	Shorter courses of therapy are frequently as effective as longer courses and they reduce the risk of emerging resistance. Individualizing route, dosing schedule, and duration of therapy promotes adherence to the drug regimen.
Consider cost and availability.	Newer, more expensive drugs do not necessarily offer advantages over tried and true therapies.
Educate patients regarding healthy drug use.	Resistance is exacerbated when individuals "share" antibiotics with friends, self-medicate with incomplete or inappropriate therapies, or fail to take medication correctly.
Educate patients about the natural history of the infection and emphasize palliative therapies and infection control measures.	Changing the attitudes, beliefs, and behaviors of the public about antibiotic use and infection control helps to avoid overuse and misuse of antibiotics.

References

1. Velicer CM, Heckbert SR, Lampe JW, Potter JD, Robertson CA, Taplin SH. Antibiotic use in relation to the risk of breast cancer. *JAMA.* 2004;291(7): 827–835.

2. Reiff-Eldridge RA, Heffner CR, Ephross SA, Tennis PS, White AS, Andrews EB. Monitoring pregnancy outcomes after prenatal drug exposure through prospective pregnancy registries: A pharmaceutical company commitment. *Am J Obstet Gynecol.* 2000; 182:159–163.

3. Hopkins L, Smaill F. Antibiotic prophylaxis regimens and drugs for cesarean section. *Cochrane Database Syst Rev.* 2000;(2):CD001136.Review.

4. Centers for Disease Control and Prevention. Sexually transmitted diseases treatment guidelines 2002. *MMWR.* 2002;51(No. RR-6).

5. Page C, Curtis M, Sutter M, Walker M, Hoffman B. *Integrated Pharmacology.* 2nd ed. Edinburgh, UK: Mosby; 2002.

6. Giannasca PJ, Warney M. Active and passive immunization against clostridium difficile diarrhea and co-litis. *Vaccine.* 2004; 22:848–856.

7. Hooten TM, Levy SB. Confronting the antibiotic resistance crisis: Making appropriate therapeutic decisions in community medical practice. [Monograph on the Internet]. Available from: http://www.medscape.com/viewprogram/618. Accessed September 10, 2005.

8. DiCarlo RP. Monitoring STD resistance to antimicrobials: Stable or rising? In: Thirteenth Meeting of the International Society for Sexually Transmitted Diseases Research. 1999 July 11–14. Denver, CO. [Monograph on the Internet]. Available from: http://www.medscape.com/viewarticle/408283. Accessed September 10, 2005.

9. Burton P, Taddio A, Aribumu O. Safety of metron-idazole in pregnancy: A meta-analysis. *Am J Obstet Gynecol.* 1995;172:525–529.

10. World Health Organization. WHO global strategy for the containment of antimicrobial resistance. Geneva: World Health Organization; 2001. Available from: http://www.who.int/csr/resources/publications/drug resist/WHO_CDS_CSR_DRS_2001_2_EN/en/.

11. Courvalin P, Davies J. Antimicrobials: Time to act! *Curr Opin Microbiol.* 2003;6:(5):425–426.

12. Hamm RM, Hicks RJ, Bemben DA. Antibiotics and respiratory infections: Are patients more satisfied when expectations are met? *J Fam Prac.* 1996;43(1): 56–63.

13. Linder JA, Stafford RS. Antibiotic treatment of adults with sore throat by community primary care physicians: A national survey, 1989–1999. *JAMA.* 2001; 286(10):1181–1186.

14. Nicolle LE, Hooten TM, Jones WK, Fisher C, Fourcroy JL, Gupta K, et al. Managing acute uncomplicated cystitis in the era of antibiotic resistance. [Monograph on the Internet]. Medscape by WebMD, Office of Women's Health at the Department of Health and Human Services, New York. September 2003. Available from: http://www.medscape.com/viewprogram/2634/.

15. Ronald A. The etiology of urinary tract infection: Traditional and emerging pathogens. *Am J Med.* 2002; 113 (Suppl 1A):14S-19S.

16. McEwen LN, Farjo R, Foxman B. Antibiotic prescribing for cystitis: How well does it match published guidelines? *AEP.* 2003;13(6):482.

17. Karlowsky JA, Jones ME, Thornsberry C, Critchley I, Kelly LJ, Sahn DF. Prevalence of antimicrobial resistance among urinary tract pathogens isolated from female outpatients across the US in 1999. *Int J Antimicrob Agents.* 2001;18:121–127.

18. Aiello AE, Larson E. Antibacterial cleaning and hygiene products as an emerging risk factor for antibiotic resistance in the community. *Lancet Infect Dis.* 2003;3:501–506.

19. Singer RS, Finch R, Wegener HC, Bywater R, Waters J, Lipstitch M. Antibiotic resistance—the interplay between antibiotic use in animals and human beings. *Lancet.* 2003;3:47–51.

Resources

American Academy of Pediatrics Committee on Drugs. The transfer of drugs and other chemicals into human milk. *Pediatrics.* 2001;108(3):776–789.

Burton GRW, Engelkirk PG. *Microbiology for the Health Sciences.* 6th ed. Philadelphia: Lippincott Williams & Wilkins; 2000.

Centers for Disease Control and Prevention. Sexually transmitted diseases treatment guidelines 2002. *MMWR*. 2002;51(No. RR-6).

Edmunds MW, Mayhew MS. *Pharmacology for the Primary Care Provider*. St. Louis: Mosby; 2000.

Edmunds MW. *Introduction to Clinical Pharmacology*. 4th ed. St. Louis: Mosby; 2003.

Rang HP, Dale MM, Ritter JM, Moore PK. *Pharmacology*. 5th ed. Edinburgh, UK: Churchill Livingstone; 2003.

Chapter 6

Obesity and Weight Management

Diane Berry

Kimberly Whitfill

Weight management requires a balance between proper nutrition and regular exercise. Midwives are in a unique position to evaluate and manage obesity in the primary care setting. Intervention in overweight and obesity for both the woman who is not pregnant and the woman who is pregnant should include accurate diagnosis and a treatment plan aimed at teaching the client to find her own personal balance in regards to nutrition and exercise. The focus is on the management of overweight and obesity in the client who is not pregnant. Assessment of overweight and obesity in pregnant women will be addressed; however, this chapter does not address the treatment of obesity and comorbidities in women who are pregnant.

The Surgeon General's Call to Action reports that overweight and obesity in the United States has reached epidemic proportions with the number of overweight children, adolescents, and adults increasing continuously and dramatically over the past four decades.[1] Overweight is defined as a *body mass index (BMI)* between 25 and 29.9 kg/m^2, and obesity is defined as a BMI >30.0 kg/m^2 (**Table 6-1**).[2] According to the Third National Health and Nutrition Examin-

ation Survey, overweight and obesity affect more than 61% (58 million) of the United States population over the age of 20.[3] Obesity is prevalent in both genders, affects all ages, crosses all ethnic groups, and has increased over the past 15 years.[4] Currently, 67% of African-American and Hispanic women are overweight compared with 46% of non-Hispanic Caucasian women.[5] Obesity increases risk factors for the development of coronary heart disease, diabetes, and certain cancers. In addition, obesity exacerbates hypertension, osteoarthritis, gallstones, dyslipidemia, and muscular problems. Obese individuals tend to suffer increased psychological effects such as depression and low self-esteem when compared with leaner individuals.[5] Currently, the direct cost of obesity has been estimated to be $70 billion, or 7% of health care expenditures in the United States.[5,6] The Healthy People 2010 statistics[7] show that overweight and obesity are major contributors to preventable causes of death and recommend reducing the proportion of children, adolescents, and adults who are overweight or obese through healthy diet and regular exercise. The National Task Force on Prevention and Treatment of Obesity[8]

Table 6-1 NON-PREGNANT WOMEN: BODY MASS INDEX AND WEIGHT STATUS

Body Mass Index	Weight Status
Below 18.5	Underweight
18.5–24.9	Normal
25.0–29.9	Overweight
≥30.0	Obese

Source: Adapted from United States Department of Health and Human Services, Public Health Service, National Center for Health Statistics. Vital and health statistics: Anthropometric reference data and prevalence of overweight United States, 1976-80. Hyattsville, MD: Department of Health and Human Services; 1987.

recommends weight loss and lasting lifestyle change through improved nutrition and increased activity.

Etiology of Obesity

Obesity is a complex problem with a multifactorial etiology; it is brought about by an interaction between predisposing genetic and metabolic factors coupled with a changing environment. Heredity, environmental, socioeconomic factors, energy intake, and energy expenditure all influence the recent increase in overweight and obesity in the United States.

Heredity plays a major role in the development of obesity with genes, gender, and population being influential. Genes passed from parents to children provide a basis for genetic inheritance, but diet and exercise provide additional variation. Identical twins are more highly correlated in body composition than fraternal twins.[9] The relationship between parental and childhood adiposity at birth is moderate, weakens during the first two years, and then strengthens at ages 3 to 4 years.[10] Overweight or obese children with overweight or obese parents have an increased risk of developing adult obesity.[10] Therefore, if both parents are of normal weight, then their child has the least risk of developing obesity as an adult.[11] Overweight and obesity in adolescence increases the risk for the development of obesity in adulthood regardless of parental weight status.[11] In addition, women have higher body fat percentages than men,[12] which may be related to an autosomal obesity gene that interacts with sex hormones to increase fat accumulation in women.[13]

Environmental influences related to the increased availability of processed food, fat, and calories coupled with a decrease in physical activity and an increase of sedentary activity over the last three decades have fueled the obesity epidemic. The importance of environment and cultural change is evidenced by Pima Indians living in Arizona who, because of their increased food intake and decreased physical activity, weigh 25 kg more than Pima Indians living in their traditional culture in Mexico.[14] Also, environmental influences upon the developing fetus have been demonstrated with evidence that proper maternal nutrition during pregnancy may minimize the risk of obesity for the developing child.[15,16] There is an association between low birth weight and the development of increased abdominal fat later in life.[17]

There is also a strong association between gender, ethnicity, socioeconomic factors, and obesity. In developed societies, women of lower socioeconomic status tend to be more obese than men or children of the same socioeconomic group.[18] The degree of socioeconomic inequality in obesity varies across gender, age, and ethnic groups. Compared with men, women have an inverse association between socioeconomic status and obesity.[19] There is a higher prevalence of obesity in ethnic minority youth with females being more obese than males.[20] Young African-American females tend to gain weight at a faster rate than African-American males or Caucasians of both genders.[21]

Energy intake includes feeding choices, dietary consumption, feeding style, and the environment. Over the last 30 years, energy intake has increased as the consumption of fast food has increased and fewer meals are eaten at home.[22] Fast food restaurants are open late into the night, and the media encourage increased intake through commercials and ads. Caloric and fat content of fast food meals is not easily available so that consumers can make intelligent choices regarding their food intake. However, this culture of overeating is slowly changing as the gravity of the obesity epidemic becomes more publicized.

Energy expenditure results from any physical activity with the greatest expenditures occurring with strenuous activities. Most studies have found that obese individuals were less physically active than those of normal weight.[23] Physical activity has decreased and sedentary activities such as television viewing and computer games have increased over the last decade.[24] Reduction of sedentary activities and an increase in physical activity has been found to reduce BMI.[24]

Pathophysiology of Obesity

Body weight regulation is complex and relates to energy intake and energy expenditure. Obesity is classified as either an exogenous condition due to an excessive intake of calories or an endogenous condition due to metabolism.[25] Structure and distribution of adipose tissue can be defined as either hyperplastic, which relates to a greater than normal number of fat cells or hypertrophic, which relates to greater than normal size of fat cells. There are multiple theories to explain the pathophysiology of obesity.

- The fat-cell theory suggests that overweight and obese individuals have an excessive number of hyperplastic fat cells, which increase whenever a positive energy balance occurs.[26]
- The lipoprotein-lipase theory proposes that enzymes regulate the size of fat cells to maintain a constant cell size, thereby thwarting weight loss attempts by obese individuals. Lipoprotein-lipase is an enzyme that is synthesized by fat cells and hydrolyzes triglycerides into free fatty acids and glycerol, which then enter fat cells and are re-esterified into triglycerides, promoting fat storage.[27] When obese individuals lose weight, lipoprotein-lipase levels rise in the cells, which stimulate the fat cells to return to their normal size, thereby preventing weight loss maintenance.
- The lipostatic theory suggests that everyone has a biological set point controlled by the ventromedial hypothalamus, which regulates appetite and maintains body weight.[28] Obese individuals have a higher set point and have more difficulty maintaining weight loss.
- The thermogenesis of brown adipose tissue theory postulates that individuals with a larger number of subcutaneous brown fat cells release excess energy through heat production instead of converting energy to fat stores, and that obese individuals have less brown fat

cells when compared with lean individuals.[29,30] Therefore, individuals with more subcutaneous fat cells expend more energy, produce fewer fat stores, and are leaner.

- The sodium-potassium-adenosine triphosphatase pump theory states that sodium is pumped out of the cell and potassium is pumped into the cell, which splits adenosine triphosphate and releases energy.[31] Obese individuals have fewer sodium-potassium-adenosine triphosphatase pumps and a decreased energy release.
- Psychological theories propose that obese individuals may be more directed by external cues, such as sight, smell, and taste of food, than by internal cues such as hunger or satiety,[32] and that eating may create a desire to eat more.[33]

Over the past decade, there has been landmark research on the genetic and metabolic control systems that regulate body weight. The central nervous system is responsible for appetite regulation through three categories of neurotransmitters, which include gamma-aminobutyric acid, monoamines, and neuropeptides.[34] Gamma-aminobutyric acid functions throughout the central nervous system as an on/off switch for neural circuits, which maintains a state of arousal. Monoamines include norepinephrine, dopamine, and serotonin, which function as a form of volume control on a variety of systems and behaviors. Dopamine has been found to be important in relation to the reward characteristics of feeding. Both norepinephrine and serotonin are present in the hypothalamus and are involved in body weight regulation. These two transmitters have a complex physiology with multiple receptor subtypes

and reuptake sites. Neuropeptides have effects on specific behaviors and body functions through receptor subtypes and interactions with other neural circuits.[34]

Other research has focused on leptin, which alters liver glucose production and fat metabolism in skeletal muscle, liver, and pancreatic beta cells.[35,36] Neuropeptide Y is a hypothalamic neurotransmitter and a potent orexigenic peptide that alters appetite, peripheral metabolism, and fat storage through alteration in adipose tissue lipoprotein lipase, thereby decreasing energy expenditure.[37] Neuropeptide Y responds to stimulation by leptin by altering its own production. Insulin production increases in response to food intake and produces satiety as a part of a coordinated response to food ingestion. Insulin acts in the brain primarily to reduce food intake, which is important in body weight regulation.[34] Excessive intake of foods rich in fat and carbohydrates stimulates hyperinsulinemia. Through a negative-feedback mechanism, excessive insulin levels decrease the number of insulin receptor sites on adipose tissue cells, thereby decreasing the amount of glucose that can enter the cell. As glucose levels rise, excess glucose is either stored as glycogen in the liver or as triglycerides in adipose cells, which enhances hypertrophy and hyperplasia of fat cells.[34,38]

Office-Based Obesity Care

Measurement of Obesity

Opportunities to work with clients who are overweight and obese present themselves to clinicians daily. A team approach with a comfortable environment and proper equipment is important for an effective plan of care. Evaluation of obesity must start with some form of measurement that quantifies the extent of the problem. The following sections describe currently available measurements.

Body Mass Index

BMI is a simple calculation that determines height to weight ratio. The index can be used to correlate the client's physical stature with mortality ratios based on actuarial studies. Overweight is defined as a BMI >25 to 29.9 kg/m^2 and obesity is defined as a BMI >30.0 kg/m^2.[2] BMI should become the fifth vital sign in assessing the client. BMI is calculated as follows[2]:

$$\text{BMI} = \text{weight (kg)/height in meters squared (m}^2)$$

To estimate BMI from pounds and inches use **Table 6-2**[39] or the following formula:

$$[\text{weight in pounds)/height (inches)}^2] \times 703$$

There are also BMI calculators available on the Internet at the Centers for Disease Control and Prevention (CDC) Web site.[40] It is important to share the number with the clients, and explain where they fall in level of risk for comorbidities and what their ideal BMI should be.

BMI only gives a general idea of obesity or excess fat. BMI may be overestimated in individuals who are very muscular or have edema, and underestimated in older clients who have lost lean body mass.

Waist Circumference

Evidence suggests that the single best predictor of adverse health effects from excess body fat is visceral adiposity through a waist circumference measurement.[41] A larger waist circumference is associated with an increased risk for type II diabetes, dyslipidemia, hypertension, and coro-

nary heart disease. Abdominal fat has three compartments: visceral, retroperitoneal, and subcutaneous fat.[42] Approximately 47% of the variance in insulin resistance among healthy subjects without diabetes can be explained by intra-abdominal fat.[43] As subcutaneous fat increases, leptin levels also increase leading to increased insulin resistance, a condition that has been found to be more prevalent in women.[43] **Figure 6-1** illustrates the correct measurement technique to assess waist circumference. A high-risk waist circumference for men is greater than 40 inches (102 cm); for women the risk is greater with a waist circumference larger than 35 inches (88 cm).[2] Waist circumference loses its predictive power in determining co-morbid conditions once the BMI reaches 35.[2] Therefore, it is not necessary to measure waist circumference in those individuals with BMIs of 35 or greater. If the woman is pregnant, then her pre-pregnancy BMI is used.

Anthropometry

The caliper method is based on the assumption that the thickness of the subcutaneous fat reflects a constant proportion of the total body fat.[44] Using hand-held calipers that exert a standard pressure, the skinfold thickness is measured in the triceps, biceps, subscapula, axilla, iliac crest, supraspinal, abdominal, front thigh, medial calf, or chest (**Figure 6-2** and **Table 6-3**). Body fat percentage based on the sum of three measurements is then calculated. Directions for performing caliper measurements include:

- Choose the site you will use for skinfold measurement.
- Firmly pinch the skinfold between your thumb and forefinger and place the calipers over the skinfold, while continuing to hold the skinfold with your other hand.

Table 6-2 BODY MASS INDEX

	Weight (lbs)																				
	120	130	140	150	160	170	180	190	200	210	220	230	240	250	260	270	280	290	300	310	320	330
4'5"	30	33	35	38	40	43	45	48	50	53	55	58	60	63	65	68	70	73	75	78	80	83
4'6"	29	31	34	36	39	41	43	46	48	51	53	56	58	60	63	65	68	70	42	75	77	80
4'7"	28	30	33	35	37	40	42	44	47	49	51	54	56	58	61	63	65	68	70	72	75	77
4'8"	27	29	31	34	36	38	40	43	45	47	49	52	54	56	58	61	63	65	67	70	72	74
4'9"	26	28	30	33	35	37	39	41	43	46	48	50	52	54	56	59	61	63	65	67	69	72
4'10"	25	27	29	31	34	36	38	40	42	44	46	48	50	52	54	57	59	61	63	65	67	69
4'11"	24	26	28	30	32	34	36	38	40	43	45	47	49	51	53	55	57	59	61	63	65	67
5'0"	23	25	27	29	31	33	35	37	39	41	43	45	47	49	51	53	55	57	59	61	63	65
5'1"	23	25	27	28	30	32	24	36	38	40	42	44	45	47	49	51	53	55	57	59	61	62
5'2"	22	24	26	27	29	31	33	35	37	38	40	42	44	46	48	49	51	53	55	57	59	60
5'3"	21	23	25	27	28	30	32	34	36	37	39	41	43	44	46	48	50	51	53	55	57	59
5'4"	21	22	24	26	28	29	31	33	34	36	38	40	41	43	45	46	48	50	52	53	55	57
5'5"	20	22	23	25	27	28	30	32	33	35	37	38	40	42	43	45	47	48	50	52	53	55
5'6"	19	21	23	24	26	27	29	31	32	34	36	37	39	40	42	44	45	47	49	50	52	53
5'7"	19	20	22	24	25	27	28	30	31	33	35	36	38	39	41	42	44	46	47	49	50	52
5'8"	18	20	21	23	24	26	27	29	30	32	34	35	37	38	40	41	43	44	46	47	49	50
5'9"	18	19	21	22	24	25	27	28	30	31	33	34	36	37	38	40	41	43	44	46	47	49
5'10"	17	19	20	22	23	24	26	27	29	30	32	33	35	36	37	39	40	42	43	45	46	47
5'11"	17	18	20	21	22	24	25	27	28	29	31	32	34	35	36	38	39	41	42	43	45	46
6'0"	16	18	19	20	22	23	24	26	27	29	30	31	33	34	35	37	38	39	41	42	43	45
6'1"	16	17	19	20	21	22	24	25	26	28	29	30	32	33	34	36	37	38	40	41	42	44
6'2"	15	17	18	19	21	22	23	24	26	27	28	30	31	32	33	35	36	37	39	40	41	42
6'3"	15	16	18	19	20	21	23	24	25	26	28	29	30	31	33	34	35	36	38	39	40	41
6'4"	15	16	17	18	20	21	22	23	24	26	27	28	29	30	32	33	34	35	37	38	39	40
6'5"	14	15	17	18	19	20	21	23	24	25	26	27	29	30	31	32	33	34	36	37	38	39
6'6"	14	15	16	17	19	20	21	22	23	24	25	27	28	29	30	31	32	34	35	36	37	38
6'7"	14	15	16	17	18	19	20	21	23	24	25	26	27	28	29	30	32	33	34	35	36	37
6'8"	13	14	15	17	18	19	20	21	22	23	24	25	26	28	29	30	31	32	33	34	35	36
6'9"	13	14	15	16	17	18	19	20	21	23	24	25	26	27	28	29	30	31	32	33	34	35
6'10"	13	14	15	16	17	18	19	20	21	22	23	24	25	26	27	28	29	30	31	32	34	35

Source: Adapted from United States Department of Health and Human Services, Public Health Service, National Center for Health Statistics. Vital and health statistics: Anthropometric reference data and prevalence of overweight United States, 1976-80. Hyattsville, MD: Department of Health and Human Services; 1987.

- Press with your thumb until you feel a click. The caliper slide will automatically stop at the correct measurement.
- After reading the measurement, return the caliper slide to the far right starting position.
- Repeat three times and use the average of your measurement.
- Refer to the body fat interpretation chart to determine body fat percentage for women (**Table 6-4**).

Skinfold measurements are easy to do and inexpensive, but may not be a valid predictor of percent body fat. However, they can be used to provide information and change in body composition over time. Reliability may be affected by the experience of the individual doing the testing and the quality of the calipers.

Near-Infrared Interactance

Near-infrared interactance uses a fiber-optic probe connected to a digital analyzer that indirectly measures fat and water tissue composition at various sites.[44] The bicep is the most often used site. The near-infrared interactance light penetrates the skin and is reflected off the bone to the detector. The data are entered into a computer using a prediction equation that includes the client's height, weight, frame size, and level of activity, and an estimate of body fat percentage is provided. The amount of pressure applied, skin color, and hydration may affect results.

Hydrodensitometry

Hydrodensiometry is based on the assumption that densities of fat mass and fat-free mass are constant. The method measures whole body density by determining body volume. The densities of bone and muscles are higher than water,

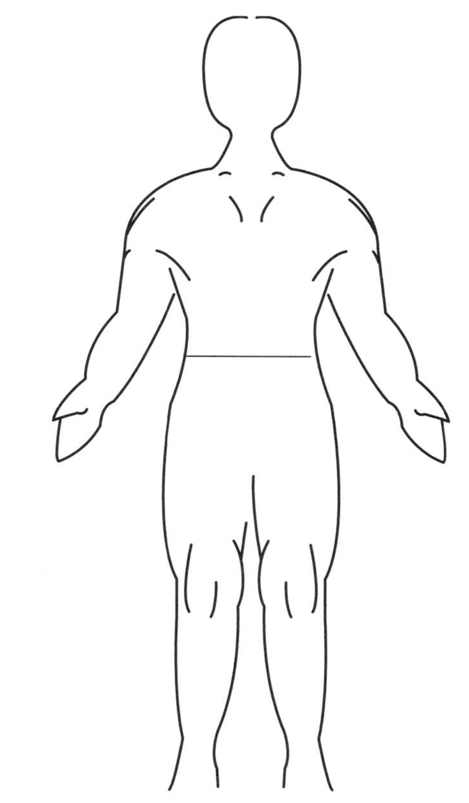

Figure 6-1 Waist circumference

To measure the client's waist circumference, palpate the upper hipbone to locate the right iliac crest. At the lateral border of the right iliac crest and the midaxillary line, the tape is placed horizontally around the waist approximately one inch above the umbilicus at normal minimal respiration.

and fat is less dense than water. A client who has more bone and muscle will weigh more in water than will a client with less bone and muscle. Therefore, the former will have a higher body

Figure 6-2 Skinfold measurement sites.

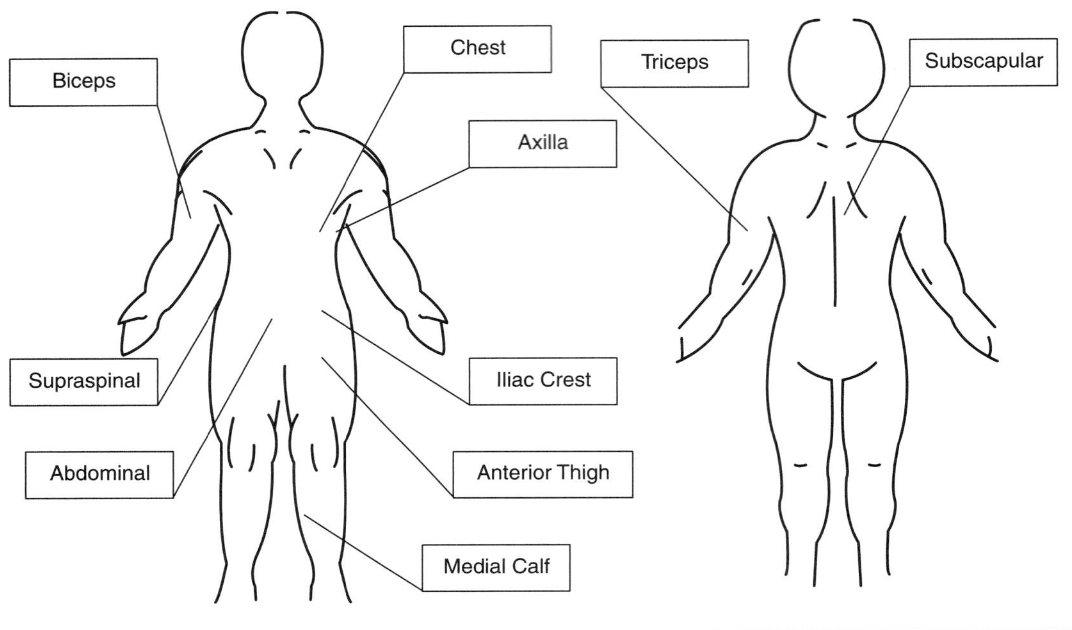

density and a lower percentage of fat. The client is weighed outside the tank in a bathing suit, and is weighed again in a chair or sling in the tank using underwater scales. A body fat percentage is calculated from the body density using either Siri or Brozek standard equations.[44,45] It is important to take into consideration the amount of air that is left in the lungs after exhaling during underwater weighing. Hydrodensitometry has been considered the gold standard for body fat measurement secondary to the level of accuracy in the majority of individuals. However, athletes have denser bones and muscles, which may lead to an underestimation of body fat. Clients with osteoporosis may have their body fat overestimated.

Air Displacement

Air displacement uses the same principles as underwater weighing.[44] The BOD POD® is a fiberglass plethysmograph that measures body volume by changes in pressure in a closed chamber. Computerized sensors are used to measure how much air is displaced. Then body density and body fat are calculated. Disadvantages include the high cost of equipment and limited exposure to radiation.

Dual Energy X-Ray Absorptiometry (DEXA)

Dual energy x-ray absorptiometry (DEXA) is based on a three-compartment model that di-

Table 6-3 SKINFOLD MEASUREMENT SITES

Site	Directions
Abdominal	5 centimeters adjacent to the umbilicus vertically.
Anterior Thigh	Mid-point of the anterior thigh, midway between the patella and inguinal fold vertically.
Axilla	Intersection of a horizontal line level with the bottom of the xiphoid process and vertical line from the mid axilla.
Biceps	Same level as the triceps on the anterior surface of the arm.
Chest	Between the axilla and nipple on the anterior axillary fold diagonally.
Iliac Crest	Above the iliac crest at the midaxillary line anteriorly and downward.
Medial Calf	The largest circumference on the medial surface of the calf vertically.
Subscapular	2 centimeters below the lower angle of the scapula laterally and downward.
Supraspinal	Intersection of the spinal and the anterior axilla and a horizontal line of the iliac crest anteriorly and downward.
Triceps	Mid-point between acromial process and proximal end of radius on the posterior surface of the arm.

Source: Adapted from United States Department of Health and Human Services, Public Health Service, National Center for Health Statistics. Vital and health statistics: Anthropometric reference data and prevalence of overweight United States, 1976-80. Hyattsville, MD: Department of Health and Human Services; 1987.

vides the body into total body mineral, fat-free lean mass, and fat tissue mass.[44] DEXA is based on the assumption that bone mineral content is directly proportional to the amount of photon energy absorbed by the bone being studied. DEXA uses a whole body scanner, which has two low-dose X-rays that read bone and soft tissue mass simultaneously, and takes between 10 and 20 minutes. DEXA is the new gold standard in body composition analysis, because it provides a higher degree of precision in one measurement and provides information about where fat is distributed throughout the body. DEXA scanning is expensive and there is a limited exposure to radiation.

Bioelectrical Impedance Analysis

Bioelectrical impedance analysis is a quick, simple, and accurate way to determine body composition. The individual removes shoes and socks, gel electrodes are placed on the hands and feet, and a mild safe electrical current (50 kHz) is sent through the body. Impedance is greatest in fat tissue, which contains only 10% to 20% water. Fat-free mass contains 70% to 75% water, which allows the current to pass easily. The differences in conduction between the two tissues provide a measure of electrical impedance, which is then applied to a formula with height, weight, gender, age, and fitness level to calculate the percentage of body fat, fat-free mass, and hydration level.[44] The Tanita leg-to-leg bioelectrical impedance analysis (BIA) scale uses two footpad electrodes that are on an electronic scale.[46] The client stands with bare feet on the electrodes, and the scale automatically measures weight and impedance. The client's height, weight, fitness level, gender, and age are entered, and the scale determines body fat percentage based on formulas. The Tanita BIA is

Table 6-4 FEMALE BODY FAT PERCENTAGE

						Skinfold Thickness, millimeters									
	⇐	Lean			⇒ ⇐	Ideal		⇒ ⇐	Average			⇒ ⇐	Overweight		⇒
Age	2–3	4–5	8–9	10–11	12–13	14–15	16–17	18–19	20–21	22–23	24–25	26–27	28–29	30–31	32–33	34–35
0–20	11.3	13.5	15.7	19.7	21.5	23.2	24.8	26.3	27.7	29.0	30.2	31.3	32.3	33.1	33.9	34.6
21–25	11.9	14.2	16.32	20.3	22.1	23.8	25.5	27.0	28.4	29.6	30.8	31.9	32.9	33.8	34.5	35.2
26–30	12.5	14.8	16.9	20.9	22.7	24.5	26.1	27.6	29.0	30.3	31.5	32.5	33.5	34.4	35.2	35.8
31–35	13.2	15.4	17.6	21.5	23.4	25.1	26.7	28.2	29.6	30.9	32.1	33.2	34.1	35.0	35.8	36.4
36–40	13.8	16.0	18.2	22.2	24.0	25.7	27.3	28.8	30.2	31.5	32.7	33.8	34.8	35.6	36.4	37.0
41–45	14.4	16.7	18.8	22.8	24.6	26.3	27.9	29.4	30.8	32.1	33.3	34.4	35.4	36.3	37.0	37.7
46–50	15.0	17.3	19.4	23.4	25.2	26.9	28.6	30.1	31.5	32.7	34.0	35.0	36.0	36.9	37.6	38.3
51–55	15.6	17.9	20.0	24.0	25.9	27.6	29.2	30.7	32.1	33.3	34.6	35.6	36.6	37.5	38.3	38.9
≥56	16.3	18.5	20.7	24.6	26.5	28.2	29.8	31.3	32.7	34.0	35.2	36.3	37.2	38.1	38.9	39.5

Source: Adapted from United States Department of Health and Human Services, Public Health Service, National Center for Health Statistics. Vital and health statistics: Anthropometric reference data and prevalence of overweight United States, 1976-80. Hyattsville, MD: Department of Health and Human Services; 1987.

quick, portable, and inexpensive. Dehydration may cause an overestimation of the body fat percentage. Clients with pacemakers or internal cardiac defibrillators should not use BIA.

In summary, the primary care provider can use several measurements of obesity to quantify the extent of the problem. BMI is the fifth vital sign and should be calculated on all clients. Waist circumference measurement is an inexpensive technique to estimate risk. Anthropometry is another cost-effective way to measure body fat percentage. Near-infrared interactance, hydrodensiometry, air displacement, and DEXA scanning are not routinely used for obesity screening because of cost and inconvenience. BIA is a cost-effective way to measure body fat percentage in the office, but currently is not commonly used in primary care. Athletes and those who exercise heavily may have a falsely elevated BMI. There is also a risk of underestimating BMI in older clients who have lost lean body mass. Therefore, it is important to evaluate each person and their level of physical activity so that accurate measurement can be accomplished.

Associated Disease Risks and Management

Every client who presents with obesity needs a thorough history taken, including family, social, dietary, and exercise history. A physical examination to rule out associated disease risks should be completed. Associated disease risks of obesity include insulin resistance syndrome, impaired glucose tolerance, type II diabetes, hypertension, and hyperlipidemia. Although hypothyroidism and Cushing's syndrome are not directly associated with obesity, their diagnosis and management may improve overweight and obesity levels and health status in those individuals.

Insulin Resistance Syndrome

Insulin resistance is the impairment of the response of insulin on glucose, lipids, protein metabolism, and vascular endothelial function.[47] Genetics and the environment interact to lead to the development of this syndrome. Individuals with a genetic predisposition to obesity who over-consume carbohydrates, fats, and calories, have decreased physical activity, and have increased sedentary activity are at an increased risk for developing insulin resistance. Insulin resistance starts with hyperinsulinemia and normal glucose tolerance. As insulin resistance progresses, β-cell function is impaired; insulin levels start to decline as impaired glucose tolerance increases.[48] The insulin resistance syndrome (syndrome X or metabolic syndrome) includes central adiposity, dyslipidemia, atherosclerosis, decreased fibrolytic activity, hypertension, acanthosis nigricans, ovarian hyperandrogenism, hyperuricemia, impaired glucose tolerance, and diabetes.[49] The diagnosis of the metabolic syndrome requires three or more of the following characteristics[1]:

- Central adiposity measured by a waist circumference greater than 40 inches in men and 35 inches in women.
- Fasting blood triglycerides greater than or equal to 150 mg/dL.
- Fasting high-density level blood cholesterol, less than 40 mg/dL in men and less than 50 mg/dL in women.
- Blood pressure greater than or equal to 130/85 mm Hg.
- Fasting glucose greater than or equal to 110 mg/dL.

Management of the insulin resistance syndrome includes diet, exercise, behavioral modification, and treatment of impaired glucose tolerance, type II diabetes, hypertension, and hyperlipidemia.

Impaired Glucose Tolerance and Type II Diabetes Mellitus

Impaired glucose tolerance is associated with obesity and the related metabolic abnormalities of hyperinsulinemia and dyslipidemia, as well as hypertension, coronary heart disease, and the development of type II diabetes.[50] Declining β-cell function, decreasing insulin levels, and increasing glucose levels describe this condition, which if untreated will progress to type II diabetes.[48] Even small reductions in weight have been found to improve blood sugar levels.[51]

Type II diabetes mellitus is increasing in direct proportion to the increase in obesity in the United States, with African Americans, Hispanics, and Native Americans at higher risk than Caucasians.[52] Risk factors for the development of type II diabetes include a family history of type II diabetes, ethnic minority group, impaired glucose tolerance, central adiposity, and obesity.[50] Acanthosis nigricans,[53] a darker pigmentation around the neck and axilla, while normal in pregnancy, is a sign of impaired glucose tolerance and a marker for type II diabetes.[54,55]

The American Diabetes Association Clinical Practice Recommendations should be used as a guide for management of impaired glucose tolerance and type II diabetes.[50] Nutrition education, exercise, and referral to both a certified diabetes educator and an endocrinologist are warranted. Chapter 16 discusses endocrine disorders and the management of impaired glucose tolerance and diabetes.

Hypertension

Overweight and obesity are risk factors for the development of hypertension. Hypertension is an independent risk factor for the development of coronary heart disease. As blood pressure increases, so does the risk of myocardial infarction, heart failure, stroke, and kidney disease. As with diabetes, hypertension increases as BMI and age increase.[56] Hypertension is more common in minority African-American and Hispanic populations. Weight loss has been found to decrease the incidence of hypertension.[2]

Chapter 14 on cardiovascular disease covers management of hypertension, including the DASH (Dietary Approaches to Stop Hypertension) eating plan.

Hyperlipidemia

The development of hyperlipidemia is an independent risk factor for the development of coronary artery disease and premature mortality.[57] Overweight or obese clients should have a lipid level drawn at least annually or more often if elevated. Lipid levels should include total cholesterol, low-density lipoprotein (LDL), high-density lipoprotein (HDL), and triglycerides.

Lifestyle changes are the first step in controlling hyperlipidemia, and one of the most important for maintenance of normal lipid levels. These include diet modification, exercise, smoking cessation, and decreased alcohol intake. Diets low in saturated fats and high in fiber are recommended. Increased exercise and dietary changes can lead to weight loss, which in itself will help to lower lipid levels in most persons. Chapter 14 provides a discussion of the management plan for hyperlipidemia.

Hypothyroidism

Screening for hypothyroidism should be performed for all overweight or obese clients. The prevalence of hypothyroidism increases with age, and it is more common in women than men.[58] Weight gain may be associated with hypothyroid states, because these slow the metabolism. Elevated levels of low-density cholesterol and increased rates of diabetes mellitus are often seen in hypothyroid patients. Management of thyroid deficiency can assist in prevention and management of other weight-related health problems. Chapter 16 offers a discussion of thyroid diseases.

Cushing's Syndrome

Cushing's syndrome is caused by the overproduction of cortisol by the adrenal glands as a result of a pituitary tumor secreting adrenocorticotropic hormone (ACTH), ectopic production of ACTH, or a tumor in one of the adrenal glands. It is difficult to evaluate clients for Cushing's syndrome because overweight and obesity can produce hypercortisolism. In addition, overweight, obesity, and symptoms such as central obesity, moon facies, supraclavicular fat pads, buffalo hump, central obesity, diabetes, and depression are similar to those of Cushing's disease.[58] Cushing's syndrome includes several specific symptoms that include proximal muscle weakness and wide violaceous striae.[58]

Screening tests include the overnight dexamethasone suppression test and the 24-hour urinary free-cortisol. The dexamethasone suppression test is conducted by having the client take a 1 mg dose of dexamethasone at 11 PM, and then at 8 AM, a serum cortisol level is drawn. A normal value is less than 5 ng/dL. The 24-hour urinary free cortisol test is collected over a 24-hour period and a value less than 100 is considered normal.[59] False-positive tests can be caused by obesity, alcohol, or depression. If either test is positive, an immediate referral to an endocrinologist is warranted.

Management of Obesity

Treatment goals for obesity include decreasing weight, improving nutrition, increasing physical activity, and decreasing sedentary activity to decrease the incidence of type II diabetes, hypertension, and hyperlipidemia.[49] Management of obesity includes dietary changes, behavioral modification, and exercise interventions to assist clients to balance their energy, lose weight, increase physical activity, and decrease sedentary activity.

Modifications to the office environment that are more comfortable for overweight and obese clients include a stable scale with a large floor plate capable of weighing heavier individuals in a private room, large gowns, large blood pressure cuffs, and armless chairs in the waiting room. Health care should be delivered using a team approach in a nonjudgmental manner.

Women's health providers need to be empathetic with clients and assume that they know they are overweight or obese. At the same time, clients should hear from their midwife or practitioner about weight control. Clients can be asked the following question. What do you think about your weight? Open-ended questions provide an opportunity to assess the client's interest and motivation for weight control in a nonjudgmental manner. The client's perspective is important to hear before making recommendations or describing the complications of overweight and obesity. The client often defines the presenting problem independent of weight. If weight is a precipitating condition, then the focus should be on factors that affect both the presenting problem and the weight issue. Working closely with the client to develop a diet and exercise plan may improve adherence. Identification of barriers to success provides insight into the client's personal struggle and provides opportunities to institute healthy behavior change. A journal of dietary intake and exercise should be brought to each visit for review. Midwives can use the detailed data in these diaries to provide specific support and encouragement without criticism. Criticism can only prevent the development of an effective therapeutic relationship. Clients will have unrealistic expectations. Midwives need to clearly describe what weight loss can accomplish, how much weight loss a patient can reasonably expect to achieve, and focus on non-weight outcomes like improved lipids, blood sugar control, and blood pressure. Empathy about dissatisfaction with weight and shape should be combined with encouragement for a weight-independent self-esteem, which reinforces that a patient's worth is not measured on a scale.

The role of the midwife with obese clients is as a consultant and coach. A good consultant recognizes that he or she is not the decision-maker, not in control, and not ultimately responsible for the outcome. A good consultant is an expert and a good listener who believes that the client has good reason for doing whatever he or she is currently doing, although the decisions may also have adverse consequences. The first step in consulting is understanding the motives for the client's actions. The next step is working with the client to appreciate the implications of behaviors on health, and moving that behavior

in a direction that would promote health. When a clinician is counseling clients about behavior change, they need to be in control, with the provider as the facilitator providing education, support, and encouragement. Behavior change takes time and is constantly evolving and changing. Overweight and obesity are life-long problems that require a strong commitment by the midwife to the client and the client to a balance of proper dietary intake, exercise, and behavioral modification.

Dietary Interventions

Dietary interventions are based on the hypothesis that overweight and obesity result when energy intake exceeds energy expenditure. A negative energy balance is needed for weight loss, and general dietary goals include reducing calorie and fat intake. Caloric restriction, developing healthier eating habits, and non-diet approaches have all been used to foster weight loss. Referral to a registered dietitian provides the client with in-depth counseling on dietary principles. Clients have to make lifestyle changes they can live with and incorporate into their daily lives. Women who are pregnant should never diet to lose weight. Refer to Chapter 6, Nutrition in Women's Health,[60] in *Varney's Midwifery*[61] and the *American Dietetic Association Complete Food and Nutrition Guide*[62] for in-depth information on nutrition and dietary guidelines.

General dietary principles include eating a healthy diet that includes five to seven servings of fruits and vegetables each day. Whole grains should take precedence over refined processed carbohydrates. Fiber intake is important to improve regularity and should be increased to 25 to 30 grams daily. Fluid intake should be increased to at least 64 ounces daily of water. Three servings of low-fat dairy products per day provide a good source of calcium. Protein should include low fat chicken and turkey, and fish at least twice a week. Sodium should be limited to no more than 2,400 mg per day.

Weight loss diets use moderate calorie reduction. A deficit of 500 to 1000 kcals per day will achieve a 1 to 2 pound weight loss per week. That is a realistic and reasonable weight loss. In the absence of exercise, a diet that contains 1400 to 1500 calories per day results in weight loss. A calorie deficit is produced through changing food choices and changing food portions. Monitoring a client's eating can be accomplished with daily food recall and journals.

Altering patterns and behaviors such as nighttime eating, binge eating, trigger foods, large portions, emotional eating, too many snacks, meal skipping, too many liquid calories, activities while eating, and dining out frequently are all areas in which the clinician can provide support. If an eating disorder is suspected, the midwife should talk with the client and make the appropriate referral to an eating disorder specialist or psychologist.

Making small, continuous, and incremental improvements in behaviors is an effective way to produce a calorie deficit and improve the overall quality of the diet and assist the client in developing a healthy dietary plan that works for them. Referral to a weight loss program sometimes works very well. Weight loss is hard work and may require long-term counseling. The clinician needs to be prepared to be flexible and provide support as the woman embarks on a journey toward improved health.

COMMERCIAL DIETS

Commercial diet programs can be useful adjuncts for clients who need nutrition education, weight monitoring, and social support (**Table 6-5**). Some programs meet weekly and others by telephone or via the Internet. Take Off Pounds Sensibly, founded in 1948, uses dietary education and a weekly weigh-in with a group meeting. Weight Watchers was founded in 1963 and uses a point system to deliver 1200 to 2200 calories per day, which are tracked in a food journal daily and brought to a weekly weigh-in and group meeting. There is an activity program and online program as well. Jenny Craig offers a program in centers, or via telephone, which includes 20 minutes weekly of a one-on-one meeting with a counselor, uses pre-prepared foods using 60% carbohydrates, 20% fat, and 20% protein, and includes an activity program. Nutrisystem is a predominately online weight loss program that provides Internet counselors, personalized exercise programs, and food journals. Pre-prepared

Table 6-5   COMPARISON OF COMMERCIAL WEIGHT LOSS PROGRAMS

Program	Meeting	Nutrition Education	Exercise Program	Pre-Prepared Foods
Take of Pounds Sensibly	Weekly	Yes	No	No
Weight Watchers	Weekly	Yes	Yes	No
Jenny Craig	Weekly	Yes	Yes	Yes
Nutrisystem	Online	No	Yes	Yes
Overeaters Anonymous	Weekly	No	No	No

food is mailed to the client's home. This program follows the same dietary guidelines as Jenny Craig. Overeaters Anonymous is patterned after the 12-Step Program of Alcohol Anonymous. Overeaters Anonymous is a weekly group recovery program that tries to address the emotional, spiritual, and physical aspects of overeating, and has no official diet. It is important to evaluate the level of support that each client needs to be successful in weight loss. Suggestions should be made that would move them toward their goals in a manner that they feel comfortable and can afford.

MEAL REPLACEMENTS

Meal replacements are an effective adjunct to diet programs that address inaccurate calorie counting and oversized portions, which lead to weight loss failure. Meal replacements include shakes, bars, soups, or frozen portion-controlled meals and provide an established caloric count. For weight loss, a 1200 to 1500 calorie meal plan is recommended. Fat calories should provide no more than 20% of total calories. Meal replacements with less than 300 calories allow fresh fruits and vegetables to be included in a meal.

SPECIFIC DIETS

Currently there are many popular diets available to the public. Many clients will seek advice on specific diets such as Atkins or South Beach. Despite incredible popularity, there is little or no long-term research to back up the claims for any of these diets except for the Ornish diet. Most popular diets are similar in structure with an introduction from the author, an idea, and then the diet plan.[63] It is important to listen to the woman's concerns and be knowledgeable about current trends, but it remains common sense to advocate balanced nutrition, better food choices, portion control, calorie counting, and exercise as research-based ways in which to lose and maintain weight loss. Each individual has to find her own nutrition and exercise balance, and the education and support provided by health care practitioners is invaluable.

The Atkins diet is based on eating a high-protein and high-fat diet with low carbohydrates.[64] In comparison, the South Beach diet is based on eating high protein chicken, turkey, and fish, and eating the right carbohydrates and fats by encouraging a balanced diet that includes plenty of fruits, vegetables, whole grains, nuts, and healthy oils.[65] The Dean Ornish diet,[66] which grew out of the Pritikin diet,[67] follows a very low-fat (10%) vegetarian diet. The Glucose Revolution diet is centered around the glycemic index.[68] The glycemic index ranks carbohydrates based on their immediate effect on blood glucose levels. Carbohydrates that break down rapidly during digestion have a higher glycemic index than carbohydrates that break down slowly and release glucose gradually. In addition, the Sugar Busters diet uses glycemic index coupled with an increased consumption of fruits, vegetables, and whole-grain foods.[69] The Zone diet advocates that the diet consist of 30% protein, 30% fat, and 40% carbohydrates.[70] The Eat Right for Your Blood Type diet is based on food that is best for your blood type and genetic make-up.[71] The Volumetrics weight control plan includes foods that are high in fiber and water.[72]

Very low calorie diets (VLCDs) can be used for severely obese (BMI >30) clients who require rapid weight loss for medical or behavioral reasons.[73] Clients on VLCDs are referred to a weight loss center and are evaluated at the clinic at least weekly. Each client requires a comprehensive history and physical exam with laboratory testing, which may include a CBC, chemistry profile, urinalysis, and an EKG. VLCDs usually last between 12 and 16 weeks and include 800 calories or less a day, high protein content (0.8–1.5 g/kg of ideal body weight per day), vitamins, minerals, electrolytes, and fatty acids, and replace usual food intake with 5 drinks a day plus an additional 64 ounces of non-caloric fluids. Adverse effects include fatigue, weakness, dizziness, constipation, hair loss, dry skin, nausea, diarrhea, change in menses, and cold intolerance. Complications include gout, gallstones, and cardiac disturbances.[73] These cannot be effectively managed in a primary care setting.

Behavioral Modification Interventions

Behavioral principles for the treatment of overweight and obesity grew out of Learning Theory.[74,75] Behavioral principles support that eating and exercise have a learned component, which can be relearned by altering environmental cues and "reinforcers" that control these behaviors.[76] Initially, behavioral programs lasted 10 weeks with weight loss averaging 4.5 kg.[77] Over the last 20 years, the length of behavioral programs has increased to 6 months with weekly meetings that focus on energy balance. Behavioral strategies include planning, self-monitoring, stimulus control, problem solving, and prevention of relapse in relation to diet and physical activity behavior, and motivational strategies.[76]

DIETARY BEHAVIOR

Weight loss requires modifying dietary intake. Calorie reduction, structured meal plans, and meal replacements with behavioral programs have all been used with varying success. Most behavioral weight loss programs encourage caloric reduction through the consumption of

1,000 to 1,500 kcal/day.[76] VLCDs providing between 400 and 800 kcal/day in a liquid formula have been found to be effective for an initial weight loss of 20 kg over 12 weeks.[78] VLCDs are expensive and necessitate continuous medical monitoring. Many clients regain weight rapidly after discontinuation of the program. Two studies found no differences in weight loss between caloric reduction diets and VLCDs.[79,80] A structured meal plan provides the client with information on how to follow a low-calorie and low-fat diet.[76] Clients learn to eat regularly and balance portions, calories, protein, carbohydrates, and fat. Meal replacements use prepared or liquid replacement meals and provide approximately 900 kcal/day, which decrease the need for medical monitoring. Providing food to clients simplifies dietary adherence.[76]

PHYSICAL ACTIVITY BEHAVIOR

Increase in physical activity has been the best predictor of long-term maintenance of weight loss.[81] The combination of changes in diet and physical activity improves weight loss and long-term maintenance. Improving exercise adherence by the use of a personal trainer and prescribing short-bout activity also improves weight loss outcomes.[76] Setting and meeting higher physical activity goals supports better weight loss and long-term weight loss maintenance.[82]

MOTIVATIONAL STRATEGIES

Motivational strategies used for weight loss and maintenance include social support and weight loss satisfaction. Social support has been found to improve long-term weight loss maintenance.[83,84] Social support from other overweight or obese individuals was instrumental in both weight loss and long-term weight loss maintenance.[83] Satisfaction with weight loss increases when clients are able to set reasonable goals to improve their health.[85]

Exercise Interventions

Exercise maintains cardiovascular health, increases flexibility and muscle strength, and improves one's sense of well-being. Exercise alone does not have a significant impact on weight loss. However, when exercise is combined with dietary changes, weight loss is enhanced. Diet and exercise interventions have been found to be effective in controlling blood glucose in 15% of clients for a few months or longer if they lost at least 7% to 10% of their body weight.[49] Less structured exercise and reducing sedentary activity appear to be more effective than higher-intensity aerobic exercise for everyone, but in particular for children and adolescents.[52]

Exercise increases flexibility and muscle strength. The benefits of exercise include improved cardiorespiratory fitness, and reduction of morbidity and mortality. Exercise has been found to reduce resting blood pressure, blood glucose levels, insulin sensitivity, and triglycerides, and increase HDL cholesterol.[86] Chapter 9, on women and exercise[87] in *Varney's Midwifery*[61] has detailed information about exercise.

DEVELOPING AN EXERCISE PROGRAM

Developing an exercise program should take into consideration the client's physical activity history, level of fitness, and whether she is normal weight, overweight, or obese. Before starting an exercise program, the client's current level of fitness must be evaluated. This information will serve as a baseline with which to compare throughout the exercise program. Clinical information such as height, weight, BMI, heart rate, and blood pressure are measured. In addition, goals, posture, flexibility, strength, past injuries, and any concerns about exercise should be assessed. Barriers to physical activity also need to be identified. A short self-reported questionnaire to use in primary care should include questions regarding leisure and exercise history. Minimum recommendations for exercise include 30 minutes of moderate intensity physical activity on most or all days of the week.[24]

The most common barriers that clients report are lack of time, convenience, or equipment. Many women work full-time and have family responsibilities. They feel pulled from many directions and have little time that they can devote to exercise. Recommendations for an initial exercise program might include starting with a 10-minute walk before breakfast, a second 10-minute walk during lunch, and a third 10-minute walk after dinner, for a total of 30 minutes of exercise a day. Lack of convenience is another problem mentioned. With every spare moment in the day spoken for, many women do not feel they can join a gym. A treadmill, stationary bicycle, or a stair climber for home use increases access. With a piece of exercise equipment in the family room, it is easier to get 30 minutes of exercise a day. Lack of enjoyment is another common concern. Physical activity should be enjoyable and each individual should try various activities to find an exercise program that they feel comfortable with and can envision themselves doing on a daily basis. Pedometers are an inexpensive way to track and challenge oneself to consistently increase activity. When assisting a client in developing an individualized exercise regimen, it is important to establish the previous level of exercise, perform a comprehensive evaluation, and medically clear a woman before starting an exercise program.

PREVIOUS LEVEL OF EXERCISE

There are several initial questions that can assist in guiding the overall assessment. What level of exercise or form of exercise did the client engage in previously? How many days a week and what duration of exercise did she engage in? This provides a foundation upon which to build a program of exercise. Activity levels can be categorized as sedentary, low activity, moderate activity, or athlete level. A sedentary level includes activities of daily living and minimal physical activity. A low activity level includes one to two 30-minute Yoga, stretching, or gentle walking sessions per week. A moderate activity level includes three or more 30-minute sessions of running, aerobics, step aerobics, or power walking. An athlete level includes daily 30-minute moderate-to-high intensity workouts.[87]

MEDICAL CLEARANCE

All clients must receive clearance from their health care provider before starting an exercise program. In addition to a comprehensive history and physical examination, an assessment of risk must be completed and may include a questionnaire (**Table 6-6**) or, if appropriate, a graded exercise test. A questionnaire provides information on the client's potential risk in participating in exercise, whereas a graded exercise test provides information on specific responses to an exercise stimulus. A graded exercise test should be conducted before starting an exercise program if the client has a medical history of coronary heart disease or a metabolic disorder. A graded exercise test consists of walking on a treadmill or riding a stationary bike while on a cardiac monitor to determine if a heart condition exists. The level of work starts out low and increases gradually until symptoms such as chest pain or shortness of breath occur or the patient reaches a prede-

termined heart rate. Low risk clients include women under the age of 55 who do not experience cardiovascular symptoms and have no more than one coronary artery disease risk factor, including obesity, sedentary lifestyle, impaired glucose tolerance, hypertension, hyperlipidemia, smoking, or a family history of coronary artery disease. Moderate risk clients include women over age 55 years and those with more than one coronary artery disease risk factor. High-risk clients include women with a history or with signs of cardiovascular, pulmonary, or metabolic disease.[23] An individual's target heart rate determines the ideal range of heartbeats per minute during exercise based on age. Morbidly obese clients may reach their target heart rate with walking alone. They should start with a gentle walking and stretching program or exercising in a pool to decrease stress on joints and muscles. As their health improves and they feel comfortable, they can increase their physical activity.

GOALS

Exercise programs with goals that are designed by the client provide a firm foundation upon which to build a program that motivates her and maintains interest. In addition, self-generated goals provide the client with an opportunity to adjust and change as her program progresses. She can evaluate her own progress with the expertise and support of a personal trainer or exercise physiologist.

POSTURE

Maintaining posture is important for all women. One of the more obvious changes in women who are overweight or obese is a change in posture. Posture changes as the weight of the abdomen

Table 6-6 MEDICAL CLEARANCE QUESTIONNAIRE

Age and Exercise
1. Are you age 46 or older? — Yes ☐ No ☐
2. How many days are you currently exercising each week? — _____________
3. How intense is the exercise you do each week on a scale from 1 to 5? — _____________
   (1 = very low, 2 = low, 3 = medium, 4 = high, 5 = very high)

Disease
1. Do you have diabetes? — Yes ☐ No ☐
2. Do you have heart trouble? — Yes ☐ No ☐
3. Have you had a stroke? — Yes ☐ No ☐
4. Do you have asthma or exercise-induced asthma? — Yes ☐ No ☐
5. Do you have chronic bronchitis or emphysema? — Yes ☐ No ☐
6. Do you have a pacemaker or cardiac defibrillator? — Yes ☐ No ☐

Symptoms
1. Do you ever have pain in your chest or heart? — Yes ☐ No ☐
2. In the last year, have you had shortness of breath, which happened when you were resting? If yes, then how often? _____________ — Yes ☐ No ☐
3. Do you faint or have dizzy spells? — Yes ☐ No ☐
4. In the last year, have you had shortness of breath at night? — Yes ☐ No ☐
5. Have you ever had back or joint pain? — Yes ☐ No ☐
6. Have you ever had a heart murmur? — Yes ☐ No ☐
7. Has your heart ever "raced" or "skipped" beats? — Yes ☐ No ☐

Risk Factors
1. Have you ever smoked? — Yes ☐ No ☐
2. Have you ever had high blood pressure? — Yes ☐ No ☐
3. Have you ever had high cholesterol? — Yes ☐ No ☐
4. Have you ever had high triglycerides? — Yes ☐ No ☐
5. Has anyone is your family had heart disease or had a heart attack before the age of 55? — Yes ☐ No ☐
   If yes, then how are you related? _____________

Medications
1. Have you ever taken medication for high blood pressure? — Yes ☐ No ☐
2. Have you ever taken medication for high cholesterol? — Yes ☐ No ☐
3. Have you ever taken medication for high blood sugar? — Yes ☐ No ☐
4. Have you ever taken medication for a heart condition? — Yes ☐ No ☐
5. Have you ever taken medication for asthma? — Yes ☐ No ☐

How would you rate your overall health?
   Excellent ☐   Good ☐   Fair ☐   Poor ☐

Medical clearance is required by your health care provider before beginning an exercise program if you answered YES to any of the previous questions.

and breast increases the curvature of the lower back (*lumbar lordosis*), and the forward rounding of the upper spine and shoulders (*kyphosis*) become more pronounced. Posture can be assessed by asking the client to stand against a wall as the health care provider reviews her body shape and angle from the side.[88] **Table 6-7** contrasts between poor and good posture. Abdominal and back muscle weakness is a contributing factor in the development of poor posture.

FLEXIBILITY

Evaluation of flexibility includes two important stretches that provide baseline information regarding level of flexibility. It is imperative to ensure that the client is not too flexible, since increased joint laxity can lead to an increased risk of injury.[89] First, ask the client to sit on the floor with her legs together and straight out in front of her. Next, with her arms stretched straight out in front of her, ask her to bend at the waist to see how far her fingertips can reach. She is very flexible if she can extend her hands past her toes. Second, ask the client to sit on the floor with her legs spread out in front of her in a "V" shape. With her back straight, ask her to bend at the waist and see how far her chest can go toward the floor. If her chest can touch the floor then she is very flexible. The client should

be sure not to overstretch and always be aware of her movements and keep control to prevent injury due to increased joint laxity. If the client is inflexible, then it is important to design a program that gently increases flexibility over time. An inflexible client would not be able to touch her toes when sitting with her legs positioned in a "V." If the client is inflexible, careful attention should be paid to ensure an adequate warm-up period and performance of exercises in a slow and controlled manner.

STRENGTH

An evaluation of the client's strength includes questioning whether she has lifted weights before. If a client has never lifted weights, or has not done so recently, she can begin by lifting either 1- or 2-pound free weights, with 10 to 12 repetitions for 2 to 3 sets, resting between sets. She may increase the sets if she is comfortable and does not feel challenged. However, if she can only manage part of the exercise sets before tiring, then she should decrease the amount of weight or resistance, and decrease the number of repetitions; she may then increase the number of sets. The client should be monitored by a trainer to make sure the exercises are being performed correctly to evaluate her weight training and increase or decrease the amount of

Table 6-7 ASSESSMENT OF POSTURE

Poor Posture	Good Posture
Head is forward with chin toward chest	Head should be aligned with body
Shoulders are rounded forward	Shoulders should be pulled back
Chest is concave	Shoulders are pulled back and chest straightens out
Pelvis is tilting forward	Pelvis should be tucked under the body
Lordosis of the back	The natural curve should remain

weight as needed. A trainer will ensure that body mechanics, breathing, and intensity level are maintained at proper levels throughout the workout.

FREQUENCY, INTENSITY, DURATION, AND TYPE OF ACTIVITY

The frequency, intensity, duration, and type of activity must be considered when starting an exercise program. The frequency of activity for women regardless of weight is that they should engage in an exercise program on most days of the week. Body weight stabilizes as energy expenditure increases.

The more vigorous the intensity of exercise, the greater the health-related benefits. Current recommendations from the CDC call for individuals to engage in moderate level activity for 30 minutes each day, most days of the week. Exercise intensity can be prescribed using different modalities, as a percentage of maximal heart rate (**Table 6-8**),[23] or by using various measures of self-perceived exertions such as the Borg Scale (**Table 6-9**).[90] Lower numbers correspond to light activities and higher numbers correspond to more strenuous activities. Clients can manually check their pulse or wear a heart rate monitor. Women should be taught how to calculate their perceived exertion or percentage of maximal heart rate to ensure that they are challenging themselves during exercise sessions.

Duration of activity is inversely related to the intensity of the activity.[23] If a client exercises moderately, she will need to exercise longer. Conversely, if a client exercises more vigorously, she does not need to exercise as long as the moderate exerciser to burn the same number of calories. The goal for overweight and obese clients is to exercise a minimum of 150 minutes per week or 30 minutes 5 days a week. If this is too difficult, then these women can begin by engaging in activity for at least 10 minutes' duration and increase, as they feel comfortable. Research demonstrates that cardiorespiratory fitness can be improved by accumulating exercise in 10-minute bouts.[91,92] Clinical evidence supports that exercise greater than the minimum recommendation of 150 minutes per week may be important in long-term weight loss and maintenance.[82]

Table 6-8 COMPUTING APPROPRIATE EXERCISE INTENSITY

Intensity Variable	Formula for Computation	Intensity Criteria	
		Moderate	Vigorous
Percentage of Maximal Heart Rate ($\%Hr_{max}$)	$\%Hr_{max} = Hr_{max} \times$ Desired $\%$	55%–69%	70%–89%
Percentage of Maximal Heart Rate Reserve ($\%HrR$)	$\%HrR = [(\%Hr_{max} -$ Resting Hr$) \times$ Desired $\%] +$ Resting Hr	40%–50%	60%–84%

Source: Reproduced with permission. Jakicic JM, Gallagher KI. Physical activity considerations for management of body weight. In: Bessesen DH, Kushner R, editors. *Evaluation and Management of Obesity.* Philadelphia, PA: Hanley & Belfus; 2002. p. 79.

Table 6-9 METHODS USED TO EVALUATE LEVEL OF EXERCISE

Goal: 30 Minutes of Moderate Intensity Exercise on Most Days of the Week

Method Used to Measure Intensity	Talk Test(1)	Pedometer	Borg Scale (2)	Metabolic(3) Equivalent Level*
Definition Based On	Ability to talk	Number of Steps per Day	Self perception of intensity of exercise using all senses (physical stress, fatigue, effort)	Measured by how hard the individual works at performing an activity.
Sedentary		2000	6 No exertion 7 Very Very Light 8	
Light Intensity	Able to sing	6000-8000	9 Very Light 10 11 Light	Walking slowly Swimming, slow treading Dusting/vacuuming
Moderate Intensity	**Able to carry on conversation comfortably**	7000–10,000	12 **13 Somewhat Hard** 14	**Walking briskly Swimming, recreational Mowing lawn Scrubbing floors**
Vigorous Intensity	Becomes winded or can not talk comfortably	11,000–15,000	15 Hard 16 17 Very Hard 18 19 Extremely Hard 20 Maximal Exertion	Jogging or running Swimming laps Mowing lawn with hand mower Moving furniture

*One MET=the energy used by the body at rest (reading, sitting quietly). 3–6 MET = moderate activity, >6 MET = vigarous activity

(1) CDC. Physical Activity for Everyone: Measuring Physical Activity Intensity: Talk Test. Available at www.cdc.gov/nccdphp/dnpa/physical/measuring/talk_test.htm

(2) CDC. Physical Activity for Everyone: Measuring Physical Activity Intensity: Perceived Exertion (Borg Rating of Perceived Exertion Scale) Available at http://www.cdc.gov/nccdhp/dnpa/physical/measuring /perceived_exertion.htm

(3) CDC. Physical Activity for Everyone: Measuring Physical Activity Intensity. Measuring Physical Activity Intensity Available at http://cdc.gov/nccdphp/dna/physical/met.htm

The type of activity suggested should provide physiologic benefits and be enjoyable for the client. When clients are overweight or obese, walking is a good activity to recommend. It requires little equipment or skill, can be performed anywhere, and the individual can select the intensity. Resistance training, Yoga, or flexibility training may improve strength and endurance when added to walking or another form of aerobic activity. Lifestyle activities to decrease sedentary activity, such as taking the stairs instead of the elevator or parking on the other side of the parking lot when going shopping provide additional physical activity. Pedometers provide visual feedback on daily activity levels and are relatively inexpensive. Clients should aim for at least 10,000 steps per day. Sedentary individuals take between 3000 and 6000 steps, moderately active individuals 7000 and 10,000, and very active individuals take between 11,000 and 15,000 steps per day.[93] Pedometer step goals should be increased by the client weekly.

Types of Exercise

A successful exercise program includes cardiovascular endurance, strength, muscular endurance, and flexibility through a cross-training program of aerobic, anaerobic, resistance, and flexibility exercises. Cardiovascular endurance depends on the system's ability to pump blood and deliver oxygen to the body. A well-conditioned heart beats between 40 to 70 beats per minute. Cardiovascular endurance is increased by aerobic activities such as walking, hiking, jogging, running, bicycling, or swimming. Strength training uses a muscle or group of muscles to exert an amount of force in a one-time burst of effort. Weight training or resistance training (which are versions of strength training) increase muscle and bone strength and muscle mass. The majority of muscles have fast and slow-twitch fibers. Fast-twitch fibers provide the explosive force used in weight lifting. Slow-twitch fibers are for endurance. When weights are lifted, muscle fibers are stretched and slightly injured and heal stronger secondary to microscopic scarring. Muscular endurance is achieved with exercise and increases the ability of the body to resist fatigue while holding a position, carrying something for a long period of time, or repeating a movement without getting tired. Flexibility is the ability of joints and muscles to achieve full range of motion.

AEROBIC

Aerobic exercise is any exercise that uses large muscles and is sustained for two minutes or longer. The heart and lungs work to supply oxygen to the body. As the heart and lungs work harder, they are conditioned and strengthened. Aerobic activities include walking, hiking, jogging, running, bicycling, or swimming. A session of aerobic activity should last from 20 to 60 minutes. At least three or more hours of aerobic activity a week will strengthen the heart. The benefits of aerobic activity include lowering the risk of heart attack by improving the cholesterol profile and increasing bone strength.

ANAEROBIC

Anaerobic exercise is any exercise that requires short bursts of power, such as weight training or sprinting, and does not require a significant increase in oxygen delivery to the muscle. Since energy supplies in the muscles are limited, anaerobic exercises can only be sustained for a short period of time. Obese women who may be in poor physical shape may not be efficient at taking in oxygen and may reach their anaerobic threshold while exercising at very low levels of intensity. As these women increase their level of fitness, they will be able to supply more oxygen to muscles and use less stored energy. Although anaerobic training improves performance, it does not provide the same health benefits as aerobic exercise. However, anaerobic training will improve oxygen delivery during training over time.

RESISTANCE

Resistance or strength training increases muscle strength and mass, bone strength, and metabolism. It is useful in improving weight loss, body image, and self-esteem. Resistance training increases muscle strength by putting a strain on the muscle, which increases the load and stimulates the growth of protein in the muscle cell, which increases the ability of the muscle to generate force. Resistance training uses free weights, weight machines, and calisthenics. When lifting free weights the client controls the bar, weights, and the body positioning through the range of motion. Weight machines allow the client to lift weight, but controls the motion performed. Calisthenics use the client's body weight as the resistance force through the motion of performing chin-ups, sit-ups, or push-ups. Resistance tubing uses an elastic band that provides resistance to active muscles. The client should do two to three 30-minute resistance workouts per week. Three sets of 8 to 15 repetitions, increasing weight with each set, will increase muscle endurance and tone. Regular weight training increases HDL and metabolic rate, burns calories, reduces fat tissue, and increases bone mineral content.

Isometric, isotonic, and isokinetic exercises are used in strength training as well. In isometric exercises, the muscles contract, but the joints do not move and muscle fibers maintain a constant length. Isometric exercises are performed against an immovable surface (wall) and have been found effective in developing total strength of a particular muscle or muscle group. In isotonic exercises, the body part is moved and the muscle shortens or lengthens. Lifting free weights, sit-ups, push-ups, and pull-ups are isotonic exercises. Isokinetic exercises require a machine that controls the speed of contraction within the range of motion and are not readily available to the public.

FLEXIBILITY

Flexibility exercises use stretching movements to increase the length of the muscles and are effective to increase joint range of motion. The goal of stretching is to lengthen the connective tissue surrounding muscle tissues and should be done only after the muscles have been warmed up by 5 to 10 minutes of gentle low-impact aerobic activity. Stretching should not be done when the muscles are cold or injuries may occur. Each stretching exercise should take between one to two minutes. Stretching at least three times a week may improve mobility, movement, and posture, and prevent injury. Yoga, Tai Chi, and dance classes provide excellent sources of stretching exercises.

Hydration and Food Intake

Current recommendations on hydration and food intake before exercise include individualizing hydration; drinking an appropriate amount of fluids before, during, and after exercise; and recognizing the signs and symptoms of dehydration.

Adequate hydration in daily exercise optimizes performance and minimizes the incidence of heat illness. Fluids are lost through perspiration and urine, and should be replaced on an individual basis. The Sweat Rate = [(pre-exercise body weight − post-exercise body weight) + (fluid intake − urine volume)] ÷ exercise time in hours.[94] The Sweat Rate allows for a calculation of a range of environmental conditions and practices. Each client drinks a different amount of fluid. She should be encouraged to monitor how much she drinks and be sure that it matches the amount that is lost. Clients who are engaged in high intensity physical activities or exercise (e.g., running) in hot humid climates can use the sweat rate to prevent dehydration.

Drinking the appropriate amount before, during, and after exercise is important in maintaining hydration and improving recovery. The woman should consume 17 to 20 ounces at least two to three hours before exercising and another 7 to 10 ounces after warming up. During exercise, she needs 28 to 40 ounces every hour of exercise or 7 to 10 ounces for every 10 to 15 minutes of exercise. After exercise, fluids lost through sweat and urine can be replaced within two hours by drinking 20 to 24 ounces for every pound lost through sweat. The optimal oral hydration solution should include water, carbohydrates, and electrolytes (70–1266 mg sodium and 14–17 g of carbohydrates) before, during, and after exercise.[94]

The signs and symptoms of dehydration include thirst, irritability, headache, weakness, dizziness, cramps, chills, vomiting, nausea, head or neck sensations, decreased performance, or general discomfort. If the client exhibits any of these symptoms, she should stop exercising immediately, lie down, increase hydration fluids, and notify medical personnel.

Food intake before exercise needs proper timing to prevent nausea, cramps in the side, and general discomfort. After eating a meal, blood is directed to the stomach to facilitate digestion.

If an individual exercises too soon after eating, the blood is redirected to the working muscles, which may cause nausea and cramps. It is best to have nothing in the stomach or intestines for two to three hours before high intensity exercise. This allows the body time to digest and avoid feeling hungry. However, exercising on an empty stomach may leave an individual feeling energy depleted. Eating a small snack with carbohydrates, such as fruits, vegetables, and grains two to three hours before exercise will provide the energy needed to complete an exercise session. An exercise program is included in the last section of this chapter.

NON-PRESCRIPTION WEIGHT LOSS PRODUCTS

Over-the-counter non-prescription herbal and alternative medicine weight loss products have developed into a multimillion dollar industry in the United States. Women may not consider these "medications" that need to be reported to their care provider. Clinicians need to be both familiar and knowledgeable regarding non-prescription weight loss products. Those currently on the market have very limited documented research supporting their claims. There are no data to suggest that the use of these products during pregnancy would be safe.

The Food and Drug Administration (FDA) recently banned ephedra alkoloids in non-prescription products. Health concerns associated with ephedra included myocardial infarction, severe hypertension, cardiac arrhthmias, hemorrhagic and ischemic strokes, and death.[95–97]

Many weight loss products continue to use caffeine. Scientific evidence suggests that caffeine increases oxygen consumption and fat oxidation.[98] Caffeine stimulates the nervous system at the cortex, medulla, and spinal cord.[99]

It has been used to treat fatigue and headaches. Caffeine is approved by the FDA at a dose of 200 mg every three hours or a total of 1600 mg per day for clients over the age of 12 years old.

Green tea catechins are widely consumed throughout Asia and are becoming popular in the United States. Green tea leaves of *Camelia sinensis* belong to the family of compounds of epigallocatechin gallate and are considered a powerful antioxidant. Catechins have been found to increase energy expenditure by enhancing the sympathetic nervous system at the level of the fat-cell adrenoreceptor.[98] It has been difficult to demonstrate the effects of green tea catechins alone. The net effect of calories burned by drinking several cups of green tea is approximately 80 calories per day.[100]

Garcina Cambogia, which is an extract from the rind of the brindall berry, contains hydroxycitric acid. Hydroxycitric acid has been found to inhibit lyase, which is the enzyme in the synthesis of fatty acid outside the mitochondrion. Hydroxycitric acid is taken in doses from 500 to 1500 mg per day.[98] Garcina cambogia has been found to have no effect on obesity.[101]

Chromium picolinate has been found to promote weight loss and enhance the effectiveness of the insulin response to glucose.[102–104] This response requires exercise while taking the supplement.[98] Chromium picolinate is taken in 200 μg per day doses and has a wide margin of safety and low incidence of toxicity. Thus far, chromium picolinate has not been found to be effective in the treatment of obesity.[105]

Beta-hydroxy-beta-methylbutyrate (HMB) is a metabolite of leucine, which burns fat and builds both strength and muscle tissue and has been found to reduce muscle catabolism and increase fat-free mass during weight lifting.[106] HMB has been taken in doses ranging from 1.5

to 3 grams per day,[98] but it has not been tested as a treatment for obesity.

Fiber has been found to decrease food intake and decrease hunger. Water-soluble fiber may support better weight loss outcomes than water-insoluble fiber.[98] Lean individuals eat more fiber when compared with obese individuals.[107] Research suggests that increasing dietary intake of fiber by 5 to 40 grams per day can improve weight loss outcomes.[98]

Chitosan has been advertised as a fat blocker. Acetylated chitin is harvested from shrimp exoskeletons and is taken in doses from 1200 to 1600 mg twice a day. Chitosan binds lipids such as cholesterol and triglycerides in the intestines. To date, chitosan has not been found to affect weight loss in doses that are recommended for human consumption.[98]

Pharmacologic Therapy

Pharmacologic therapy should be guided by the principles of *beneficence* (benefits) and *nonmalfeasance* (risks).

Benefits may include the reduction in health risks such as hyperlipidemia, hypertension, and coronary artery disease, and improvement in psychosocial benefits such as an improved quality of life or decrease in depression. Each client prescribed pharmacologic therapy for weight loss must be fully competent, independent, and in a position to make decisions relevant to his or her health. As a part of the informed consent, the risks, benefits, possible side effects, and course of treatment should be discussed and questions answered.

Centrally acting anorexiants increase satiety and decrease hunger, thereby reducing calorie intake and providing a greater sense of control (**Table 6-10**). They target the ventromedial and lateral hypothalamic regions in the central

Table 6-10 PHARMACOLOGIC AGENTS

Generic (Trade Name)	Dosage (DEA Schedule)	Class/Action
Phenylpropanolamine (Acutrim)	75 mg SR qd (OTC)	Centrally acting adrenergic; alpha-1 agonist
Phenylpropanolamine (Dexatrim)	75 mg SR qd or 25 mg tid (OTC)	
Phenylpropanolamine (Prolamine)	37.5 mg qd (OTC)	
Phentermine (Adipex-P)	37.5 mg qd (IV)	Centrally acting adrenergic; stimulates norepinephrine release
Phendimetrazine (Bontril)	105 mg SR qd (III)	
Benzphetamine (Didrex)	25-50 mg qd-tid (III)	
Phenteramine (Fastin)	30 mg qd (IV)	
Phenteramine (Ionamin)	15–30 mg qd (IV)	
Phendimetrazine (Plegine)	105 mg SR qd (III)	
Phendimetrazine (Prelu-2)	105 mg SR qd (III)	
Diethyloproprion (Tenuate)	75 mg SR qd or 25 mg tid (IV)	
Mazindol (Mazonor)	1 mg tid (IV)	Centrally acting adrenergic; blocks norepinephrine reuptake
Mazindol (Sanorex)	1 mg qd (IV)	
Sibutramine (Meridia)	5–15 mg qd (IV)	Centrally acting adrenergic and serotonergic serotonin and norepinephrine reuptake inhibitor
Orlistat (Xenical)	120 mg tid (not scheduled)	Lipase inhibitor; gastric and pancreatic lipase inhibitor

Abbreviations are: DEA, Drug Enforcement Agency; OTC, over-the-counter; qd, every day; tid, three times a day; SR, sustained release.

Sources: 1) NHLBI Obesity Education Initiative Practical Guide: Identification, Evaluation, and Treatment of Overweight and Obesity in Adults. U.S. Department of Health and Human Services, Public Health Service, National Institutes of Health, National Lung, and Blood Institute. NIH Publication No. 00-4804. October 2000.
2) Halpern A, Mancini MC. Treatment of obesit: an update on anti-obesity medications. *Obesity Reviews.* 4(1):25–42.

nervous system and augment the neurotransmission of norepinephrine, serotonin, and dopamine, thereby decreasing food intake.[108] Adrenergic drugs either stimulate norepinephrine release or block its reuptake, which results in improved appetite control. Two centrally acting serotonergic drugs (fenfluamine, dexfenfluramine), which were selective for stimulating serotonin release and blocking its reuptake, were withdrawn from the market in September 1997, because of an increased risk of valvular heart disease.[109]

Adrenergic and serotonergic drugs function as serotonin and norepinephrine reuptake inhibitors (SNRI). The only two drugs approved for long-term use are sibutramine and orlistat. Sibutramine is not chemically related to the amphetamine class. Sibutramine cannot be used with clients with a history of coronary artery disease, arrhythmias, uncontrolled hypertension, or stroke but can be used in clients with controlled hypertension. SNRIs should not be used in clients taking monoamine oxidase inhibitors, other centrally acting appetite suppressants, selective serotonin reuptake inhibitor antidepressants, SNRIs (venlaxafine), or P450 (3A4) cytochrome inhibitors such as ketaconazole and erythromycin.[108,109]

Orlistat is the first nonsystemic drug that acts directly in the gastrointestinal tract for weight loss. As a pentaenoic acid ester, orlistat forms a covalent bond with the active serine residue site of gastric and pancreatic lipases, inhibiting their activity and preventing reabsorption of about 30% of dietary fat. On a 2000 calorie, 30% fat diet, orlistat would block 22 grams of fat or 200 calories per day. Orlistat also negatively reinforces clients when they eat a high fat meal by the appearance of side effects such as anal leakage and diarrhea. Orlistat has been found to decrease total cholesterol, LDL, blood pressure, glucose and insulin.[108,109] Malabsorption of vitamins A, D, E, K, and beta-carotene are a concern. Patients on orlistat should take a supplement including these vitamins at bedtime. Both sibutramine and orlistat should be started in parallel with lifestyle modifications when a client has a BMI of 30 or above, or 27 or above in the presence of other risk factors. Lifestyle modifications including a low fat, low cholesterol diet and exercise increase weight loss and minimize the side effects of orlistat. The drugs should be discontinued for any side effects, when the client's BMI is within normal limits, or within two years.[108,109]

Surgical Treatment

Surgical treatment of obesity or bariatric surgery should only be considered for clients with severe obesity (BMI >40), or those with a BMI above 35 associated with serious co-morbidities such as coronary artery disease or diabetes. A multidisciplinary team that incorporates medical, nutritional, and psychological care should thoroughly examine the client before a decision is made. Bariatric surgery clients require long-term follow-up to maintain success and treat any complications as they may arise.

Currently, there are two surgical approaches: vertical banded gastroplasty (VBG) and Roux-en-Y gastric bypass (RYGB) surgery. By reducing stomach storage capacity to between 30 and 50 centimeters and reducing the stomach's emptying rate by narrowing the stomach exit to 10 millimeters in diameter, the volume and rate of food consumed is decreased.[110,111] Both surgeries are effective in producing an average loss of approximately 50% of excess body weight that is maintained in 60% of clients for at least five years.[110] The RYGB further limits caloric intake by inducing a dumping syndrome whenever sugar is consumed. There are more vitamin deficiencies associated with RYGB than VBG surgery.[111] Up to 25% of bariatric surgeries fail because of over-consumption of food, which effectively stretches the stomach and allows an increased intake of calories and volume.[110] Reducing the failure rate of bariatric surgery requires a team approach with close follow-up over time.

Weight Loss Maintenance

The National Weight Control Registry (NWCR) was founded in 1994 by Doctors Wing and Hill to follow clients who succeeded at long-term weight loss.[112] The NWCR now includes over 3,000 subjects who have maintained a minimum weight loss of 30 pounds for at least one year. Successful weight loss was accomplished by eating a low-fat, high carbohydrate diet, monitoring their weight and food intake, and regularly engaging in high levels of exercise.[112]

Currently, there are many obesity resources available on the Internet for both clients and midwives to assist in both weight loss and maintenance.[113] These include general information such as nutrition, exercise, surgery, and organizations dedicated to the treatment of obesity (**Table 6-11**).

Obesity and Pregnancy

Obesity in pregnant women is also increasing at an alarming rate. The prevalence of obesity in women aged 18 to 29 years old has increased by 70% compared to 47% for women overall.[114] Young women with obesity have been found to have higher rates of insulin resistance, impaired

Table 6-11 OBESITY WEB SITES

Sponsor	Web Site Address
American College of Sports Medicine	http://www.acsm.org
American Council on Exercise	http://www.acefitness.org
American Obesity Association	http://www.obesity.org
American Society of Bariatric Physicians	http://www.asbp.org
American Society for Bariatric Surgery	http://www.abs.org/html/ration.html
Centers for Disease Control and Prevention	http://www.cdc.gov
National Institute of Diabetes, Digestive, and Kidney Disease; National Institutes of Health (NIH)	http://www.hiddk.nih.gov/health/nutrit/pubs/presmed
NAASO, The Obesity Society	http://www.naaso.org
National Agricultural Library, United States Department of Agriculture	http://nutrition.gov
Partnership for Healthy Weight Management	http://www.consumer.gov/weightloss/
The American Dietetic Association	http://www.eatright.org

NASSO, The Obesity Society

glucose tolerance, type II diabetes, hypercholesterolemia, and polycystic ovarian syndrome.[115] According to Institute of Medicine (IOM) guidelines, women who become pregnant are overweight if their baseline BMI ranges from 26.1 to 28.9 and obese if their BMI is 29 or above (**Table 6-12**).[116] Recommendations from the IOM suggest that BMI before pregnancy be used as a guide to calculate the amount of weight to be gained during pregnancy. Obese women are more likely to develop preeclampsia and to require a cesarean section.[117] In addition, their pregnancies are more likely to end in miscarriage or antepartum fetal death[118]; their babies are more likely to be macrosomic and to develop obesity later in childhood.[10,117] In addition, excessive gestational weight gain increases the likelihood that women will retain weight postpartum, with minority women who have lower incomes retaining the most weight.[119,128]

Management of Obesity During Pregnancy

Treatment goals for overweight and obese pregnant women include stabilizing weight gain, improving nutrition, increasing physical activity, and decreasing sedentary activity. It is important for women who are pregnant to not diet, but to follow a nutritious dietary plan that provides healthy whole foods that encourage weight stabilization.

Dietary Interventions

Pregnant women who are overweight or obese should follow the same basic guidelines of proper nutrition as the non-pregnant overweight or obese women with the following differences. Women who are pregnant should consume sufficient calories to gain the proper amount of weight and sustain the growing child. Approximately 300 additional calories a day are suggested to meet this goal. Women require about 64 to 80 ounces of fluid per day, and more in hot weather and when exercising. Nutrients are best in their natural form, so enriching the diet with whole grains, fruits, and vegetables also will increase fiber and help prevent constipation. Simple things such as looking for labels on foods reading 100% whole wheat or whole grain, drinking 100% fruit juice, eating more fruits and vegetables, and substituting 2 egg whites for 1 whole egg in recipes decrease both fat and cholesterol content.[86]

Table 6-12 PREGNANCY WEIGHT GAIN RECOMMENDATIONS

Weight Before Pregnancy	BMI	Suggested Gestational Weight Gain, *pounds*
Underweight	<19.8	28–40
Normal	19.9–26.0	25–35
Overweight	26.1–28.9	15–25
Obese >29.0		15, Upper limit unspecified

Source: Used with permission from the National Academy of Sciences. Nutrition during pregnancy: Part I, Weight gain and nutrient supplements. Washington, DC: National Academy Press; 1990.

Behavioral Modification Interventions

Behavioral modification interventions during pregnancy include dietary and exercise behaviors and motivational strategies to encourage proper weight gain during pregnancy. Dieting during pregnancy is not recommended. Pregnancy is a time in most women's lives when they are willing to make healthy behavior change for both themselves and their unborn child. Assisting women in learning portion control, adding an additional 300 calories per day, eating whole grains, fruits, and vegetables, and drinking an adequate amount of fluid are all important ways to positively modify dietary behavior. Foods that should be avoided during pregnancy include soft unpasteurized cheese, processed food, and raw or undercooked meat or fish. If the pregnant woman is healthy and has received clearance from her midwife, she should be encouraged to partake in exercise daily. Motivation should include a healthy pregnancy for both the woman and her unborn child, proper weight gain, and general feeling of well-being.

Exercise Interventions

As reviewed earlier in this chapter, exercise alone does not have a significant impact on weight stabilization. However, when regular exercise is combined with healthy dietary changes, weight stabilization is enhanced. Exercise during pregnancy can assist in achieving a healthy weight gain, determined by the pregnant woman's pre-pregnancy BMI.[116] Exercise should never be used for weight loss during pregnancy.

There are very few standards of care regarding exercise and pregnancy. Each woman enters pregnancy with an individual medical and exercise history, and each pregnancy progresses differently. To date, there have been few studies in women who exercise during pregnancy, and a large majority of these studies have demonstrated results that have been either equivocal or contradictory.[121] Therefore, women have difficulty integrating their pre-pregnant exercise routine into a pregnant exercise routine. Most healthy women can continue their pre-pregnant routine with some adaptations throughout their entire pregnancy as long as there are no medical complications. The American College of Obstetricians and Gynecologists (ACOG) supports that exercising at least 30 minutes on most, if not all, days provides clear benefits to both the mother and unborn child.[122] The Society of Obstetricians and Gynecologists of Canada has released guidelines that suggest it may be detrimental not to exercise during pregnancy.[123]

Some exercise activities that a woman engages in pre-pregnancy are contraindicated during pregnancy; these include scuba diving and sky-diving. ACOG suggests exercises that put the pregnant woman at risk of falling or receiving a blow to the abdomen should be avoided.[122] However, Clapp[124] suggests that knowing the client's gestation, goals, experience, and potential for injury should all be considered before advising a woman to avoid a particular exercise. Therefore, a thorough evaluation and careful program design can provide a safe exercise regime that will support a women's desire to remain physically active throughout her entire pregnancy. Please refer to *Varney's Midwifery*[87] for an excellent review of exercise in pregnancy.

Health care providers who are not familiar with current absolute and relative contraindications[125] regarding exercise and pregnancy may not provide the client with proper counsel (**Table 6-13**). However, relative and absolute

Table 6-13 CONTRAINDICATIONS TO EXERCISE IN PREGNANCY

Absolute Contraindications	Relative Indications
Hemodynamically significant heart disease	Severe anemia
Restrictive lung disease	Unevaluated maternal cardiac arrhythmia
Incompetent cervix or cerclage	Chronic bronchitis
Multiple gestation at risk for premature labor	Poorly controlled type 1 diabetes
Persistent second or third trimester bleeding	Extreme morbid obesity
Placenta previa after 26 weeks of gestation	History of extremely sedentary lifestyle
Premature labor during the current pregnancy	Intrauterine growth restriction in current pregnancy
Hypertension	Poorly controlled hypertension
	Orthopedic limitations
	Poorly controlled seizure disorder
	Poorly controlled hyperthyroidism

Source: Adapted from America College of Obstetricians and Gynecologists. Committee Opinion No. 267, Exercise during pregnancy and the postpartum period. *Obstet Gyneco* 2002;99:171–173.

contraindications to exercise are very restrictive and may cause some women to refrain from exercising or continue to exercise but keep this information from their midwife for fear the provider will tell her to stop. Clapp[124] states that pregnancy is normal and except in certain conditions, healthy pregnant women should continue their pre-pregnant levels of exercise.

Exercise does not need to be continuous to be beneficial.[126] Short (10 min) periods of moderate activity will produce health benefits and may burn more than 150 calories. Moderate activities include pushing a stroller for one mile in 30 minutes, swimming laps for 20 minutes, stair walking for 15 minutes, or walking briskly for 30 minutes. If the client regularly engaged in weight training before pregnancy, then she may continue to do so during pregnancy, provided she is comfortable and doing it correctly.

Education about Exercise for Pregnant Women

Women who are pregnant should maintain a comfortable level of exercise, but they should be taught about adaptations needed in order to exercise safely in pregnancy. These adaptations include avoiding the use of the valsalva maneuver, sitting and back lying positions while exercising; using appropriate measures to determine a safe level of exertion; and using correct body mechanics, proper posture, and exercise techniques in order to prevent worsening of backache and diastasis recti commonly found in pregnant women.

VALSALVA MANEUVER

The valsalva maneuver is performed when an individual exhales forcibly against a closed glottis while no air enters through the nose or mouth.[25] Individuals can perform the valsalva maneuver while lifting heavy weights, straining during a bowel movement, or strenuous coughing. During the valsalva maneuver, return of venous blood to the heart is decreased and the client may feel lightheaded. The woman needs to breathe without holding her breath and unintentionally doing the valsalva maneuver, which can decrease oxygenation to the fetus.

The woman can be taught to count aloud while exercising.

HEART RATE VERSUS PERCEIVED EXERTION

It is no longer an accepted standard that a heart rate of 140 beats per minute is appropriate for pregnant women. A target heart rate of 140 beats per minute may be too low for a novice who has never exercised before or too high for an avid exerciser. There are many changes to the cardiovascular system during pregnancy, so that use of a target heart rate may be unreliable in determining physical exertion. Currently, most texts recommend using the Borg's scale of the Rate of Perceived Exertion a scale ranging from 0 to 10, with 0 being no exertion and 10 being very, very strong exertion (Table 6-9).[127]

SITTING VERSUS STANDING

During pregnancy, extended periods of motionless standing are not advisable, even during the course of exercise. Motionless standing can decrease venous return and cause edema in the lower extremities. The tailor sit position is a much better position in which to exercise (**Figure 6-3**). The tailor sit places the woman is in a seated position, with her weight on her buttocks, legs crossed in front of her and her back extended and relaxed. Most exercises can be modified to a seated position. For the seated exercises detailed later in this section, the tailor sit is the desired start position.

BACK LYING

There is debate whether a pregnant woman can exercise safely while lying on her back. The back lying position can cause a decrease in cardiac output by putting pressure on the inferior vena cava. Pressure from the weight of the uterus and fetus decreases blood flow to the uterus, placenta, and fetus. ACOG suggests avoiding exercise in a

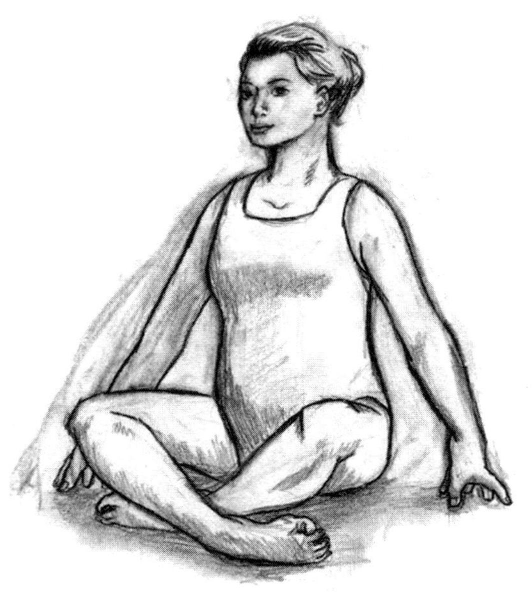

Figure 6-3 Tailor seated position, ideal for pregnant women.

Drawing courtesy of Kai Hackley-Baker

back lying position after the first trimester.[122] In contrast, Clapp[124] states that if the pregnant woman is back lying while exercising, but her torso and legs are moving, then there should not be a problem with the vena cava syndrome. Moreover, Tupler[89] supports that short periods of exercise while back lying should not be problematic. If any signs or symptoms of dizziness occur, then the woman can roll into a side lying position. Exercising in the back lying position is acceptable throughout pregnancy provided the client stays attuned to the possible warning signs of the vena cava syndrome.

BODY MECHANICS AND POSTURE

One of the more obvious changes during pregnancy is a change in posture and adjustment in center of gravity. Posture changes as the weight of the uterus, breasts, and fetus increases, which increases both the curvature of the lower back and forward rounding of the upper spine and shoulders. During pregnancy, the client's center of gravity shifts upward and forward. The client should always be aware of her posture and should try to stand with her feet hip width apart and her weight evenly distributed with her knees held softly and not locked. Her head should be centered over her shoulders and her chest should be pointed upward. Lastly, her shoulders should be relaxed and not shifted upward, and her umbilicus should be pulled back toward her spine.

DIASTASIS RECTI

A separation of the rectus abdominus muscle is known as diastasis recti. Weak abdominal muscles in relation to back muscles may contribute to poor posture. Abdominal muscles that are stronger during pregnancy assist the women during labor and the birthing process.

The main abdominal muscles involved in diastasis recti are the rectus abdominus and the transverse muscle. The rectus abdominus is a longitudinal muscle that is divided in two halves and connected by a soft, fibrous band called the linea alba. The transverse muscle wraps around the body at the level of the umbilicus. Assessment for diastasis recti begins with asking the client to lie flat on her back, feet flat on the ground with her knees bent. Her arms should rest at her sides and abdominal muscles should be relaxed. Fingers are placed on the client's mid-abdominal area at the level of the umbilicus facing toward the client's head. With the forefinger, middle, and ring fingers just below the umbilicus, the woman is asked to raise her head about 4 inches off the ground. With the client's head raised, a separation of the

recti can be palpated. If there is a separation, the fingertips should fit easily into the opening. If there is more than a 2-$\frac{1}{2}$ finger separation, the client would benefit from seeing a prenatal fitness trainer before doing abdominal exercises to ensure she is performing the exercises correctly. Common actions such as coughing, sneezing, getting up from an examination table, or any other movement that pushes the transverse muscle against the recti can cause further separation.

Several precautions can help prevent the development of diastasis recti. First, when coughing or sneezing, the abdominal muscles should be held in a contracted position while internally pulling the umbilicus toward the spine, and then released once the cough or sneeze is finished. This contracted position should be held while taking a slow deep breath and not bearing down. Second, when a client is rising from a horizontal position, she should be encouraged to roll into a side lying position and push up with both arms, not using the abdominal muscles. Third, when moving from a floor sitting position to standing position, the client should roll onto her hands and knees position and bring one foot forward to the floor with hands on her knee. Then she should push up with the arms to a standing position. Fourth, when exercising, each stretch and exercise should begin with diaphragmatic breathing, which will bring the transverse muscle back toward the spine during exhalation.

Specific Exercises for Pregnant Women

AEROBIC EXERCISES

There are many low-risk aerobic exercises such as dancing, cycling, swimming, and walking. Aerobic dancing or low-impact aerobics provide a complete workout, which should include a warm-up, aerobic exercise, and cool-down period. Cycling is an excellent exercise, but stationary or recumbent bikes are suggested toward the latter part of pregnancy because increased joint laxity and changes in the center of gravity may place the client at risk of falling.[120] Swimming uses many different muscles and is safe throughout pregnancy; the water supports the client as she gets a full body workout. Walking is another exercise that can be gentle or more vigorous depending on how the client is feeling and her level of fitness.

WEIGHT TRAINING

Free weights are an excellent way in which to strengthen muscles. The client should start out with 1 to 2 pound weights and increase the weight, as she feels comfortable. If she does not feel challenged, then she should use the next heavier weight. Free weights are usually found in 0.5, 1, 2, 3, 5, and 10 pound sizes. Adding weight should be done according to what feels comfortable. However, the exercises should be challenging, slow, and controlled. If the prescribed number of repetitions and sets is comfortable, additional weight may be added. If additional weight makes the exercises performed uncomfortable and uncontrolled, then the weights should be decreased to the previous level. If at anytime it becomes painful, the amount of weight needs to be reduced. If free weights are not available, the client may try items found in her own home, such as soup cans or bottles of water.

RESISTANCE

Resistance training is a specialized method of conditioning designed to increase muscle strength, muscle endurance, and muscle power. Resistance training can be performed by using resistance bands, resistance machines, or the client's own body weight. Resistance bands are easy to use, inexpensive, and can be easily adjusted to increase or decrease the amount of resistance desired. It is important to remind the client that her wrists should remain straight without applying pressure on the wrist. The increase in relaxin can cause increased laxity and may injure the wrists. During exercise with resistance bands, the wrists should be kept neutral with thumbs pointing out straight and in line with the hand.

Hydration and Food Intake

Pregnant women need to keep well hydrated during exercise. In addition to the daily 8-ounce glasses of water, pregnant women should drink 14 to 22 ounces of fluid two hours before exercise, 6 to 12 ounces every 15 to 20 minutes during exercise, and 16 to 24 ounces for every pound lost after exercise.[128,129] In addition, women who are pregnant need to eat before exercising so the body does not burn fat, since weight loss is not a goal. Eating approximately two to three hours before exercise will ensure adequate availability of calories for a workout. Light, high water content fruits (peaches or watermelon), fruited yogurt, cottage cheese, raisins, a bagel with low fat cheese, a bowl of cereal with low fat milk, yogurt with graham crackers, fruit smoothie with nonfat yogurt, or whole-wheat toast are good choices.

Warning Signs

If at any time during exercise a woman experiences chest pain or tightness, dizziness, headache, increased shortness of breath, muscle weakness or tingling pain, or redness, warmth, or swelling of the calf, then she should stop exercising immediately and seek medical attention. If the woman is pregnant and feels decreased fetal movement, fluid leakage from the vagina, one-sided headache, blurred vision, uterine contractions (not Braxton Hicks), or vaginal bleeding, she should stop exercising immediately and seek medical attention. After the woman is examined by her midwife and medically cleared, she may resume her exercise regime. She may need to alter, decrease, or discontinue certain activities.

SCIATICA

Pain from sciatica is caused at the point where the sciatic nerve passes through and emerges from the lumbar vertebrae. A prolapsed intervertebral disc or a herniated nucleus pulposus may cause sciatica. During pregnancy, the enlarging uterus coupled with a change in posture and center of gravity may cause the woman to experience these symptoms. The pain travels below the knee and may involve the foot. In addition, there may be numbness or weakness of the lower leg muscles. It is important for the client to be evaluated to rule out any disc involvement before exercising. Refer to the chapter on musculoskeletal disorders (Chapter 21) for a further description of the signs and symptoms associated with herniated discs. Comfort measures for women with non-pathologic presentations include stretching and bending the affected leg at the knee, while keeping the opposite leg extended, and pulling the affected leg across the body.[89] Another exercise includes stretching the lower back by getting in the knee chest position to change the pressure of the uterus and baby.[88]

Program Evaluation

A program evaluation is performed to evaluate whether the client's goals are being met and whether she is satisfied with her current exercise regimen. Second, it provides an opportunity to determine how the client should proceed with her exercise regimen and make adjustments if she is pregnant. Third, this helps determine if the number of repetitions and the amount of weight or resistance is appropriate. Lastly, if the client is pregnant, it allows monitoring her exercise program for changes and assessing for development of diastasis, low back strain, sciatica, or other pregnancy-related discomforts.

Example of an Exercise Program

Warm-up

A ten-minute warm-up period should always occur before active exercise begins. During the warm-up period, low resistance exercises and light activity prepare the muscles for vigorous activity. Then the client should gently stretch in order to avoid muscle stiffness and soreness. Stretching should feel good and should not be painful. The client should stretch until the point of mild discomfort and then release.[130] Stretches should be held for 10 to 20 seconds without bouncing, as this can be harmful as the muscles may shorten reflexively.[131,132] The client should use diaphragmatic breathing by slowly inhaling through the nose as the abdomen expands. During exhalation through the mouth, the abdomen falls back into a neutral position and the body relaxes.[88,89]

Stretching

Below are examples of stretching techniques for the neck, shoulders, chest and upper body, lower back, and lower body. To prevent soreness and injury, all muscles should be stretched.

NECK AND SHOULDERS

Women who are overweight, obese, or pregnant have an increased strain in their neck and shoulders due to the increased weight of their breasts. Strain and tension can be relieved by using the following stretches. All of the following stretches can be done in the tailor sit position.

Neck Rotation   Ask the client to relax her neck and shoulders. Have her lower her head forward with her chin toward her chest, and slowly rotate her head to the right, back to center, and to the left. Do five slow and gentle rotations on each side.

Shoulder Shrug   Ask the client to raise her shoulders slightly toward her ears and then drop her shoulders down slowly. Do five repetitions.

Ear to Shoulder   Ask the client to tilt her left ear to her left shoulder until resistance is felt. She should hold that position for 10 seconds and then bring her head back to center. Repeat on the right side. Do five repetitions on each side.

Shoulder Circles   With a straight back and arms at her sides, slowly have the client move her shoulders forward, upward, backward, and downward in a controlled full circle. Do five circles in each direction.

Shoulder Stretch   Ask the client to pull the elbow of her left arm across her chest toward the opposite shoulder. She should press at the point of her arm between the elbow and shoulder, making sure she does not put pressure directly on her elbow. When resistance is felt, then have her hold that position for 10 seconds and release. Repeat on the opposite side. Do 2 shoulder stretches on each side (**Figure 6-4**).

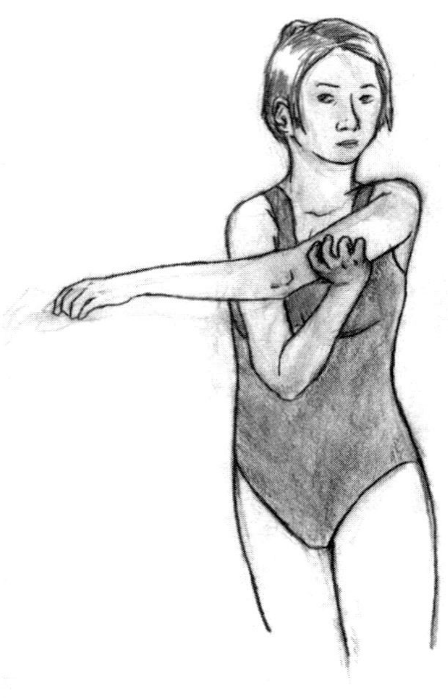

Figure 6-4 Shoulder stretch.

Drawing courtesy of Kai Hackley-Baker

CHEST AND UPPER BODY STRETCHES

Women who are overweight and obese or pregnant tend to bring their shoulders forward due to the increased weight of their breasts. All of the following stretches can be done in the tailor sit position.

Arms Behind the Back   Ask the client to grab her hands behind her back and pull up and back with her hands. Do two stretches (**Figure 6-5**).

Towel Stretch   Ask the client to grab a towel with both hands behind her head. Have her squeeze her shoulder blades together, pulling the towel tight as she expands her chest, keeping her elbows behind her shoulders. Make sure that her back is not arched. She should try to hold the stretch for 20 seconds and do at least 10 chest stretches per day. This exercise will also strengthen the upper back (**Figure 6-6**).

Arms Overhead   Ask the client to raise her arms over her head. Then have her put the back of her

palms together, as she expands her chest. Do two stretches (**Figure 6-7**).

Triceps Stretch   Ask the client to bring her arms overhead, and grab the elbow of one arm with the hand on the opposite arm. Have her gently and slowly pull her elbow behind her head until there is resistance. When resistance is felt, have her hold the position for a few seconds, release and repeat on the other side (**Figure 6-8**).

LOWER BACK STRETCHES

Women who are overweight and obese or pregnant tend to tilt their pelvis forward and accentuate their natural lumbar curve. The following

---

Figure 6-5 Arms behind the back stretch.

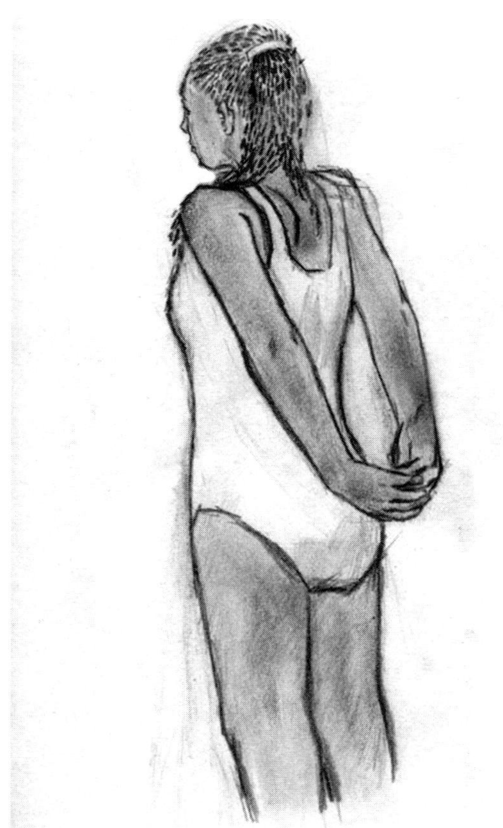

Drawing courtesy of Kai Hackley-Baker

Figure 6-6 Towel stretch.

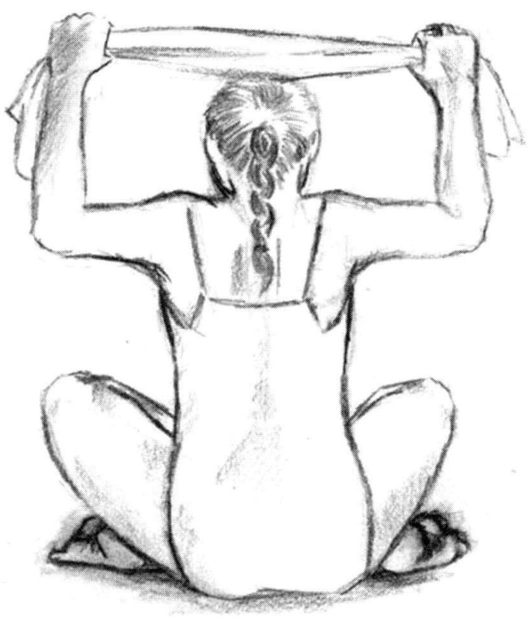

Drawing courtesy of Kai Hackley-Baker

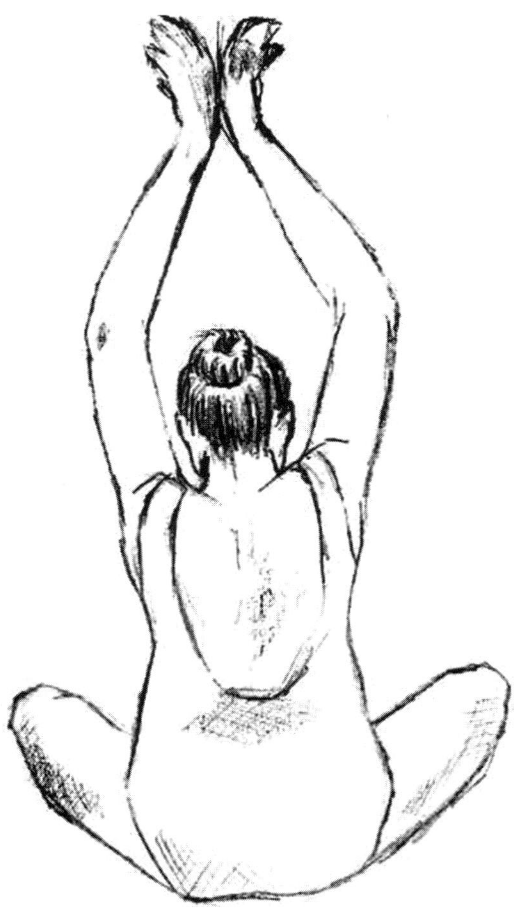

Drawing courtesy of Kai Hackley-Baker

two stretches provide relief and comfort to lower back strain.

C-Curve or Kneeling Pelvic Tilt with Chair   Ask the client to kneel on the floor with her elbows resting on a pillow laid on a chair in front of her for support. Have the client exhale and contract the abdominal muscles (pull the umbilicus to-

ward the spine) while creating a c-shape with her spine. Relax back to the starting position (**Figure 6-9**).

Child's Pose   Ask the client to get on her hands and knees position and then move her hips and buttocks backward (slowly) while keeping her hands on the floor. If she is pregnant, she may widen her knees to allow her abdomen to lie between her legs. Do not attempt if the client has a history of knee problems (**Figure 6-10**).

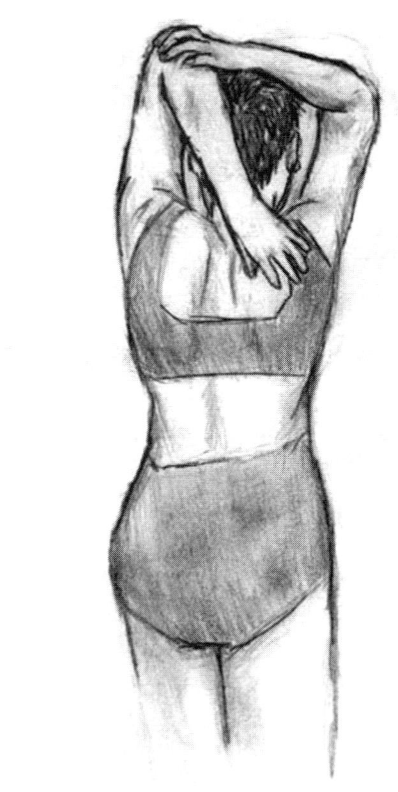

Drawing courtesy of Kai Hackley-Baker

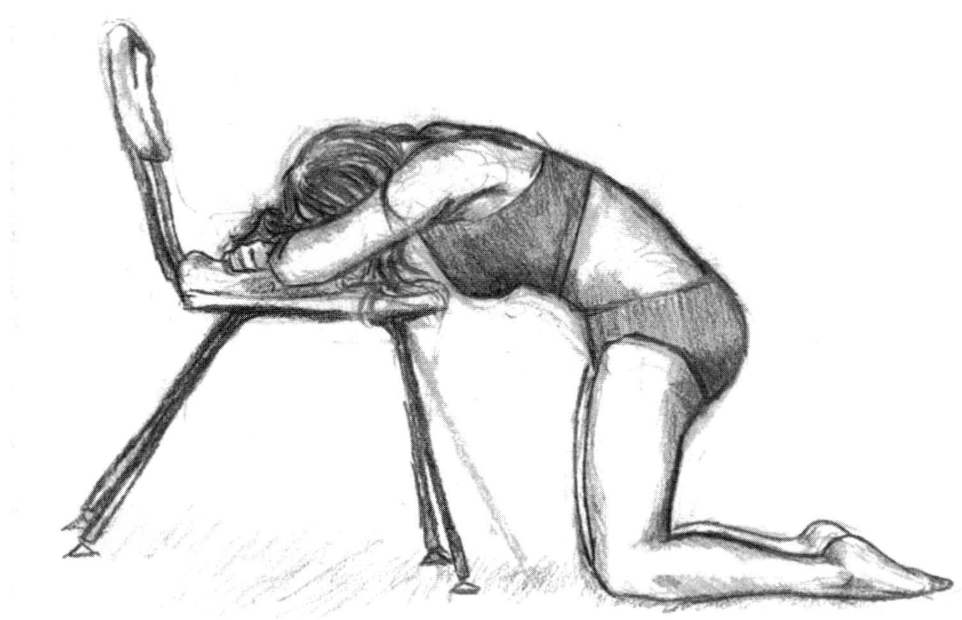

Figure 6-9 Using a chair for the C-curve or kneeling pelvic tilt position.

Drawing courtesy of Kai Hackley-Baker

LOWER BODY STRETCHES

Stretches to the lower body include the gastrocnemius, ankle, quadriceps, hip adductors, and gluteus maximus muscles. Most are done in the tailor sit position unless otherwise noted.

Ankle Rotation   Ask the client to sit on the floor or in a chair and rest the left ankle on the right leg's knee (partial tailor sit). Have her rotate her ankle clockwise. Do a few circles in this direction, using the entire foot and ankle. Repeat with the opposite ankle.

Calf Stretch   Have the client sit on the floor with one leg extended out and the other leg bent at the knee, foot to opposite knee (inverted hurdler's stretch). Have her pull the toes of the extended leg toward her shin until she feels a stretch in the calf. Hold the stretch for a count of 10 and repeat. Repeat on opposite leg. This stretch can be done using a towel around the front of the leg and pulling the towel toward the shin or using the wall in a standing position (**Figure 6-11**).

Sitting Butterfly (Hip Adductors)   Ask the client to put the soles of her feet together and hands on her ankles or shins. Have her gently press her elbows downward onto her inner thigh without bouncing. (**Figure 6-12**).

Seated Gluteal Stretch   Ask the client to bring her left (bent at knee) leg over the thigh of her right (extended) leg. Have her lean back slightly

Figure 6-10 Child's pose.

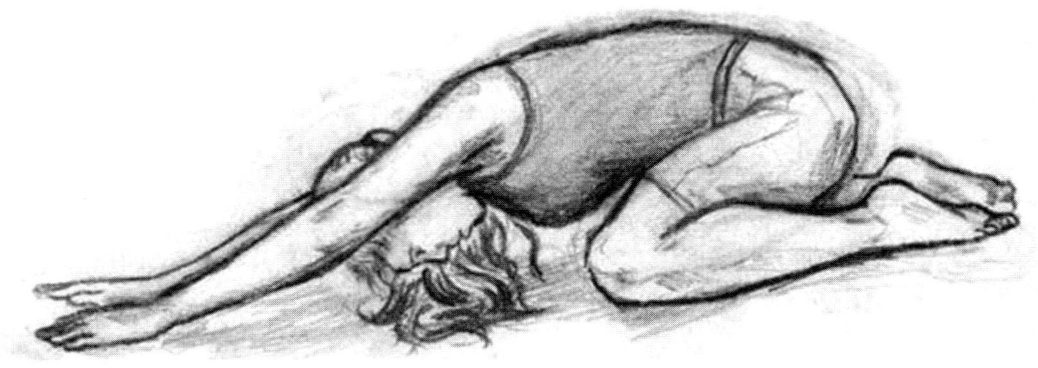

Drawing courtesy of Kai Hackley-Baker

while bending the straight leg while keeping that heel on the floor. Have her grab her foot and knee and lean forward slightly, feeling a stretch in the gluteus. Hold for 15 to 20 seconds and then switch legs (**Figure 6-13**).

Stair Calf Stretch   Ask the client to hold onto a railing or wall for balance and position her toes and balls of her feet on a stair with her arches and heels extended off. Have her shift her weight to one foot and hold for 15 to 20 seconds. Repeat with opposite leg (**Figure 6-14**).

Quadriceps Stretch   Ask the client to lean against a wall with one hand. She should reach back and grab her leg just above her ankle with her other hand and gently bring her foot toward her buttocks to feel a stretch in her quadriceps.

Lying Gluteal Stretch   Ask the client to lie on her back with her feet on the floor with knees bent. She should lift one leg toward her torso while placing her hands behind her thigh to increase the stretch (**Figure 6-15**).

SQUATS

Squatting stretches the hip adductor, gluteal, and quadriceps muscles. Squats are difficult to maintain and must be practiced. If the client has knee problems, pelvic pain, or varicose veins, squatting may not be a good stretch for her.

Ask the client to begin on the floor in a seated position. Have her bring one foot up and place it on the floor with her knee in line with her ankle. She can bring both hands in front of her on the floor for support as she brings the other foot up and places it on the floor. To stand from a squatting position, the woman should sit on the floor, then move to the hands and knees position and then to a standing position. This puts less stress on the knees and abdominal muscles.

Holding onto an immovable object may make squats more comfortable to practice. Ask the client to stand with feet in the straddle position, holding onto an immovable object and slowly lower herself to the floor, keeping her knees in line with her toes. Having her knees forward and out

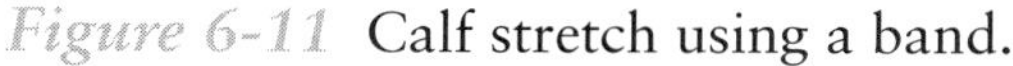

Figure 6-11 Calf stretch using a band.

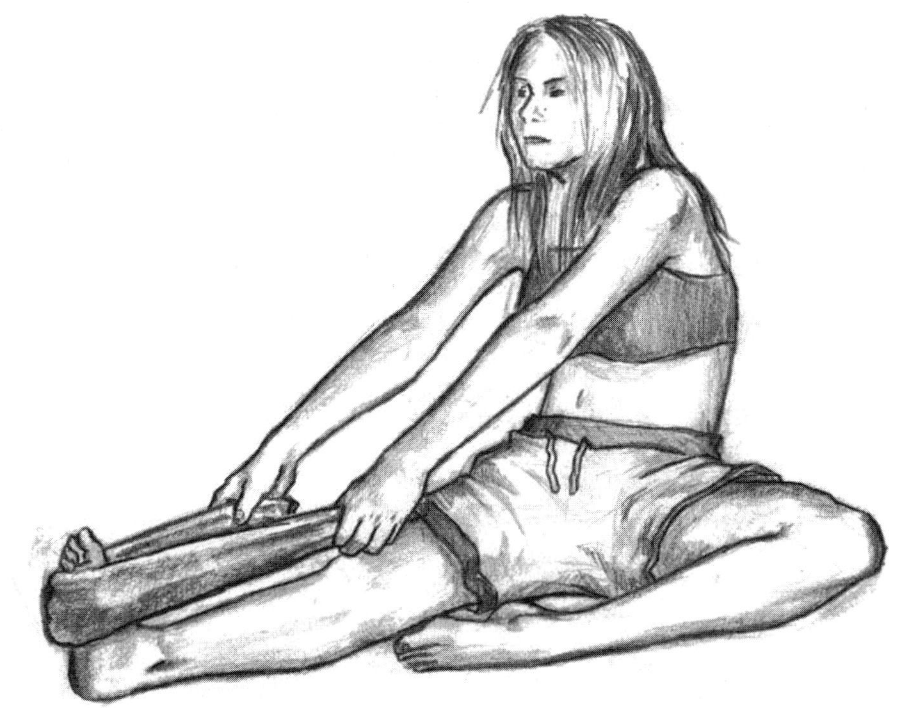

Drawing courtesy of Kai Hackley-Baker

over her toes can strain the knee. Make sure her heels are on the floor with her weight on the outside of her feet. Her arms should be straight out in front of her at shoulder level as she continues to hold firmly onto the immovable object. If she experiences any discomfort, she should stop immediately. She should be able to hold the position for 15 to 20 seconds and do squats several times a day. Within a few weeks, she should be able to increase the amount of time in the squat position to at least one minute. The woman can also squat with the support of one or two individuals standing on each side of her. The individuals providing support for the woman squatting should put their hands under her arms while avoiding putting pressure on her axilla or elbows.

Exercises

UPPER BODY

All exercises are done in a seated position unless otherwise noted.

Front Raises (Anterior Deltoid) Ask the client to take free weights in each hand. Have her raise her left arm forward with the elbow bent at 30 degrees and raise until the arm is parallel to the floor. Continue with alternate arm. Do ten repetitions on each side.

Figure 6-12 Sitting butterfly position.

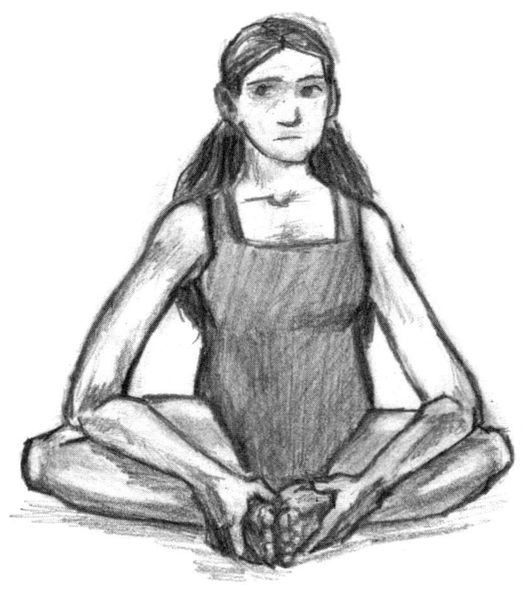

Drawing courtesy of Kai Hackley-Baker

Squeeze (Upper Back)   Ask the client to place the palms of her hands on the back of her head, bringing the elbows away from the body as she squeezes her shoulder blades together.

Arm Press (Chest)   Ask the client to hold the dumbbells in each hand. Starting position should be arms bent at the elbow at shoulder height. Have the client press upward until her arms are fully extended. Have her hold for a second and then slowly and, in a controlled motion, have her lower her arms to the starting position.

Resistance (Latissimus Dorsi): Lat Pull Downs   Ask the client to hold the resistance band in each hand at the level of her neck, elbows bent as she extends her arms overhead. She should lower her elbows downward toward her sides as she adducts her shoulder blades.

Resistance (Upper Back and Shoulders): Forward Pull   While sitting, have the client place the resistance band in each hand with arms out to the sides at shoulder level. The band should feel comfortable across her chest. She should squeeze her shoulder blades together as she brings her arms behind her shoulders, while keeping her back straight. Repeat ten times.

Resistance (Upper Back and Shoulders): Overhead Pull   Ask the client to grab the resistance band in each hand and put the band behind her head with her arms extended out to the side. The client should pull the band until it is tight between her hands. Slowly have her lower her arms to shoulder height and back to the starting position. She should exhale on the downward movements. Repeat ten times.

Ask the client to place her hands on the floor, while her knees assist in supporting her body. Her palms should be a little more than shoulder width apart. Have her keep her body straight, as she lowers herself to the floor, then pressing into the floor as her arms extend just before the point where her elbows are not locked. Repeat 10 times.

Weighted One Arm Row (Rhomboids, Trapezius, and Posterior Deltoid)   Ask the client to stand and hold onto a wall for support. Ask her to lean slightly forward, grab the free weight in her right hand and extend that arm behind her. Have her raise her right arm, bending at the elbow, and lift the elbow toward the ceiling.

Shrugs (Trapezius)   Ask the client to stand with her arms at her sides and holding free weights in each hand. Have her elevate or raise her

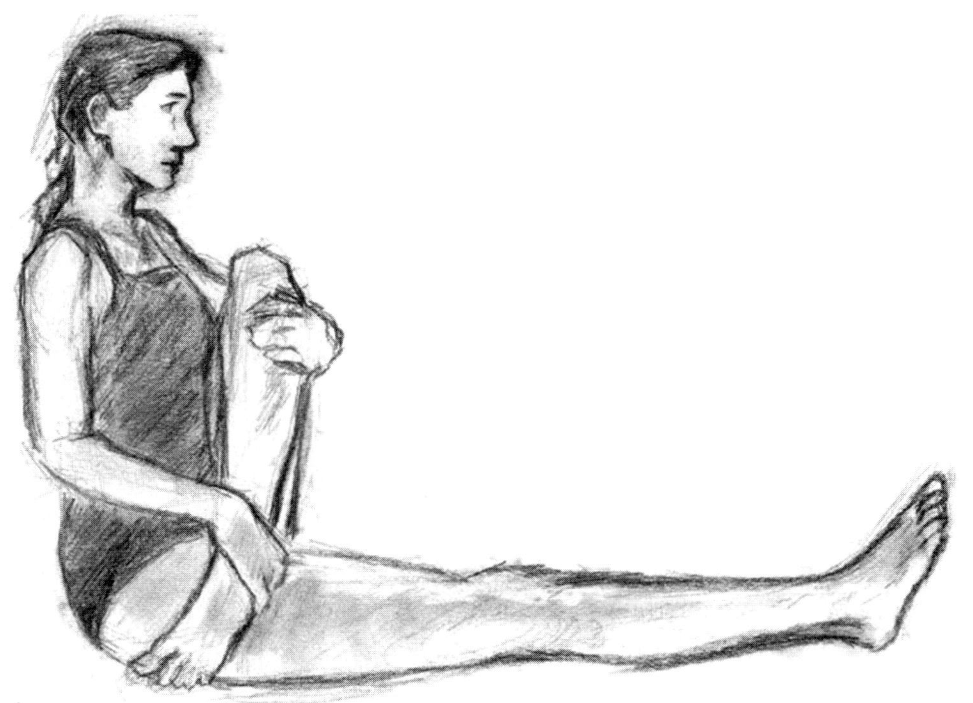

Drawing courtesy of Kai Hackley-Baker

shoulders to her ears and slowly lower. She should keep her back straight, and her knees should not be locked. Repeat ten times.

ARMS

Bicep Curls Biceps are the muscles located in the front and upper portion of each arm. Ask the client to put a free weight in each hand with palms facing inward toward each other. Have the client bend her arm at the elbow as she slowly raises the weights toward her shoulders. Have the client keep her shoulders still, hold for a second, and slowly lower the weights. Repeat ten times with each arm.

Triceps Triceps are the muscles in the back of the arm directly opposite the bicep. Ask the client to put a free weight in her hand and lean slightly forward as she brings her right elbow back behind her with the weight at her waist. As she squeezes her triceps muscle, have her extend her arm at the elbow, keeping the elbow stationary and push the weight away from her body. Release and return to the starting position. Repeat ten times with each arm.

ABDOMINAL MUSCLES

Strengthening the Transverse Muscles Ask the client to sit with her back supported and

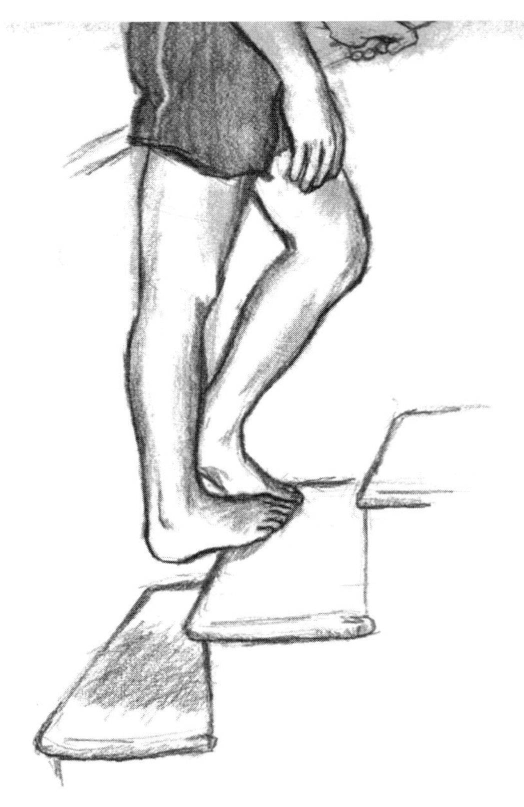

Drawing courtesy of Kai Hackley-Baker

expand her abdomen as she inhales through her nose. As she exhales through her mouth, she should bring her transverse muscle (umbilicus) back toward the spine. Hold for a count of 30. Remind the client to count and to not hold her breath.

Transverse Abdominis Raise   Ask the client to get on both hands and knees on a soft surface. Her knees should be in line with her hips, and her hands directly in line with her shoulders with her head in line with her body. Slowly draw the transverse muscle (umbilicus) to the spine. Do not move the body and keep the spine in a neutral position. Hold while breathing normally and then relax. Repeat ten times.

LOWER BODY

Lower Leg Lifts (Inner Thigh)   Ask the client to lie on her left side with her right (top) leg resting on the floor in front of her. Her left (bottom) leg should be extended straight with her foot flexed. Her head can be resting on a pillow or on her hand. The right arm or hand should be resting in front of her on the floor for support. Working the inner thigh, the client should raise her left (bottom) leg off the floor at a 45-degree angle. As she lowers the leg, make sure it does not touch the floor. Continue until the muscle feels fatigued and then repeat on the opposite side (**Figure 6-16**).

Doggies or Fire Hydrants (Outer Thigh)   Ask the client to get on her hands and knees with her knees hip width apart and hands on the floor a little further apart than her shoulders. Her back should be straight and she should look straight ahead. Have her bend her leg at a 90-degree angle and raise it to the side, hold for a second, and slowly lower to the ground. Do 20 and switch sides (**Figure 6-17**).

Upper Leg Lift (Outer Thigh)   Ask the client to lie on her left side with left (bottom) leg bent. Working the outer thigh, have her lift her right (top) leg to a 45-degree angle. While bringing the leg down, make sure not to rest the leg on the floor. Continue until the muscle feels fatigued and then repeat on the opposite side (**Figure 6-18**).

Supported Plie (Quadriceps, Hamstrings, Gluteus Maximus)   Ask the client to use a wall for balance and support. She should put her feet in a straddle position (toes pointing toward 10 and

Figure 6-15 Supine gluteal stretch.

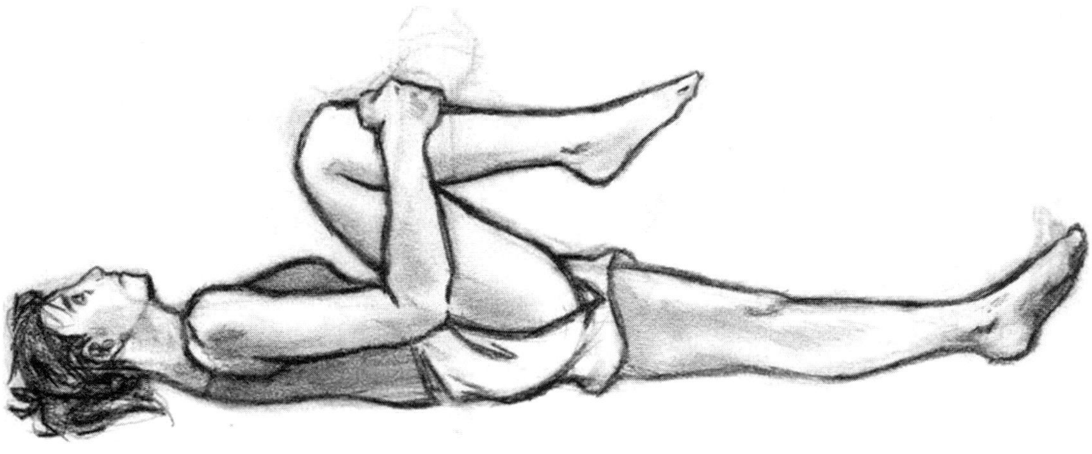

Drawing courtesy of Kai Hackley-Baker

2 position on a clock). Ask her to do a pelvic tilt and plié or squat down. She should then extend her legs back to her starting position.

PELVIC FLOOR

Kegel Exercises   Kegel exercises strengthen the muscles of the pelvic floor and the muscles that support the bladder, uterus, and intestines. Kegal exercises should not be done while urinating because that can cause a urinary tract infection. Kegal exercises should be done in a slow and controlled manner with repetitions determined by the client. She should start by doing ten repetitions of each kegel exercise two to

Figure 6-16 Lower leg lifts.

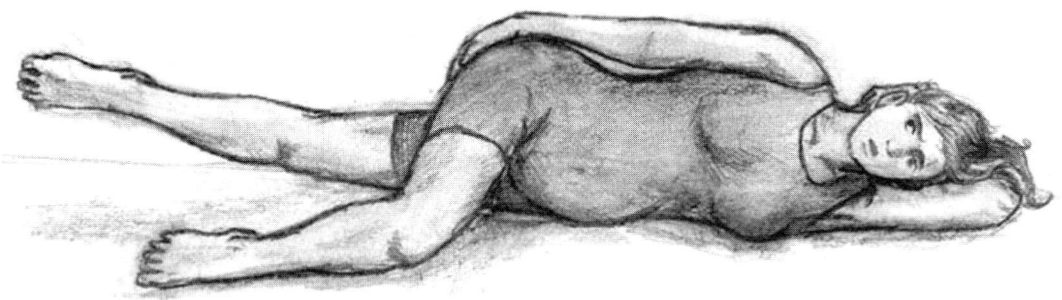

Drawing courtesy of Kai Hackley-Baker

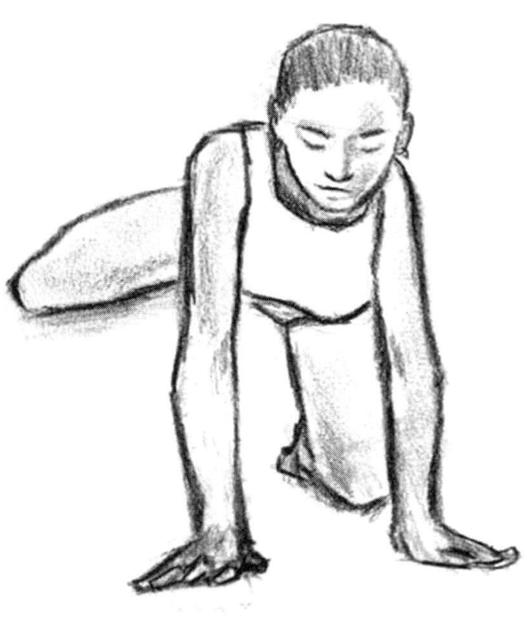

Figure 6-17 Doggie leg lifts or fire hydrant lifts.

Drawing courtesy of Kai Hackley-Baker

three times per day. As she feels comfortable, she can increase to 50 repetitions twice a day. There are two ways to do Kegel exercises, which include holds or progressions or elevators. Holds start by releasing the abdomen, thigh, and buttock muscles, and then contracting the pelvic floor muscles while holding for a count of ten. The client relaxes and then repeats. Remind client not to hold breath or to bear down, which can cause a valsalva maneuver. Progressions or elevators start by releasing the abdomen, thigh, and buttock muscles, and then contracting the pelvic floor muscles progressively tighter for a count of five. Then the muscles are slowly released for a count of five. The client relaxes and then repeats.

Cool Down

A five-minute cool down should follow every exercise session. This is when the client reduces the exercise and allows the heart rate to return to normal. Stretching is done again to prevent muscle soreness and to increase flexibility. Diaphragmatic breathing with visualization during the cool-down period is suggested. Diaphragmatic breathing allows the breathing to slowly return to normal. During the cool-down period, have the client close her eyes as she breathes slowly. Have her visualize pleasant things (her baby, a fast labor, a place she enjoys) while her entire body relaxes with the lights dimmed and calming music playing. It is during this time that she can reconnect with her body.

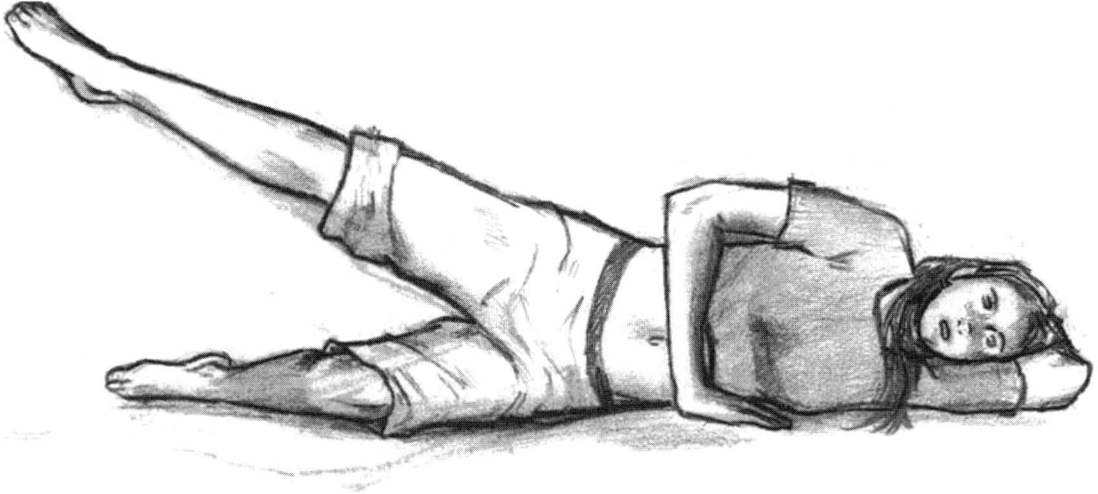

Figure 6-18 Upper leg lifts.

Drawing courtesy of Kai Hackley-Baker

References

1. United States Department of Health and Human Services. The Surgeon General's call to action to prevent and decrease overweight and obesity. Washington, DC: U.S. Department of Health and Human Services, Public Health Services, Office of Surgeon General, Government Printing Office; 2001.

2. United States Department of Health and Human Services, National Heart, Lung, and Blood Institute, National Institute of Diabetes Digestive and Kidney Diseases. Clinical guidelines on the identification, evaluation, and treatment of overweight and obesity in adults: Public Health Services. NIH Publication No. 98-4083. Bethesda, MD: National Institutes of Health. National Heart, Lung, and Blood Institute; 1998.

3. Allison DB, Engel CN. Predicting treatment outcome: Why have we been so unsuccessful? In: Allison DB, Pi-Sunyer FX, editors. *Obesity Treatment: Establishing Goals, Improving Outcomes, and Reviewing the Research Agenda.* New York, NY: Plenum Press; 1995.

4. Flegal MS, Carroll MD, Kuzarski RJ, Johnson CL. Overweight and obesity in the United States: Prevalence and trends. *Int J Obes Relat Metab Disord.* 1998;22:39–47.

5. Field AE, Barnoya J, Colditz GA. Epidemiology and health and economic consequences of obesity. In: Wadden TA, Stunkard AJ, editors. *Handbook of Obesity Treatment.* New York: The Guilford Press; 2002.

6. National Heart, Lung, and Blood Institute, National Institute of Diabetes and Digestive and Kidney Diseases. Clinical guidelines on the identification, evaluation, and treatment of overweight and obesity in adults. NIH Publication No. 98-4083. Washington, DC: National Institutes of Health; 1998.

7. United States Department of Health and Human Services. Healthy People 2010: National health promotion and disease prevention objectives. Washington, DC: Government Printing Office, U.S. Department of Health and Human Services, Public Health Service; 2000.

8. National Institute of Diabetes and Digestive and Kidney Diseases. Overweight, obesity, and health risk: National task force on prevention and treatment of obesity. *Arch Intern Med.* 2000;160:898–904.

9. Stunkard AJ, Harris JR, Pederson NL, McClearn GE. The body-mass index of twins who have been reared apart. *N Engl J Med.* 1990;322:1483–1487.

10. Whitaker RC, Wright JA, Pepe MS, Seidel KD, Dietz WH. Predicting obesity in young adulthood from childhood and parental obesity. *N Engl J Med.* 1997;337(13):869–873.

11. Berkowitz RI, Stunkard AJ. Development of childhood obesity. In: Wadden TA, Stunkard AJ, editors. *Handbook of Obesity Treatment.* New York: The Guilford Press; 2002.

12. Bray GA. Obesity. *Curr Ther Endocrinol Metab.* 1994;5:465–474.

13. Chehab FF. Leptin as a regulator of adipose mass and reproduction. *Trends Pharmacol Sci.* 2000;21(8):309–314.

14. Esparza J, Fox C, Harper IT, Bennett PH, Schulz LO, Valencia ME, et al. Daily energy expenditure in Mexican and USA Pima Indians: Low physical activity as a possible cause of obesity. *Int J Obes.* 2000;24:55–59.

15. Ravelli AC, van der Meulen JH, Osmond C, Barker DJ, Bleker OP. Obesity at the age of 50 in men and women exposed to famine prenatally. *Am J Clin Nutr.* 1999;70:811–816.

16. Ravelli GP, Stein ZA, Susser MW. Obesity in young men after famine exposure. *N Engl J Med.* 1976;295:349–353.

17. Barker M, Robinson S, Barker D. Birthweight and body fat distribution in adolescent girls. *Arch Dis Child.* 1997;77:381–383.

18. Sobal J, Stunkard AJ. Socioeconomic status and obesity: A review of the literature. *Psychol Bull.* 1989;105:260–275.

19. Zhang Q, Wang Y. Socioeconomic inequality of obesity in the United States: Do gender, age and ethnicity matter? *Soc Sci Med.* 2004;58:1171–1180.

20. Gordon-Larsen P, Adair LS, Popkin BM. The relationship of ethnicity, socioeconomic factors, and overweight in U.S. adolescents. *Obes Res.* 2003;11:121–129.

21. Ambrosius WT, Newmans SA, Pratt JH. Rates of change in measures of body size vary by ehnicity and gender. *Ethn Dis.* 2001;11:303–310.

22. Schlosser E. *Fast Food Nation.* New York: Houghton Mifflin; 2002.

23. Jakicic JM, Gallagher KI. Physical activity considerations for management of body weight. In: Bessesen DH, Kushner R, editors. *Evaluation and Management of Obesity.* Philadelphia, PA: Hanley & Belfus; 2002. pp. 73–87.

24. Jakicic JM, Clark K, Coleman E, Donnelly JE, Foreyt JP, Melanson E, et al. American College of Sports Medicine position stand: Appropriate intervention strategies for weight loss and prevention of weight gain for adults. *Med Sci Sports Exerc.* 2001;33:2145–2156.

25. Huether SE, McCance KL, Tarmina MS. Alterations of digestive function. In: McCance KL, Huether SE, editors. *Pathophysiology: The Biologic Basics for Diseases in Adults and Children.* 4th ed. St. Louis, MO: Mosby; 2001. pp. 1320–1375.

26. Faust IM, Johnson PR, Stern JS, Hirsch J. Diet-induced adipocyte number increases in adult rats: A new model for obesity. *Am J Physiol.* 1978;235:E279–286.

27. Schwartz RB, Brunzell JD. Increase of adipose tissue in lipoprotein lipase activity with weight loss. *J Clin Invest.* 1981;67:1425.

28. Keesey RE. A set-point theory of obesity. In: Brownell KD, Foreyt JP, editors. *Handbook of Eating Disorders.* New York: Basic Books; 1986. pp. 63–87.

29. Himms-Hagen J. Brown adipose tissue metabolism and thermogenesis. *Annu Rev Nutr.* 1985;5:69–84.

30. Miller DS. Thermogenesis and obesity. *Bibliotheca Nutritio et Dieta.* 1979;27:25–32.

31. De Luise M, Blackburn GL, Flier JS. Reduced activity of the red cell sodium-potassium pump in human obesity. *N Engl J Med.* 1980;303:1017.

32. Wadden TA, Stunkard AJ. Social and psychological consequences of obesity. *Ann Intern Med.* 1985;103:1062–1067.

33. Stunkard AJ. *Obesity.* Philadelphia: Saunders; 1980.

34. Bessesen DH. Regulation of appetite by the central nervous system. In: Bessesen DH, Kushner R, editors. *Evaluation and Management of Obesity.* Philadelphia: Hanley and Belfus; 2002. pp. 155–166.

35. Elmquist JK, Elias CF, Saper CB. From lesions to leptin: Hypothalamic control of food intake and body weight. *Neuron.* 1999;22:221–232.

36. Ahima RS, Flier JS. Leptin. *Ann Rev Physiol.* 2000;62:413–437.

37. Schwartz MW, Woods SC, Porte D, Deely RJ, Baskin DG. Central nervous system control of food intake. *Nature.* 2000;404:661–671.

38. Kushner R. Defining the scope of the problem of obesity. In: Bessesen DH, Kushner R, editors. *Evaluation and Management of Obesity.* Philadelphia: Hanley and Belfus, Inc.; 2002. pp. 1–8.

39. Matz R. Calculating body mass index. *Ann Intern Med.* 1993;118:232.

40. Centers for Disease Control and Prevention. BMI – body mass index: BMI for adults. [Monograph on the Internet]. Atlanta, GA. [updated daily] Available from: http://www.cdc.gov/nccdphp/dnpa/bmi/bmi-adult.htm.

41. Snijder MB, Zimmet PZ, Visser D, Dekker JM, Seidell JC, Shaw JE. Independent and opposite associations of waist and hip circumferences with diabetes, hypertension and dyslipidemia: The Aus Diab Study. *Int J Obes Relat Metab Dis.* 2004;28(3):402–409.

42. Lean ME, Han TS, Morrision CE. Waist circumference as a measure for indicating need for weight management. *BMJ.* 1995;311:158–161.

43. Cnop M, Landchild MJ, Vidal J, Havel PJ, Knowles NG, Carr DR, et al. The concurrent accumulation of intra-abdominal and subcutaneous fat explains the association between insulin resistance and plasma leptin concentrations: Distinct metabolic effects of two fat compartments. *Diabetes.* 2002;51(4):1005–1015.

44. Davies PSW, Cole TJ. *Body Composition Techniques in Health and Disease.* New York: Cambridge University Press; 1995.

45. Burke L, Deakin V. *Clinical Sports Nutrition.* 2nd ed. Rosehill, Australia: McGraw-Hill Publishers; 2000.

46. Nunez C, Rubiano M, Horlick J, Thornton J, Heymsfield SB. Leg-to-leg bioimpedance system validity in children. In: *Experimental Biology.* New York: Federation of American Societies for Experimental Biology; 1999.

47. Farkus-Hirsch R. *Intensive Diabetes Management.* 2nd ed. New York: American Diabetes Association; 2003.

48. Saltiel AR, Olefsky JM. Thiazolidinediones in the treatment of insulin resistance and type II diabetes. *Diabetes.* 1996;45:1661–1669.

49. Rosenbloom AL, Silverstein JH. Type 2 diabetes in children and adolescents: A guide to diagnosis, epidemiology, pathogenesis, prevention, and treatment. Alexandria, VA: American Diabetes Association; 2003.

50. American Diabetes Association. Clinical practice recommendations 2004. *Diabetes Care.* 2004;27(S1): S1–150.

51. Sudi KM, Gallistl S, Trobinger M, Payerl D, Aigner R, Borkenstein MH. The effects of changes in body mass and subcutaneous fat on the improvement in metabolic risk factors after short-term weight loss. *Metabolism.* 2001;50(11):1323–1329.

52. Wadden TA, Stunkard AJ. *Handbook of Obesity Treatment.* New York: The Guilford Press; 2002.

53. Pan XR, Li GW, Hu YH, Wang JX, Yang WY, An ZX, et al. Effects of diet and exercise in preventing NIDDM in people with impaired glucose tolerance. The Da Qing IGT and Diabetes Study. *Diabetes Care.* 1997;20(4):537–544.

54. Stoddart ML, Blevins KS, Lee ET, Wang W, Blackett PR. Association of acanthosis nigricans with hyperinsulinemia compared with other selected risk factors for type 2 diabetes in Cherokee Indians: The Cherokee Diabetes Study. *Diabetes Care.* 2002; 25(6):1009–1014.

55. Arslanian SA. Metabolic differences between Caucasian and African-American children and the relationship to type 2 diabetes mellitus. *J Pediatr Endocrinol Metab.* 2002;15[suppl 1]:509–517.

56. National High Blood Pressure Education Program, National Institutes of Health, National Heart, Lung, and Blood Institute. JNC 7 Express: The Seventh Report of the Joint National Committee on Prevention, Detection, Evaluation, and Treatment of High Blood Pressure. Washington, DC: United States Department of Health and Human Services; 2003.

57. United States Department of Health and Human Services, Public Health Service, National Institutes of Health, National Heart, Lung, and Blood Institute. Third Report of the National Cholesterol Education Program Expert Panel on the Detection, Evaluation, and Treatment of High Blood Cholesterol in Adults (Adult Treatment Panel III). Washington, DC: United States Department of Health and Human Services; 2002.

58. Goroll AH, May LA, Mulley AJ. *Primary Care Medicine: Office Evaluation and Management of the Adult Patient.* 4th ed. Philadelphia, PA: J.B. Lippincott; 2000.

59. Fischbach F. *A Manual of Laboratory and Diagnostic Tests.* 7th ed. Philadelphia: J.B. Lippincott; 2003.

60. Fahey JO. Nutrition in women's health. In: Varney H, Kriebs JM, Gregor CL, editors. *Varney's Midwifery.* 4th ed. Boston, MA: Jones and Bartlett; 2004. pp. 99–133.

61. Varney H, Kriebs JM, Gregor CL. *Varney's Midwifery.* 4th ed. Boston, MA: Jones and Bartlett; 2004.

62. Duyff RL. *American Dietetic Association Complete Food and Nutrition Guide.* 2nd ed. Hoboken, NJ: John Wiley & Sons; 2002.

63. Bessesen DH. Talking to patients about popular diet books. In: Bessesen DH, Kushner R, editors. *Evaluation and Management of Obesity.* Philadelphia, PA: Hanley & Belfus; 2003. pp. 59–69.

64. Atkins RC. *Dr. Atkins' New Diet Revolution.* New York: M. Evans and Company; 2002.

65. Agatston A. *The South Beach Diet.* Emmaus, PA: Rodale Press; 2003.

66. Ornish D. *Dr. Dean Ornish's Program for Reversing Heart Disease: The Only System Scientifically Proven to Reverse Heart Disease Without Drugs or Surgery.* 2nd ed. New York: Ballantine Books; 1996.

67. Monte T, Pritikin I. *Pritikin: The Man Who Healed America's Heart.* Emmaus, PA: Rodale Press; 1988.

68. Brand-Miller J, Wolever TMS, Foster-Powell K, Colagiuri. *The New Glucose Revolution: The Authoritative Guide to the Glycemic Index—The Dietary Solution for Lifelong Health.* New York: Marlowe & Company; 2003.

69. Steward HL, Bethea MC, Andrews SS, Balart LA. *The New Sugar Busters: Cut Sugar to Trim Fat.* New York: The Ballantine Publishing Group; 2003.

70. Sears B. *A Week in the Zone.* New York: HarpersCollins Publishers; 2000.

71. D'Adamo PJ, Whitney C. *Eat Right for Your Blood Type.* New York: G.B. Putnam's Sons; 2003.

72. Rolls BJ, Barnett RA. *The Volumetrics Weight-Control Plan.* New York: HarperCollins Publishers; 2000.

73. Bessesen DH, Kushner R. *Evaluation and Management of Obesity.* Philadelphia, PA: Hanley & Belfus; 2003.

74. Ferster CB, Nurnberger JI, Levitt EB. The control of eating. *J Math.* 1962;1:87–109.

75. Stuart RB. Behavioural control of overeating. *Behav Res Ther.* 1967;5:357–365.

76. Wing RA. Behavioral weight control. In: Wadden TA, Stunkard AJ, editors. *Handbook of Obesity Treatment.* New York: The Guilford Press; 2002. pp. 301–316.

77. Wing RR, Jefferey RW. Outpatient treatments of obesity: A comparison of methodological and clinical results. *Int J Obes.* 1979;3:261–279.

78. Wadden TA, Stunkard AJ, Brownell KD. Very low calorie diets: Their efficacy, safety, and future. *Ann Intern Med.* 1983;99:675–684.

79. Wadden TA, Foster GD, Letizia KA. One-year behavioral treatment of obesity: Comparison of moderate and severe caloric restriction and the effects of

80. Wing RR, Blair E, Marcus MD, Epstein LH, Harvey J. Year-long weight loss treatment for obese patients with Type II diabetes: Does inclusion of an intermittent very low calorie diet improve outcome? *Am J Med.* 1994;97:354–362.

81. Pronk NP, Wing RR. Physical activity and long-term maintenance of weight loss. *Obes Res.* 1994;2:587–599.

82. Klem ML, Wing RR, McQuire MT, Seagle HM, Hill JO. A descriptive study of individuals successful at long-term maintenance of substantial weight loss. *Am J Clin Nutr.* 1997;66:239–246.

83. Berry D. An emerging model of behavior change in women maintaining weight loss. *Nurs Sci Q.* 2004; 17:242–252.

84. Wing RR, Jeffery RW. Benefits of recruiting participants with friends and increasing social support for weight loss maintenance. *J Consult Clin Psychol.* 1999;67:132–138.

85. Hill JO, Wyatt H, Phelan S, Wing R. The National Weight Control Registry: Is it useful in helping deal with our obesity epidemic? *J Nutr Educ Behav.* 2005;37:206–210.

86. Blair SN, Leermakers EA. Exercise and weight management. In: Wadden TA, Stunkard AJ, editors. *Handbook of Obesity Treatment.* New York: The Guilford Press; 2002. pp. 283–300.

87. Cowlin A. Women and exercise. In: Varney H, Kriebs JM, Gregor CL, editors. *Varney's Midwifery.* 4th ed. Boston, MA: Jones and Bartlett; 2004. pp. 187–247.

88. Myers-Smith C. *Perinatal Fitness.* Tuscon, AZ: Desert Southwest Fitness; 2000.

89. Tupler J. *Maternal Fitness: Preparing for the Marathon of Labor.* New York: Simon and Schuster; 1996.

90. American College of Sports and Medicine. *Guidelines for Exercise Testing and Prescription.* 7th ed. Philadelphia, PA: Lippincott, Williams and Wilkins; 2005.

91. Jakicic JM, Winters C, Lang W, Wing RR. Effects of intermittent exercise and use of home exercise equipment on adherence, weight loss, and fitness in overweight women: A randomized trial. *J Am Med Assoc.* 1999;266:1535–1542.

92. Jakicic JM, Wing RR, Butler BA, Robertson RJ. Prescribing exercise in multiple short bouts versus one continuous bout: Effects on adherence, cardiorespiratory fitness, and weight loss in overweight

women. *Int J Obes Relat Metab Disord.* 1995; 19(12): 893–901.

93. Schneider PL, Crouter SE, Bassett DR. Pedometer measures of free-living physical activity: Comparison of 13 models. *Med Sci Sports Exerc.* 2004;36: 331–335.

94. Eston R, Reilly T. *Kinanthropometry and Exercise Physiology Laboratory Manual: Tests, Procedures, and Data.* London, UK: Chapman & Hall; 1996.

95. Knight J. Safety concerns prompt US ban on dietary supplement. *Nature.* 2004;427:90.

96. Lenz TL, Hamilton WR. Supplemental products used for weight loss. *J Am Pharm Assoc.* 2004;44(1): 59–67.

97. Chen C, Biller J, Willing SJ, Lopez AM. Ischemic stroke after using the counter products containing ephedra. *J Neurol Sci.* 2004;217(1):55–60.

98. Heber D. Non-prescription weight-loss products. In: Bessesen DH, Kushner R, editors. *Evaluation and Management of Obesity.* Philadelphia, PA: Hanley & Belfus; 2002. pp. 89–95.

99. Smith AP, Caffeine at work. *Hum Psychopharmacol.* 2003;20:441–445.

100. Dulloo AG, Seydoux J, Girardier L, Chante P, Vandermander J. Green tea and thermogenesis: interactions between catechin-polyphenols, caffeine and sympathetic activity. *Int J Obes Relat Metab Dis.* 2000;24:252–258.

101. Bell SJ, Goodrick GK. A functional food product for management of weight. *Crit Rev Food Sci Nutr.* 2002;42(2):163–178.

102. Porter DJ, Raymond LW, Anastasio GD. Chromium: friend or foe? *Arch Fam Med.* 1999;8:386–390.

103. Hasten DL, Rome EP, Franks BD, Hegsted M. Effects of chromium picolinate on beginning weight training students. *Int J Sport Nutr.* 1992;2:343–350.

104. Grant KE, Chandler RM, Castle AL, Ivy JL. Chromium and exercise training: Effect on obese women. *Med Sci Sports Exerc.* 1997;29:992–998.

105. Anderson RA, Bryden NA, Polansky MM. Lack of toxicity of chromium chloride and chromium picolinate in rats. *J Am Coll Nutr.* 1997;16:273–279.

106. Nissen S, Sharp R, Ray M, Rathmacher JA, Rice D, Fuller JC, et al. Effects of leucine metabolite beta-hydroxy-beta-methylbutyrate on muscle metabolism during resistance-exercise training. *J Appl Physiol.* 1996;81(5):2095–2104.

107. Alfieri MA, Pomerleau J, Grace DM, Anderson L. Fiber intake of normal weight, moderately obese and severely obese subjects. *Obes Res.* 1995;3:541–547.

108. Staff PDR. *Physician's Desk Reference.* Montvale, NJ: Medical Economics Company; 2005.

109. Kushner R. Pharmacologic therapy. In: Bessesen DH, Kushner R, editors. *Evaluation and Management of Obesity.* Philadelphia, PA: Hanley & Belfus; 2002. pp. 97–106.

110. Kushner R. Surgical treatment of obesity. In: Bessesen DH, Kushner R, editors. *Evaluation and Management of Obesity.* Philadelphia, PA: Hanley & Belfus; 2002. pp. 115–124.

111. Balsiger BM, Luque-de Leon E, Sarr MG. Bariatric surgery for weight control in patients with morbid obesity. *Med Clin North Am.* 2000;84:477–489.

112. Wyatt HR, Wing RR, Hill JO. The national weight control registry. In: Bessesen DH, Kushner R, editors. *Evaluation and Management of Obesity.* Philadelphia, PA: Hanley & Belfus; 2002. p. 119–124.

113. Primak LE. Obesity Web resources for health professionals. In: Bessesen DH, Kushner R, editors. *Evaluation and Management of Obesity.* Philadelphia, PA: Hanley & Belfus; 2002. pp. 145–154.

114. Mokdad AH, Serdula MK, Dietz WH, Bowman BA, Marks JS, Koplan JP. The spread of the obesity epidemic in the United States, 1991–1998. *JAMA.* 1999;282(16):1519–1522.

115. Hu FB. Overweight and obesity in women: Health risks and consequences. *J Women's Health* (Larchmt). 2003;12(2):163–172.

116. National Academy of Sciences. Nutrition during pregnancy: Weight gain and nutrient supplements. Washington, DC: National Academy Press; 1990.

117. Castro LC, Avina RL. Maternal obesity and pregnancy outcomes. *Curr Opin Obstet Gynecol.* 2002; 14(6):601–606.

118. Stephansson O, Dickman PW, Johansson A, Cnattingius S. Maternal weight, pregnancy weight gain, and the risk of antepartum stillbirth. *Am J Obstet Gynecol.* 2001;184(3):463–469.

119. Olson CM, Strawderman MS, Hinton PS, Pearson TA. Gestational weight gain and postpartum behaviors associated with weight change from early pregnancy to 1 y postpartum. *Int J Obes Relat Metab Disord.* 2003;27(1):117–127.

120. Rooney BL, Schauberger CW. Excess pregnancy weight gain and long-term obesity: One decade later. *Obstet Gynecol.* 2002;100(2):245–252.

121. Wang TW, Apgar BS. Exercise during pregnancy. *Am Fam Phys.* 1998;57(8):1846–1852.

122. The American College of Obstetricians and Gynecologists. Exercise during pregnancy: ACOG Education Pamphlet AP119. Washington, DC: The American College of Obstetricians and Gynecologists; 2003.

123. Davies GA, Wolfe LA, Mottola MF, MacKinnon C, Arsenault MY, Bartellas E, et al. Exercise in pregnancy and the postpartum period. *J Obstet Gynaecol Can.* 2003;25(6):516–529.

124. Clapp JF. *Exercising Through Your Pregnancy.* 3rd ed. Omaha, NE: Addicus Books; 2002.

125. The American College of Obstetricians and Gynecologists. Exercise during pregnancy and the postpartum period: ACOG Committee Opinion Number 267. Washington, DC: The American College of Obstetricians and Gynecologists; 2002.

126. United States Department of Health and Human Services. Historic Surgeon General's Report offers new moderate view of physical activity. Washington, DC: United States Department of Health and Human Services; 1996.

127. American Council on Exercise. *Monitoring Exercise Intensity Using Perceived Exertion.* San Diego, CA: American Council on Exercise; 2001.

128. Coleman E. *Exercise and Fitness.* Ashland, OR: Nutrition Dimension; 1990.

129. Convertino VA, Armstrong LE, Coyle EF, Mack GW, Sawka MN, Senay LC, Jr., et al. American College of Sports Medicine position stand. Exercise and fluid replacement. *Med Sci Sports Exerc.* 1996;28(1):i–vii.

130. Anderson BJ, Auslander WF, Jung KC, Miller JP, Santiago JV. Assessing family sharing of diabetes responsibilities. *J Pediatr Psychol.* 1990;15(4): 477–492.

131. The American College of Obstetricians and Gynecologists. *Exercise and Fitness: A Guide for Women.* Washington, DC: The American College of Obstetricians and Gynecologists; 1998.

132. Anderson RA, Anderson JE. *Stretching.* Bolinas, CA: Shelter Publications; 2003.

Chapter 7

Violence Against Women and Children

Patricia A. Paluzzi

Violence against women is common and has far-reaching and long-lasting effects. The Federal Bureau of Investigation estimates that between one-third to one-half of all women in the United States will experience some form of physical violence during their lifetime.[1] Long time family violence researcher Murray Straus stated that the American household is perhaps the most violent institution in the country, and that Americans generally face a greater risk of violence among people they know as opposed to strangers.[2] This is especially true for women. While only 5% of violent crimes against men involve family and friends, 33% of violent crimes against women fit this description.[3]

Both men and women can be victimized as children or adults, and by family, friends, and strangers. Women, however, experience more sexual assault and more violent intimate partner violence (IPV). Violence can be emotional, physical, sexual, or financial and often includes more than one type. No one is safe from abuse; it affects women of all ages, racial and ethnic groups, sexual orientations, and socioeconomic status. Survivors of violence, in all of its forms, are at risk for long-lasting physical and/or psychological effects.

Midwives care for women across the life span and therefore will evaluate all types of violence, including abuse experienced as a child, adolescent, or adult, date or stranger rape, and ongoing IPV or family violence. This chapter describes each of the types of violence that may occur in women's lives and their potential clinical sequelae, including child abuse and neglect, sexual assault, and IPV. Theoretical explanations for why abuse occurs are presented along with guidelines for assessing and managing abuse in midwifery practice.

Child Abuse and Neglect

Current U.S. law mandates the response to reports of child abuse and neglect. This has not always been the case. It was not until 1973 that a federal law was passed to protect children from abuse and neglect. The first recorded child abuse court case, brought against foster parents in New York City, was won on the argument made by Henry Bergh, founder of the Society for the Prevention of Cruelty to Animals in 1866, that children were part of the animal kingdom and deserved the same protection. This case led to the development of the New

York Society for the Prevention of Cruelty to Children in 1874, allowing legal protection for children for the first time. Over time other states followed suit, implementing laws to offer children some protection against abuse and neglect.[4]

Child abuse and neglect were "rediscovered" after a seminal work by Dr. C. Henry Kempe and Dr. Ray Heller in their article entitled, "The Battered Child Syndrome," which appeared in the *Journal of American Medical Association* in 1962. This article described the types of injuries often found in abused children under age three. This work focused attention on the issue and eventually led to legal protections for children under federal law.

By the time the Child Abuse Prevention and Treatment Act (CAPTA) was passed in 1973, every state had some law regarding reporting of and response to child abuse and neglect. Federalizing the issue provided more funding for states and provided model laws for states to follow. All state laws have at least three similarities: they share the same general definitions of abuse and neglect; include mandated reporting requirements; and provide for anonymity and confidentiality. CAPTA defines *abuse and neglect* as "any recent act or failure to act on the part of a parent or caretaker which results in death, serious physical or emotional harm, sexual abuse or exploitation, or an act or failure to act which represents an imminent risk of serious harm."[5] The definition further defines statutory rape as carnal knowledge occurring between persons having reached the age of majority with persons who have not yet reached the age of majority.

Though there are commonalities across state laws for definition of abuse and neglect, these definitions remain problematic. Cultural dif-ferences regarding what constitutes punishment versus abuse are not easy to discern. Further, who is a mandated reporter and under what circumstance can differ from state to state. Professionals, however, are generally mandated reporters and are required to report even suspicious (as opposed to proven) abuse. **Table 7-1** lists resources available on the Internet that outline each state's reporting requirements.

Prevalence

Estimates of child abuse and neglect rely primarily on reports to the Department of Health and Human Services. In 2003, an estimated 2.9 million referrals for child abuse and neglect were accepted by social service agencies, representing some 5.5 million children. Based on these reports, more than 2 million children were estimated to have suffered abuse, and of those cases 60% were neglect by parents or caretakers; almost 20% involved physical harm; 10% involved sexual abuse; 5% involved emotional abuse. In addition to these categories, 20% represented abandonment, chronic drug abuse, threats, or other forms of abuse. Some children fall into multiple categories. The largest numbers of reported cases occurred in children between 0 and 3 years; slightly more reported cases involved girls than boys. One out of four reports includes more than one type of abuse.[6]

Fatality statistics from both abuse and neglect of children show similar trends. The National Child Abuse and Neglect Data System reported an estimated 1,500 child fatalities in 2003.[6] This translates to 1.98 per 100,000 children in the general population. Children ages 0 to 3 represent the majority of the deaths (76.1%), with 41.2% occurring in children less than one year old. Boys suffer

Table 7-1 RESOURCES

Organization	Web Site Address	Focus
American College of Nurse Midwives	http://www.midwife.org	Position statement on violence against women; training video on IPV; office resources for IPV.
Family Violence Prevention Fund	http://www.endabuse.org	National clearinghouse primarily focused on IPV, but addresses all forms of violence; training materials for providers.
Prevent Child Abuse America	http://www.preventchildabuse.org	Membership organization with state and local chapters; home of the National Center on Child Abuse Prevention Research; educational resources for providers.
Child Abuse Prevention Network	http://www.child-abuse.com	Membership organization with resource materials for providers.
National Clearinghouse on Child Abuse and Neglect Information	http://nccanch.acf.hhs.gov	International child abuse network; resource clearinghouse; fact sheets, information on emerging practices, prevention, research; state by state laws for reporting child abuse.
Rape, Abuse and Incest National Network	http://www.rainn.org	Nation's largest anti-sexual assault organization; operates the national hotline at 1-(800) 656-HOPE; data source including FBI Crime Reports and NCVS.
Men Can Stop Rape	http://www.mencanstoprape.org	Empowers men to work with women to stop rape, change prevailing attitudes about women and girls, and incorporate healthy views of gender equality.
National Center for Injury Prevention and Control	http://www.cdc.gov/ncipc	Facts, publications, and funding sources; publications are free.

(continues)

Table 7-1 RESOURCES *(continued)*

Organization	Web Site Address	Focus
United States Department of Justice	http://www.ojp.usdoj.gov	Links to sites about violence against women and family violence; provides data, programs, and funding opportunities.
Wild Iris Medical Education	http://www.nursingceu.com	Online nursing trainings with pre- and post-tests on several forms of abuse.

more fatalities than girls until age two, after which there is no gender difference in fatality rates. Neglect is the most common cause of death, and this is followed by physical, mental, emotional, and then sexual abuse. Perpetrators are most often the mother alone, followed by mothers and fathers together, and then fathers alone. Due to underreporting, abuse and neglect reporting and fatalities data represent only the tip of the iceberg.

Etiology

Several theories have been posited to explain childhood abuse and neglect:

- *Psychodynamic Theory* stems from Freud's psychoanalytic approach; that much of mental disorders and adult behavior stems from childhood experiences; therefore, abusers were most likely abused or witnessed abuse as children.
- *Transaction Model* poses that stress is what makes most families vulnerable to conflict, potentially increasing the risk of child abuse. This model generally follows three stages: Stage 1, in which the parent is stressed by life circumstances and is unable to fully cope with the child's behavior; Stage 2, when the parent has increasing difficulty managing and begins to blame the child; and Stage 3, when the parent begins to abuse the child.
- *Intergenerational Transmission Theory* borrows from social learning theory and posits that children learn to be abusive by growing up with abuse.
- *Cognitive-Behavioral Theory* also describes four stages of behavior rooted in unrealistic parental expectations that lead finally to abuse.
- *Ecological Model* relies on the four levels of individual, family, community, and cultural/society to explain the dynamics that lead to abuse.[7]

What underlies each of the theories that are fairly well substantiated in the literature and makes this issue relevant for midwives is that abusive parents often were abused themselves. When a positive history of abuse is obtained from an adult client, the clinician must be mindful of the possibility for that client to abuse her own child(ren).

Sequelae

Sequelae may include psychosocial effects such as problems with socialization and interpersonal relationships; depressive and anxiety disorders; self-mutilation and suicide attempts; alcohol and drug abuse; eating disorders, posttraumatic stress disorder (PTSD); and other risky behaviors. These may include teen delinquency and adult criminal behavior, and unsafe sexual behaviors that may result in unintended pregnancies, including teen pregnancy and/or sexually transmitted diseases (STDs). Further, women growing up with abuse either as direct victims or witnesses are more likely to abuse their own children as well as be re-victimized during their lifetimes.[8]

Rape or Sexual Assault

Rape has traditionally been defined by the Bureau of Justice Statistics as "carnal knowledge (penile-vaginal penetration only) of a female forcibly and against her will." Over the past two decades, the federal code and most states have broadened this definition by:

- including sexual penetration of any type, including vaginal, anal, and oral, and by penis, fingers, or objects;
- focusing on the offender's behaviors rather than the survivor's;
- restricting the use of a survivor's previous sexual history as evidence.

Many states have also removed marital status as an exemption. Some states and the U.S. Code have replaced the term "rape" with other terms such as sexual abuse, sexual assault, or sexual battery. Every midwife is responsible for knowing the legal definition of rape or sexual assault in her/his state. This information is essential in order to provide appropriate counseling as well as to comply with reporting requirements. Web resources to gain information regarding rape reporting can be found in Table 7-1.

Prevalence

Only about 39% of rapes are reported. Victims, most often women, may be fearful of exposure of other parts of their lives. While rape shield laws have been imposed to prevent a woman's previous sexual activity from entering into a courtroom, this does not afford full protection. Victims often doubt themselves and question if they were partially at fault, perhaps thinking they were dressed provocatively, had too much to drink, or had placed themselves in a risky situation. Today, professionals recognize that rape is a crime of violence and not of passion; the victim's behavior does not warrant this assault. However, societal messages are often mixed, and victims themselves may have conflicted emotions. In 2002, there were 247,730 reported cases of rape, attempted rape, or sexual assault.[9] These data do not include victims younger than age 12. The statistics describing rape are not accurate and the incidence is grossly underestimated.

Estimates are that one of every six women in the United States has experienced an attempted or completed rape in their lifetime. Teenagers aged 16 to 19 are more than twice as likely as any other age group to experience rape or sexual assault. Two-thirds of survivors know their assailants. Approximately 48% are raped by friends or acquaintances, 34% by strangers or an unknown assailant, 16% by intimate partners, and 2% by another relative.[10]

Etiology

Several theories attempt to explain why rape occurs:

- *Sexual Assault and Male Dominance Theory* states that rape is the result of social inequality between men and women. Men rape women to assert their male dominance and ensure female subordination. This theory claims that pornography and prostitution encourage rape because they degrade women and portray them as subservient.

- *Cultural Norm Theory* posits that rape is learned behavior and is linked to a larger societal pattern of violence. According to this theory, rape is more prevalent in cultures where male physical prowess and honor are revered.
- *The Biological Bases Theory of Sexual Assault* suggests that reproductive drives, not violence, lead to rape. This theory states that rape is part of a biological norm in that men are driven to have sex with as many women as possible to advance the species and their status. Women resist because they are biologically driven to mate with only a few chosen males. This latter theory is highly controversial because it relieves any responsibility for rape from the assailant.[11]

The first two theories are the more generally accepted, because they view rape as an act of aggression and violence rather than an act of passion. This view underlies current rape laws as well. Regardless of the circumstances—where a woman was at the time of the rape, how she was dressed, or whether or not she was under the influence of any substances—no one has the right to force a woman into unwanted sexual activity.

Sequelae

After a rape, most women go through four emotional stages that evolve over time:

- Phase 1 includes the immediate emotional responses that may include shock, denial, crying, or other emotional release.
- Phase 2 begins when the woman feels safe and begins to share her experience. Rape can be very difficult to talk about and is often complicated by feelings of guilt and shame.
- Phase 3 may last for weeks, months, or years, and is a calm period during which the woman thinks she has adjusted to the experience.
- Phase 4 can be triggered by a word, image, or event that brings back the thoughts about the event. This time the thinking is obsessive, but the survivor is usually able to discuss her deeper feelings and come to a place of comfort with the event.

A client may present for care during any of these phases. Recognizing them and responding appropriately can assist the woman in getting the care she needs at that moment. The survivor needs a safe and supportive environment to speak about the incident during each of these phases. Long-term therapy or support groups may be most effective once the survivor reaches the fourth phase. Each client interaction will most likely be different and what is most important is to offer the client appropriate referrals to meet her needs.

Other sequelae to rape include PTSD; depressive and anxiety disorders; other phobias; lowered self-esteem, social adjustment problems, and sexual dysfunction.[12] This constellation of symptoms is sometimes referred to as the rape trauma syndrome. Chapter 9 contains a full discussion of PTSD and other related mental health issues.

Intimate Partner Violence

IPV is defined as a pattern of assaultive or coercive behaviors, including physical, sexual, and psychological attacks as well as economic coercion that adults or adolescents use against their intimate partners.[13] Intimate partners include individuals who are currently in dating, cohabitating, or marital relationships, or those who have been in such relationships in the past. Heterosexual, gay, or lesbian couples can experience IPV. IPV usually consists of multiple episodes over time and includes a range of tactics that may or may not be injurious and/or illegal. This combination of physical attacks, terrorist acts, and controlling tactics results in fear as well as physical and psychological harm to the victim and her children. IPV sets up a dynamic of power and control in the relationship. **Table** 7-2 contrasts healthy and unhealthy behaviors in relationships.

Prevalence

The prevalence of IPV is difficult to state with certainty because studies have used different definitions, populations, and data collection techniques. National estimates generally are lower than those from clinical sites. While one in four women in the United States report having been physically abused by a husband or boyfriend at some point in their lives,[14] estimates are much higher for women cared for in hospital emergency rooms. In one report, 37% of women seeking care in an emergency room for violence-related injuries were injured by a current or former intimate partner.[15] While IPV cuts across all racial/ethnic; age; socioeconomic, and cultural lines, certain groups have an increased risk: teens, minorities, and poor women.

Etiology

IPV often follows a pattern that begins with social isolation and emotional degradation that leads to physical, sexual, and/or financial abuse and assault. In classic situations, the victim of the abuse has been manipulated and isolated to the point that she cannot recognize the abuse as such, so she minimizes the behavior or blames herself.

The first description of a cycle of violence was developed in 1978. It delineates a pattern of tension building, leading to the abusive episode, which is followed by a "honeymoon" phase. The tension building phase describes a period when the abuser's behavior begins to change and tension builds in the relationship. This phase can last for hours or days. Eventually, the survivor learns to recognize this phase and may alter his or her own behavior to attempt to delay or further provoke the abusive incident. The abusive incident then follows and can vary greatly in intensity and duration. The honeymoon phase then begins, during which the abuser apologizes for his or her behavior, asks forgiveness, and tries to reconcile with the survivor. This phase appears to be critically important in the beginning to maintain the abusive relationship, because the abuser appears appropriately apologetic and the survivor wants to believe that everything will be okay again.

After 20 years of research, a group of nurse researchers amended this cycle to recognize dynamics that are consistent over time in abusive relationships. They offered a new cycle that incorporates a heightened tension building phase, followed by increasingly dangerous abusive incidents, and a shortened honeymoon phase, which decreases and disappears altogether over time. This amended cycle takes into account that abusive relationships generally become increasingly abusive and thus more dangerous over time. The abuser no longer feels the need to apologize and indulge

Table 7-2 COMPARING CHARACTERISTICS OF HEALTHY AND UNHEALTHY RELATIONSHIPS

Unhealthy Characteristics	Healthy Characteristics
Coercion and threats: threatens harm, to leave, commit suicide, report her to welfare, makes her do illegal things.	*Negotiation and fairness:* seeks mutually satisfying resolutions to conflict, accepts change, is willing to compromise.
Intimidation: creates fear through looks, actions, gestures, smashing things, hurting pets, displaying weapons, or threatening the children.	*Non-threatening behavior:* talks and acts in a manner that makes her feel safe when expressing herself.
Economic abuse: prevents her from getting or keeping a job, controls the money.	*Economic partnership:* money decisions are made together.
Male privilege: defines gender roles as male dominant/female subservient; makes all decisions; is the "head of the household."	*Shared responsibility:* work is fairly distributed through mutual agreement.
Emotional abuse: humiliates her, makes her think she's crazy, plays mind games.	*Respect:* Listens non-judgmentally, is supportive and affirming.
Uses children: uses the children as emotional pawns, makes her feel guilty about the children.	*Responsible parenting:* shares duties, is a responsible non-violent role model.
Isolation: controls her behavior in and outside of the home; severely limits her contact with family and friends; no or limited outside activities.	*Trust and support:* supportive of her life goals, respectful of her friends and activities.
Minimizes, denies, blames: does not take responsibility for abusive behavior, shames her, and makes the abuse her fault.	*Honest and accountable:* takes responsibility for own behavior, admits to being wrong, communicates openly and honestly.

Source: Adapted with permission from the Domestic Abuse Intervention Project. 202 East Superior Street, Duluth, Minnesota, 55802. www.duluth-model.org/.

in a honeymoon phase as the survivor becomes more and more disempowered by the relationship. Understanding this cycle is important to appropriately recognize the abusive pattern and counsel survivors.

As with other forms of violence, many theories have been proposed:

- *Feminist Theory* developed in the 1970s with the advent of the Women's Movement and increased attention to IPV. This theory posits that abuse is strictly about male dominance over women and the etiology lies in a patriarchal society.
- *Family Violence Theory* states that IPV is just one type of violence that occurs within families. Because families spend a great deal of time together, family matters may be kept private from the outside world and family members know each other's vulnerabilities.

Abuser(s) within families are expert at exploiting other family members' vulnerabilities, while those that are abused learn how to avoid provoking the abuser(s) and by doing so prevent confrontation.

- *Learned Behavior Theory* argues that violence is learned in the home; therefore, children who are themselves abused or saw abuse in their family of origin are more likely to be abusive adults.
- *Pathology and Psychodynamic Theories* argue that abusers are mentally ill or have a substance abuse or other problem that causes the violence. These theories hold up for only a small amount of abusers who are truly ill. The majority of abusers are not mentally ill, nor do they have a neurological disorder that makes them prone to violence.[7,16]

Most advocates and researchers subscribe to either the Feminist or Family Violence Theories, because these seem most congruent with what is known about violence. The abuse that occurs within intimate relationships and fits the pattern of IPV is usually executed in a private manner and with controlling behavior from the abuser. Also, abusive partners are often quite charismatic and never display their abusive tendencies toward others. This part of the dynamic can be used to reinforce guilt to the survivor: that it is her fault as it only happens with her. An individual with a true psychological disorder cannot control his or her behavior in such a manner.

SEQUELAE

As with child abuse or sexual assault, women currently living with or having a history of abusive intimate relationships may experience common sequelae. These include gastrointestinal conditions such as irritable bowel syndrome, chronic pain (particularly pelvic pain), depression, suicide attempts, drug or alcohol use, eating disorders, repeated unintended pregnancies, miscarriages, STDs, various forms of sexual dysfunction, and vulvar or labial bruising. **Table 7-3** lists the four types of IPV and examples of what constitutes abuse within each type.

Table 7-3 **FOUR TYPES OF INTIMATE PARTNER VIOLENCE AND EXAMPLES OF EACH TYPE**

Physical	Slapping, punching, biting, kicking, spitting, poking, choking, burning; controlling access to health care.
Emotional	Humiliating, name calling, put downs, infanticizing, threatens to leave, or hurt family, children, pets, or expose her for something such as drug use or being gay, stalking, or other controlling activities.
Financial	Prevents her from getting a job or sabotages a current job; controls how all money is spent; doesn't contribute financially.
Sexual	Rapes; forces acts with which she is uncomfortable; calls her lewd names; exposes her sexually.

Assessment

GENERAL GUIDELINES

Assessing for abuse of any type is more effective when certain parameters and guidelines are followed. Because of the prevalent and non-discriminating nature of abuse, all clients should be screened for all types of abuse, past and present. Recommendations are to assess every client during every annual visit as well as every prenatal visit during pregnancy. A few studies have demonstrated that repeated assessment seems to be more effective for gaining disclosure, especially during pregnancy.[17] Problem visits, especially if the client is presenting with an STD or repeated complaints of a pelvic problem, gastrointestinal problems, or other stress-related diseases should also be used as a time for assessment. Because anyone can be abused and because repeated screening is more effective, universal screening is the preferred practice.

Special emphasis should be placed on assessing those clients who demonstrate any of the sequelae listed in this chapter. **Table 7-4** provides a succinct overview of the types of violence and sequelae discussed here.

It is best to use clear language and ask questions directly; however, carefully chosen wording is important. For example, it is not recommended to ask the client if she or he has been abused because she may not see the situation as abusive. It is best to ask if the client has ever been forced to participate in sexual activity that made her uncomfortable, or has been hit, slapped, kicked, and so forth. The seminal question for assessing IPV, in particular, is to ask the client if she is ever afraid of her partner. Being fearful of one's partner is what separates the normal arguments that couples have from a dynamic involving coercion and fear.

It is important to generalize the questioning so the client does not feel singled out for any

Table 7-4 OVERVIEW OF TYPES OF VIOLENCE AND SEQUELAE

Type of Violence	Sequelae
Child Abuse	Relationship difficulties, sexual dysfunction, difficulty with pelvic exams, disassociation during exams, teen pregnancy, repeat unintended pregnancies and/or STDs, depressive or anxiety disorders, suicide attempts, eating disorders, drug and alcohol abuse, other risky behaviors such as delinquency or adult criminal activities.
Sexual Abuse and Assault	All of the above plus signs of posttraumatic stress disorder dependent on the time of the assault, lowered self-esteem, problems with social adjustment, and phobias.
Intimate Partner Violence	All of the above plus fearful affect, chronic disorders such as chronic pain and particularly chronic pelvic pain, gastrointestinal disorders, particularly irritable bowel syndrome, late entry to or sporadic prenatal care, non-adherence to treatments, repeat abortions, poor weight gain during pregnancy, history of low birth weight and premature infants, vulvar or labial bruising, bruising in various stages of healing.

reason. For example, if abuse assessment questions are on the history form, then simply follow up on them. If they aren't on the form, it is good to preface these questions with an introduction explaining why all clients are assessed. This can also be a time for assessing for other sensitive issues such as drug use.

What follows is a suggested list of questions that can be used for assessing violence of all types:

- Generalize with an introduction, such as: *"Because of the pervasiveness of violence against women in our society, I ask all women in my practice if they have ever been hurt by someone. These questions can be sensitive, but they are important and I am asking them because they can affect your health."*
- Specific Questions:
  - Child Sexual Abuse/Sexual Assault: *"Has anyone ever forced you to take part in any sexual activities that made you uncomfortable?"*
  - IPV, past or present: *"Has anyone ever slapped, punched, kicked, bitten, or otherwise hurt you? Are you in a relationship now? Are you satisfied with the relationship? Everyone has arguments when they are in a relationship and sometimes fights can be physical and with a lot of name-calling and anger. When you and your partner fight, are you ever afraid of him/her? Does he/she ever do anything to make you feel bad about yourself, like humiliate you in public?*

It is essential that clients are always screened in private for abuse. This is especially important when screening for IPV because you do not know who the perpetrator is or the relationships to the perpetrator of anyone accompanying the client. It is also significant for assessing past abuse, because the client may be more willing to be open if no one else is in the room. It may be helpful to establish a clinic or office protocol that allows alone time for every client to screen for abuse as well as other sensitive issues.

CHILD ABUSE

The importance of knowing state laws regulating reporting of suspected or disclosed child abuse has been discussed. Since midwives will be mandated reporters in all states, another important aspect of the law includes the time limits that may exist for prosecution. Many adults may begin to have memories of child abuse, particularly sexual abuse, later in life. The midwife should be prepared to advise the client as to her rights in this matter, or at least be able to access that information easily. The midwife must also let the client know, before assessing for child abuse, that he or she are mandated to report and what that could mean. This, of course, poses some difficulties because fewer clients may disclose abuse if they do not want to face potential legal involvement. Each midwife will need to develop a personal approach to this type of assessment, balancing the risks and benefits of assessment with full disclosure.

SEXUAL ASSAULT AND RAPE

Midwives may be the first providers to care for a rape survivor. If this is the case, the midwife needs to counsel the client about the usefulness of having a sexual assault exam during which evidence can be collected. The client should be counseled that going through this type of exam does not mean that she must participate in legal activities but does have that option, should that be her decision. It may take awhile to convince the client to do this, but it is worth the time and effort. Sexual Assault Recovery Centers (SARCs) are generally available in communities, often within a hospital setting, with SARC trained personnel and counselors.

Anticipatory guidance for a SARC exam includes counseling that evidence collection can be done for up to 72 hours after the incident using a Physical Evidence Recovery Kit. This involves: collecting clothing worn at the time of the assault; combing through pubic and head hair to collect samples; taking swabs from all orifices that were involved in the assault; and perhaps performing a toxicology screen if the assailant used drugs. If the incident occurred more than 72 hours ago, the kit is no longer used. Evidence can still be collected, however, and important services rendered. Another important aspect is taking baseline tests for pregnancy, STDs, and human immunodeficiency virus (HIV). The client should be seen again in six weeks for a repeat pregnancy test and STD screens, and six months for the repeat HIV screen. Emergency contraception should be offered. Current guidelines for HIV/STD prophylaxis are available from the Centers for Disease Control and Prevention on the Internet (http://www.cdc.gov). The client should know that she must give written consent to have this exam; she must also consent to contact the police and turn over the evidence.

If the client refuses to have a SARC exam, then the midwife should assess and document injuries, perform baseline pregnancy, STD, and HIV screens and offer emergency contraception. The client's mental status should be examined and appropriate measures taken. Finally, the midwife should document all available details of the incident that might be used later should the client decide to pursue legal action. Photos and/or use of a body map (**Figure 7-1**) will be helpful with this type of documentation.

Past Sexual Abuse/Assault   Including a question about previous sexual abuse can cover ac-

quaintance or stranger rape and should be a part of every annual history. If the woman acknowledges rape or sexual assault, then exploring when the rape occurred, or if she has previously disclosed this event, whether she wants support at this time are all relevant issues. If the woman seeks support, it is probably best to refer her to someone with this expertise. Repeated exploration of sexual abuse and rape should occur when red flags are present (Table 7-4).

Bruising and Behavior Changes   Two additional considerations when assessing for IPV include the appearance of bruises and behavior of the client's partner. Any bruising should be questioned as to how it occurred. Important to note are:

- Bruises that appear to be defensive; for example, on the inside of the forearm, or across the palms of the hands.
- Bruises that are incongruent with the client's history. Accidental bruising usually involves the hands, knees, shins, and top of the head. Bruises on the inside of the arms, on the back, or around the upper arms are probably intentional.
- Bruises that carry characteristic marks such as those that look like a hand grabbing an upper arm, or carry an outline of a weapon such as an iron or cigarette.
- Bruises in various stages of healing. Just as with child abuse, a woman who is being repeatedly battered may have several bruises in various stages of healing on her body.

A more subtle indication of an abusive intimate relationship is a partner who appears overprotective. This type of partner wants to be present at every minute of every visit and may even speak for the woman. When such a partner is present, it is critical to find some time alone with the woman to assess the relationship.

Figure 7-1 Example of an injury location chart or body map.

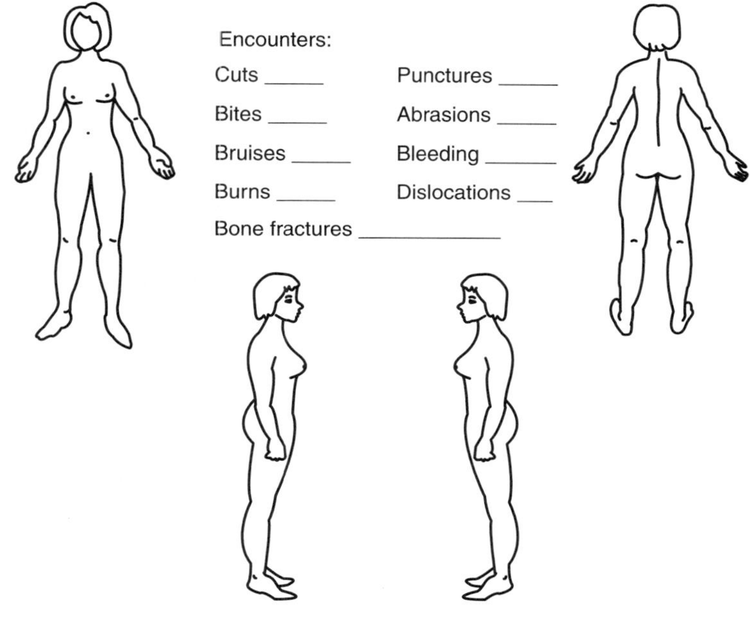

Source: Used with permission from the Family Violence Prevention Fund. Adapted from Warshaw C, Ganley AL, Salter PR. *Improving the Health Care Reponse to Domestic Violence: A Resource Manual for Health Care Providers.* San Francisco: The Family Violence Prevention Fund; 1995.

Management

When assessing for abuse of any kind, the midwife must be prepared with a nonjudgmental and empathetic response that shows unequivocal support for the survivor. If the client has chosen to disclose abuse of any kind, the midwife must listen thoughtfully, show empathy, remind the client that it is not her fault, and offer appropriate resources and referrals.

If the client chooses not to disclose abuse and the midwife feels fairly certain that abuse is ev-ident, it is acceptable to state that doubt to the client while not implying that she is lying. This type of response must be thought out. For example, if the woman describes a situation that is clearly abusive but doesn't acknowledge it as such, the midwife can say something like, "What you have described sounds like abuse to me. I would like to give you some resources that tell you more about abuse. Please know that I am here for you and we can talk more about this at a later date if you'd like." Even in the face of compelling evidence to the contrary, it is essential to meet the woman where she is in her process and not try to "force" her to see things that she is not yet ready to face.

Each client needs time to talk about her experience when she is ready to do so. The woman must be allowed the time to talk about her experiences and feelings, and offered further opportunity to do so with the appropriate professional. It is important for the midwife to understand her/his limits in caring for abuse survivors who may need professional counseling. If memories of abuse are just re-emerging, as can happen when a woman is questioned during an outpatient visit or during the course of a pregnancy, she may need professional support while she acknowledges her history. Each midwife, therefore, should be knowledgeable about professional and community resources to support the survivor of both past and current abuse.

Another aspect of management, particularly with rape and sexual assault, is being sensitive to the client's potential unwillingness to disclose a perpetrator who is familiar to them. Keep in mind that someone known to the survivor perpetrates most sexual abuse of children, teens, and adults. This may hinder their willingness to disclose the abuse or take legal action. Clients deserve full information about what it means to take legal action as well as the time to consider all of the implications of disclosing a family member or friend as a sexual assaulter. Providing a referral to a counselor or abuse center is probably the best way to handle this situation.

The Stages of Change Model, originally developed to assess the process of change in behaviors such as addictions, provides an effective way to form a response and offer appropriate stage-based counseling and resources for women living with abuse. **Table 7-5** provides a framework for using this model to assess and respond to abuse, past or present, in a manner that may be most effective for assisting the survivor in moving to the next phase of change. Using this model meets the survivor where she/he is emotionally, allows them to hear what is being offered, and assists the client in moving to the next stage.

Abuse during Pregnancy

Abuse during pregnancy poses its own special risks and dynamics. The incidence and risks associated with IPV in pregnancy is unclear. Incidence rates vary dramatically from study to study, reflecting differences in the definitions used to describe abuse, sample sizes, and characteristics as well as the method, timing, and frequency of screening. One summary of the literature on the rates of abuse during pregnancy reported a range between 0.2% and 20%.[19]

Additional factors such as culture and pregnancy intendedness can affect the risk of abuse during pregnancy. For example, one study found that pregnancy protected women against abuse among some Latino cultures whereas it seems to increase the risk of abuse among white women.[19] Why pregnancy would be protective in some circumstances and risky in others is unclear. Some theorists believe that because abuse is a situation of power and control, the abuser may feel as if he or she is losing some control over the pregnant woman. Abusers are thought to be immature and narcissistic. They may also be jealous of the attention a pregnant woman gives to her unborn baby. This jealousy may increase the risk of IPV. Why pregnancy may be a protector against abuse among some Latino cultures is not completely understood, but may be, in part, because of the role pregnancy plays in that culture.

Table 7-5 STAGES OF CHANGE MODEL: ABUSE ASSESSMENT AND RESPONSE

Stage	Evidence of Stage	Counseling Stage Appropriate	Stage Appropriate Resources
Pre-contemplation: Does not acknowledge that there is a problem.	Denies any abuse, past or present, even in the face of compelling evidence. For example, she may say that the bruises are a result of an accident.	"What you are describing to me would be considered abuse. If you ever want to discuss this with me further, I am always ready to listen."	Materials that define and describe abuse are helpful to give her a name for what is happening to her. The materials may contain links to more resources.
Contemplation: Beginning to acknowledge a problem exists but not ready to do anything about it.	May state something like, "I know there is a problem but what can I do? I can't leave because of the kids."	Respond with acceptance of the difficulties with leaving. Perform a safety assessment as part of counseling on how to remain safe within the relationship.	Phone numbers for a hotline and/or shelter or other community-based resources available if she needs to leave or wants more information.
Preparation: Is considering taking action and is gathering information to prepare for the action.	Client may say something like, "I am interested in seeking help with this situation. Do you have any contacts you can share?"	Warn the client that leaving can be the most dangerous time and counsel how to leave safely (if that is what she is considering).	Give names and numbers for community resources that address her issue (domestic violence shelters, therapists for child abuse, etc.).
Action: Client is taking action to change or address her situation.	She may report that she has left the situation and is staying with friends or at a shelter.	Support her decision and remind her what she needs to do to stay safe; repeat safety planning given her new situation.	Offer support groups; offer to see her more often if needed; referrals for any other assistance she may need for her and her family.
Maintenance	She may report that she has been back and forth but has been out of the situation for a month now and is feeling positive.	Offer support, remind her that relapse is a normal part of the process. Discuss what triggers relapse, offer comments accordingly.	Offer support groups and any resource materials that address the difficulties with staying away.

There have been at least two studies demonstrating a relationship between pregnancy intendedness and IPV.[20,21] While it is difficult to ascertain which came first, there is more reported abuse among women with unintended pregnancy. This is particularly true for teens. In a seminal study of medical examiners' records of autopsies of women during their childbearing years, there was a statistically significant higher rate of murder in pregnant teenagers (15–19 years) than non-pregnant teenagers. Most of the teens were less than 21 weeks pregnant.[22] While the study design did not enable the authors to determine causality, the risk of homicide for pregnant teens seems apparent. Therefore, disclosing the results of a positive pregnancy test, to anyone, but particularly to teens should always be done in private.

Sequelae

Indications of abuse during pregnancy may include low birth weight, prematurity, depression (including postpartum depression), excessive weight gain or loss, and a lack or sporadic use of prenatal care. Women with these pregnancy histories or who have difficulty with weight gain and general attendance to prenatal care during the pregnancy should be carefully screened and observed for abuse. As with non-pregnant survivors, smoking, drug, and alcohol use, repeated STDs, unintended pregnancies, pregnancy losses, "non-compliance" with treatment, and the other sequelae stated earlier all may be present.

Memories of child sexual abuse may begin to emerge during pregnancy. It is beneficial to assess for such an abuse history at least once each trimester or more often if red flags begin to emerge. Signs of an abuse history can emerge during pregnancy and may include poor attendance at prenatal visits, unrealistic fears, or, in extreme cases, total denial of the reality of labor and delivery. During the physical exam, the midwife should pay attention to signs of weight fluctuations, which can be either weight loss or gain, difficulty with pelvic exams, including disassociation, and scarring from potential self-mutilation or suicide attempts.

Danger Assessment and Safety Planning

While it is critical to be empathetic and respectful of the woman's view of her relationship, keeping the client safe remains of utmost importance. If the woman discloses a situation that sounds abusive, even if she is unwilling to label it as such, a safety assessment must be conducted to assist her in planning how to keep herself and her children safe should the situation escalate.

Safety planning is a critical aspect of caring for a woman in an abusive relationship. Safety planning can be lengthy and assess every aspect of the woman's life as well as her children's or more succinct with an emphasis on recognizing increased danger and having a plan of response. The goal of safety planning is to maximize the safety of the woman and her children in any given situation that is abusive or threatens to be abusive. Therefore, safety planning includes reviewing various situations where abuse may occur and identifying a plan to either avoid or respond to the situation in the safest way possible.

Safety planning may include a fair amount of disclosure about the abuse, and not every woman will be comfortable with providing that information. For example, safety assessment may mean letting neighbors know about the abuse and asking them to call police if they hear sounds of loud fighting or physical altercation. Similarly, protecting children may involve disclosure to schools or day care centers. While every woman will have her own comfort level that can help assess the risk of lethality among women living with abuse, asking these questions when abuse is revealed can help both the midwife and client see if the abuse is escalating. If the woman answers yes to one or more of the questions in **Table 7-6**, we must advise her of her risk and assist her with appropriate safety planning.

Finally, for all women living with abuse, a plan to leave the situation safely should be developed. Each woman should have a bag prepared that includes a change of clothing for everyone in the family, identification for all members of the family, comfort items for children, keys to the house and car, other important items such as driver's license, insurance cards, and credit cards along with some cash. Each woman should identify someone she can go to if she and her children must leave quickly. She may keep her bag with that person or outside the house somewhere that is both hidden and accessible. The process of safety planning is often helpful in that it allows the woman to acknowledge and address the abuse.

Abuse generally increases in frequency and severity over time, which increases the risk of lethality. Women must know that the act of leaving is potentially the most dangerous time in the relationship. If the abuser feels that he/she is losing control, then his/her need to control will escalate and this can translate into more severe forms of violence and even homicide. Therefore, leaving is something that must be taken very seriously. Women, of course, should leave immediately if they believe their life or their children's lives are threatened. Otherwise, having a plan for a safe place to go and having a "safety bag" prepacked will make leaving

safely easier if it becomes necessary. Table 7-6 suggests the types of assessments that should be part of danger assessment and safety planning.

Other Important Aspects of Caring for Abuse Survivors

There are two additional areas for consideration when responding to survivors of abuse of any kind: legal issues and documentation. Each will be considered briefly with resources including where more detailed information can be found.

Legal Issues

It is the midwife's responsibility to become familiar with all of the laws in her/his state regarding violence of all kinds including the reporting requirements for potentially illegal activity such as rape, statutory rape, and assault. In addition, each clinician should either be familiar with client rights or have a ready referral source where clients can gain accurate information regarding the legal protection and recourse.

As an example, California has a mandatory reporting requirement for clinicians detecting IPV among their clients. While well intended, this law has made disclosure less likely to occur in some situations. Clinicians are obligated to let their clients know that they are required to report suspected cases of abuse. However, women who know that their midwife or practitioner is a mandated reporter may not be comfortable revealing IPV. This is particularly likely when dealing with statutory rape among teens, or with a woman who has experienced previous child abuse or IPV. Each professional must decide on a "script" for abuse assessment that includes proper disclosure regarding reporting require-

Table 7-6 QUESTIONS FOR DANGER ASSESSMENT AND SAFETY PLANNING

Assess the immediate safety of the victim.	Is there imminent danger? Where is the perpetrator now? Does the client want or need security at this time?
Assess the pattern and history of abuse.	What type of abuse has occurred? When does it happen?
Counsel regarding safety based on abuse patterns.	Make client aware that increased episodes and severity of abuse as well as certain types of abuse (specifically: sexual, use of weapons, and abuse of children) increases the risk of lethality.
Assess the client's plans at this time.	Is the client planning to stay in the relationship? Does she have adequate safety mechanisms in place? Is her "safety bag" packed? Does she have a plan for escape?
Assess the client's knowledge of resources.	Does she know about local support groups or shelters? Does she know about her legal rights and where to get an _ex parte_ should she want one?
Assess the safety of the children.	Are the children being abused? Are they witnessing the abuse? Is she aware of resources for them? Has she noticed changes in their behavior? Does she have a safety plan that includes them?

ments and yet promotes the best possible situation for client disclosure. Discuss this issue with peers and other experts in the field.

Many cities and jurisdictions have police and judges trained in IPV issues, and court advocates may be available for the woman. The local battered woman's shelter, IPV coalitions, or police departments can provide this information as well as knowledge about the _ex parte_ system in the area. _Ex parte_ refers to a safety or keep away order prohibiting contact between the parties.

Documentation

Documentation of any kind of abuse should be well thought out and approached in a manner that advocates for the client in both the medical and legal arenas. Medical records can be subpoenaed. Clear and thorough documentation offers more support for the client in the court-

room. Confidentiality, however, is a major concern and care must be taken not to expose the client to more danger by having others view something in her medical records that is potentially harmful. Think of how often medical records are faxed to labor and delivery staff, for example, and the risk this poses if the perpetrator sees evidence of abuse in the record. In rural areas with little anonymity, even more care must be taken to protect a client who has admitted to any kind of abuse.

This may require some alterations to procedures. Medical records may need to be separated so that notes documenting the abuse are kept separate from the rest of the medical record. The chart can be marked in a manner that tells other clinicians to look for the additional notes. These notes are then available for court support as necessary and help clinicians provide ongoing support and care for the survivor but pose less of a risk of breaching confidentiality.

There are two other tools for documentation of physical abuse that can be helpful: a body map and taking photographs. The body map can be used to record the location of bruises or other marks (Figure 7-1), and photographs can serve a similar purpose with even more detail and clarity. Keeping a Polaroid camera or a digital camera in the clinic or office setting is useful. Certain guidelines, such as taking pictures from different angles, labeling each photo with the woman's name and date, and placing an object near the bruise or wound (i.e., a ruler or coin) before shooting the photograph will help with determining scale. It is important that a third party (or court) could be able to accurately view the immediate physical aftermath of the abuse long after the woman has healed.

A Final Note for Clinicians

Working with abuse survivors can be challenging on several fronts. Adopting a universal screening policy and developing an open and accepting style will lead to identifying more abuse survivors. Clearly, this is desirable for the good that can come to the clients, but it may be chal-

lenging for the provider. It can be a heavy emotional burden to know this level of detail about clients' lives. Additionally, the midwife may feel some responsibility and concern for clients who are not yet ready to end an abusive situation or start legal action against a rapist or molester. It is important to maintain a client-centered focus, regardless of personal beliefs about what someone "should" do.

How one defines success in working with survivors is important. Success may not mean that the woman leaves the abusive relationship or seeks legal recourse for a rapist or perpetrator of previous incest. These may be long-term goals for some clients and not goals at all for others. It is the client's choice. The clinician's role is to actively listen and reflect, and add professional objective information that assists the client in her/his decision-making process.

It is helpful to think of every possible action as successful. Consider the Stages of Change Model (Table 7-5) and what it takes for humans to move through painful situations. Having a long-term client finally admit to abuse is success. Getting someone to accept a brochure or phone number for a rape crisis center or IPV shelter is success. Maintaining an open, honest conversation with a client about her/his past or current abuse is success.

References

1. Federal Bureau of Investigation, United States Department of Justice. *Uniform Crime Report for 1996 and 1997.* Washington, DC: U.S. Government Printing Office; 1998.

2. Straus MA, Gelles RJ. *Behind Closed Doors. Violence in the American Family.* New York: Anchor Press; 1981.

3. Office of Justice Programs, United States Department of Justice. *Violence by Intimates.* Analysis of Data on Crimes by Current or Former Spouses, Boyfriends and Girlfriends. Washington, DC: U.S. Government Printing Office; 1998.

4. New York Society for the Prevention of Cruelty to Children. Internet site available from: http://www.nyspcc.org/beta_history/index_history.htm.

5. U.S. Department of Health and Human Services. Administration for Children and Families. Legal citation on the Internet. Available from: http://www.acf.hhs.gov/programs/cb/laws/capta/.

6. U.S. Department of Health and Human Services. Administration for Children and Families. Child Maltreatment 2003. [Monograph on the Internet]. Washington, DC. Accessed September 11, 2005. Available from: http://www.acf.dhhs.gov/programs/cb/publications/cm03/index.htm/.

7. Flanagan AY. *Child Abuse and Neglect. What Healthcare Providers Need to Know.* Wild Iris Medical Education, Nursing Continuing Education, Compton, CA. [December 2002]. Previously available from: http://www.nursingceu.com.

8. Holz K. A practical approach to clients who are survivors of childhood sexual abuse. *J Nurse Midwifery.* 1994;39(1):13–18.

9. United States Department of Justice. *National Crime Victimization Survey.* 2000. Monograph available on the Internet from: http://www.icpsr.umich.edu/ NACJD/NCVS.

10. National Institute of Justice and Centers for Disease Control. Prevalence, Incidence, and Consequences of Violence Against Women Survey. 1998. Monograph on the Internet. Available from: http://www.nij.ncjrs.org/publications.

11. Thornhill R, Palmer CT. Why men rape. *The Sciences.* 2000:Jan/Feb:30–36.

12. Bell R, Duncan M, Eilenberg J, Fullilove M, Hein D, Innes L, et al. *Violence Against Women in the United States: A Comprehensive Background Paper.* The Commonwealth Fund Commission on Women's Health. New York; November 1995.

13. Ganley A. *Improving the Health Care Response to Domestic Violence: A Trainer's Manual for Health Care Providers.* San Francisco: Family Violence Prevention Fund; 1998.

14. Tjaden P, Thoennes N. *Prevalence, Incidence and Consequences of Violence against Women: Findings from the National Violence against Women Survey.* Washington DC: National Institute of Justice, research in Brief. U.S. Department of Justice; 1996.

15. Frank JB, Rodowski MF. Review of the psychological issues in victims of domestic violence seen in emergency settings. *Emerg Med Clin North Am.* 1999;17:657–677.

16. Crowell NA, Burgess AW, editors. *Understanding Violence Against Women.* National Research Council. Washington, DC: National Academy Press; 1996.

17. Bohn DK. Domestic violence and pregnancy, implications for practice. *J Nurs Midwife.* 1990;35:86–89.

18. Gazmararian JA, Lazorick S, Spitz A, Ballard TJ, Saltzman LE, Marks JS. Prevalence of violence against pregnant women. *JAMA.* 1996;(275):1915–1919.

19. Torres S, Campbell J, Campbell D, Ryan J, King C, Price P, et al. Abuse during and before pregnancy: Prevalence and cultural correlated. *Violence and Victims.* 2000;15:303–321.

20. Goodwin MM, Gazmararian JA, Johnson CH, Cilbert BC, Saltzman LE, the PRAS Working Group. Pregnancy intendedness and physical abuse around the tie of pregnancy: Findings from the Pregnancy Risk Assessment Monitoring System, 1996-1997. *Matern Child Health J.* 2000;4(2):85–92.

21. Paluzzi P. *The Relationship between Drug Use and the Experience of Physical Violence among Inner City Pregnant Women.* Doctoral Thesis. Johns Hopkins School of Public Health; 2001.

22. Krulewitch CJ, Pierre-Louis ML, de Leon-Gomez R, Guy R, Green R. Hidden from view: Violent deaths among pregnant women in the district of Columbia, 1988–1996. *J Midwifery Women's Health.* 2001;46(1):4–10.

Substance Abuse

Chapter 8

Thomas J. Kidder
Barbara Hackley

Have you had your "fix" today of the world's most popular psychoactive drug? In fact, "if you regularly get a hefty dose, you [will continue to] need it for your brain to function normally." These are the words of Wake Forest University researcher Paul Laurienti, describing daily coffee consumption. Studies have shown that coffee drinkers who normally consume three 12-ounce cups of coffee daily (650 mg of caffeine) experienced low visual and auditory brain activity when they stopped their intake for just one day. Regular caffeine consumers needed to reintroduce one cup (250 mg) of caffeine in order for their visual and auditory brain activity to equal that of individuals who had no caffeine.[1]

The reality is that we live—and have always lived—in a drug culture. Even seemingly benign substances, such as caffeine, are in reality drugs. Substances have been used from the earliest civilizations for medicinal, recreational, and spiritual purposes[2,3] to cure illness, manage pain, and to "feel" different or "better." Prehistoric peoples ingested and inhaled products made of berries, leaves, and weeds in their search for food and nourishment and in the process discovered that some had psychotropic properties. The Hittites of Central Turkey first brewed and used beer in 7000 BC, and the civilizations of the Middle Ages used beer as a major source of nutrition. India and other Far Eastern societies have long used marijuana, which is derived from hemp, as an intoxicant and as medication. Central and South American cultures have grown and chewed coca leaves (from which cocaine is made) and peyote (a strong hallucinogen) for religious ceremonies and spiritual purposes.[2,3]

Throughout human history, the underlying drive for the use (and excessive use) of substances has been the desire to reduce pain and to increase pleasure. People use drugs to feel different, to change their mood, to produce feelings of happiness, and to numb physical, emotional, and/or social pain. They are used for recreation and, in some instances, as a coping strategy. However, excessive use can pose immediate risks of injury due to impaired judgment and physical coordination, cause end-organ damage with prolonged heavy use, and can lead to addiction for a few.

Today, chemical substances from caffeine, nicotine, and alcohol to over-the-counter medications to prescription medicines are widely used and accepted as "legal drugs." While legal, they still can lead to abuse and addiction. A large national survey conducted in 2003 estimated that 22% of individuals 12 years or older participated in binge drinking, and 6% in heavy drinking, in the previous month.[4] Approximately 20% of all Americans smoke cigarettes; young adults between 18 and 25 years of age report the highest rate of current use of any tobacco product.[5] Even some over-the-counter products, such as cough medications containing alcohol, can be problematic. Prescription drugs, particularly tranquilizers, sedatives, and pain killers, are commonly misused. In 1999, four million people reported use of prescription drugs for non-medicinal purposes.[6] Illegal drugs widely used in our culture include marijuana, cocaine, crack cocaine, opiates like heroin and methadone, and oxycontin, hallucinogens like phencyclidine (PCP, or Angel Dust), and amphetamines. Over 19 million people reported using illicit drugs in 2003.[4]

Given the prevalence of drug use and abuse, it is imperative that providers working in primary care settings be able to recognize, manage, and refer as appropriate, substance abuse problems for the clients in their care. This chapter discusses three areas: the differences between excessive use, abuse, and addiction; the physiology of commonly abused drugs; and how to identify drug use in women. More importantly, this chapter provides a framework that midwives can use with drug-using women, regardless of the substance used, to help women recognize the negative impact that drug use has on their lives and more effectively motivate them to consider and implement healthier patterns of behavior.

Use, Abuse, or Addiction? A Continuum

Initial or casual use of drugs is described as experimental or recreational and sometimes as medicinal if used as a home remedy. This level of use may be experienced as a social bonding experience with friends or peers, as a way of relaxing, as an exciting or mind-expanding experience, or as a non-prescription home remedy pain killer. Casual or recreational use may continue at short and random intervals over the course of a lifetime. Although brain functioning is altered temporarily through social use, the cumulative negative effect of social use on the brain may be short-lived and cause no long-term neurological harm because of abbreviated and/or noncontinuous use.

Abuse of any legal or illegal substance is characterized by frequent and regular use that results in intoxication, an altered ability to reason and function physically, a state of craving for more substance, and failure to follow through on personal and professional responsibilities. Substance use becomes substance abuse when minimal, limited, random use changes to increased regular use. Initially, this increased use may take place with others in the same or similar social situations. However, the abuse of substances often progresses to solitary use, outside of previous social contexts. Abusive use is characterized by progressive interference with the ability to think and act as an individual had done prior to the abuse. An increased desire to prolong the altered physical state and mood is followed by drug-seeking behaviors that take up more of the individual's time and resources. At this point, drug use is becoming a disease state.

Addiction is the next stage of the use–abuse continuum and is present when withdrawal of the substance produces more intensive and frequent cravings, more extensive drug-seeking and substitution behaviors, and symptoms of physical and/or psychic discomfort if consumption declines. At this point, the individual seems to be "controlled" by the substance, and may not be able to limit or stop its use. Failure to use more substance may produce withdrawal symptoms. Withdrawal symptoms are not seen with all drugs of abuse but, if they occur, can include intense and erratic changes in body temperature, chills, fever; sweating and increased pulse rate; hand tremor; insomnia or hypersomnia; increased appetite; nausea, vomiting, diarrhea, head and muscle aches, body ache, or cramps; psychomotor retardation or agitation; dysphoric mood; fatigue; pupillary dilation; and anxiety. Whether withdrawal symptoms develop, and the extent to which they bother individuals, depends on the specific substance and the usual dose consumed as well as the duration of abuse. For example, withdrawal from alcohol can be life-threatening, while heroin withdrawal— although extremely uncomfortable with severe flu-like symptoms—is not. Withdrawal from methadone may take longer and be more painful than heroin withdrawal.

Addicts commonly focus increasing amounts of time and attention on obtaining drugs and use ever-higher amounts of drugs in order to prolong the "high." Addiction alters brain chemistry and interferes with a user's ability to reason, to use judgment, and to act in accordance with personal and social customs, norms, and values. It is also characterized by increased social isolation and decreased ability to perform routine activities of daily living and/or personal, family, or work obligations and responsibilities.

Common Drugs of Abuse and Their Impact

Addiction leads to permanent changes in brain functioning. All drugs of abuse except the benzodiazepines have been found to cause changes in the mesolimbic dopamine system in the brain and affect dopamine release. The mesolimbic dopamine system mediates the body's response to "rewards" and is activated by such pleasurable experiences as eating, sex, or receiving praise.[6] Dopamine is thought to provide positive reinforcement by inducing feelings of immediate pleasure and may also play a role in establishing links between environmental cues and anticipated pleasure. For example, cocaine used in an environment where it was previously used seems to increase dopamine levels more than cocaine used in a new environment.[7] However, long-term use seems to negatively affect dopaminergic function and is associated with reduced levels of dopamine transporters and receptors, leading to lower levels of dopamine.[8] These changes may explain why addicts develop tolerance as well as why dysphoria is a common symptom of withdrawal.[7] Chronic use seems to induce other changes in neurotransmitters and receptors, signaling pathways, and structural changes that affect synaptic plasticity. These changes can ultimately affect many cognitive functions such as motivation, emotion, and decision making.[8]

While many substances seem to affect dopamine levels, other physiologic affects differ according to the specific substance used by an individual. Heroin, morphine, and other opiates are highly addictive because their molecular structures are similar to dopamine and other chemicals naturally produced by the brain; therefore, their use leads to a sensation of intense pleasure.[9] Marijuana interferes with the part of the brain that controls emotions, memory, and judgment.[10] Intake of marijuana weakens short-term memory and problem-solving ability. It also blocks the uptake of information into long-term memory. Inhalants, such as glue, gasoline, hair spray, and paint are sniffed, making the effect on the brain almost immediate. Inhaling vapors (also called "huffing") destroys the fatty tissue that protects the nerve cell, slowing or stopping neural transmissions.[11] Effects include diminished ability to learn, remember, and problem-solve. **Table 8-1** describes other commonly used drugs and their effects.

The health of women using substances is adversely affected not only from the physical damage caused by the abused drug, but also by the social context in which substance abuse often occurs. Alcohol and drug use blocks the brain's attempt to think clearly, to have good judgment, to plan, and to foresee the consequences of one's actions. It may also lead to lower inhibitions and increase the possibility of unsafe sexual practices, and or intravenous (IV) drug use. Unsafe or unprotected sex, without the use of a condom, often occurs when judgment is impeded. Unsafe sex can also be the result of drug-seeking behavior in an attempt to exchange services (sex) for goods (drugs). Having sex with a partner who is an active IV drug user increases the risk of transmission of sexually transmitted diseases (STDs) and human immunodeficiency virus/acquired immunedeficiency syndrome (HIV/AIDS).

Substance Abuse during Pregnancy

Substance abuse in pregnancy poses significant risks to women and their fetuses. Because almost all substances consumed by the mother pass freely through the placenta, the fetus as well as the mother experiences substance use, abuse, and addiction. In addition, the process of obtaining and using drugs often increases the chance that women may engage in other risky behaviors such as unsafe sexual practices and the exchange of sex for drugs and/or money, or experience domestic violence. Drug-using women also are less likely to be adequately nourished or to have safe, stable housing and are more likely to experience depression.[26]

Substance-using women are at higher risk of contracting STDs, which may increase the pregnant woman's risk of spontaneous abortion, premature birth, and intrapartum or neonatal infections.[27] Maternal infection with HIV, hepatitis B or C, and syphilis can be transmitted during pregnancy, at birth, and potentially through breastfeeding.[28,29]

Substance-abusing women are more likely to have unplanned pregnancies and receive late prenatal care. A study of postpartum women who were substance abusers[30] found that only 2 of 20 had planned pregnancies. Other studies have shown that women who use alcohol and drugs are more likely than non-using women to have irregular menstrual cycles.[31] Consequently, pregnancies are often unrecognized until the second trimester when fetal movement and other pregnancy-related physical changes make the pregnancy evident to these women.[31,32] Late prenatal care places the fetus at greater risk for developmental problems, especially to those due to nutritional insufficiency.

Nutrition in a pregnant woman is vital to the normal and healthy growth and development of the fetus. The use of alcohol and other drugs can cause decreased appetite, change the woman's metabolism, and decrease the availability of

Table 8-1 COMMONLY USED SUBSTANCES

Substance	Prevalence	Street Name	How Ingested	Maternal Effect	Fetal Effect
Alcohol	• 33% of adults report last-month binge drinking (defined as 5 or more drinks on one occasion).[12] • 4.5% of women report heavy drinking in the last month (defined as more than 1 drink per day on average for women).[12] • 44% of students in grades 9–12 have had one or more drinks in the preceding 30 days.[16]		Oral	Craving, not being able to stop; once begun, physical dependence and tolerance.[13] Causes liver damage, heart disease, blackouts and seizures, esophagitis, gastritis, cirrhosis, GI hemorrhage, and increased risk for breast, oral, esophageal, and rectal cancers.[14]	Fetal alcohol syndrome; facial abnormalities, growth retardation, brain damage.[15]
Amphetamines	7% of students in grades 9–12 have tried them.[16]	Ice, crystal, crank, meth, oz.[17]	Oral, smoke, inject	Highly addictive. Increases energy and alertness. Intense rush. Can cause stroke, seizures, brain damage, anxiety, insomnia, arrhythmias, and increased blood pressure, temperature, and respiratory rate. Chronic use can lead to psychotic behavior including paranoia, hallucinations, and overwhelming rage.[17]	Increased risk for preterm delivery and neonatal irritability. May cause congenital anomalies.[17]

(continues)

Table 8-1 COMMONLY USED SUBSTANCES *(continued)*

Substance	Prevalence	Street Name	How Ingested	Maternal Effect	Fetal Effect
Cocaine	• 4% of students in grades 9–12 have used a form of cocaine within the preceding 30 days.[16] • 11%–12% of general public report any lifetime use; 0.5% report use in preceding month.[19]	Coca, Aspirin, Snow white, Gold dust, Happy dust, Zip.[18]	Sniffed, snorted, injected	High followed by restlessness, anxiety, irritability, paranoia, and rebound depression. Causes constricted blood vessels, dilated pupils, and increased temperature, heart rate, and blood pressure. If large amounts are ingested, can experience tremors, vertigo, and paranoia. Use increases risk of arrhythmias, heart attacks, respiratory failure, stroke, seizures, abdominal pain, and nausea. If heroin is snorted, it can cause loss of smell, nose bleeds, difficulty swallowing, and chronic runny nose.[18]	Decreases uterine blood flow and induces contractions leading to increased risk of preterm labor, abruption, premature ruptured membranes, and fetal stress.[18]
Crack	• 2.4%–2.8% of general public report any lifetime use. • 0.1%–0.2% report any use in preceding month.[19]	Freebase, Rock, Roxanne, Twinkie, Yam, Kool-Aid.[18]	Smoked	Same as cocaine, but a more intense and faster high.[18]	Same as cocaine.

Ecstasy (methylenedi-oxymetham--phetamine)	• 11% of students in grades 9–12 have tried it.[16] • 2.9% of general public report any lifetime use.[19]	Adam, Hug, Bens, Love, B-bombs, Dex, Sweeties, X, XTC.[20]	Oral	Stimulant with psyche-delic effects. Can cause confusion, depression, insomnia, anxiety, and paranoia for weeks; muscle tension, involuntary teeth clenching, blurred vision, rapid eye movements, increased heart rate and BP, increased risk of kidney and CV failure.[20]	
Heroin	• 3% of students in grades 9–12 have tried it.[16] • 1.2%–1.4% report any lifetime use. • 0.1% report use in preceding month.[19]	Big H, Crop, Hell dust, Smack, Thunder. If mixed with marijuana, A-bomb. If mixed with crack, dragon rock.[21]	Snorted, injected, smoked	Initial feeling of euphoria, warm flushing of skin, dry mouth, and heavy extremities. Patient then feels drowsy, may "nod off," experiences clouded mental functioning. Chronic users can develop endocarditis, abscesses, cellulitis, pneumonia, and liver disease.[21]	Possible congenital anomalies. Increased risk of low-birth weight and small for gestational age babies.[21] Withdrawal 24–72 hours after birth. Long-term cognitive and behavioral problems.[18]
Marijuana	• 22% of students in grades 9–12 have used it one or more times in the preceding 30 days.[16] • 34%–36% of general public report any lifetime use. • 5% report use in preceding 30 days.[19]	Mary Jane, Boom, Gangster[22]	Smoked	Long-term use changes brain chemistry, damages lungs; impaired attention, memory, and learning with heavy use.[22]	Evidence conflicts; unclear impact.[22]

(*continues*)

Table 8-1 Commonly Used Substances *(continued)*

Substance	Prevalence	Street Name	How Ingested	Maternal Effect	Fetal Effect
Oxycodin	5% of 12th graders and 2.6% of young adults aged 19–28 years report using it within the last year.[23]	40, 80, Blue, Hillbilly heroin, Kicker, Oxy.[23]	Chew tablets; crush tablets and snort the powder or mix with water and inject[24]	Prescription pain killer. Depressant. When used inappropriately can cause euphoria. Similar effects to heroin.[24]	
PCPs	2.6% of general public report any lifetime use.[19]	Angel Dust, Boat, Tic tac, Zoom.[25]	Snorted, smoked, oral.[25]	Hallucinogen. Effects are unpredictable. Increases blood pressure, heart rate, and temperature. Can cause nausea, blurred vision, dizziness, and decreased awareness. High doses can lead to convulsions, coma, and hyperthermia.[25]	
Tobacco	• 21% of students in grades 9–12 have smoked it within previous 30 days.[16] • 22.5% of adults are current smokers.[5]		Smoking, oral	Cardiovascular disease, lung disease, and cancer	Increased risk of preterm labor, low birth weight, stillbirth, and miscarriage.[15]

essential nutrients.[33] The focus on obtaining and using drugs, and the intense need to maintain a "high" override internal messages to attend to nutritional needs, leading to self-neglect and poor diet.[34] While a woman may be able to tolerate poorer nutrition, the fetus may experience nutritional insufficiency and be at risk for intrauterine growth retardation and other complications.

Fetal Health Consequences

Fetal vulnerability to drugs is much greater because the fetus has not developed the enzymatic system needed to metabolize drugs.[35] Although not all infants or children show the negative effects of prenatal exposure to alcohol and drugs, maternal drug use increases the risk for short- and long-term physical, cognitive, behavioral, and developmental damage.[36–38] Predicting whether maternal drug use will lead to these problems in a particular case is impossible. Whether damage occurs, and to what extent, depends on the type and combination of drugs used, the amount and frequency of use, and the fetus's genetic susceptibility to alcohol and drugs.[39,40] Research also suggests that the trimester in which drug use occurred can influence outcomes: first trimester exposure to alcohol and drugs may result in congenital anomalies whereas exposure during the second or third trimesters seems to affect fetal growth.[41] For some substances fetal damage occurs throughout gestation (Table 8-1).

Neonatal Addiction

Fetuses exposed to alcohol and drugs, especially heroin, may experience withdrawal symptoms within 72 hours of birth, because access to the drug is cut off after physical separation from the mother at birth. Most cases of neonatal withdrawal are not life-threatening and are termed *neonatal abstinence syndrome (NAS)*. NAS affects the central nervous system (as evidenced by tremors, irritability, abnormal suck, or poor feeding), the autonomic system (sneezing and yawning), the gastrointestinal system (diarrhea and vomiting), and the pulmonary system (increased apnea).[34,42] Mothers must be taught that withdrawal changes neonatal behavior. For example, a baby who displays irritability and non-responsiveness could be mistakenly thought by the mother to be rejecting her, when in reality the infant is experiencing withdrawal symptoms.

Alcohol and drug exposure for the mother and fetus is harmful and dangerous; however, maternal detoxification should be approached with caution. Maternal detoxification can be extremely harmful to the fetus depending on the substance involved. It can cause placental vasoconstriction leading to increased rates of abruption, placental insufficiency, intrauterine growth restriction, and stillbirth.[43] While the process of opioid withdrawal is less life-threatening to the mother than the fetus, acute withdrawal from alcohol and other sedatives and hypnotic drugs may result in life-threatening danger for mother and fetus. Withdrawal from cocaine and other stimulants is less severe for both the mother and fetus, and often can be accomplished without the use of other drugs/medications.[34]

The detoxification process for pregnant women is usually done in an inpatient setting where the woman and fetus can be monitored by a medical team. The tapering of dependent sedative/hypnotic drugs is vital for the mother and the fetus, so that the drug-free state is slowly achieved without the experience of uncontrolled withdrawal.[34] Although withdrawal from heroin may be managed by replacing heroin use with methadone, methadone maintenance is often preferable to heroin detoxification because of the potential for lethal harm to the fetus from detoxification.[34,44]

Historical Understanding of Addiction: Explanatory Models

Public understanding of drug use has evolved over time. Prior to our current knowledge of the relationship between brain functioning and addiction, when substance use "got out of hand," men were criticized for public drunkenness and women were isolated or "sent away" to sanatoriums. Abuse and addiction was thought to be a result of weak human nature, inadequate psychological or personality development, and/or poor moral and ethical character. Moral rejection of drunken behavior progressed to a legal/criminal interpretation, popularized through television in the 1960s in shows like "The Andy Griffith Show," where Otis, the town drunk, was transported to the local jail to sleep off the effects of imbibing. During the 1970s and 1980s, substance abuse became perceived as a medical problem. In those two decades, "Otis-type" characters were gathered up and taken to the local emergency rooms for evaluation and possibly treatment referrals. Substance abuse was thought to be a progressive disease. For example, alcoholism progressed from early controlled drinking to less controlled drinking with resulting negative consequences at home, work, and in public; to total loss of control with severe personal, professional, and social consequences. The likelihood of developing alcoholism was theorized to be due to a combination of genetics and environment. Multigenerational genetic personality characteristics (e.g., being argumentative, weak-willed with low impulse control, and selfish), were thought to be transmitted to the alcoholic via inherited and learned family behavioral influences. All of these early models proposed that personality and genetic defects were essential factors in the development of abuse and addiction. In fact, substance abuse was considered a mental illness.

Parallel to these social interpretations of substance use as a form of indulgence was the development of the self-help movement, most notably Alcoholics Anonymous (AA). AA combined the concepts of religious forgiveness and the saving power of personal repentance with a highly structured peer group. The peer group process developed by AA uses personalized story telling as a basic mechanism by which participants acknowledge their substance abuse, commit to change, and receive support for making change. It also provides a "24/7/365," anywhere–anytime–for-anyone personal support network worldwide. The self-help movements that began with AA have assisted millions of individuals with abuse problems, and the model developed by AA has been adapted for use with many other substance abuse problems including other drugs (Narcotics Anonymous; NA), food (Overeaters Anonymous), and emotional effects on family members (Al-Anon).

Many theories have been developed on the causes and best treatment approaches for substance abuse based on the experiences of alcoholics and drug addicts. One approach thought to be effective is the need for at least some addicts to "hit bottom," with the premise that by doing so, the addicts develop an internal motivation to change. A basic tenet of the self-help movement is the need for absolute abstinence in order for recovery to occur and to be sustained. Self-help organizations such as AA have developed multiple tools to help individuals stay in recovery including using motivational stories found in the *Big Book*, sharing responsibilities for meeting tasks, using memory reminders like "easy does it" and "one day at a time." The structure of AA uses self help/support groups, substance avoidance, and behavioral cues to reform behavior patterns. The alcoholics involved in developing the AA program knew that continued substance abuse would ultimately result in death and that abstinence could prolong life. Although this approach has advanced the understanding of substance abuse by promoting the disease concept, and continues to help many individuals, it does not work for every substance abuser.

Over the past 20 years, science has identified addiction as a state that is distinct from the process of substance use and excessive use/abuse. Addiction has been used to describe a process of self-destructive behaviors in combination with substance use/abuse of one or more substance. Today many models of addiction have been proposed. They include:

- *Social/environmental.* Emphasizes the role of societal influences; peer pressure, social policies, availability (e.g., crack and crack houses), and family systems on the development of substance use/abuse.[45,46]
- *Genetic/physiological.* Stresses the importance of genetic predisposition ("the apple does not fall far from the family tree").[47] Physical dependence and addiction are seen as synonymous, with markers of drug abuse being the development of tolerance with continued use and withdrawal symptoms when substance use declines.
- *Personality/intrapsychic.* Links personality/intrapsychic dysfunction and psychological problems to juvenile delinquency and antisocial behavior disorders, including substance use and abuse.[48,49]
- *Coping/social learning.* Associates abuse with inadequate coping skills or critical personality deficits. Substances are used to cope with stress and to manage anger, frustration, and depression.[50–54]
- *Conditioning/reinforcement behavioral.* Focuses on the direct effects of addictive behavior, such as tolerance, withdrawal, and other physiological responses and rewards.[55]
- *Compulsive/excessive behavioral.* Conceptualizes addictions as due to "excessive appetites."[56] Increasing appetite leads to excess and the developmental process of increasing attachment similar to a social learning model.
- *Biopsychosocial behavioral.* Integrates biological, psychological, and sociological (biopsychosocial) explanations. Donovan and Marlatt suggest that, "addiction appears to be an interactive product of social learning in a situation involving physiological events as they are interpreted, labeled, and given meaning by the individual."[57]

The biopsychosocial behavioral model has emerged as the predominant model for understanding and treating substance abuse and addiction. The biological aspect refers to our ever-growing understanding of addiction as a chemical interaction with the brain that takes control of brain functioning. Psychological, social, and behavioral aspects of an individual each play a significant role in the development of and recovery from abuse and addiction. Use, abuse, and addiction are distinct stages in a long and complex process. The biopsychosocial behavioral model helps to identify where the individual is in this process, for example, whether she is experiencing any physiological changes, withdrawal symptoms, or any social or behavioral consequences from substance use. Further, it helps gauge where the individual is with regard to changing her pattern of behavior and provides guidance on which treatment approaches may be most effective for an individual. **Table 8-2** compares three different treatment modalities that address various psychosocial and behavioral aspects of addiction.

Drug Addiction: A Treatable Brain Disease

The Partnership for a Drug-Free America has stated that, "Drug abuse is a preventable behavior; drug addiction is a treatable disease."[59] This statement emphasizes two facts: 1) drug abuse is fundamentally different from addiction; and 2) drug addiction is a disease. While addiction may be the result of heavy and sustained drug use, it is fundamentally different from frequent drug use. Drug use and drug addiction are not simply two points on a continuum beginning with drug use, progressing to drug abuse, heavy and sustained drug abuse, and then addiction. The user cannot move back and forth along such a continuum at will. Addiction is a qualitatively different state because the addicted brain is, in fact, different in its neurobiology from the non-addicted brain.[59]

People use drugs because they like what it does to their brain. Drugs modify mood, perception, and psychological state by altering brain chemistry. Prolonged use changes the brain in profound and long-lasting ways; this appears to be a major component of addiction.[59] However, addiction is not necessarily dependent on the amount or length of time that a substance has been used. While heavy and prolonged use increases the chance that addiction may occur, addiction can also occur at lower

Table 8-2 ADDICTION: BEHAVIORAL CONSTRUCTS AND TREATMENT FOCUS[58]

Addictive Component	Behavioral Construct	Treatment Focus
Pleasure	Positive reinforcement	Motivational therapy
Self-medication	Negative reinforcement	Self-help (AA, NA)
Habit	Conditioned positive	Cognitive behavioral reinforcement
Habit	Conditioned negative	Cognitive behavioral reinforcement

levels of use that have been present for a shorter period of time. Leshner suggests that it is as if a "switch was thrown in the brain" at some point during drug use.[59] The exact factors that cause the switch to be thrown are unclear, but when the switch is thrown, it changes a user/abuser of drugs into an addict and alters the brain forever. Current scientific research suggests that the brain's mesolimbic dopamine system is activated by all drugs of abuse and may play a role in the conversion from abuse to addiction.

When answering the question "Is this drug addictive?" two possibilities must be considered:

1. Does this particular drug cause compulsive, uncontrollable, drug-seeking behavior?
2. Does it cause physiological addiction?

Physical symptoms are less significant than whether the drug causes compulsive drug-seeking behavior. Crack cocaine and methamphetamine, which do not have dramatic withdrawal symptoms, are among the most addictive substances known.[59] Addiction is a powerful motivator. The overwhelming need to obtain substances can lead to crime, family abandonment, job loss, and loss of life.

Addiction occurs in an interdependent set of contexts—environmental, historical, and physiological—and these contexts affect the way in which drug use interacts with the brain. Biology and behavior are both essential to understanding addiction. Biology cannot be explained by behavioral or social context any more than behavior or social context can be explained by biology. Therefore, in dealing with addicts, we are dealing with a person who is in an altered state. The task for treatment becomes not to change the brain back, but to compensate for, or even reverse the brain changes in some form, whether pharmacologically or behaviorally. Behavioral treatments can produce a functionally changed brain. The most effective treatments attend simultaneously to the biological, behavioral, and social contexts.

Addiction can be treated by removing access to the substance, allowing the brain to recover, and by helping the individual to change her behaviors and beliefs about continued substance use. Since the continued use of substances causes the brain to develop and maintain an addiction state, the first and most important step in treating this disease is to cut off the supply of the substance to the brain. The second step is to stabilize the body systems, which may require detoxification and medical monitoring for adverse side effects.

Once the brain is actively substance-free, the motivation for long-term change can be assessed. At this point, the recovering addict may envision a new and healthy life, and begin to plan the steps toward achieving this new life. This is followed by motivational, cognitive, behavioral, social, emotional, and spiritual interventions aimed at moving the addict away from unhealthy addictive behaviors and toward a newly envisioned lifestyle of recovery, personal success, and fulfillment.

Diagnosis of Substance Abuse

Drug use affects all segments of society and has devastating consequences. Therefore, midwives should have a high index of suspicion and carefully evaluate all women under their care. One of the more common approaches is to try to determine whether a problem exists by quantifying the amount of drugs consumed by asking "How many cigarettes, how much alcohol…do you consume daily, weekly…?" Drinking more than one drink a day for women is considered to be at-risk drinking; binge drinking for women is defined as consuming more than 4 to 5 drinks on any one occasion. Because alcohol content varies greatly between alcohol products and within drink types, it is not possible to generalize about the quantity of alcohol ingested by an individual. In addition, using a counting method to determine if substance abuse is present is problematic because this approach is subject to recall bias and, more importantly, does not gauge how substance use affects an individual's life.

Several screening questionnaires have been suggested for general use in ambulatory settings, but many focus primarily on alcohol abuse. **Table 8-3** shows some examples. However, one short questionnaire appears to effectively screen for multiple substances, is easy to administer, and has been designed to focus primarily on the impact of drug use on an individual's life. The two-item conjoint screening test asks:

1. In the last year, have you ever drunk or used drugs more than you meant to?
2. Have you felt you wanted or needed to cut down on your drinking or drug use in the last year?

A positive response to either question was found to have a sensitivity and specificity of 81% in detecting polysubstance use disorders.[63]

Other problems elicited in a careful history can also provide clues that a particular woman may be having problems with drug use. Women using substances may be more likely to report insomnia, sexual dysfunction, and to

have multiple vague complaints. Inconsistent health care, frequent infections, problems with holding jobs, a history of being involved in the legal system or incarceration, or family discord can be due to or worsened by substance abuse. Substance abusing women are also more likely to suffer from depression, experience domestic violence or other mental health conditions, and to self-medicate with drugs. Therefore, midwives should always include a social history and mental health evaluation as part of a standard health visit. Chapters 7 and 9 provide further details on those topics.

A careful physical examination, while less effective at identifying drug use than a thorough history, can also provide clues to substance abuse (**Table 8-4**). Specific physical findings can be seen in withdrawal from various substances (**Table 8-5**).

Laboratory tests are infrequently used in primary care settings, but may be helpful in select circumstances. Urine drug screens are one of the most commonly ordered tests. A typical panel screens for amphetamines, cocaine, opiates, PCP, and tetrahydrocannabinol, and will detect drugs used within the last 24 to 48 hours.[65] These five drugs have standardized cutoff values for positive and negative tests based on federal guidelines for employee testing programs. Other drugs may be added to this panel but are less likely to have standardized normative values, so their results must be interpreted with caution. Other tests can detect drug levels in saliva, sweat, or hair, but these tests are offered by only a few laboratories and are not commonly used. If alcohol abuse is suspected or present, liver function tests may be helpful in detecting and monitoring the extent of the disease. Liver function tests, specifically the γ-glutamyl transpeptidase (GGT), aspartate

Table 8-3 SCREENING QUESTIONNAIRE AND TOOLS

Drug Abuse Screening Test (DAST)	TWEAK Tool	CAGE Tool
Have you abused prescription drugs?	*Tolerance:* How many drinks can you hold (>6 indicates tolerance = 2 points) or How many drinks does it take to make you feel high? (>3 drinks indicates tolerance = 2 points).	*Cut down:* Have you ever felt you should cut down on drinking?
Do you abuse more than one drug at a time?		*Annoyed:* Have people annoyed you by criticizing your drinking?
Can you get through the week without using drugs (other than those required for medical reasons)?	*Worry:* Have close friends or relatives worried or complained about your drinking in the past year? (1 point).	*Guilty:* Have you ever felt guilty about your drinking?
Are you always able to stop using drugs when you want to?	*Eye opener:* Do you sometimes take a drink in the morning when you first get up? (1 point).	*Eye opener:* Have you ever had a drink first thing in the morning to steady your nerves or get rid of a hangover?
Do you abuse drugs on a continuous basis?	*Amnesia:* Has a friend or family member ever told you about things you said or did that you could not remember? (1 point).	Score of 1 to 3 = high likelihood of alcohol abuse.
Do you try to limit your drug use to certain situations?	(K) *Cut down:* Do you sometimes feel the need to cut down on your drinking? (1 point)	
Have you had "blackouts" or "flashbacks" as a result of drug use?	Score of ≥3 points = positive for alcoholism/heavy drinking.	
Do you ever feel bad about your drug abuse?		
Does your spouse (or parents) ever complain about your involvement with drugs?		
Do your friends or relatives know or suspect you abuse drugs?		
Has drug abuse ever created problems between you and your spouse?		
Have you had problems related to your drug use?		
Have you ever lost friends because of your use of drugs?		

(continues)

Table 8-3 SCREENING QUESTIONNAIRE AND TOOLS *(continued)*

Drug Abuse Screening Test (DAST)	TWEAK Tool	CAGE Tool
Have you ever been arrested because of unusual behavior while under the influence of drugs?		
Have you engaged in illegal activities to obtain drugs?		
Have you ever been arrested for possession of illegal drugs?		
Have you experienced withdrawal symptoms as a result of heavy drug intake?		
Have you had medical problems as a result of your drug use (e.g., memory loss, hepatitis, convulsions, or bleeding)?		
Have you ever gone to anyone for help for a drug problem?		
Have you ever been involved in a treatment program specifically related to drug use?		
Have you been treated as an outpatient for problems related to drug abuse?		
Score of ≥ 6 positive responses = substance use problem.		

Sources: DAST[60]; TWEAK[61]; and CAGE[62].

Table 8-4 PHYSICAL EXAMINATION IN THE EVALUATION OF SUBSTANCE ABUSE

System	Findings
Affect	Depressed, anxious, nervous, mood lability
	Inability to focus
	Impaired judgment and coordination
	Paranoid and/or suicidal ideation
Mental Status Changes	Slurred, incoherent, or too rapid speech
	Unsteady gait and/or tremors
	Blackouts or periods of memory loss
	Nodding off, dozing or falling asleep
	Agitation and/or delirium tremens
	Seizures
	Changes in levels of consciousness
	Visual or auditory hallucinations
Skin	Jaundice
	Sensation of insects crawling on the skin resulting in scratching and skin ulcerations
	Needle track marks
	Skin abscesses
	Swollen lymph nodes
Eye	Nystagmus (sedative/hypnotics, cannabis)
	Mydriasis (stimulants, hallucinogens, or withdrawal from opiates)
	Miosis (opioid use)
Nose and Throat	Dental (caries, gingivitis)
	Perforated septum
	Rhinorrhea
Cardiac	Murmurs
	Arrhythmias
	Chest pain
	Increased blood pressure
Respiratory	Shortness of breath
	Chronic cough
	Pneumonia
Abdominal	Diarrhea, constipation, hepatolmegaly, splenomegaly, ascites
Gynecologic/ Urologic	Palpable lymph nodes
	Signs and symptoms of sexually transmitted infections

aminotransferase (AST), and alanine aminotransferase (ALT), are markers of tissue damage.[65] GGT is the most specific indicator of alcohol abuse. Other tests that should be considered when substance abuse is of concern are triglycerides and high-density lipoprotein, which are elevated with moderate levels of alcohol intake as well as a complete blood count,

Table 8-5 COMMON SYMPTOMS SEEN IN DRUG WITHDRAWAL

Opioid	Alcohol	Cocaine	Nicotine
Dysphoria mood	Autonomic hyperactivity	Dysphoric mood	Dysphoric or depressed mood
Nausea or vomiting	Hand tremor	Unpleasant dreams	Insomnia
Muscle aches	Insomnia	Insomnia or hypersomnia	Irritability
Lacrimation	Nausea or vomiting	Increased appetite	Anxiety
Rhinorrhea	Hallucinations	Psychomotor retardation or agitation	Difficulty concentrating
Pupillary dilation	Illusions		Restlessness
Piloerection	Psychomotor agitation		Decreased heart rate
Sweating	Anxiety		Increased appetite
Diarrhea	Seizures		Weight gain
Yawning			
Fever			
Insomnia			

Sources: American Psychiatric Association. *Diagnostic and Statistical Manual of Mental Disorders IV-TR.* Washington, DC: American Psychiatric Association; 2000.

Al-Sanouri I, Dikin M, Soubani AO. Critical care aspects of alcohol abuse. *Southern Medical Journal.* 2005. 98(3):372–381.

O'Connor PG, Fiellin DA. Pharmacologic treatment of heroin-dependent patients. *Annals of Internal Medicine.* 2000. 133(1):40–54.

Etter JF. A self-administered questionnaire to measure cigarette withdrawal symptoms: The Cigarette Withdrawal Scale. *Nicotine & Tobacco Research.* 2005. 7(1):47–57.

renal function tests, and a complete lipid panel. However, these tests can be elevated in other diseases; therefore, abnormal results need further evaluation and cannot be assumed to be due to substance use. Substance users are also at higher risk for HIV and hepatitis B and C. Screening for these infections should also be considered (**Table 8-6**).

Treatment Options

Change Is the Goal

Although the biopsychosocial behavioral model has become the most accepted model explaining the underlying antecedents of addiction, there is no universal agreement regarding the etiology or optimal treatment approach for addiction. There is simply no single developmental model that can explain the acquisition of or recovery from addiction.[66–68]

The Transtheoretical Model (TTM) of intentional behavioral change attempts to merge these divergent perspectives by focusing on how individuals change behavior and by identifying key change dimensions involved in this process.[69,70] According to the TTM Model, understanding who is likely to become addicted and the environments in which these higher-risk individuals live and work is less important

Table 8-6 LABORATORY EVALUATION

Test	Findings
Complete Blood Count	Nutritional anemias common if intake affected, MCV increased if heavy drinking (6–8 drinks a day)
Hepatitis B Antigen and Antibody	At risk if engaged in unsafe sexual practices or using needles
Hepatitis C Antigen	At risk if using needles
Human Immuno-deficiency Virus	At risk if engaged in unsafe sexual practices or using needles
Gonorrhea and/or Chlamydia	At risk if engaged in unsafe sexual practices
Lipid Profile	High density lipoprotein can be elevated with alcohol abuse
Liver Function Tests Renal tests	Elevated in alcohol abuse, particularly the GTT
Purified protein derivative of tuberculin	May be at increased risk of tuberculosis depending on exposure environment

than understanding how these multiple influences converge to lead to addiction for a specific individual. Thus, the best way to understand addiction is to understand an individual's personal pathway to addiction. Each person's choices are influenced by internal and external forces, by an individual's character, and by social factors. The interaction between the individual and her risk and protective factors influence whether an individual will become addicted and whether she leaves the addiction. Addiction does not occur without the participation of the individual. Everyone must process the influences upon them and choose whether these influences will be strong enough to overcome healthier contrary values. Addiction and recovery take place through a personal and individual journey through an intentional change process that is influenced at many points by a multitude of biological, psychological, social, and spiritual factors.[45]

Stages of Change

The change process described by the TTM model evolved from earlier work by Prochaska and DiClemente, Miller, and Rollnick on the stages of change.[71,72] These stages of change can be visualized as a pie with five slices (**Figure 8-1**).

The first slice represents the change stage of precontemplation. In this stage, the person does not believe that she has a problem. The second slice represents the contemplation stage of change. This is the stage that contains the "Aha!" moment. The individual realizes or begins to realize, perhaps for the first time, that she does (or may have) a problem. However, the person may say, "OK, so I have a problem but it is not a big deal to me and I am not going to change."

Throughout the precontemplation and contemplation stages, the primary interventions are engagement and persuasion. The tasks of continued engagement and persuasion serve to motivate the individual and to move her through the change stages.

Active contemplation may also bring the individual along to a conscious position of, "You are right. I do have a problem. So now what do I do?" Once this person has moved to this phase, she will often progress into the third stage of change: the action stage. This phase of the change process is where the individual may become actively involved in treatment programs. Referral to formal treatment programs prior to this point, although a necessary and indicated step, may not prove successful. However, once a person acknowledges that she wants to change and is willing to take steps to make change a reality, the effectiveness of formal treatment interventions and programs increases rapidly. These strategies and therapies may include detoxification (medically monitored outpatient or inpatient), behavioral health interventions, and self-help therapies.

The fourth change stage is relapse prevention. This stage involves formal (program based and monitored) and informal (self-help, peer-to-peer, and family based) behavioral skills training and implementation of new healthier behaviors focused on harm reduction and abstinence, leading toward or to a new substance-free lifestyle. This new lifestyle may be the beginning of achieving the once only "envisioned" desired ideal life. If the individual is successful in this stage, she can exit the cycle and live her new substance free life of recovery. If, however, she is unsuccessful in this relapse prevention stage, or in recovery, she may continue with prevention efforts with occasional slips or abstinence lapses followed by a renewed attempt to implement relapse prevention skills.

Figure 8-1 Five stages of change

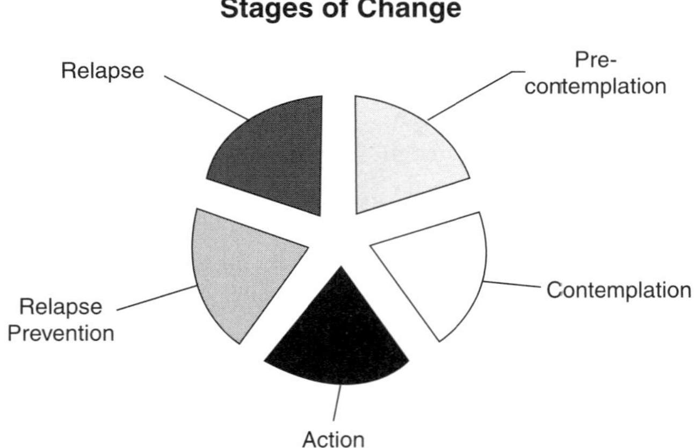

The fifth stage of change is the relapse stage. Relapse is the full-blown return to the former abusive and addictive behaviors. This may be short-lived or a longer term problem. Relapse may result from an inability to cope with the negative influences and factors that originally helped push an individual into inappropriate drug use. These might include an inability to remove herself from her personal drug environment, to deal effectively with co-existing domestic violence or with a strong previous addiction, and the lack of adequate personal resources to support the new changes as well as many other factors. Whatever the reason for the relapse, this brings the person back to the beginning of the change process. In her renewed addictive state, she may revert to preconscious denial of any problem and choose not to deal with her renewed substance abuse problem. Once again, the outpatient treatment response can be a nonjudgmental engagement and persuasion to motivate her through the stages of change again. **Table 8-7** summarizes the stages of change and has corresponding recommended therapeutic approaches.

Typically, people do not present in a state of readiness for change and are not actively seeking treatment. They more commonly present in a precontemplative or contemplative state of mind, do not believe that they have a problem, and have no intention to act in ways that can help resolve the problem. *Motivational Enhancement Therapy (MET)* describes one common reaction, the "righting reflex," as a maladaptive approach used to try to help motivate these individuals toward healthy change. Helpers, clinicians, and more well-adjusted individuals in the addict's life use the "righting reflex" to push, pull, or drag the abuser or addict over the divide between illness and health, and into a way of life more likely to promote wellness and happiness. However, the impulsive use of the righting reflex often results in the opposite effect—resistance to suggestions and to change. A better approach is to use engagement and persuasion interventions. These interventions are intended to share responsibility and power for change with the clients and to assist them in movement from precontemplation through contemplation into action. Once the action stage is entered, higher levels of successful treatment outcomes will result.

Motivational Enhancement Therapy

Caring for women who cannot acknowledge that they have a substance abuse problem can be frustrating for providers. Education alone is not generally enough. While education is a necessary condition for change, knowledge is not a sufficient condition for change. In fact, many women who abuse alcohol and drugs continue to do so after having received the information on the negative health and life-threatening consequences of continued use. Often these women, while able to intellectually understand the consequences of drug use, are not yet ready to make necessary changes. While some women will be able to recognize that their level of drug use requires treatment, others will deny that help is needed. In this circumstance, the goal of changing substance abuse risk behaviors can be best achieved through MET, using engagement, persuasion, and treatment-planning strategies to assist individuals in embracing treatment as a means of achieving a healthier life.

Table 8-7 STAGES OF CHANGE: THERAPEUTIC SUGGESTIONS USING MOTIVATIONAL ENHANCEMENT THERAPY

Stages of Change	Treatment Strategies					
Precontemplative	Engagement and persuasion					
Contemplative	Engagement and persuasion	Psycho-education	Data sharing, lab work, etc.	Psychosocial data	Natural consequences	Social network interventions
Action	Detoxification	Outpatient individual and group	Intensive outpatient 3 hours a day program	Partial hospital 4–8 hours a day program	Short-term inpatient hospital or program	Self-help; social and family supports; long-term shelter programs (some are faith-based)
Relapse Prevention	Cognitive behavioral skills training	Group support	Self-help network			
Relapse and Addiction	Outreach	Harm reduction	Engagement and persuasion			

Specific approaches can be employed in a primary care setting. Getting women into care—of any type—is an essential first step. The following qualities and strategies employed by health care facilities can help engage women in care and provide opportunities for staff to encourage women to consider changing their behavior:

- Staff are perceived as warm and welcoming.
- Staff are willing to meet patients in their own environments, including home, street, hospital, or other setting.
- Clinicians make use of Rogerian client-centered therapeutic skills, such as reflective listening and accurate empathy to affirm collaboration (partnership with the client), evocation (draw on the client's perceptions, goals, and values), and autonomy (client right and capacity for self-direction) as opposed to confrontation, education, and authority.[66]
- Patients are not prejudged. Rather, they are accepted as they are, with whatever baggage they bring.
- Barriers to care are minimized by improving access. These include: nonjudgmental response, protocols for walk-ins, limited waiting time, telephone contact between scheduled sessions, supportive outreach, and rapid linkage to ancillary services.
- Staff members act as good hosts by offering physical comforts, such as water and coffee, a welcoming physical space, and by providing clear communication.
- The facility provides accurate and clear messages about available services. For example, established linkages to treatment providers, wait times, contingency plans, costs and consequences, and professional referrals as opposed to a name and number with the expectation of client follow-through. These are motivational enhancement tools, not enabling of dependency.
- Clients receive case management assistance early in the course of their care.
- Transportation problems are identified and resolved early.
- Clear verbal and nonverbal messages are given that invite the individual into a partnering relationship with a multidisciplinary team. Partnering is important because it shifts the power dynamic to one of shared responsibility between the patient and the team.

A multidisciplinary team approach is essential to the successful engagement of the patient. While primary care providers, nurses, social workers, and case managers provide the bulk of care that women receive in a health facility, all staff including receptionists and referral staff who have contact with drug using/abusing women may have opportunities to help motivate and engage women into care. This multidisciplinary team needs to be trained to serve as greeters, "treaters," and ambassadors between drug using/abusing women and specialty clinics (obstetrics/gynecology, dental, nutrition, pediatric, ophthalmology, podiatry clinics, etc.), treatment programs (mental health, substance abuse treatment, and detoxification centers), and community sites (prisons, homeless shelters, and elderly and low income housing projects).

Once a woman is engaged in care at a facility, staff can employ persuasion strategies to provide information that women need in order to recognize the extent of their problem and consider treatment. Women need general information about substance abuse and treatment and more specific information on the substance(s) of personal concern to the individual woman, especially information on risk behaviors and how addiction develops, treatment and how treatment is delivered, the importance of treatment adherence, and the consequences of poor decisions. However, in order to be effective, information on drug use and addiction must be delivered in a nonjudgmental manner that allows for a woman to hear and understand the information being given.[40] Discussing drug behaviors in a judgmental manner only increases anxiety and the use of defense mechanisms, such as denial, projection, intellectualization, and the defense of drug behaviors.[45] Other persuasion techniques that should be used include:

- Involving family and social supports.
- Helping the patient to understand and accept a social/family/financial plan that is linked to a primary care plan.
- Sharing laboratory values, which can provide concrete "measures" of the negative health impact of substance use.
- Explaining the difference between addictions.
- Helping substance-abusing individuals see the link between their substance abuse and the development of comorbidities from physical or psychological damage caused by substance use.
- Integrating treatment planning and implementation by a team of nurses, social workers, case managers, and primary care providers who work together to ensure the successful engagement of

the patient, even if the "treaters" are community, not center, based and represent multiple programs and services.

The following are specific therapeutic tasks that must be accomplished before an abusing or addicted individual will be ready to accept treatment and should be a focus in patient-provider encounters:

1. To help the individual accept herself as she is, in the spirit of positive self regard.[45,73] Positive self regard is a prerequisite for positive growth and development. It is acceptance of the person but does not indicate acceptance or tolerance of unhealthy behaviors. Substance abusers often feel extreme guilt about their drug behavior and the negative impact it has had on their friends and family. Even then, they may continue their addictive behaviors; they may feel and act in a self-punishing way, feeling undeserving of care or kindness, even from within themselves. Positive self regard should be modeled by the provider and encouraged in the substance abuser.

2. To clarify the discrepancy between where the abusing individual is and where she would like to be in life. This can be done by asking the following questions:

- How do you like how your life is going?
- Do you enjoy the complications or consequences of your substance use?

AND

- Would you like your life to be different? In what ways?

- When you dream about how you want your life to be, what does it look or feel like?

The difference or distance between these two visions is the discrepancy. Pointing out this discrepancy by stating, "So this is how it is for you and this is how you would like it to be" can make concrete the impact substance abuse has on an individual's life.

3. To clarify and resolve the ambivalence over maintaining risk behaviors. This can be evaluated by focusing on two areas: the pros and cons of various options (decisional balance) and the individual's capacity and willingness to change today (self-efficacy).

The following set of questions can help evaluate decisional balance.

- List the reasons why continued use is good, important, or valued. (The advantages of continued use.)
- List the reasons why discontinued use is good, important, or valued. (The disadvantages of continued use.)
- List the reasons why quitting use is good, important, or valued. (The advantages of quitting use.)
- List the reasons why not quitting use is good, important, or valued. (The disadvantages of quitting use.)
- "On a scale of 1 (low) to 10 (high), how do you value your use?" and "On a scale of 1 (low) to 10 (high), how do you value quitting your use?"
- "On a scale of 1 (low) to 10 (high), how much do you want to make these changes?"

- If you visualize a balance scale with the value of continued use on one side and ending use on the other, both the provider and the patient can see the weight of these options. Until the values list on the quitting use side outweighs the continued use side, it is unlikely that the person will change her behavior.

Self-efficacy (which answers the question, does the person feel she can/will make the necessary change to achieve her desired life?) can be assessed by the following questions:

- How likely are you to make these changes?
- On a scale of 1 (low) to 10 (high), rate yourself on how likely you are to make these changes.
- Do you feel/think you can make these changes?

The person's own assessment of her ability to change is often the best indicator of whether change will occur.

4. To elicit "change talk" and "change behaviors" from the individual. "Change talk" helps users concretely visualize what a healthier life would be like and contemplate what "change behaviors" would be needed to move toward the envisioned life. "Change talk" can be encouraged by:
   o Identifying statements and behaviors that indicate movement toward healthier behavior.
     - I see that you have picked up the brochures on detox and treatment.
     - I see that you have scheduled an appointment with your medical doctor.

- ○ Providing affirmation for health choices and identifying change talk when it occurs.
  - I noticed that you asked if I thought you could do this, [change]?
  - I have heard your concern about being around long enough to see your kids grow up.

Harm Reduction Model

Although abstinence is the best treatment option, this is not an immediately achievable option for many addicts, abusers, or users. The public health approach of harm reduction is a far more achievable goal for many. This model of recovery seeks to reduce and/or limit addictive behaviors and, therefore, limit the negative consequences and the destructive deterioration of the addict. The premise of this model is that some change is better than no change. Small steps toward more healthy behaviors can lead to less risk and open up the possibility of other potential changes. It can buy time for the addict to reconsider other, more healthy options.

Methadone maintenance treatment for heroin addicts is an example of a harm reduction option for those who cannot stay clean after detoxification. Methadone, which is always administered through very structured programs, replaces heroin, an unstable drug, with a maintenance dose of methadone, a much more stable drug. This maintenance dose allows the addict to maintain a nonintoxicated stable state and be able to function normally, while preventing craving and withdrawal.

Self Help

Self help in this chapter is defined as AA or NA. This group process is enormously helpful for many users and is a free, universal, nonprofessional approach to recovery. It involves self-declaration of addiction and telling of one's story about problems with alcohol or drugs. Peer support is offered. Participants can attend as many meetings as necessary in order to remind themselves of their addiction and to strengthen their resolve not to give in to it. It also offers a mentor or sponsor system as a means of maintaining abstinence. Although extremely helpful, self-help groups do not enjoy universal acceptance or success; however, if used in conjunction with other professional treatment, they can be very beneficial.

Rehabilitation

Historically, treatment for substance abuse was primarily developed for and directed to men.[44,74] Although women were secluded in sanatoriums in the early to mid-1900s, treatment specifically developed for women became available only in the late 1900s. Federally funded initiatives targeting substance-abusing women were developed in the 1990s. Overall, treatment programs for substance-abusing women increased by 53% by the late 1990s; however, few programs exist that are designed specifically for substance-abusing pregnant women.[75]

Post-detoxification treatment traditionally has been provided in long-term inpatient residential treatment facilities. These programs were typically three or more months in duration. Because of changes made as a result of the institution of managed care, these programs were reduced in length to 60 days and reduced again to three to five days of treatment. These shorter treatment programs were only possible because of the development of the four-hour per day partial hospital and three-hour per day intensive outpatient programs. Current treatment models recommend offering the least restrictive setting first, and then moving to a more restrictive setting as needed.

Nicotine Addiction

The midwifery role in the management of most substances is primarily to identify whether use poses problems for the individual woman and, if so, to help her recognize these problems, assess her willingness to engage in treatment, and facilitate her entry into care. Actual management of withdrawal from a substance will generally be managed by a team of experts in the care of addicted women. However, nicotine addiction is the exception to this rule. It is common, legal, and poses few social, but substantial health risks. Therefore, midwives need to employ all of the techniques discussed early in the chapter on helping women recognize and be willing to change their addictive behaviors. In addition, midwives must be intimately familiar with the medication options available to help women stop smoking and be comfortable using them in their practice.

Nicotine is an addictive drug and negatively affects the fetus if exposed during pregnancy. Nicotine addiction directly affects the central nervous system. Specifically, nicotine affects the C-6 receptor sites and other transmitter systems, especially norepinephrine, which is believed to be significantly related to some of the negative aspects of withdrawal.[76] Nicotine stimulates the release of acetylcholine and triggers electroencephalographic changes. Nicotine causes the releases of endorphin and dopamine and seems to inhibit monoamine oxidase in the brain. These are components of the brain's motivational system.[76]

Nicotine can be introduced to the body in multiple formats. It can be smoked in ciga-rettes, snuffed (inhaled) orally, or chewed and spit. The most common use among women is smoking. Smoking (cigarettes) has the highest potential to cause nicotine addiction because it produces marked increases in arterial blood concentration of nicotine. Within 7 to 10 seconds of inhaling cigarette smoke, a bolus of nicotine is delivered to the cerebral arteries in the brain.[76]

The *Diagnostic and Statistical Manual of Mental Disorders*, version IV (DSM-IV) describes the physical and psychological symptoms of nicotine withdrawal. Psychological symptoms include: dysphoria, depression, anxiety, irritability, frustration, and anger. These symptoms can develop after quitting "cold turkey" and will completely subside within two to three weeks. The physical symptoms, however, may be more prolonged and even persistent. Physical symptoms may include: sleep disruption from poor quality sleep, increased appetite, and weight gain. These symptoms have been reported to occur for as long as one to six months after quitting. Reports of craving vary between individuals, regardless of whether they are "thinking" of returning to smoking.

What is more consistent among ex-smokers is that relapse is positively correlated with exposure to any amount of tobacco, even after long periods of being abstinent.

Exposure to a substance, even after detoxification and periods of abstinence, will often result in relapse or return to substance use. Patients who relapse often return to a level of use equivalent to whatever level of use was their previous highest level. The addicted brain recalls the drug, and when the drug is re-introduced the brain craves the level of the last use. Users who detoxify from a substance and then attempt to ease back into minimal use are shocked to discover that they pick up from where they left off. This explains why relapse can be deadly in some cases. Whereas the first level of addiction resulted from a gradual buildup, the relapse event returns the brain to its prior addicted/altered state. Cigarette smoking is no exception.

Treatment consists of three approaches: nicotine replacement therapy, antidepressants used to minimize cravings, and behavioral interventions. Many options are available for nicotine replacement. Nicotine gum was the first available option; others include transdermal nicotine (the patch), nasal sprays, and inhalers. Nicotine treatment studies using antidepressants such as nortriptyline and bupropion, which increases central dopaminergic activity, have generally been found to increase the numbers who successfully stop smoking (of note, subjects enrolled in these studies generally do not have comorbid depression; **Table 8-8** lists commonly used medications for smoking cessation).

Clients often benefit from using a variety of behavioral interventions in addition to medication. Clients can be asked to keep a smoking diary to monitor both the amount and the circumstances surrounding the choice to smoke. Some individuals prefer to wean slowly and others to quit "cold turkey." For those interested in weaning, two suggestions may make reducing the daily number of cigarettes easier: 1) smoke a different brand of cigarette of the same strength but different taste; or 2) remove the daily quota of cigarettes from the pack and place in an obvious spot, thereby reducing the temptation to smoke more. At the agreed-upon quit date, other techniques may be helpful, including: throwing away ashtrays, matches, and lighters; changing or laundering curtains, bedspreads, or clothing because they retain the smell of cigarette smoke; or identifying an "antismoking buddy" who can lend support im-

mediately as needed. Keeping the money that has been spent on cigarettes in a special money jar or bank provides small rewards for success at quitting.

Combining approaches is more effective. People who are treated with medications are twice as likely to quit smoking as those whose therapy did not include pharmacology. Strong behavioral treatment strategies double the long-term quit rates. A factor in nicotine relapse is whether the person who quit took a puff within two weeks of ending the treatment program. In one study, 90% of the "puffers" were renewed smokers at six months while 40% of "nonpuffers" were nonsmokers in the same time period.[76] Therefore, the clinical goal is to develop a strong commitment to abstinence from day one.[76]

Conclusion

Substance abuse is a result of a confluence of many variables and is best understood as a personal pathway of change toward and away from addiction. Addiction results in permanent changes in the brain and is treatable through detoxification, intensive formal and informal counseling, relapse prevention, cognitive behavioral skills training, and self-help support systems.

Successful treatment can be enhanced through the application of MET. Early intervention can serve to begin a change process that can empower the person to clarify lifestyle discrepancies, and by doing so increase the individual's ambivalence about her behavior, which is a necessary first step in the change process. This change process can ultimately alter the addiction, stop the abuse, and improve the health and social/emotional status of the individual.

Table 8-8 MEDICATIONS FOR SMOKING CESSATION

Category	Drug Type	Dose	Comments
Nicotine Replacement	Patch	21, 14, and 7 mg available as 24-hour patch. 15 mg patch available for 16 hours.[77]	• Start with 21 mg patch if smokes $\frac{1}{2}$ PPD or more; use 24-hour patch particularly if smokes in the morning. May use lower doses if smokes less than $\frac{1}{2}$ PPD. • Rotate patch sites. • Side effects: nausea, insomnia, headache, itching, erythma, and rash with patch use.[77,78] • Local treatment of skin reactions with hydrocortisone cream 1% or triamcinolone cream 0.5% and rotating sites may help.[79,80]
	Gum	1–24 cigarettes/d: use 2 mg gum up to 24 pieces/d.[77] ≥25 cigarettes a day: use 4 mg gum up to 24 pieces/d.[77]	• Chew gum until taste is strong, and then park between the check and gum. Chew again when taste has faded. • Continue this pattern for about 30 minutes or until flavor is gone.[78] • Side effects: mouth soreness, dyspepsia, hiccups.[77] • Acidic beverages (coffee, juice, soft drinks) interfere with absorption, so eating and drinking anything but water should be avoided for 15 minutes before or after chewing.[81] • Often patients do not use enough pieces to be effective. May consider advising to follow a schedule of at least one piece every 1–2 hours.[81]
	Nasal Spray	8–40 doses/d.[77] Deliver with head tilted slightly back.[82]	• One spray each nostril as needed.[78] • Side effect: Nasal irritation, congestion, transient changes in smell and taste.[82]
	Nicotine Inhaler	One dose equals one puff. Each cartridge contains 4-mg nicotine delivered over 80 inhalations.	• Side effect: Local irritation of mouth and throat.[77] • Coughing and rhinitis common.[83] • Cold air decreases medication availability, so carry in an inside pocket or keep warm. Do not eat or drink anything except water for 15 minutes before or after use, because buccal absorption may be impaired by certain foods and beverages.[83]

(continues)

Table 8-8 MEDICATIONS FOR SMOKING CESSATION *(continued)*

Category	Drug Type	Dose	Comments
		Use 6–16 cartridges/d.[62,81] Best effect achieved with frequent use.	
Antidepressants	Bupropion (Wellbutrin or Zyban)	150 mg PO qd for 3 days, then increase to 150 mg PO BID.	• Start medication one week before the quit date. • Contraindicated if at risk for seizures: do not use for those with epilepsy, extreme caution in patients at higher risk of having a lower seizure threshold (those with history of head trauma, alcohol misuse, diabetes treated with hypoglycemic agents or insulin, or if on drugs such as antipsychotics, antidepressants, and systemic corticosteroids). Also contraindicated for use in those with anorexia or bulimia, hepatic necrosis, bipolar disorder, or who are taking monamine oxidase inhibitors. • Common side effects include dry mouth, skin rash, pruritus, and hypersensitivity.[84]
Other second line medications	Clonidine	Oral doses of 0.15 mg/d. Transdermal doses of 0.10–0.20 mg/d.[85]	
	Nortriptyline	Initial dose of 24 mg/d, increasing to 75–100 mg/d.[86]	

Key: d - day; PPD - packs per day; PO - by mouth; qd - every day; BID - twice a day.

Table 8–9 INTERNET RESOURCES

Organization	Web Site
National Clearinghouse for Alcohol and Drug Information	http://www.health.org
National Institute on Drug Abuse	http://www.nida.nih.gov
Treating Tobacco Use and Dependence— Clinician's Packet. A How-To Guide For Implementing the Public Health Service Clinical Practice Guideline; March 2003. U.S. Public Health Service.	http://www.surgeongeneral.gov/tobacco/clinpack.html

Using the perspective of intentional human behavior change as the integrating concept for understanding and promoting substance abuse and addiction treatment is useful for several reasons. First, human behavioral change implies human development. Personal change takes place over time, at different points in the life cycle, most often through a sequence of events. Likewise, addiction and recovery occur in the context of human development, and in an individual's life space through physiological and psychological events and transitions.[13,67,87] In addition, the change-process perspective moves us away from thinking about constant variables to a focus on an active process. Substance addiction and recovery are dynamic in nature with periods of disruption as well as stability. This process is also vulnerable to acceleration and deceleration through intervening physiological, social, and psychological factors. Finally, the change perspective allows for use, abuse, and addiction to be understood and treated as a continuum of biopsychosocial-behavioral-spiritual behaviors similar to other health and mental health behaviors that also change over time. Midwives who employ these techniques will help women change unhealthy behaviors and, by doing so, help them create a better, more fulfilling life. Those desiring more information can refer to the Internet resources listed in **Table 8-9.**

References

1. Reid T. What's the buzz? *National Geographic.* 207(1): 2–33.

2. Mueser K, Glynn S. *Behavioral Family Therapy for Psychiatric Disorders.* 2nd ed. Oakland, CA: New Harbinger; 1999.

3. Drake R. Dual diagnosis disease management. In: Trafton JA, Gordon WP, editors. *Best Practices in Behavioral Management of Chronic Disorders.* Los Altos, CA: Institute for Brain Potential/Institute for Disease Management; 2003(10). pp. 1–12.

4. Substance Abuse and Mental Health Services Administration. *Results from the 2003 National Survey on Drug Use and Health: National Findings.* NSDUH Series H–25, DHHS Publication No. SMA 04–3964. Rockville, MD: Office of Applied Studies; 2004.

5. Anonymous. Cigarette smoking among adults, United States, 2002. *MMWR* 2004;53(20):427–431.

6. Research Report Series. *Prescription Drugs: Abuse and Addiction.* NIH Publication Number 01-4881. Rockville, MD: National Institute on Drug Abuse; 2001.

7. Lingford-Hughes A. There is more to dopamine than just pleasure. Commentary on Volkow et al. Role of dopamine in drug reinforcement and addiction in

humans: Results from imaging studies. *Behav Pharmacol.* 2002;13(5-6):367–370.

8. Self D. Dependence and addiction: Neural substrates. *Am J Psychiatry.* 2004;161(2):223–232.

9. Research Report Series. *Cocaine Abuse and Addiction.* NIH Publication Number 99-4342. Rockville, MD: National Institute on Drug Abuse; 1999.

10. Research Report Series. *Marijuana Abuse.* NIH Publication Number 02-3859. Rockville, MD: National Institute on Drug Abuse; 2002.

11. Research Report Series. *Inhalant Abuse.* NIH Publication Number 05-3818. Rockville, MD: National Institute on Drug Abuse; 2005.

12. National Center for Chronic Disease Prevention and Health Promotion. General Alcohol Information. 2004. [Monograph on the Internet.] Centers for Disease Control, Atlanta, GA. Available from: http://www.cdc.gov/alcohol/factsheets/general_information.html.

13. Kandel D, Davis M. Progression to regular marijuana involvement: Phenomenology and risk factors for near daily use. In: Glantz M, Picken R, editors. *Vulnerability to Drug Use.* Washington, DC: American Psychological Association; 1992. pp. 211–254.

14. Anonymous. Alcoholism. In: Baronial E, Fuci A, Kasper D, Hauser S, Longo D, Jameson L, editors. *Harrison's Manual of Medicine.* 15th ed. New York: McGraw Hill; 2002. pp. 921–922.

15. Henderson C. Alcohol and substance abuse. In: Cohen W, editor. *Cherry & Market's Complications of Pregnancy.* 5th ed. Philadelphia: Lippincott Williams & Wilkins; 2000. pp. 147–155.

16. Grunbaum J, Kann L, Kinchen S, Ross J, Hawkins J, Lowry R, et al. Youth Risk Behavior Surveillance-United States, 2003. *MMWR Surveil Sum.* 2004; 53(SS-2):1–29.

17. Lloyd J. Methamphetamine. November 2003. Office of National Drug Control Policy. *Drug Policy Information Clearinghouse Fact Sheet;* 2003. [Monograph on the Internet.] Available from: http://www.whitehousedrugpolicy.gov/publications/factsht/methamph/index.html.

18. Lloyd J. Cocaine, November 2003. Office of National Drug Control Policy. *Drug Policy Information Clearinghouse Fact Sheet;* 2003. [Monograph on the Internet.] Available from: http://www.whitehousedrugpolicy.gov/publications/factsht/cocaine/index.html.

19. Office of Applied Studies. 2001 National Household Survey on Drug Abuse: Detailed Tables. Table H.1. Estimated Numbers (in Thousands) of Lifetime, Past Year, and Past Month Users of Illicit Drugs among Persons Aged 12 or Older: 2000 and 2001. [Monograph on the Internet.] U.S. Department of Health and Human Services Substance Abuse and Mental Health Services Administration, Washington, DC [2004]. Available from: http://www.drugabusestatistics.samhsa.gov/NHSDA/2k1NHSDA/vol2/appendixh_1.htm#tableh.1.

20. Spiess M. MDMA (Ecstasy), February 2004. Office of National Drug Control Policy. *Drug Policy Information Clearinghouse Fact Sheet.* 2004. [Monograph on the Internet.] Available from: http://www.whitehousedrugpolicy.gov/publications/factsht/mdma/index.html.

21. Anonymous. Drug Facts Heroin. Office of National Drug Control Policy; 2005. [Monograph on the Internet.] Available from: http://www.whitehousedrugpolicy.gov/drugfact/heroin/index.html.

22. Anonymous. Marijuana, February 2004. Office of National Drug Control Policy. *Drug Policy Information Clearinghouse Fact Sheet;* 2004. [Monograph on the Internet.] Available from: http://www.whitehousedrugpolicy.gov/publications/factsht/marijuana/index.html.

23. Anonymous. *Drug Facts Oxycontin.* Office of National Drug Control Policy; 2005. [Monograph on the Internet.] Available from: http://www.whitehousedrugpolicy.gov/drugfact/oxycontin/index.html.

24. Anonymous. *Oxycontin Diversion and Abuse.* Johnstown, PA: U.S. Department of Justice Product Number 2001-L0424-001; 2001.

25. Anonymous. Drug Facts Hallucinogens (LSD, psilocybinmushrooms, mescaline, DMT, AMT, Foxy, DXM). Office of National Drug Control Policy; 2005. U.S. Department of Justice Product Number 2001-L0424-001. [Monograph on the Internet.] Available from: http://www.whitehousedrugpolicy.gov/drugfact/hallucinogens/index.html.

26. Finch B, Vega W, Kolody B. Substance abuse during pregnancy. *Social Sci Med.* 2000;52(4):571–583.

27. Carey P. Sexually transmitted diseases, pregnancy, and the drug user. In: Siney C, editor. *The Pregnant Drug Addict.* Hale, Cheshire, England: Books for Midwives Press; 1995. pp. 42–50.

28. Carey P. Human immunodeficiency virus, pregnancy, and the drug user. In: Siney C, editor. *The Pregnant Drug Addict.* Hale, Cheshire, England: Books for Midwives Press; 1995. pp. 58–82.

29. Cohen M. *Counseling Addicted Women: A Practical Guide.* Thousand Oaks, CA: Sage Publications; 2000.

30. Carten A. Mothers in recovery. *Soc Work.* 1996;41:214–233.

31. Boyd S. *Mothers and Illicit Drugs: Transcending the Myths.* Toronto: University Press of Toronto; 1999.

32. Siney C. Management of pregnant women who are drug dependent. In: Siney C, editor. *The Pregnant Drug Addict.* Hale, Cheshire, England: Books for Midwives Press; 1995. pp. 1–8.

33. Treatment Child and Family Services Agency (CFSA). *Pregnant Substance Abusing Women.* DHHS Publication No. (SMA) 95-3056. Rockville, MD: U.S. Department of Health and Human Services; 1995.

34. Sparey C, Walkinshaw S. Obstetric problems for drug abusers. In: Siney C, editor. *The Pregnant Addict.* Hale, Cheshire, England: Books for Midwives Press; 1995. pp. 24–33.

35. Geller A. The effects of drug use during pregnancy. In: Ruth P, editor. *Alcohol and Drugs Are Women's Issues.* Meutechen, NJ: Scarecrow Press; 1991. pp. 101–106.

36. Little B, Yonkers K. Treatment of substance abuse during pregnancy: An overview. In: Yonkers K, Little B, editors. *Management of Psychiatric Disorders in Pregnancy.* London, UK: Arnold; 2000.

37. Streissguth A. *Fetal Alcohol Syndrome: A Guide for Families and Communities.* Baltimore: Paul H. Brookes; 1997.

38. VanBeveren T, Little B, Spence M. Effects of prenatal cocaine exposure and postnatal environment on child development. *Am J Hum Biol.* 2000;12(3):417–428.

39. Kropenske V, Howard J. *Protecting Children in Substance-Abusing Families.* Circle Solutions, McLean, VA: U.S. Department of Health and Human Services; 1994.

40. Little B, Gilstrap L. Counseling and evaluation of the drug exposed pregnant patient. In: Little B, Gilstrap L, editors. *Drugs and Pregnancy.* New York: Chapman and Hall; 1998. pp. 25–31.

41. Coles C. Critical periods for prenatal alcohol exposure. *Alcohol Health Res World.* 1994;1994(1):22–29.

42. Walkinshaw S, Shaw B, Siney C. Neonatal abstinence syndrome. In: Hilary K, Jackson M, Lewis S, editors. *Drug Misuse and Motherhood.* London, UK: Routledge; 2002. pp. 213–233.

43. Curet L, Hsi A. Drug abuse during pregnancy. *Clin Obstetr Gynecol.* 2002;45(1):73–88.

44. Blume S. Addictive disorders in women. In: Frances R, Miller S, editors. *Clinical Textbook of Addictive Disorders.* New York: Guilford Press; 1998. pp. 413–429.

45. DiClemente C. *Addiction and Change.* New York: The Guilford Press; 2003.

46. Johnson B. *Toward a Theory of Drug Subcultures.* DHHS publication number (ADM) 80–967. Rockville, MD: Department of Health and Human Services, Public Health Service, Alcohol, Drug Abuse, and Mental Health Administration, National Institute on Drug Abuse; 1980.

47. Hesselbrock M, Hesselbrock V, Epstein E. Theories of etiologies of alcohol and other drug use disorders. In: McCrady B, Epsteing E, editors. *Addictions: A Comprehensive Guidebook.* New York: Oxford University Press; 1999. pp. 50–74.

48. Robins L. *The Natural History of Drug Abuse.* DHHS publication number (ADM) 80-967. Rockville, MD: Department of Health and Human Services, Public Health Service, Alcohol, Drug Abuse, and Mental Health Administration, National Institute on Drug Abuse; 1980.

49. Weiss R. The role of psychopathology in the transition from drug use to abuse to dependence. In: Glantz M, Picken R, editors. *Vulnerability to Drug Abuse.* Washington, DC: American Psychological Association; 1992. pp. 137–148.

50. Willis T, Shiffman S. Coping and substance use: A conceptual framework. In: Shiffman S, Willis T, editors. *Coping and Substance Use.* Orlando, FL: Academic Press; 1992.

51. Pandina R, Johnson V, LaBouvie E. Affectivity: A central mechanism in the development of drug dependence. In: Glantz M, Picken R, editors. *Vulnerability to Drug Abuse.* Washington, DC: American Psychological Association; 1992. pp. 179–210.

52. Bandura A. *Social Foundations of Thought and Action: A Social Cognitive Theory.* Englewood Cliffs, NJ: Prentice-Hall; 1986.

53. DiClemente C, Fairhurst S, Pitroski N. The role of self-efficacy, adaptation, and adjustment. In: Maddux J, editor. *Self Efficacy, Adaptation, and Adjustment: Theory, Research and Application.* New York: Plenum Press; 1995. pp. 109–142.

54. Maisto S, Carey K, Bradizza C. Social learning theory. In: Ke L, Blane H, editors. *Psychological Theories of Drinking and Alcoholism.* New York: Guilford Press; 1999. pp. 106–123.

55. Barrett R. Behavioral approaches to individual differences in substance abuse: Drug taking behavior. In: Galizio M, Maisto S, editors. *Determinants of Substance Abuse: Biological, Psychological, and Environmental Factors.* New York: Plenum Press; 1985. pp 125–178.

56. Orford J. *Excessive Appetites.* New York: Wiley; 1985.

57. Donovan D, Marlatt G. *Assessment of Addictive Behaviors.* New York: Guilford Press; 1988.

58. Fiore M, Jorenby D, Baker T, Kenford S. Tobacco dependence and the nicotine patch. *JAMA.* 1992; 268(19):2687–2694.

59. Leshner A. Drug abuse and addiction are bio-medical problems. *Hosp Pract.* 1997; April Special Issue.

60. Gavin D, Ross H, Kinner H. Diagnostic validity of the drug abuse screening test in the assessment of DSM-III drug disorders. *Br J Addict.* 1989;84(3): 301–307.

61. Chan A, Pristach E, Welte J, Russell M. Use of the TWEAK test in screening for alcoholism/heavy drinking in three populations. *Alcohol Clin Exp Res.* 1993;17(6):1188–1192.

62. Ewing J. Detecting alcoholism, the CAGE questionnaire. *JAMA.* 1984;252(14):1905–1907.

63. Brown R, Leonard T, Saunders L, Papasouliotis O. A two-item screening test for alcohol and other drug problems. *J Fam Pract.* 1997;44(2):151–160.

64. American Psychiatric Association. Diagnostic and Statistical Manual of Mental Disorders Version 4 (DSM-IV). Washington, DC: APA; 1995. pp. 201–202.

65. Anonymous. Laboratory studies. In: Gitlow S, editor. *Substance Use Disorders: A Practical Guide.* Philadelphia: Lippincott Williams & Wilkins; 2001. pp. 54–66.

66. Chassin L, Presson C, Sherman S, Edwards D. Four pathways to young adult smoking status. *Health Psychol.* 1991;10:409–419.

67. Jessor R, Van Den Bos J, Vanderryn J, Costa F, Turbin M. Protective factors in adolescent problem behavior: Moderator effects and developmental change. *Dev Psychol.* 1995;31:923–933.

68. Schulenberg J, Maggs J, Steinman K, Zucker R. Development matters: Taking the long view on substance abuse etiology and interventions during adolescence. In: Monti P, Colby S, Ta O, editors. *Adolescents, Alcohol, and Substance Abuse.* New York: Guilford Press; 2001. pp. 19–51.

69. DiClemente C, Prochaska J. Toward a comprehensive trans-theoretical model of change: Stages of change and addictive behavior. In: Miller W, Heather N, editors. *Treating Addictive Behavior.* 2nd ed. New York: Plenum Press; 1998. pp. 3–24.

70. Prochaska J, DiClemente C. *The Trans-Theoretical Approach: Crossing the Traditional Boundaries of Therapy.* Malabar, FL: Kreiger; 1984. pp. 1–24.

71. Miller W, Rollnick S. *Motivational Interviewing: Preparing People to Change Addictive Behaviors.* New Yory: Guilford Press; 1991.

72. Prochaska J, DiClemente C. Toward a comprehensive model of change. In: Miller W, Heather N, editors. *Treating Addictive Behaviors: Process of Change.* New York: Plenum Press; 1986. pp. 3–27.

73. Rogers C. (1959) A theory of therapy, personality, and interpersonal relationships as developed in the client-centered framework. Reprinted in Kirschbaum H, Herderson V, editors. *The Carl Rogers Reader.* Boston: Houghton-Mifflin; 1989. pp. 219–236.

74. Finkelstein N. Treatment issues for alcohol and drug dependent pregnant and parenting women. *Health Soc Work.* 1994;19(3):7–15.

75. Breitbart V, Chavkin W, Wise P. The accessibility of drug treatment for pregnant women: A survey of programs in five cities. *Am J Pub Health.* 1994;84(10): 1658–1661.

76. Jorenby D. Effects of nicotine on the central nervous system. *Hosp Pract.* 1997; Special Issue:17–21.

77. Anonymous. Suggestions for the clinical use of pharmacotherapies for smoking cessation. In: *U.S. Public Health Service;* 2003. Available from: http://www.surgeongeneral.gov/tobacco/clinicaluse.htm.

78. Molyneux A. Nicotine replacement therapy. *BMJ.* 2004;328(7438):454–456.

79. Fiore M, Bailey W, Cohen S, et al. Table 37. Suggestions for the clinical use of the nicotine patch. In: ACHPR, editor. *Treating Tobacco Use and Dependence Clinical Practice Guideline.* Rockville, MD: U.S. Department of Health and Human Services. Public Health Service; 2000.

80. Fiore M, Bailey W, Cohen S, et al. Smoking cessation. *Clinical Practice Guideline No 18,* Agency for Health Care Policy and Research (AHCPR) Publication No 96-0692. Rockville, MD: U.S. Department of Health and Human Services, Public Health Service, Agency for Health Care Policy and Research; 1996.

81. Fiore M, Bailey W, Cohen S, et al. Table 34. Suggestions for the clinical use of nicotine gum. In: Agency for Health Care Policy and Research (ACHPR), editor. *Treating Tobacco Use and Dependence Clinical Practice Guideline.* Rockville, MD: U.S. Department of Health and Human Services. Public Health Service; 2000.

82. Fiore M, Bailey W, Cohen S, et al. Table 36. Suggestions for the clinical use of the nicotine nasal spray. In: Agency for Health Care Policy and Research (ACHPR), editor. *Treating Tobacco Use and Dependence Clinical Practice*

Guideline. Rockville, MD: U.S. Department of Health and Human Services. Public Health Service; 2000.

83. Fiore M, Bailey W, Cohen S, et al. Table 35. Suggestions for the clinical use of the nicotine inhaler. In: Agency for Health Care Policy and Research, editor. *Treating Tobacco Use and Dependence Clinical Practice Guideline.* Rockville, MD: U.S. Department of Health and Human Services. Public Health Service; 2000.

84. Roddy E. Bupropion and other non-nicotine pharmacotherapies. *BMJ.* 2004;328(7438):509–511.

85. Fiore M, Bailey W, Cohen S, et al. Table 38. Suggestions for the clinical use of clonidine. In: Agency for Health Care Policy and Research (ACHPR), editor.

Treating Tobacco Use and Dependence Clinical Practice Guideline. Rockville, MD: U.S. Department of Health and Human Services. Public Health Service; 2000.

86. Fiore M, Bailey W, Cohen S, et al. Table 39. Suggestions for clinical use of nortriptyline. In: Agency for Health Care Policy and Research, editor. *Treating Tobacco Use and Dependence Clinical Practice Guideline.* Rockville, MD: U.S. Department of Health and Human Services. Public Health Service; 2000.

87. Deas D, Riggs P, Langenbucher J, Goldman M, Brown S. Adolescents are not adults: Developmental considerations in alcohol users. *Alcohol Clin Exp Res.* 2000;24(2):232–237.

Chapter 9

Mental Illness in Primary Women's Health Care

Ruth Johnson

Mental illness causes profound suffering among women and their families. The most widespread psychiatric diagnoses are the anxiety disorders and the mood disorders, and these disorders are diagnosed more frequently in women than in men. In women, depression alone has a lifetime prevalence of about 21% and is believed to be the leading cause of disease-related disability for women worldwide.[1]

Patients with mental illness often suffer from other medical conditions and tend to be frequent utilizers of outpatient care.[2,3] Mental illness can complicate the treatment of other conditions by clouding the patient's thought processes, impairing her ability to make good decisions and act in her own best interest.

Mental disorders are currently conceptualized as being stress-induced illness. Most psychiatric disorders—from depression and anxiety to bipolar disorder and schizophrenia—are now believed to have a genetic component. An environmental trigger is also needed to start the cascade of neurologic events that result in mental illness.[4] The relative importance of biology versus environment seems to vary among the different illnesses: Bipolar disorder requires a genetic predisposition to the illness, while the personality disorders are regarded as developing from learned behaviors. Psychiatric disorders tend to run in families, partly because of genetic vulnerability but also because of the situational stress created by family members who are ill.

Women appear to be more vulnerable than men to environmental stress, and not only when faced with life-threatening trauma. Women who have a biological susceptibility to mental illness are likely to become symptomatic when they encounter the stressful events of a typical life. The hormonal shifts of puberty, menstruation, and childbearing, or the stress of parenthood and intimate relationships can be devastating to the neurological and immune systems of these women.[5] Women are also more likely than men to experience somatic symptoms when they are anxious or depressed. Patients often report appetite changes, sleep disturbances, fatigue, and pain rather than emotional distress.[6]

Mental illness significantly impairs a woman's relationships with others, and maternal mental illness, in particular, threatens a woman's interactions with her children. Maternal mental illness adversely affects even very young infants.

Depressed mothers do not engage with their infants as fully as healthy mothers. With limited maternal feedback, their babies are less likely to seek interaction with others.[7] According to recent meta-analyses, children of depressed mothers show developmental and cognitive delays, and more conduct and behavior disorders later in childhood. These problems persisted in children studied up to age 18 and were in direct proportion to the severity of the mother's illness.[8,9]

The effects of maternal anxiety are less well documented. In a 2003 study, infants of mothers with panic disorder showed more sleep disorders and higher levels of stress hormones than did infants of control mothers. It is as if the babies were anxious, too.[10] The effects of maternal stress and anxiety may begin before birth: animal research shows that prenatal stress can affect learning, anxiety, and social behavior in the offspring.[11]

Even mothers with a history of mental illness who feel well after childbirth tend to show more disengaged behavior toward their infants than do mothers without such a history. It is this disruption in the mother–infant bond that is believed to affect the infant's neurochemical and neuroendocrine development, with lasting effects.[12] It is possible, however, to teach depressed mothers how to interact with their babies and coach them to elicit the responses that babies need.[13] When a mother's mental illness is treated to remission, it appears that her interactions with her baby are not impaired, and the infants of treated mothers appear to develop normally.[14]

Each episode of mental illness makes the patient more vulnerable to the next. The term *kindling* describes the neurologic process whereby an individual's threshold for illness becomes progressively lower with each succeeding exposure to stress or trauma.[15] The first episode of illness may be triggered by a sexual assault, the death of a loved one, or the hormonal shifts of pregnancy. The patient may recover with time, but the next trauma will likely produce more distress than the first. Over a woman's lifetime, kindling causes episodes to become more frequent, more severe, and more resistant to treatment.[16,17] Untreated—or inadequately treated—mental illness will lead to increasing disability over the patient's lifetime. Clinicians must identify signs of illness and engage their patients in effective treatment.

Presentations of Mental Illness Throughout the Life Cycle

Women's reproductive landmarks—pregnancy, childbirth, menarche, menopause—are often the very events that can trigger or worsen mental illness. Midwives may be the primary providers of care during these times and need to be aware of how mental illness may present throughout a woman's life in order to appropriately identify, treat, and refer their patients. Mental disorders discussed in this chapter include those most often seen in primary women's health care. A number of well-known diagnoses (i.e., schizophrenia and dissociative disorders) are much more rare, and the reader is referred to the psychiatric literature for more information.

Menstruation

Premenstrual symptoms are most commonly reported by women in their 20s and 30s, but may appear at any time. Emotional distress that varies through the menstrual cycle includes the familiar gynecological diagnosis of *premenstrual syndrome (PMS)* as well as the psychiatric condition known as *premenstrual dysphoric disorder*. These conditions are discussed more fully later in this chapter. Women who experience cyclic emotional distress are more likely to have an exacerbation of an underlying mental illness than a "pure" premenstrual disorder.

A woman with a known psychiatric illness may request help from her primary or gynecologic provider in managing menstrual symptoms. In such a case, co-management of illness with a mental health provider will validate the patient's experience and provide her with coordinated care.

Contraception and Sexual Behavior

Mental illness can affect a woman's ability to engage in safe sexual and contraceptive practices. Any of the mental illnesses can impair cognition and increase confusion about making choices, and an affected patient may require lengthy visits and repeated explanations. She may then still make decisions that lead to a pregnancy or sexually transmitted infection that are—to the patient—unexpected.

Thus, when a patient reports that she is participating in risky sexual behavior, it is important to consider that an underlying mental illness may be impairing her judgment. In addition to the cognitive slowing that is a hallmark of depression, bipolar disorder or personality disorders may lead to impulsive behaviors, while eating disorders and posttraumatic stress disorder (PTSD) often feature self-injurious behavior.

The Childbearing Years: Pregnancy and Postpartum

Women are especially at risk to develop mood disorders and anxiety disorders during their childbearing years. The first year postpartum, in particular, is the time when a woman is most likely to be hospitalized for psychiatric illness. With an estimated incidence between 5% and 25% of all recently delivered mothers, postpartum depression is the most common medical problem following childbirth.[18] Postpartum psychosis occurs once or twice in each 1,000 births and carries a significant risk of infanticide or suicide.

The strongest predictor of mental illness in pregnancy and postpartum is a history of previous mental illness in the patient or her family. Bipolar disorder in the patient or a family member is the single strongest predictor of psychosis in the postpartum period. The initial patient history is the most powerful tool for identifying risks. Because illness during pregnancy predicts postpartum illness, clinicians need to continue screening for symptoms as pregnancy progresses as well as throughout postpartum care.

Menopause

The decade *before* menopause is another time of vulnerability for development of mood disorders, particularly depression. As women mature, the accumulated stresses of life begin to wear down the neurologic defenses. A woman who gives a history of premenstrual distress, dysphoric mood with hormonal contraceptives, postpartum illness, or any prior episode of mental illness is particularly at risk to develop psychiatric illness in middle age. Women can also experience a new onset of mental illness (including bipolar disorder and schizophrenia) as they enter middle age.

Mental Disorders Commonly Seen in Primary Care

Psychiatric diagnoses are based primarily on observations of behavior. Unlike the disciplines of medicine and surgery, which can base diagnoses on measurable phenomena and laboratory or imaging studies, psychiatry describes the behavior of its patients. To minimize the subjectivity and confusion that can result from such a diagnostic process, the American Psychiatric Association publishes standard diagnostic criteria and minutely detailed descriptive codes of recognized of disorders. The *Diagnostic and Statistical Manual of Mental Disorders, Fourth Edition* (*DSM-IV*) is used by mental health professionals to describe and diagnose psychiatric disorders. A summary of the diagnostic categories appears in **Table 9-1**, Classification of Mental Disorders.

The *DSM-IV* diagnostic codes are different from those in the *International Classification of Diseases* (*ICD-9-CM*), which are used by other health clinicians to codify diseases for research or billing. An example of this difference can be seen by comparing the ways in which an obstetric clinician and a mental health clinician would describe a depressed new mother. The obstetric clinician may diagnose "postpartum depression" and use the *ICD-9* obstetric code for "mental postpartum condition" or "complication."

The mental health clinician, however, would diagnose major depressive disorder using a *DSM-IV* code that specifies the severity of impairment and whether it is a first episode or a re-

currence of previous illness. If the most recent episode begins in the first four weeks postpartum, the verbal descriptor "with postpartum onset" would be added. Where the obstetric clinician describes "postpartum" depression as an obstetric problem, the mental health clinician sees it as depression, with the same symptoms, treatment choices, and prognosis as any other episode of depression.

This chapter uses the *DSM-IV* terminology and descriptions because it is the standard used by the mental health clinicians with whom midwives will consult. Learning a common language of description and diagnostic terminology will make it easier to communicate and to provide the best patient care.

Mood Disorders

These disorders are grouped into unipolar and bipolar diagnoses and are described in the table of Mood Disorders in the *DSM-IV* (**Table 9-2**). *Unipolar mood disorders* include major depression and dysthymia, which are characterized by episodic or chronic periods of depressed mood. In *bipolar* illness, depression alternates with periods of irritable or manic highs. When diagnosing and treating depression, it is imperative to distinguish between unipolar and bipolar depression because the medications used for unipolar depressive illnesses can trigger acute mania or psychosis if the patient actually has a bipolar illness.

Major Depressive Disorder

The phrase "I'm depressed" is probably the most frequently heard psychiatric complaint. In addition to feeling sad or low, the patient suffering from depression may also report sleep disturbances, lack of energy, appetite changes, digestive difficulties, headaches, and

Table 9-1 CLASSIFICATION OF MENTAL DISORDERS

Category	Includes
Disorders Usually First Diagnosed in Infancy, Childhood, or Adolescence	Mental retardation, learning DO*, communication and developmental DO, attention deficit and disruptive behavior DO, feeding and elimination DO
Delirium, Dementia, and Amnesial and Other Cognitive Disorders	Delirium; Dementias including Alzheimer's, vascular, and HIV-related; amnesias; other cognitive DO
Mental Disorders Due to a General Medical Condition	Catatonic, personality change, or mental DO due to a medical condition not elsewhere classified
Substance-Related Disorders	Substance dependence, intoxication, and withdrawal
Schizophrenia and other Psychotic Disorders	Schizophrenia; schizoaffective DO; brief psychotic DO with postpartum onset
Mood Disorders	Major Depression, Dysthymia, Bipolar DO. "With Postpartum Onset" may be added as a descriptor.
Anxiety Disorders	Panic DO, Phobias, Posttraumatic Stress DO, Obsessive-Compulsive DO, Generalized Anxiety DO
Somatoform Disorders	Somatization, conversion, and pain DO; hypochondriasis; body dysmorphic DO
Factitious Disorders	Factitious symptoms are intentionally produced or feigned; popularly called Munchausen's Syndrome
Dissociative Disorders	Dissociative amnesia and fugue states; Dissociative Identity, formerly Multiple Personality, DO, Depersonalization DO
Sexual and Gender Identity Disorders	Sexual Dysfunction, Paraphilias, Gender Identity DO
Eating Disorders	Anorexia Nervosa, Bulimia Nervosa
Sleep Disorders	Dyssomnias: Insomnia, Hypersomnia. Parasomnias: Nightmare, sleep terror, sleep-walking DO
Impulse-Control Disorders Not Elsewhere Classified	Intermittent Explosive DO; kleptomania; pyromania; gambling; trichotillomania
Adjustment Disorders	Adjustment DO with Mixed Emotional Features
Personality Disorders	Borderline Personality DO

Source: Reprinted with permission from the *Diagnostic and Statistical Manual of Mental Disorders, Fourth Edition*, 2000, American Psychiatric Association.

*"DO" is the abbreviation for Disorder. Those appearing in boldface are included in this chapter.

unexplained bodily pains. Anxiety frequently accompanies depression, and patients may report feeling irritable, worried, or frustrated rather than blue.

PRESENTATION

Depressed women often do not report changes in mood, but instead seek help for memory loss, weight gain or loss, or decreased libido. They

Table 9-2 Mood Disorders

Disorder	Selected Diagnostic Criteria	Presentations	Evidence-Based Treatment	Notes
Major Depression	>4 symptoms during the same 2-week period, representing a change from previous functioning: 1. Depressed mood noticed by patient or others 2. Diminished interest or pleasure in activities 3. Decrease or increase in appetite, or unplanned weight gain or loss 4. Insomnia or Hypersomnia 5. Psychomotor agitation or retardation, noticed by others 6. Fatigue or loss of energy nearly every day 7. Feelings of worthlessness or guilt 8. Diminished ability to think or concentrate, or indecisiveness 9. Recurrent thoughts of death, with or without a plan for suicide	Patient may complain of "stress" and fatigue or low mood, somatic symptoms; clinicians notice poor decision making or history of prior mood episodes; thoughts of self-injury usually have to be elicited by direct questioning.	Psychotherapy plus *antidepressant*; adjunct medication may be needed.	Episodes become more severe over time; untreated or undertreated episodes make the patient more likely to relapse with increasing severity.
Dysthymia	Depressed mood for most of the day, more days than not, for at least 2 years, with at least 2 of the following: 1. Poor appetite or overeating 2. Insomnia or hypersomnia 3. Low energy or fatigue 4. Low self-esteem 5. Poor concentration or difficulty making decisions 6. Feelings of hopelessness	A chronic pattern, more often noticed by the clinician; patients think that this is how life has to be.	Psychotherapy plus *antidepressant*.	Stressful events may trigger major depressive episodes, which become worse over time.
Bipolar Disorder I	At least one manic episode, which features abnormally or persistently elevated, expansive, or irritable mood for at least 1 week, with at least 3 of the following: 1. Inflated self-esteem or gradiosity	Patients often have depressive complaints during a "low" time; family history of bipolar illness, substance abuse,	Psychotherapy plus *mood stabilizer*; adjunct medication may be required, especially if comorbid	Must be kept in the differential diagnosis of every mood disorder. Comorbidities include atten-

Table 9-2 MOOD DISORDERS *(continued)*

Disorder	Selected Diagnostic Criteria	Presentations	Evidence-Based Treatment	Notes
	2. Decreased need for sleep 3. More talkative than usual or pressure to keep talking 4. Flight of ideas or feeling that thoughts are racing 5. Distractibility 6. Increase in goal-directed activity or psychomotor agitation 7. Excessive involvement in pleasurable activities that have a high potential for painful consequences Mood disturbance may require hospitalization to prevent harm to self or others; psychotic features may be present.	or suicide raises the index of suspicion. Patients often stop treatment between episodes, thinking they are "cured." Cycles become shorter and more severe over time.	disorders are present. Antidepressant medication typically triggers mania.	tional disorders, substance, and impulse-control issues. Most patients with postpartum psychosis are eventually diagnosed as bipolar. Patients usually have had at least one episode of major depression; mood may be normal between episodes.
Bipolar Disorder II	At least one major depressive episode AND at least one hypomanic episode, lasting at least 4 days and featuring at least 3 of the criteria for mania but are not so severe as to cause marked impairment or require hospitalization.	Depressive episodes predominate; patients often report unsuccessful use of antidepressants.	Psychotherapy plus *mood stabilizer*; antidepressant and other adjunct medications are often needed.	Often a diagnosis of exclusion when antidepressant therapy triggers a manic episode.
Mood Disorder Specifier: With Postpartum Onset	Onset of symptoms within 4 weeks postpartum.	More common is onset or recurrence of illness *during pregnancy* with worsening postpartum.	Stress reduction; psychotherapy; medication for sleep, depression, or mood stabilization.	Strongest predictors of postpartum illness are prior illness, situational stress.
Specifier: With Seasonal Pattern	Describes a pattern of episodes that recur during a particular time of the year and are in remission during other times.	Patients most often report depressive symptoms in the fall; bipolar illness may destabilize in the spring as well.	Serotonergic antidepressants; bright light therapy; aerobic exercise as adjunct therapy.	Milder symptoms are more likely to respond to light and exercise.

may become preoccupied with physical complaints, feelings of guilt or hopelessness, and—as the illness deepens—suicidal thoughts or hallucinations. The clinician may notice a woman's slowed thinking, poor concentration and retention, confusion, and vague or contradictory decision making during the course of a routine visit. A sad or tearful appearance, slowed speech and delayed responses to questions, or an anxious look with agitated gestures are signs that the patient is not well. She may also demand frequent, lengthy visits and multiple workups for problems that others would take in stride.

A history of depression in response to a previous trauma or change is a warning that recurrence is likely. Patients often dismiss their prior depressive episodes as "situational" or "stress related," and discount the likelihood that they will ever be troubled again. But any episode of depression indicates that the patient has a biological vulnerability that may well cause a recurrence during subsequent periods of life stress. The clinician must keep in mind that depression is qualitatively the same no matter what triggered it, and any prior episode requires vigilance to anticipate a relapse.

DIAGNOSIS

A careful clinical interview may be all that is needed for diagnosis. Several screening tools suitable for office use are listed in Appendix 9-A.

TREATMENT

Major depression is an episodic disease that tends to recur throughout a lifetime. But it can be treated, often to full remission of symptoms. The evidence-based best practice is to use both psychotherapy and antidepressant medication to achieve the fastest remission of illness with the least likelihood of relapse.[19–21] Although combined therapy is the most effective, one approach or the other may be favored by the patient. Some women find that medication alone makes them feel as if they can handle life's problems and that they don't want to talk to anyone. Others prefer to "talk things through" with someone but consider medication to be a sign of weakness.

The most crucial differential diagnosis to be made before initiating treatment for depression is the distinction between unipolar depression and the depressive phase of a bipolar illness. Antidepressant drugs typically trigger manic episodes in bipolar patients.[22] Any depressed woman with a history suspicious of previous manic states or family bipolar illness must have a medication evaluation by a mental health clinician who is skilled in the management of mood stabilizing medication regimens.

Dysthymia

While major depression is an acute illness that runs an episodic course, *dysthymia* is characterized by chronic low-grade symptoms. Dysthymia can include sleep and appetite disturbances, poor concentration, and fatigue; but the symptoms are not severe enough to meet the diagnostic criteria for major depression and the patient has no thoughts of self-injury. In some cases, the patient's mood may become normal temporarily in response to positive environmental circumstances, then return to the usual low mood and energy when events are less favorable.

PRESENTATION

Dysthymic women typically do not report feeling depressed. Rather, they take for granted their low energy, poor sleep, weight gain, chronic pains, and feelings of isolation and low self-esteem. It is the chronic pattern over years—of never quite feeling up to life, even when offered support and opportunity—that reveals the underlying disorder.

DIAGNOSIS

A diagnosis of dysthymia is more likely to be suggested by the observant clinician than by the patient herself. The patient thinks of her dysthymia as a normal state because that is how she has always felt. She may seek treatment for an acute depressive or anxious episode, then discontinue treatment when she feels "better" and sink back into a familiar state of low mood and somatic discomforts. This familiarity can make the dysthymic woman resist diagnosis and treatment more adamantly than if she was acutely depressed.

Dysthymic women are particularly vulnerable to developing major depressive episodes and anxiety disorders (including PTSD) in response to life crises. Hormone changes can also trigger severe symptoms. Dysthymia, like major depression, is often seen in women who have thyroid disease, migraine, chronic fatigue syndrome, fibromyalgia, and chronic pelvic pain.

TREATMENT

Treatment of dysthymia is similar to that of major depression: psychotherapy plus medication. But dysthymia differs from an acute mood episode in that medication may be a lifelong undertaking. Discontinuation may leave the patient vulnerable to acute relapses, or recurring and varied somatic illness. Some women realize quickly that they feel better with treatment and eagerly ask how long they can stay on the medication. Others discontinue medication as soon as they feel a little better and then slide back into

their usual state. They may go through several cycles of treatment, discontinuation, and relapse before accepting a diagnosis of dysthymia and making a commitment to effective treatment.

Bipolar Disorder I

Formerly called manic depression, bipolar disorder I is a familial illness characterized by episodes of both low (depressed) and high (manic) mood, usually alternating with periods of normal mood. It is less common than unipolar depression, affecting perhaps 1% of the population.[23] Bipolar disorder I occurs equally often in men and women, but several variants of the illness are more common in women. Women tend to experience more depressive episodes and "mixed mania," in which depressive symptoms are present during a manic episode. Bipolar women are also more likely to develop "rapid cycling," with four or more mood episodes each year, and to experience seasonal destabilization of mood.[24]

In women who have a genetic predisposition to bipolar illness, symptoms can be triggered by hormonal shifts in pregnancy and postpartum. Postpartum psychosis is currently believed to be a manifestation of bipolar illness.[25,26] Among bipolar patients, the most common cause of premature death is suicide. Drug overdose and accidental injury also contribute to morbidity and mortality.[27]

PRESENTATION

Episodes of mania involve an elevated, expansive mood accompanied by impaired decision making and poor insight. The patient may forget to eat and get little sleep, perceiving herself to be productive and inspired. Women may engage in compulsive shopping, gambling, sexual activity, or substance use while they are manic.

Irritability and self-centeredness may lead to interpersonal conflicts and impaired functioning at work, especially if the illness deepens to include paranoid or psychotic features. Acute mania usually comes to the attention of the health care system when the patient requires control of symptoms or treatment of injuries.

A woman in the midst of a manic episode is unlikely to appear in the office for a primary care appointment. She has too many other, more exciting, things to do. She will instead come in during a period of normal mood, or when she needs to deal with the consequences of risky behavior. During a depressed episode, the woman may recall her manic times as productive and positive and seek help to regain her "high functioning."

It may be helpful to think of the manic "high" as an addiction: the woman is almost certain to cling to her symptoms and behavior. In truth, manic symptoms are the most dangerous, destructive part of the illness.[28] Patients in the grip of mania believe that they are experiencing brilliant inspirations or profound revelations that exempt them from the rules of ordinary behavior.

Bipolar patients often consider themselves cured once an acute episode has passed. They may discontinue medication and psychotherapy, and describe their illness as something in their past. Clinicians must remember that bipolar disorder, if correctly diagnosed, is a lifelong and potentially deadly illness that never remits spontaneously. Untreated, episodes become more severe and mood changes more frequent over time. The clinician must be prepared for the next episode even if the patient is not.

DIAGNOSIS

Bipolar illness frequently goes unrecognized for years. Mania with psychotic features may be confused with schizophrenia, while depressive episodes are often mistaken for unipolar depression. It is usually the alert clinician, rather than the patient, who will identify the illness in the primary care setting.

A history of substance use, including alcohol dependence, may indicate attempts to self-medicate mood or irritability; episodic substance use is associated with periods of mania. The patient may also describe a history of school difficulties, frequent employment conflicts, and inappropriate relationships. Reproductive health clinicians will notice a history of risky sexual behavior, poor contraceptive choices, and ill-timed pregnancies. Extreme irritability or irrational behavior around menses may also be reported. Bipolar patients often give a history of unsuccessful antidepressant medication. Antidepressants typically trigger mania, irritability, and sleeplessness in bipolar individuals. Since bipolar illness has a strong genetic component, any family history of suicidal behavior, substance abuse, or psychiatric hospitalization suggests a vulnerability to bipolar illness.

Bipolar illness often occurs with other psychiatric illness, including anxiety, eating, and personality disorders. Bipolar disorder can be difficult to differentiate from attention deficit disorder (ADD) and is often present in disorders of impulse control and conduct. Medical conditions that can trigger mania include: multiple sclerosis, cerebrovascular accidents, thyroid disease, and postpartum status. The causal mechanisms for this are unclear.

TREATMENT

The cornerstone of treatment for bipolar disorder is mood-stabilizing medication. The illness is biological, and treatment is a lifelong necessity. While a patient may be stable on a single medication most of the time, usually several medications are needed to control acute episodes.

Lithium revolutionized the treatment of bipolar illness in the middle of the last century, and it remains the classic mood stabilizer today. Several other medications, notably the anticonvulsants, are also used to stabilize mood and as adjunct therapy. Antidepressants also may be used as adjunct therapy; they must not be prescribed without a mood stabilizer because of the risk of triggering manic episodes.

Patient compliance with treatment is a particular challenge with bipolar illness. During periods of normal mood, the patient typically wants to discontinue treatment and consider herself "cured." During a depressive episode, she may ask her primary provider for an antidepressant prescription. And when the emergency room psychiatrist restarts a mood stabilizer (or neuroleptic), there will be a risk of treatment resistance. Whenever mood stabilizers are discontinued, there is a significant risk that they will be ineffective when resumed.

Bipolar illness is the single strongest predictor of postpartum psychosis, as described in **Box 9-1**. If a pregnant woman's history includes bipolar illness in herself or a first-degree relative, she must be followed by a psychiatric provider who is skilled in the treatment of bipolar illness in pregnancy. Discontinuing medication during pregnancy or postpartum increases the risk of relapse with mania or psychosis.

Bipolar Disorder II

Bipolar disorder II is of particular importance to clinicians who care for women. While men are more likely to be diagnosed with bipolar disorder I, women are more likely to suffer from bipolar disorder II. The clinical course of this disorder is dominated by periods of depression that alternate with episodes of hypomania, which involves elevated mood or irritability that does not qualify as fully manic. Like bipolar disorder I, it is a heritable condition of lifelong duration with a significant risk of morbidity and mortality.

Presentations

Hypomanic episodes tend not to attract the professional intervention that full-blown mania requires, and such times may be perceived by the patient as "normal" and productive. A woman may experience hypomania as a time when she feels energized and alert. Needing less sleep and "comfort food" than when she is depressed, she may finally be able to lose weight or finish her dissertation. She lives in dread of the next bout of depression and tries to accomplish as much as possible before it flattens her again.

The patient probably recognizes her depression when an episode arrives. She may seek help for the depression and may have tried a number of antidepressant medications without relief. A woman may experience only depressive episodes of her illness for years, until a strong environmental stressor such as childbirth triggers a hypomanic episode.

Diagnosis

Bipolar disorder II can be a diagnosis of exclusion. It is frequently identified when a depressed patient responds to antidepressant medication by becoming irritable or acting irrationally. She may describe the effect of an antidepressant as "it made me crazy" or "I wanted to jump out of my skin all the time." Sometimes, patients refuse to discuss their reaction to an antidepressant, saying only "I just wasn't myself" and quickly changing the subject. Findings in the patient history and family history will be similar to those of bipolar disorder I, and the same screening criteria may be used.

Box 9-1 Postpartum Psychosis and Bipolar Disorder

Postpartum psychosis is the most severe form of postpartum psychiatric illness. It is believed to occur once or twice in every 1000 deliveries. Symptoms include delusions and irrational beliefs, a sense of unreality, insomnia, hallucinations, and obsessive thoughts. Psychotic illness usually begins in the first days or weeks following childbirth and constitutes a psychiatric emergency that requires hospitalization. The risks of suicide and of infanticide are each believed to be about 5%.

A prior patient or family history of bipolar illness is the strongest predictor of postpartum psychosis. Most women with postpartum psychosis are eventually diagnosed as bipolar. Prenatal and preconception interviews must include an effort to identify a history of bipolar illness in the patient and her family. Bipolar women should be co-managed with psychiatric providers who are expert in the treatment of bipolar disorder through pregnancy and postpartum. Prophylactic medication may reduce the likelihood of recurring illness.[29]

An episode of postpartum psychosis or mania is virtually guaranteed to recur after subsequent births, and possibly during pregnancy. A woman with a history of postpartum psychosis or mania must be followed by psychiatric providers during every subsequent pregnancy.

Bipolar disorder II presents the same differential diagnoses and comorbidities as bipolar disorder I. Bipolar disorder II most often masquerades as a unipolar depressive disorder. Women usually have somatic or medical problems that may, initially, present more prominently than do their shifting moods.

TREATMENT

Mood stabilization is key to successful treatment, as discussed in the section on bipolar disorder I. Antidepressants should not be prescribed for women with bipolar disorder II, even when depression is the presenting symptom, since they typically trigger hypomanic episodes.

Anxiety Disorders

Anxiety is a state of apprehension and arousal that warns of impending danger; it is a lifesaving response that tells a person in danger to prepare for fight or flight. Anxiety is a universally experienced human emotion, and the anxiety disorders are probably the most common psychiatric diagnoses.

Anxiety becomes pathological when it occurs without an impending threat or apparent danger. The anxious person is "on edge" under ordinary circumstances, and what begins with periodic episodes of intense panic or irritability can eventually become a constant state of worry that needs no provocation to trigger autonomic arousal and physical symptoms. Anxious people demand constant reassurance from those around them, especially family and caregivers.

Anxiety typically presents in the primary care office as digestive disturbance, disordered sleep, headache, or chest pain. Anxious patients tend to be heavy utilizers of emergency services, incurring multiple workups that show no physical cause of symptoms.

The biological predisposition to anxiety runs in families, and women appear to be particularly vulnerable to developing anxiety with depression. Early childhood abuse tends to cause anxiety in children, although years may pass before symptoms are recognized and correctly diagnosed.

Like the mood disorders, anxiety disorders can be triggered by medical conditions, substance use, and many medications. Whenever new symptoms appear, it is important to check for changes in the patient's health, habits, and medications. It is also possible to have more than one anxiety disorder: a patient with PTSD may develop phobias and obsessive-compulsive behavior. Anxiety also accompanies other psychiatric conditions, and may be the distressed patient's impetus for seeking treatment.

Some of the anxiety disorders, such as the specific phobias, can be readily treated to full remission. Others, including obsessive-compulsive disorder (OCD) and generalized anxiety disorder, can cause lifelong impairment despite multiple treatment strategies (**Table 9-3**).

PANIC DISORDER

Perhaps the most common of the anxiety disorders is panic disorder. The hallmark of panic disorder is the panic attack, as described in **Box 9-2**. A first panic attack can be triggered by a physical stimulus such as noise or vibrations, or by emotional stress as in stage fright. The sufferer's overwhelming fear coupled with the intense physical discomfort makes a panic attack unforgettable. Anyone who has experienced a panic attack dreads the possibility of ever having another one.

In panic disorder, the initial panic attacks are triggered by specific circumstances, but over time the attacks begin to appear spontaneously. The patient becomes increasingly fearful that another attack will appear and begins to structure her life around anticipating the next attack.

Panic disorder is categorized as occurring either with or without *agoraphobia* (**Box 9-3**). Agoraphobic fears can cause patients to lead increasingly restricted lives, as they hesitate to participate in normal activities. In extreme cases, they are unable to leave the house at all.

The benzodiazepine drugs are commonly prescribed for occasional panic attacks, but these drugs are habituating and a patient with panic disorder will require long-term therapy. The selective serotonin reuptake inhibitor (SSRI) antidepressants are most commonly used to suppress panic attacks over time. Psychotherapy focuses on behavioral interventions to help the patient control her symptoms.

Phobias

A phobia is an excessive fear of a particular object or situation. Phobias may begin after a traumatic experience—such as a fear of dogs after having been bitten—but then evolve into a pattern of avoidance that the patient recognizes as being excessive or unreasonable.

Common specific phobias include: fears of heights, storms, or other environmental stimuli; invasive medical procedures or contamination; and certain situations such as being in an enclosed space. Phobias frequently occur with other anxiety disorders and can lead to a life with severely restricted activities and choices.

A woman with social phobia avoids situations in which she fears that others may judge her to be inadequate. The physical signs of anxiety (trembling hands, shaky voice, muscle tension, and blushing) may be so embarrassing that

Table 9-3 ANXIETY DISORDERS

Disorder	Selected Diagnostic Criteria	Presentations	Evidence-Based Treatment	Notes
Panic Disorder May be with or without Agoraphobia	Recurrent unexpected Panic Attacks *and* An attack has been followed by 1 month of persistent worry about having another attack and its implications; significant change in behavior about the attacks.	—Patient may fear that physical symptoms are caused by a medical illness and pursue multiple workups. —In pregnancy, may be triggered by normal cardiac and respiratory changes.	—Medication for acute attacks. —Antidepressants helpful for long-term prevention and treatment of comorbid disorders. —Behavioral approaches to self-control of symptoms and triggers.	—Panic attacks are fairly common in the general population; the psychiatric disorder is diagnosed when attacks are frequent, unprovoked, and cause significant impairment. —Onset is usually in young adulthood.
Phobias	1. Marked and persistent excessive fear, cued by the presence of a specific object or situation. 2. Exposure to the stimulus provokes an anxiety response that may include Panic Attacks. 3. The person avoids exposure to the feared stimulus, knowing that the fear is unreasonable.	—"Needle phobia" and other fears of medical intervention lead patients to demand reassurance that they will not be exposed to such stimuli.	—Behavioral interventions teach patients how to control their symptoms and tolerate increasing exposure to the stimulus. —Anti-anxiety drugs may be used for short-term treatment of acute anxiety.	—Patients who resist treatment may be using their phobias for secondary gain. —Phobias can develop after a traumatic experience. —Comorbid conditions must be considered and treated.
Obsessive-Compulsive Disorder (OCD)	—Obsessions are recurrent, persistent thoughts or impulses that are intrusive and cause marked distress. —Compulsions are repetitive behaviors or mental acts, driven by obsessions in an attempt to reduce distress or prevent a dreaded event.	—Patients may be embarrassed or ashamed about their thoughts or behavior. —Postpartum obsessions may center around the baby's safety; mothers may be afraid to be left alone with the baby.	—Long-term medication plus psychotherapy. —Antidepressant drugs are used for OCD; high doses are often necessary.	—Among the most disabling of mental illnesses. Delayed treatment means poorer prognosis. —Treatment-resistant OCD is among the few modern indications for psychosurgery.

Table 9-3 ANXIETY DISORDERS *(continued)*

Disorder	Selected Diagnostic Criteria	Presentations	Evidence-Based Treatment	Notes
Posttraumatic Stress Disorder	The response of intense fear, helplessness, or horror to an event that threatened death or serious injury to self or others: —The traumatic event is persistently re-experienced. —Persistent avoidance of stimuli associated with the event, with emotional numbing. —Persistent symptoms of arousal.	—Intrusive, distressing memories of the trauma. —Intense distress at being reminded of the trauma in any way. —Avoiding activities, places, or people related to the trauma. —Constricted emotions, estrangement from others. —Hypervigilance: difficulty sleeping, easily startled, difficulty concentrating, irritability, and anger.	—Control of intrusive symptoms is paramount to avoid deepening neurological damage. —Psychotherapy focuses on avoiding re-triggering trauma and teaching patient to control symptoms. —Medications may help sleep problems, anxiety, depression, and comorbid medical illness.	—Expressive therapies that encourage talking about or reliving the trauma can be harmful. —Traumatic stimuli can become addicting. — Substance abuse and risk-seeking behaviors are common.
Acute Stress Disorder	During or immediately after the trauma, the person experiences at least 3 dissociative symptoms: 1. A sense of numbing or detachment 2. Reduced awareness of surroundings 3. Derealization 4. Depersonalization 5. Inability to remember parts of the trauma	The disturbance begins within 4 weeks of the trauma, and may prevent the person from telling others about the experience or obtaining assistance and resources.	Current research suggests that prophylactic use of beta blockers may prevent the neurological damage that leads to post-traumatic stress.	It is important to take the initiative when a patient is faced with a traumatic event, such as serious illness, a loss, or a difficult birth. She may be unable or unwilling to report her symptoms, so ASK. Do not pursue details that may re-trigger the trauma.

(continues)

Table 9-3 ANXIETY DISORDERS *(continued)*

Disorder	Selected Diagnostic Criteria	Presentations	Evidence-Based Treatment	Notes
Generalized Anxiety Disorder	Chronic, excessive worry about a number of activities. At least 3 symptoms are present: 1. Feeling restless or on edge 2. Being easily fatigued 3. Difficulty concentrating 4. Irritability 5. Muscle tension 6. Sleep disturbance	—Patients often admit that they "worry about everything." —Anxiety is free-floating and out of proportion to the feared object. —Interpersonal relations are strained by the constant need for reassurance. —Insight is often limited.	—Medication plus psychotherapy. —Antidepressant medications are used; short-term anxiolytics and sleep aids may be helpful for acute episodes. —Therapy can include behavioral control of symptoms.	—Anxiety can provide an effective means of controlling family and caregivers. —Chronically anxious people often self-medicate with alcohol.

Source: Reprinted with permission from *Diagnostic and Statistical Manual of Mental Disorders, Fourth Edition* of the American Psychiatric Association.

she declines social invitations or even hesitates to engage in ordinary conversation with others. A vicious cycle may develop in which the woman's anticipation of anxiety leads to symptoms, which impair her social functioning, leading to further anxiety and avoidance.

Anxiolytic medications are used to treat phobic attacks that occur under predictable circumstances, such as stage fright. See the section, *Psychotropic Medications*, later in the chapter for a fuller description of medications commonly used in primary care. As noted below in the section on "talk" psychotherapies, cognitive and behavioral interventions teach patients to control their symptoms and tolerate increasing exposure to the feared stimulus.

Obsessive-Compulsive Disorder

Obsessive thoughts are persistent, intrusive ideas or impulses that are inappropriate and cause dis-

tress. Most patients recognize that their obsessions are unreasonable and try to control such thoughts, often by repeating certain behaviors that aim to soothe their anxiety. *Compulsive repetitions* can include washing, checking, hoarding, and counting. Compulsive behaviors may evolve into elaborate rituals that lead to very rigid and limited lifestyles. Patients are often deeply ashamed of their thoughts and behaviors, and very secretive about their habits.

OCD is usually recognized in late adolescence or early adulthood, but it may begin in childhood and tends to run in families. It is among the most disabling mental illnesses and can be highly resistant to treatment of any kind. The longer it remains untreated, the poorer the prognosis.

The serotonergic antidepressants are useful in treating OCD; long-term medication and psychotherapy are usually needed. Electroconvulsive

Box 9-2 Panic Attacks

Diagnostic criteria for panic attack, adapted from DSM-IV, is a discrete period of intense fear or discomfort, in which at least four of the following symptoms develop abruptly and peak within ten minutes:

- Palpitations, pounding heart, or accelerated heart rate
- Sweating, trembling, or shaking
- Sensations of shortness of breath or smothering
- Feeling of choking
- Chest pain or discomfort
- Nausea or abdominal distress
- Feeling dizzy, unsteady, lightheaded, or faint
- Feelings of unreality or of feeling detached from oneself

- Fear of losing control or going crazy
- Fear of dying
- Paresthesias (numbness or tingling sensations)
- Chills or hot flashes

Note: Intravenous (IV) infusions of Ringer's lactate (RL) can induce panic attacks in susceptible individuals.[30,31] It is questionable whether the amount of lactate infused in the course of a typical labor or surgery is enough to trigger panic,[32] but many clinicians choose to avoid using RL for patients with a history of panic attacks. If a patient receiving IV RL has a panic attack, it makes sense to change her IV fluid immediately.

---

therapy or surgery may be helpful to patients with severe and treatment-resistant illness.

Posttraumatic Stress Disorder

Most people who are exposed to life-threatening shock or stress will recover in due time, but vulnerable individuals can incur a lifetime of emotional and physical disability. PTSD begins with a triad of symptoms: 1) the constant emotional re-experiencing of the traumatic event; 2) avoidance of stimuli that are associated with the event; and 3) a persistent state of anxious vigilance after the stressful time has passed.

Each aspect of PTSD causes problems. Intrusive thoughts of the trauma cause disordered sleep and nightmares, and may compel the sufferer to talk obsessively about her experience, thereby reinforcing the trauma. To avoid stimuli that are related to the traumatic event, patients can develop phobic or compulsive patterns of behavior. Avoidance can include emotional numbing, which leads to impaired and distressing personal relationships. *Dissociation*, that is, mentally detaching oneself from the present, is another means of escape. Dissociative disorders (including multiple personalities) may develop in response to traumatic stress.

Perhaps the most life-threatening aspect of PTSD is the constant state of autonomic arousal, the hypervigilance that is so familiar among war veterans and abuse survivors. Attempts to relieve the distress of constant anxiety can lead to substance use and other risk-seeking behavior.

Box 9-3 Agoraphobia

Agoraphobia is not a disorder in itself, but its presence or absence is used to describe or qualify other disorders.

As described in the DSM-IV, agoraphobia is anxiety about being in places or situations from which escape might be difficult, or in which help might not be available in case a panic attack occurs. Fear usually has to do with being outside the home alone, being in a crowd, or being in places where a panic attack has previously occurred.

The constant alertness can precipitate the onset of hypertension, cardiovascular disease, and other chronic health problems.

The treatment of PTSD starts with symptom control. Initial medication seeks to prevent the deepening of neurological trauma that happens with repetition of symptoms. Research suggests that early treatment with beta blockers such as propranalol (Inderol) may be able to prevent the PTSD triad from becoming established.[33] Medications used in other anxiety disorders (i.e., anxiolytics, antidepressants, and sleep aids) may be helpful in controlling symptoms to the point where the patient can learn effective behavioral interventions.

Psychotherapy also emphasizes symptom control first. Patients must learn coping behaviors that help them manage their symptoms and avoid triggering stimuli. Dialectical behavioral therapy provides a structured program that is widely used for survivors of profound trauma.[34]

Well-intentioned people often encourage trauma victims to "talk it through" as a way to resolve their feelings and move on. This can be disastrous. Particularly in women who have suffered early and repeated abuse, expressive or supportive therapies can be re-traumatizing and lead to further destabilization. It is important to reassure patients that they need not divulge the details of their trauma to anyone, including their therapist.

Acute Stress Disorder

Acute stress disorder is diagnosed during or immediately following a traumatic experience. Symptoms include emotional numbing, a reduced awareness of surroundings, a sense of unreality, and an inability to remember parts of the trauma. These disturbances in perception often prevent the patient from recognizing and seeking help for her problem. It is important for clinicians to take the initiative in observing a patient's response to a traumatic event and inquiring about symptoms. As noted above, there is some evidence to support the prophylactic use of beta blockers to prevent full-blown PTSD from developing. Intensive case management includes ensuring adequate nutrition and sound sleep for the patient, and initiating stress-reduction measures throughout the period of recovery.

Generalized Anxiety Disorder

Many women with *generalized anxiety disorder (GAD)* readily describe themselves as "worriers" and report that they have felt "nervous" for as long as they can remember. They may seek treatment for their physical symptoms for years without relief. They usually appear in the primary care office rather than the psychotherapist's practice and are prescribed psychotropic drugs more often than patients with other anxiety disorders.[35] When life crises and transitions occur, these women may develop more acute problems that require emergency mental health services; they then return to their usual level of functioning, with free-floating anxiety as a constant companion.

GAD tends to run a chronic, persistent course that is remarkably resistant to treatment over time. Even when appropriately treated—usually with long-term antidepressant medication—it has a lower likelihood of remission than other anxiety disorders.[36] Even a mild state of pervasive anxiety can disable the patient and impair her family life, becoming a lifelong pattern.

Menstrual Disorders

Women commonly report both physical and emotional changes around the time of their menses. When a patient's symptoms are severe enough to interfere with her daily life, the clinician must determine whether the situation represents the familiar gynecologic problem known as PMS, the psychiatric disorder tentatively named premenstrual dysphoric disorder (PMDD), or the cyclic worsening of another mental illness around the time of menses. The differences between these three diagnoses are summarized in **Table 9-4.**

Women often blame their symptoms on abnormal "hormones." On the contrary, women with severe premenstrual mood swings tend to have normal hormone levels but an extreme neurological sensitivity to fluctuations across their cycles. It is the neurochemical vulnerability, rather than any abnormality in gonadal functioning, that causes the troubling symptoms.[37]

Women with severe premenstrual mood changes are also likely to experience psychological trouble around other reproductive events, such as pregnancy and postpartum, and to de-velop psychiatric disorders in the years prior to menopause. A patient's report of PMS should be taken seriously and treated aggressively to prevent the progression of neurological vulnerability that can result from years of monthly cycles.

PREMENSTRUAL SYNDROME: A GYNECOLOGIC DIAGNOSIS

The gynecologic literature recognizes a "premenstrual syndrome" that includes a myriad of symptoms such as migraine, weight gain, appetite alterations, disordered sleep, mood changes, and irritability. The diagnosis of PMS, a gynecologic disorder in the *ICD-9-CM*, requires that symptoms be documented prospectively through at least two menstrual cycles and show complete remission of symptoms during some portion of the cycle.[38]

While the majority of women are believed to experience some premenstrual symptoms, most neither request nor need any specific treatment. A minority, however, do experience symptoms such as migraine or emotional distress that impair their ability to carry on normal activities. It is also possible for other illnesses, such as seizure disorders or diabetes, to destabilize around the time of menses. Gynecologic treatment of premenstrual distress usually begins with trying to stabilize the woman's well-being by interventions in nutrition, exercise, and general stress management. More aggressive treatment focuses on controlling the menstrual cycle, either by minimizing hormonal fluctuations or suppressing ovarian function altogether.

PREMENSTRUAL DYSPHORIC DISORDER: A PROPOSED PSYCHIATRIC DIAGNOSIS

PMDD is not yet a fully recognized psychiatric disorder in the *DSM-IV.* Current research indicates that its incidence in the general population

Table 9-4 MENSTRUAL DISORDERS

Disorder	Diagnostic Criteria	Prevalence	Presentations	Evidence-Based Treatment	Notes
Premenstrual Syndrome A gynecologic diagnosis with *ICD-9* code	Per ACOG: At least 1 physical and at least 1 emotional symptom; symptoms remit with menses	May include >50% of women to some degree; most require no treatment.	• "PMS" or "hormones" may be the chief complaint. • Somatic symptoms may be most troublesome (e.g., headache or joint pain). • Many women do not offer symptoms unless asked specifically.	• Aerobic exercise. • Stress management skills. • Calcium or magnesium supplements. • Medication includes SSRI or tricyclics. • Hormonal therapy aims at suppressing ovulation.	• Symptoms may not be present during every menstrual cycle. • Symptoms generally worsen over time and are relieved at menopause.
Premenstrual Dysphoric Disorder A proposed psychiatric diagnosis, included in *DSM-IV* Appendix B, Research Criteria	Per *DSM-IV:* At least 5 symptoms: 1. Depressed mood 2. Anxiety or tension 3. Affective lability 4. Anger or irritability; increased interpersonal conflicts 5. Decreased interest in usual activities 6. Difficulty concentrating 7. Lethargy	Currently being studied; ≥3%–5%. Other mood, anxiety, substance, and personality disorders are more prevalent and must be ruled out.	• Anger, irritability, and interpersonal conflicts are most prominent symptoms. • Problems may be noted by family members or law enforcement officials.	Medications: SSRI, tricyclic antidepressants are first line; benzodiazepines to be avoided, especially with substance history. Differences from other mood disorders: • Expect prompt response in 1–2 cycles. • Cyclic dosing may be just as effective as continuous.	• Believed to be an abnormal response to normal hormone cycles. • High comorbidity with mood and anxiety disorders; associated with increased risk of mental illness around other reproductive events.

Table 9-4 **MENSTRUAL DISORDERS** (*continued*)

Disorder	Diagnostic Criteria	Prevalence	Presentations	Evidence-Based Treatment	Notes
	8. Change in appetite 9. Insomnia or hypersomnia 10. Feeling overwhelmed 11. Other physical symptoms, e.g., headache or joint pain				
Premenstrual Exacerbation of Underlying Mental Disorder *DSM-IV* diagnosis of the mental disorder	*DSM-IV* criteria for the mental disorder	Consistent with the prevalence of mental disorders among women; probably accounts for most complaints of PMS.	Symptoms do not fully remit at any time in the cycle; suppressing menstrual cycle does not cure symptoms.	The underlying disorder must be treated first; minimizing hormonal fluctuations may be adjunct therapy.	PMS or "hormone trouble" is a more acceptable diagnosis for many patients.

Abbreviation: ACOG, American College of Obstetricians and Gynecologists.

is probably low, affecting perhaps 5% of women. Because other mental illnesses are far more prevalent, a woman reporting premenstrual emotional distress is more likely to be experiencing an exacerbation of another mental illness around the time of menses.

The *DSM-IV* criteria for diagnosing PMDD are more stringent than the gynecologic criteria for PMS, requiring at least five symptoms severe enough to disrupt normal functioning, only one of which may include physical complaints. Symptoms need not be present every month, but must be documented prospectively through at least two cycles and show complete remission during some portion of each cycle.

Psychiatrists studying PMDD currently describe several ways in which it appears to differ from mood disorders. The most common symptoms of PMDD are irritability and lability of mood, rather than feeling depressed or anxious. Impaired social functioning may be the most common reason for seeking treatment, rather than subjective emotional distress. Antidepressant medication appears to relieve symptoms more quickly in PMDD than when treating other disorders, and may be effective when taken only in the second half of the menstrual cycle rather than daily.

Like other mental illnesses and PMS, PMDD seems to predict vulnerability to other psychiatric diagnoses. PMDD also appears to have a high comorbidity with mood and anxiety disorders.

MENTAL ILLNESS WITH PERIMENSTRUAL WORSENING OF SYMPTOMS

There are two common situations in which a woman with an underlying mental disorder presents with premenstrual distress. First, a woman who has a known mental illness may seek help for the management of perimenstrual exacerbation of her illness. She may not have told her psychiatric provider about her PMS, or her provider may have dismissed her complaints as being irrelevant to the management of her mental illness. More commonly, women seek treatment only for the period of exacerbation, blaming PMS or "my hormones" rather than acknowledging the possibility of a mental illness.

Three strategies are helpful in differentiating a "pure" premenstrual disorder from an underlying or comorbid mental illness:

1. Ask the patient to record her symptoms daily on a calendar, just as she would for any investigation of PMS. Emotional symptoms that are severe enough to impair functioning or cause distress and that do not abate for more than a few days at a time are not a premenstrual disorder.

2. Administer a standard depression screening tool, such as the Edinburgh Postnatal Depression Scale,[39] during the early part of the patient's menstrual cycle, or weekly throughout the cycle. If the patient scores positive for depression at times not related to menses, a premenstrual disorder is not her primary diagnosis.

3. Suppress her ovulation, perhaps with several weeks of hormonal contraception. Symptoms that persist in the absence of an ovulatory cycle are not, by definition, premenstrual.

It is often abundantly clear to the clinician that the patient suffers from a mental illness, but the patient may only accept a diagnosis of PMS and be unwilling (or not yet ready) to acknowledge the full scope and implications of her problem. Happily, the evidence-based treatment of PMS, PMDD, and disorders of anxiety and depression is very similar.

TREATMENT

Pharmacological treatment of premenstrual emotional distress has two aspects:

1. Control of cycles, thereby limiting hormonal fluctuations that trigger neurologic dysfunction.
2. Enhancing neurologic resilience to hormonal changes via psychotropic medication.

Control of Menstrual Cycles   Hormonal contraceptives effectively eliminate ovulatory cycles. Hormone fluctuations can be minimized by using a monophasic product in a continuous-therapy regimen. *Tricycling*, whereby the patient takes nine continuous weeks of active pills or nine weekly patches or three monthly vaginal rings, followed by a withdrawal for four days, provides a more steady state than does a monthly withdrawal. Some women withdraw only twice a year. Continuous therapy, that is, without planned withdrawals, will eventually result in occasional irregular bleeds that may be quite acceptable to the patient.

Mood changes on hormonal contraceptives are generally due to the progestin component of the pill. Medroxyprogesterone acetate, the first synthetic progestin and still widely available in both oral and injectable form, has been reported for years to trigger depressive symptoms.[40] Of the newer progestins, levonorgestrel and drospirenone tend to be the least likely to trigger adverse moods.[41] Drospirenone additionally can minimize fluid retention and other PMS symptoms and may be the first-choice oral contraceptive (OC) formulation for women with mood disorders as well as for PMDD.[42]

When hormonal products are used to minimize neurochemical stress, effective contraception becomes a side effect rather than the primary intent of the therapy and must be discussed with the patient. Mental illness, especially depression, can slow cognition and impair decision making, leading the patient to make vague or contradictory plans around managing her fertility and sexual behavior. Discussing hormonal therapy to manage premenstrual complaints may provide a way to focus a woman's thinking around contraception and help her to clarify her decisions.

Psychotropic Medication Psychiatric research has established that the SSRI and tricyclic antidepressants are effective treatments for PMDD.[43] The Food and Drug Administration (FDA) has recently approved sertraline (Zoloft) specifically for PMDD, although the other SSRIs appear to be equally useful. (See the section *Psychotropic Medication* later in the chapter for further details about medication management.) It may be hard to convince a woman that she may be helped by an antidepressant when she conceptualizes her illness as being caused by "hormones" and may fear taking medicine. She may reasonably suspect that an antidepressant is being suggested because the clinician thinks she is "crazy" or "it's all in my head." It is important to emphasize that antidepressant medications are also useful for a variety of other conditions, including migraine prevention and smoking cessation. Their use for premenstrual disorders differs from their use for depression in two significant ways:

1. They appear to be effective during the first month or two that they are taken, but when used as an antidepressant, they may take longer for a full effect.

2. They are often effective when taken cyclically, for the last week or two before expected menses, whereas they must be taken continuously for antidepressant effect. This regimen may also reduce the incidence of side effects such as sexual dysfunction. A woman may more readily accept the idea of taking medication for the week or two prior to menses (the weekly time-release form of fluoxetine [Prozac] requires only two pills, taken on days 14 and 21 of the cycle), than the prospect of daily medication for the foreseeable future.[44]

Adjustment Disorders

When a life crisis causes more distress than expected, an *adjustment disorder* may be diagnosed. The *DSM-IV* specifies that symptoms begin within three months of a specific stressor and cause a significant impairment in daily functioning. Symptoms are expected to resolve within six months unless the stressor becomes chronic, as with a long-term medical illness. By definition, the symptoms of adjustment disorder do not represent bereavement, nor are they severe enough to meet criteria for PTSD. An adjustment disorder can include depressive or anxious symptoms, or disturbed behavior such as reckless driving or vandalism.

The practical usefulness of an adjustment disorder is that most people don't mind having it as a diagnosis on their medical record. It is considered to be a biologically based illness for purposes of insurance coverage. Women fear being labeled with a psychiatric diagnosis—with good reason—but generally accept the idea that their disturbing symptoms are stress-induced and temporary. The idea of an adjustment disorder allows the patient to begin supportive treatment, including psychotherapy and medication if appropriate, and see what happens. If her symptoms do not resolve as expected, or if she begins to meet the criteria for another psychiatric disorder, her diagnosis can be reconsidered.

Eating Disorders

The *eating disorders* involve a disturbance in eating behavior combined with a distorted perception of body shape and weight. Eating disorders are diagnosed far more frequently in women than in men, for reasons that seem to include social and cultural expectations as well as biological vulnerability. Also, eating disorders and distorted self-image commonly follow early sexual abuse, which is believed to be more common in women than in men. Women with eating disorders share a deep preoccupation with a self-image and self-esteem based on body shape and size, usually with extreme shame and secretiveness around their eating and purging habits. The major types of eating disorders are summarized in **Table 9-5**.

Women with *anorexia nervosa* refuse to maintain a normal weight and obsessively fear becoming fat. They perceive themselves as being overweight even when their emaciated state is obvious to others. Patients restrict their food intake to lose even more weight. They may also induce vomiting or use diuretics, purgatives, or enemas. Untreated anorexia is among the most reliably lethal of all psychiatric diagnoses, with an estimated premature mortality rate of 10% to 15%.[45,46] Lifelong disability or death can result from the medical complications of starvation.

Women with *bulimia* may be of normal weight or overweight, and they do not have the amenorrhea that accompanies anorexia. The alternating of binge eating and purging behaviors causes damage to a number of body systems, including teeth and gums, esophagus, and the gastrointestinal (GI) tract. The long-term outcome of bulimia is less well researched than that of anorexia, but studies suggest that it may have a very guarded prognosis because of its comorbidity with mood and personality disorders and the likelihood of recurrence throughout the patient's life.[47]

The diagnosis of *eating disorder not otherwise specified* is applied to a number of conditions that involve distorted body image and disturbed eating habits. Some patients have all the signs of anorexia except amenorrhea, or engage in binge eating without the compensatory purging or restrictive behavior.

It is not unusual for different eating disorders to appear at different times in a woman's life. A teenage athlete may recover from anorexia only to resort to binge eating in college, and then

Table 9-5 **EATING DISORDERS**

Disorder	DSM-IV Diagnostic Criteria	Presentations	Co-morbidities and Medical Complications	Treatment	Notes
Anorexia Nervosa	1. Refusal to maintain a minimally normal body weight 2. Intense fear of gaining weight, even though underweight 3. Disturbed perception of body shape and weight 4. Amenorrhea	–Weight loss to <85% of normal body weight. –In teens, failure to gain with growth. –Amenorrhea, infertility. –Physical signs: see Exam section.	–High co-morbidity with depression, anxiety disorders including OCD, personality disorders. –Cardiac and renal complications of starvation can be lethal.	–Weight restoration is crucial; requires inpatient stabilization. –Medication includes SSRI antidepressants. –Pregnancy should be co-managed with psychiatric providers.	–Usual onset is in adolescence. –Patients may conceal and deny their symptoms for years. –"Female Athlete Triad" of eating DO, amenorrhea, osteoporosis is increasingly seen.
Bulimia Nervosa	1. Recurrent episodes of binge eating 2. Recurrent inappropriate compensatory behavior: induced vomiting, fasting, excessive exercise, use of diuretics or laxatives 3. Self evaluation is unduly influenced by body shape and weight	–May be normal weight or overweight. –Patients believe their weight or eating interferes with work and social relationships. –Physical signs: see Exam section.	–High comorbidity with depression, anxiety disorders including OCD, personality disorders. –Purging behavior can be destructive to teeth, GI tract.	–Outpatient psychotherapy includes cognitive-behavioral and interpersonal approaches. –SSRI antidepressants are used; ondansetron (Zofran) and topiramate (Topamax) are being studied.	–Thought to be less lethal than AN, but outcome even with treatment is uncertain.

(continues)

Table 9-5 EATING DISORDERS *(continued)*

Disorder	DSM-IV Diagnostic Criteria	Presentations	Co-morbidities and Medical Complications	Treatment	Notes
Eating Disorder Not Otherwise Specified	Includes disturbed eating or compensatory behaviors that do not meet all AN or BN criteria	—May include all signs of AN except amenorrhea	Same as for corresponding eating disorders	Same as for corresponding eating disorders	Patients will have the distorted self-image and preoccupation with eating as for other ED.
"Binge-Eating Disorder"	An Eating DO NOS with research criteria: Uncontrolled binge eating without compensatory behaviors	—Overweight or obese —Long history of dieting and weight fluctuations. —Feels distressed and guilty about eating habits.	—Probable co-morbidity with mood and personality disorders and substance use —Medical risks of obesity apply and can be lethal.	Treatment is being researched.	Overeating is frequently seen with an acute episode of major depression.

Source: Reprinted with permission from *Diagnostic and Statistical Manual of Mental Disorders, Fourth Edition* of the American Psychiatric Association.
Abbreviations are: AN, anorexia nervosa; BN, bulimia nervosa; DO, disorder; ED, eating disorder; NOS, not otherwise specified; OCD, obsessive compulsive disorder; SSRI, selective serotonin reuptake inhibitor.

alternate cycles of bingeing and purging behaviors in later years. A pregnant woman with a history of an eating disorder should be followed very carefully, because the normal weight gain of pregnancy may cause issues around body image and a relapse of dangerous eating behaviors.

PRESENTATION

Eating disorders typically appear with other psychiatric illness, most often mood and anxiety disorders, personality disorders, or substance abuse. These other problems, along with the physical complications of bulimia and anorexia, are the most common presentations of eating disorders in primary care. Families may bring in the underweight teenager because of her amenorrhea; a depressed smoker may request an infertility workup; dental caries and damage may be noted on a routine exam; obesity may lead to a discussion that reveals alternating bingeing and restricting behaviors.

An increasingly frequent presentation of eating disorders is the *female athlete triad*, which includes disordered eating, amenorrhea, and osteoporosis.[48,49] It is most common in disciplines that require a very slender appearance, such as gymnastics and ballet. Amenorrhea can be masked by OCs, which are frequently taken by young women to avoid bleeding during competition or performances.

DIAGNOSIS

Physical signs and symptoms and the laboratory workup for eating disorders are covered in the section on Assessment of Mental Illness that follows. A thorough history is the most powerful screening tool. Two questions that can be integrated into routine interviews have been shown to be helpful in detecting bulimia:[50]

1. Are you satisfied with your eating habits?
2. Do you ever eat in secret?

Anorexia should be suspected in underweight young women with delayed menarche, failure to menstruate other than with hormone withdrawal, or failure to gain weight as expected in adolescence or during pregnancy. The section on assessment describes laboratory testing, including electrocardiogram (EKG) and bone density. Consultation with the patient's primary care physician or pediatrician is essential.

TREATMENT

The treatment of eating disorders is complicated by the patient's secrecy around her behavior and the frequent comorbidity with other psychiatric illness. Although treatment regimens for all of the eating disorders involve psychotherapy and medication, anorexia and bulimia require different approaches depending on the patient's medical condition.

Women with active anorexia nervosa require a structured inpatient treatment program to restore weight and stabilize medical complications. A comprehensive program involves a multidisciplinary team to provide both individual and family therapy, with continued outpatient follow-up after the treatment program. Medication may be helpful for comorbid mood and anxiety disorders. Because eating disorders tend to recur, clinicians caring for "recovered" patients must remain alert for signs of relapse during periods of life stress.

An anorexic woman is generally infertile, but if her illness remits and she begins to gain weight, she may unexpectedly begin to ovulate and become pregnant. Usually menses return when the patient regains 90% of her normal body weight. Recent studies find that anorexic women experience more miscarriages, caesarian sections, premature births, and small-for-dates babies than do controls.[51,52] Pregnant women with a history of eating disorder will require comprehensive co-management between obstetric and psychiatric personnel for optimal outcome.[53]

While anorexia requires inpatient care, bulimia may be treated on an outpatient basis. Psychotherapy involves individual or group cognitive-behavioral interventions designed to normalize patients' self image and eating habits. SSRI antidepressants have been shown to be helpful, and fluoxetine (Prozac, Sarafem) may be the best-tolerated drug.[54] Bupropion (Wellbutrin, Zyban) has been associated with increased likelihood of seizures in bulimic patients and is contraindicated in patients with a history of this eating disorder.

Personality Disorders

Personality disorders cause serious and complex impairments in the patient's ability to function in society, especially in interpersonal relationships. Distorted perceptions of people and events, combined with impulsive behavior and labile moods, are disabling even though the patient may appear to be high-functioning on a superficial level. Personality disorders have a high comorbidity with other psychiatric diagnoses and can impair the patient's ability to recognize and participate in treatment of her other illnesses.

Personality disorders, as defined by the criteria in **Box 9-4**, are categorized in several ways. They include many types and subtypes, several

---

Box 9-4 Personality Disorders

According to the DSM-IV, a personality disorder is an enduring pattern of inner experience and behavior that is markedly different from the expectations of the individual's culture. This pattern is manifested in at least two of the following areas:

- Cognition: impaired perception of self and others, interpretation of events
- Affect or mood: tends to be intense and labile, often inappropriate to circumstances
- Interpersonal functioning
- Impulse control

The pattern of behavior can usually be traced to adolescence and is stable over years, leading to impairment in social and occupational functioning.

---

of which are more frequently diagnosed in women.

Women represent about 75% of patients diagnosed *with borderline personality disorder*,[55] which features unstable relationships, intensely labile moods, feelings of emptiness, and impulsive behavior. Borderline patients frequently have a history of childhood physical and sexual abuse, with inconsistent or neglectful parenting. Such children often develop posttraumatic stress symptoms or obsessive-compulsive behaviors that are resistant to treatment. Eating disorders and dissociative disorders, including multiple personalities, may develop. By adolescence the patient may begin cutting or burning herself, engaging in risky sexual behavior, and using substances. Chronic feelings of helplessness, guilt, and loneliness drive suicidal gestures that can be highly dramatic. The rate of suicide among patients with borderline personality is close to 10%; premature mortality from all causes is about 18%.[56]

Borderline can also be an informal term used by clinicians to describe patients who are demanding and manipulative, and who push the boundaries of professional relationships as they move from crisis to crisis and from provider to provider. When a psychiatric problem list includes the notation "with borderline features," it generally refers to behavior patterns that have tried the patience of caregivers, whether or not formal diagnostic criteria are met.

In the primary care setting, personality disorders can prevent the development of a trusting clinician–patient partnership. "Staff splitting" describes the patient's practice of being friendly and flattering to one staff member and argumentative or insulting to another. The patient may accept and cooperate with treatment one day while rejecting it the next. Such patients also tend to present "boundary" issues: they may ask that clinicians be available to them beyond regular work hours, seek reassurance that only certain people will be involved in their care, reject referrals to psychotherapy, and demand treatment or prescriptions that are outside the normal scope of primary care practice.

Treatment of personality disorders historically has been difficult. Personality structure is regarded as a learned behavior rather than being biologically determined, and medication has not been predictably helpful. Medication of comorbid illness (typically including depression, PTSD, substance use, or bipolar disorders) can be compromised by the patient's impulsive behavior. Insight-oriented or supportive psychotherapy is not consistently useful. Psychotherapy approaches have been developed specifically for the treatment of borderline personality disorder, notably the psychologist Marsha Linehan's Dialectical Behavior Therapy (DBT). DBT provides a structured program that can be used in individual or group therapy to help the patient learn new, more useful ways of perceiving herself and controlling her impulses.

Substance-Related Disorders

The *DSM-IV* disorders related to substances include deliberate drug abuse, side effects of medication use, and toxin exposure. Drug abuse can cause or be comorbid with psychiatric disturbances during intoxication or withdrawal. Several substances, notably the volatile inhalants, can be either toxins or drugs of abuse (see Chapter 8). Whenever a patient reports the new onset of troubling symptoms, a detailed history of possible substance exposure should be explored.

Assessment of Mental Illness

A careful clinical interview is the most powerful diagnostic tool for identifying current mental illness and risk factors that predict vulnerability to future illness. Along with the physical examination and laboratory investigations, the interview can be integrated into a routine office visit. Table 9-6 summarizes how to gather information about the patient's mental health at each phase of an office visit.

Women often avoid talking about their illness for fear that clinicians will be judgmental or unsympathetic. A clinician who is comfortable asking questions about mental illness and encourages the patient to tell her story will obtain the most useful information and be most helpful to her patient. The knowledge base and perspective that a midwife offers may be uniquely useful, because many mental health providers are not expert in women's health issues.

Chief Complaint

The current health status and emotional distress reported by the patient should be documented, even if it is not the stated reason for her visit. Life events, including recent surgery or current medical illness, often trigger or exacerbate psychiatric symptoms. **Table 9-7** includes factors that can be either comorbid with or causes of psychiatric illness. Even some over-the-counter (OTC) medications and antibiotics have been known to trigger symptoms. A patient's report of emotional disturbance while taking a particular medication should be considered to be just as serious as a report of drug allergy.

It is also important to document the use of herbs, hormones, supplements, and vitamin preparations; use a standard reference [e.g., the National Center for Complementary and Alternative Medicine Web site: http://www.nccam.nih.gov] to check for possible drug effects and interactions. Substance use can be either a cause or an effect of mental illness. Direct questioning elicits the best information on alcohol and nicotine use (i.e., "How many cigarettes per day?" or "When was your last drink?"), because many people tend to minimize their reported use of these substances.

Review of Systems

Such problems as chronic headaches, GI disturbances, fatigue, disordered sleep, changes in cognition or memory, appetite derangements, or chronic pain may be signs of psychiatric

Table 9-6 ASSESSMENT OF MENTAL ILLNESS: ELEMENTS TO BE INCLUDED IN THE PRIMARY CARE OFFICE VISIT

Area of Assessment	Data	Rationale
Chief Complaint: Current Health Status	Emotional distress	Patients may report their own illness.
	Stressful events	Stress can trigger mental illness.
	Medications and prescribers; diagnosis and duration of use	Medications can trigger mental symptoms.
	Habits	Use of or withdrawal from substances can trigger mental symptoms.
Review of Systems	Headaches, GI disturbances, fatigue, disordered sleep, changes in cognition or memory, appetite derangements, chronic pain	Can be somatic or neurochemical manifestations of psychiatric illness.
Patient History	1. Have you ever had trouble with feeling anxious or depressed? 2. Have you ever been in therapy? 3. Have you ever taken medication for emotional troubles? 4. Have you ever been hospitalized or gone to the emergency room for emotional troubles? 5. Have you ever thought of hurting yourself? 6. Have you had any thoughts like that recently?	When taking the patient's history, ask about physical health first to build rapport, and then begin asking about mental health. The questions are in order of increasing intrusiveness and specificity for serious mental illness. Ask them in the order given; a positive response to one should be followed by the next.
Family History	1. Have any of the women in your family had emotional troubles after childbirth? 2. Has anyone in your family had trouble with mental illness? 3. Do you think that anyone in your family may have been bipolar or manic depressive? 4. Has anyone in your family attempted suicide? 5. Does anyone in your family have a substance problem?	Mental illness can be familial and the history should include grandparents, aunts, uncles, cousins, nieces, and nephews. Proceed as for the patient history, above.
Physical Exam	Physical appearance: grooming, gait, tics, speech	Changes or inconsistencies can suggest emotional distress or neurological disturbance.

Table 9-6 ASSESSMENT OF MENTAL ILLNESS: ELEMENTS TO BE INCLUDED IN THE PRIMARY CARE OFFICE VISIT *(continued)*

Area of Assessment	Data	Rationale
	Mental Status: appearing sad or anxious; impaired cognition, insight, memory	These are key indicators of mental functioning.
	Body mass index, especially changes since last visit	Body mass index can be a marker for eating disorders, depression, drug use, and other problems.
	HEENT: thyroid, dental condition	Thyroid disease can trigger psychiatric symptoms; women with sex abuse histories often avoid dental exams.
	Skin: signs of self-injury	Scars, burns, cuts, or extensive piercings may indicate parasuicidal behaviors.
	Pain or "difficult exam"	May be a sign of previous abuse; may be somatization of emotional distress.
Laboratory Studies	Complete blood count	Rule out anemia.
	Thyroid function tests	Thyroid disease can cause psychiatric symptoms.
	Glucose tolerance screening	Diabetes has a high comorbidity with depression.
	Drug screening; metabolic screening for liver, adrenocortical, and renal function	If history indicates, order these tests to check on toxicity or malfunction that could cause symptoms.
	Blood levels of psychotropic meds, as indicated by the prescriber	Check with the prescriber and follow serum levels where indicated.
	If an eating disorder is suspected: serum electrolytes, liver function tests, bone density assessment, and EKG	Blood tests can reveal metabolic malfunction if eating disorder is suspected; work in consultation with the patient's primary providers if the diagnosis is known.

illness. If workups have not shown physical causes for the patient's distress, particularly if she's been told that, "it's all in my head," she may be experiencing psychomotor, cognitive, or somatic manifestations of an underlying mental disorder.

Patient History

The single strongest predictor of future mental illness is past mental illness. Although medical history forms typically include a standard query about whether the patient has a history of

---

Table 9-7 CONDITIONS AND MEDICATIONS THAT MAY BE ASSOCIATED WITH PSYCHIATRIC ILLNESS

Medical Conditions	Endocrine: thyroid disorder, adrenocortical disorder, diabetes mellitus
	Neurologic: migraine, multiple sclerosis, epilepsy
	Rheumatologic: fibromyalgia, chronic fatigue, lupus, rheumatoid arthritis
	Cancers
	Gastrointestinal: irritable bowel syndrome
	Cardiovascular disease
	Substance use
	Medications
	Hormonal preparations, including contraceptives and hormone replacement therapy
	Psychotropic medications, including benzodiazepines and neuroleptics
	Cardiac drugs, including beta blockers and antihypertensives
	Corticosteroids, either systemic or topical preparations
	Isoretinoin (Accutane)

Note: A patient history of emotional disturbance while taking a particular medication is just as serious as a drug allergy, and should be documented in the medical record.

mental illness, these items produce many false negative responses. Rather than rely on such standard histories, clinicians should include direct and specific questions in every patient interview. Following the principle of beginning with less intrusive questions, the patient's history of physical illness and treatment should come first. As the patient and clinician become more comfortable with each other, the following six questions should be asked. These questions are in increasing order of intrusiveness and specificity for serious mental illness. A positive response to one question should be followed by the next.

1. *Have you ever had trouble with feeling anxious or depressed?*
Depression and anxiety are common problems and relatively easy to talk about. Start there and continue inquiring about other problems. Ask about diagnoses and whether they seemed reasonable to the patient.

2. *Have you ever been in therapy?*
Ask whether the therapy was helpful and why (or if) it was stopped. Ask for dates, duration, type of therapy, and provider(s) seen.

3. *Have you ever taken medication for emotional troubles?*
Ask whether the medicine was helpful, and whether there were any problems with it. List all medications, dosages, duration, and reasons why (or if) discontinued. It is also helpful to know the prescriber's credentials.

4. *Have you ever been hospitalized or gone to the emergency room to treat emotional troubles?*
Hospitalization indicates a serious episode. Ask about diagnosis, treatment, institution, duration, and outcome.

5. *Have you ever thought of hurting yourself?*
Did she have a plan? What method(s) did she try? What stopped her?

6. *Have you had any thoughts like that recently?*
This provides an opening to talk about how likely she is to hurt herself or someone else. A woman who admits to having "bad thoughts" must contract for safety. **Box 9-5** explains how to approach this topic.

Box 9-5 A Contract For Safety

If a patient reports that she is having thoughts of hurting herself or others, you must ask her to contract for safety. In this context, "safety" means that she will not act upon an urge to hurt herself or another person. A woman who has been in therapy or been hospitalized for psychiatric illness understands what is meant by "contracting for safety," but you may have to explain what you mean very specifically to a patient who has not been in treatment before. Ask these questions in the order given:

1. *Are you safe now?*
2. *If you have any thoughts of hurting yourself or others, you must call me. If you can't wait for me to call back, you must call 9-1-1 and go to the hospital. Can you promise me you will do that?*
3. *Can you promise that you will not act on any urge to hurt yourself or someone else?*

A negative answer to any of these questions requires your immediate action to ensure the patient's safety. Psychiatric emergency protocols for your practice should be spelled out and adhered to just as they would be for any other medical emergency.

Even in the absence of a formal diagnosis, the clinician should also take note of behavior and events that suggest mental illness. This includes risky sexual behavior and poor decision making, interpersonal conflicts, and inappropriate relationships.

Family History

As with the patient history, the family history should begin with inquiries about physical health. Many mental illnesses have a strong genetic component, and a family history of mental illness should be as wide-ranging as any other genetic history. Before asking about mental health issues, the clinician should clarify to the patient that these questions include grandparents, aunts, uncles, cousins, nieces, and nephews. Be specific and include these questions in the order given:

1. *Have any of the women in your family had emotional troubles after childbirth? (For a gynecologic visit, a good opening might be to ask if other women have had trouble with PMS or menopausal symptoms.)*
   This is the least intrusive inquiry about mental illness, especially in the context of an obstetric or preconceptional visit. Family members may have used such terms as "nervous breakdown," "nerve trouble," or "that postpartum" in describing their difficulties. The patient should be encouraged to describe such episodes in her own way.
2. *Has anyone in your family had trouble with emotional problems? Been hospitalized for mental illness?*
   As above, the patient should be encouraged to describe diagnoses and treatment however she can. When a serious illness is described, it is important to

sympathize with the devastating effect it has had on the family.

3. *Do you think anyone in your family might have been bipolar or manic depressive?* In previous generations, bipolar illness was often not diagnosed or treated as such. If an older relative had times of high energy, sleeplessness, and grand ideas that alternated with periods of feeling low and miserable, bipolar illness can be presumed.

4. *Has anyone in your family attempted suicide? Succeeded?* This question is a very sensitive indicator of a history of severe illness, especially undiagnosed or untreated bipolar disorder. A family history of suicide is troubling to family members, and patients are generally grateful when a clinician opens the topic for discussion.

5. *Does anyone in your family have a substance problem? How about alcohol?* Alcoholism is normal in some families. Be sure to include it in any substance abuse history.

Physical Examination

Women with longstanding mental illness often look worn down and older than their age. Their appearance may be unkempt and their grooming inconsistent with their resources. Such outward signs of distress are particularly significant if they are a change from the patient's previous appearance; such changes may indicate a new onset of psychiatric illness.

Women who are depressed may look sad and withdrawn, or they may present with psychomotor slowing and confusion. Anxious women may be physically tense and fidgety, asking many questions and demanding constant reassurance. For presentations of specific disorders, see the sections on commonly encountered illnesses.

Changes in body mass index (BMI) can also raise suspicions of possible mental illness. Significant weight loss in an adult or a failure to gain in a growing teenager suggest anorexia nervosa, which ranks among the deadliest of psychiatric disorders. Obesity may indicate bulimia or another eating disorder. Weight gain can also accompany depression; hypomanic or manic episodes may be associated with weight loss. Anxiety can either suppress appetite or trigger overeating of "comfort" foods.

An enlarged thyroid gland should be noted and followed by thyroid function testing, as noted in the section on laboratory workup. Thyroid disease can trigger psychiatric symptoms and should be suspected whenever a woman complains of emotional distress. Thyroid function can also change during pregnancy and especially postpartum; a woman with a history of psychiatric or thyroid disease in herself or her family should have thyroid testing during each trimester and postpartum.

Poor dental condition is associated with eating disorders. Acidic vomitus wears away dental enamel and can inflame mucosal tissue. Women who have experienced oral sexual abuse typically avoid dental examinations and treatment.

Physical signs of self-injury are varied. The forearms and anterior thighs are the most frequent sites for cuts, burns, and self-tattoos. Multiple short, straight scars are typical of razor cuts. Scars or tattoos on the wrists may be concealed by decorative cuffs or bracelets. Genital self-injury can include cutting and piercing, or the peri-anal injuries resulting from purging behaviors. It is reasonable to ask about such signs during the course of an examination: "How did this happen?" The patient may readily explain an accidental injury, or she may be embarrassed and hesitant to answer. She may honestly not know how the injuries happened if they occurred when she was not conscious of her actions. The patient may discount the seriousness of self-injuries, but they are considered to be para-suicidal gestures associated with a guarded long-term prognosis.[57]

A woman who somaticizes her emotional distress may show signs of pain or guarding during a general physical exam, even if no cause for the pain is apparent. It is important to acknowledge the patient's discomfort and not to dismiss it with, "I can't find anything wrong."

If a woman cannot tolerate a routine pelvic exam, she may have suffered previous sexual trauma or injury. It is best not to pursue questioning after a "difficult" exam, especially if the patient has already given a negative response to routine queries about abuse. If the woman does, in fact, suffer from PTSD, talking about it can re-trigger her symptoms, including panic and dissociation. It is well to remember that many instances of vaginismus and vulvodynia, for example, are not at all related to abusive experiences.

Laboratory Studies

Unfortunately, there are no reliable diagnostic studies for mental illness. Laboratory findings can be helpful, however, in detecting metabolic disorders and other conditions that can cause or masquerade as mental illness. Certain tests can be done as indicated:

- Complete blood count (CBC) to rule out anemia as a cause of fatigue.
- Thyroid function tests (TFT) should be done when any mental illness is suspected; TFTs should be followed

through pregnancy and postpartum, especially in women with a history of psychiatric or thyroid illness.
- Glucose tolerance screening should be performed to detect diabetes.
- Drug screening, liver, adrenocortical, and renal function tests are needed when indicated by history.
- If the patient is on psychotropic medication, check with her prescriber to determine whether blood levels should be followed, especially during pregnancy.
- If an eating disorder is suspected, then perform test for serum electrolytes, liver function tests (LFTs), and bone density assessment, in consultation with the primary providers.

Diagnostic Tools

A number of concise screening tools are available for use in the office. Information on obtaining and using them is contained in Appendix 9-A.

Midwifery Management of Common Mental Disorders

Given the frequency with which mental illness is encountered in the primary care setting, it is clear that midwives need to be familiar with a range of management options to offer their patients. The extent to which the midwife will be involved in the care of a woman experiencing psychiatric symptoms will vary with the severity of the current episode, the availability of mental health resources, the practice structure and its place in the local health system, and the individual skills and comfort level of the midwife. To the extent that safe care can be ensured, the patient's wishes should also be considered when developing a plan of care.

Treatment of mental illness is multifaceted, and midwifery practice includes several elements that can be crucial aspects of a comprehensive patient care plan:

- Educating the patient and family about the condition and the treatment plan.
- Communication and collaborative practice with other clinicians.
- Implementation of self-care practices, including: sleep hygiene, nutrition, and exercise regimens.
- Managing reproductive health events (fertility, pregnancy, menopause) in ways that minimize stress to the patient and her family and maximize healthy adjustment and development.

Midwives also provide the following aspects of care to any patient with a history or symptoms of mental illness:

- Assessment and screening.
- Supportive counseling and referral to appropriate resources.
- Teaching and encouragement to promote compliance with the treatment plan.

In addition, midwives may also participate in:

- Developing and implementing a treatment plan in consultation with mental health clinicians.
- Medication management.
- Case management and care coordination.

These aspects of patient care require that the midwife have access to appropriate consultants and be trained in the use of psychotropic medications. The remainder of this section presents information and management protocols to facilitate this expansion of midwifery practice.

Referral and Consultation with Mental Health Clinicians

Several situations require that the patient be referred to one or more mental health clinicians (**Table 9-8**). If a patient presents with severe symptoms or if she is unable to contract for safety, the situation must be treated as a medical emergency and psychiatric treatment obtained to ensure her safety.

Patients with severe mental illness who are taking any of the medications listed in Table 9-8 or who take multiple medications should be in the care of a psychiatric clinician. Such a patient may describe herself as being "between providers" and ask for a medication refill or re-start, or say that she is "more comfortable" getting her care from her primary women's health providers. This is not good practice. She should be referred to an appropriate mental health clinician.

A woman with a history of major mental illness should be referred for a psychiatric consultation before or during pregnancy, even if she has been stable without treatment for years. Her risk of a relapse during pregnancy or postpartum is significant, and establishing a therapeutic relationship will decrease her anxiety and lessen her stress during pregnancy.

Patients are often unaware of the different credentials and scope of practice of their providers, and it is important for primary clinicians to know the range of available mental health practitioners. **Table 9-9** describes the categories of mental health providers, how they are trained and licensed, and whether they prescribe medication. This information can be used

Table 9-8 WHEN TO REFER

Referral Requirement	Examples	Reason
Psychiatric conditions	Severe depression Bipolar Disorder Eating Disorder, especially Anorexia Psychotic illness Substance abuse	Risk of self-harm is significant, also risk to others; impulsive acts; possible need for inpatient stabilization with team outpatient follow-up.
Psychotropic medications	Mood stabilizers Antipsychotics Stimulants Non-benzodiazepine Anticonvulsants	These drugs have potential for severe and complex side effects and interactions, unsuitable for independent primary management.
History of major mental illness and pregnant or considering pregnancy	Asymptomatic and off medication	Risk of recurrence during pregnancy or postpartum is significant; consultation and evaluation are needed even without active treatment.

Medical emergency: Whenever a patient is unwilling to contract for safety, the situation must be considered a medical emergency and appropriate care ensured. These patients may need immediate evaluation in the psychiatric emergency room.

These situations require referral to appropriate mental health providers, even if the patient requests that her care be managed in the primary setting.

to help a patient decide which clinicians will provide her with the most appropriate care.

Just as a patient may have more than one clinician following her physical health, she may have several mental health providers involved in her care. A therapeutic team may include a "talk" therapist, a prescriber, a case manager, a family or couples therapist, and a support group. **Table 9-10** summarizes several therapies that are used for different conditions, which can be used when considering various treatment plans.

Another referral consideration is financial. Insurance coverage for mental illness is often much more limited than for other medical conditions. A few states have mental health parity laws, but these affect only the treatment of biologically based illnesses such as depression and anxiety. Personality disorders and marital troubles are not considered to be biologic illnesses, and their treatment is not generally covered by insurance. Patients who can afford to pay out-of-pocket for psychotherapy frequently choose not to use their insurance to pay for mental health care, because doing so requires that a mental health diagnosis appear on their insurance claims.

When referring a patient or consulting with her mental health clinicians, it is crucial to document the patient's permission to discuss her

Table 9-9 MENTAL HEALTH PROVIDERS

Provider	Description	State License	Eligible for 3rd Party Payment*	Prescribes Psychotropic Medication
Psychiatrist	MD with psychiatric residency and specialty board certification. May specialize in treating children, adults, families, or specific illnesses	MD	Yes	Yes; practice increasingly focuses on medication rather than talk.
Clinical Nurse Specialist	Masters and ANCC certification as either Adult or Child Psychiatric Mental Health Clinician or Nurse Practitioner	Advanced practice RN	Yes	Yes; some choose not to prescribe.
Psychologist	Doctorate, usually PhD or EdD. Psychotherapy with various specialties, psychometric testing	Psychologist	Yes	Varies by state.
Social Worker	Masters degree in social work or related field. Psychotherapy and case management may include couples and families	Licensed Independent Clinical Social Worker (MSW, LCMSW)	Yes	No.
Licensed Mental Health Counselor	Varies; usually master's degree in counseling or education	Title varies by state and insurance plan	Yes, depending on state	No.

| Counselors | Varies: marital, family, or clergy training Certification may be from various organizations | None | No; some employers will subsidize | No. |
| Peer Groups, e.g., Overeaters Anonymous, Depressive-Bipolar Support Alliance | Support programs for various conditions | None | No; some programs are free; employers some-times subsidize | No. |

* Clinicians may choose not to accept insurance or to accept only some plans. Insurance benefits for mental health conditions typically are different from physical health coverage. Patients need to check their coverage by calling the number on their insurance card. Coverage is typically limited to a certain number of visits with a limited panel of providers. In states covered by mental health parity laws, mental health benefits will still be limited to coverage for *biologically based* diagnoses only.

Abbreviation: ANCC, American Nurses Credentialling Center

Table 9-10 SELECTED PSYCHOTHERAPEUTIC APPROACHES

Type of Therapy	Practice Approach	Type of Therapy	Notes
Psychodynamic Therapy ("The Talking Cure")	Focus is on gaining insight into how behaviors and beliefs developed	Individual, couple, family, group; may be short- or long-term	Insight can lead to changing beliefs and behaviors. This approach originated with the early psychoanalysts and still informs much therapeutic practice today. It can be combined with medication and other biological approaches.
Cognitive-Behavioral Therapy (CBT)	A structured approach to challenging and changing behaviors	Individual or group; short-term programs for specific problems	Commonly used to treat phobias and other anxiety disorders; behavioral approaches are often incorporated into therapy for many other disorders. Often, medication is used initially until symptoms can be controlled by CBT intervention.
Interpersonal Therapy (IPT)	Focuses on the patient's relationships with others as both a source of illness and resource for healing	Individual or group; couple and family members may be included	Can be particularly helpful for women who often experience their lives as being based on relationships with others. A body of research documents IPT's usefulness, particularly with postpartum illness.
Dialectical Behavioral Therapy (DBT)	Combines cognitive, behavioral, and mindfulness approaches	A structured curriculum teaches skills that can be taught in both individual and group format	Developed by psychologist Marsha Linehan to treat borderline personality disorder in women. The skills include increasing mindfulness, emotion regulation, and psychosocial functioning. DBT is the basis for many treatment programs for severe and complex illnesses including posttraumatic stress disorder, dissociative disorders, drug use, and self-injurious behaviors.

care with her mental health clinicians. Some patients hesitate, fearing that intimate details of their psychotherapy will be shared. When it is explained that this would not happen, because clinicians are interested only in discussing the treatment plan and not the narrative content of visits, and the consent form specifies "to discuss treatment plan," receiving informed consent should not be a problem.

The professional culture of mental health clinicians encourages interdisciplinary cooperation. Once assured of the patient's consent to communicate, psychiatric providers welcome a team approach in planning for their patient's total care.

Psychotropic Medications

Midwives need to be familiar with the use of psychotropic medications. These medications are commonly prescribed for a variety of situations, including acute grief reactions and episodic anxiety. In addition, psychotropics—either prescribed alone or in combination with hormonal products—are becoming first-line treatment for perimenstrual disorders and mid-life problems such as vasovagal symptoms and disordered sleep.

Table 9-11 presents common medications that can be included in midwifery practice. Table 9-12 provides further details on the various types of antidepressants that primary-care patients may be taking. The information that follows is intended to supplement the detailed prescribing information and patient instructions that can be found in Appendix 9-A. These references describe side effects, warning signals, medical and laboratory follow-up, and specific instructions for patients and prescribers.

ANTIHISTAMINES

These inexpensive OTC drugs are probably the most commonly used sleep aids. They can also relieve nausea and soothe some of the somatic symptoms of mild anxiety. Patients may take diphenhydramine (Benadryl, Unisom SleepGels) 25 to 50 mg up to three times a day; occasional paradoxic reactions may require a change to a prescription drug of another category. Diphenhydramine has been used for many years and is considered to be largely benign during pregnancy and lactation.

SELECTIVE SEROTONIN REUPTAKE INHIBITOR (SSRI) ANTIDEPRESSANTS

Drugs in this category include fluoxetine (Prozac, Sarafem), sertraline (Zoloft), paroxetine (Paxil), citalopram (Celexa), and escitalopram (Lexapro). Originally developed to treat depression, the SSRIs have been found to be useful for a number of other conditions, including anxiety and menstrual disorders, posttraumatic stress, migraine prophylaxis, and vasovagal symptoms. Although pharmaceutical manufacturers market specific SSRIs for specific disorders, in actual practice "individual results vary," and any of the SSRIs may be used for any diagnosis.

The initial choice of SSRI can depend on the patient's history of previous response, availability and price, expected side effect profile and tolerability, and the plans for pregnancy or lactation in the near future. As with any antidepressant medication, the medical record should document that the patient has no personal or family history suspicious of bipolar disorder, and that she has been warned of the possibility that the medication may trigger agitation or manic symptoms.

Initial side effects of SSRI use include nausea or other GI upset, constipation or loose stools, headaches, irritability or jumpiness, and vivid dreams. These effects generally fade within two weeks and should disappear by two months of use. Possible sexual side effects include decreased libido and delayed orgasm; these effects tend to persist after two months and may require management or a medication change.

Each SSRI has a somewhat different side effect profile. Fluoxetine, for example, tends to be somewhat stimulating while sertraline and paroxetine tend to be sedating. Paroxetine also

Table 9-11 PSYCHOTROPIC DRUGS USED IN PRIMARY CARE

Category	Availability	Examples	Commonly Used for	Dependency Risk	Overdose Danger	Notes
Antihistamine	Over-the-counter	Diphenhydramine (Benadryl, Unisom SleepGels)	Sleep aid, nausea	Low	Low	Commonly used in pregnancy.
Selective serotonin reuptake inhibitor (SSRI)	Prescription	Fluoxetine (Prozac, Sarafem), sertraline (Zoloft) citalopram (Celexa)	Depression, anxiety disorder, menstrual disorder, migraine prophylaxis, hot flashes	None; Sudden withdrawal may cause symptoms	Low	Takes 2–4 weeks to take effect; 3–6 months minimum recommended treatment. Sertraline most extensively studied in breastfeeding.
Benzodiazepine (Benzo)	Controlled substance	Clonazepam (Klonopin), lorazepam (Ativan)	Panic attacks, anxiety, sleep aid	High; Withdrawal syndrome and rebound can be severe.	High when taken with other drugs, including alcohol	Short-term or occasional use, until long-term medication takes effect; avoid in patients with substance abuse history. Avoid in first trimester of pregnancy.
Tricyclic Antidepressant	Prescription	Imipramine (Tofranil), amitriptyline (Elavil), doxepin (Sinequan)	Depression, anxiety, menstrual disorder, sleep aid	Low	High; cardiac arrhythmia can be fatal	Low doses at bedtime are used for sleep; prescribe limited quantities

						without refills. Used in pregnancy and lactation.
Atypical antidepressant	Prescription	Trazodone (Desyrel)	Sleep aid	Low	Low	Low doses at bedtime; common adjunct to SSRI. Considered benign in pregnancy.
Imidazopyridine	Prescription	Zolpidem (Ambien)	Sleep aid	?Low	?Low	A new drug class; few data and high co-pay. No data on safety on pregnancy or lactation.

Psychotropic drugs that should not be prescribed in the primary care setting include mood stabilizers, neuroleptics (antipsychotics), stimulants, and anticonvulsants other than benzodiazepines. Patients sometimes request a refill, a re-start after time off medication, or renewal of a prescription. They should be referred to their mental health prescriber.

Table 9-12 ANTIDEPRESSANT MEDICATIONS

Category	Examples	Common Uses	Use in Pregnancy and Lactation
Selective serotonin reuptake inhibitors (SSRIs)	Fluoxetine (Prozac, Sarafem), Sertraline (Zoloft), Paroxetine (Paxil), Citalopram (Celexa), Escitalopram (Lexapro)	Depressive, anxiety, menstrual, eating disorder; migraine prophylaxis; smoking cessation; vasomotor symptoms; chronic pain	Data support use of fluoxetine in pregnancy; data on other SSRIs are more limited but reassuring. Doses will probably need to be raised across pregnancy to maintain adequate serum concentrations. Sertraline is the most studied in lactation with reassuring data emerging.
Tricyclics (TCA)	Imipramine (Tofranil), Nortriptyline (Pamelor), Amitriptyline (Elavil), Doxepin (Sinequan)	Depressive, anxiety menstrual disorder; bulimia; migraine prophylaxis; chronic pain	Early studies led to FDA Category C-D ratings; more recent studies are exonerating. Widely used and considered safe in pregnancy and lactation. Doses probably will need to be raised across pregnancy to maintain serum concentrations.
Monoamine oxidase inhibitors	Phenelzine (Nardil), Tranylcypromine (Parnate)	Depression, dysthymia, panic disorder; bulimia; chronic pain	Avoid use in pregnancy and lactation. Dangerous interaction with meperidine (Demerol) or fentanyl (Sublimaze).
Atypicals	Venlafaxine (Effexor)	Depression, anxiety disorder, vasomotor symptoms	Recent small studies are reassuring; published data are insufficient to support use in pregnancy or lactation.

Table 9-12 ANTIDEPRESSANT MEDICATIONS *(continued)*

Category	Examples	Common Uses	Use in Pregnancy and Lactation
	Bupropion (Wellbutrin, Zyban)	Depression, smoking; adjunct in bipolar and attention deficit disorders	No published data.
	Trazodone (Desyrel)	Hypnotic	Considered safe as a sleep aid.
	Mirtazapine (Remeron)	Depression, anxiety	No published data

tends to trigger significant weight gain, particularly in women, while fluoxetine and citalopram are more likely to cause some weight loss. Fluoxetine has a half-life of several days (other SSRIs are cleared in about 24 hours), which can make it a good choice for a patient who has trouble taking medication regularly.

Patients often stop their medication if they have side effects or do not get prompt relief. Stopping medication suddenly can lead to withdrawal symptoms that are misinterpreted as meaning that the drug is addictive, which the SSRIs are not. If a patient experiences uncomfortable side effects, the initial dose can be kept low for two to four weeks, until the side effects begin to fade. The dose can then be increased as tolerated for maximum symptom relief.

Antidepressants, including the SSRIs, are not a quick fix. They typically take two to four weeks to become effective (longer if the initial dose must be kept low), and at least two months for neurochemical healing to begin. Patients often want to discontinue medication as soon as they begin to feel better. It is important to stress the value of continuing treatment until a full remission of symptoms is achieved, usually a trial of several months. Stopping medication too soon also increases the likelihood of a relapse that may require even more aggressive treatment. Research indicates that the longer a patient takes an antidepressant medication, the less likely she is to relapse later.[58]

Information on the use of SSRIs during pregnancy and lactation continues to emerge, so the latest research should be consulted before prescribing these drugs to pregnant or breastfeeding women. In general, fluoxetine and sertraline have been on the market the longest and have been the most extensively studied. Overall, the evidence to date suggests that there is no relationship between SSRI use and birth defects or other long-term damage to infants.[59] A retrospective epidemiological study of 3581 women released in October 2005 found higher rates of congenital anomalies (OR 2.20, CI 1.34-3.63) in women using paroxetine (Paxil) compared to women using other SSRIs; other studies have not seen this association.[60] The use of the SSRIs may also be associated with serotonin withdrawal syndrome. Several case reports have described symptoms such as jitteriness, hypothermia, and irritability in infants born to mothers who used paroxetine and fluoxetine during pregnancy.[61] These findings need to be verified before firm clinical conclusions can be drawn. Providers need to keep abreast of these changes, because they provide guidance about safe medication use in pregnancy. At the same time, given the devastating impact that depression can have on women and their families, they should not deny medications to women who need them. While there are some reports of transient neurobehavioral changes and potentially an increased risk of more serious complications in exposed infants,[60–62] these risks may be acceptable when compared to the effects of untreated maternal illness.[63] If antidepressant medication is needed, the SSRIs are thought to be among the safest in pregnancy.[62]

Sertraline has been the most extensively studied SSRI during lactation and is probably the most widely prescribed for breastfeeding women. Blood levels of sertraline in nursing infants have been found to be minute, and no ill effects in the infants have been seen. Breast milk levels of sertraline are highest about eight to nine hours after the mother's daily dose, and women who wish to further minimize infant drug exposure can pump and discard at that time.[64]

BENZODIAZEPINES: THE "BENZO" ANXIOLYTICS

Although categorized as anticonvulsants, the so-called "benzos" are widely used to relieve anxiety, stop panic attacks, and induce sleep. Partly because of their strong potential for habituation and abuse, they are no longer favored as first-line therapy. However, they continue to be useful for prompt symptom relief until long-term medication begins to take effect. A patient with a newly identified illness or crisis may be prescribed one of the longer-acting benzodiazepines, such as clonazepam (Klonopin) or lorazepam (Ativan) at the time she is started on an SSRI. She can then taper off the benzodiazepine as the SSRI starts to relieve her symptoms. A typical dose would be 0.50 mg clonazepam up to three times a day. The patient may take 1 to 2 mg at bedtime and break the scored tablets into 0.25 mg doses during the day, as needed to control her symptoms.

Benzodiazepines should be avoided in treating patients with a history of substance abuse. All patients should be warned of the risk of habituation and possible withdrawal symptoms. Clinicians should be wary of any situation in which the patient appears to be "shopping" for benzodiazepine refills.

It is common for patients to present with long-term benzodiazepine use under relatively benign circumstances. These drugs were once the most widely prescribed drugs in America (the notorious "mother's little helpers") and some women have been taking them for many years. Patients who have tried to cut back or quit may have decided that "it's not worth it" to endure the symptoms of withdrawal. It may be neither useful nor safe to try to discontinue these medications in the primary care setting. However, it is reasonable to tell the patient that she should receive her prescription renewals from her original prescriber rather than from her midwife.

Early studies of benzodiazepine use in pregnancy identified risks of cleft palate when taken in the first trimester and a newborn withdrawal syndrome when taken at the end of pregnancy; hence, it has an FDA category rating of D. Recent studies have found no serious adverse infant outcomes,[65,66] but liability can be an issue in prescribing these drugs. They are considered "probably safe" in lactation, making their short-term use for postpartum disorders a viable choice.

TRICYCLIC ANTIDEPRESSANTS

Formerly the mainstay of antidepressant therapy, the tricyclics (TCAs) have been largely replaced by the SSRIs for first-line therapy. They remain useful, however, for patients who do not respond to SSRIs and they are often prescribed for chronic pain conditions such as vulvodynia and fibromyalgia. Low doses are used to induce sleep, especially when anxiety is present. TCAs are inexpensive and available in generic form. The most familiar TCA is amitriptylene (Elavil), which is typically prescribed for 25 to 50 mg at bedtime.

The TCAs are not habituating and can be used by patients with a history of substance problems. TCAs are dangerous in overdose, causing potentially fatal cardiac arrhythmias. This is unlikely to be an issue in primary care patients who have a low risk of self-harm, but it is best to prescribe limited quantities and document the patient's contract for safety.

The TCAs are often used during pregnancy and lactation despite their FDA category ratings of C or D, which are based on very old data. They have been included in studies of fetal and infant outcomes as noted above with the SSRIs and should be subjected to the same risk/benefit considerations.

ATYPICAL ANTIDEPRESSANT: TRAZODONE

Trazodone (Desyrel) is marginally effective as an antidepressant, but it is very useful as a hypnotic. It is generally well tolerated, provides good quality sleep, and is inexpensive. Its most concerning side effect is the risk of priapism (continuous erection) in men. It can also cause vulvar pain in women from clitoral priapism, which resolves after discontinuation.[67] Trazodone is compatible with the use of SSRI or TCA antidepressants, and is often prescribed to counteract stimulating side effects of these other drugs. Bedtime dosing is typically 50 to 100 mg, and patients may break the tablets in half for a lower dose.

Trazodone use during pregnancy has not been well studied, so it would not be the first choice of hypnotic medication then. It is considered "probably safe" during lactation, although the American Academy of Pediatrics classifies this drug as one in which the effect is unknown but may be of concern.[68]

A NOVEL HYPNOTIC: ZOLPIDEM

Zolpidem (Ambien) is a new and heavily marketed hypnotic that is intended for short-term treatment of insomnia. The manufacturer claims that it is non-habituating, but the literature has identified a risk for habituation and abuse with long-term use or high doses that is similar to that of the benzodiazepines.[69] Zolpidem is an expensive drug because it is new, and it is often not covered by insurance or requires a high co-pay. Given the number of less expensive and well-studied hypnotics available, zolpidem should not be considered a first choice sleep aid.

There are no data to date on the safety of Zolpidem during pregnancy or lactation.

GENERAL INFORMATION ABOUT ANTIDEPRESSANTS

The FDA has directed that all antidepressants carry a "black box" warning on their packaging and instructions for use that cites an increased suicide risk in children and adolescents taking these medications.[70] Prozac is currently the only medication approved to treat depression in children and adolescents.

Antidepressant medications can trigger agitation or mania in individuals who have an underlying bipolar disorder. The medical record should document that the patient has no personal or family history suspicious of bipolar illness and that she has been told to discontinue medication if agitation or manic symptoms appear.

The National Committee for Quality Assurance (NCQA) is a nonprofit agency that sets standards for performance measurement and accrediting of managed care organizations. To meet NCQA standards for effective antidepressant therapy, patients must be seen for follow-up at least three times in the first 12 weeks after the initial prescription, and the patient should remain on medication for at least six months.[71]

Adjunct Therapies

In addition to psychotherapy and psychotropic medication, several other approaches to the treatment of mental illness are currently under study. **Table 9-13** summarizes evidence-based information on the use of four therapies used as adjuncts to standard psychiatric treatment described below.

1. *Essential Fatty Acids:* New research suggests that the omega-3 fatty acids, especially as those present in fish oils, can be helpful in a number of psychiatric disorders, and they may prove safe and effective in pregnancy and lactation. Doses used are significantly higher than recommended for nutritional use. Sources of essential fatty acids are subject to the same cautions described below in the discussion of American food supplements.

2. *Bright Light Therapy:* Particularly when combined with physical exercise, morning bright light therapy appears to im-

Table 9-13 **ADJUNCT THERAPIES**

Intervention	Evidence for Use In	Regimen	Notes
Essential fatty acids	Depression, bipolar disorder, schizophrenia.[72–75]	Starting dose of 1 ω-eicosapentoic acid (EPA)/day.	Concentrated fish body oils are best source of EPA.[76]
Bright light therapy	Depression.[77–79]	Varies with study; 100,000 lux × 30 minutes in am is common.	Usually used for seasonal affective changes.
Exercise	Depression, anxiety, fatigue syndromes.[80,81]	Various aerobic and resistance training approaches have been used in combination with other therapies.	Controlled trials are needed for further study.
Alternative biologicals: St. John's Wort	Meta-analyses show questionable effectiveness in mild-to-moderate depression.[82]	Preparations vary; no regulation of quality in U.S.[83]	Side effects can be significant;[84] can decrease action of other drugs, including oral contraceptives and statins.[85,86]

prove mood and can be used during pregnancy.

3. *Physical Exercise:* Aerobic exercise and weight training have been used to improve mood and energy in various programs. Controlled trials of specific regimens are lacking, however.
4. *Alternative Biologicals:* St. John's Wort is probably the most extensively studied herbal preparation. Some studies have found St. John's Wort to be more effective than placebo in mild-to-moderate depression, but more recent meta-analyses question the biases of these studies. Side effects of St. John's Wort include headache, jitteriness, and worsening mood or mania. It also appears to reduce the bioavailability of several common prescription drugs, including cholesterol-lowering agents, cyclosporines, and OCs. It can dangerously potentiate the action of other psychotropic drugs. There are no current data on the safety of St. John's Wort during pregnancy or lactation.

Many patients are attracted to using "natural" remedies rather than prescription medication, but such products present problems with both efficacy and safety.

The 1994 Dietary Supplement Health Education Act exempts products sold as herbals or "supplements" from regulation by the FDA. Manufacturers are not required to prove safety or efficacy of these products, unlike the laws governing food, drug, and cosmetic products. The FDA can take action against a "supplement" only by proving that it is harmful, rather than requiring that the manufacturer prove it is safe, as is the case with prescription drugs. Consequently, it is easy to recommend the use of unproven and unregulated products that are not covered by insurance.

Perhaps the greatest risk to the patient who tries "natural" substances is the risk of delaying effective treatment. A patient who chooses to treat her depression with, for example, St. John's Wort can spend months using products of unproven usefulness. In the meantime, her symptoms can worsen and she may eventually require more aggressive treatment than if she had used a standard regimen from the beginning. "Natural" remedies can be useful, however, as a first step toward self-care for patients who have difficulty accepting any treatment at all.

Hormone Therapy and Mental Illness

The gonadal steroids affect neurotransmission, and clinicians who prescribe hormones should be mindful of their potential effects on patients' mental status. Estrogen, progesterone, and testosterone all affect mood for good or ill, and hormone metabolism can also interact with psychotropic medications. Hormonal products, either as contraceptives or hormone replacement therapy (HRT), should be initiated cautiously in women with mental illness. While the illness may be helped by inducing a steady hormonal state and postmenopausal women may respond to medication better while on HRT,[87] hormone products have the potential to destabilize psychiatric illness. Patients should be informed of potential effects on mood and encouraged to report any changes promptly.

Contraceptive preparations and hormone replacement products can interact with psychotropic medications, requiring special attention to the management of the patient. Drug interactions with OCs have been more extensively studied than other hormone preparations, and their effects are summarized in **Table 9-14**.

Estrogen appears to potentiate the effect of SSRI and tricyclic antidepressants. Estrogen is also being studied for use as an antidepressant itself, either as monotherapy or as an adjunct to antidepressant medication, particularly for midlife women.[88,89] Conversely, the SSRI antidepressants, tricyclics, venlafaxine (Effexor), and possibly trazodone (Desyrel) appear to potentiate the effectiveness of OCs.

Anticonvulsants used as mood stabilizers that reduce the effectiveness of OCs include: phenytoin (Dilantin), phenobarbitol, primidone (Mysoline), carbamazapine (Tegretol), topiramate (Topamax), and oxcarbazepine (Trileptal). For women on these drugs and an OC, consider using

---

Table 9-14   INTERACTION OF PSYCHOTROPIC DRUGS AND HORMONE THERAPIES

Effects of Psychotropic Drugs on Combination Oral Contraceptives

Drugs That **Decrease** OCP Efficacy*	Drugs That **Increase** OCP Efficacy
Anticonvulsant-mood stabilizers	Antidepressants
Phenytoin (Dilantin)	Fluoxetine (Prozac)
Phenobarbitol	Sertraline (Zoloft)
Primidone (Mysoline)	Paroxetine (Paxil)
Carbamazepine (Tegretol)	Venlafaxine (Effexor)
Topiramate (Topamax)	?Trazodone (Desyrel)
Oxcarbazepine (Trileptal)	
Stimulant	
Modafinil (Provigil)[91]	

Effects of Oral Contraceptives on Psychotropic Drugs

Drugs with Increased Serum Levels	Drugs with Decreased Serum Levels
Tricyclic antidepressants	Some Benzodiazepines
SSRI antidepressants	Lorazepam (Ativan)
Some Benzodiazepines	Oxazepam (Serax)
Diazepam (Valium)	Anticonvulsant-Mood Stabilizer
Alprazolam (Xanax)	Lamotrigine (Lamictal) [92]

*For women who are on oral contraceptive pills (OCPs) and taking these drugs, consider using a 50-μg pill, tricycling, and taking 1 gm. Ascorbic acid with OC. Depo-Provera should be given every 10 weeks instead of every 12. Breakthrough bleeding should be considered a sign of decreased efficacy.[93,94]

Anticonvulsants that do not appear to affect OCP effectiveness: valproic acid (Depakote, Depakene), lamotrigine (Lamictal), and gabapentin (Neurontin).[95]

Anticonvulsants are known teratogens; neural tube defects are among their effects. Women of childbearing age who take these medications should also take 2 to 3 mg of folic acid daily in case of contraceptive failure.

a 50 μg pill, tricycling, and taking 1 gram of ascorbic acid with their contraceptive pill. Depo-Provera should be given every 10 weeks instead of every 12 weeks. Breakthrough bleeding should be considered a sign of decreased efficacy.

Several of the newer anticonvulsants do not appear to significantly reduce the effectiveness of OCs. They are: valproic acid (Depakote, Depakene), lamotrigine (Lamictal), and gabapentin (Neurontin). OCs have been found to reduce plasma levels of lamotrigine, so it is important to talk to the mental health prescriber when initiating or changing hormone therapy.

If a patient who is taking OCs plans to start anticonvulsant medication, discuss the contraceptive implications with the prescriber. The prescriber may then choose to try one of the drugs that have no interaction with OCs. However, if a patient is already on anticonvulsant medication and wishes to start hormonal contraception, it is better to adjust the contraceptive regimen than to risk destabilizing the patient by changing her psychiatric medications.

Management of Mental Illness during Pregnancy and Postpartum

It is important to establish management protocols for mental illness, just as for any other medical condition. All pregnant women need an initial assessment as described in this chapter, with subsequent screening in each trimester and postpartum using one of the tools listed in Appendix 9-A. The degree to which a provider will manage depression and anxiety varies depending on the severity of the presentation, the resources available to the clinician, and their level of expertise. Given that depression is common and often undertreated and that there is a shortage of mental health providers, particularly for low income minority women, some advocate that management of many mental health conditions by primary care providers is essential, while others advocate that these issues are best managed by mental health providers. Each provider will need to balance these two approaches in his or her own practice. There are five situations that are likely to appear in the course of obstetric care (**Table 9-15**):

1. *Patient's diagnosis is known and treated to remission by appropriate providers; the patient fully participates in her care.*
   The clinician should obtain the patient's written permission to communicate with her mental health providers about her care plan; names, credentials, and contact information should be recorded in the patient chart. The obstetric and mental health clinicians should discuss: the expected course of illness during pregnancy and postpartum; plans for breastfeeding and implications for care; and laboratory or other surveillance that can be done during prenatal visits. In general, mental health providers are unfamiliar with the physiologic changes of pregnancy, and this information can be crucial to their treatment plans.

2. *Known or suspected diagnosis; partial treatment with continued symptoms; or the patient is between providers or reluctant to continue care.*
   Many women have the mistaken belief that they will get better during pregnancy, and they are often eager to discontinue treatment. It is imperative to

Table 9-15 MANAGEMENT OF MENTAL ILLNESS DURING PREGNANCY

History and Symptoms	Initial Plan	Interval Surveillance
• Known diagnosis. • Treated to remission by appropriate providers. • Patient participating fully in her care.	• Get patient's written permission to communicate with mental health providers. • Discuss expected course of illness and treatment during pregnancy and postpartum with patient and mental health providers. • Record plan in the chart.	• Follow labs, including thyroid function, medication levels as requested by mental health prescriber. • Screen for symptoms, somatic complaints at each visit. • Plan with patient and family for postpartum support.
• Known or suspected diagnosis. • Partial treatment with continued symptoms. • Patient between providers or reluctant to continue care.	• Discuss with patient risks of worsening illness in pregnancy and postpartum. • Refer to mental health provider for evaluation and treatment plan. • Record plan in the chart.	• Revisit mental health provider each trimester and postpartum, or according to plan, and as needed.
• History of previous diagnosis and treatment. • Currently asymptomatic.	• Discuss the risks of recurring illness; illness tends to worsen with each pregnancy. • Refer to mental health provider for evaluation and treatment plan as appropriate.	• Screen and follow with mental health provider as appropriate.
• History of previous illness. • Recurring symptoms.	• Contract for safety. • Assess severity of symptoms and need for referral. • Consider initiating treatment; see text.	• Patient and family support for compliance with care. • Case management support as needed. • Treatment follow-up as indicated.
• New onset of symptoms in a patient without prior history of mental illness.	• Contract for safety. • Assess severity of symptoms and need for referral. • Ask patient about history again; ask family members as well. • Consider initiating treatment, see text. • Consult with mental health provider as needed.	• As above.

All pregnant patients need an initial assessment as described in this chapter, with re-screening at least every trimester and postpartum.

discuss the risks of continued or worsening symptoms during pregnancy and postpartum, and to support the patient's obtaining appropriate care. The clinician should be as straightforward as in talking to a woman whose glucose screening or thyroid function tests are abnormal. Managing her situation is crucial to the health of her pregnancy. The patient should be referred to a mental health provider who is skilled in treating pregnant women and followed as appropriate for her specific circumstances.

3. *History of previous diagnosis and treatment; the patient is currently asymptomatic.*
   This can be a delicate situation. The patient wants very much to believe that she will remain healthy through pregnancy and postpartum, but she will have to be told that her risk of relapse is at least 50% for depressive or anxiety disorders, and higher for bipolar illness. Without treatment, previous postpartum mania or psychosis is virtually guaranteed to recur after subsequent births, and symptoms may begin in pregnancy.[96,97] Minimally, the patient must be evaluated by a provider who is skilled in the mental health treatment of pregnant women, with follow-up visits in each trimester. Each prenatal visit should include questions about mood and cognitive functioning, and laboratory surveillance will include thyroid function testing in each trimester.

4. *History of previous illness with recurring symptoms.*
   The recurring symptoms may be reported by the patient or noticed by the alert clinician. This is when the value of a thorough initial history pays off: the clinician has a good idea of "how bad it can get" and what treatment has been helpful in the past. It is essential to establish the patient's safety first and then evaluate the severity of symptoms and need for referral or consultation. The midwife can consider initiating treatment with previously useful antidepressant or anxiolytic medication, pending the patient's evaluation by her mental health provide.

5. *New onset of symptoms in a patient without prior history of mental illness.*
   A family member may be the first to notice the patient's distress and notify the clinician. As in the situation above, establishing safety for the patient as well as the family comes first. If the patient is not safe, then emergency services should be arranged just as for any other medical emergency. It is also useful to review the patient's history, including family input if available, to see if any prior episodes are remembered. While consultation with a mental health provider is often helpful in this situation, the availability of expert resources is uneven. The treatment approach can be individualized depending on the needs and wishes of the client, the expertise of the provider, and the characteristics of the practice setting. In any case, treatment should not be delayed. Some women will accept immediate referral to a mental health specialist. Others will prefer to return for counseling with their primary provider. Medication treatment should also be considered and consultation with

a psychiatric prescriber should be obtained as appropriate.

When considering psychotropic medication, it is important to discuss with the patient the current literature, which is summarized in **Table 9-16**. In addition, the texts and Web sites listed in Appendix 9-A can provide the most recent information.

Table 9-16 PSYCHOTROPIC MEDICATIONS IN PREGNANCY AND LACTATION

Medication Category	Examples	Pregnancy	Lactation
Mood stabilizer	Lithium (Eskalith, Lithobid)	Safest mood stabilizing agent; absolute risk of cardiac anomalies low; follow fetal ultrasound and echo.[98,99]	Becomes concentrated in breast milk and can cause toxicity in baby; generally contraindicated.
Anticonvulsants used as mood stabilizers	Carbamazepine (Tegretol) Valproic acid (Depakote, Depakene) Oxcarbazepine (Trileptal) Gabapentin (Neurontin)	Teratogenic; long-term neurologic syndromes seen in children of epileptic moms.	Some are considered safe if infant; CBC and liver function tests are followed.
Typical antipsychotics	Chlorpromazine (Thorazine) Haloperidol (Haldol)	No teratogenic effects. Avoid in first trimester. Extrapyramidal side effects noted in newborns.	Limited data available.
Atypical antipsychotics	Olanzapine (Zyprexa) Clozapine (Clozaril) Risperdone (Risperdol) Quetiapine (Seroquel)	Very limited data are available on these newer drugs; no teratogenic effect.[100,101]	Very limited data.
Stimulants	Methylphenidate (Ritalin, Concerta) Amphetamine-dextroamphetamine (Adderall) Modafinil (Provigil)	Very limited data, mostly from drug-abusing populations; animal studies under way.	Safety unknown.

See Tables 9-11, 9-12, and 9-13 for antidepressant medications, and the text for detailed information on medications prescribed in primary care.

It is important to stabilize the pregnant woman before she gives birth. In mental health, as in football, the best defense is a good offense. Clinicians who take a thorough mental health history for every patient and are vigilant for signs of illness during pregnancy rarely will be surprised by any new onset illness postpartum.

MOOD STABILIZERS

Mood stabilizers are crucial for the management of bipolar illness in pregnancy and prevention of postpartum mania and psychosis. Lithium is the safest mood-stabilizing agent during pregnancy, although it was formerly believed to have a high incidence of fetal cardiac malformations. The absolute risk of anomalies is now known to be low, and patients can be reassured by fetal echocardiogram examinations. Lithium has a narrow therapeutic window, and maternal serum levels should be monitored during pregnancy. Hyperemesis in early pregnancy and hemodilution in later pregnancy can cause toxic high and subtherapeutic low levels of lithium, respectively. Serum levels should also be followed during labor and postpartum, and maternal hydration status should be kept optimal.

Prevention of Postpartum Illness

Researchers have identified several reliable risk factors for postpartum mental illness, particularly depression, in multiple studies of many populations.[102–105] The strongest predictors of psychiatric illness in the postpartum period are summarized as follows:

- The presence of psychiatric symptoms during pregnancy is the strongest predictor of postpartum illness. It doesn't get better after the baby is born.
- Any prior episode of mental illness indicates a biologic vulnerability to becoming symptomatic under stressful conditions.
- Psychosocial stress, including marital conflict and unemployment, combined with biologic vulnerability yields illness.
- Infant illness in the newborn period, including feeding problems and colic, is strongly associated with maternal mental illness.

Three of these four risk factors can be readily identified during pregnancy, and preventive strategies have been shown to greatly reduce postpartum morbidity. Preventive strategies can be both biological and environmental in approach.

For women whose histories place them at elevated risk, there is evidence that starting prophylactic antidepressant medication in pregnancy or immediately postpartum can dramatically reduce the likelihood of postpartum illness.[106] Many women try to get through pregnancy without medication, even to the point of denying that they are ill, but they may be receptive to the idea of *preventing* postpartum illness. Obtaining a consultation and prescription in the third trimester can help the patient feel prepared and in control, even if she ultimately decides to "see how it goes" rather than take active preventive measures.

Disordered sleep is common in late pregnancy, but it is not benign and should be taken seriously. In fact, sleep deprivation has been identified as the probable trigger of postpartum mania and psychosis as well as depression.[107,108] A woman who is unable to fall asleep at bedtime, has difficulty going back to sleep after getting up to urinate, or wakes very early in the morning and can't get back to sleep may be experiencing somatic signs of anxiety or depression. Simple sleep hygiene measures, along with an OTC antihistamine such as diphenhydramine (Benadryl) can prevent sleep deprivation from increasing the patient's vulnerability to postpartum stresses. If the patient reports poor sleep *but does not feel tired during the day*, hypomania or mania may be emerging (Box 9-1).

Prevention of postpartum illness requires active measures for stress reduction. Depending on the severity of the woman's illness or risk, the following measures should be implemented:

- *No visitors, only helpers* may enter the new family's home. Phones are off the hook or on the answering machine with the ringer turned off. Doors are locked and the window shades closed so no one can see who is at home.
- The new mother needs five consecutive hours of sleep in every 24-hour period, plus at least three additional hours. Arrangements for ensuring adequate sleep should be worked out during pregnancy. Some women will choose to bottle feed completely in order to safeguard their sleep time, and this decision should be supported. Some women may plan to breastfeed and pump milk for someone else to give the baby; if pumping is too stressful for the mother to cope with, formula feeds are preferable to maternal depression or mania.
- Regular communication with the family is important. Call-in times, visiting nurses, or additional office visits can be arranged according to the available community resources.

Treatment Considerations during Pregnancy and Postpartum

Treatment of maternal mental illness is complicated by the vulnerability of the fetus and newborn to the risks of both maternal illness and treatment regimens. Treatment decision making should consider the risks of maternal mental illness, which include:

- Women who are emotionally impaired are less likely to care for themselves during pregnancy and more likely to use substances such as nicotine and alcohol.
- Recent research suggests that the disruption of the hypothalamic-pituitary-adrenal axis that occurs in depressive and anxiety disorders may directly affect fetal development in subtle ways and increase uterine irritability.[109,110]
- Discontinuation of psychotropic medication during pregnancy is associated with high rates of relapse, particularly if the medication is stopped abruptly. Especially in bipolar disorder, medication discontinuation is associated with elevated risk of suicide. Even "maintenance" medication taken by a woman who appears symptom-free cannot be stopped without increasing her risk of worsening illness.[111]

Patient assessment and treatment planning are complicated by physiologic changes in pregnancy that can be confused with or exacerbate psychiatric symptoms (**Table 9-17**). Mental health clinicians may not be aware of these changes and so not consider them in their treatment planning. Conversely, clinicians may

Table 9-17 PHYSIOLOGIC CHANGES OF PREGNANCY THAT CAN AFFECT PRESENTATION AND TREATMENT OF MENTAL ILLNESS

Change	Effects	Management
Expanding blood volume	Dilution of medication; recurring or worsening illness despite continued medication.	May need to follow medication blood levels; dosage may need to be increased across pregnancy.[112,113]
Thyroid function shifts	Can cause mood symptoms or destabilization of illness.	Thyroid function tests checked each trimester or as recommended by mental health clinician.
Anemia	Can cause fatigue, depressive symptoms, orthostatic symptoms.	Follow CBC and prevent anemia.
Fluid balance: hyperemesis, edema, labor hydration	Can affect metabolism and blood levels of medication.	Maintain optimal hydration and follow serum drug levels as indicated.
Disordered sleep	Increases stress and vulnerability to illness; *can trigger mania or psychosis.*	Prevent sleep deprivation with measures outlined in text.
Somatic discomforts	Can be difficult to distinguish from somatic manifestations of depression, anxiety.	Maintain a high index of suspicion; use screening tools and discuss with patient.
Cardiovascular and respiratory system changes	Palpitations, shortness of breath, orthostatic symptoms can trigger or be confused with panic attacks.	Patient education and reassurance are key; behavioral treatment may be sufficient; medication can be considered.

discount a patient's moodiness or physical distress by attributing symptoms to pregnancy rather than worsening illness. This is where the midwife's information about pregnancy and the patient's condition become crucial to the treatment of mental illness. Inter-disciplinary communication is crucial for comprehensive patient care.

Resources

It is important that health care providers stay current with the latest research and governmental policies in women's mental health. Appendix 9-A lists selected books and Web sites that may prove helpful in this continuously evolving field.

References

1. Kessler RC. Epidemiology of women and depression. *J Affect Disord.* 2003;74(1):5–13.

2. McWilliams LA, Cox BJ, Enns MW. Mood and anxiety disorders associated with chronic pain: An examination in a nationally representative sample. *Pain.* 2003;106(1–2):127–133.

3. Ford JD, Trestman RL, Steinberg K, Tennen H, Allen S. Prospective association of anxiety, depressive, and addictive disorders with high utilization of primary, specialty, and emergency medical care. *Soc Sci Med.* 2004;58(11):2145–2148.

4. Kornstein SG, Clayton AH, editors. *Women's Mental Health: A Comprehensive Textbook.* New York: The Guilford Press; 2002. p. 3.

5. Kiecolt-Glaser JK, McGuire L, Robles TF, Glaser R. Emotions, morbidity and mortality: New perspectives from psychoneuroimmunology. *Annu Rev Psychol.* 2002;53:83–107.

6. Silverstein B. Gender differences in the prevalence of somatic versus pure depression: A replication. *Am J Psychiatry.* 2001;159(6):1051–1052.

7. Weinberg MK, Tronick EZ. The impact of maternal psychiatric illness on infant development. *J Clin Psychiatry.* 1998;59(Suppl 2):53–61.

8. Beck CT. The effects of postpartum depression on child development: A meta-analysis. *Arch Psychiatr Nurs.* 1998;12(1):12–20.

9. Beck CT. Maternal depression and child behavior problems: A meta-analysis. *J Adv Nurs.* 1999;29(3):623–629.

10. Warren SL, Gunnar MR, Kagan J, Anders TF, Simmens SJ, Rones M, et al. Maternal panic disorder: Infant temperament, neurophysiology, and parenting behaviors. *J Am Acad Child Adolesc Psychiatry.* 2003;42(7):814–825.

11. Kofman O. The role of prenatal stress in the etiology of developmental behavioural disorders. *Neurosci Biobehav Rev.* 2002;26(4):457–470.

12. Cirulli F, Berry A, Alleva E. Early disruption of the mother-infant relationship: Effects on brain plasticity and implications for psychopathology. *Neurosci Biobehav Rev.* 2003;27(1-2):73–82.

13. Horowitz JA, Bell M, Trybulski J, Munro BH, Moser D, Hartz SA, et al. Promoting responsiveness between mothers with depressive symptoms and their infants. *J Nursing Scholarsh.* 2001;33(4):323–329.

14. Clark R, Tluczek A, Wenzel A. Psychotherapy for postpartum depression: A preliminary report. *Am J Orthopsychiatry.* 2003;73(4):441–454.

15. Kaplan HI, Sadock, BJ. *Synopsis of Psychiatry.* 8th ed. Baltimore: Williams and Wilkins; 1998. p. 542.

16. Kendler KS, Thornton LM, Gardner CO. Genetic risk, number of previous depressive episodes, and stressful life events in predicting onset of major depression. *Am J Psychiatry.* 2001;158(4):582–586.

17. Kendler KS, Thornton LM, Gardner CO. Stressful life events and previous episodes in the etiology of major depression in women: An evaluation of the "kindling" hypothesis. *Am J Psychiatry.* 2000;157(8):1243–1251.

18. Richards JP. Postnatal depression: A review of recent literature. *Br J Gen Pract.* 1990;40(340):472–476.

19. Nierenberg AA, Petersen TJ, Alpert JE. Prevention of relapse and recurrence in depression: The role of long-term pharmacotherapy and psychotherapy. *J Clin Psychiatry.* 2003;64(Suppl 15):13–17.

20. Sutherland JE, Sutherland SJ, Hochnas JD. Achieving the best outcome in treatment of depression. *J Fam Pract.* 2003;52(3):201–209.

21. Thase ME. Achieving remission and managing relapse in depression. *J Clin Psychiatry.* 2003;64(Suppl 18):3–7.

22. Arnow BA, Constantino MJ. Effectiveness of psychotherapy and combination treatment for chronic depression. *J Clin Psychol.* 2003;59(8):893–905.

23. Kessler RC, Rubinow DR, Holmes C, Abelson JM, Zhao S. The epidemiology of *DSM-III-R* bipolar disorder in a general population survey. *Psychol Med.* 199;27(5):1079–1089.

24. Arnold LM. Gender differences in bipolar disorder. *Psychiatr Clin North Am.* 2003;26(3):595–620.

25. Chaudron LH, Pies RW. The relationship between postpartum psychosis and bipolar disorder: A review. *J Clin Psychiatry.* 2003;64(11):1284–1292.

26. Jones I, Craddock N. Familiality of the puerperal trigger in bipolar disorder: Results of a family study. Am J Psychiatry. 2001;158(6):913–917.

27. Tondo L, Isacsson G, Baldessarini R. Suicidal behavior in bipolar disorder: Risk and prevention. *CNS Drugs.* 2003;17(7):491–511.

28. Garberson LH. Personal correspondence. 2004.

29. Sharma V. Pharmacotherapy of postpartum psychosis. *Expert Opin Pharmacother.* 2003;4(10):1651–1658.

30. Gorman JM, Goetz RR, Dill D, Liebowitz MR, Fyer AJ, Davies S, et al. Sodium d-lactate infusion in panic disorder patients. *Neuropsychopharmacology.* 1990; 3(3):181–189.

31. Shekhar A, Keim SR. The circumventricular organs form a potential neural pathway for lactate sensitivity: Implications for panic disorder. *J Neurosci.* 1997; 17(24):9726–9735.

32. Tsen LC, Datta S. Panic attacks and lactated Ringer's solutions: Is there a relationship? *Anaesth Analg.* 1999;88(4):795–796.

33. Vaiva G, Ducrocq F, Jezequel K, Averland B, Lestavel P, Brunet A, et al. Immediate treatment with propranalol decreases posttraumatic stress disorder two months after trauma. *Biol Psychiatry.* 2003;54(9): 947–949.

34. Linehan MM. *Cognitive-Behavioral Treatment of Borderline Personality Disorder.* New York: The Guilford Press; 1993.

35. Wittchen HU. Generalized anxiety disorder: Prevalence, burden, and cost to society. *Depress Anxiety.* 2002;16(4):162–171.

36. Yonkers KA, Warshaw MG, Massion AO, Keller MB. Phenomenology and course of generalised anxiety disorder. *Br J Psychiatry.* 1996;168(3):308–313.

37. Roca CA, Schmidt PJ, Altemus M, Deuster P, Danaceau MA, Putnam K, et al. Differential menstrual cycle regulation of hypothalamic-pituitary-adrenal axis in women with premenstrual syndrome and controls. *J Clin Endocrinol Metab.* 2003;88(70): 3057–3063.

38. American Medical Association. *International Classification of Diseases ICD-9-CM.* Chicago: American Medical Association; 2003.

39. Cox JL, Holden JM, Sagovsky R. Detection of postnatal depression: Development of the 10-item Edinburgh Postnatal Depression Scale. *Br J Psychiatry.* 1987;150:782–786.

40. Facts about injectable contraception. *Contracept Rep.* 1994;5(1):1–2.

41. Rapkin A. A review of treatment of premenstrual syndrome and premenstrual dysphoric disorder. *Psychoneuroendocrinology.* 2003;28(Suppl 3):39–53.

42. Freeman EW, Kroll R, Rapkin A, Pearlstein T, Brown C, Parsey K, et al. Evaluation of a unique oral contraceptive in the treatment of premenstrual dysphoric disorder. *J Women's Health Gend Based Med.* 2001; 10(6):561–569.

43. Luisi AF, Pawasauskas JE. Treatment of premenstrual dysphoric disorder with selective serotonin reuptake inhibitors. *Pharmacotherapy.* 2003;23(9):1131–1140.

44. Halbreich U, Kahn LS. Treatment of premenstrual dysphoric disorder with luteal phase dosing of sertraline. *Expert Opin Pharmacother.* 2003;4(11): 2065–2078.

45. Lowe B, Zipfel S, Buccholz C, Dupont Y, Reas DL, Herzog W. Long-term outcome of anorexia nervosa in a prospective 21-year follow-up study. *Psychol Med.* 2001;31(5):881–890.

46. Ratnasuriya RH, Eisler I, Szmukler GI, Russell GF. Anorexia nervosa: Outcome and prognostic factors after 20 years. *Br J Psychiatry.* 1991;158:495–502.

47. Keel PK, Mitchell JE, Miller KB, Davis TL, Crow SJ. Long-term outcome of bulimia nervosa. *Arch Gen Psychiatry.* 1999;56(1):63–69.

48. Kleposki RW. The female athlete triad: A terrible trio implications for primary care. *J Am Acad Nurse Pract.* 2002;14(1):26-31; quiz 32–33.

49. Kazis K, Iglesias E. The female athlete triad. *Adolesc Med.* 2003;14(1):87–95.

50. Freund KM, Boss RD, Handleman EK, Smith AD. Secret patterns: Validation of a screening tool to detect bulimia. *J Women's Health Gend Based Med.* 1999; 8(10):1281–1284.

51. Bulik CM, Sullivan PF, Fear JL, Pickering A, Dawn A, McCullin M. Fertility and reproduction in women with anorexia nervosa: A controlled study. *J Clin Psychiatry.* 1999;60(2):130–135; quiz 135–137.

52. Franko DL, Blais MA, Becker AE, Delinsky SS, Greenwood DN, Flores AT, et al. Pregnancy complications and neonatal outcomes in women with eating disorders. *Am J Psychiatry.* 2001;158(9):1461–1466.

53. Little L, Lowkes E. Critical issues in the care of pregnant women with eating disorders and the impact on their children. *J Midwifery Women's Health.* 2000; 45(4):301–307.

54. Bacaltchuk J, Hay P. Antidepressants versus placebo for people with bulimia nervosa. *Cochrane Database Syst Rev.* 2003;(4):CD003391.

55. Skodol AE, Bender DS. Why are women diagnosed borderline more than men? *Psychiatr Q.* 2003;74(4): 349–360.

56. Paris J. Implications of long-term outcome research for the management of patients with borderline personality disorder. *Harv Rev Psychiatry.* 2002;10(6): 315–323.

57. Zahl DL, Hawton K. Repetition of deliberate self-harm and subsequent suicide risk: Long-term follow-up study of 11,583 patients. *Br J Psychiatry.* 2004; 185;70–75.

58. Shelton RC. Steps following attainment of remission: Discontinuation of antidepressant therapy. *Prim Care Companion J Clin Psychiatry.* 2001;3(4):168–174.

59. Nonacs R, Cohen LS. Assessment and treatment of depression during pregnancy: An update. *Psychiatr Clin North Am.* 2003;26(3):547–562.

60. News Release FDA GlaxoSmithKline Dear Health Care Professional Letter. Available at http://www.fda.gov/medwatch/SAFETY/2005/Paxil_dearhcp_letter.pdf.

61. Stiskal J, Kulin N, Koren G, Ho T, Ito S. Neonatal paroxetine withdrawal syndrome. *Arch Dis Child Fetal Neonatal Ed.* 2001; 84:134–135. Available at http://fn.bmjjournals.com/cgi/reprint/84/2/F134?ijkey=9e50bd9024fae0be32b6599c6e7030dce64bd302.

62. Kallen B. Neonate characteristics after maternal use of antidepressants in late pregnancy. *Arch Pediatr Adolesc Med.* 2004;158(4):312–316.

63. Cohen LS, Heller VL, Bailey JW, Grush L, Ablon JS, Bouffard SM. Birth outcomes following prenatal exposure to fluoxetine. *Biol Psychiatry.* 2000;15;48(10): 996–1000.

64. Stowe ZN, Hostetter AL, Owens MJ, Ritchie JC, Sternberg K, Cohen LS, et al. The pharmacokinetics of sertraline excretion into human breast milk: Determinants of infant serum concentrations. *J Clin Psychiatry.* 2003;64(1):73–80.

65. Weinstock L, Cohen LS, Bailey JW, Blatman R, Rosenbaum JF. Obstetrical and neonatal outcome following clonazepam use during pregnancy: A case series. *Psychother Psychosom.* 2001;70(3):158–162.

66. Birnbaum CS, Cohen LS, Bailey JW, Grush LR, Robertson LM, Stowe ZN. Serum concentrations of antidepressants and benzodiazepines in nursing infants: A case series. *Pediatrics.* 1999;104(1):e11.

67. Medina CA. Clitoral priapism: A rare condition presenting as a cause of vulvar pain. *Obstet Gynecol.* 2002;100(5 Pt 2):1089–1091.

68. Trazodone. In: *Drugs in Pregnancy and Lactation,* 7th ed. Editors: Briggs G, Freeman R, Yaffe S. New York: Lippincott Williams & Wilkins. pp. 1609–1610.

69. Hajak G, Muller WE, Wittchen HU, Pittrow D, Kirch W. Abuse and dependence potential for the non-benzodiazepine hypnotics zolpidem and zopiclone: A review of case reports and epidemiological data. *Addiction.* 2003;98(10):1371–1378.

70. FDA launches a multi-pronged strategy to strengthen safeguards for children treated with antidepressant medications. *FDA News.* 15 Oct 2004. [Monograph on the Internet.] Food and Drug Administration, Rockville, MD. Available from: http://www.fda.gov/bbs/topics/news/2004/NEW01124.html.

71. Koback KA, Taylor L, Katzelnick DJ, Olson N, Clagnaz P, Henk HJ. Antidepressant medication management and the Health Plan Employer Data Information Set (HEDIS) criteria: Reasons for nonadherence. *J Clin Psychiatry.* 2002;(63):727–732.

72. Colin A, Reggers J, Castronovo V, Ansseau M. [Lipids, depression and suicide]. *Encephale.* 2003; 29(1):49–58. [in French].

73. Peet M. Eicosapentaenoic acid in the treatment of schizophrenia and depression: Rationale and preliminary double-blind clinical trial results. *Prostaglandins Leukot Essent Fatty Acids.* 2003;69(6):477–485.

74. Freeman MP. Omega-3 fatty acids in psychiatry: A review. *Ann Clin Psychiatry.* 2000;12(3):159–165.

75. Haag M. Essential fatty acids and the brain. *Can J Psychiatry.* 2003;48(3):195–203.

76. Stoll AL. The psychopharmacology reference card 2004. Self published. Available from astoll@mclean.harvard.edu.

77. Loving RT, Kripke DF, Schucter SR. Bright light augments antidepressant effects of medication and wake therapy. *Depress Anxiety.* 2002;16(1):1–3.

78. Epperson CN, Terman M, Terman JS, Hanusa BH, Oren DA, Peindl KS, et al. Randomized clinical trial of bright light therapy for antepartum depression: preliminary findings. *J Clin Psychiatry.* 2004;65(3): 421–425.

79. Tuunaimen A, Kripke DF, Endo T. Light therapy for non-seasonal depression. *Cochrane Database Syst Rev.* 2004;(2):CD004050.

80. Dunn AL, Trivedi MH, O'Neal HA. Physical activity dose-response effects on outcomes of depression and anxiety. *Med Sci Sports Exerc.* 2001;33(6 Suppl): S587–S597.

81. Leppamaki S, Haukka J, Lonnquist J, Partonen T. Drop-out and mood improvement: A randomised controlled trial with light exposure and physical exercise. *BMC Psychiatry.* 2004;4(1):22.

82. Werneke U, Horn O, Taylor DM. How effective is St John's Wort? The evidence revisited. *J Clin Psychiatry.* 2004;65(5):611–617.

83. Rousseau CG, Schacter H. Regulatory issues concerning the safety, efficacy and quality of herbal remedies. *Birth Defects Res Part B Dev Reprod Toxicol.* 2003; 68(6):505–510.

84. Rodriguez-Landa JF, Contreras CM. A review of clinical and experimental observations about antidepressant actions and side effects produced by *Hypericum perforatum* extracts. *Phytomedicine.* 2003; 10(8): 688–699.

85. Zhou S, Chan E, Pan SQ, Huang M, Lee EJ. Pharmacokinetic interactions of drugs with St. John's Wort. *J Psychopharmacol.* 2004;18(2):262–276.

86. Mills E, Montori VM, Wu P, Gallicano K, Clarke M, Guyatt G. Interaction of St. John's Wort with conventional drugs: Systematic review of clinical trials. *BMJ.* 2004;3;329(7456):27–30.

87. Cohen LS, Soares CN, Poitras JR, Prouty J, Alexander AB, Shifren JL. Short-term use of estradiol for depression in perimenopausal and postmenopausal women: A preliminary report. *Am J Psychiatry.* 2003; 160(8):1519–1522.

88. Westlund TL, Parry BL. Does estrogen enhance the antidepressant effects of fluoxetine? *J Affect Disord.* 2003;77(1):81–92.

89. Shors TJ, Leuner B. Estrogen-mediated effects on depression and memory formation in females. *J Affect Disord.* 2003;741(1):85–96.

90. Shenfield GM, Griffin JM. Clinical pharmacokinetics of contraceptive steroids. An update. *Clin Pharmacokinet.* 1991;20(1):15–37.

91. Robertson P Jr, Hellriegel ET, Arora S, Nelson M. Effect of modafinil on the pharmacokinetics of ethinyl estradiol and triazolam in healthy volunteers. *Clin Pharmacol Ther.* 2002;71(1):46–56.

92. Sabers A, Ohman I, Christensen J, Tomson T. Oral contraceptives reduce lamotrigene plasma levels. *Neurology.* 2003;61(4):570–571.

93. Crawford P. Interactions between antiepileptic drugs and hormonal contraception. *CNS Drugs.* 2002; 16(4):263–272.

94. Back DJ, Orme ML. Pharmacokinetic drug interactions with oral contraceptives. *Clin Pharmacokinet.* 1990;18(6):472–484.

95. Elwes RD, Binnie CD. Clinical pharmacokinetics of newer antiepileptic drugs. Lamotrigine, vigabatrin, gabapentin, and oxcarbazepine. *Clin Pharmacokinet.* 1996;30(6):403–415.

96. Viguera AC, Nonacs R, Cohen LS, Tondo L, Murray A, Baldessarini RJ. Risk of recurrence of bipolar disorder in pregnant and nonpregnant women after discontinuing lithium maintenance. *Am J Psychiatry.* 2000;157(2):179–184.

97. Altshuler LL, Hendrick V, Cohen LS. Course of mood and anxiety disorders during pregnancy and the postpartum period. *J Clin Psychiatry.* 1998;59(Suppl 2):29–33.

98. Cohen LS, Friedman JM, Jefferson JW, Johnson EM, Weiner ML. A reevaluation of the risk of in utero exposure to lithium. *JAMA.* 1994;271(2):146–150.

99. Yonkers KA, Wisner KL, Stowe Z, Leibenluft E, Cohen L, Miller L, et al. Management of bipolar disorder during pregnancy and the postpartum period. *Am J Psychiatry.* 2004;161(4):608–620.

100. Gentile S. Clinical utilization of atypical antipsychotics in pregnancy and lactation. *Ann Pharmacother.* 2004;38(7-8):1265–1271.

101. Ernst CL, Goldberg JF. The reproductive safety profile of mood stabilizers, atypical antipsychotics, and broad-spectrum psychotropics. *J Clin Psychiatry.* 2002;63(Suppl 4):42–55.

102. O'Hara MW, Schlechte JA, Lewis DA, Varner MW. Controlled prospective study of postpartum mood disorders: Psychological, environmental, and hormonal variables. *J Abnorm Psychol.* 1991;100(1): 63–73.

103. Warner R, Appleby L, Whitton A, Faragher B. Demographic and obstetric risk factors for postnatal psychiatric morbidity. *Br J Psychiatry.* 1996; 168(5):607–611.

104. Glasser S, Barell V, Boyko V, Ziv A, Lusky A, Shoham A, Hart S. Postpartum depression in an Israeli cohort: Demographic, psychosocial and medical risk factors. *J Psychosom Obstet Gencol.* 2000; 21:99–108.

105. Beck CT. Revision of the postpartum depression predictors inventory. *J Obstet Gynecol Neonatal Nurs.* 2002;31(4):394–402.

106. Wisner KL, Wheeler SB. Prevention of recurrent postpartum major depression. *Hosp Community Psychiatry.* 1994;45(12):1191–1196.

107. Swain AM, O'Hara MW, Starr KR, Gorman LL. A prospective study of sleep, mood, and cognitive function in postpartum and nonpostpartum women. *Obstet Gynecol.* 1997;(3):381–386.

108. Sharma V, Mazmanian D. Sleep loss and postpartum psychosis. *Bipolar Disord.* 2003;5(2):98–105.

109. Sandman CA, Glynn L, Wadhwa PD, Chicz-DeMet A, Porto M, Garite T. Maternal hypothalamic-pituitary-

adrenal dysregulation during the third trimester influences human fetal responses. *Dev Neurosci.* 2003;25(1):41–49.

110. Dole N, Savitz DA, Hertz-Picciotto I, Siega-Riz AM, McMahon MJ, Buekens P. Maternal stress and preterm birth. *Am J Epidemiol.* 2003;157(1):14–24.

111. Viguera AC, Nonacs R, Cohen LS, Tondo L, Murray A, Baldessarini RJ. Risk of recurrence of bipolar disorder in pregnant and nonpregnant women after discontinuing lithium maintenance. *Am J Psychiatry.* 2000;157(2):179–184.

112. Hostetter A, Stowe ZN, Strader JR Jr, McLaughlin E, Llewellyn A. Dose of selective serotonin uptake inhibitors across pregnancy: Clinical implications. *Depress Anxiety.* 2000;11(2):51–57.

113. Wisner KL, Perel JM, Wheeler SB. Tricyclic dose requirements across pregnancy. *Am J Psychiatry.* 1993;150(10):1541–1542.

Appendix 9-A SELECTED RESOURCES

Type	Resource
Screening Tools	*The Edinburgh Postnatal Depression Scale*[39] Has been shown to be valid and reliable in multiple populations, can be used in late pregnancy, and has been translated into several languages. The authors permit copying and use free of charge. *The Mood Disorder Questionnaire* (http://www.DBSAlliance.org) A brief self-administered screen for bipolar illness. Patients can go to the Web site and complete the questionnaire themselves, then print a copy and show it to a clinician. *The Postpartum Depression Screening Scale and Postpartum Depression Predictors Inventory*[8,9,105] Developed by Cheryl Beck, CNM, DNSc, for routine screening in primary clinical practice. The PDSS is also available in Spanish.
Psychotropic Prescribing Information	*Clinical Handbook of Psychotropic Drugs* Authored by Kalyna Bezchlibnik-Butler, J. Joel Jeffries, and Barry Martin, it is the standard complete prescriber's reference. It is revised annually and quarterly; updates are available by subscription. *ePocrates* (http://www.epocrates.com) Drug information databases that can be downloaded to PDAs and PCs. Prescribing information includes dosage, interactions, side effects, prices, and FDA category ratings. Upgrades include herbals, several calculators, and treatment protocols for various illnesses. *Essentials of Clinical Psychopharmacology* Authored by Alan F. Schatzberg and Charles B. Nemeroff, this is a distillation and update of their classic comprehensive textbook, published by American Psychiatric Press; 2001.
Drugs in Pregnancy and Lacation	Thomas Hale, M.D., maintains a Web forum for health professionals at http://neonatal.ttuhsc.edu/lact/. He authored *Medications and Mothers' Milk* and keeps several registries of drug use during lactation. The Canadian Health Network (http://www.motherisk.org) Web site provides evidence-based information on medications, environmental toxins, and occupational safety concerns during pregnancy and lactation. *Drugs for Pregnant and Lactating Women* Authored by Carl P. Weiner and Catalin Buhimschi, available as a PDA CD-ROM, downloadable to handheld devices. Updates are issued several times per year.
Patient Information and Support	*Women's Moods*, Quill Editions, 2000. Authored by Deborah Sichel and Jeanne Watson Driscoll, could be called, "Our Brains, Our Selves," This book describes the interaction of hormones and neurochemistry throughout the life cycle in straightforward language. Individual women's stories illustrate how mood disorders can emerge; offers a comprehensive self-care program for prevention and treatment.

(continues)

Appendix 9-A SELECTED RESOURCES *(continued)*

Type	Resource
	The National Depressive and Bipolar Support Alliance (NDBSA) (http://www.DBSAlliance.org) A nonprofit group that offers information, resources, and local support groups. Postpartum Support International (http://www.postpartum.net) A national nonprofit group that provides information and support; Web site offers articles and self-screening tools as well as a list of local groups. *More Than Baby Blues* (http://www.paraclete-press.com) A 30-minute videotape on postpartum depression, featuring the stories of two women and their experiences. It is an eloquent introduction for patients and providers. The Reproductive Psychiatry practice of the Massachusetts General Hospital (http://www.womensmentalhealth.org) One of the major centers for research in women's mental illness; Web site contains articles about various disorders and links to other sources of information.
Treating Mental Illness in Primary Care	It is difficult to find texts that discuss treating mental illness in the primary care setting. A comprehensive handbook is *Massachusetts General Hospital Guide to Primary Care Psychiatry,* by Theodore Stern, John Herman, and Peter Slavin. Its 700+ pages include the care of patients with many conditions not included in this chapter, plus management of violent patients, family crises, and medically complex situations. Sections on infertility, PMS, and other conditions affecting women are well done.

Chapter 10

Headache

Diane Viens

Almost everyone has had a headache. Approximately 99% of women and 93% of men report having had at least one headache in their lifetime.[1] For some, however, these headaches are disabling and have a negative impact on all aspects of their lives. The person who cannot achieve relief from headache with over-the-counter (OTC) medication may often have migraine or tension-type headache (TTH). This chapter addresses the pathophysiology, signs and symptoms, and management of these types of headaches. Other headaches, such as cluster headaches or headaches that relate to other sources (eyes, sinuses, jaw) are not addressed here.

Definitions and Epidemiology

Migraine and TTH are both classified as primary headache disorders (**Tables 10-1, 10-2, and 10-3**). They are separate disorders with their own pathophysiology, rather than being symptomatic of an underlying condition. Migraine is characterized by episodes of head pain and associated symptoms, including but not limited to nausea, and sensitivity to light and sound. TTH causes pain that radiates in a band-like, non-pulsatile pattern, is of mild-to-moderate intensity, lasts anywhere from 30 minutes to 7 days, and is not aggravated by activity.[2]

In 1988, The International Headache Society (IHS) published diagnostic criteria for a wide range of disorders.[3] These criteria have been extensively utilized in research and in clinical practice to accurately diagnose headaches. In 2004, a second edition of the International Classification of Headache Disorders was published.[4]

Migraine Prevalence

In 2001, the American Migraine Study II estimated that there were 28 million Americans suffering from migraine.[5] This number represented 25% of all American women, as well as 8% of men. With 1 out of 4 women suffering from migraine, the condition is more common than asthma and diabetes combined, more common than osteoarthritis and rheumatoid arthritis.[6] Migraine varies by age and gender, with migraine being more prevalent in boys before puberty and more prevalent in girls after puberty. Prevalence rises through early adult life

---

Table 10-1 MIGRAINE WITHOUT AURA

Diagnostic Criteria

A. At least five attacks fulfilling criteria B–D
B. Headache lasting from 4–72 hours (untreated or successfully treated)
C. Headache has at least two of the following characteristics:
   1. Unilateral location
   2. Pulsating quality
   3. Moderate or severe intensity
   4. Aggravation by or causing avoidance of routine physical activity (e.g., walking, climbing stairs)
D. During the headache at least one of the following:
   1. Nausea and/or vomiting
   2. Photophobia and phonophobia
E. Not attributed to another disorder

Source: Used with permission from Cephalalgia: An International Journal of Headache. The International Classification of Headache Disorders, 2nd ed. *Cephalalgia*. 2004:24 Suppl 1; 26.

Table 10-2 MIGRAINE WITH AURA

Diagnostic Criteria

A. At least two attacks fulfilling criteria for Migraine without Aura (Table 10-1) as well as B and C.
B. At least three of the following four characteristics:
   1. Fully reversible aura symptoms
   2. Aura symptoms develop over more than 4 minutes
   3. Aura that does not last more than 60 minutes
   4. Headache follows within 60 minutes of aura termination
C. Not attributed to another disease

Source: Used with permission from Cephalalgia: An International Journal of Headache. The International Classification of Headache Disorders, 2nd ed. *Cephalalgia*. 2004:24 Suppl 1; 27.

Tension-Type Headache Prevalence

TTH, formerly called tension or muscle contraction headache, has been researched less than migraine; however, it is believed to be a common condition that is most frequently self-treated with OTC analgesics.[2] Schwartz et al.[8] found that the prevalence of episodic tension-type headache (ETTH) was 38%, with women having a higher incidence than men in all age, ethnicity, and educational levels, and with white women having a significantly higher incidence of ETTH than African-American women (47% vs. 31%). A strong positive correlation between ETTH and education was reported. The same study examined chronic tension-type headache (CTTH) and found these are also more frequent in women than men (3% vs. 1.4%).

and increases until age 40, when it begins to decline.[3,5] In the American Migraine Studies I and II, migraine prevalence was inversely related to household income, with rate of migraine falling as household income rose.[3] Although it had been suggested in earlier studies, the American Migraine Studies did not find a direct relationship between migraine, intelligence, or social class.

It is estimated that 52% of those with migraine remain undiagnosed.[5] Many individuals who suffer from severe headaches continue to rely on episodic care in emergency or urgent care settings.[7]

<table>
<tr><td colspan="2">Table 10-3 Tension-Type Headache</td></tr>
<tr><td colspan="2" align="center">Diagnostic Criteria</td></tr>
</table>

A. At least 10 episodes occurring on ≥ 1 but <15 days per month for at least 3 months (≥ 12 and <180 days per year) and fulfilling criteria B–D.

B. Headache lasts from 30 minutes to 7 days.

C. Headache has at least two of the following characteristics:
1. Bilateral location
2. Pressing/tightening (non-pulsating) quality
3. Mild or moderate intensity
4. Not aggravated by routine activity such as walking or climbing stairs

D. Both of the following:
1. No nausea or vomiting (anorexia may occur)
2. No more than one of photophobia or phonophobia

E. Not attributed to another disorder

Source: Used with permission from Cephalalgia: An International Journal of Headache. The International Classification of Headache Disorders, 2nd ed. *Cephalalgia.* 2004:24 Suppl 1; 38.

Burden of Headache

Headaches cause a significant impact for both the individual and society. For the individual, one must take into consideration not only the suffering caused by the pain and associated symptoms during the headache, but also the disruption caused in the person's personal and work life. Studies have projected that headache, especially migraine, causes a total of 112 million bedridden days per year; 93% of female migraineurs have reported lost work days due to migraine. These numbers do not account for the diminished ca-pacity of a woman who is at work with the pain and associated symptoms of headache. It is esti-mated that migraine costs American employers approximately $13 billion dollars a year as a re-sult of missed days and reduced functioning on the job. Further, there is the reduced time spent with family, friends, and in social and recreational activities that is a result of headache.[9] Over half of migraineurs have reported missing family, so-cial, and recreational activities.[5]

Headache is one of the top ten complaints mentioned by patients who visit their health care provider and accounted for 4% of visits to physicians' offices (over 10 million visits in one year).[10] Headaches also account for a vast num-ber of visits to the emergency departments and urgent care centers.[5]

Pathophysiology

Migraine

Migraine is a neurovascular headache. Histori-cally, various theories have been advanced as to the cause. Once considered to have a strictly vas-cular origin, experts now agree that both the vascular and nervous systems are involved in a complex interaction that results in migraine. The five components identified as being in-volved in migraine include: a genetic basis; a sensitive brain; migraine triggers; migraine aura; and migraine pain structures.[11]

While the specific genes have yet to be iden-tified, it is well accepted that migraineurs have a strong family history, suggesting an inherited susceptibility. Additionally, the migraineur's brain has an increased sensitivity or hyperex-citability that contributes to the susceptibility for headache. The periodicity of migraine also suggests some involvement of the hypothalamus.[12] Persons with migraine headache have exaggerated responses to normal sensory stimuli such as light and sound. Several central nervous system manifestations point to the sensitivity of the brain as part of the pathogenesis. About one quarter of patients will report yawning, elation, irritability, hunger, and thirst hours before the onset of the headache pain. These are referred to as premonitory symptoms and are likely to originate in the hypothalamus, indicating a sensitivity of the central nervous system.

The concept of the sensitive brain is also important in understanding migraine triggers. Migraine triggers have long been recognized as events such as stress, or substances such as nitrates, which are part of the migraine syndrome. Many of these triggers are known to directly affect cranial blood vessels, which may then cause excitation of the craniovascular system that leads to pain. Understanding triggers has helped in understanding the complex phenomenon known as migraine headache.

Migraine aura also has provided some clues to the pathophysiology. Approximately 15% of migraineurs have an aura that precedes the actual pain of headache. The visual symptoms of aura (scintillating scotoma, flashing lights) or other focal neurological symptoms have been associated with a decrease in cerebral blood flow that moves across the cerebral cortex. However, aura is believed to be a symptom of neuronal hyperexcitability rather than an ischemic event.[3]

The predominant feature of the migraine attack—pain—also has received significant attention. There are several important pain-producing intracranial structures: the large cranial vessels, proximal cerebral vessels, dural arteries, and the large veins and venous sinuses. There is also trigeminal innervation of the blood vessels, which causes the activation of the pain fibers of the trigeminocervical complex. Given the areas that the trigeminal nerve innervates, this explains the typical pattern of migraine pain.[12] Pain is also produced by the many complex neurohormonal and neurochemical substances that are released and contribute to the headache pain. One neurochemical substance that has received a great deal of attention and has led to the development of specific pharmacotherapeutic intervention is serotonin. Serotonin is released abnormally from platelets during migraine.[13] Rich supplies of serotonin nerve endings are abundant in the meningeal vasculature.

To summarize, migraine is a neurovascular pain syndrome with referred pain from vascular structures in the brain and involves the release of numerous neurohormonal and neurochemical substances that cause a headache with unique symptoms and severe pain.

Tension-Type Headaches

Although TTHs are very common, their pathophysiology is not yet well understood. It has been postulated that the pain is muscular in origin. Muscular pain is often described as achy, poorly localized, and radiating. The pain of TTH was thought to be related to increased muscle tension in the neck and shoulder muscles. It has been suggested that persons with CTTH have permanently altered muscles that may be in continuous spasm mode.[2] However, other research has concluded that those with migraine headaches have as many, if not more, muscle spasms in their necks as persons who suffer from TTH. It seems that TTH is likely a manifestation of abnormal neuronal sensitivity and pain facilitation but not necessarily abnormal muscle contraction. There may be some abnormal modulation of the trigeminal nerve to the motor neurons that results in TTH.[3]

Assessment of the Woman with Headache

In collecting the history of a woman presenting with headache, the primary care provider not only wants to ferret out the type of headache the patient is having, but also to be sure to exclude a headache from a secondary source. The history should be conducted in a systematic fashion, beginning with an in-depth description of the pattern of headache. Questions should include the onset, quality, duration, location, and progression of the headache over time. It is important for the woman to describe any prodromal or symptoms of aura that she might experience. Associated symptoms such as nausea, vomiting, or other constitutional symptoms must be carefully explored. Once the provider has a good picture of the headache, there are several other important components to the history. The first of these is prior medication use. Typically, when a patient presents with a chronic headache, she may have tried many OTC or herbal preparations that were not effective in relieving the headache pain. It is important for the provider to ask questions in a nonjudgmental way so that the patient relates accurately what type of analgesics or other drugs she has taken, the dosage, and frequency. It is usual for the woman with unrelieved headache pain to be taking large quantities of nonsteroidal anti-inflammatory drugs (NSAIDs) and/or other analgesics, and she may be reluctant to share this with the primary care provider.

Other parts of the history should not be excluded. It is important to explore the past medical history, psychosocial history, allergies, and medications. The family history is particularly valuable in establishing a pattern of migraine headaches in the patient's family. The psychosocial history may shed some clues as to stressors in the patient's life that are potential triggers for migraine. A review of systems provides clues to potential secondary cause for the headache. As the clinician begins to develop an understanding of the characteristics of the headache that the patient is describing, then this picture can be compared to the IHS's classification system to determine the type of headache and whether it may be from a secondary and less benign cause, such as a brain tumor or infection of the central nervous system.

Assessment of the Woman with Headaches

The primary care provider needs to be alert to red flags in the history that might indicate a serious cause of the headache pain. These can be easily remembered by the mnemonic "SSNOOP" (**Table 10-4**).

Pattern recognition can be invaluable to the midwife who is evaluating the woman with chronic headaches. **Table 10-5** details additional criteria to consider. Although they are not included in the IHS criteria, there is a strong correlation between these characteristic features and the migraine syndrome.

Physical Examination in a Woman with Headache

The patient who complains of recurrent headaches should receive a screening physical

Table 10-4 RED FLAGS IN THE HEADACHE HISTORY: THE SSNOOP ACRONYM

Systemic symptoms (fever, weight loss)
OR
Secondary risk factors (HIV, systemic cancer)
Neurologic symptoms or altered mentation (confusion, impaired alertness, or consciousness)
Onset: sudden, abrupt or split second
Older: new onset of headache, especially in middle age (over 50)
Previous headache history: worst headache has ever had, or different (change in pattern, frequency, severity of symptoms)

Source: Adapted from the American Headache Society and American Academy of Neurology. Ambassador Program™. Mt. Royal, NJ; 2003. Available from: http://www.ahsnet.org/ambass and used with permission.[14]

Table 10-5 ADDITIONAL FEATURES OF MIGRAINE

- Predictable timing around menstruation (or ovulation)
- Stereotyped prodromal symptoms (change in mood, hunger, feeling unwell)
- Characteristic triggers (foods, stressors, etc that bring on headache for individual)
- Abatement with sleep
- Positive family history
- Childhood precursors (motion sickness, episodic vomiting, episodic vertigo)
- Osmophobia (strong reaction to odors)

Source: Adapted from the American Headache Society and American Academy of Neurology and used with permission.[14]

examination. This includes a thorough examination of the head, eye, ear, nose, and throat systems, and respiratory, cardiovascular, and abdominal systems. This examination helps to rule out any systemic abnormalities. Organic causes of severe headache include brain tumors, aneurysms, brain injuries, and brain infections, among many others. The focus of the physical examination is a thorough neurological evaluation. This screening examination should include the following:

- *Assessment of mental status.* If there is any question as to the patient's mental status, a mini-mental status examination can easily be performed.
- *Assessment of cranial nerves.* II–XII. Both optic discs are visualized to assess for papilledema, for any ptosis bilaterally, and to ensure that pupils are equal, round, react to light, and accommodate.

- *Assessment of motor function.* It is necessary to assess for muscle bulk, symmetry, tone, and strength of muscles. The clinician also assesses for pronator drift, and for any tremors in upper and lower extremities.
- *Assessment for coordination.* For the neurological examination to assess the patient's general coordination, the Romberg Test must be performed. To assess coordination in both upper and lower extremities, the examiner should perform the finger to nose test and the heel-shin test, with both tests being performed on both sides of the body. The examiner should be looking for abnormalities of movement, comparing one side of the woman's body to another as she performs these tests. The patient should also be observed as she rises from a chair, to identify abnormalities of gait and posture.

- *Assessment for sensory function.* Both upper and lower extremities are evaluated for light touch, pain, position sense, and vibration.
- *Assessment of deep tendon reflexes.* The biceps, triceps, brachioradialis, patellar, ankle, and plantar reflexes are assessed bilaterally.

The findings on physical examination of the patient with headache are typically normal. However there are some red flags in the physical examination that should alert the provider to a possible secondary cause of headache (**Table 10-6**).

If there are any abnormalities identified in the physical examination, **Table 10-7** contains some signs and symptoms that may help point to the cause of the headache. Any abnormal finding relating to the headache on the history or physical examination warrants a referral to a neurologist.

Table 10-6 RED FLAGS IN THE PHYSICAL EXAMINATION

- Abnormal vital signs (increased blood pressure, increased pulse or temperature)
- Change in higher intellectual function or cognition
- Alterations in consciousness
- Signs of meningeal irritation (stiff neck)
- Papilledema
- Presence of focal neurological signs (hemiparesis, sensory loss, ataxia, aphasia, signs of brain stem dysfunction, or abnormal reflexes)

Source: Adapted from the American Headache Society and American Academy of Neurology and used with permission.[14]

Diagnostic Tests for the Woman with Headache

Because headache is such a common complaint, the list of differential diagnoses can be lengthy. However, the cause of most headaches can be determined using a careful and detailed health history and a comprehensive physical examination including a thorough neurological screening examination. In 90% of the cases, the type of headache the woman has will be clear by the end of the health assessment. What then, are the essential diagnostic tests for the patient with a complaint of headache?

If the history and physical examination has not uncovered any of the red flags, there is no need for further diagnostic testing.[11,14] It is imperative, however, to recognize any of these warnings since these may be suggestive of a secondary cause for the headache. These patients should be referred as soon as possible to a neurologist. For most headaches, the IHS criteria for migraine with or without aura and TTHs along with characteristic features of migraine (Table 10-7) are sufficient for making the diagnosis.

Chronic Daily Headache (CDH)

Many terms found in the literature are used interchangeably with chronic daily headache (CDH), particularly because this phenomenon has received more attention recently.

Mathew[15] was the first to coin the term *transformed migraine*, which refers to a migraine that went from being episodic to chronic. Cady et al.[16] propose that while persons with episodic headaches return to normal neurologic function

---

Table 10-7 SIGNS AND SYMPTOMS OF OTHER CAUSES OF SEVERE HEADACHE

- Subarachnoid Hemorrhage: Sudden, dramatic, "explosive" headache, accompanied by nausea and vomiting. There are visual disturbances, neck stiffness, focal neurological dysfunction, and alterations in consciousness. The alteration in consciousness can quickly move to loss of consciousness which is directly related to a dramatic raise in intracranial pressure from the leaking blood that is acting like a space-occupying lesion.
- Pseudotumor Cerebri: Very rare, constant, unremitting headache that is worse in the morning and often presents with papilledema. Physical exam is normal. Computed tomography scan and lumbar puncture show elevated pressure and may improve head pain. Cause may be related to increased production of cerebrospinal fluid or inadequate absorption.
- Tumor (Primary or Metastatic): Triad of symptoms: headache, vomiting (without nausea), and papilledema. Associated focal neurological symptoms or signs. Changes in cognition, loss of interest, difficulty with numbers, clumsiness, seizures.
- Temporal Arteritis: Over the age of 55, onset of headache in the temple that is severe, constant, and accompanied by a burning pain. Can be unilateral or bilateral. Client complains of generalized malaise, and anorexia, weight loss, fever, sweating, and myalgias. There is marked tenderness at the temple of the side(s) involved. Diagnostic test: Erythrocyte Sedimentation Rate.

Source: Adapted from the American Headache Society and American Academy of Neurology and used with permission.[14]

between migraines, those with chronic headaches may not do so. This decline in function may be characterized by an increase in nonspecific complaints such as headache, gastrointestinal complaints, and muscle syndromes. This is the period when, according to the authors,[16] some patients may overuse acute headache medications in an attempt to relieve their discomfort and may develop excessive use patterns; the mechanism behind this phenomenon is not known.

It is conceivable that poorly controlled migraines may contribute to this phenomenon. Retrospective studies focusing on patients who have chronic headaches estimated that the average time to transform episodic headache to a CDH often exceeds 10 years.[16] It is suggested that more aggressive treatment of episodic headaches with preventive pharmacology by in-

tervening earlier may slow the process leading to CDH.[16]

CDH is defined as a primary headache disorder with 15 or more headaches per month, lasting less than 4 hours, for 4 months or more. CDH accounts for approximately 4.1% of headaches in the general population, but this number rises dramatically to 80% of patients seen in headache centers.[11]

The history presented in CDH is one of having episodic migraines that increase over time until they occur almost daily. Periodic, acute attacks of migraine occur and the day-to-day pain is described more as resembling TTH. Thus, the question is whether the woman is suffering from two distinct types of headaches or her headache is a variation of the same process with a changing manifestation of two types of headache.[14] The answer to this question is not yet known, but for the woman suffering with CDH, the answer is irrelevant.

It is believed that episodic migraines transform into CDH in two ways. For 30% of sufferers, CDH occurs rapidly after head and neck trauma, flu-like illness, traumatic life events, medical illness that is neurological in nature such as aseptic meningitis, and surgical procedures such as epidural injections. For the other 70%, the change is more gradual and insidious, and happens over years. Head trauma may be the culprit, but more commonly, analgesia overuse is the source. Drugs, such as caffeine, analgesic/caffeine/butalbital combination drugs, opioids, ergotamines, and triptans, sleep disturbances, and traumatic life events are also risk factors.[17]

The woman with CDH may also be the woman with rebound headache, who takes increasing doses of analgesic medication with less and less pain relief. As this happens, tolerance to medication develops and the patient must increase the dose of medication to get the same effect. A self-sustaining cycle of headache-medication develops in which medication becomes a necessity.

Headache specialists continue to debate whether analgesia overuse or abuse is the cause of CDH. Some argue that analgesia abuse is a consequence of CDH. Regardless, it is well recognized that analgesia overuse perpetuates CDH, making it difficult to treat.[17] Of interest is that chronic use of analgesics for other chronic conditions (e.g., patients with rheumatoid arthritis) does not lead to increased headaches.

The health history is of extreme importance in the care of the woman who complains of a headache almost every day. Vital clues that will help diagnose CDH will be found in the patient's history, including a family history of migraine headache. A family history of comorbid conditions, particularly depression, anxiety, and alcoholism, and whether these are or have been present in the patient are essential to identify, as these are strongly linked to CDH. It is also important to carefully explore when the woman's migraine headaches first started, what they were like, how often they occurred, when that changed, and how. A comparison of past headaches to how the headaches are now is very helpful to determine if the patient has CDH.[11] If this is the first visit to the provider, the woman most likely will not have a headache diary (**Figure 10-1**). However, if there is difficulty in ferreting out the diagnosis, a headache diary is essential work for the woman to complete to bring to the second visit. Recording the frequency and duration of her headaches as well as all aspects of how she feels will provide much-needed information to help with the diagnosis of CDH.

The physical examination and diagnostic testing are the same for the woman with CDH as with migraine and TTHs.

Treatment of the Woman with CDH

The goals of treatment are twofold: appropriately treat each acute migraine headache episode with abortive medication and attempt to reduce the use of analgesics to two or fewer days per week and two doses per headache. Medications that the woman has been taking in the past must be discontinued and replaced with other medications. Her headaches initially escalate in severity and frequency as the analgesia is tapered off, and it may take several months for the headaches to subside. Because

Figure 10-1 Sample headache diary and instructions.

Diary Instructions:

You and your midwife need to work together to fine-tune the treatment of your headaches. The diary is one way of recording important factors that are happening around you when you are having a headache.

For each attack, please fill out the information in the diary. It is very important that you bring the diary to your next visit. You and the midwife will review the diary together to look for triggers that might be factors in your headaches.

HEADACHE DIARY

DATE OR HOURS	HEADACHE INTENSITY (1–10)	MEDS & DOSE TAKEN	LENGTH OF H/A	ACTIVITY BEFORE H/A	CHANGE IN ACTIVITY D/T H/A	ASSOCIATED SX	TX RESULT OUTCOME

Key: H/A = headache; D/T = due to; SX = symptoms; TX = treatment.

this is such a prolonged and difficult process, it is strongly suggested that once the diagnosis of CDH is suspected, the woman be referred to the nearest headache and pain center for expert management.

Treatment of the Woman with Migraine

Effective treatment of migraine and TTH requires a comprehensive approach. The principles of headache management include: client education, pharmacotherapy, and other types of preventive therapy such as behavioral and physical treatments.

Client Education

The key to successful management is a sound primary care provider–client relationship. The midwife–client relationship is important in any encounter, but this is even more important when treating the woman with migraine and TTHs. By the time she comes to the primary care provider with a complaint of headache, she has probably tried many remedies to ease the pain and discomfort. She may have tried home or herbal remedies and most certainly OTC analgesics. This patient may be reluctant to share with the midwife exactly how much medication she has taken in an attempt to ease the headache pain.

There are several key points that the woman needs to understand. These points may need to be repeated several times before they are heard clearly by the client.

First, migraine and probably TTH are genetic disorders. Enough research points to a genetic basis, the provider can reassure the woman that her headache has a biological basis. This can be stressed by referring to the history of migraine or TTH in her family. The patient should be counseled about the pathophysiologic basis for the headaches in a simple, straightforward manner, using language that she can understand. It should be stressed that the sufferer most likely inherited a sensitive brain and nervous system, and that having migraine headaches is no different and no less respectable than having another heritable condition like diabetes or hypertension.

Another important message is that migraine headaches are a chronic illness. While there are now effective medications that will relieve the pain, migraine headaches cannot be cured. Working together as partners, the clinician and the patient can achieve management of the pain of headache and its associated symptoms.

Some women may have heard that their headaches are the result of too much stress in their lives, but migraines are not necessarily due to ineffective stress management. While stress is a factor or trigger in migraine and TTHs, it is not the only factor. Migraines are biologically based, so effective management of stress will not "cure" the headaches. Women with migraine also may have concomitant co-morbidities that are related to the inherited sensitivity of the woman's nervous system. Conditions such as depression, irritable bowel syndrome, and panic disorders are manifestations of the sensitive nervous system. It is true

that there are triggers that set off the cycle that leads to migraine. These can be identified and some can be avoided to decrease the frequency and intensity of the headaches. However, identification of all triggers is difficult, if not impossible. Usually there is a combination of triggers that must come together to cause the headache attack, so identification of triggers, while very helpful to the patient, will rarely completely resolve the headaches.

Educating the woman on lifestyle changes that can ameliorate migraine headaches is also important. The initiation of a headache diary as a therapeutic tool is essential. Once the diagnosis has been established, the patient can be asked to record activities, diet, stress level, mood, and amount of sleep as well as presence or absence of headache, intensity of pain, and associated symptoms. It is also helpful for the woman to note in the diary where in the menstrual cycle she is. This diary can be a helpful tool for the patient to identify factors or triggers that are occurring at the time of the headache. It is also useful for the midwife as she reviews the diary with the patient, because the diary will offer clues to various triggers and give a glimpse into the patient's lifestyle. Often the provider can ascertain from the diary that the woman is skipping meals or not getting enough sleep or exercise. The diary also affords a starting point for discussion on the importance of not skipping meals, getting regular exercise, getting enough sleep, and trying to establish a regular time to go to sleep and to wake up. Simple measures such as these can make a difference in the frequency of migraine headaches.

The diary can be maintained through several visits or until the headaches are under better control. The diary becomes especially important after abortive therapy has been prescribed. The patient can record when the medication was taken, how long it took to alleviate the headache, the need for a second dose, and whether she used another medication at the time.

A useful headache diary should include at least the following categories: date of each headache, intensity of headache (on a scale of 0–10), total length of headache (in hours or days or both), activity preceding headache, change in activity necessitated by headache, associated symptoms (nausea, vomiting, photophobia), medications taken for each headache (prescription and nonprescription), and treatment result outcome. A sample diary and instructions are in Figure 10-1.

In summary, education of the migraineur is essential in order for the client to participate in her own management effectively. The more the person knows about migraine and its treatment options, the more likely she will participate in the management of her care. Based on the woman's input, the treatment plan can be altered to achieve relief as quickly as possible with a minimum of adverse effects. Obviously, the need for client education is ongoing. Encouraging questions can help the provider to determine what the woman understands about her headaches and what more she needs to know.

Pharmacotherapeutic Management of Migraine

A comprehensive plan for treatment of migraine headaches typically includes pharmacological agents. Pharmacotherapeutic management includes abortive (acute) or prophylactic (preventive) management. *Abortive treatment* is used to abort the attack, stop the pain, and reverse the progression of a migraine attack. *Prophylaxis* is utilized when the migraine headaches are frequent (>2–3 times a week) and/or when they

occur, the headaches are disabling so that the migraineur misses work and family activities.

General Guidelines for Treatment

The goals for the management plan are to relieve pain, disability, and impairment and to relieve accompanying symptoms. The following principles are important in choosing the medications that will achieve these goals.

1. The intensity level of the individual's headache pain needs to be considered. For example, a migraine headache of less severity may resolve with NSAIDs, and headaches of greater severity may need migraine specific medications (triptans and ergotamine) for treatment. Generally, however, when headache sufferers come to a primary care provider, they have tried several OTC analgesics in varying doses and need migraine-specific treatment for abortive therapy.

2. Concurrent symptoms must be considered when prescribing abortive medication. If the client has nausea and vomiting with migraine attacks, a route other than oral should be considered. Triptans come in nasal spray and injectable as well as oral preparations.

3. The client's expectations of the treatment plan are explored. Once the provider understands the client's goals, the client and provider can work together to discuss expected benefits of the prescribed therapy, and how long it will take to achieve the benefit.

4. A headache diary may be beneficial in the treatment phase as well. In addition to the information mentioned earlier,

the diary is a visible way for the client to see that progress is being made, that she is missing less work, and that the medication is aborting the headache earlier, allowing her to return to work more quickly.

Principles for the Use of Abortive Therapy

Abortive therapy may range from OTC medications (nonspecific pain management medications) to triptans (specific to the treatment of migraine headaches). The goals of abortive therapy are to relieve the migraine attacks rapidly and consistently without recurrence, and to restore the client's ability to full functioning as quickly as possible. Remembering the principles listed below for use of abortive therapy will enhance meeting these goals.

1. All patients with migraine headaches should have abortive therapy available at all times.
2. The headache is treated as soon as the first symptoms appear. For migraineurs with aura, this would be when the aura first appears. Research has demonstrated that treatment with triptans during mild pain produces extremely high pain-free rates (85%–90%).[18]
3. The headache must be treated at a dosage high enough to prevent recurrence of the headache. Migraines inadequately treated may lead to so-called "rebound" headaches. *Rebound* or *drug-induced headaches* are believed to result from overuse of ergotamine, triptans, opiates, simple analgesics, and mixed analgesics (those containing butalbital and caffeine). The woman takes more

doses of her medication because the initial dose did not provide complete relief. Continuing this practice is thought to lead to rebound headache. It is best therefore to instruct the client to limit abortive therapy to two days per week.

4. The choice of medication is made to offer the minimum adverse effects and to address any comorbid conditions the client may have. In some instances, a medication may be contraindicated because of other existing conditions or, in other cases, a medication may actually ameliorate a comorbid condition. It is also always important to consider the cost of the medication to the patient. Certain medications in the same category may be covered by the woman's insurance carrier while others may not.
5. Women should minimize the utilization of "rescue" medication. *Rescue medications* are those drugs that are prescribed for the client to take should the abortive therapy fail. The sole purpose of a rescue medication is to allow the client to achieve some relief without the discomfort or expense of going to an emergency room or urgent care. Rescue medications often offer pain relief so that the woman can sleep in order to escape the headache. Now that reliable and specific abortive therapy for migraines is readily available, rescue medications such as opiates have limited use. The client who uses rescue medications on a regular basis may be a candidate for preventive therapy.
6. *Preemptive treatment* is a form of abortive therapy used when a known headache trigger exists, such as engaging in

exercise or sexual activity, and when individuals will experience a time-limited exposure to a trigger, such as menstrual migraine or migraine due to exposure to high altitude.

7. Headache relief should be complete within two hours. If this does not occur or there is only partial relief, the clinician should consider switching to another triptan. If trying different triptans does not achieve the desired outcome, the client should be referred to a headache specialist.

8. Optimizing self-care reduces the subsequent use of health care resources. Again, education of the client plays a crucial role. The more the woman understands the expected outcomes of the abortive therapy and is involved in her care, the more likely she is to be an active participant.

Understanding the mechanisms of drugs ordered can not only relieve the patient's pain but may also contribute directly to a decrease in utilization of health care resources.

Acute Migraine Medications

A recent government-funded meta-analysis of acute migraine therapies permits the categorization of treatments (**Table 10-8**).[19] Group 1 demonstrated the best evidence for efficacy-consistent statistical significance and moderate-to-large effect size. Group 1a includes migraine-specific therapies such as: triptans, dihydroergotamine, and nonspecific prescription therapies, including ibuprofen, naproxen sodium, intravenous, and prochlorperazine.

These therapies show substantial empirical evidence and pronounced clinical benefit in migraine.

Group 1b includes OTC analgesics (aspirin, acetaminophen, caffeine). These therapies show substantial empirical evidence of clinical benefit in restricted populations. OTC trials excluded individuals who usually required bed rest or who vomited 20% or more of the time. Therefore, the results are not fully applicable to the broad spectrum of patients.

Group 2 agents had evidence of less significant clinical effect and include a number of opioids, several nonsteroidal agents, prochlorperazine, and intranasal lidocaine. In addition to those groups noted above, additional medications were reviewed. In the case of butal-bital-containing agents, there were no migraine studies. Although these agents are effective in migraine treatment, the possibility of drug-induced headache (rebound) is an indication that use should be restricted. The effects of the use of steroids in migraine treatment are unknown.[19]

When To Use Prophylaxis

There are no hard and fast rules as to when a client should be placed on medication for migraine prophylaxis. Recommendations are somewhat arbitrary and dependent upon the individual's need and their pattern and frequency of headaches. The presence of one or more of the following factors merits consideration of initiating prophylaxis medication.

- Migraines that significantly interfere with the woman's daily routine despite treatment with abortive medication (≥ 2 headaches/month with significant disability for ≥ 3 days).

Table 10-8 ACUTE MIGRAINE MEDICATIONS

Group (evidence)	Medications

Group 1a
Substantial empirical evidence and pronounced clinical benefit
In migraine treatment
	Migraine specific
	   Triptans, DHE
	   (SC, IM, IN, IV, plus antiemetic)
	Nonspecific prescription
	   Butorphanol (IN)
	   Ibuprofen/Naproxen sodium
	   Prochlorperazine IV
	   Droperidol

Group 1b
   Substantial empirical evidence of clinical benefit in restricted populations
	OTC analgesics
	   Aspirin
	   Acetaminophen + aspirin + caffeine
	   Naproxen

Group 2 Evidence of less significant clinical effect	Isometheptene Metoclopramide (IV) Lidocaine Chlorpromazine (IM, IV) Ketorolac (IM) Diclofenac K Meperidone (IM, IV) Methadone (IM, IV) Prochloroperazine (IM, PR)

Key: DHE, dihydroergotamine mesylate; OTC, over-the-counter; SC, subcutaneous; IM, intramuscular; IN, intranasal; IV, intravenous; PR, per rectum.

Source: Adapted from the American Headache Society and American Academy of Neurology and used with permission.[14]

- Failure of, contraindication to, or troublesome adverse effects from abortive medications.
- Overuse of acute or abortive treatment.
- Special circumstances (hemiplegic migraine, basilar migraine).
- Patient preference such as the client's desire to have as few migraines as possible.
- Frequent migraines, usually defined as two or more per week.

Principles for Use of Prophylaxis or Preventive Therapy

Preventive/prophylactic therapy requires that the woman take medication on a daily basis. Goals for prophylaxis for migraine headaches are to reduce frequency by at least 50% and to reduce severity and duration of headaches when they occur. The following principles should be kept in mind when the primary care provider contemplates placing the client on preventive therapy. As with all medications, it is important to start at a low dose and increase the dose slowly until clinical benefits are achieved, the ceiling dose is reached, or the adverse effects become intolerable. Each pharmacological agent must be given an adequate trial of two to four months. Clients and providers must understand this concept and not stop medication after one to two weeks, thinking that the medication has not been effective. It is important to use long-acting formulations whenever possible. This helps to increase compliance because the client needs to take the medication less frequently. Available medications should be discussed, and a drug should be chosen based on its proven efficacy and the woman's preference once she understands her choices (**Table 10-9**).

Abortive therapy is also prescribed, so that the client has relief for an acute headache in the early phase of preventive therapy. It is important for the client to understand that she must avoid certain medications as much as possible (i.e., overuse of certain analgesic medications, such as ergot preparations, triptans, and analgesics) because these may lead to rebound and CDHs. For the woman who has comorbid conditions such as hypertension, anxiety, or depression, the therapy for prophylaxis may be beneficial to both conditions. For example, the drug atenolol can be used for migraine prophylaxis and can concurrently be used to treat hypertension. The woman with childbearing potential must clearly be made aware of any potential risks. If preventive therapy becomes necessary for a pregnant client, it is imperative to consult a headache specialist who can tailor the best treatment options. Client education includes: rationale for treatment; expected benefit for particular drug chosen; potential adverse effects; client expectations of the prophylaxis; and how long it will take for the medication to take effect.

A formal plan of care should be developed as the client begins this medication. She should maintain a diary so that both provider and client can see results of the medication on her headaches.

Prophylaxis does not prevent all headaches. There will occasionally be breakthrough acute attacks that will require abortive treatment. Abortive treatment needs to be limited to two days per week to prevent drug-induced rebound headache. Abortive medication may work more effectively when the client is taking prophylaxis. In six months, the midwife should re-evaluate the therapy. If the headaches have been completely controlled during that time, it is time to consider slowly decreasing the dose of prophylaxis.[20]

Whenever there is a discussion of the use of triptans, there is concern for women who have a family history and/or any risk factors for car-

Table 10-9 PREVENTIVE MEDICATIONS BY DRUG CLASSES

Antiepileptics	Other
Antidepressants	• Vitamins
β-Blockers	• Minerals
Ca^{2+} channel blockers	• Herbs
NSAIDs	• Angiotensin
5-HT antagonists	antagonists
Neurotoxins	

Key: 5-HT, 5-hydroxytryptamine; NSAIDs, nonsteroidal anti-inflammatory drugs.
Source: Adapted from the American Headache Society and American Academy of Neurology and used with permission.[14]

diovascular disease. Women often go without abortive treatment for their migraines because providers fear that the vasoconstrictive effects of triptans will have deleterious effects.

In 1992, the American Headache Society convened the Triptan Cardiovascular Safety Expert Panel to "evaluate the evidence on triptan-associated cardiovascular risk and to formulate consensus recommendations for making informed decisions for patients with migraine."[21] Because of the risk of vasospasm, triptans are contraindicated in women with known cardiovascular disease.[22] Furthermore, the consensus panel conclusions were as follows:

- Chest symptoms occurring during use of triptans are usually nonserious and usually not attributed to ischemia.
- While serious cardiovascular adverse events have occurred after use of triptans, their incidence in both clinical trials and practice appears to be extremely low.
- Cardiovascular risk-benefit profile of triptans favors their use in the absence of contraindications.
- Most clinical trials and clinical practice on triptans has been based on patients without known coronary artery disease. These data support the conclusion that, in patients at low risk of coronary artery disease, triptans can be prescribed confidently without the need for prior cardiac status evaluation.[21]

Behavioral and Physical Treatments

Nonpharmacologic treatment encompasses a broad category of therapeutic modalities including biofeedback and relaxation and cognitive-behavioral (stress management) therapy. Physical treatments may include acupuncture, cervical spine manipulation, and mobilization therapies. Nonpharmacologic treatment should be considered in all patients with chronic headaches. These treatments are usually used as adjuncts to abortive and prophylactic therapy, but some patients may prefer to try these treatments first before beginning pharmacologic treatments. In fact, these therapies may be preferred as the first choice in women who have poor tolerance or medical contraindications for pharmaceutical treatments, experience insufficient relief from pharmacological treatment, have a history of analgesia-rebound headaches, or simply prefer to avoid medication use.[23]

Before recommending these therapies, it is important to consider that some insurance carriers do not cover the cost, and these alternative modalities can be expensive. However, if these services are covered, participating in these alternative treatments can give the woman a sense of control over the headaches in that she can do something to stop the headache from getting worse. For the woman whose insurance may not cover these modalities, it is important to discuss these choices so that the client is aware of the options and the costs.

The question often arises of whether a woman with migraines, especially if they are frequent and severe, ought to be advised to seek psychological counseling. Again, this requires a individualized response. Depression often accompanies migraine headache as a co-morbidity. The woman whose quality of life has been impacted by frequent and severe headaches indeed may have depression. It is often useful for the patient to discuss the issues that have arisen over the course of the illness for herself and her family. The family also may benefit from some intervention. They have lived with this illness vicariously and may feel helpless or angry. Often it is helpful for families to have the opportunity to express their feeling about this chronic illness that has affected their family life.

Treatment for Tension-Type Headache

Episodic TTH is very common. Almost everyone has them at some time or other, but for some women these headaches can be frequent and disabling. Most women have been self-medicating with OTC or herbal remedies before they seek help from their primary care providers. Treatment goals should include recommending effective medications that will relieve the headaches and discovering potential circumstances that might trigger TTH in the individual.[2]

The same multidimensional approach utilized for migraine headaches ought to be utilized for TTH. Behavioral and physical treatment modalities such as physical therapy, acupuncture, and relaxation therapy/stress management may provide some relief for the TTH sufferer.[3]

The principles listed under client education for the migraineur also apply to the woman with TTH. Developing healthy eating and sleeping habits, adding regular exercise, and avoiding alcohol and tobacco are also helpful to the woman with TTH. Depression and anxiety are often consequences of TTH. Combining pharmacotherapeutics that may ameliorate both the headaches and depression or anxiety with short-term counseling can make a great deal of difference for the life of a woman with TTH.

Pharmacotherapy

Abortive therapy for TTH consists of utilizing simple analgesics alone or in combination with caffeine, anxiolytics, or codeine, and NSAIDs. Research has confirmed that NSAIDs and acetaminophen are effective in reducing headache symptoms.[24,25] Some studies have indicated that NSAIDs are more effective at relieving TTH than acetaminophen. The combination analgesics, which combine acetaminophen or aspirin with butalbital, work well. One concern is that these drugs are often implicated in rebound headache that can lead to CDH. There is also a risk of dependency and abuse, so their use must be limited to twice a week. **Table 10-10** lists acute medications for TTH and their efficacy.

Prophylaxis

Prophylaxis should be considered for the same reasons as for migraine headaches: frequency

---

Table 10-10 ACUTE MEDICATIONS FOR TENSION-TYPE HEADACHE[3]

Drug
Analgesics
Aspirin
Acetaminophen
Nonsteroidal
Indomethacin (Indocin)
Ibuprofen (Motrin)
Naproxen (Anaprox)
Fenoprofen (Nalfon Pulvules)
Ketoprofen (Orudis)
Ketorolac (Toradol)
Combination
Aspirin and/or acetaminophen plus caffeine (Anacin)
Aspirin and/or acetaminophen plus butalbital with caffeine (Fiorinal, Fioricet)

($>$2/week); duration ($>$3–4 hour); and severity that leads to significant disability and disruption of daily living or overuse of abortive medication.[3]

Any of the preventive medications used for migraine headaches can be used for TTH, but the class of tricyclic antidepressants has the most research data on its effectiveness[2] and is the pharmaceutical therapy most commonly used for TTH.[3] Of the tricyclics, amitriptyline is the most commonly utilized. It is most commonly prescribed in dosages from 10 to 75 mg at bedtime because of its sedating effects and to minimize grogginess upon awakening. Selective serotonin reuptake inhibitors have also been utilized for prevention of TTH and have proven to be effective.[2]

Smoking also has been implicated in patients with CTTH, so smoking cessation should be considered when planning prevention techniques. Payne et al.[25] discovered that the number of cigarettes smoked were "significantly related" to the headache index score and the number of days with a headache each week. The woman may be motivated for smoking cessation if she knows that cigarettes have been implicated in the frequency of headaches.

In summary, care of the woman with TTH needs to be as comprehensive as the plan for the woman with migraines. This diagnosis can be as disabling and disruptive, but with proper care, the client can return to a normal life.

Women and Headaches

Based on epidemiological data, it is obvious that headache is predominantly a woman's affliction. The appearance of all types of headaches peaks after menarche, and the frequency and intensity of headaches dissipate after menopause. How female hormones are involved is not known, but there does appear to be some correlation with the fluctuation of hormones.

Migraines Related to the Menstrual Cycle

Several theories have been proposed that may shed light on the relationship between hormonal cycles and migraine headaches. One theory suggests that during the menstrual cycle, vasospasm occurs as a response to fluctuations in hormones and results in migraine headache. MacGregor comments that the menstrual cycle is so complex that it is unlikely that one event leads to migraine headache during the menstrual cycle. She suggests that the likely cause of premenstrual migraine is the falling levels of estrogen, particularly after there has been an abundance of estrogen in the late luteal phase of the normal menstrual cycle.[26] Prostaglandin release may play a role in the migraines that occur during the first few days of the menstrual cycle. There is a threefold increase in prostaglandin release from the follicular to luteal phase with a further increase during menstruation. These headaches are often accompanied by menorrhagia and/or dysmenorrhea.

Migraines during Pregnancy

Women with pre-existing migraine without aura who become pregnant may notice an increase in migraine, usually during the first trimester.[27] However, 60% to 70% of pregnant women who have migraine without aura report a great improvement in their migraines during the second and third trimesters. The reason is often thought to be due to the stable estrogen levels during the latter parts of pregnancy; however, MacGregor[26] believes that it is unlikely that the reasons are that simple. Again, it is probably a complex interaction of a variety of biochemical, physical, and psychological mechanisms.

Perimenopausal and Menopausal Migraines

The general rule is that migraine headaches decrease with age; however, the perimenopausal period with its fluctuation and changes in hormones may signal an increase in migraine headaches. In addition, uncomfortable symptoms may be introduced such as hot flashes, irritability, and insomnia. Changes in the menstrual cycle during the perimenopause include more anovulatory cycles and a shortened follicular phase. Declining levels of estrogen and episodes of estrogen fluctuations occur. This is followed by increases in estradiol, and an accompanying increase in progesterone.[27] As Moloney et al. state, this "chaotic hormonal pattern" may produce more frequent migraine headaches.[27] The irregularity of menses at this time of life may make it harder to predict when the menstrual migraines will occur and be one of many disruptive events at this stage of the woman's life.

Treatment for Menstrual Migraine

Many women complain that their migraines seem to cluster around the menstrual cycles, and 50% of women report their menses as a trigger for migraines. They may report having several headaches during their cycle, but the association of the migraines and their menstrual cycle and headaches is usually inconsistent, that is, it is not necessarily the same each month.[26] "True 'menstrual' migraine is defined as attacks of migraine without aura that occur regularly on day 1 of menstruation ±2 days and at no other time." These are less than 10 percent of all migraines in women.[26; p.33]

Once the diagnosis of migraine headache has been made, and abortive therapy has been prescribed, the midwife will want to ascertain whether these are menstrual migraines. This is when the headache diary can help to make a diagnosis. After a minimum of three months, it will be clear whether the migraines are related only to the menstrual cycle. At three months, many women will have their headaches under control with the abortive therapy, so there is no need for further intervention other than continued follow-up.

Some women with menstrual migraine may get relief with OTC medications. Women can be advised to take aspirin or acetaminophen for mild to moderate headaches. They should also be advised to take these medications with food and warned against taking no more than two to three doses per week to avoid rebound headaches.

There have been sporadic reports in the literature of herbal remedies and vitamin supplements for headache relief,[27] but to date there has been no systematic review of the research to assess the benefits of these products in order to recommend them for use for headache treatment. Some preliminary work has also been done with the use of low dose triptans on a daily basis around the time of menses for menstrual migraines, but this work is early and experimental and is not recommended.[6]

For the woman who has established menstrual migraines and whose menses are regular, the following prophylaxis is recommended (**Table 10-11**). The medication should be taken beginning two to three days prior to the menses and continuing for five to six days. This should be given a trial of three months before a re-evaluation is done.

If this regimen does not decrease the frequency and intensity of the headaches or if the menses are not regular, then another approach must be considered. If menstrual cycles are irregular and the above strategies have not relieved the migraines sufficiently, hormonal manipulation can be tried. Using estrogen or combined hormonal contraceptives for stabilization of estrogen levels may improve migraine for women in whom hormones are a significant trigger.[28] Women already on the birth control pill may simply need to eliminate the pill-free week to achieve decreased headache frequency and intensity. A transdermal estrogen skin patch can also be of benefit when applied three days before the onset of menses is expected, replaced 2 days later and on day 3 of the cycle, and worn throughout the period. Adding a low dose of oral estrogen (estradiol 1 mg) during the pill-free week may also help prevent or decrease the frequency and intensity of menstrual migraines.[27]

Estradiol and ethinyl estradiol are generally preferred to conjugated estrogens. The latter are more likely to exacerbate, rather than relieve, the headache. Other estrogens, including micronized 17-β estradiol and esterified estrogen can also be used, as can danazol. Both tamoxifen and raloxifene are under investigation for possible future use with resistant migraine.[26]

Table 10-11 Management of Menstrual Migraine

NSAID	Dose per day
Naproxen sodium (Anaprox, Aleve)	375–750 mg
Ibuprofen (Motrin)	600–800 mg

Other nonsteroidal anti-inflammatory drugs also may be used to identify the most effective medication for the individual.

Previously discussed preventive/prophylactic medications have also been used for menstrual migraines. Although many of these pharmacotherapeutic agents have not specifically been researched for this purpose, some anecdotal reports have supported their effectiveness in the treatment of menstrual migraines.[29] Some clinicians have used the preventive medications by having the women utilize the same regime that is recommended and described above. There is, however, no scientific evidence to support this management plan.

Treatment for Peri-/ Menopausal Migraine

For a small percentage of women, the first migraine may occur during perimenopause. For others, fluctuating hormone levels can increase the severity or frequency of attacks. A continuous low-dose, estrogen-progestin combination regimen is sometimes effective in preventing migraines because it provides a consistent hormone level.[27] Maloney et al.[27] state that current American College of Obstetricians and Gynecologists guidelines support a regimen of continuous estrogen for three months followed by progestin to initiate withdrawal menses. This treatment is controversial. Some are concerned that this therapy may increase ischemic stroke risk. This risk is believed to be greater in women in migraine with aura than in woman in migraine without aura. Therefore, women in migraine with aura should not take oral contraceptives.[27]

When women reach menopause, migraines should begin to subside but this takes time (the length may vary, just as perimenopause does). Women ought to be cautioned that this will not happen overnight, just as menopause does not happen overnight. However, the woman often begins to realize that she has not had a migraine for some time.

Since the Women's Health Initiative was released in 2002,[30] there has been increased controversy about hormone therapy (HT) when women reach menopause. However, there will still be women whose menopausal symptoms are severe enough that HT is an acceptable choice to them, given the risk/benefit ratio. For a few of these women, a worsening of their migraines may occur. HT can both exacerbate and relieve migraine headaches. Switching to a transdermal route of administration may lessen the headaches. Reducing the estrogen dose, changing the type of estrogen, using continuous dosing, and adding an androgen are also other possible approaches that may help.[27]

Progesterone must be prescribed along with estrogen for the woman with an intact uterus in order to minimize the risk of endometrial cancer. Unfortunately, progesterone may also precipitate migraine headaches. In this case, the provider can try micronized progesterone or megastrol, which may be less predisposing to headaches than other progesterones.[27]

Finally, if the woman is still having headaches and all the above strategies have been attempted, the provider can try the preventive therapies described earlier in the chapter or consider referral to a headache clinic.

Migraine and Pregnancy

Some women who have migraine headaches give thought to how they will manage their headaches when they become pregnant. However, the periconceptional period is also of concern.[29] Some headache specialists suggest tapering off preventive medications if a woman is planning to become pregnant. This can be started one to two weeks before attempting pregnancy. The woman should consult with her provider as she is doing this.[29] Some migraineurs who have very severe headaches are unable to taper their medications. These women often have been referred previously to a headache specialist and should see that clinician when they are contemplating a pregnancy. Many preventive medications, such as beta-blockers and tricyclics, have been utilized, and the woman can be reassured that it is unlikely that these will harm the fetus. Other preventive medications, such as sodium valproate, are known to cause birth defects. **Table 10-12** lists acute/abortive and preventive/prophylactic medications, fetal risk, and transmission in breast milk.

It is difficult to reassure women about any medication prescribed during pregnancy, because it is not ethically justifiable to test medications on pregnant women. The background rate of malformations or congenital deformities of infants is 1% to 2%, so it can be difficult to determine whether adverse outcomes are due to the medications or to other causes. However, long-term experience with some types of medications has produced evidence suggesting that they are relatively safe. As noted in Table 10-12, acetaminophen and some narcotics (oxycodone, hydrocodone) can be used in pregnancy for relief of pain. If narcotics are used, overuse, dependency issues, and rebound headaches should be addressed.

The Food and Drug Administration classifies triptans as medications that should be used during pregnancy only if the potential benefit to the mother outweighs the potential risk to the fetus. Triptans then should only be used in pregnancy in consultation with a headache specialist. Severe headaches with nausea and vomiting

Table 10-12 MEDICATIONS USED IN PREGNANCY AND BREASTFEEDING

	First Trimester	Second Trimester	Third Trimester	Lactation
Aspirin	(3)	(3)	avoid	avoid
Codeine	(3)	(3)	(3)	3
Ibuprofen	(3)	(3)	avoid	(3)
NSAIDs	ID	ID	avoid	(3)
Paracetamol	3	3	3	3
Buclizine	ID	ID	ID	ID
Cyclizine	ID	ID	ID	ID
Domperidone	(3)	(3)	(3)	3
Metoclopramide	(3)	(3)	(3)	avoid
Prochlorperazine	(3)	(3)	(3)	(3)
Ergotamine	C/I	C/I	C/I	C/I
Dihydroergotamine	C/I	C/I	C/I	C/I
Triptans	ID	ID	ID	ID*
Amitriptyline	avoid	(3)	avoid	avoid
Methysergide	C/I	C/I	C/I	C/I
Pizotifen	(3)	(3)	(3)	(3)
Propanolol	(3)	(3)	(3)	(3)
Valproate	C/I	C/I	C/I	C/I
Verapamil	C/I	(3)	(3)	3

Abbreviations: ID, insufficient data; C/I, contraindicated; (3), probably safe; 3, no evidence of risk; (*), Rizatriptan data sheet recommends avoiding breastfeeding for 24 hours after treatment.
Source: Adapted from MacGregor A. Headaches and women: Treatment of the pregnant and lactating migraine headache. *The Journal of Head and Face Pain.* 1993;43(1):533–540.

can cause dehydration, which is not healthy for the fetus.[31] When this occurs, consultation with a specialist is warranted.

After the woman with migraine has delivered her baby, management may be affected by issues specific to the postpartum period. Headache during the first week after delivery occurs in over one-third of all women, but in nearly two-thirds of women with migraine.[29] A postpartum headache may not be as severe as one's typical headache. Estrogen levels fall very quickly and dramatically after delivery; this rapid hormonal change may precipitate headache in women predisposed to migraine. How the postpartum migraine is treated will depend on whether the mother is breastfeeding her infant. Once again, there are no research studies done with breastfeeding mothers and pharmacotherapeutics. The effect on the infant through the breast milk of any medication prescribed for the mother to take for migraine medications must be considered. Table 10-12 rates acute/abortive and preventive/

prophylactic medications for compatibility with breastfeeding.

Advantages of breastfeeding for the infant and the mother have been well documented. Concerns about migraine headaches should not deter the mother from considering breastfeeding after her baby is born.[29] For women with menstrual migraines, the delay of menses that occurs with breastfeeding may delay the return of her menstrual headaches as well. Life with a newborn baby means an erratic schedule with sleep deprivation and the stresses of becoming a new parent and adjusting to a new member in the family. However, between the new mother, the midwife, the headache specialist and the many modalities of therapy available, it is possible for the woman with migraine to breastfeed and still receive relief from her headaches. For example, since the triptans (sumtriptan, rizatriptan, and zolmitriptan) have half-lives of about two to three hours and should be essentially gone from the mother's system in 8 to 12 hours, pumping and discarding the breast milk during the 8 to 12 hours after using the triptans for a migraine would allow the mother to treat her headaches and still continue breastfeeding her baby.[29]

Behavioral and physical therapies should also always be considered during any phase of preconception, pregnancy, and postpartum as a part of the treatment plan for the woman with headaches. Marcus[32] researched the use of biofeedback training to treat migraines during pregnancy and found this form of therapy to be very helpful. Local anesthetic injections into trigger points in the neck have also been found to bring relief.

In summary, while migraine headaches may present more of a challenge to the pregnant woman and her primary care provider, therapies are available. The midwife will want to consult with a headache specialist in some circumstances. Working together with a team can help make this time of life as headache free as possible.

When to Consult

When evaluating the woman with headache, it is essential in the assessment and management processes to consider if a consultation with a specialist is necessary. This is usually a neurologist who specializes in headaches. These neurologists are versed in the treatment of headaches and will be of the most help to the client. **Table 10-13** lists instances when a referral should be considered.

Conclusion

Migraine is a complex illness that disrupts millions of women's lives every day. A number of therapies can be utilized to alleviate the pain and the accompanying symptoms of migraine.

Table 10-13 WHEN TO CONSULT

- If there is any red flag in the patient's history or physical exam
- If any atypical features are present
- If the diagnosis is uncertain
- If additional risk factors are present (e.g., immunodeficiency)
- If there are daily chronic headaches
- If there is known cardiac disease
- If the treatment regimen has been given adequate trial and is ineffective
- If there is escalating use of analgesics, preparations, and/or prescription medications
- If the commonly used abortive and preventive treatment fails
- If there is a history of status migrainus

A combination of assessment and initial management in the primary care office with a reliable specialty referral is effective; midwives and other women's health providers may find that this area of primary care is a particularly helpful one for the women they see.

References

1. Rasmussen BK. Epidemiology of headache. *Cephalalgia*. 1995;15(1):45–68.

2. Millea PJ, Brody JJ. Tension-type headache. *Am Fam Physician*. 2002;66:797–804.

3. Silberstein SD, Lipton RB, Goadsby PJ. *Headache in Clinical Practice*. 2nd ed. London, UK: Martin Dunitz; 2002.

4. US Headache Consortium. The International Classification of Headache Disorders. *Cephalalgia*. 2004;24 Suppl 1:6–160.

5. Lipton RB, Diamond S, Reed M, Diamond M, Stewart WF. Migraine diagnosis and treatment: Results from the American Migraine Study II. *Headache*. 2001;41:638–645.

6. 2000 United States Census. Online data available at http://census.gov.

7. Vinson DR. Treatment patterns of isolated benign headache in US emergency departments. *Ann Emerg Med*. 2002;39:215–222.

8. Schwartz BS, Stewart WF, Simon DMS, Lipton RB. Epidemiology of tension-type headache [brief report]. *JAMA*. 1998; 279:381–383.

9. Stewart WF, Lipton RB, Simon D. Work-related disability: Results from the American Migraine Study. *Cephalalgia*. 1996;16(4):231–238; discussion 215.

10. Hu XH, Markson, LE, Lipton RB, Stewart WF, Berger ML. Burden of migraine in the United States: Disability and economic costs. *Arch Intern Med*. 1999; 159:813–818.

11. Griffin NJ, Ruggiero L, Lipton RB, Silberstein SD, Tvedskov JF, Olesen J, et al. Premonitory symptoms in migraine: An electronic diary study. *Neurology*. 2003;60:935–940.

12. Goadsby PJ, Lipton RB, Ferrari MD. Drug therapy. Migraine—current understanding and treatment. *N Engl J Med*. 2002;346:257–270.

13. Weitzel KW, Thomas ML, Small RE, Goode J-V R. Migraine: a comprehensive review of new treatment options. *Pharmacotherapy*. 1999;19:957–973.

14. American Headache Society and the American Academy of Neurology. Headache Diagnosis and Treatment in the Neurology Ambassador Program. Mt. Royal, NJ. 2003. Available from http://www.ahsnet.org/ambass.

15. Mathew N. Migraine transformation and chronic daily headache. In: Cady R, Fox AW (editors). *Treating the Headache Patient*. New York: Marcel Decker; 1995. pp. 75–100.

16. Cady RK, Schreiber CP, Farmer KU. Understanding the patient with migraine: The evolution from episodic headache to chronic neurologic disease. A proposed classification for patients with headache. *Headache*. 2004;44:426–435.

17. Matthew N. When headache is a daily occurrence. *National Headache Foundation Headlines*. 2003:1–3.

18. Cady RK, Hall C, Stewart WF, O'Quinn S, Gutterman D. Treatment of mild headache in disabled migraine sufferers: Results of the Spectrum study. *Headache*. 2000;40:792–797.

19. Silberstein S. Practice parameter: Evidence-based guidelines for migraine headache (an evidence-based review). Report of the Quality Standards Subcommittee of the American Academy of Neurology. *Neurology*. 2000;55:754–762.

20. Silberstein SD, Goadsby PJ. Migraine: Preventive treatment. *Cephalalgia*. 2002; 22:491–512.

21. Dodick DW. Introduction: Cardiovascular safety and triptans in the acute treatment of migraines. *Headache*. 2004;44 Suppl 1:S1–4.

22. Papademetriou V. Cardiovascular risk assessment and triptans. *Headache*. 2004;44 Suppl 1:S31–S39.

23. Goslin R, Gray RN, McCrory DC, et al. Behavioral and physical treatment for migraine headache. U.S. Department of Health and Human Services, Agency for Health Care Policy and Research. Durham, NC: Duke University; 1999.

24. Millea PJ, Brodie JJ. Tension-type headaches. *Am Fam Physician*. 2002; 66:797–804, 807.

25. Payne T, Stetson B, Stevens VM, Johnson CA, Penzien DB, Van Dorsten B. The impact of cigarette smoking on headache activity in headache patients. *Headache.* 1991;54:395–402.

26. MacGregor A. *Migraine in Women.* London, UK; Martin Dunitz; 2003.

27. Moloney MF, Matthews KB, Scharbo-DeHaan M, Strickland OL. Caring for the woman with migraine headaches. *Dimens Crit Care Nurs.* 2001;20:17–25.

28. Anonymous. Women and headache (part 2). The life stages of migraine. *NHF Headlines.* 2002;July/August:1–2. Monolog on the Internet. Available at http://www.headaches.org/consumer/education index.html.

29. ACHE: Women and Migraines. In: *Preventive Treatments.* Mt. Royal, NJ: Merk, American Council for Headache Education. Available from: http://www.achenet.org/women/.

30. Cushman M, Kuller LH, Prentice R, Rodabough RJ, Psaty BM, Stafford RS, Sidney S, et al. Estrogen plus progestin and risk of venous thrombosis. *JAMA.* 2004;13:1573–1580.

31. Aube M. Migraine in pregnancy. *Neurology.* 1999;54:S26–S28.

32. Marcus D. Focus on primary care diagnosis and management of headache in women. *Obstet Gynecol Surv.* 1999;54:395–402.

Chapter 11

Common Conditions of the Eye and Ear

Mary Ellen
Bouchard

While conditions of the eye and ear are relatively uncommon in most women's health practices, they can, and do, occur. Many of these conditions are self-limited, such as allergies or infections, but some symptoms may herald more serious or more chronic conditions. This chapter is not meant to cover all of these conditions in depth; rather, it provides the background needed by midwives and women's health providers to recognize and treat self-limited and milder versions of chronic conditions, and to recognize and refer appropriately more serious problems.

The Eye

Clinical Presentation

Patients with acute onset of eye problems often complain of ocular itching or irritation, watery or purulent eye discharge, and/or redness. They also may present with a "bump" or swelling of the eyelid and infrequently with eye dryness. Changes in vision are less commonly reported, but if acute in onset may be a sign of more significant medical problems. Each of these symptoms requires an understanding of basic eye anatomy as well as careful evaluation.

Redness can be caused by inflammation, infection, or irritation of the conjunctival membranes that line the posterior surface of the lids and anterior surface of the sclera. In primary care practice, one of the most common causes is conjunctivitis, which can result from infection or allergy. Infection of the conjunctiva, whether due to viruses or bacteria, is often accompanied by inflammation and discomfort. Allergic conjunctivitis may present with these same symptoms, but in addition cause the eyes to be itchy. Redness can also result from rupture of the blood vessels within the conjunctiva (subconjunctival hemorrhage), which is commonly caused by valsalva maneuvers such as vomiting and can be seen after childbirth secondary to pushing. Other causes of eye redness include styes, corneal abrasion, foreign object, chalazion, cellulitis of the eyelid or skin around the eye, blepharitis, injury, or (more rarely) serious eye disorders and systemic diseases.

Patients presenting with a "bump" need to be evaluated for conditions related specifically to the eye as well as more general conditions that can affect the skin anywhere on the body. **Table 11-1** lists the differential diagnoses that should be considered during the evaluation of common eye problems.

Table 11-1 DIFFERENTIAL DIAGNOSIS OF EYE PROBLEMS

Symptom and Condition	History and Associated Symptoms	Physical Findings	When to Refer
Stye			
Stye	Non-abrupt onset.	• Normal vision • Red, tender eyelid • Boil-like lesion on eyelid • May have conjunctival erythema • Normal fundoscopy exam	No resolution after 10–14 days.
Chalazion	Non-abrupt onset. May have history of previous occurrence.	• Normal vision unless vision blurred by cyst on upper lid • Nontender cyst • Normal fundoscopy exam	Persists despite soaking. Surgical incision and drainage may be needed. Symptoms recur several times, or evaluation findings suggest sebaceous gland neoplasia.
Flaky Skin and Irritation Along Eyelid Margins			
Blepharitis	Often has history of allergy, seborrhea, or other dermatologic condition.	• Normal vision • Normal fundoscopy exam • Conjunctival inflammation • Erythema and edema of eyelid • May have crusting of lid from discharge • Eyelash loss or pointing in opposite directions of other eyelashes	Condition unresponsive to treatment or initial presentation is severe.
Watery Eyes			
Allergic conjunctivitis	Exposure to known trigger including: environmental, medication, cosmetics.	• Diffuse redness • Eyelid edema • Itching • Tearing • Stringy, white discharge • Nasal congestion • Normal vision • Normal fundoscopy exam	No response to treatment.

Table 11-1 **DIFFERENTIAL DIAGNOSIS OF EYE PROBLEMS** *(continued)*

Symptom and Condition	History and Associated Symptoms	Physical Findings	When to Refer
Bacterial conjunctivitis	Exposure to others with similar complaints.	• Sudden onset • Diffuse redness • Purulent discharge • Edema of the conjunctiva • Normal vision • Normal fundoscopy exam	Unresponsive to treatment, suspect chlamydia or gonnorheal infection, or if accompanied by a sensation of foreign body (to rule out keratitis).
Viral conjunctivitis	Concomitant upper respiratory infection. Exposure to others with similar complaint.	• Diffuse redness • Edema of the conjunctiva • Blurry vision due to clear watery discharge, otherwise normal vision • Edema of the eyelid • Normal vision • Normal fundoscopy exam • May start in one eye and spread to other eye • Possible pre-auricular lymph node edema	No improvement in 14 days.
Irritant	Complaint of splash to eye or to contact with irritating substances.	• Diffuse redness • Possible irritation • Normal vision • Normal fundoscopy exam	Irritation continues or associated eye pain or lesions are noted.
Eye Dryness			
Idiopathic	Most common in aging women.	• Burning • Foreign body sensation or sensation of grittiness • May have over-reactive mucin production	No response to treatment or symptoms persist (to prevent progressive tissue damage and/or to evaluate for underlying systemic disease such as Sjogren's disease or sarcoidosis). White spots noted on cornea.
Medication side effect	Common with use of antihistamines. Can rarely occur with use of hormone therapy.	• Ceases with cessation of medication	Symptoms persist after medication discontinued.

(continues)

Table 11-1 DIFFERENTIAL DIAGNOSIS OF EYE PROBLEMS *(continued)*

Symptom and Condition	History and Associated Symptoms	Physical Findings	When to Refer
Eye Pain			
Corneal abrasion	History of trauma or prolonged contact lens use.	• Redness concentrated around limbus • Photophobia • Exam with penlight across cornea may demonstrate abrasion • Fluoroscein exam may be necessary to see abrasion: refer	Condition suspected or present. Warrants evaluation by an ophthalmologist.
Foreign body	History of sudden onset of symptoms with or without exposure to known substance.	• Redness • Excessive tearing • Sense of presence of irritant • Photophobia • Fundoscopy is normal, but may be difficult to do	Condition suspected or present. Warrants evaluation by an ophthalmologist.
Chemical splash	History of splash.	• Eye pain • Erythema • May have ulcers or blisters	Condition suspected or present. Warrants evaluation by an ophthalmologist.
Trauma	History of injury to eye ("black eye").	• Bruising of eyelid • Otherwise normal eye and fundoscopy exam • Normal vision	Injury accompanied by blurred vision or vision loss, possible infection, painful orbit, headache, bleeding, unequal pupils, suspected injury to surrounding tissue, flashing lights, bleeding, or injury to sclera.
Acute angle-closure Glaucoma	Symptoms often occur in evening; usually in older person. May report history of anticholinergic or sympathomimetic agents (some antidepressants, nasal decongestants). Precipitated by incident of pupilary dilation such as in darkened room.	• Eye redness • Moderate to severe pain • Symptoms usually occur in one eye • Reports halos around lights • Dilated pupil • Cornea appears "steamy" • Eye feels hard to palpation due to increased intraocular pressure	Condition suspected or present. Warrants evaluation by an ophthalmologist.

Table 11-1 **DIFFERENTIAL DIAGNOSIS OF EYE PROBLEMS** *(continued)*

Symptom and Condition	History and Associated Symptoms	Physical Findings	When to Refer
		• Possible headache, nausea, and vomiting	
Herpes zoster and herpes simplex	History of varicella or herpes simplex.	• Painful lesions noted on face, eyelid, nose	Condition suspected or present. Warrants evaluation by an ophthalmologist.
Scleritis, iritis, uveitis	History of chronic disease such as inflammatory bowel disease, autoimmune disorders, or infections such as cytomegalovirus or toxoplasmosis.	• Irritation or itchiness • Erythema of sclera, iris • Painful orbit to palpation • Photophobia	Condition suspected or present. Warrants evaluation by an ophthalmologist.
Red Eye			
Subconjunctival hemorrhage	History of coughing, or vigorous physical activity or valsalva maneuver such as pushing in labor.	• Erythema • Painless • Normal vision • Normal fundoscopy	No spontaneous healing seen within ~2 weeks.
Flashes and Floaters			
Age-related floaters	Spots before the eyes. Chronic floaters unassociated with flashing lights.	• Otherwise normal vision • Normal eye exam • Normal fundoscopy	Condition suspected or present. Warrants evaluation by an ophthalmologist unless previously evaluated.
Retinal detachment	Spots before the eyes. Flashes of light. Sudden loss of vision. Sudden or progressively blurry vision. No pain or redness.	• Loss of portion or whole visual field • "Hanging" retina or irregular retinal surface	Condition suspected or present. Warrants evaluation by an ophthalmologist.
Migraine	Visual disturbances. Loss or alterations in vision field that seem to "dance." Flashes of light. Usually precedes headache.	• May have diminished visual acuity	For assessment of migraine headache, refer to Chapter 10.
Vision Loss			
Refractive error	Slow onset. Blurry or double vision. Headache.	• Painless • Decrease of visual acuity • Normal fundoscopy	Condition suspected as corrective lenses are needed.

(continues)

Table 11-1 DIFFERENTIAL DIAGNOSIS OF EYE PROBLEMS (*continued*)

Symptom and Condition	History and Associated Symptoms	Physical Findings	When to Refer
Vision Loss			
Cataracts	Slow onset. Most frequently occurs in older population and persons with a history of diabetes mellitus.	• Painless • Decreased visual acuity • Lens over pupil appears hazy or cloudy when examined with penlight • In late disease, unable to do fundoscopy due to cloudy lens • May be unilateral	Condition suspected or present. Warrants evaluation by an ophthalmologist.
Glaucoma	Occurs most frequently in older population. History of ophthalmic or systemic corticosteroid medication use for several weeks.	• May be symptom free • Usually found on routine ophthalmic examination • Fundoscopy: cupping of disc	Condition suspected or present. Warrants evaluation by an ophthalmologist.
Age-related macular degeneration	Gradual loss of vision, blurry vision, or "holes in vision."	• Unilateral • Distortion of vision using Amsler's grid	Condition suspected or present. Warrants evaluation by an ophthalmologist. Requires urgent referral if sudden onset.

Essential History, Physical, and Laboratory Evaluation

HISTORY

A few essential questions can help differentiate common relatively benign conditions from more serious problems requiring evaluation by a specialist. Positive responses to questions about vision being affected, the presence of photophobia or a sensation of "something being under the eyelid," or a history of trauma all warrant urgent referral to an ophthalmologist. However, careful questioning is sometimes needed to distinguish the discomfort commonly found with conjunctivitis, styes, or dry eye syndromes from the pain due to corneal involvement from abrasions or a foreign body. Discomfort from conjunctivitis and dry eye is often described as irritation, grittiness, or scratchiness. Patients with corneal involvement often report that they have difficulty opening or keeping open their eyes as well as pain, photophobia, and a sensation of "something in my eye."[1] Deep-seated or severe pain is indicative of more serious problems. Further questioning about the suddenness and severity of any associated visual changes is also important. Sudden vision loss can be due to vitreous hemorrhage, retinal detachment, or vascular occlusion, and requires immediate referral. Gradual loss can be associated with changing refractive error, cataract, glaucoma, and macular degeneration and will also need—albeit less urgent—evaluation.[2]

Asking about the presence of eye discharge and its timing can also help differentiate between possible sources of the discomfort. Eye discharge that is heaviest in the morning upon awakening and minimal later in the day can be seen with allergy, styes, viral or allergic conjunctivitis, and dry eyes. Discharge that persists throughout the day is more consistent with a diagnosis of bacterial conjunctivitis or bacterial keratitis. Bacterial conjunctivitis requires treatment, but bacterial keratitis, which should be suspected if the patient also has photophobia or foreign body sensation, requires emergent referral.[3]

Questions about trauma or chemical splash also should be asked. Contact lens overuse or a blow to the eye can lead to redness and irritation. Rarely will subconjunctival hemorrhages be a symptom of hypertension or blood dyscrasias.[1] If they recur frequently, an evaluation for systemic disease should be considered.

PHYSICAL EXAMINATION

Patients with benign conditions can comfortably hold their eyes open during an examination and are not disturbed by ambient light.[3] A complete examination of the head, neck, and respiratory system may be necessary to evaluate associated symptoms such as rhinorrhea, cough, or lymphadenopathy, because infections of the upper respiratory tract and allergies can cause eye-related symptoms.

External exam of the eye includes evaluation of the lids, conjunctiva, pupils, and extraocular movements. Inflammation and injection of the conjunctival membranes should be noted as well as any opacities of the sclera and cornea.

A penlight evaluation is essential. The pupil should be examined to determine its reaction to light and its size. The pupil can be fixed, for example, in glaucoma or pinpoint with corneal abrasion, infectious keratitis, or iritis. The cornea should be evaluated for opacity and the presence of an abrasion or foreign body. The pattern of redness also should be noted. Benign conditions usually cause redness affecting the entire conjunctiva equally, but redness concentrated centrally at the limbus and fading toward the periphery can indicate problems such as corneal injury, iritis, or acute glaucoma. These latter conditions require emergent referral.

Fundoscopy is a difficult skill to master unless done regularly and so may be more accurately performed by an ophthalmologist in questionable cases. Therefore, normal findings should be confirmed by an ophthalmologist in patients with symptoms suggestive of serious eye injury or disease. Findings indicative of more serious disease include abnormal cup-disc ratios seen in glaucoma, retinal hemorrhages and cotton wool spots in diabetes, and depigmented areas in the macula in macular degeneration.[2] These findings also require follow-up by an ophthalmologist.

LABORATORY

No laboratory tests are available in the primary care setting that can help differentiate the diagnosis under consideration. Additional tests can be employed by an ophthalmologist. Referral is appropriate for tests of visual acuity and evaluation of more significant presentations. **Tables 11-3 and 11-4** describe various eye tests.

Changes in Pregnancy

During the third trimester, there are changes in the cornea that may cause corneal edema, which can make it difficult for the pregnant woman to wear contact lenses. The pregnant woman wearing contact lenses may experience blurring of vision because of a temporary change in the composition of her tears. Slight thickening of the cornea prevents accurate refractive error assessment and correction.[4] Thus, an exam for new contact lenses or glasses should be avoided until several weeks after delivery. The hormonal changes during pregnancy may produce chloasma and spider hemangiomas around the eyelids. In addition, the intraocular pressure decreases midway through pregnancy and returns to pre-pregnancy pressure approximately eight weeks after delivery.[4] Occasionally, other visual changes can occur due to pregnancy. These cannot be assumed to be due to normal pregnancy changes, because obstetrical complications such as pre-eclampsia can present with ocular manifestations. Women with underlying systemic disease such as diabetes, hypertension, autoimmune disease, and pre-existing glaucoma must continue examinations as determined by an ophthalmologist to ensure preservation of vision.

Systemic absorption of ophthalmic medications is minimal but can be reduced further by employing certain techniques during administration. Pregnant women being treated for ophthalmic conditions with antibiotic solutions should be instructed to hold the nasolacrimal duct closed for three to five minutes after drops are placed to minimize absorption. Antibiotic solutions should be prescribed for the shortest effective period to limit exposure in pregnancy.[4]

Management of Specific Conditions

STYE

A stye is a common local infection of the eyelid. The patient presents with a pustule-like lesion on the eyelid. The lid is typically edematous, red, and tender to touch. Occasionally, the adjacent conjunctiva may also be red. Vision is only affected if the upper lid is infected and causes blurry vision. Treatment consists of the application of warm compresses to the affected area for 15 minutes four times per day. Styes often spontaneously rupture and drain within several days, but an antibiotic ointment can be applied until it is healed.[5,6] If there is no resolution after 10 to 14 days, or if cellulitis of the eyelid develops, the patient should be referred. **Table 11-2** lists some commonly used eye medications.

CHALAZION

The patient may present with a previous history of a chalazion or a localized eyelid infection. In this condition, which may become chronic, the meibomian gland develops a granulomatous inflammation.[6,7] The palpable area may feel cystic but nontender. The visual exam is normal. Using warm compresses may help resolve the inflammation; however, surgical intervention for incision and drainage is usually needed.[5,7] If the chalazion reoccurs several times or remains unhealed after drainage, referral for evaluation of underlying sebaceous gland neoplasia is warranted.[7,8]

BLEPHARITIS

Blepharitis is a chronic condition of the eyelid that usually presents with flaky or scaly skin and irritation along the lid margins. The visual exam is normal. The midwife may see erythema and edema of the eyelid along the margin. Crusting of the lid, conjunctival inflammation, and eyelash loss or displacement may be noted.[8,9] The irritation may be caused by a staphylococcus infection[5,6,8] or a skin condition such as rosacea or seborrhea.[6] Treatment consists

Table 11-2 COMMONLY USED EYE MEDICATIONS

Drug	Trade Name	Dose	Notes
Antibiotic Eye Drops			
Erythromycin 0.5% ophthalmic ointment	Ilotycin, generic	$1/_2$″ to conjunctiva up to 6 times daily for 7–10 days	
Bacitracin 500 units/gm ointment	Thin ribbon to conjunctiva every 3–4 hours for 7–10 days		
Sulfacetamide ophthalmic drops	Sulamyd	1–2 drops every 3 hours while awake × 7–10 days	
Fluoroquinolone ophthalmic drops 0.3%	Ocuflox	Day 1 and 2: 1–2 drops to affected eye every 2–4 hours Day 3–7: 1–2 drops 4 × per day	Read specific administration instructions for other trade names of this medication, as they will vary
Natural Tears			
Eye lubricant	Refresh, Hypotears	1–2 drops 4 times per day May use hourly with increased irritation	Used in the treatment of viral or allergic or irritant-induced conjunctivitis and dry eye
Antihistamine Drops			
See Chapter 12 for medications and management.			Used for the treatment of allergic conjunctivitis

initially of eyelid hygiene. The lid margins should be washed with baby shampoo on a clean cotton-tipped applicator two times per day. If there is no resolution, or the crusting or irritation is significant and suggests an infection, a culture should be done and the condition treated with an antibiotic ointment. If resolution does not occur, or if the condition is severe, the patient should be referred to an ophthalmologist.[5,8]

CONJUNCTIVITIS

Conjunctivitis specifically refers to the inflammation of the conjunctiva and is relatively commonly seen in the primary care setting. However, the source of this inflammation and therefore the treatment can vary. Steroid use is contraindicated in the treatment of conjunctivitis due to the possible masking of significant viral infections such as herpes.[8] Treatment options for conjunctivitis are listed in Table 11-2.

Allergic Conjunctivitis The patient presenting with allergic conjunctivitis presents with diffuse redness of the conjunctiva, eyelid edema, tearing, occasional itching, and normal vision.[6] The eye exam is normal. Stringy, white,[5,6,8] mucus,[9] or mucoserous discharge[10] is also seen with this form of conjunctivitis. However, in chronic conditions, white spots may develop on the cornea indicating keratitis, requiring a referral for evaluation. The patient also may have other symptoms of allergies such as nasal congestion, asthma, or dermatitis, and may benefit from treatment with antihistamines (see Chapter 12 for more information). Occasionally, allergies to medications, cosmetics, or other substances cause conjunctivitis; this possibility should be suspected if the onset of symptoms occurs with exposure to the offending agent and resolves when exposure ceases. Instillation of artificial tears, without preservatives, may provide comfort by diluting and washing out the offending agent.[8,9]

Bacterial Conjunctivitis The patient with bacterial conjunctivitis typically presents with sudden onset of watery eyes with diffuse redness and edema of the conjunctiva and purulent discharge. The patient may complain of difficulty in opening the eye in the morning due to the voluminous production of thick discharge. The patient's vision is normal. This condition is highly contagious and the patient may be aware of exposure to others with this condition. The most common infecting agents are *Staphylococcus aureus*, *Streptococcus pneumonia*, and *Hemophilus*.[5,6] *Pseudomonas* can also be found.[6,8] The patient should be treated with an antibiotic ophthalmic solution. The patient should be referred for evaluation if there is eye pain or loss of vision, no improvement within 72 hours, or

worsening symptoms. Because this condition is highly contagious, the patient should avoid close contact with others and be diligent in using effective hand washing. In sexually active individuals, a vaginal or penile discharge should raise the suspicion of a chlamydia or gonoccocal infection. In this situation, the eye symptoms often have rapid onset and are severe. Cultures and treatment for these infections are indicated, and the patient should be referred to an ophthalmologist.[5,6,9,11]

Viral Conjunctivitis The patient with viral conjunctivitis often presents with a history of a recent or concomitant viral or upper respiratory infection. There is diffuse redness and edema of the conjunctiva (hence the name "pink eye"). The discharge may be less than in bacterial conjunctivitis and typically is clear and watery. Because of the discharge, the vision may be blurry but is otherwise normal. Palpable pre-auricular lymph nodes are often present.[9,11] This condition is self-limiting and treatment with antibacterial eyedrops is used for secondary bacterial infections.[6] Cool compresses may ease discomfort. Refer for evaluation if there is not resolution in 10 to 14 days, if a change in or loss of vision occurs, or if symptoms worsen. White spots noted on the cornea are also cause for referral to evaluate for keratitis. As in bacterial conjunctivitis, this condition is highly contagious and close contact with others should be avoided until symptoms are resolved. The provider should also remind the patient of effective hand washing techniques to avoid infecting others.[5,6,8,9]

EYE IRRITATION

The patient with eye irritation may report a recent splash to the eye or exposure to irritating substances. The patient also may experience diffuse redness of the conjunctiva; vision will be normal. The patient who calls for advice should be told to rinse immediately with cool or room temperature water under a faucet to dilute the irritant and then to come to the office to be evaluated. If the irritation continues or if eye pain or lesions are noted, the patient should be referred.

EYE DRYNESS

Eye dryness occurs because of a decrease in tear production. Tears serve as a lubricating agent and as a protective mechanism from bacteria. Decreased production most commonly occurs in women as they approach their 50s, but can also result from using medications such as antihistamines and rarely from use of hormone

Table 11-3 **IN-OFFICE EYE EXAMS**

Tests	Procedure	Notes
Visual Acuity	Snellen Chart: The patient stands 20 feet from the chart, with glasses if usually worn, covers one eye, and reads the smallest line that can be read accurately. The other eye is then tested. Special charts using hand directions are available for patients who are illiterate.	Vision should be 20/20 with corrective lenses. Acuity less than 20/30 is considered abnormal. Legal blindness: 20/200.
Visual Fields	The examiner stands 3 feet in front of the patient and is at eye level of the patient. The patient closes one eye and focuses on the examiner's nose. The examiner closes the opposing eye and holds up one or two fingers and asks the patient to count the fingers. This is repeated in all 4 quadrants. The test is then performed on the patient's opposite eye.	Normal central vision extends for 30 degrees from the central point of focus. Holes or distortions in the field are called scotoma.
Amsler's Grid	This is a rapid screening test for patients complaining of blurry vision. The patient stares at the spot in the middle of the grid and identifies any "holes" or distortions seen.	This can identify abnormal areas of vision for patients with possible retinal or neurologic disease. If areas of distortion are seen, the patient should be referred to an ophthalmologist.
Pinhole Test	This is a rapid screening test for patients complaining of blurry vision. A small pinhole is placed in an index card. The patient looks through the pinhole with one eye, while closing the opposite eye.	If the patient sees clearly through the pinhole, the cause of blurry vision is a refractive error and she can be referred for a non-urgent ophthalmic exam. If the vision is still blurry, the patient should be referred urgently.

replacement therapy. Patients with underlying autoimmune diseases such as sarcoidosis, or more notably Sjögren's disease, may report eye dryness as one of the initial presenting symptoms of their disease.[5–7] The patient presents with a burning sensation and reports the sensation of the presence of a foreign body, although there is none upon exam. The lack of tears may result in an overproduction of mucin resulting in a stringy discharge. Vision is normal. If the cause is medication, the symptoms will abate with cessation of the drug, and artificial tears can be used during therapy to provide relief. If the cause is idiopathic, symptoms can be relieved by using artificial tears without preservatives three to four times per day. Longer-acting solutions containing methylcellulose are also helpful (Table 11-2). The patient should be referred if symptoms are unrelieved or if underlying disease is present or suspected.[6,12]

CORNEAL ABRASION

The patient presenting with corneal abrasion is typically aware of the offending agent and may have experienced trauma to the eye, such as an object touching the eye while the lid is open. The patient may have symptoms from edema of the cornea that can occur, for example, from wearing contact lens for too long a time. Patients particularly at risk are those with extended wear lenses. Abrasion due to contact lens overuse may quickly evolve into an ulceration and has the potential to cause blindness. An exam reveals redness concentrated around the limbus and irritation or pain of the cornea. In the event of trauma, the midwife should examine the cornea to ensure that no residual irritant or foreign body is present. The presence of significant pain and photophobia require a referral for examination.

Abrasions caused by trauma or wearing contact lenses require an examination with fluoroscien, which is most often performed by an ophthalmologist but can be performed by other providers who have received training in this technique. Patients diagnosed with corneal abrasions are generally treated with antibiotic ophthalmic medication and patching of the eye. However, not all authorities agree that patching is useful and some believe that patching may increase the risk of infection.[13] Others think that patching should be avoided if the abrasion is caused by a contact lens or vegetable matter.[5] Therefore, consultation may be warranted in questionable cases. The patient should be re-examined in 24 hours.[5–8] If the patient is receiving care from her primary care provider and no improvement is seen in 24 hours, then the patient should be referred to an ophthalmologist. If a laceration or ulceration is suspected, or if white spots are noted on the cornea indicating keratitis, the patient should be referred immediately. Use of contact lenses should be resumed only after the cornea is completely healed.[5,7,8]

FOREIGN BODY

The patient with a foreign body presents with a complaint of redness, excessive tearing, presence of an eye irritant, and mild photophobia. The patient may or may not be aware of the cause of the sudden onset of these symptoms. The eye should be examined using a cotton-tipped applicator to evert the eyelid. With the nondominant hand, the midwife should place the cotton-tipped applicator on the outer eyelid margin, gently rolling the eyelid back. The cornea and surrounding areas should be examined with a penlight. The foreign body should be removed with a cotton-tipped applicator held in the dominant hand. The eye also can be

Table 11-4 SPECIALIZED TESTS GENERALLY PERFORMED BY AN OPHTHALMOLOGIST

Test	Notes
Fluorescein exam	Used for suspected abrasions, fluorescein is placed in the eye and then examined under a blue light to expose defects in the surface of the eye.
Dilated exam	Medications are used to dilate the pupil, making it non-reactive to light. This allows a clearer and more extensive examination of the interior eye and the retinal area.
Tonometry	Used to measure intraocular pressure for the diagnosis and management of glaucoma. Normal pressure is 10–24 mm Hg.
Magnetic resonance imaging or computed tomography scan	Used to identify lesions, tumors, or pockets of fluid.

rinsed with saline. To do this, the patient should sit in a chair, preferably leaning to the injured side over a sink or large container. A large needleless syringe can be filled with saline and the fluid gently released over the open, affected eye. Intravenous (IV) tubing attached to a 1 liter bag of saline can be used as well. Removal should result in relief of symptoms. If the object cannot be flushed or removed easily, prompt referral to an opthalmologist should be considered. If injury to the cornea or sclera is suspected, the foreign body appears imbedded in the eye tissue, or there is known exposure to a penetrating foreign body such as metallic or wood fragments, or if there is no improvement in 24 hours, referral is required.[5,8,11]

CHEMICAL SPLASH

The patient presenting to the office with a history of a chemical splash and complaints of burning and redness of the eye should immedi-

ately have the eye rinsed with 1 liter of saline.[8] The patient is then referred for immediate ophthalmic evaluation. If the splash took place at the patient's place of work, Occupational Safety and Health Administration guidelines mandate that there be available a description of the composition of the substance (Material Data Safety Sheets), which should be available to the patient and the examining provider and can provide guidance about appropriate treatment.

TRAUMA

The patient presenting with trauma to the eye may simply have a bruised eyelid requiring no treatment, such as a black eye, or may have significant injury. The vision exam, eye exam, and fundoscopy should be normal in those who present with a black eye. Any blunt trauma resulting in blurred vision or vision loss, headache, flashing lights, suspected infection, unequal pupils, painful orbit, bleeding, or injury to the sclera is cause for immediate referral.[6,8] A blue sclera may be indicative of bleeding into the vitreous and also requires immediate referral.

HERPES ZOSTER AND HERPES SIMPLEX

The patient who has herpes zoster or simplex infections of the eye requires immediate referral. The patient typically has a prior history of varicella or herpes simplex infections, and may report a history of periorbital pain and itching or headache. In *herpes zoster*, the patient may have a history of fever or malaise and lesions along the division of the trigeminal nerve that leads to the eye. In *herpes simplex*, the patient may have had a recent viral infection or upper respiratory infection (URI). Lesions may be noted on the nose, face, or eyelid in addition to the cornea. Damage to the cornea may occur in both if not appropriately treated.[5,6,8]

EPISCLERITIS, SCLERITIS, IRITIS, AND UVEITIS

Episcleritis is an inflammation of the tissue between the sclera and the conjunctiva. The eye appears red, suggesting conjunctivitis, but there is no discharge. Inflammation of the deeper tissue, termed *scleritis*, presents with redness of the eye and a pink sclera. This is often accompanied by deep ocular pain. Inflammation of the anterior portion of the eye is termed *iritis* or *anterior uveitis*. Symptoms include photophobia, ocular pain, constricted pupil, and redness of the circumcorneal area. An ophthalmologic exam of the anterior eye reveals inflammatory cells in the vitreous humor or on the cornea. Inflammation of the posterior portion of the eye, or *posterior uveitis*, typically has as the primary symptom decreased vision. It may occur alone or along with inflammation of the anterior eye. Patients with a history of chronic disease such as inflammatory bowel disease or autoimmune disorders, and infections such as Lyme disease, cytomegalovirus

(CMV), or toxoplasmosis are particularly at risk.[7,14] In some cases, ophthalmic manifestations may be the presenting symptom of underlying disease. A patient with any of these suspected conditions requires immediate referral to avoid permanent vision impairment.[5,7,8,14]

Subconjunctival Hemorrhage

Subconjunctival hemorrhage results from bleeding from the blood vessels between the conjunctiva and the episclera. The eye appears red from the bleeding, but there is no pain and vision is normal. The patient frequently reports a history of trauma to the eye such as rubbing the eye roughly, coughing, vigorous activity, or valsalva maneuver such as pushing in the second stage of labor. Healing occurs spontaneously within two weeks.

REFRACTIVE ERROR

Refractive errors are usually slow in onset resulting in decreased or blurry vision over time. These errors may result from the eye globe being too long (*myopia*), too short (*hyperopia*), or not perfectly round (*astigmatism*). All of these prevent the light entering the eye from being focused directly onto the retina. Also, as humans age, the lens loses its refractive abilities and thus diminishes the ability to see close objects clearly (*presbyopia*). Referral for evaluation for corrective lenses is necessary. The "pinhole test" is a rapid screening tool to determine if blurry vision is due to refractive error.[7]

Cataracts

Cataracts affect approximately 20.5 million individuals more than 40 years old in America.[15] The patient with cataracts may complain of progressive blurred vision without pain or evidence of erythema. Upon exam, the lens is cloudy and can be seen with a penlight in advanced cases.

The cause may be congenital, metabolic, acquired, or senile.[8] Congenital cataracts are often caused by viral infections such as CMV. Metabolic causes include systemic diseases, such as diabetes which causes changes to the lens because of episodes of hyperglycemia. Acquired cataracts can be due to damage to the lens from injury such as burns. Senile cataracts occur in aging patients as the lens gradually becomes denser with age. Corrective glasses may compensate for the change in the lens, thus delaying surgery or making it unnecessary. Referral for full eye evaluation and assessment of surgical intervention is essential. Clinicians should advise all patients to wear sunglasses with ultraviolet (UV) protection in the sunlight. Exposure to UV light has been shown to increase the risk of certain types of cataracts.[16]

GLAUCOMA

Glaucoma is a disease in which the optic nerve becomes damaged leading to visual field loss and eventually blindness; this usually occurs because of increased intraocular pressure. The damage may also occur with normal intraocular pressure, possibly because of extreme tissue sensitivity. On fundoscopy, the physiologic cup holding the optic disc appears to enlarge. This is thought to occur as the nerve fibers holding the optic disc are destroyed, causing the disc to become smaller. This appearance is called *cupping*. The exact physiology of this process is unknown. The cup-to-disc ratio, intraocular pressure, and assessment of the visual field are followed to indicate progression of disease. Glaucoma may occur abruptly and acutely or progressively over time. Both situations require referral. While a thorough evaluation is best done by an ophthalmologist, some screening tests can be done in the office. Treatment includes the management and reduction of the intraocular pressure. Patients

with this condition are typically older, but glaucoma can occur at any age.

Primary open-angle glaucoma is the most common type of glaucoma. *Open-angle glaucoma* occurs without structural blockage of fluid movement through the eye. It is more common as individuals age and may be genetic. Glaucoma is three to four times more common in African Americans; it is the leading cause of blindness in this population.[7,17] Often it is identified on a routine ophthalmic exam in the early stages without patient-perceived symptoms. The initial sign found on examination by the ophthalmologist may be increased intraocular pressure with or without cupping. In the case of normal pressure glaucoma, cupping may be seen without elevated intraocular pressure. The disease worsens progressively over time, so if it is undiagnosed or untreated, loss of peripheral vision results in tunnel vision and eventually blindness. Management is focused on reduction of the intraocular pressure and may include medications and/or surgery.

Secondary glaucoma can have several causes, including trauma, uveitis, diabetes mellitus, and vascular disease, among other conditions. In addition, the recent administration of ophthalmic or systemic steroid medications can also cause secondary glaucoma. The increased intraocular pressure usually abates over several months after the medication is stopped. However, the loss of vision that occurs during medication use may not resolve.[8] The symptoms and management of secondary glaucoma are similar to primary open angle glaucoma. Treatment and management of the underlying conditions causing secondary glaucoma can also affect the patient's outcome. These patients should be evaluated by an ophthalmologist.[8]

Acute angle-closure glaucoma is rare and occurs if the flow of aqueous fluid through the anterior chamber angle is blocked. This process is initiated by dilation of the pupil causing the border of the iris to block the angle and disrupt the movement of fluid through the angle, resulting in an abrupt rise in intraocular pressure. Acute increases in intraocular pressure can occur with use of some medications, such as anticholinergic or sympathomimetic agents (e.g., some antidepressants or nasal decongestants).[6] The acute episode is usually precipitated after pupilary dilation such as can occur in a darkened room or cinema. Symptoms include moderate-to-severe pain, eye redness, halos around lights, and a dilated pupil, usually in only one eye. The eye feels hard to palpation. The patient may also have headache, nausea, and vomiting. These latter systemic symptoms may confuse the clinical picture, making it easier to ignore or downplay the ocular symptoms, and result in a delay in diagnosis. Individuals of Asian descent are at higher risk for this type of glaucoma. Immediate referral is necessary in order to institute treatment and prevent permanent loss of vision.[6–8, 18]

Congenital glaucoma is caused by conditions, including congenital rubella, and genetic defects or congenital syndromes producing a structural defect or condition that leads to glaucoma during infancy or childhood.[19] Treatment by a pediatric ophthalmologist may be surgical as well as medical.

AGE-RELATED MACULAR DEGENERATION

Age-related macular degeneration is the primary cause of loss of vision for older individuals. Atrophic or "dry" macular degeneration occurs when hard yellow deposits (termed *drusen*) form on the macular area of the retina. The resulting atrophy causes progressive loss of central vision and may be severe. In early disease, the patient may complain of "holes" in her vision. Screening with the Amsler's grid (Table 11-3) may reveal distortion of vision in early disease.[20] Although there is no treatment, referral for evaluation is necessary to accurately identify the cause of the vision loss. Exudative or "wet" macular degeneration occurs when blood or serous fluid seeps into the retina, separating the delicate layers and resulting in sudden visual loss. Urgent referral is needed to prevent permanent loss of vision.[6–8,13]

Women with macular degeneration and other eye conditions leading to loss of vision are at risk for depression with even a small reduction of vision.[17] In addition, patients are at risk for limited mobility and decreased ability to perform activities of daily living.[21] The provider can be particularly helpful in referring the patient to services for low-vision.

Smoking is a known risk factor for age-related macular degeneration. All clinicians should advocate smoking cessation at an early age to diminish the risk of developing this condition (**Table 11-5**).[16]

FLOATERS AND FLASHES

Reports by patients of "spots before my eyes" or floating spots are often a benign manifestation of aging. The vitreous fluid may develop small opacities that can interfere with vision, which often resolve over time. The eye exam is normal. Sudden development of floaters or flashes of light should be referred to rule out retinal detachment.[6,8,11]

RETINAL DETACHMENT

Patients with a history of cataract extraction, myopia, or trauma are most at risk for retinal detachment. Symptoms include floaters or flashes of light in the visual field, sudden loss of vision, and blurry or progressively blurry vision. These symptoms occur without pain or redness of the eye. Thinning or weakness in the retina

---

Table 11-5 PRIMARY CARE TEACHING POINTS FOR PATIENTS FOR THE
PRESERVATION OF VISION

1. Prevention of eye infections:
   - Change eye makeup, particularly mascara, every 3 months
   - Do not share eye makeup or applicators
   - Wash hands prior to touching eye, changing contact lenses, or applying makeup
2. Use protective eye wear when working with tools, potentially caustic liquids, and during recreation.
3. Wear sunglasses to protect eyes from harmful ultraviolet rays when out in natural sunlight or using
   tanning beds. Limiting exposure can decrease the risk of developing some types of cataracts.
4. Stop smoking to decrease risk of developing cataracts and age-related macular degeneration.
5. If diabetic, keep blood glucose levels in control to decrease risk of developing diabetic retinopathy.
6. Have regular routine screening to identify and treat potentially serious problems such as glaucoma.

---

can lead to a hole causing leakage of vitreous fluid. The fluid build-up behind the retina leads to detachment. Upon ophthalmic exam, the retina will appear to be "hanging."[7,8]

Another type of detachment is due to diabetic retinopathy or retinal vein occlusion. In this type of detachment, the underlying disease causes development of fibrous tissue that causes traction on the retina and eventually causing detachment. Ophthalmic exam reveals an irregular retinal surface. Immediate referral to an ophthalmologist is necessary.[6] If the patient presents to the office with these complaints, the patient should be transported lying down and with minimal movement to prevent further damage; doing so allows the retina to fall back into place.[6]

MIGRAINE

Patients with migraine headaches may present with a prodromal visual aura lasting approximately 20 minutes before the onset of the headache. The patient may present with visual disturbances, complaints of loss of or alterations in visual field that move or "dance," or flashes of light. See Chapter 10 for further information on headaches.

The Ear

Patients presenting with ear-related symptoms in midwifery practices most commonly complain of ear pain, although some will also report loss of hearing, vertigo, or tinnitus. These symptoms can indicate an array of problems ranging from local and systemic infections to malfunctions of the inner ear to age-related or environmentally induced hearing loss. This section of the chapter discusses the evaluation and management of these common symptoms in the women's health setting.

Clinical Presentation

PAIN

Two of the most common causes of ear pain in adults are otitis externa (OE) and otitis media (OM). Although otitis media is typically thought of as a pediatric diagnosis, it can occur in persons over the age of 15. According to the National Ambulatory Medical Care Survey conducted between 1975 and 1990, approximately 20% of ambulatory physician visits because of otitis media were made by persons over the age of 15.[22] Pain results from localized swelling, inflammation, or infection, which can be caused by a variety of other conditions such as myringitis, mastoiditis, cysts, or furuncles. Pain can also be a result of trauma, neoplasm, or temporomandibular joint dysfunction. Eliciting a history of the initial presentation, associated symptoms, and progression of the problem can help limit the possibilities under consideration. For example, individuals who have had trauma to the ear often initially experience hearing loss, but may also report dizziness or pain, and even facial weakness if nerve damage has occurred.[23] *Mastoiditis*, an infection of the mastoid bone, is rare today, but was common in the pre-antibiotic era as a complication after infections such as otitis media. Today those presenting with an antecedent and inadequately treated otitis media are at risk for mastoiditis. Cancers of the oral cavity and throat can also cause ear-related pain or affect hearing, but are rare in ambulatory care and are usually accompanied by other more prominent signs and symptoms such as difficulty swallowing, muffled speech, oral lesions, and palpable masses in the neck.[24]

VERTIGO, DIZZINESS, AND TINNITUS

Women experiencing *vertigo* describe it as movement, most commonly as "the room is spinning." Vertigo should be differentiated from *dizziness* and fainting, which is more often described as "feeling light-headed." Not all patients with vertigo or dizziness will be able to describe their symptoms clearly. True vertigo tends to wax and wane. Those with continuous symptoms usually do not have vertigo. Head movement usually exacerbates vertigo; therefore, if symptoms do not worsen with head movement, vertigo is unlikely. Other movements, such as sneezing, coughing, or valsalva

maneuvers, which can change pressure in the middle ear or result in movement of the head, often precipitate vertigo.[25] Mimicking these movements may help diagnose vertigo and differentiate vertigo from *presyncope*, which is much more common in women seen in midwifery practice, particularly in women who are dehydrated from excessive blood loss or hyperemesis. Vertigo can be severe enough that women may be unable to maintain enough balance to walk and is often accompanied by nystagmus. Nystagmus can be subtle and may not be clinically obvious, requiring the use of specialized tests in order to identify its presence.

The duration of vertigo can offer a clue as to its cause. Vertigo that lasts less than one minute can be seen in disorders of the peripheral vestibular system such as benign paroxysmal positional vertigo. Episodes lasting from a few minutes to several hours can be due to Ménière's disease, transient cerebral hypoperfusion, or phobic/anxiety disorders, although vertigo in Ménière's disease can be longer-lasting. Viral infections can present with a complaint of acute rotational vertigo that can last for several days before improving gradually.[26]

A sense of balance is achieved by the integration in the brain stem of neural messages from the vestibular system, information from proprioceptive receptors in the joints, skin, and muscles (particularly the neck and ankles), and visual inputs. Nerve impulses are stimulated by the movement of cilia in the fluid-filled spaces of the semicircular canals of the inner ear and are sent to the vestibular nuclei in the brain stem and cerebellum. The semicircular canals are arranged so that each lies in a different plane at right angles to each other. They are responsible for helping the body sense movement from side to side, up and down, and tilting. The utricle and the saccule, which are connected to the lower ends of the semicircular canals, are responsible for helping the body determine if it is still and to sense acceleration (movement forward in a straight line) and gravity. The visual system provides a reference to the horizon. The proprioceptive system gives feedback on the position of the legs in space and detects movement of the feet. Approximately 70% of balance is due to visual input, 15% from proprioception, and 15% from the vestibular system.[27] Vertigo can be caused by problems in any of these pathways, by central conditions such as multiple sclerosis, brain tumors, or cerebrovascular disease, and by peripheral conditions such as trauma or infection in the ear. It can also be caused by physiological changes such as hyperventilation.

Tinnitus is often described as "ringing in the ear," but any sensation of sound is considered to be tinnitus. It can be intermittent or continuous, in one or both ears, or seem to be caused by a source outside of the body. The cause is unknown. It is a nonspecific finding and is common in many ear-related conditions, particularly those that result in hearing loss, but it also may be a manifestation of systemic diseases such as cardiovascular disease (hypertension, cardiac failure), a hyperdynamic circulation (anemia, fever, drugs), and neurological conditions (multiple sclerosis, neuropathy).[28]

Few women report symptoms of vertigo, dizziness, or tinnitus in ambulatory settings in which midwives practice, but they can be seen in women who have postural hypotension from severe anemia or dehydration and in those who have had a recent viral infection.

PRURITIS

Pruritis of the outer and inner ear can occur with OE, but can also be due to other skin conditions such as seborrhea, contact dermatitis, eczema, or psoriasis, which can affect the skin of the outer ear and ear canal as well as other parts of the body.[29] Seborrhea is commonly found on the scalp and nasolabial folds, and presents as red, greasy scales. It can be seen on the external ear, outer ear canal, or most commonly behind the posterior auricle and along the hairline behind the ear.[30] Psoriasis can be found in these same locations and classically has a silver-white scale. Eczema is typically found along the cubital and popliteal fossae of the extremities. In the ear, it presents as a dry scale on an inflamed base.[30] Oozing can occur. Contact dermatitis can develop after exposure to metal (often from earrings), hair products, perfume, medications, or soap. Exposure leads to pruritis, edema, vesicles, and erythema.[31]

HEARING LOSS

Hearing loss is caused by conditions that block sound from passing into the inner ear (*conductive hearing loss*) or by conditions that disrupt the processing of sound in the brain (*sensorineural loss*). In ambulatory practice, one of the most common causes of hearing loss is blockage of the ear canal from cerumen impaction. Conductive hearing loss can also be caused by a swollen ear canal as in OE, the buildup of debris in the ear canal found with psoriasis or other skin conditions, and fluid buildup in the inner ear or a ruptured ear drum commonly seen with otitis media. Sensorineural hearing loss can be a result of a stroke, tumor, viral cochleitis, noise, and aging, among other conditions. An accurate and complete history and physical as well as hearing tests can help differentiate these possibilities.

Distinguishing the underlying cause(s) of ear pain, vertigo, dizziness, and hearing loss can be difficult. However, certain patterns of symptoms and physical findings may indicate a specific diagnosis. **Tables 11-6, 11-7, and 11-8** describe the presentation of various conditions that can present with ear pain, vertigo, or loss of hearing. Many of these conditions present with some or all of these symptoms in varying degrees and are listed by their most common presenting symptom.

Essential History, Physical, and Laboratory Evaluation

HISTORY

The history should focus initially on the symptom of greatest concern to the patient. If a patient complains primarily of pain, she should be asked: 1) to identify which part of the ear is in pain; 2) when and where the pain originated; 3) the characteristics of the pain, particularly if it has increased in the affected area; and 4) whether the onset of pain was associated with a specific precipitating event such as trauma, illness, or allergic exacerbation. If the patient reports discharge, further questions include its color, odor, timing, and duration. Discharge from the ear can occur with otitis externa as well as with infections or trauma if the tympanic membrane has ruptured or bleeding has occurred. Midwives should also inquire about other associated symptoms. These may include a cough, sore throat, swollen glands, or fever, which could indicate an infection; nausea, vomiting, or vertigo, which could indicate a neurological problem such as a tumor; and recent dental work or toothache, which cause referred pain from the oral cavity. Ear pain may result from damage to the ear canal, the eardrum, and the inner ear. Inquiry is made for exposure to extreme cold, barotraumas from flying and diving,

or excessive noise; whether headphones or noise-muffling protective gear have been used appropriately for work or recreation; and whether gentle nonabrasive methods are employed for cleansing the ear. The use of cotton-tipped applicators can lead to OE by causing microabrasions of the ear canal that become secondarily infected.

If a patient complains primarily of hearing loss, then she should be questioned on the acuity of the presentation. Sudden hearing loss is most often associated with viral infections, but may also present with acoustic neuroma, perilymphatic fistula, Ménière's disease, vascular insufficiency, multiple sclerosis, and other central etiologies. More gradual hearing loss can be due to damage from excessive noise exposure and is also seen with aging.

A full history should be obtained to determine if the patient has other conditions such as prior hospitalizations and antibiotic use; previous surgery of, injury, or radiation to the head or neck, pregnancy, or other medical problems that could impact the presentation or management of ear-related problems.

PHYSICAL EXAMINATION

A complete physical examination of the head, eyes, ears, nose, and throat is required in the investigation of ear-related symptoms. Depending on which diagnoses are most likely, additional testing such as an examination of the heart and lungs or hearing evaluation may also be needed.

A thorough ear examination should include all of the following components:

- *External Ear:* Note all areas of the auricle for size, shape, color, lesions, edema, and injury including evidence of trauma, frostbite, or burns. Gently pull

Table 11-6 **Differential Diagnosis Table: Ear Pain**

Condition	Associated Findings	History and Physical Findings	Refer If
Inner Ear Pain			
Acute otitis media (AOM)	Fever. Otalgia (if history of sudden relief from pain, suspect perforation). Tinnitus. Vertigo. Otorrhea (if perforation). More likely if recent history of upper respiratory infection (URI), influenza, or pneumonia.	External ear canal: normal. Ear canal: discharge in canal indicates perforation of tympanic membrane. Otoscopy: omit pneumatic otoscopy if suspect perforation. Tympanic membrane: bulging, red, opaque, yellow indicates purulent discharge. Reduced or absent mobility.	Persistent or repetitive episodes of AOM. History of trauma. Blue tympanic membrane: indicative of presence of blood. Facial paralysis or weakness. Cholesteatoma. Post-auricular edema, redness. Suspected mastoiditis or meningitis. Co-existing disease such as diabetes or prior radiation of head or neck.
Otitis media with effusion (OME)	Fullness in ear. Tinnitus on affected side. Hearing loss. Pain. Can be asymptomatic. More common if a history of recent allergy, URI, or AOM. Other risk factors: exposure to passive smoke, structural defect of Eustachian tube, barotraumas.	External ear: normal. Ear canal: no discharge. Tympanic membrane: bulging; may be mobile or immobile; clear, cloudy or gray; presence of air bubbles.	Persistent hearing loss or tinnitus. Persistent OME for more than 3 months. Suspicion of carcinoma. Persistent perforated tympanic membrane with or without suspected infection.
Bullous myringitis	Severe otalgia of inner ear or external ear canal. Possible serous or blood otorrhea. Hearing loss. Tinnitus.	Otoscopy: intra-epithelial fluid pockets of tympanic membrane or external ear canal. Tympanic membrane: mobile and clear or presence of pockets of intraepithelial fluid.	Lancing of fluid pockets required for pain relief. Persistent hearing loss or tinnitus.

(continues)

Table 11-6 DIFFERENTIAL DIAGNOSIS TABLE: EAR PAIN *(continued)*

Condition	Associated Findings	History and Physical Findings	Refer If
Inner Ear Pain			
Herpes zoster	Severe otalgia of inner or outer ear. Herpetic lesions. Facial palsy. Vertigo.	Otoscopy: herpetic lesions visible or not visible. Tympanic membrane: mobile; may or may not have lesions; may not be able to examine because of pain.	Suspect this etiology. Must refer if lesions present or facial palsy.
Herpes simplex	May or may not have pain. Facial palsy (Bell's palsy). Possible history of recent viral infection.	Otoscopy: herpetic lesions usually not visible. Tympanic membrane: mobile, clear.	Suspect this etiology.
Cerumen impaction	Hearing loss on affected side. Tinnitus on affected side. Feeling of fullness in ear.	Difficult or unable to do otoscopy due to impacted cerumen. Tympanic membrane: unable to see.	Unable to remove wax or suspect perforated tympanic membrane.
Foreign body	Hearing loss. Feeling of fullness in ear. Tinnitus. After removal of foreign body, may see symptoms of otis externa.	Otoscopy: presence of maggot, tick, or other insect is common. Can also see other organic or inorganic foreign body.	Unable to remove foreign body.
Perforation of tympanic membrane	Vertigo. Hearing loss and/or tinnitus on affected side. History of ear pain with sudden relief associated with perforation. Can be seen with otitis media or with sudden change in inner ear pressure due to barrotrauma such as air travel or scuba diving. Suspect if history of ear trauma. Can occur if ear was cleaned with a foreign object.	Otoscopy: clear, slightly bloody, yellow discharge in external canal. Do not perform pneumatic otoscopy. Tympanic membrane: perforation with clear, slightly bloody, or yellow otorrhea.	Persistent perforation with or without otorrhea. Persistent hearing loss or vertigo. Suspect associated mastoiditis. Cholesteatoma.

Table 11-6 **DIFFERENTIAL DIAGNOSIS TABLE: EAR PAIN** (*continued*)

Condition	Associated Findings	History and Physical Findings	Refer If
Temporo-mandibu-lar joint disorder	Feeling of ear fullness. Tinnitus. Dizziness. Difficulty or pain with eating. Associated with bruxism or grinding teeth at night and dental disorders.	External ear: normal. Otoscopy: normal. Palpation of the joint produces pain. May hear "click" with opening mouth. Tympanic membrane: mobile, clear.	Patient has dental disorders or if symptoms persist despite treatment by a dentist.
Outer Ear Pain			
Otitis externa	Pruritis of outer or inner ear. Pinna pain. Otorrhea. Hearing loss and/or tinnitus on affected side if canal with significant edema. Prolonged exposure to water or moisture. Local irritation or trauma.	Exam of external ear and canal: white, green, or foul smelling discharge in canal. Discharge may not be present. Edema and redness of canal. Edema may block canal. Foreign body. Pain elicited by movement of pinna. Tympanic membrane: clear, non-bulging.	Condition does not resolve or suspect abscess formation.
Furunculosis	Discharge. Tenderness limited to the affected area.	Pustule and erythyma noted in outer third of ear canal. Tympanic membrane: mobile, clear.	Symptoms persist despite treatment or suspect abscess formation.
Trauma	History of injury to external ear. Vertigo.	External ear may be injured. If blunt trauma, otoscopy may reveal blood in canal. Tympanic membrane: may appear blue due to presence of blood behind membrane. If ruptured, may be clear or bloody.	Suspect trauma has occurred.

Table 11-7 DIFFERENTIAL DIAGNOSIS FOR VERTIGO

Symptom and Condition	History and Associated Symptoms	Physical Findings	When to Refer
Orthostatic hypotension	Dizziness or faintness upon standing without "spinning." Suspect if severe or sudden anemia, dehydration, or recent illness.	Positive findings for orthostatic hypotension.	Persistent anemia or dehydration without known cause.
Hypoglycemia	Dizziness or feeling "faint," without "spinning." Suspect if inadequate nutrition or has underlying diabetes mellitus.	Neurological, physical, and otoscopic exam normal.	Abnormal glucose testing.
Hyperventilation syndrome	Dizziness or lightheadedness with rapid breathing during stress.	Normal exam or may be hypotensive during episode of hyperventilation.	
Cardiac	May report episodes of faintness or actual syncope with or without palpitations or pain.	Normal neurological and otoscopic exams. May hear palpitations as skipped beats on auscultation of heart. Refer for evaluation.	Abnormal EKG and/ Holter monitoring results. Consult as needed.
Benign paroxysmal positional vertigo	Occasionally, head trauma. Often pattern of sleep on affected side.	Normal neurological exam. Positive or negative Romberg test. Normal gait. Dix-Hallpike maneuver: positive.	May require Electronystagmography or MRI to rule out more serious causes. Consult as needed.

Table 11-7 **DIFFERENTIAL DIAGNOSIS FOR VERTIGO** *(continued)*

Symptom and Condition	History and Associated Symptoms	Physical Findings	When to Refer
Labyrinthitis (vestibular neuronitis)	Episodes of vertigo as "spinning" and then mild vertigo lasting several days. Tinnitus: unilateral. Hearing loss: unilateral. Nausea and vomiting. History of recent upper respiratory infection, AOM, OME.	Normal neurological exam. Romberg test may be positive. Balance can be normal or can fall to affected side. Otoscopic exam to note lesions, inflammation, or perforation of the tympanic membrane. Refer for perforation, presence of blood or cholesteatoma.	Condition suspected.
Drug induced	Vertigo. Tinnitus. Hearing loss. History of using ototoxic drugs, in particular aminoglycosides. Other common medications/substances: salicylates, indomethacin, gargamazepine, propanolol, mesalamine, caffeine, alcohol, nicotine.	Balance may be normal or patient may fall to affected side.	Condition persists. May need audiogram. Often resolves with cessation or decrease in medication or substance.

(continues)

Table 11-7 **DIFFERENTIAL DIAGNOSIS FOR VERTIGO** *(continued)*

Symptom and Condition	History and Associated Symptoms	Physical Findings	When to Refer
Ménière's disease	Symptoms are not continuous, has episodes of vertigo, described as "spinning." Tinnitus described as like "roaring" and clanging. Feeling of fullness in the ear during episodes. Loss of balance. Nausea and vomiting. Usually unilateral hearing loss. If hearing loss bilateral, one ear often more affected than the other.	During episode: abnormal gait and positive Romberg test. Between episodes may have normal exam.	Condition is suspected. May need audiogram, Electronystagmography, or MRI.
Vertebrobasilar insufficiency	Frequent cause of vertigo in elderly. Initiated by hyperextension of neck or postural change.	Normal neurological, otoscopic, and physical exam. May be able to elicit response during exam.	Condition suspected.
Ischemia due to vertebrobasilar insufficiency	Severe vertigo. Nausea. Vomiting. May have visual disturbances or hallucinations. Drop attacks without faintness.	Usually accompanied by abnormal neurological exam, but may exist as only symptom of stroke.	Condition suspected.

Table 11-7 **DIFFERENTIAL DIAGNOSIS FOR VERTIGO** *(continued)*

Symptom and Condition	History and Associated Symptoms	Physical Findings	When to Refer
Multiple sclerosis	Intermittent vertigo with persistent imbalance without precipitating event. May report accompanying neurologic dysfunction such as visual disturbances, hearing loss, unsteady gait. Tinnitus: generally bilateral, pulsatile with clicking but presentation varies. Hearing loss.	Normal or abnormal neurological screen. May have abnormal gait.	Condition suspected. May need MRI.
Intracranial lesions or tumors	Persistent severe vertigo. Nausea and/or vomiting. Unilateral hearing loss. Tinnitus.	Usually accompanied by abnormal neurological exam.	Condition suspected.
Acoustic neuroma	Vertigo may be mild or nonexistent. Unilateral hearing loss.	Abnormal office hearing exam with normal otoscopic exam.	Condition suspected. May need audiogram or MRI.
Migraine	History of migraine headaches. Vertigo can occur with or without headache and can be transient or persistent.	See Chapter 10 for evaluation of migraine syndrome.	Headaches not relieved with standard management or become progressively worse over time.
Clinical depression or anxiety	Often associated with other somatic complaints. May be accompanied by hyperventilation syndrome.	Normal physical, otoscopic, and neurological exam.	See Chapter 9 for details on management of these conditions.

Table 11-8 DIFFERENTIAL DIAGNOSIS TABLE: HEARING LOSS

Symptom and Condition	History and Associated Symptoms	Physical Findings	Management
Presbycusis (age-related)	Bilateral hearing loss. Tinnitus.	Otoscopy: normal. External ear: normal. Neurological exam: normal. Physical exam: normal.	Audiogram. Refer for evaluation for hearing aid.
Congenital or genetic disease	Family history of hearing loss. Intrauterine anoxia, infection, metabolic, or endocrine disorder.	Otoscopy: normal unless presence of congenital malformation. External ear: normal unless presence of congenital malformation.	Refer for evaluation.
Osteosclerosis	Hearing loss. Tinnitus: roaring or hissing.	External ear normal. Otoscopy normal. Physical exam normal. Neurological exam normal.	May need audiogram. Refer for evaluation and possible surgical repair.
Environmental noise	Damage can occur with episodic or chronic exposure. Hearing loss and/or tinnitus may be unilateral or bilateral.	External ear normal. Otoscopy normal. Neurological exam normal.	May need audiogram. Symptoms usually resolve over time if exposure diminishes to safe levels or ceases. Refer for evaluation if persistent symptoms.

Refer to Tables 11-6 and 11-7 for other conditions that cause hearing loss.

up on the auricle and move the tragus, noting any pain. Palpate the mastoid area for tenderness and edema. Examine the external auditory canal, noting any signs of discharge, odor, edema, lesions, and foreign objects.

- *Otoscopic Exam:* Use the largest ear speculum that the ear will accommodate and is tolerated by the patient to examine the ear canal and the middle ear. Place the patient in a comfortable sitting-up position. Gently, but firmly, hold the auricle, pulling it up and backwards to straighten the ear canal. With the opposite hand, hold the otoscope with the handle pointing upward, inserting the speculum gently. Cerumen may need to be removed prior to proceeding with the exam. Note the condition of the canal including redness, lesions, foreign objects, discharge, cerumen, and edema. Examine the tympanic membrane noting color (red, white, opaque, clear, pearly gray, yellow); presence of air bubbles, lesions, or masses; contour (bulging, flat, retracted), identification and position of landmarks. For orientation, note particularly the position of the short process and handle of the malleus, the umbo, and the cone of light. Move the speculum to clearly see the entire membrane. It can be common to see thick, white plaques on the membrane called tympanosclerosis in the patient with a history of ventilation tubes. Note perforations and any discharge. If perforated, note location of perforation, discharge, and the presence of any lesions. During pregnancy there is an increase in vascularity due to increased levels of estrogen. Slight redness in the canal or noted on the tympanic membrane is not in and of itself a significant finding, especially in the pregnant woman because of the increase in vascularity.

- *Pneumatic Otoscopy:* This test is essential for the diagnosis of otitis media. For an accurate exam, ensure that the speculum seal is tight within the ear canal, thus preventing outside air from entering. A soft-tipped speculum works best for this exam. Gently press the pneumatic bulb attachment, forcing air into the ear canal. The normal tympanic membrane will move inward. The abnormal membrane will be sluggish or immobile. Do not perform this test if a perforation of the tympanic membrane is noted. Practice will increase the provider's skill and ease with this exam.

- *Other Tests:* Other physical examination techniques are also helpful when evaluating specific symptoms. **Table 11-9** describes maneuvers that can be performed in the office.

More sophisticated tests for which referral is required can be performed when the diagnosis is unclear. For example, tympanometry and acoustic reflectometry can confirm middle ear fluid and can help pinpoint a specific diagnosis. During tympanometry, changes in movement of the tympanic membrane (compliance) are measured in response to various air pressures in the ear canal. In addition to detecting if fluid is in the inner ear, tympanometry can help determine if the tympanic membrane is scarred or ruptured, if a tumor is present, and if there is a dysfunction of the Eustachian tube. Acoustic reflectometry is used to measure the contractions of the stapedial muscle in response to varying levels of sound. The response of the muscle to specific levels of sound indicates the presence or absence of disorders of the ear, cranial nerves, and the brainstem. These tests, while useful, do not replace a thorough basic examination including an office evaluation of the tympanic membrane using pneumatic otoscopy.

LABORATORY

Few laboratory tests are helpful in the evaluation of ear pain. A complete blood count with differential may be helpful in selected cases if underlying infection is thought to be a contributing factor in ear pain but is usually not

Table 11-9 PHYSICAL EXAMINATION: EVALUATION OF VERTIGO

Test	Procedure	Results
Romberg's Test	The patient 1. Stands with feet together with heels and toes touching. 2. Closes her eyes. 3. Extends both arms with palms facing the floor.	Normal/negative: The patient stands without swaying or repositioning the feet. Abnormal/positive: The patient is unsteady or must reposition the feet to maintain balance.
Gait	The patient is instructed to: 1. Walk normally in a straight line. 2. Walk on tiptoes. 3. Walk in a straight line heel to toe with one foot placed ahead of the other. 4. Turn around and return.	Normal/negative: If the patient is able to complete the walks as instructed with erect posture. Abnormal/positive If the patient loses balance or performs steps using an abnormal gait such as dragging a foot, stepping unevenly, or favoring one side.
Dix-Hallpike Maneuver	The patient is placed in a recumbent position. The head is turned toward the affected side. Wait 60 seconds.	Positive: vertigo induced when head in turned position for several seconds. Lasts less than 60 seconds. Nystagmus can be noted toward the affected side as vertigo is induced.
Nylen-Br'r'ny Maneuvers	The patient is instructed to: 1. Sit on the exam table with head turned to side. 2. The midwife lowers the patient to the supine position, head over the edge of the table and 30 degrees lower than the rest of the body. 3. The midwife observes for vertigo and nystagmus. 4. The procedure is repeated with the head turned to the opposite side and then for a third time with the head facing straight ahead.	Abnormal/positive: If the patient reports a worsening of vertigo during the procedure.

Source: Jackler R, Kaplan M. Ear, nose, and throat. In: Tierney LM, McPhee SJ, Papadakis MA, editors. *Current Medical Diagnosis and Treatment.* New York: McGraw-Hill; 2005;[29] and Swartz M. The eye. In: Swartz M, editor. *Textbook of Physical Diagnosis.* 4th ed. Philadelphia: W.B. Saunders; 2002.[32]

needed. Hearing tests may help to distinguish conductive or sensineurologic hearing loss and can help narrow the etiologies being considered. **Tables 11-10** and **11-11** describe various conditions that lead to hearing loss. Other tests are used by specialists in the evaluation of vertigo but are not commonly ordered by primary care providers (**Table 11-12**).

Management of Specific Conditions

OTITIS MEDIA

Patients with *otitis media* usually report abrupt onset of severe, usually unilateral ear pain with or without fever and often request an urgent visit due to the severity of symptoms. The patient may also report symptoms of vertigo, hearing loss, or tinnitus, although these symptoms are much less common. Patients who note a bloody or purulent discharge should be evaluated for the possibility of a perforated tympanic membrane, which can occur in more severe infections.

Otitis media frequently occurs after a recent URI, either viral or bacterial in origin. It may also occur after more severe infections such as influenza or pneumonia, or after an allergy exacerbation. The resulting inflammation of the Eustachian tube creates an obstruction, usually at the isthmus, causing negative pressure and an increase in middle ear fluid. Initially, the negative pressure causes air to become trapped in the middle ear. When this happens, air bubbles can be visualized behind the tympanic membrane, but as the air is absorbed by minute blood vessels, the membrane can appear flat or retracted. The volume of fluid in the middle ear then increases and becomes trapped, causing bulging of the tympanic membrane or effusion, with or without pain.

Although the pathophysiology is unclear, it is thought that *acute otitis media (AOM)* results from a viral or bacterial colonization in the usually sterile middle ear. Negative pressure in the Eustachian tube caused by obstruction allows the middle ear to be contaminated by pathogens pulled in from the nasopharynx. The most common bacteria causing AOM are *Streptococcus pneumoniae*, *Haemophilus influenzae*, and *M. catarrhalis*.[34–37]

Less common pathogens are *Staphylococcus aureus*, *Streptococcus pyogenes*, *Proteus*, and *Pseudomonas*.[38] These pathogens, especially *Pseudomonas*,[39] are more frequently found with chronic suppurative otitis media, which is a chronic infection associated with perforation of the tympanic membrane.[29]

Otitis media can be difficult to distinguish from *otitis media with effusion (OME)*. Misdiagnosis can lead to excessive and inappropriate treatment with antibiotics and contributes to the increase of drug-resistant bacteria. Diagnosis criteria and appropriate treatment are more completely studied in children, as AOM is significantly more common in this population, especially in younger children. However, the disease process is thought to be the same in both children and adults, and thus much of the research in children is applicable to adults. The American Academy of Pediatrics and the American Academy of Family Physicians recently published a clinical practice guideline on diagnostic criteria and suggested management of AOM that is consistent with recommendations made by other authorities.[34,35]

Diagnostic criteria for AOM include:

- History of acute onset of signs and symptoms

Table 11-10 **HEARING TESTS**

Test	Description	Findings
Whisper Test	The examiner stands to the side of the patient, covers their mouth to prevent the patient from anticipating the sound, and speaks an easily understood word in a soft whisper into the ear being tested. The patient covers the opposite ear during the test and repeats the word spoken.	The threshold of normal hearing is 0–20 dB or the equivalent of a soft whisper.
Weber Test	The examiner strikes a 512 Hz tuning fork against the palm of the hand while holding the fork by its stem. The examiner then places the stem of the fork on the center of the patient's forehead and asks if the patient hears or feels the sound in the middle, or to the side.	This tests bone conduction and hearing. Feeling the sound in the middle is the normal response. If there is hearing loss, sound is heard on the affected side.
Rhine Test	The examiner strikes a 512 Hz tuning fork and places the stem at the mastoid tip. The examiner asks the patient if she can hear the sound, and if so, to indicate when it stops. The examiner then places the vibrating tuning fork tines in front of the auditory canal without touching the patient. The patient is asked if she can still hear the tuning fork. If the patient can still hear the vibrations, the test is positive. If the patient can no longer hear the vibrations, the test is negative.	This test compares air conduction with bone conduction. A positive test is normal and indicates better air conduction than bone conduction. A negative test indicates better bone conduction than air conduction.
Audiogram	Performed by a trained audiologist, this test measures the threshold of tonal and speech sounds heard by the patient. Earphones are placed over the patient's ears, and sounds of differing intensity are emitted. The patient indicates when she can hear the sound.	Mild hearing loss: 20–40 dB or the equivalent of a soft spoken voice. Moderate hearing loss: 60–80 dB or the equivalent of a loud spoken voice. Profound loss: 80 dB or the equivalent of a shout within 1 foot.

Table 11-11 COMMON HEARING TEST FINDINGS

Condition	Whisper Test	Weber Test	Rhine Test	Speech
Conductive Loss				
Cerumen impaction	Diminished or absent	Heard on affected side	Positive	May be louder
Foreign body in ear	Diminished or absent	Heard on affected side	Positive	May be louder
Otitis media with effusion	Diminished	Heard on affected side	Negative	May be louder
Perforation of tympanic membrane	Diminished or absent on affected side	Heard on affected side	Negative	May be louder
Moderate-to-severe otitis externa if significant edema of ear canal	Diminished or absent on affected side	Heard on affected side	Negative	May be louder
Bullous myringitis	Diminished or absent on affected side	Heard on affected side	Negative	May be louder
Sensorineural Hearing Loss				
Labyrinthitis	Diminished or absent on affected side	Heard on less affected side	Positive	Louder than usual
Ménière's disease (Weber test)	Diminished or absent on affected side	Heard on unaffected on less affected side	Positive	Louder than usual
Ototoxic medications	Diminished	Not heard or heard on less affected side	Positive	Louder than usual
Presbycusis (age-related)	Diminished or absent	Heard on less affected side	Positive	Louder than usual
Congenital or genetic disease	Absent or diminished	Absent or heard on less affected side	Positive	Louder than usual
Central Hearing Loss				
Ischemia Neoplasia Compression hematoma	Absent or diminished	May be abnormal	May be abnormal	May be normal or abnormal

Table 11-12 VERTIGO: SPECIALIZED TESTS USED TO DIFFERENTIATE PERIPHERAL AND CENTRAL LESIONS

Test	Description
Electronystagmography	Records presence and type of nystagmus after stimulation by movement, vision, or caloric testing.
Caloric testing	With patient recumbent at a 30-degree angle, warm and cold water is used to irrigate the ear to induce nystagmus.
Rotary Chair or "Spin Testing"	Nystagmus is recorded by electronystagmography while the patient is in a computer-driven rotary chair.
CT scan or MRI	Notes tumors or lesions.

Source: Jackler R, Kaplan M. Ear, nose, and throat. In: Tierney LM, McPhee SJ, Papadakis MA, editors. *Current Medical Diagnosis and Treatment.* New York: McGraw-Hill; 2005.[29] Seidman M, Simpson G, Khan M, Common problems of the ear. In: Noble J, editor. *Textbook of Primary Care Medicine.* 3rd ed. St. Louis: Mosby; 2001.[33]

- Presence of *middle ear effusion (MEE).* Findings on exam indicating MEE include any of the following: a bulging tympanic membrane; decreased or absent tympanic membrane mobility; an air-fluid level visualized on otoscopy; and otorrhea.
- Signs and symptoms of middle-ear inflammation. Evidence suggesting inflammation includes a complaint of significant otalgia (defined as discomfort clearly referable to the ear(s) that results in interference with or precludes normal activity or sleep) or erythema of the tympanic membrane.

The decision to treat a patient with AOM is based on accurate diagnosis and the severity of symptoms. Studies in children note that only 70% of AOM episodes appear to be caused by bacteria and that 10% to 15% of these infections are unresponsive to antibiotic therapy.[37] In addition, AOM symptoms do not appear to be directly dependent on the presence of bacteria and may resolve without treatment. Spontane-ous resolution of symptoms has been reported to occur in two to seven days in 80% to 90% of children without intervention.[35,37]

In the adult, it is acceptable to delay treatment with antibiotics for 48 to 72 hours to observe for spontaneous resolution of mild symptoms or if the diagnosis of AOM is in question. The patient can be treated with over-the-counter analgesics such as acetaminophen or ibuprofen. If symptoms are severe, particularly for those with otalgia, treatment with an antibiotic is appropriate. In addition, if the pain is severe, narcotics may be necessary for analgesia. The first-line choice of antibiotic is a single five-day course of high-dose amoxicillin. Amoxicillin has been demonstrated to be superior in effectiveness and resolution of symptoms, and is relatively low-cost. It is effective against most of the offending agents including penicillin resistant *S. pneumoniae*, which responds to high dose amoxicillin or IM ceftriaxone (Rocephin). If there is no relief from symptoms in 72 hours, a single course of amoxicillin/clavulanate (Augmentin) is appropriate. If there is still no relief, then one to three doses of intramuscular ceftriaxone should be given.[37] If the patient is allergic to penicillin, treatment with trimethoprim/sulfamethoxazole (Bactrim), azithromycin (Zithromax), or a second-generation cephalosporin is appropriate (**Table 11-13**).[37]

The patient should be referred to an otolarnygologist if symptoms are unresponsive to treatment. Multiple courses of antibiotics should be avoided to prevent an increase of resistant bacteria, ineffective treatment, and possible complications such as mastoiditis, meningitis, and intracranial abscess. Immediate referral is indicated for patients with symptoms of mastoiditis including post-auricular edema and redness, facial nerve palsy or weakness, meningitis, history of trauma to the area, blood noted behind the tympanic membrane, vertigo, suspicion of carotid or sinus thrombosis, or a history of significant co-existing disease or history of treatment such as neck or head radiation or surgery.

Patients with AOM should be followed every four to six weeks until the effusion resolves, which often takes three months, but may take as long as one year. Repeated or preventative courses of antibiotics have not been demonstrated to be effective. Recurrent episodes of AOM, as well as persistent hearing loss despite treatment, should be referred for investigation of underlying causes.

Otitis Media with Effusion

OME can present in several ways. The patient may be asymptomatic and the finding incidental; the patient may have otalgia with or without fever; or may complain only of a feeling of fullness in the middle ear, tinnitus, vertigo, or hearing loss. OME is more common in patients with a history of a recent or concurrent URI, allergy symptoms, or who have previous episodes of AOM. On examination middle ear effusion is seen but there are no signs of acute inflammation.

OME will usually resolve without intervention. If the patient has underlying allergy symptoms, treatment with appropriate medications to control the allergies may be helpful. However, in the absence of allergy symptoms, antihistamines, decongestants, and corticosteroids have not been found to provide any demonstrated benefit. Antibiotics are recommended only if MEE persists for more than three months. A single course of high-dose amoxicillin/clavulanate may then be used and a referral made to an otolaryngologist if symptoms persist (Table 11-13).[37] Patients with persistent MEE need an evaluation in order to exclude neoplasm as a possible etiology, to identify if an anatomical defect is causing obstruction, and to prevent possible damage to the bones of the middle ear, specifically the ossicles, from chronic MEE.

Patients with OME should be advised to avoid activities that can increase the pressure in the inner ear, such as diving and airplane travel. If it is necessary to fly in an airplane, use of a decongestant can decrease the risk of perforation. Gum chewing, swallowing liquids, and "popping the ears" can also help the Eustachian tube remain open during descent. If perforation should occur, the ear should be examined and treated. See the section on perforation of the tympanic membrane below.

Patients with both AOM and OME should avoid smoking and exposure to secondhand smoke to prevent aggravation of symptoms and to promote healing. Those at higher risk of developing AOM and OME can be offered the influenza and pneumonococcal vaccines,[40] although whether the use of these vaccines helps

Table 11-13 COMMONLY USED EAR MEDICATIONS

Indication	Drug	Trade Name	Dose	Notes
Acute Otitis Media				
	Amoxicillin		875 mg po TID × 5 days	
	Amoxicillin/ Clauvulanate	Augmentin	875 mg po BID × 7 days	
	Ceftriaxone	Rocephin	1 g IM per day × 1–3 days	
	Trimethoprim/ Sulfametho- xazole	Bactrim, Septra	1 DS tab po BID for 7–10 days	
	Azithromycin	Zithromax	500 mg × 1 dose then 250 mg per day × 4 days	For patients with penicillin allergy.
	Cefuroxime	Ceftin	500 mg po BID 7 days	
Otitis Externa				
Bacterial	Ofloxacin	Floxin Otic	10 drops qd into affected ear × 7 days	If systemic antibiotic is needed, Ciprofloxacin (Cipro) 500 mg po BID × 7 days. Avoid Benzocaine as a topical anes- thetic because of significant al- lergic response. Use Acetaminophen or NSAID for pain relief.
	Ciprofloxacin with hydro- cortisone	Cipro HC Otic	3 drops BID × 7 days	
	Polymyxin B neomycin, hydrocorti- sone	Cortisporin	4–6 drops 3 times per day	Do not use with perforated tympanic membrane.

prevent otitis media is debatable and seems increasingly unlikely (Chapter 2).[41,42]

PERFORATION OF THE TYMPANIC MEMBRANE
Perforation of the eardrum can occur as a sequalae of conditions that can increase inner ear pressure (otitis media, OME, barotraumas) or from trauma. When perforation of the tympanic membrane occurs, the patient often describes pain that initially crescendos and then diminishes abruptly as the tympanic membrane ruptures. Purulent or slightly bloody

discharge from the ear canal may then be noted. The practitioner may see drainage in the ear canal and a hole in the tympanic membrane on otoscopy. Pneumatic otoscopy should not be performed. Debris and blood should be gently wiped from the canal, analgesics advised, and topical ofloxacin or ciprofloxacin/hydrocortisone prescribed. Systemic antibiotics are not indicated in this situation unless there are concurrent systemic symptoms indicating that systemic treatment is needed. If needed, amoxicillin is the drug of choice.[37]

The tympanic membrane generally heals in three to four weeks, but may take longer. Until the tympanic membrane heals, patients should be advised to avoid swimming and to use earplugs when showering or washing their hair. The patient should also be advised to avoid barotrauma such as scuba diving and flying in airplanes. The patient should be re-examined to evaluate whether healing has occurred. Patients with persistent perforation should be referred to an ear-nose-throat physician. Incomplete or delayed healing can occur if a cholesteatoma or keratoma has formed along the edge of the perforation, which can potentially damage the ossicles of the middle ear. Therefore, referring to a specialist in this situation is essential in order to prevent permanent hearing loss.

BULLOUS MYRINGITIS

Bullous myringitis is a relatively uncommon acute infection of the tympanic membrane that causes intraepithelial fluid pockets (bullas) to develop on the tympanic membrane. These patients present with severe otalgia and on exam may have serous or bloody otorrhea. Treatment generally consists of otic antibiotic and corticosteroid medications, oral antibiotics, and oral analgesics such as acetaminophen or non-steroidal anti-inflammatory drugs. Lancing of the bulla may be helpful in relieving pain and thus will require referral.[43]

OTITIS EXTERNA

OE, which is a bacterial, viral, or fungal infection of the ear canal, is one of the most common causes of ear pain in adults. The patient may also report pruritis, edema, or discharge, which may have a foul odor. Manipulation of the pinna exacerbates the pain. The ear canal may be swollen and if significant edema is present may cause hearing loss or a feeling of fullness in the ear. Presentations can range from slight irritation of the skin lining the external ear canal and auricle to significant inflammation. In the most extreme cases, OE can spread to the soft tissue, involve the underlying bone, and develop into a very rare but possible fatal complication, necrotizing or malignant otitis externa, which is usually caused by *Pseudomonas* and is most common in immunocompromised and diabetic patients.[43,44] Immediate referral is required for these patients in order to receive life-saving early treatment.

Most cases of OE are bacterial or viral, but a few can be caused by fungi and can be more difficult to treat. One study noted yeast and fungi in less than 2% of the isolated organisms in OE.[45] They are more common in the presence of persistent moisture and are more frequently found in individuals living in tropical climates. A more serious fungal infection may be suspected if OE does not respond to the usual treatment, or if the patient is immunocompromised or diabetic. The patient may complain of a white or green discharge, and white and black debris may be noted on physical examination. A culture may be required; the most common fungal infections are caused by *Aspergillus* and *Candida*.[44–46] *Rhizopus*, *Alternaria*, *Penicillium*, and *Tinea* dermatophytes can also be cultured.[47]

OE occurs when the usual protective mechanisms of the ear fail. The skin lining the external ear canal is protected by an "acid mantle," which develops through the production of cerumen. This acidic environment is thought to impair the growth of pathogenic bacteria and fungi. The cerumen, which consists of desquamated epithelial tissue and secretions from the glands lining the ear canal, is thick and tacky, thus trapping debris and preventing its entrance into the middle ear. Cerumen coats the ear canal and protects the skin from excessive water exposure. Hair follicles in the ear canal help trap the cerumen until it can be pushed out of the ear canal through the action of the muscles involved in chewing and talking, and provide a further barrier to debris and foreign objects from reaching the middle ear.

OE is often called "swimmer's ear" because it is associated with a history of recent and/or frequent swimming. Exposure to water can strip the ear canal of the protective coating of cerumen and cause breakdown of the skin due to repeated exposure to moisture. The condition is common in hot, humid environments and occurs most frequently during the summer months or year round in tropical locations. Excessive use of protective headgear, headphones, or earplugs can raise the humidity locally in the ear canal, which contributes to the development of OE. Individuals with psoriasis, seborrhea, or other skin conditions affecting the skin of the ear are more susceptible to OE. Excessive itching or cleaning of the ear, including the use of cotton swabs or hairpins, can cause microabrasions and also predispose individuals to infection.[46,47] The most common pathogenic organisms are *Pseudomonas aeruginosa*, *Staphylococcus aureus*,[45,46] and *Staphylococcus epidermidis*.[45]

Cleaning the ear with a cotton swab or cerumen ear loop will increase visualization of the canal and tympanic membrane and greatly aid in the healing process if OE is present. Irrigating the ear with a 1:1 solution of hydrogen peroxide and water can promote healing if the tympanic membrane is intact.[46] The solution should be slightly warm or at room temperature to avoid inducing vertigo. However, OE can be very painful, and some patients may not be able to tolerate irrigation. In this case, treatment with otic drops can provide relief. If only slight erythema of the ear canal is present, the patient can be treated with either combined acetic acid/corticosteroid or combined antibiotic/corticosteroid otic drops. In mild disease, the effectiveness of these two types of medications are equal.[48] However, the use of acetic acid drops alone is more painful and less effective than the use of otic drops containing a corticosteroid. In a moderate infection, edema is present and partially occluding the canal, making a combined antibiotic/corticosteroid otic drop the better choice. In severe cases, the canal will be occluded and require the insertion of a wick (either a cotton wick or a commercially available sponge wick such as Oto-wick). Antibiotic/corticosteroid otic drops should be placed on the wick for two days following the normal recommended schedule. After two days, usually the edema has subsided enough that the wick can be removed and medication can be directly applied to the ear. If the wick cannot be easily inserted or if symptoms do not improve after two days of treatment with the wick in place, the patient should be referred to a specialist. Symptoms should improve within 48 to 72 hours of initiation of treatment. Patients should be evaluated 7 to 14 days after initiation of treatment to confirm that the infection has resolved.[41,45,46]

When choosing the appropriate medication for the treatment of OE, several issues need to be considered (Table 11-13). First, the use of ototoxic antibiotics should be avoided, particularly if perforation is suspected or confirmed. Second, because it is difficult to determine the causative agent in most cases of OE, the use of medications that target the most commonly implicated organisms is preferred. Third, OE can be extremely painful and use of a corticosteroid containing otic drop can provide prompt relief. Benzocaine, a topical anesthetic, should be avoided because allergies are common with use of this product. Acetaminophen or nonsteroidal anti-inflammatory medications can also be offered. If pain is severe enough that narcotics are necessary, more serious infections may be present and the patient should be re-evaluated and a referral considered.

Some of the better medication choices for bacterial infections are the fluoroquinolones, otic solutions such as ofloxacin (Floxin Otic), and ciprofloxacin with hydrocortisone (Cipro HC Otic). These have been demonstrated not to be ototoxic, are less likely to cause an allergic response, and cover both Gram-negative and Gram-positive organisms. The combination of polymyxin and neomycin (Cortisporin) is another commonly used medication. It effectively treats both *Staphylococcus aureus* and *Pseudomonas aeruginosa*, but may result in more allergic responses and is considered ototoxic in the presence of a perforated tympanic membrane.[45,46,48] Allergies can occur after the use of any otic medication and should be suspected if significant pruritis, persistent edema, appearance of vesicles, and increased erythema develop after their use. If an allergic response occurs, the ear should be cleaned and then treated with an acidic solution to re-acidify and heal the ear canal.

Corticosteroid solution can be used to decrease the inflammation.[46] A combination solution containing both an acidic solution and a corticosteroid, such as VoSol HC, can be easier to use for the patient.

Very mild fungal infections may respond to treatment with cleaning the ear well and applications of an acidifying agent such as VolSol HC. Other treatment consists of cleaning the ear well and applying topical sulfanilamide, clotrimazole, or miconozole. Patients who do not respond to treatment or are immunocompromised or diabetic should be referred for treatment.[46,49]

Patients requiring treatment with otic drops should be counseled on the correct technique for administration. The patient should lie on her side with the affected ear up. The medication should be warmed to body temperature by holding the bottle in the hand for a few minutes. Placing the bottle under hot water or in the microwave should be avoided as it may overheat the medication. The medication should be well shaken. The auricle is pulled up and back, to allow instillation of the prescribed number of drops into the ear. The patient should remain in that position for at least two minutes. It is normal for the medication to sting initially. An allergic response in the form of a contact dermatitis can occur with any otic medication. Patients should be counseled to report symptoms of persistent edema and significant pruritis, and given the warning signs that indicate a worsening infection.[33,44]

After treatment for OE, the patient should avoid swimming until healed. The ear should remain clean and dry during this time. Earplugs or cotton coated with petroleum jelly should be used for shampooing or showering. Drying the ear can be accomplished by holding a blow dryer 12 inches from the ear. Plain cotton should not be used to avoid worsening symptoms by absorbing moisture. Patients who swim frequently or who had recurrences of OE may benefit from using prophylactic measures to prevent infection. The patient may instill two to three drops of a commercial product such as acetic acid (VoSol) or a homemade solution of 1:1 isopropyl alcohol and white vinegar after swimming.[45,46] A more mild solution of 1:1:1 homemade solution of isopropyl alcohol/water/white vinegar may also be used.[44] This will allow for re-acidification and prevent tissue breakdown.

The patient should be instructed that the ear does not need "cleaning" as ears are self-cleaning. Cotton swabs inside the ear canal should be avoided; the swab can push debris farther into the canal, cause microabrasions, and deposit debris. Hairpins and other homemade instruments should not be used, in order to prevent causing infection, damage to the tympanic membrane, and permanent hearing loss.

Patients with symptoms indicative of more severe disease or the development of complications should be referred to a specialist. Patients with cellulitis, fever, or lymphadenopathy usually require systemic medications and should be referred. Immediate referral is warranted if pain and swelling are found over the mastoid area. Individuals with recurrent or persistent infection should also be referred to a specialist to rule out underlying pathology such as cancer. Very rarely, OE occurs after the tympanic membrane perforates as a result of an AOM infection. If this situation is suspected or confirmed, ototoxic otic drops should be avoided and care should proceed as discussed in the section, *Perforation of the Tympanic Membrane.*

FURUNCULOSIS

Furunculosis of the ear canal is uncommon but does occur. It typically presents as a pustule in the outer third of the ear canal where hair follicles are present. The patient may report otalgia, discharge, and tenderness limited to the affected area. Management consists of gently cleaning the outer ear canal with 1:1 solution of hydrogen peroxide and warm water, topical antibiotics, and warm, moist compresses. If the infection does not clear or if symptoms increase or spread to surrounding tissue, referral is indicated.

IMPACTED CERUMEN

On occasion, wax can build up and occlude the ear canal, causing pain, pressure, and hearing loss in the affected ear. Adherent wax can be softened by instilling drops of a commercially available ear wax remover for a few days. If this is not sufficient to remove the wax, the ear can be gently irrigated to flush out the wax. However irrigation is contraindicated when a perforated tympanic membrane is suspected. The following is one technique that can be used:

1. Fill a 5 cc or 10 cc syringe with either normal saline or a solution of 1:1 hydrogen peroxide and warm water.
2. Remove the needle from an 18 or 20 gauge IV angiocatheter and attach the catheter to the solution-filled syringe.
3. Position the patient in a chair with the head tilted slightly toward the affected side and visualize the ear canal and ear drum to confirm that no other pathology is suspected. Note whether there is any area that is wax free.
4. Place a receptacle, such as an emesis basin, under the ear.

5. Introduce the catheter into the ear canal using care not to injure the sidewall of the ear canal or perforate the tympanic membrane. Attempt to direct the catheter so that the fluid will be directed toward any wax-free areas of the canal so that the fluid can get around the plug and flush the plug out.

6. Gently flush the ear canal. Stop immediately if the patient reports pain.

7. Examine the ear with the otoscope and see if flushing removed all the ear wax. If there is residual ear wax, use an ear curette to gently remove the wax.

8. Refer if the wax is severely hardened and unable to be removed or if perforation is suspected.

FOREIGN BODY

The presence of a foreign body can cause irritation and pain. Before attempting to remove the object, it is important to try to determine what it could be. For example, if the material is organic, such as rice thrown at a wedding, it is important not to attempt to flush the ear with fluid as the object might swell. In this case, removal using a cerumen ear loop or forceps is preferred. Care should be taken not to lodge the object deeper in the canal. If an insect is suspected, special care is also needed. Applying drops of oil, alcohol, or anesthetic will drown most insects and make them easier to retrieve. Many, if not most of these situations, should be referred to a specialist.[50]

Performing gentle irrigation with a solution of 1:1 hydrogen peroxide and water or saline at room temperature will flush out most inorganic foreign bodies. However, if the object appears impacted or cannot be easily removed, referral to a specialist is warranted. Treatment after removal of the object may be necessary for OE if the presence of the foreign body led to localized infection.

Patient Education, Lifestyle, and Prevention

Patients undergoing treatment for infections of the outer or inner ear should be educated about their particular diagnosis and treatment as well as instructed to anticipate the relief of symptoms within 48 hours of the onset of treatment. Patients at risk of infection should minimize exposure of the ear to water and avoid cigarette smoke.

Pregnancy and Lactation

In pregnancy, increased estrogen levels cause an increase in vascularity and thus increased mucus production. A complaint of fullness in the ears is common in pregnancy and may be normal; it could also indicate underlying infection. Pregnancy is associated with mild immunosuppression, making infections of all types more common. To minimize this possibility, pregnant women should be offered the influenza vaccine. The identification and management of ear-related problems is otherwise unchanged during pregnancy and lactation. Topical medications have minimal absorption. The fluoroquinolones should be avoided whenever possible; they are considered to be Category C medications, but other safer alternatives are available.

Referral

Patients with persistent or severe presentations may need to be referred to a specialist. Women who report transient vertigo, hearing loss, or tinnitus may be watched conservatively, but if symptoms recur, become more severe, or are persistent, they will benefit from an evaluation by an otonologist.

References

1. Farnath D. The red eye. In: Rubin R, Voss C, Derksen D, Gateley A, Quenzer R, editors. *Medicine: A Primary Care Approach.* Philadelphia: W. B. Saunders Company; 1996. pp. 80–84.

2. Farnath D. Common disorders of vision. In: Rubin R, Voss C, Derksen D, Gateley A, Quenzer R, editors. *Medicine: A Primary Care Approach.* Philadelphia: W. B. Saunders Company; 1996. pp. 84–88.

3. Jacobs D. Evaluation of the red eye. In: *2005 UpToDate®.* [Monograph on the Internet; subscriber-only site.] Waltham, MA. Available from: http://www.uptodate.com/index.

4. Mogul L, Friedman A. Ocular complications. In: Cohen WR, editor. *Cherry & Merkatz's Complications of Pregnancy.* 5th ed. Philadelphia: Lippincott Williams & Wilkins; 2000.

5. Kamoun L. The red eye. *Top Emerg Med.* 2000;22(4): 37–51.

6. Riordan-Eva P. Eye. In: Tierney LM, McPhee SJ, Papadakis MA, editors. *Current Medical Diagnosis and Treatment 2004.* 43rd ed. New York: Lange Medical Books/McGraw-Hill; 2004.

7. Horton J. Disorders of the eye. In: Kasper DL, Braunwald E, Fauci A, Hauser S, Longo D, Jameson L, editors. *Harrison's Principles of Internal Medicine.* 16th ed. New York: McGraw-Hill; 2005.

8. Crouch E, Berger A. Ophthalmology. In: Rakel R, editor. *Textbook of Family Medicine.* 6th ed. Philadelphia: W.B. Saunders; 2001.

9. Leibowitz H. Primary care: The red eye. *N Engl J Med.* 2000;343(5):345–351.

10. Jacobs D. Conjunctivitis. In: *2005 UpToDate®.* [Monograph on the Internet; subscriber-only site.] Waltham, MA. Available from: http://www.uptodate.com/index.

11. Goroll A, Mulley A. *Primary Care Medicine Recommendations.* New York: Lippincott Williams & Wilkins; 2001.

12. Foulks G. What is dry eye and what does it mean to the Contact Lens Wearer? *Eye Contact Lens: Science and Clinical Practice* 2003;29 Suppl 1: S96–100.

13. Neher J. Eye problems of aging: Cataracts, glaucoma, and macular degeneration. In: Taylor RB, editor. *Manual of Family Practice.* 2nd ed. New York: Lippincott Williams & Wilkins; 2002.

14. Mintz R, Feller E, Bahr R, Shah S. Ocular manifestations of inflammatory bowel disease. *Inflam Bowel Dis.* 2004;10(2):135–139.

15. Congdon N, Friedman D, Lietman T. Important causes of visual impairment in the world today. *JAMA.* 2003;290:2057–2060.

16. Rowe S, MacLean C, Shekelle P. Preventing visual loss from chronic eye disease in primary care: Scientific review. *JAMA.* 2004;291:1487–1495.

17. Horowitz A. The prevalence and consequences of vision impairment in later life. *Topics in Geriatric Rehabilitation.* 2004;20(3):185–195.

18. Jacobs D. Primary open-angle glaucoma. In: *2005 UpToDate®.* [Monograph on the Internet; subscriber-only site.] Waltham, MA. Available from: http://www.uptodate.com/index.

19. Traboulsi E, Maumenee I. Eye problems. In: McMillan JA, Deangelis CD, Feigin RD, Warshaw JB, Oski FA, Warshaw JB, editors. *Oski's Pediatric: Principles and Practice.* 3rd ed. Philadelphia: Lippincott Williams & Wilkins; 1999.

20. Shingleton B, O'Donoghue M. Primary care: Blurred vision. *N Engl J Med.* 2000;343:556–562.

21. Goldzweig C, Rowe S, Wenger N, MacLean C, Shekelle P. Preventing and managing visual disability in primary care: clinical applications. *JAMA.* 2004; 291:1497–1502.

22. Schappert S. *Office Visits for Otitis Media: United States, 1975–1990.* Report No. 214. Hyattsville, MD: Advance Data from Vital and Health Statistics National Center for Health Statistics; 1992.

23. Kamerer D, Thompson S. Middle ear and temporal bone trauma. In: Bailey B, Healy G, Johnson J, Jackler R, Calhoun K, Pillsbury H, et al., editors. *Head & Neck Surgery-Otolaryngology.* 3rd ed. Philadelphia: Lippincott Williams & Wilkins; 2001. pp. 1774–1785.

24. Anonymous. Laryngeal carcinoma. In: Roland N, McRae RDR, McCombe AW, editors. *Key Topics in Otolaryngology.* 2nd ed. Abingdon, Oxfordshire, UK: BIOS Scientific Publishers Ltd; 2000.

25. Barton J, Branch W. Approach to the patient with vertigo. In: *2005 UpToDate®.* [Monograph on the Internet; subscriber-only site.] Waltham, MA. Available from: http://www.uptodate.com/index.

26. Roland P, Eaton D, Meyerhoff W. Aging in the auditory and vestibular system. In: Bailey B, Healy G, Johnson J, Jackler R, Calhoun K, Pillsbury H, et al., editors. *Head & Neck Surgery-Otolaryngology.* Philadelphia: Lippincott Williams & Wilkins; 2001.

27. Lesser T. Vertigo. In: Roland N, McRae RDR, McCombe AW, editors. *Key Topics in Otolaryngology.* 2nd ed. Abingdon, Oxfordshire, UK: BIOS Scientific Publishers Ltd; 2000.

28. Anonymous. Tinnitis. In: Roland N, McRae RDR, McCombe AW, editors. *Key Topics in Otolaryngology.* 2nd ed. Abingdon, Oxfordshire, UK: BIOS Scientific Publishers Ltd; 2000.

29. Jackler R, Kaplan M. Ear, Nose, and Throat. In: Tierney LM, McPhee SJ, Papadakis MA, editors. *Current Medical Diagnosis and Treatment.* New York: McGraw-Hill; 2005.

30. Anonymous. Seborrheic Dermatitis, Acne, and Rosacea. In: Hall JC, editor. *Sauer's Manual of Skin Diseases.* 8th ed. Philadelphia: Lippincott Williams & Wilkins; 2000. pp. 114–126.

31. Anonymous. Dermatologic Allergy. In: Hall JC, editor. *Sauer's Manual of Skin Diseases.* Philadelphia: Lippincott Williams & Wilkins; 2000. pp. 67–90.

32. Swartz M. The eye. In: Swartz M, editor. *Textbook of Physical Diagnosis.* 4th ed. Philadelphia: W.B. Saunders; 2002.

33. Seidman M, Simpson G, Kan M. Common problems of the ear. In: Noble J. *Textbook of Primary Care Medicine.* 3rd ed. St. Louis: Mosby; 2001.

34. Hendley J. Otitis media. *N Engl J Med.* 2002;247: 1169–1174.

35. Fendrick A, Saine S, Brook I, Jacobs M, Pelton S, Sethi S. Diagnosis and treatment of upper respiratory tract infections in the primary care setting. *Clin Ther.* 2001;23:1683–1706.

36. Ferro T. Overview of national treatment guidelines for common respiratory tract infections. *Am J Ther.* 2004;11 Suppl 1:S9–14.

37. Otitis Media Guideline Team. Guidelines for Clinical Care: Otitis Media. In: *University of Michigan Health System,* 2002. Available at http://cme.med.umich.edu/pdf/guideline/om.pdf.

38. Strohl, K. Upper airway diseases. In: Goldman L, editor. *Cecil Textbook of Medicine,* 22nd ed. St. Louis: W. B. Saunders, 2004, pp. 2432–2435.

39. Roland P, Stewart M, Hannley M, Friedman R, Manolidis S, Matz G, et al. Consensus panel on role of potentially ototoxic antibiotics for topical middle ear use: Introduction, methodology, and recommendations. *Otolaryngol Head Neck Surg.* 2004;130 Suppl 3:S51–56.

40. Edwards K, Griffin M. Great expectations for a new vaccine. *N Engl J Med.* 2003;349:1312–1314.

41. Straetemans M, Sanders E, Veenhoven R, Schilder A, Damoiseaux R, Zielhuis G. Review of randomized controlled trials on pneumococcal vaccination for prevention of otitis media. *Pediatr Infect Dis J.* 2003; 22:515–524.

42. Brouwer C, Maille A, Rovers M, Veenhoven R, Grobbee D, Sanders E, et al. Effect of pneumococcal vaccination on quality of life in children with recurrent acute otitis media: A randomized, controlled trial. *Pediatrics.* 2005;115:273–279.

43. Shah R, Blevins N. Otalgia. *Otolaryngol Clin N Am.* 2003;36:1137–1151.

44. Felis M. Acute otitis externa. *Lippincott Prim Care Pract.* 2000;4:529–533.

45. Beers S, Abramo T. Otitis externa review. *Pediatr Emerg Care.* 2004;20:250–256.

46. Goguen L. External otitis. In: *2005 UpToDate®.* [Monograph on the Internet; subscriber-only site.] Waltham, MA. Available from: http://www.uptodate.com/index.

47. Rosenfeld J, Clarity G. Otitis media and otitis externa. In: Taylor R, editor. *Family Medicine: Principles and Practice.* 5th ed. New York: Springer-Verlag, Inc; 1998.

48. Van Balen F, Smit W, Zuithoff N, Verheij T. Clinical efficacy of three common treatments in acute otitis externa in primary care: Randomized controlled trial. *BMJ.* 2003;327:1201–1205.

49. Curry R, Hall K. Selected Disorders of the Ear, Nose, and Throat. In: Taylor RB, David AK, Johnson TA Jr, Phillips M, Scherger JE, editors. *Family Medicine: Principles and Practice.* 5th ed. New York: Springer Verlag; 1998.

50. Roland, NJ. *Acute Suppurative Otis Media, Key Topics in Otolaryngology,* 2nd ed. Oxford: BIOS Scientific Publishers Ltd.

Chapter 12

Asthma and Allergy

Barbara Hackley

Asthma

Asthma is a common chronic condition, estimated to affect more than 14 million individuals or more than 7% of all Americans.[1] It affects more children than adults, more women than men, and is more common among African Americans and the economically disadvantaged.[2] In 2001, asthma accounted for over 4400 deaths, 450,000 hospitalizations, 1.8 million emergency room visits, and 10 million outpatient visits.[1]

Clinical Presentation

Asthma is characterized by episodes of inflammation and narrowing of the airways. Attacks vary in severity and commonly present with wheezing, cough, shortness of breath, or chest pain and tightness. These symptoms result from exposure to triggers such as allergens, exercise, infections, and airway irritants and are at least partially reversible. Evidence of reversibility is defined as an increase of $>12\%$ or >200 cc in FEV1 (forced expiratory volume in one second, in liters) on spirometry testing after treatment with a short acting bronchodilator.[3] Exposure to triggers results in a cascade of events including denudation of airway epithelium, collagen deposition, mast cell inflamma-

tion, and inflammatory cell infiltration, which lead to bronchospasm, mucosal edema, and increased mucus production, all of which narrow the airway and cause breathlessness and wheezing (**Figure 12-1**).[3]

Chronic inflammation leads to hyper-responsiveness to a variety of stimuli and for some individuals, to airway remodeling. In general, for those with milder asthma, airway obstruction is completely reversible either spontaneously or with treatment. Those with more severe asthma may develop airway remodeling and have only partial resolution of airway obstruction. Chronic inflammation can result in fibrosis, hypertrophy, and hyperplasia of airway smooth muscle cells, and increased mucous gland mass, making asthma difficult to distinguish from chronic obstructive pulmonary disease (COPD).[4] Patients complaining of persistent cough need to be evaluated not only for chronic respiratory conditions such as COPD, but also conditions that cause postnasal drip such as allergies, sinusitis, and upper respiratory infections, underlying cardiac disorders that lead to pulmonary edema and dyspnea, and common co-existing conditions such as gastro-esophageal reflux. Wheezing is also a symptom of other obstructive respiratory tract disorders

Figure 12-1 Mechanisms underlying the definition of asthma.

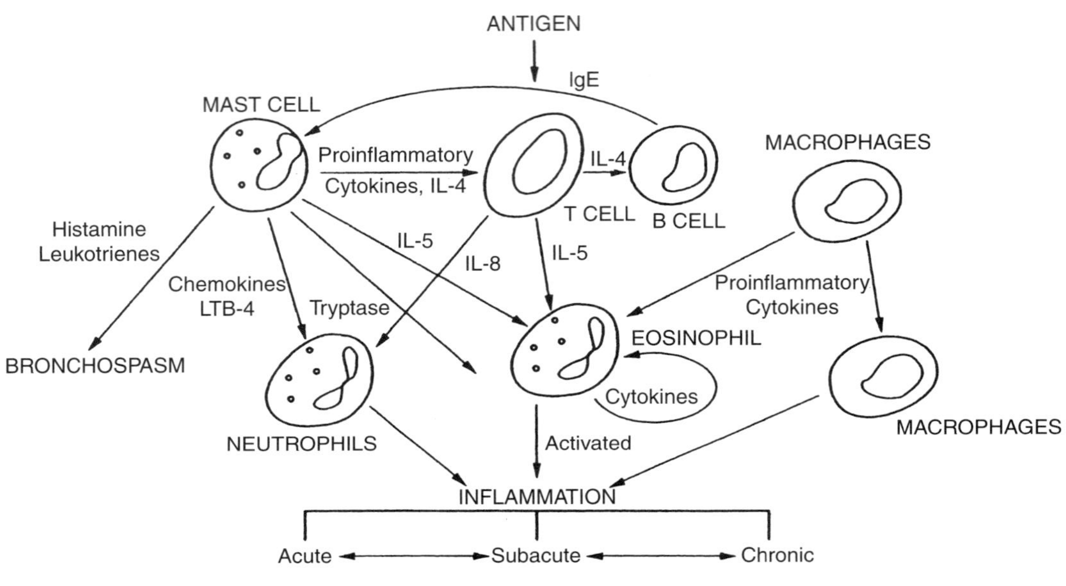

Source: From the National Asthma Education and Prevention Program.[3]

such as cystic fibrosis, vocal cord dysfunction, and mechanical obstruction from aspiration or tumors. Therefore, careful history, physical examination, and laboratory evaluation are necessary in order to differentiate asthma from other diagnostic possibilities. **Table 12-1** provides diagnostic clues that can help distinguish asthma from other conditions.

Essential History and Physical and Laboratory Evaluation

HISTORY

A thorough history is essential in helping to diagnose asthma, stage its severity, and monitor the effectiveness of treatment. Patients who present with recurrent episodes of wheezing, chest tightness, and shortness of breath and whose symptoms respond appropriately to treatment or to the removal of offending triggers can be assumed to have asthma. **Table 12-2** lists common asthma triggers.

Patients should be asked about the frequency of daytime and nighttime symptoms, because these questions allow the provider to stage asthma severity and guide treatment choices. The four states of asthma correspond to increasing severity and frequency of symptoms. **Table 12-3** outlines the asthma classifications and corresponding medication recommendations.[5] Providers should also determine what types of exposures trigger symptoms, and note whether

Table 12-1 DIFFERENTIAL DIAGNOSIS FOR ASTHMA

Condition	History	Physical	Laboratory
Asthma	• Nonproductive cough • Recurrent SOB and chest tightness • Symptoms worsened or triggered by exposure to allergens and irritants • Symptoms worse at night and may awaken patient • Commonly presents in childhood, although may develop at any age • Associated with allergies, atopy, and nasal polyps	• Wheezing (Note, in severe attacks no wheezing may be heard due to reduced air flow) • Use of accessory muscles, retractions • Breathing easier in upright position • Cyanosis • Hyperinflated chest • Pale nasal mucosa or "allergic shiners" seen in those with allergies	• Diurnal variation in peak flow measures of 20% or more • Spirometry findings demonstrate reversible airway obstruction
COPD	• Exertional dyspnea • Productive cough • Associated with cigarette smoking • Recurrent URIs • Usually presents in mid-life	• Wheezing and rhonchi • Hyperinflated chest • Use of accessory muscles • Decreased breath sounds	• Spirometry findings demonstrate airway restriction <70% of predicted value and more rapid loss of lung function than expected for age
URI	• Cough, occasionally productive • Abrupt and specific onset • Fever and chills • Symptoms resolve within 2 weeks	• Thick opaque nasal secretion • Red and watery conjunctivae	• No changes are seen in spirometry findings
Pneumonia	• Fever and chills • Chest discomfort • Cough • Dyspnea	• Toxic appearance • Tachypnea, tachycardia • Rales • Respiratory consolidation	• PA and lateral chest x-ray show localized opacification from infiltrates
Sinusitis	• Usually antecedent URI • URI symptoms for longer than 10–14 days	• Sinus tenderness and congestion	
GERD	• Heartburn, dysphagia • Sour or bitter taste in mouth • Use of antacids • Cough • Symptoms worse after meals, better with sitting	• Normal lung sounds	

Abbreviations are: SOB, shortness of breath; COPD, chronic obstructive pulmonary disease; URI, upper respiratory infection; GERD, gastroesophageal reflux disease; PA, posterior-anterior.

Table 12-2 LIST OF COMMON TRIGGERS FOR ASTHMA

- Exercise
- Cold air
- Weather changes
- Allergens (i.e., mold, dust, pollen, animal dander)
- Viral infections
- Cigarette smoke
- Laughing/crying
- Airborne chemicals (i.e., cleaning products and perfumes)
- Medications (i.e., aspirin, nonsteroidal anti-inflammatory drugs, beta-blockers, eye drops)
- Food and food additives (i.e., sulfites)

---

symptoms are sporadic or continual, what approaches the patient has used in the past, and whether these approaches were successful.

Appropriate asthma treatment allows a patient to maintain her normal activities with minimal or no symptoms. Providers should question patients on whether their symptoms cause them to limit their physical activity, miss school or work, or require the use of quick relief medications. Providers also should routinely question patients about the frequency and consistency of use of all their asthma medications as well as monitor for common side effects. In addition, providers should determine whether or not their patients are at risk for severe exacerbations of asthma by asking about such risk factors as those listed in **Table 12-4**. Many of these individuals—particularly those with unstable asthma or who require high dosages to control their symptoms—may require consultation with an asthma specialist.

PHYSICAL EXAMINATION

The physical examination for an individual suspected of having asthma should not only look for data to confirm the diagnosis of asthma, but also for signs of other conditions that can mimic asthma and common comorbidities (**Table 12-5**).

LABORATORY STUDIES

Chest x-rays, arterial blood gases, and other laboratory tests have only a limited role in the evaluation of asthma. Pulmonary function testing is the gold standard, useful in both diagnosis and management. Lung function in asthmatics tends to vary throughout the day and is usually poorest on arising in the morning and peaks mid-day. Asthma also is reversible with treatment. A variation of more than 20% between early morning and mid-day measurements, or improvement in lung volumes of 12% after treatment, is indicative of asthma. The two most commonly used testing modalities are *spirometry*, most commonly used for diagnosis, and *peak flow meters*, usually used to monitor response to treatment.

Spirometry is generally performed in a dedicated laboratory, although office models are becoming increasingly common. Spirometry testing is not universal because of cost and access issues. Many providers do not order spirometry if the diagnosis is clear, if the patient is young with no other comorbidities, and if the patient responds as expected to treatment. However, spirometry always should be ordered for patients who do not react appropriately to medications, whose course is atypical, or who have comorbidities that complicate the diagnosis or management of asthma.

Spirometry is helpful in distinguishing whether or not the patient has restrictive lung disease (where the patient has difficulty getting sufficient air into the respiratory tract) or obstructive lung disease (where the patient has difficulty getting air out of the respiratory tract).

Table 12-3 ASTHMA STAGES AND MAINTENANCE THERAPY

Stage	Symptoms		Pulmonary Function		Preferred Treatment Alternative Treatment
Step 4 Severe Persistent	Day: Night:	Continual Frequent	PEF or FEV1 Variability	$\leq$60% >30%	**High-dose inhaled corti-costeroids plus long-acting inhaled beta$_2$ agonists** And if needed, cortico-steroid tablets long term
Step 3 Moderate Persistent	Day: Night:	Daily >1 night/week	PEF or FEV1 >60%–80% Variability	 >30%	**Low- to medium-dose inhaled corticosteroids and long-acting in-haled beta$_2$ agonists** Increase inhaled cortico-steroids within medium-dose range OR low-to-medium dose corticosteroids and ei-ther leukotriene modi-fier or theophylline
Step 2 Mild Persistent	Day: Night:	>2 days/week but Not daily >2 nights/ month	PEF or FEV1 Variability	$\geq$80% 20–30%	**Low-dose inhaled corti-costeroids** Cromolyn, leukotriene modifier, nedocromil, or substained release theo-phylline
Step 1 Mild Intermittent	Day: Night:	$\leq$2 days/week $\leq$2 nights/ month	PEF or FEV1 Variability	$\geq$80% <20%	**No daily medication needed**

Key: Bold = preferred treatment. *Abbreviations are:* PEF, peak expiratory flow; FEV1, forced expiratory volume in one second, in liters.

Source: Adapted from National Asthma Education and Prevention Program.[5]

Measures used to differentiate restrictive and obstructive lung disease are: 1) FVC (forced vital capacity); 2) FEV1; and 3) the FEV1/FVC ratio (**Table 12-6**). Normal values for these tests vary by a patient's height, weight, age, and sex. Therefore, results are reported by the "expected value" for a specific patient. **Figure 12-2** shows different measurements used to describe various lung volumes. **Figure 12-3** provides a pictorial example of a spirometry test.

Table 12-4 RISK FACTORS FOR DEATH FROM ASTHMA

- Prior intubations
- Prior admission to intensive care unit
- Two or more hospitalizations in last year
- Three or more ER visits in last year
- Use of more than two canisters of rescue inhalers per month
- Current use of systemic corticosteroids
- Difficulty perceiving severity

Source: Adapted from the National Asthma Education and Prevention Program.[6]

Spirometry findings differ for patients with restrictive and obstructive lung disease (**Tables 12-7 and 12-8**). Patients with restrictive lung disease will have lower than expected lung volumes and so will have lower than expected FVC, because the airway will not allow normal filling to occur on inspiration. However, because exhalation is not impeded in patients with restrictive disease, expiration can occur at a normal rate and their FEV1 will be normal. Lung findings in patients with obstructive disease have the reverse pattern. Their FVC will be normal because airway filling is not hindered, but they will have lower than expected FEV1 because obstruction delays the emptying of the lung with expiration.

Peak flow meters provide less data than spirometry but are easy to use. They are most useful in monitoring response to treatment in the office or at home. Individuals with more severe asthma have greater diurnal variation in lung function. Peak flow meters can be used to document this variation and can help stage the severity of the asthma and confirm treatment success. Appropriate treatment should mini-

Table 12-5 PHYSICAL EVALUATION TO DIAGNOSE ASTHMA

Test	Description
Vital signs	P, RR, BP
	(Acute asthma symptoms can increase P, RR, and cause Pulsus paradoxus)
Pulse oximetry	Normal if >95% SaO_2 on room air
Appearance	Observe posture patient assumes for comfortable breathing
Voice	Nasal quality
	Able to speak in full sentences with comfort
Skin	Cyanosis, diaphoresis, eczema
HEENT	Allergic shiners
	Sinus tenderness
	Presence of nasal polyps
	Pale, boggy, nasal mucosa and nasal discharge
Respiratory	Wheezing
	Diminished breath sounds with the absence of wheezing in severe attacks
	Respiratory effort: use of accessory muscles, retractions
	Evidence of hyperinflation: barrel chest, hyper-resonance

Source: Adapted from the National Asthma Education and Prevention Program.[3]

Table 12-6 PULMONARY FUNCTION TESTS

Measurement	Tool	Definition	Normal Value	Notes
Forced vital capacity (FVC)	Spirometry	The maximal volume of air exhaled using maximal effort, following maximal inspiration	>80% of predicted value	Most useful measurement for diagnosing restrictive lung disease.
Forced expiratory volume-1 (FEV1)	Spirometry	Volume of air exhaled in the first second	>80% of predicted value	Most important measurement for following obstructive lung disease; determines the severity of airway obstruction.
FEV1/FVC ratio	Spirometry	Expressed as a percentage and reflects how much of the total lung volume can be exhaled in the first second	Ratio <70% indicates an obstructive disorder in middle aged adults	Ratio is used to detect airway obstruction.
Peak expiratory flow (PEF; measured in L/sec or L/min)	Peak Flow Meter	Largest expiratory flow achieved using maximal forced effort, following maximal inspiration	<80% of personal best suggests obstruction	

mize the diurnal pattern seen in asthmatics, so measuring peak flows at various times through the day can help a provider decide whether the patient is on an appropriate preventive regimen. Peak flow measurements before and after treatment of an acute attack also can document effectiveness of quick relief measures.

Peak flow measurements differ from spirometry in several key ways. First, peak flow measurements do not give as complete a picture of pulmonary function. They do not provide information about vital capacity or measure the level of "obstruction" as well as spirometry. There is no time element as there is with FEV1 measurements, and peak flow meters measure only obstruction found in the large airways. Spirometry can measure obstruction in both the large as well as the small airways. Second, proper technique is vital in getting accurate pulmonary function tests. Spirometry has the capacity to confirm whether or not the patient used maximal effort,

Figure 12-2 Lung volumes.

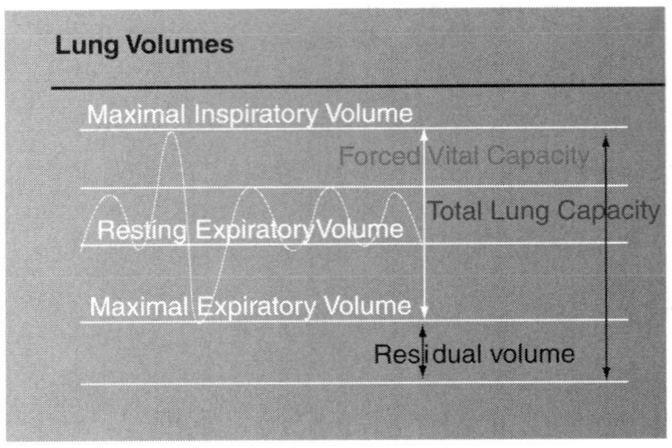

whereas peak flow meters do not. **Table 12-9** describes the proper technique to obtain accurate peak flow measurements.

Management of Asthma

Since 1991, the National Asthma Education and Prevention Program (NAEPP) has issued a series of Expert Panel Reports meant to improve the clinical management of asthma and to stimulate research.[3,5,7] These Expert Panel Reports, which have been seminal in setting standards for the diagnosis and management of asthma, have classified the stages of asthma by severity, linked recommended pharmacologic therapies to these stages, and advocated active patient involvement in developing treatment plans and monitoring their effectiveness.

The stages of asthma are based on measurable objectives, such as the frequency and timing of symptoms and the degree of variation in pulmonary function throughout the day. Providers looking for an easy way to remember these stages should remember the principle of "two." Patients with infrequent symptoms are classified as Stage 1 Mild Intermittent. Patients experiencing more than two episodes of wheezing a week during the day or more than two episodes of wheezing a month at night are deemed Stage 2 Mild Persistent. Patients with Stage 3 Moderate Persistent asthma have symp-

Figure 12-3 Sample spirometry volume time and flow volume curves.

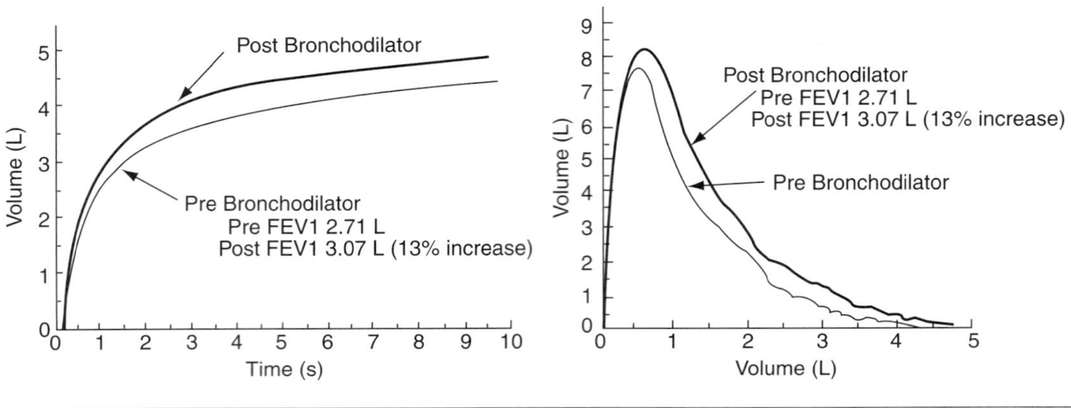

Source: Adapted from the National Asthma Education and Prevention Program.[3]

Table 12-7 SPIROMETRY FINDINGS IN OBSTRUCTIVE AND RESTRICTIVE LUNG DISEASE

Test	Obstructive Disease	Restrictive Disease
FVC	Normal	Reduced
FEV-1	Reduced	Normal
FEV-1/FVC	Reduced	Normal

Abbreviations are defined in Table 12-6.

toms daily and twice a week or more at night; those with Stage 4 experience symptoms almost continually during the day and frequently at night. Patients whose symptoms fall into two different steps should be treated at the higher step. For example, if a patient meets the criteria for Stage 2 based on daytime symptoms, but meets the criteria for Stage 3 based on night-time symptoms, he or she should receive treatment corresponding to Stage 3. Table 12-3 outlines these four steps.[5]

MEDICATIONS

The two principal categories of medications used in the management of asthma are quick relief medications, such as albuterol (Proventil, Ventolin) or another short-acting bronchodilator inhaler, and controller medications, usually steroidal inhalers. **Table 12-10** lists some common medications used for the relief of immediate symptoms, and **Table 12-11** contains those used for long-term control needed to prevent symptoms from re-occurring. Patients with Stage 1 Mild Intermittent asthma need to use only short-acting beta-agonist inhalers as symptoms arise. Patients with more persistent asthma will need to continue to use short-acting bronchodilators, but should add controller medication(s). The need to increase the use of quick relief inhalers may indicate the need to add on or increase the dose of controller medications (**Table 12-12**).

There are four basic types of controller medications: systemic or inhaled steroids; nonsteroidal anti-inflammatory inhalers; leukotriene modifiers; and long-acting inhaled β_2-agonists. Each type plays a role in asthma management, but the mainstay therapy is inhaled corticosteroids.

CORTICOSTEROIDS

The inhaled corticosteroids minimize inflammation and may prevent long-term airway remodeling.[7,10] They also provide the best control of all the maintenance medications and

Table 12-8 EXAMPLES OF OBSTRUCTIVE AND RESTRICTIVE LUNG DISEASE

Obstructive Lung Disease	Restrictive Lung Disease
Asthma	Obesity
Chronic obstructive pulmonary disease	Fibrosis (idiopathic or radiation induced)
Cystic fibrosis	Sarcoidosis
Bronchiectasis	Pneumonia
Bronchial foreign body	Congestive heart disease
	Pleural effusions

Table 12-9 CORRECT PEAK FLOW TECHNIQUE

Peak Flow Meter	Proper Technique
	• Push indicator button to the bottom • Stand up, and take a deep breath • Blow out as hard and fast as you can in a single blow • Use the best measurement out of 3 tries

have fewer side effects than oral corticosteroids.[7,11] Oral corticosteroids are avoided wherever possible because long-term exposure is associated with hypothalamic-pituitary-adrenal suppression, osteoporosis, immunosuppression, and other adverse systemic effects. Their use may be necessary for the management of more severe asthma and during exacerbations. The adverse effects of corticosteroid use are dose-dependent and worsen as the total dose and length of exposure increase. Inhaled corticosteroids seem to be safer than oral formulations. Bone loss is less than with oral products but may still occur. While the data are not conclusive, inhaled corticosteroids in the medium-to-high dose range may be associated with significant bone loss, prompting some authorities to recommend routine bone mineral density testing and calcium/vitamin D supplementation for all adults on long-term oral or inhaled corticosteroids.[12] Few data exist on the relative effectiveness and safety profiles of specific inhaled corticosteroids.[13] Further studies are needed to determine whether significant differences exist between the inhaled corticosteroids.

To minimize inconvenience, inhaled corticosteroids are generally prescribed to be taken twice a day, although some women will require more frequent dosing to gain good control. However, a recent review of the literature found that many patients can be adequately controlled on a once-daily regimen.[14] Once- to twice-a-day dosing may improve adherence by making regimens easier to follow.

LONG-ACTING INHALED β_2 AGONISTS

According to the NAEPP, patients who do not achieve adequate control on low-dose inhaled corticosteroids should add a long-acting inhaled β_2 agonist inhaler.[5] β_2 agonists relax smooth muscle and reduce bronchoconstriction. Long-acting inhaled β_2 agonists have a 12-hour duration of action after a single dose. They are NOT used for quick relief. Rather, they are used to control nighttime symptoms, to prevent exercise-induced asthma, and to enhance the effect of corticosteroid inhalers. Combining corticosteroid inhalers with long-acting β_2 agonist inhalers results in greater improvement in lung function and symptom control than the use of either agent alone.[13] In one study, doubling the dose of inhaled corticosteroids resulted in poorer control than did the use of low-dose inhaled corticosteroids plus a long-acting inhaled β_2 agonist.[13] Not only does combination therapy lead

Table 12-10 MEDICATIONS USED FOR QUICK RELIEF

Drug	Trade Name	Dose
Albuterol MDI	Ventolin HFA MDI Proventil HFA MDI	2 puffs tid to qid.
	200 puffs/canister	For acute exacerbation in home. Begin with MDI: 2-4 puffs every 20 min, up to 3 treatments. Patient should refer to instructions given by provider in this circumstance. Therapy individualized thereafter.
		For acute exacerbation in emergency room. Begin with MDI: 4–8 puffs every 20 min for 3 doses. Therapy individualized thereafter.
Albuterol Rotahaler	DPI 200 mcg/capsule	1–2 capsules every 4–6 h.
Albuterol Nebulizer Solution	5 mg/mL	For acute exacerbation. 2.5–5 mg every 20 min for 3 doses. Dilute with a minimum of 3 cc normal saline with oxygen flow of 6–8 L/min. Therapy individualized thereafter.
Levalbuterol Nebulizer Solution	Xopenex 0.31 mg/3 mL, 0.63 mg/3 mL, 1.25 mg/3 mL vial, single use vials	For acute exacerbation. Nebulizer. 0.63–2.5 mg every 4–8 h.
Pirbuterol MDI	Maxair Autoinhaler Breath actuated MDI	2 puffs tid to qid.

Abbreviations are: MDI, metered dose inhaler; HFA, hydro fluoroalkane; TID, three times daily; QID, four times daily; H, hour; DPI, dry powder inhaler.
Source: Adapted from the National Asthma Education and Prevention Program.[5,6,8]

to better control because it allows lower doses of steroids to be used, but it is also less likely to lead to the development of sequelae associated with long-term steroid use.

LEUKOTRIENE MODIFIERS

Leukotriene modifiers inhibit mediators released from mast cells, esoinophils, and basophils that contract airway smooth muscle, increase vascular permeability, increase mucus production, and activate inflammatory cells.[7] They are the newest class of medications being used for the management of asthma and are popular with patients because, as oral agents, they are much easier to use. They are less effective than inhaled corticosteroids or long-acting β_2 agonist inhalers, whether they are prescribed as adjunctive or monotherapy.[13,15] Adjunctive treatment with long-acting β_2 agonist inhalers results in better symptom control and lung

Table 12-11 MEDICATIONS FOR LONG-TERM CONTROL

Drug	Type/Trade Name/Dose/Number of Inhalations per Canister	Low Dose: Daily dose Number of daily inhalations	Medium Dose: Daily dose Number of daily inhalations	High Dose: Daily dose Number of daily inhalations
Inhaled corticosteroids pregnancy category C				
Beclomethasone Depropionate	MDI Qvar HFA (CFC free) 40 or 80 mcg/puff, /100 inhalations	MDI 80–240 mcg daily 40 mcg: 2–6 puffs daily 80 mcg: 1–3 puffs daily	MDI 240–480 mcg daily 40 mcg: 6–12 puffs daily 80 mcg: 3–6 puffs daily	MDI >480 mcg daily 40 mcg: Use higher dose 80 mcg: >6 puffs
Budesonide	DPI Pulmicort Turbuhaler 200 mcg/inhalation/ 200 inhalations Nebulizer Pulmicort Respules	DPI 200–600 mcg daily 1–3 inhalations daily Recommended for use in children and elderly only	DPI 600–1200 mcg daily 3–6 inhalations daily	DPI >1200 mcg daily >6 inhalations daily
Flunisolide	MDI Aerobid 250 mcg/puff, 100 inhalations	MDI 500–1000 mcg daily 2–4 puffs daily	MDI 1000–2000 mcg daily 4–8 puffs daily	MDI >2000 mcg daily >8 puffs daily
Fluticasone	MDI Flovent 44, 110, or 220 mcg/puff, 60–120 inhalations	MDI 88-264 mcg daily 44 mcg: 2–6 puffs daily 110 mcg: 1–2 puffs daily 220 mcg: 1 puff daily	MDI 264–660 mcg daily 44 mcg: Change to 110+ 110 mcg: 2–6 puffs daily 220 mcg: 1–3 puffs daily	MDI >660 mcg daily 44 mcg: Use higher dose 110 mcg: >6 puffs 220 mcg: >3 puffs
	DPI Flovent Rotadisk 50, 100, or 250 mcg/ inhalation	DPI 100-300 mcg daily 50 mcg: 2–6 inhalations daily 100 mcg: 1–3 inhalations daily	DPI 300–600 mcg daily 50 mcg: Use higher dose 100 mcg: 3–6 inhalations daily	DPI >600 mcg daily 50 mcg: Use higher dose 100 mcg: >6 inhalations daily

		250 mcg: Use lower dose	250 mcg: 1–2 inhalations daily	250 mcg: >2 inhalations daily
Triamcinolone Acetonide	MDI Azmacort 100 mcg/puff, 240 inhalations	MDI 400–1000 mcg daily 4–10 puffs daily	MDI 1000–2000 mcg daily 10–20 puffs daily	MDI >2000 mcg daily >20 puffs daily

Long Acting β_2-Agonist Inhalers pregnancy category C

Formoterol	DPI Foradil 12 mcg/single use capsule, 18 or 60 capsules	DPI 1 capsule every 12 h
Salmeterol	MPI 21 mcg/puff	MPI 2 puffs q 12 h May use one dose for control of nighttime symptoms
	DPI Serevent Diskus 50 mcg/ blister, 60 blisters	DPI 1 blister q 12 h

Nonsteroidal Anti-Inflammatory (mast cell stabilizer) pregnancy category B

Cromolyn Sodium	MDI Intal 1 mg/puff 200 inhalations per 14 g inhaler	MDI 2–4 puffs tid to qid

(continues)

Table 12-11 MEDICATIONS FOR LONG-TERM CONTROL *(continued)*

Drug	Type/Trade Name/ Dose/Number of Inhalations per Canister	Low Dose: Daily dose Number of daily inhalations	Medium Dose: Daily dose Number of daily inhalations	High Dose: Daily dose Number of daily inhalations
Leukotriene Modifiers pregnancy category B				
Montelukast Sodium	Tablet Singulair 10 mg	1 tab PO q HS		
Zafirlukast	Tablet Accolate 10 mg and 20 mg	20 mg PO bid		
Zileuton	Tablet Zyflo 300 or 600 mg	600 mg PO qid		
Combination Products pregnancy category C				
Salmeterol and Fluticasone	DPI Advair Diskus 100/50, 250/50, 500/50, 60 blisters in a pack	Fluticasone 100 mcg/ Salmeterol 50 mcg per inhalation, 1 inhalation bid	Fluticasone 250 mcg/ Salmeterol 50 mcg per inhalation, 1 inhalation bid	*High Dose* Fluticasone 500 mcg/ Salmeterol 50 mcg per inhalation, 1 inhalation bid

Abbreviations are: CFC, chlorofluorocarbon; H, hour; q, every; tid, three times daily; qid, four times daily; bid, two times daily; hs, at night; po, orally; HFA, hydrofluoralkane; MDI, metered dose inhaler; DPI, dry powder inhaler.

Sources: National Asthma Education and Prevention Program.[5,9]

<table>
<tr><td colspan="2">Table 12-12 Level of Use Triggering Re-evaluation of Maintenance Medication</td></tr>
<tr><td>Asthma Level</td><td>Dose</td></tr>
<tr><td>Step 1
mild–intermittent
  asthma</td><td>>2 times a week</td></tr>
<tr><td>Steps 2–4
mild-to-severe
  persistent asthma</td><td>Daily or increasing use</td></tr>
</table>

Source: From the National Asthma Education and Prevention Program.[5]

function than adjunctive treatment with leukotriene modifiers.[13] Similarly, patients on monotherapy with leukotriene modifiers are 60% more likely to suffer exacerbations requiring systemic corticosteroids, to have poor FEV1 measurements, and to have more nocturnal awakening than patients treated with medium-dose inhaled corticosteroids.[11]

Other NonSteroidal Anti-Inflammatory Inhalers

The two agents in this category—cromolyn and nedocromil—affect mast cell mediator release and inhibit early and late asthmatic response triggered by allergens and exercise. Both compounds seem to be equally effective in reducing bronchospasm induced by allergens, but nedocromil appears to be more effective than cromolyn in the management of bronchospasm induced by non-allergen triggers.[3] However, whether these two products differ significantly in their clinical action is controversial; both cromolyn and nedocromil have long been used in the control of exercise-induced asthma.[16] Both agents are less effective than inhaled corticosteroids and less convenient, requiring dosing three or four times a day. However, their safety profile is better. These properties make these agents most appropriate for use in patients with milder asthma, particularly if allergens are a primary trigger, and for those patients concerned about the safety of inhaled corticosteroids. Nedocromil inhalers (Tilade) are not currently available in the United States.

All patients, regardless of stage, need to be prescribed a quick relief medication. The drug of choice for the treatment of acute bronchospasm is a short-acting inhaled β_2 agonist. Systemic routes are not recommended because they are less effective, have a longer onset of action, and are associated with more side effects. The most commonly prescribed agent is albuterol. Recently, levalbuterol, which is a derivative of albuterol, has been under investigation to determine whether it is more effective with a better side effect profile than albuterol. To date, controversy remains about whether the use of this more expensive medication is warranted.[17] Other less selective β_2 agonists, such as isoproterenol, metaproterenol, isoetharine, and epinephrine, are not recommended; they can cause excessive cardiac stimulation, especially at high doses.[3] Patients who overuse quick relief medication should be evaluated for the need to either add-on or increase the dose of controller medication(s).

Medication Delivery Systems: Inhalers, Spacers, and Nebulizers

Inhalers   There are two types of inhalers in use: dry powder inhalers (DPI) (**Figure** 12-4) and metered dose inhalers (MDI) (**Figure** 12-5). MDI inhalers are pressurized and need a propellant to push the medication out of the attached canister. Until recently, most MDIs were actuated by chlorofluorocarbon (CFC) propellants. However, when the United States signed the Montreal Protocol in 1987, it agreed to help protect the ozone layer by phasing out CFCs, which has stimulated the development of alternative propellants.[18] One alternative propellant currently available is hydrofluoroalkane, which is used in some MDIs, although CFC based inhalers are still readily available. Implementation of the Montreal Protocol has also stimulated the development of new systems, such as the DPIs, which do not require the use of any propellant. The DPIs contain individually packaged doses of dry powder medication, which are loaded into a reservoir. Each dose is dispensed into the breathing chamber just before use. Deposition of the medication into the lungs is triggered by inhalation for the majority of DPIs, although a few use another mechanism such as compressed air to activate the device.

DPIs use an entirely different delivery system than MDIs. Most DPIs are *breath-actuated*, meaning that a deep inhalation pulls the med-ication into the lungs, whereas MDIs use a propellant to force medication into the lungs. The technique needed for the correct use of DPIs is very different than the technique needed for MDIs. Therefore, it is essential that the midwife review with patients the correct steps in how to use their particular medication (**Table 12-13**). Correct use of a DPI requires rapid forceful inhalation as opposed to a coordinated slow breath with an MDI. Unlike the MDI, patients should never shake a DPI before use because this will cause the dose to be spilled and lost. In addition, patients using DPIs may not feel, smell, or taste the medication.

Correct use of an MDI inhaler requires the patient to push down on the canister to dispense the medication at the very beginning of a slow, deep inhalation. DPIs are easier to use for those who find the coordination required by this technique too difficult. However, some patients may not be able to breathe in deeply or quickly enough as the correct use of a DPI requires.

Figure 12-4 Dry powder inhaler.

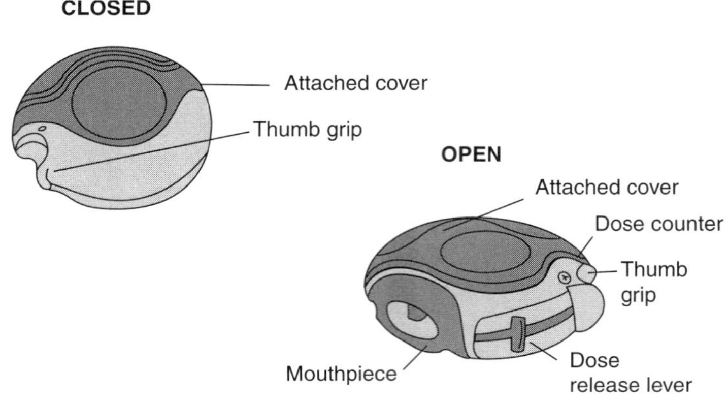

Soruce: Used with permission from the Asthma Society of Canada (http://www.asthma.ca).

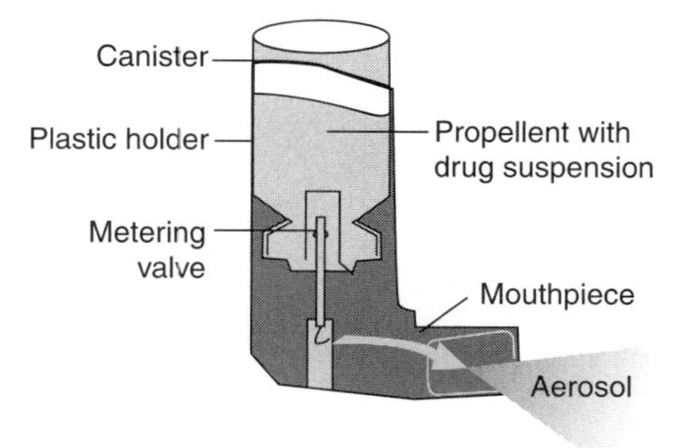

Figure 12-5 Metered dose inhaler.

Source: Used with permission from the Asthma Society of Canada (http://www.asthma.ca).

Correct technique is critical because it is one of the major determinants of whether a patient receives a full prescribed dose.[19] Therefore, the patient should be prescribed an inhaler type that she finds the easiest to use correctly.

Spacers   *Spacers* are used with MDI inhalers only (**Figure 12-6**). The MDI attaches to the spacer; medication is released into the spacer, and the patient inhales the medication through the spacer. Using an MDI inhaler in combination with a spacer provides many of the same advantages of DPI inhalers. Like DPIs, they do not require a patient to inhale at the same moment that they push down on the canister to release the medication. In a literature review evaluating over 50 studies on inhaler technique, Cochrane et al. reported that only about 7% to 23% of any drug delivered by an MDI reaches the lungs.[19] Use of a spacer can almost double the deposition of medication in the lungs and significantly reduces deposition into the oropharynx. Not only does a spacer improve medication delivery, but

it can minimize side effects of medications dispensed by MDIs. They help prevent the development of oral thrush, which is a common side effect of corticosteroid-containing inhalers, and minimize the systemic absorption of MDI-dispensed medications.[19] **Table 12-14** describes the proper spacer technique.

The major disadvantage of spacers is that they are bulky and awkward to carry. Therefore, they are best used with dosing patterns, such as daily or twice a day frequencies, which allow the patient to keep the spacer at home. Another approach is to prescribe several spacers so that the patient can leave one at home and another at school or work.

Nebulizer   A *nebulizer* is a T-shaped cylinder with a mouthpiece at one end, a cup to hold medication in the middle, and a port at the other end. Tubing attaches to this port and connects either to an oxygen tank or nebulizer machine. Medication and saline are added to the cup; oxygen bubbles through this solution and provides an aerolized medicated mist to the patient. Nebulizers are popular with patients due to their ease of use. However, they are less practical than inhalers because they are not portable. Nor do they provide any added benefit; studies have shown that using MDI inhalers with a spacer is as effective as a nebulizer treatment, as long as the patient uses good inhaler technique.[20] **Table 12-15** describes the proper nebulizer technique.

MANAGEMENT OF EXERCISE-INDUCED ASTHMA

Exercise-induced asthma is common and thought to affect 10% to 50% of recreational and elite athletes.[16] It can occur solely with exercise and therefore meet the definition of exercise-induced asthma or may be a manifestation of chronic

Table 12-13 CORRECT INHALER TECHNIQUE

Inhaler	Correct Usage

Metered dose inhaler	Canister
	Plastic holder
	Propellent with drug suspension
	Metering valve
	Mouthpiece
	Aerosol
	• Hold the inhaler upright and shake several times
	• Hold the mouthpiece in any of the following 2 correct positions
	  1) Seal your mouth around the mouthpiece
	  2) Hold the mouthpiece 1 to 2 inches away from your lips (a spacer may also be used; see Table 12-14)
	• Do not block the inhaler opening with your tongue
	• Press down on the inhaler as you start to breathe in
	• Breathe in slowly and steadily over 3 to 5 seconds
	• Remove the inhaler from your mouth
	• Hold your breath for 10 seconds
	• Breathe out slowly
	• Rinse your mouth if using an inhaler containing corticosteroids
	• Store in dry place

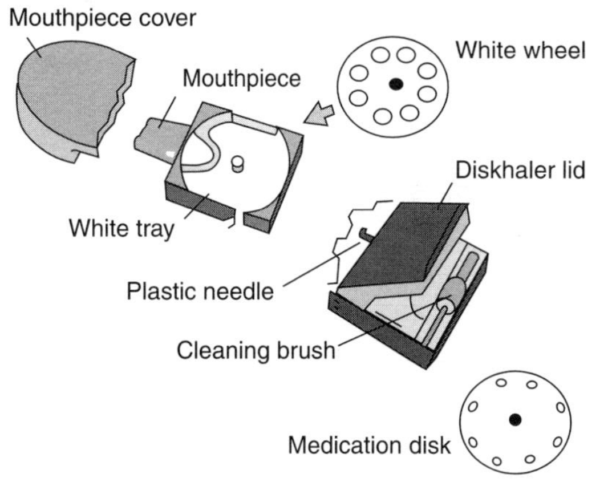

- Hold the inhaler upright
- Load your inhaler
- Do NOT shake the inhaler or your medication will spill
- Seal your lips around the inhaler
- Do not block the inhaler opening with your tongue
- Breathe in quickly and forcefully to release the medication
- Remove the inhaler from your mouth
- Hold your breath afterward for 10 seconds
- Breathe out slowly
- Do not breathe out through the inhaler, because the humidity from your breath in combination with the dry powder medication can clog the device
- In general, do not wash DPI. Use a dry cloth to wipe out the device.
- Do not use a DPI with a spacer
- Rinse your mouth if using an inhaler containing corticosteroids
- Each DPI is different; refer to the operating instructions for further details governing the patient's specific medication

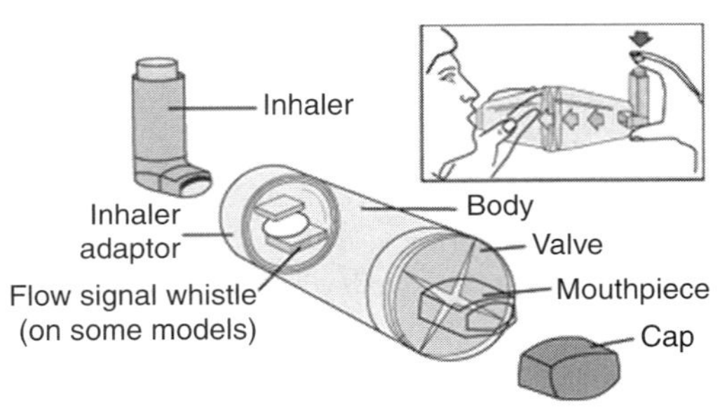

Figure 12-6 A spacer.

Source: Used with permission from the Asthma Society of Canada (http://www.asthma.ca).

asthma if the patient only recognizes asthma symptoms while exercising. Typically, exercise-induced asthma presents with coughing, wheezing, chest tightness, or shortness of breath after six to eight minutes of exercise.[16] Symptoms tend to resolve in 20 to 30 minutes after exercise is stopped.[6] A careful history is needed to determine the diagnosis because the management of exercise-induced asthma and chronic asthma worsened by exercise differs. Those with chronic asthma may require daily medications plus pretreatment before exercising, whereas those with exercise-induced asthma will need only pretreatment.

The preferred pretreatment for exercise-induced asthma is the use of short-acting inhaled β_2 agonists 15 minutes before the onset of exercise. The effect of this pretreatment should last two to three hours.[7] If this regimen provides only partial relief, then inhaled cromolyn given in a higher dose than that required for maintenance therapy (4–10 puffs) may be added.[16] Inhaled nedocromil given in a dose of two to four puffs may also be used.[16] The long-acting inhaled β_2 agonists are another alternative and may be particularly helpful for those who participate in marathons or other activities of long duration.[16] Long-acting inhaled β_2 agonists should be taken a minimum of 30 minutes before exercising and will last 10 to 12 hours.[6] Patients who still experience symptoms after trying these options may need to be placed on daily maintenance medication.

Other non-pharmacologic approaches can help. Pre-exercise warm-ups are essential. Avoiding exposure to cold air by using a scarf outdoors or exercising indoors may help. Exercising indoors may

Table 12-14 **CORRECT SPACER TECHNIQUE**

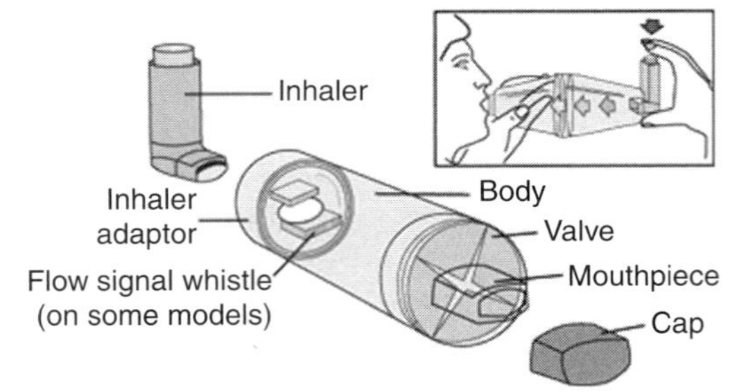

- Use only with an MDI inhaler
- Shake the inhaler
- Attach the spacer to the mouthpiece of the inhaler
- Press down on the inhaler and release one puff into the spacer
- Place the mouthpiece into your mouth and inhale slowly
- Hold your breath for 10 seconds and exhale

Source: Figure is used with permission from the Asthma Society of Canada (http://www.asthma.ca).

Table 12-15 CORRECT USE OF A NEBULIZER

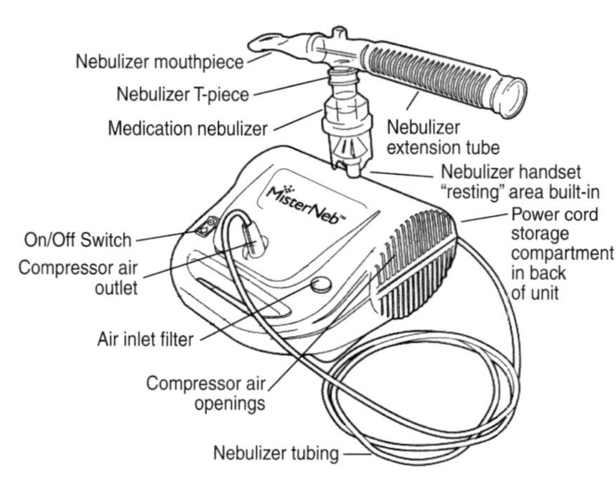

- Measure the correct amount of normal saline and add to the cup
- Measure the correct amount of medication and add to the cup
- Fasten the mouthpiece to the T-shaped cylinder
- Connect the T-shaped cylinder to the oxygen tank or nebulizer
- Turn on the oxygen tank
- Seal your mouth around the mouthpiece
- Take slow deep breaths
- Hold each breath for one to two seconds
- Continue until all of the medication is gone
- Turn off the oxygen source
- For home machines, disconnect the tubing
- Rinse the mouthpiece and T-shaped cylinder in warm running water. Do not rinse the tubing.
- Reconnect the mouthpiece, T-shaped cylinder, and tubing
- Run the oxygen for a few minutes to air dry the nebulizer
- Disconnect and store in dry place

also help those whose asthma is triggered by outdoor allergens or air pollution. The type of exercise also can make a difference. Sports such as long-distance running, cycling, basketball, soccer, ice hockey, ice skating, and cross-country skiing are more likely to trigger asthma than swimming, diving, sprinting, boxing, wrestling, karate, tennis, gymnastics, baseball, downhill skiing, isometrics, and water polo.[16]

MANAGEMENT OF ACUTE EXACERBATIONS

All patients need to be educated on how to manage worsening asthma symptoms and when to come to the hospital or clinic for emergency management. The NAEPP strongly recommends that providers give all patients a written asthma action plan, which describes a specific individualized plan to follow based on changes in symptoms and/or pulmonary function. A written action plan breaks down symptoms and peak flow measurements into three categories:

- *Red Zone:* Requires immediate treatment and emergent evaluation by a health care provider.
- *Yellow Zone:* Requires immediate treatment and urgent evaluation by a health care provider if symptoms do not resolve with yellow zone management.

- *Green Zone:* Normal pulmonary function that requires continuation of maintenance medication.

This "Red-Yellow-Green Stoplight" format presents a clear visual image for the patient to follow. **Figure 12-7** is an example of a written action plan. Action plans are based on the treatment recommendations made by the NAEPP and can be found in the **Figure 12-8** algorithm.[6]

Midwives are most likely to encounter women experiencing acute asthma exacerbations in the triage area on Labor and Delivery, as it is common for hospitals to send all pregnant women to Labor and Delivery for evaluation regardless of the nature of their presenting problem. A prompt and focused evaluation is essential to provide symptomatic relief and prevent worsening of the attack. In this situation, the history should focus primarily on asthma-related questions. It is essential to determine what medications the patient is currently prescribed, adherence to her prescribed regimen, recent use of any quick relief medications at home, known triggers, and history of prior exacerbations requiring intubations or hospitalization. The midwife should obtain vital signs, pulse oximetry, and a peak flow if readily available and observe how comfortable the patient is with talking and breathing. Pulse oximetry should be obtained on room air BEFORE giving the patient supplemental oxygen. The midwife should begin immediate emergency treatment with a nebulizer using a short-acting β_2 agonist and consult for further management with a provider skilled in asthma management. The goal is to administer medications without delay in order to prevent pulmonary deterioration; therefore all midwives must be skilled in the emergency management

of asthma. **Figure 12-9** provides an algorithm for managing asthma attacks in the emergency department.

Patients with severe exacerbations may require oral or intravenous corticosteroids and a change in their maintenance medications in order to regain control. Patients are often given a steroid "burst" of 40 to 60 mg of oral prednisone for three to ten days and are continued on a higher dose of their controller medication(s). After discharge, patients should be seen within three to five days by their primary asthma provider.[6] The burst dose of steroids should continue until the patient is symptom free or the patient achieves 80% of her personal best peak flow.[5] Patients should remain on a higher level inhaled corticosteroid dose for a minimum of several weeks to a month and then can be slowly weaned down if they maintain good asthma control.

Impact of Pregnancy and Lactation

Debate exists about whether pregnancy improves or worsens asthma. However, studies based on asthma severity indicate that those women with milder disease experience little change in their asthma status in pregnancy, whereas those with more severe asthma do.[21,22] Debate also exists about whether, and if so how, asthma affects fetal or maternal outcomes. Older retrospective studies indicated that women with asthma were more likely to experience preeclampsia, premature births, or other complications, and their babies were more likely to need neonatal intensive care management. However, prospective case-matched studies indicate that women with actively managed asthma who achieve good control have rates of perinatal complications similar to women without asthma.[21,22]

Figure 12-7 Sample asthma action plan.

ASTHMA ACTION PLAN FOR _________________________ Doctor's name _________________ Date _________

Doctor's Phone Number _________________ Hospital Emergency Room Phone Number _________________

GREEN ZONE: Doing Well
- No cough, wheeze, chest tightness, or shortness of breath during the day or night
- Can do usual activities

And, if a peak flow meter is used, Peak flow: more than _________ (80% or more of my best peak flow)

My best peak flow _________

Take These Long-Term-Control Medicines Each Day (include an anti-inflammatory)

Medicine	How much to take	When to take it

Before exercise ☐ _________________ ☐ 2 or ☐ 4 puffs   5 to 50 minutes before exercise

YELLOW ZONE: Asthma is Getting Worse
- Cough, wheeze, chest tightness, or shortness of breath, or
- Waking at night due to asthma, or
- Can do some but not all usual activities

-Or-

Peak flow: ____ to ____ (50%–80% of my best peak flow)

[FIRST] **Add: Quick-Relief Medicine—and keep taking your GREEN ZONE medicine**

_________________ ☐ 2 or ☐ 4 puffs, every 20 minutes for up to 1 hour
(short-acting beta-agonist)   ☐ Nebulizer, once

[SECOND] If your symptoms (and peak flow, if used) return to *GREEN ZONE* after 1 hour of above treatment:
- ☐ Take the quick-relief medicine every 4 hours for 1 to 2 days.
- ☐ Double the dose of your inhaled steroid for _______ (7–10 days).

-Or-

If your symptoms (and peak flow, if used) *do not return to GREEN ZONE* after 1 hour of above treatment:
- ☐ Take: _________________ ☐ 2 or ☐ 4 puffs or   ☐ Nebulizer
  (short-acting beta-agonist)
- ☐ Add: _________________ _______ mg. per day For ____ (3–10) days
  (oral steroid)
- ☐ Call the doctor ☐ before ☐ within _________ hours after taking the oral steroid

RED ZONE: Medical Alert!
- Very short of breath, or
- Quick-relief medicines have not helped, or
- Cannot do usual activities or
- Symptoms are same or get worse after 24 hours in Yellow Zone

-Or-

Peak flow: less than _________ (50% of my best peak flow)

Take this medicine:

☐ _________________ ☐ 4 or   ☐ 6 puffs or Nebulizer
(short-acting beta-agonist)

☐ _________________ _______ mg
(oral steroid)

Then call your doctor NOW.   Go to the hospital or call for an ambulance if:
- You are still in the red zone after 15 minutes AND
- You have not reached your doctor

DANGER SIGNS
- Trouble walking and talking due to shortness of breath
- Lips or fingernails are blue

- Take 4 or 6 puffs of your quick-relief medicine *AND*
- Go to the hospital or call for an ambulance (_________) *NOW!*

Source: National Asthma Education and Prevention Program.[6]

Figure 12-8 Home treatment management for exacerbations of asthma in non-pregnant women.

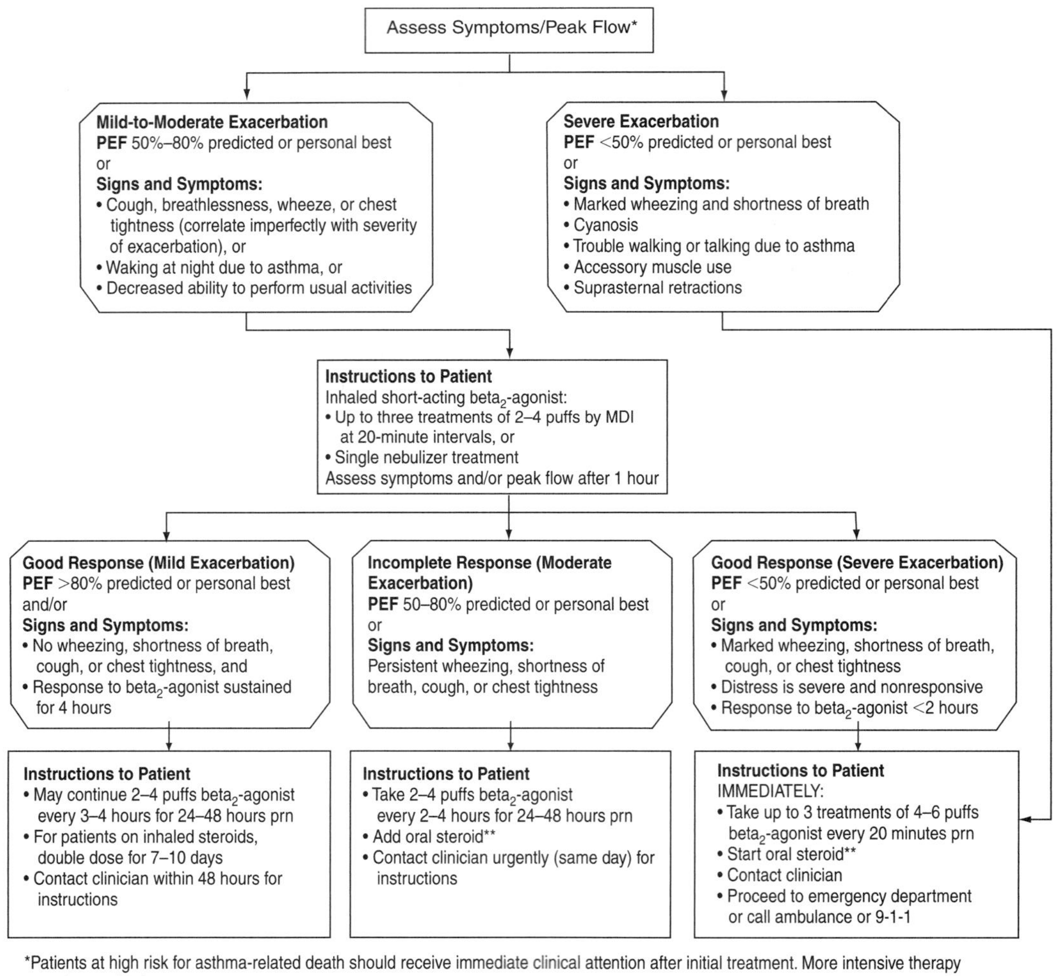

Abbreviations are: MDI, metered dose inhaler; PEF, peak expiratory flow; prn, as needed.

Source: National Asthma Education and Prevention Program.[6]

One potential confounding variable in these studies may be the use of oral corticosteroids. A recent study of over 2000 pregnant and non-pregnant women supports this premise.[23] In that study, women using oral corticosteroids delivered two weeks earlier than women not using

Figure 12-9 Emergency department and hospital-based management for exacerbations of asthma for non-pregnant women.

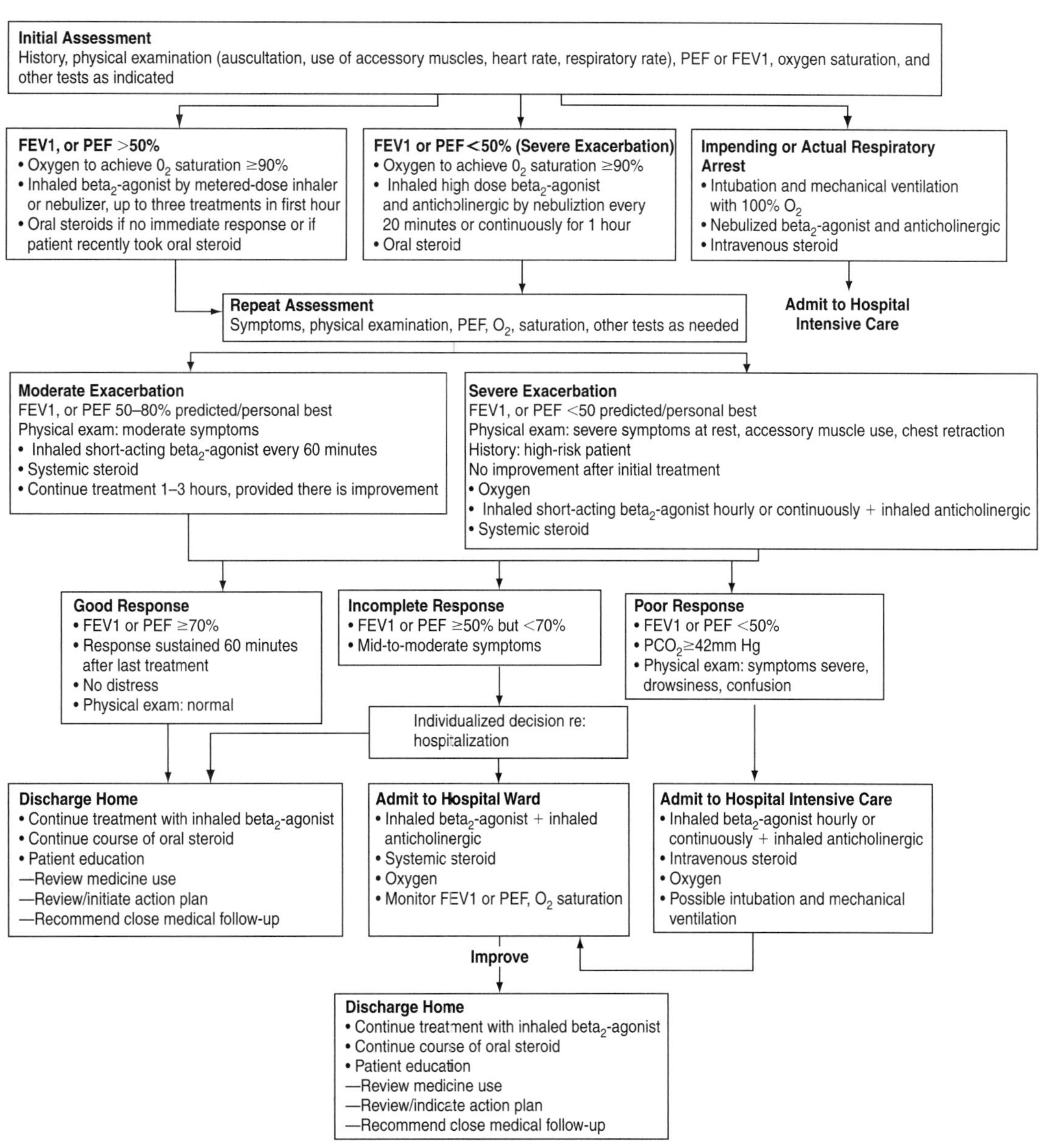

Abbreviaitons are: PEF, peak expiratory flow; FEV1, forced expiratory flow in 1 second.
Source: National Asthma Education and Prevention Program.[6]

systemic corticosteroids ($P = 0.001$). Asthma severity was not associated with preterm birth, but was associated with intrauterine growth restriction (IUGR). Each increased step of asthma severity was associated with a 24% increased risk of delivering an IUGR infant.

All of the medications used in the treatment of asthma can be used during pregnancy and lactation.[24] Any of the corticosteroid inhalers are acceptable, although budesonide (Pulmicort) is recommended by the NAEPP as the preferred treatment—not because budesonide is thought to be any safer than other corticosteroid inhaler choices, but because it has more extensive safety data. Therefore the NAEPP recommends beginning with budesonide for women initiating corticosteroid inhaler use in pregnancy, but does not advocating switching to budesonide for women already using other products. Oral corticosteroids can also be used in pregnancy. While the use of oral corticosteroids may be associated with some adverse outcomes,[22,23] their use is mandatory for severe asthma given the grave consequences of uncontrolled asthma. Of the other medications commonly used for asthma management, the leukotriene modifiers have the least available data, but are still thought to be safe.[24] Therefore, the approach to management of asthma is unchanged by pregnancy or lactation. Unfortunately, pregnant women are often reluctant to use enough medication to achieve control. Providers also tend to under prescribe. The end result is that pregnant women are much more likely to seek emergency care in pregnancy and to experience relapse after emergency treatment. In a study investigating the care received by pregnant and non-pregnant women with similar pretreatment asthma profiles, pregnant women received a similar number of nebulized β_2 agonist treatments in the emergency room, but were less likely to receive systemic corticosteroids or be prescribed steroids on discharge. At the two-week follow-up interview, pregnant women were three times more likely to report ongoing exacerbation of their asthma.[25]

Acute asthma attacks are rare during labor and birth. Women should continue on their usual medications but may require systemic corticosteroids if they are on an oral regimen before labor. The NAEPP recommends that women receive a stress dose of corticosteroids during labor and the early postpartum period if oral steroids were used within the four weeks prior to admission (**Box 12-1**).[24] Women with asthma should be asked about their sensitivity to aspirin or nonsteroidal anti-inflammatories, which are commonly used for pain management postpartum. These pain relievers have been found to provoke exacerbations in a small subset of asthmatics.[22]

Patient Instructions

Patients need to know that asthma is a lifelong condition requiring ongoing care. Acceptance of this is a prerequisite for a patient to be able to appropriately manage her asthma. Even those women who recognize the need for treatment may have difficulty adhering to a daily medication regimen, particularly when they feel well. Studies have documented that 24% to 69% of patients

---

Box 12-1 Stress Dose of Steroids[24]

A. Give if the woman has received oral steroids within previous four weeks

B. Start in labor and continue until 24 hours after delivery

C. Regimen: Hydrocortisone 100 mg IV every 8 hours.

fail to take all of their prescribed medications.[19] However, education, regular follow-up, and use of adjunctive tools such as patient diaries and peak flow meters can significantly improve adherence. In one randomized study of 100 urban Latino and African-American families, those families participating in an intervention using all of these techniques had significantly better adherence and fewer symptoms than the control group. Patients in the intervention group were more likely to take their medications regularly (82% intervention vs. 40% control group), refill their medications before they ran out (68% intervention vs. 48% control group), and report less activity restriction (20% decrease in the intervention group, 2% increase in control group).[26]

Midwives must make certain that all of their patients with asthma understand the physiology of asthma, how and when to take their medications, and what to do if their symptoms worsen. Written action plans can provide a structured approach for patients. These plans give patients guidance on how to monitor their symptoms, how to change their medications if symptoms worsen, and when to notify their provider (Figure 12-7).

Written action plans are recommended by the NAEPP for use with all asthmatics, regardless of the severity of their disease. According to the NAEPP, a written action plan[5] should include:

- Explicit patient-specific recommendations for environmental control and other preventive efforts that may be necessary to avoid or reduce exacerbations.
- An algorithm of procedures that clearly describes how to use long-term control and rescue medication, given a set of specific circumstances and conditions, and clear instructions on how to make medicine adjustments when conditions change.
- Steps the patient should take when medicines are ineffective or if an emergency arises.
- Contacts for securing urgent care if needed.

To be effective, written action plans require patient monitoring of their symptoms, which can be done subjectively based on patient perceptions or objectively based on peak flow measurements. The NAEPP does not recommend long-term daily use of peak flow measurements in those asthmatics with milder disease, although their use may be helpful during exacerbations. Patients with more severe disease or who cannot recognize worsening symptoms can benefit from more consistent use of peak flow meters. Daily peak flow monitoring in patients can be helpful in detecting early changes in disease status that require changes in medication management, evaluate the effectiveness of medication changes, provide objective measurements, and give guidance to those patients who cannot perceive air flow obstruction.[5] While the NAEPP recommends daily monitoring for patients with moderate to severe persistent asthma, patients who cannot adhere to long-term monitoring may benefit from daily monitoring over a two- to three-week period, particularly when maintenance medications are changed or when evaluating possible environmental triggers. Short-term monitoring when a patient feels well can also establish a "personal best" measurement, which can be used as an objective basis for comparison during the treatment of any future exacerbations.

Complementary and Alternative Medicine

Studies on the use of complementary and alternative medicines in asthma suffer from the same methodological weaknesses found generally in the field, in particular small sample sizes, heterogeneous designs, and lack of randomization. Two large reviews of over 50 studies concluded that the use of acupuncture and herbs cannot be recommended, based on the quality and quantity of available evidence.[27,28] However, the use of relaxation techniques, breathing exercises, and vitamin C supplementation may warrant further investigation; a few small nonrandomized studies suggest that these methods may be minimally effective.[28,29]

Lifestyle

The goal in asthma therapy is to allow the patient to be symptom-free by using appropriate medications and environmental controls. Environmental control is particularly helpful in those patients whose asthma is triggered by allergens. Numerous studies have documented significant increases in symptom-free days with control of dust mite allergies.[6] Studies have also found that appropriate treatment of allergic rhinitis can reduce the risk of asthma exacerbations by one-third to one-half.[30] Therefore, all asthmatics should be evaluated to determine to what extent allergens affect their asthma; if a link is found between asthma symptoms and allergens, environmental controls and appropriate medications should be recommended. The section on allergies below details the evaluation, treatment, and lifestyle modifications required for the control of allergies.

Consultation

Asthma care needs to be provided in a system that allows for emergency evaluation and treatment. Therefore, the role of midwives in the care of asthmatic women will vary according to the system in which they practice as well as by the prevalence of this condition in their particular patient population and by their own particular interests. At a minimum, all midwives should be able to evaluate whether women are receiving appropriate care, using their medications correctly, and have an emergency plan in place if an exacerbation occurs. All midwives should also be able to initiate care during an asthma attack, as prompt treatment is critical in preventing a severe episode. However, midwives can also provide more direct and independent care. Those who function in a system that can provide ready access to emergency care can independently manage women with mild intermittent, mild persistent, and well-controlled moderate persistent asthma. Midwives should consult with an asthma specialist if a patient does not respond appropriately to care or if a patient requires numerous medication changes and/or high doses in order to achieve control. All women with severe persistent asthma should be under the care of an asthma specialist.

Allergies

Allergies are common in the general population, but the incidence is particularly high in individuals with asthma and atopy. Allergic rhinitis has been reported to occur in approximately 10% to 20% of the general population compared to 75% of asthmatics.[31] Good control of allergy symptoms not only significantly improves asthma symptoms[31] but may also delay or prevent the development of future asthma in individuals affected by allergic rhinitis.[32] Studies have shown allergies also adversely affect patients' professional and personal lives. Over 90% of those with allergic rhinitis have reported severe-to-moderate impairment in their ability to be productive at school, work, and in their activities of daily living.[33] Skillful management of these conditions not only may improve health but also significantly improve the quality of life for those with allergies.

Clinical Presentation

Exposure to allergens can lead to allergic rhinitis, food allergies, or contact dermatitis depending on which organ system is affected. Those with allergic rhinitis will report rhinorrhea, sneezing, nasal obstruction, itchy watery eyes, or sneezing. Those with food allergies may report oral irritation and tightness; some will report gastrointestinal (GI) upset and diarrhea, and others will develop hives or contact dermatitis. Allergic contact dermatitis often presents as an itchy rash where exposure occurred. Many of these same symptoms are also present with other conditions. However, the hallmark finding with allergies is that symptoms develop after exposure to an offending trigger and remit once the trigger is removed. Diagnosis is easiest when the exposure to a trigger is episodic, such as in seasonal allergies, and is hardest when exposure is chronic, such as with indoor allergens, where it is difficult to remove the offending trigger. **Table 12-16** provides differential diagnoses for common allergies. Refer to Chapters 17 and 22 for GI and dermatological disorders, which can help distinguish between those diagnostic possibilities, especially in those who have persistent symptoms.

Despite the variety of ways that allergies can present, they all seem to be the result of similar impairments in the immune system.[35] In allergic rhinitis, exposure to allergens trigger CD4 T lymphocytes to release interleukin and other T helper 2 (Th2) cytokines. Cytokine release leads to inflammation through immunoglobulin E

(IgE) production, mucosal infiltration, and the release of mediators caused by degranulation of mast cells. Like asthma, the chemical cascade in the early phase of allergic rhinitis leads to the release of mediators that damage blood vessels and stimulate the sensory nerves, leading to watery nasal discharge, mucosal edema, nasal congestion, and itching. During the late phase response, which occurs six to eight hours after exposure, symptoms recur as the Th2 lymphocytes release cytokines, resulting in chronic nasal and sinus congestion. While the pathophysiology of food allergies and allergic contact dermatitis is less well understood, they also seem to be at least partially a result of IgE production and mediator release similar to that in allergic rhinitis.[35]

Essential History and Physical and Laboratory Evaluation

HISTORY

Patients should be asked about the range of symptoms that may accompany allergies, because this will help identify all possible triggers and guide treatment choices. Environmental controls and medication management should be chosen to provide the greatest relief from the specific allergen(s) suspected of causing the patients' symptoms.

Patients should be asked not only about their specific symptoms, but also about the timing of the onset of these symptoms in relation to exposure to suspected triggers. Symptoms typically develop shortly after exposure to episodic triggers, making it easiest to identify these triggers. Questions focusing on whether symptoms occur year round or only in certain seasons can help pinpoint which specific allergens are problematic for an individual patient. Patients with symptoms only in the spring should be suspected of having allergies to pollen; those who experience symptoms only in the fall may have

Table 12-16 DIFFERENTIAL DIAGNOSIS FOR ALLERGY

Symptom	Condition	History	Physical	Laboratory
Rhinorrhea	Allergic rhinitis	• Watery rhinorrhea, sneezing, nasal obstruction, nasal itching, conjunctivitis • Symptoms episodic or continuous depending on trigger • Itchy mouth and ears • History of other atopic conditions such as asthma and eczema	• Usually pale, boggy nasal mucosa, occasionally purple • Increased vascularity • Clear watery nasal discharge • Edematous swollen turbinates • Significant congestion can lead to darkening of tissue below the eye (allergic shiners)	• Elevated serum eosinophils although this is nonspecific and of little clinical utility • Positive skin testing for allergies
	Common cold	• Symptoms with identified onset and resolution within 10 to 14 days, including rhinorrhea, watery eyes • Possibly accompanied by myalgia, fever, and malaise	• Thick mucopurulent nasal discharge • Nasal mucosa normal or red and inflamed	• Not helpful
Watery eyes	Allergic conjunctivitis	• Red watery eyes • Bilateral presentation • Itchy	• Red and watery conjunctiva	• Not helpful
	Bacterial conjunctivitis	• Usually unilateral onset, possibly spreading to other eye • Acute onset • Classic discharge with complaint of irritation and tearing	• Classically thick yellow discharge gluing the eye to the lower lid, most noticeable upon arising	• Culture and sensitivity not necessary unless diagnosis unclear or if symptoms are pronounced

Table 12-16 **Differential Diagnosis for Allergy** *(continued)*

Symptom	Condition	History	Physical	Laboratory
Watery eyes	Viral Conjunctivitis	• Usually unilateral onset, possibly spreading to other eye	• Classically clear watery discharge with conjunctival redness • Transient blurred vision, no photophobia	• Culture and sensitivity not necessary unless diagnosis not clear or if symptoms are pronounced
Skin rash	Allergic contact dermatitis	• Onset after exposure to offending trigger • Symptoms consistent upon re-exposure	• Acute exposure leads to erythematous macules, papules, or vesicles at site of exposure or adjacent areas • Chronic exposure leads to lichenification, scaling, or fissures	• Skin testing
	Atopic dermatitis	Refer to Chapter	22	
Diarrhea and stomach pain	Food allergies	• Symptoms occuring after consumption of offending food • Symptoms consistent upon re-exposure • Predominantly GI tract symptoms, including oral itching, swelling of the airway, abdominal pain and diarrhea	• Not helpful	• Not helpful
	Gastroenteritis Other GI conditions	Refer to Chapter 17		

Source: Bousquet J, van Cauwenberge P, Khaltaev N, Aria Workshop Group, World Health Organization. Allergic rhinitis and its impact on asthma. *Journal of Allergy & Clinical Immunology* 2001; 108(5 Supplement):S14–S334.

allergies to ragweed or mold. The onset and duration of allergies can also vary by geographic location depending on climate zones and elevations. For example, dust mite levels tend to be lower at higher elevations, and pollen counts tend to be higher earlier in the spring in the South.

Patients with year-round symptoms should be queried about exposure to animals, cockroaches, indoor molds, and house-dust mites. Asking a patient whether symptoms occur only in certain indoor living spaces (bedroom, basement) or times of day (nighttime or daytime) can help differentiate potential indoor triggers. For example, patients with dust mite allergies typically complain of symptoms upon arising in the morning because dust mite levels tend to be highest in pillows, mattresses, and bedding. Patients whose allergens may be triggered by chronic exposures should be asked whether eliminating these triggers (such as avoiding suspected foods or living in a home without pets for several weeks) has ever improved their symptoms. **Table 12-17** has further details on common allergy triggers.

Patients suspected of having food allergies or allergic contact dermatitis should be queried about timing of symptoms in relationship to exposures. These conditions often mimic other GI and dermatological disorders; this line of questioning is critical in uncovering potential allergens. Resolution of symptoms with food avoidance or with cessation of use of specific products supports the diagnosis, as does a return of symptoms with resumption of use of these products or with consumption of offending foods.

PHYSICAL

Patients suspected of having allergies need a complete physical evaluation of the head, ear, eye, nose, throat, skin, and respiratory systems, because allergies commonly affect these systems. Patients suspected of having allergic contact dermatitis need a careful skin inspection, looking for rashes that originate at the exposure site. The physical exam is of little help when evaluating potential food allergies. However, individuals with food allergies or allergic contact dermatitis can infrequently experience symptoms of allergic rhinitis and need the same evaluation as those with primary allergic rhinitis. All patients with persistent allergic rhinitis symptoms need a thorough nasal exam to evaluate the nasal anatomy, the color of the mucosa, and the quality and quantity of the mucus. This exam is best facilitated with the use of a nasal speculum. Findings suggestive of allergies are outlined in Table 12-16.

LABORATORY

In general, laboratory testing is of limited value in the evaluation of allergies, with the exception of skin testing. Individuals with allergies may have elevated serum eosinophils, but this is a nonspecific finding also seen in some cancers, parasitic infections, skin disorders, and drug reactions, so it has little clinical utility in the diagnosis of allergies. A few authorities recommend nasal cytology, which can identify high levels of eosinophils in the nasal exudates of allergic individuals. In contrast, neutrophils tend to predominate in the nasal cytology of individuals with infection. However, eosinophils can also be seen on cytology smears of individuals with asthma, nasal polyps, and aspirin sensitivity. The poor specificity of nasal smears limits their usefulness, although some clinicians use them to monitor the effectiveness of anti-inflammatory treatment.[36]

Table 12-17 ALLERGY TRIGGERS

Trigger	Indications	Environmental Controls
Dust mites	Symptoms worse in the morning after sleeping all night in bed.	• Wash all bedding in hot water every week and blankets/comforters at least 4 times a year. • Whether using polyester filled pillows as opposed to feather or down is helpful is unclear, although this traditionally has been recommended. • Encase mattress and in particular pillows with allergy-proof covers. Use specially designed allergy covers, not "dust covers." Dust covers do not filter out dust mites, only larger particle dust. • Minimize use of soft materials by replacing carpets with linoleum or wood flooring, drapes with blinds or washable curtains, and upholstered furniture with leather furniture. • Hot wash or freeze soft toys. • Vacuum daily using a vacuum equipped with a HEPA filter or special allergen-proof vacuum cleaner bags or connected to a duct system. • Do not use humidifiers; they increase the growth of dust mites.
Dust	Symptoms worsen with dusting and sweeping.	All of the measures listed under dust mites and in addition: • If forced air heat or air conditioning is used, cover the vents with a filter and wash or change this filter every month. • Where possible, have non-allergic household members be responsible for dusting and vacuuming. • Air filtration systems and ionizers are controversial and are not thought to significantly reduce symptoms for many individuals. • Keep dust-collecting items inside of cupboards.

Pet allergens	Symptoms begin or worsen after pet introduced into household and are relieved when away from household.	• Remove pet from household if possible.
		• If pet removal is not possible, try:
		  • Keeping pet out of bedroom, especially off of the bed
		  • Keeping pet off furniture in all rooms and out of doors as much as possible
		  • Washing pet weekly
		  • Sweeping regularly with a vacuum equipped with HEPA filter or special allergy-proof bags

(continues)

Table 12-17 ALLERGY TRIGGERS *(continued)*

Trigger	Indications	Environmental Controls
Indoor molds	Symptoms worsen in areas of high humidity (basement, areas of water damage) or when area smells musty.	• Use dehumidifiers in damp areas of household. • Do not lay carpeting directly on concrete basement flooring. • Do not use humidifiers anywhere in the household.
Outdoor allergens	Suspect allergy to pollen and grasses if symptoms worse in the spring and early summer. Suspect allergies to ragweed and mold if symptoms worse in the fall. Fall allergies usually subside after the first hard frost.	• Use air conditioners even if not needed for cooling to filter outdoor air. Wash filters regularly. • Have air conditioners professionally cleaned to remove mold. • Avoiding outdoor activities between 11 AM and 3 PM when pollen counts are highest, or in early morning and late evening if mold allergies are a problem.

Skin testing (also called puncture, prick, or epicutaneous skin testing) is considered to be the gold standard and is useful in identifying the specific allergens that produce symptoms. Individuals being tested receive multiple small skin punctures; each one is inoculated with a different extract containing a single antigen of such common allergens as dust mite, mold, and pollen. Allergic individuals develop a wheal to their specific offending allergens within 20 minutes of being inoculated. A positive test will result in a wheal 3-mm or greater in diameter than the negative control reaction and is accompanied by erythema.[37] Women scheduled for skin testing should be advised to avoid the use of first generation antihistamines for three days and the use of second generation antihistamines for a minimum of 10 days before their skin testing appointments; the use of these drugs can inhibit the wheal and flare reaction of these tests and lead to false negative results.[37]

Most skin panels test for 10 to 20 common allergens. Skin testing is particularly helpful in developing environmental control strategies designed to minimize exposure. They also can help determine whether or not treatment with allergen immunotherapy may be helpful in controlling symptoms. Serum tests are also available that can help identify problematic IgE for allergic individuals, but are of limited usefulness because they are more expensive and less sensitive than skin testing.

MANAGEMENT

Allergic Rhinitis According to ARIA-WHO (Allergic Rhinitis Impact on Asthma-the World Health Organization), management of allergic rhinitis relies on three main principles: 1) instituting environmental controls to minimize exposure to offending allergens; 2) prescribing anti-inflammatory agents to halt the chemical cascade leading to IgE production, cytokine release, and mast cell activation; and 3) providing symptomatic relief through the use of antihistamines and decongestants.[34]

The most recent guidelines published by ARIA-WHO in 2001 changed the classification system used to describe allergic rhinitis.[34] Traditionally, allergic rhinitis had been subdivided into seasonal and perennial categories. However, these categories do not adequately reflect the extent to which allergic rhinitis can negatively affect individuals. The new classification system subdivides allergic rhinitis into four categories based on the frequency of symptoms and the impacts these symptoms have on the lives of affected individuals. ARIA-WHO linked these classifications to recommended treatment guidelines based on a review of the evidence by a panel of international experts. The ARIA-WHO categories are as follows.[34]

1. *Mild Intermittent:* Symptoms occur less than 4 days per week or less than 4 weeks at a time. Symptoms do not affect sleep or interfere with daily activities. Recommended treatments include oral antihistamines, intranasal antihistamines, or intranasal decongestants.

2. *Severe Intermittent:* The frequency of symptoms is the same as in Category 1 ($<$4 days/week or $<$4 weeks at a time) but are more problematic. Symptoms are severe enough to lead to at least one of the following: disrupted sleep, troublesome symptoms, or impaired work, school, sport, or leisure time performance. Treatments include those recommended for Category 1 (oral or intranasal antihistamines) with the exception of intranasal decongestants. However, other medications such as the intranasal corticosteroids or mast cell stabilizers may provide more relief. Immunotherapy can also be considered.

3. *Mild Persistent*: Although symptoms occur more frequently (at least 4 days in a week lasting for more than 4 weeks at a time), they are mild and do not interfere with sleep or daily activities. Treatment options consist of all of those listed for Category 2: oral and intranasal antihistamines, oral decongestants, intranasal corticosteroids or mast cell stabilizers, and possibly immunotherapy. The patient should be re-evaluated in two to four weeks and medications adjusted as needed. Those thought to have perennial symptoms may need to continue medications indefinitely. Those thought to have symptoms from exposure to episodic or seasonal triggers may be able to have their medication(s) titrated downward; usually intranasal corticosteroids doses are reduced by 1/2 until the patient is weaned off.

4. *Moderate to Severe Persistent:* Symptoms in this category are severe enough to disrupt sleep, are generally bothersome, or can interfere with an individual's ability to perform well in school or at work, as well as at home. They also occur frequently: at least 4 days a week and for more than 4 weeks at a time. Intranasal corticosteroids are considered to be first line treatments. Immunotherapy also can be helpful. The patient should be re-evaluated in 2–4 weeks. If symptoms have improved, treatment can be stepped down but continued for a minimum of three months or for the duration of the pollen season. Some patients may require continuous treatment with low-dose intranasal corticosteroids. If the initially prescribed regimen does

not afford relief, the provider should check that the patient is compliant (taking all prescribed doses using correct technique) as well as reconsider whether the initial diagnosis was correct. If the initial diagnosis is correct, then the following treatment options may be helpful: increase the intranasal corticosteroid dose, add an antihistamine if itchiness or sneezing is present, or prescribe adjunctive medications that target the most problematic symptom (intranasal ipratropium for rhinorrhea, oral decongestants for nasal congestion). If none of these approaches provide relief, referral may be warranted.

Environmental Controls Environmental controls vary according to the allergen(s) found to be problematic. One of the most difficult triggers to control is pet dander. Removing the pet from the home will result in the greatest clinical response. Families who give up the family pet should be counseled that it may take three or more months of cleaning after the pet is removed before enough pet allergens have been removed for symptoms to subside.

However, pets are beloved family members in many households and many families are reluctant to give their pets away, particularly if they have been in the family for years. While removing the pet from the home will afford the greatest relief, other measures may provide some relief for families unwilling to give up their pets. Because pet allergens increase fivefold when the pet is in the room, the pet should be kept out of the bedroom, preferably out of doors as much as possible. Washing pets thoroughly also seems to reduce allergen levels, as does removing upholstered furniture and carpeting. Animal allergens accumulate to levels up to 100 times higher in carpets than on polished floors.[38]

Regular sweeping with a vacuum equipped with a high efficiency particulate air (HEPA) filter or special allergen-proof bags or connected to a duct system can remove significant amount of pet dander as well as dust-mite allergens, which are another common trigger. Women should be advised that use of vacuums without these special features may increase allergy symptoms because regular vacuums cannot filter out allergens, which tend to be of very small particle size and will make allergens airborne when they are exhausted out of the vacuum. Individuals with dust mite allergies also should avoid using indoor humidifiers because these are difficult to clean well; their use may increase the prevalence of indoor mold as well as dust mites that thrive in higher humidity environments. Dust mites are ubiquitous and are present in all households regardless of their cleanliness. Patients should be reassured that measures needed to control dust mites or other allergens are not a reflection of any judgment made about their standards of cleanliness but are necessary to minimize exposure to triggers. Table 12-17 contains specific suggestions on control measures for various common allergens.

Medication Choices Anti-inflammatory medications, such as corticosteroids and mast-cell stabilizers, are commonly used in the treatment of allergic rhinitis. Other medications used include decongestants and antihistamines. Which of the available options is best for an individual patient will depend on the severity and frequency of symptoms. In general, second generation antihistamines are the preferred treatment for intermittent allergic rhinitis, and intranasal corticosteroids are preferred for those with more persistent symptoms.

Anti-Inflammatory Agents   The two main categories of anti-inflammatory medications used in the treatment of allergic rhinitis are mast cell stabilizers, and corticosteroids, both of which are available in topical formulations. Intranasal corticosteroids are more effective in relieving symptoms than intranasal mast cell stabilizers and have fewer systemic side effects than oral agents. Between 5% and 10% of patients using intranasal corticosteroids report nasal dryness and irritation; 5% report mild epistasis. Patients who experience these side effects may be able to minimize these problems if a saline nasal spray is used prior to using an intranasal corticosteroid or if the dose of corticosteroid is reduced. Nasal septal perforation has been reported with use of these drugs, so patients should be instructed in correct positioning of the device. Evidence of superficial erosions, significant crusting, or bleeding should prompt the patient to immediately discontinue use of these medications.[39]

Patients with ocular symptoms may find relief with antihistamine or mast cell stabilizer eye drops or a combination of the two, or with the use of oral antihistamines. Steroidal eye drops should **NEVER** be used in the treatment of ocular itching secondary to allergies because of the risks associated with ocular steroids and the availability of other safer alternatives (**Table 12-18**).

Symptomatic Relief   Patients may choose various types of medications for symptomatic relief (either antihistamines or decongestants) and delivery routes (topical or systemic), depending on the presentation of their particular allergic reactions. In general, topical agents will have the fewest side effects, but patients who present with multiple symptoms, such as allergic conjunctivitis and rhinitis, may respond better to oral agents. Decongestants are best for those suffering primarily from nasal congestion; antihistamines are better for those with rhinorrhea and itchiness. Patients who have all of these symptoms may do best with combined products. These products can be used episodically for those with intermittent or seasonal allergies and daily for those with persistent symptoms. Midwives should prescribe intranasal decongestants with caution because overuse of these products can lead to a rebound effect and worsening of the patient's symptoms with extended use. Table 12-18 contains common available medications.

OTHER OPTIONS

Allergen immunotherapy is another treatment option. Immunotherapy has several benefits. It can reduce the dose of medication(s) needed to achieve control for asthmatics patients with allergies, may protect against the future development of asthma for those with allergic rhinitis, and may reduce the likelihood that allergic individuals will develop additional allergies.[41,42] It is indicated in the treatment of allergic rhinitis, allergic conjunctivitis, allergic asthma, and insect stings, but not for food allergies or atopic dermatitis. Immunotherapy is most effective if initiated early in the course of the disease in childhood or early adulthood.

All patients receiving immunotherapy need skin testing in order to identify their particular allergens. During the course of immunotherapy, patients receive slowly increasing subcutaneous doses of extracts to allergens that are particularly problematic for them. This desensitizes the patient and improves symptoms. In order to be

Table 12-18 COMMON ALLERGY MEDICATIONS

Indication	Drug	Trade Name	Dose	Effective Against	Notes
Decongestants					
Allergic conjunctivitis	Levocabastine hydrochloride 0.05%	Livostin	1 gtt each eye qid	Eye symptoms	Rapidly effective with minor side effects
Allergic rhinitis	Pseudoephedrine 30 mg tab	Sudafed	2 tabs PO qid	Nasal congestion and blockage, less effective against rhinorrhea	Good relief of nasal congestion but can develop insomnia, headache, dry mucous membranes, exacerbation of glaucoma or thyrotoxicosis
Allergic rhinitis	Intranasal decongestants Oxymethazoline hydrochloride	Afrin	2–3 sprays each nostril BID for 3 days	Nasal congestion	Rapid relief but rebound effect with prolonged use. Limit treatment to <5 days; maximum length of treatment is 10 days. Do not repeat more than twice a month
Antihistamines					
First Generation					
Allergic rhinitis	Diphenhydramine	Benadryl	25–50 mg PO tid or qid	Pruritis, rhinorrhea, eye symptoms. Less effective	More likely to be sedating, to potentiate alcohol, and to have

Table 12-18 **COMMON ALLERGY MEDICATIONS** *(continued)*

Indication	Drug	Trade Name	Dose	Effective Against	Notes
	Clemastine	Tavist	1 mg PO bid	against nasal congestion	anti-cholin-ergic side effects than second generation anti-histamines
	Chlorphen-iramine	Chlor-Trimeton	4 mg PO qid		
	Hydroxyzine	Atarax, Vistaril	25 mg PO tid or qid		
	Cyproheptadine	Periactin	4 mg PO tid		
Second Generation					
Allergic rhinitis	Azelastine	Astelin 137 mcg/spray	2 sprays each nostril bid	Nasal congestion and blockage	Rapidly effective but bitter taste
Allergic rhinitis	Cetirizine	Zyrtec	5 or 10 mg PO daily	Pruritis, rhinorrhea, eye symptoms. Little effect against nasal congestion	Recommended over first generation antihistamines because of less sedation and fewer side effects. More convenient because of once-daily dosing
	Desloratadine	Clarinex	5 mg daily		
	Fexofenadine	Allegra	60 mg PO bid		
	Loratadine	Claritin	10 mg PO daily		

Intranasal Corticosteroids

Indication	Drug	Trade Name	Dose	Effective Against	Notes
Allergic rhinitis	Beclomethasone	Beconase AQ (42 mcg)	1–2 sprays in each nostril bid	Pruritis, rhinorrhea, and nasal congestion Partial relief from eye symptoms	Intranasal corticosteroids recommended for persistent symptoms
	Budesonide	Rhinocort Aqua	Max 4 sprays each nostril daily		
	Flunisolide	Nasarel	2 sprays each nostril bid to tid		
	Fluticasone propionate	Flonase	1 spray in each nostril bid initially, then daily		
	Mometasone furoate	Nasonex	2 sprays in each nostril daily		

(continues)

Table 12-18 COMMON ALLERGY MEDICATIONS *(continued)*

Indication	Drug	Trade Name	Dose	Effective Against	Notes
Allergic rhinitis (cont'd)	Triamcinolone	Nasacort AQ	2 sprays in each nostril daily		
Mast Cell Stablizers					
Allergic conjunctivitis	Pemirolast potassium 0.1%	Alamast	1–2 gtts affected eye qid	Ocular itching	Provides effective relief with minor side effects
	Nedocromil sodium 2%	Alocril	1–2 gtts affected eye bid		
Allergic rhinitis	Cromolyn sodium 5.2 mg/spray	Nasalcrom	1 spray each nostril qid	Pruritis and rhinorrhea	Less effective than intranasal corticosteroids but excellent safety profile
Combined					
Allergic conjunctivitis	Antihistamine/ mast cell stabilizer: olopatadine hydorochloride 0.1%	Patanol	1 gtt affected eye bid	Ocular itching	
	Antihistamine/ mast cell stabilizer Azelastine 0.05%/	Optivar	1 gtt affected eye bid		
Allergic rhinitis	Antihistamine/ Decongestant Fexofenadine 60mg/ Pseudoephedrine 120 mg	Allegra-D	1 tab PO bid	Pruritis, nasal congestion and blockage, rhinorrhea, eye symptoms	
	Antihistamine/ decongestant Loratadine 10 mg/pseudoephedrine 240 mg	Claritin D	1 tab PO daily		

Table 12-18 **COMMON ALLERGY MEDICATIONS** (*continued*)

Indication	Drug	Trade Name	Dose	Effective Against	Notes
Topical Anti-Cholingerics					
Allergic Rhinitis	Ipratropium bromide 0.03%	Atrovent Nasal Spray 0.03% 21 mcg per spray	2 sprays each nostril daily or up to tid	Rhinorrhea only	Use as adjunctive therapy if insufficient response with oral antihistamine or intranasal corticosteroid use

Abbreviations are: gtt, drop; qid, 4 times daily; tab, tablet; po, orally; tid, three times daily; mcg, microgram; bid, twice daily; max, maximum.

Sources: Bousquet J, van Cauwenberge P, Khaltaev N, Group AW, World Health Organization. Allergic rhinitis and its impact on asthma. *J Allergy Clin Immunol.* 2001; 108 Suppl 5:S147–334.

Nurse Practitioner Prescribing Reference. New York: Prescribing Reference, Inc.; 2004.[8]

Salib R, Howarth P. Safety and tolerability profiles of intranasal antihistamines and intranasal cortocosteroids in the treatment of allergic rhinitis. *Drug Safety.* 2003;26:863–893.[40]

effective, doses needed to be increased to reach a target level and then repeated at weekly to monthly levels, usually for three years. Failure to reach the target dose level or to receive doses as scheduled or for treatment to last a sufficient length of time will reduce the effectiveness of immunotherapy.[32] Serious side effects, such as severe asthma or anaphylaxis, are rare but do occur. Therefore, immunotherapy should only be prescribed by allergists.

Occasionally, patients with allergic rhinitis may also be prescribed intranasal ipratropium (Atrovent), a topical anticholingeric, as an adjunctive therapy. It is typically added to the medication regimen for those patients who, despite adequate treatment with intranasal corticosteroids and oral antihistamines, continue to have significant rhinorrhea or for those whose primary symptom is rhinorrhea. It is ineffective against many other common symptoms, such as sneezing, congestion, or itching, that accompany allergic rhinitis. Common side effects include nasal irritation, crusting, and occasional mild epistaxis.[39]

FOOD ALLERGIES

In general, food allergies are thought to be more common in children than in adults. For adults, the most common triggers causing severe reactions are milk, eggs, fish, and shellfish, although nuts (peanuts, almonds, walnuts, pecans, hazelnuts), soya beans, some fruit such as apples and peaches, sesame, celery, and other foods can also cause problems.[43] Many individuals with food allergies also demonstrate cross-reactivity to inhalant allergens (ragweed and grass/banana and melon, birch pollen/apples). Most of these reactions are mild, but occasionally severe cross-reactions do occur.

The treatment for food allergies is avoidance. Patients exposed to food allergens may experience a range of symptoms ranging from oral itching to GI upset to anaphylaxis. **Table 12-19** lists symptoms of anaphylaxis. Patients at risk should wear an alert bracelet and carry diphenhydramine (Benadryl) and injectable epinephrine (Epi-Pen) for use in an emergency. The Epi-Pen comes in two strengths: adult (Epi-Pen) and pediatric (Epi-Pen Jr). Midwives should order the adult dose (1:1000 dilution, 0.3 mg) and make sure the patient, and ideally another family member, is trained in its use.[44]

ALLERGIC CONTACT DERMATITIS

Allergic contact dermatitis is difficult to distinguish from other eczematous disorders. Initial exposure typically presents as erythematous macules, papules, or vesicles. Chronic exposure results in lichenification, scaling, or fissured dermatitis. These findings are not distinctive; consequently, the most important diagnostic clues are the location and evolution of the rash. For example, allergies to poison ivy often begin as linear lesions and occur on more

exposed areas. However, textile-related allergens tend to occur in areas covered by clothing. Skin testing can be particularly helpful in differentiating allergen based from non-allergen based dermatitis. Treatment is directed at avoidance as well as symptom management.[45] Weeping lesions are best treated with drying agents and lichenified lesions with emollients. Pruritis can be relieved with the use of topical antipruritics or oral antihistamines. Topical corticosteroid creams and lotions can also help. Refer to Chapter 22 for details about dermatological conditions.

Individuals with allergic contact dermatitis may also experience symptoms of allergic rhinitis. Management for these individuals should follow the guidelines outlined earlier in this chapter.

Management in Pregnancy

ALLERGIC RHINITIS

Nasal congestion is common in pregnancy, and distinguishing this finding from allergic rhinitis can be difficult. Patients with nasal congestion due to estrogen increase during pregnancy will not have itchiness or rhinorrhea, only stuffiness. In addition, treatment for allergic rhinitis will not afford relief. In this case, the use of nasal saline, which has no side effects, may help.

Treatment of allergic rhinitis is essentially unchanged in pregnancy. Allergen avoidance is the primary treatment modality of allergic rhinitis in pregnancy. Medications should be prescribed only if environmental measures fail to provide sufficient relief. However, if medications are needed, authorities differ in their opinion about which ones are most appropriate for use in pregnancy. Most authorities recommend the use of intranasal mast cell stabilizers as the preferred treatment in pregnancy due to their

Table 12-19 SYMPTOMS OF ANAPHYLAXIS

Listed from most to least common
- Hives
- Upper airway edema
- Wheezing/shortness of breath
- Flushing
- Dizziness
- Nausea, vomiting, diarrhea, cramping

Source: Tang A. A practical guide to anaphylaxis. *Am Fam Physician.* 2003;68:1325–1332 and Greenberger P. Anaphylaxis. In: Adelman D, Casale T, Corren, J, editors. *Manual of Allergy & Immunology,* 4th ed. Philadelphia: Lippincott Williams & Wilkins; 2002. pp. 200–207.

excellent safety profiles.[34,39] However, pregnant women who do not respond completely to these products may be offered other options. Studies of the safety in pregnancy of antihistamines, decongestants, and intranasal corticosteroids are generally based on small non-randomized samples. Based on their evaluation of the evidence, both the NAEPP and ARIA recommended using specific medications in the various classes: in particular, the intranasal corticosteroids beclomethansone and budesonide (ARIA), and the oral antihistamines cetirizine and loratadine (ARIA, NAEPP).[24,34] Other authorities recommend different options such as the oral antihistamine chlorpheniramine and the decongestant pseudoephedrine as well as intranasal mast cell stabilizers and corticosteroids.[39] The use of oral decongestants is controversial. NAEPP recommends against their use since exposure in the first trimester has been associated with gastroschisis, although the risks appear to be low.[24] Because of minimal systemic absorption, topical agents, except for the intranasal decongestants, are safest in pregnancy. Good control of allergic rhinitis may also reduce the need for medications in asthmatics, and these women should receive aggressive treatment of allergic rhinitis in pregnancy.

ARIA also recommends against initiating immunotherapy in pregnancy.[34] Women already on immunotherapy before the pregnancy may safely continue. The allergen extract doses used should not be increased in order to minimize the risk of anaphylaxis in pregnancy, although this risk is extremely rare during immunotherapy.

FOOD ALLERGIES

Management of food allergies is unchanged by pregnancy. The primary treatment modality is avoidance. All women, whether pregnant or not, need to be prepared in case of exposure by having ready access to appropriate emergency medications.

ATOPIC DERMATITIS

Management of atopic dermatitis is also essentially unchanged by pregnancy. Chapter 22 offers further details.

Patient Instructions

Patients with allergies need to understand how to adapt their environment to meet their particular needs. No other management technique will provide as much relief as implementing effective environmental controls. Midwives should tailor their suggestions to match the lifestyle needs of the individual client. For example, asking a woman with limited financial resources to cover the bed and pillows with allergy-proof covers or invest in a HEPA vacuum, all of which are expensive, will be ineffective because it is unlikely that she will be able to comply with these suggestions. In this case, asking her to cover only the pillows on her bed in allergy-proof covers, to wash all of her bedding in hot water every week, and to ask another family member to wet mop her bedroom floor may provide enough environmental control to help minimize her symptoms and still be within her financial means. Similarly, asking a woman to give up a household pet may not be reasonable, but instituting other control measures (Table 12-2) may be effective.

Women also need to understand how to choose medications that are effective and easy to use, given their particular situation. Individuals with intermittent symptoms with known triggers (i.e., exposure to animals, pollen, or mold) can institute therapy several days to weeks before the exposure and stop medications once exposure ceases. For example, those with ragweed allergies can start medications several weeks before the beginning of the ragweed season and stop with the first hard frost. Those with more persistent symptoms will need to choose products with dosing regimens or delivery systems that are acceptable to them. Some women will find intranasal sprays to be uncomfortable and will prefer oral medications. Others will prefer topical agents with fewer systemic side effects. Because allergies are a chronic condition, midwives will need to develop a partnership with their patients and help women choose appropriate medication(s) and environmental control measures as their needs change.

Women with food allergies need to be taught how to read food packages to identify possible allergens, and to understand manufacturing processes that can lead to cross contamination and potential exposure to problematic allergens.

Women who could experience anaphylaxis reactions should be counseled to carry Benadryl, as well as an Epi-Pen, and be skilled in their use. In addition, individuals who have severe reactions to various foods or insect bites should wear an identification band to alert others in the event of an anaphylactic episode.

References

1. Anonymous. Self-reported asthma prevalence and control among adults—United States 2001. *MMWR.* 2003;52(17):381–384.

2. Anonymous. *Asthma Prevalence: Health Care Use and Mortality, 2000–2001.* National Center for Health Statistics; 2003.

3. National Asthma Education and Prevention Program. *Expert Panel 2: Guidelines for the Diagnosis and Management of Asthma.* NIH Publication No. 97-4051. Bethesda, MD: National Institutes of Health; 1997.

4. Ryu J, Scanlon P. Obstructive lung diseases: COPD, asthma, and many imitators. *Mayo Clin Proc.* 2001;76:1144–1153.

5. National Asthma Education and Prevention Program. *Guidelines for the Diagnosis and Management of Asthma—Update on Selected Topics 2002.* NIH Publication No. 02-5074. Bethesda, MD: National Institutes of Health; 2003.

6. National Asthma Education and Prevention Program. *Practical Guide for the Diagnosis and Management of Asthma.* NIH Publication No. 97-4053. Bethesda, MD: National Institutes of Health; 1997.

7. National Asthma Education and Prevention Program. *Expert Panel Report: Guidelines for the Diagnosis and Management of Asthma.* NIH Publication No. 91-3642. Bethesda, MD: National Institutes of Health; 1991.

8. *Nurse Practitioner Prescribing Reference.* New York: Prescribing Reference, Inc; 2004.

9. *Drugs in Pregnancy & Lactation.* 6th ed. Philadelphia: Lippincott Williams & Wilkins; 2002.

10. Beckett P, Howarth P. Pharmacotherapy and airway remodeling in asthma? *Thorax.* 2003;58:163–174.

11. Ducharme F. Inhaled glucocorticoids versus leukotriene receptor antagonists as single agent asthma treatment: Systematic review of the current evidence. *BMJ.* 2003;326:621.

12. Goldstein M, Fallon J, Harning R. Chronic glucocorticoid therapy-induced osteoporosis in patients with obstructive lung disease. *Chest.* 1999;116:1733–1749.

13. Martin R. Considering therapeutic options in the real world. *J Allergy Clin Immunol.* 2003;112:S112–115.

14. Boulet L. Once-daily inhaled corticosteroids for the treatment of asthma. *Curr Opin Pulmonary Med.* 2004;10:15–21.

15. Ducharme F. Anti-leukotrienes as add-on therapy to inhaled glucocorticoids in patients with asthma: Systematic review of current evidence. *BMJ.* 2002;324:1545.

16. Storms W. Exercise induced asthma: Diagnosis and treatment for the recreational or elite athlete. *Med Sci Sports Exerc.* 1999;31 Suppl 1:S33–38.

17. Apter A. Clinical advances in adult asthma. *J Allergy Clin Immunol.* 2003;111(3, part 2) Suppl: S780–784.

18. Newman S, Busse W. Evolution of dry powder inhaler design, formulation, and performance. *Respir Med.* 2002;96:293–304.

19. Cochrane M, Bala M, Downs K, Mauskopf J, Ben-Joseph R. Inhaled corticosteroids for asthma therapy: Patient compliance, devices, and inhalation technique. *Chest.* 2000;117:542–550.

20. Cates C, Bara A, Crilly J, Rowe B. Holding chamber versus nebulizers for beta-agonist treatment of acute asthma. *Cochrane Rev.* 2003;3:CD000052.

21. Teirstein A, Schilero G, Lesser M. Respiratory disease. In: Cohen W, editor. *Cherry & Merkatz's Complications of Pregnancy.* 5th ed. Philadelphia: Lippincott Williams & Wilkins; 2000. pp. 234–262.

22. Nelson-Piercy C. Asthma in pregnancy. *Thorax.* 2001;564:325–328.

23. Bracken M, Triche E, Belanger K, Saftlas A, Beckett W, Leaderer B. Asthma symptoms, severity, and drug therapy: A prospective study of effects on 2205 pregnancies. *Obstetr Gynecol.* 2003;102:739–752.

24. National Asthma Education and Prevention Program. *Working Group Report on Managing Asthma During Pregnancy: Recommendations for Pharmacologic Treatment, Update 2004.* US Department of Health and Human Services, National Institutes of Health, National Heart, Lung, and Blood Institute, NIH Publication No. 05-3279, January 2005.

25. Cydulka R, Emerman C, Schreiber D, Molander K, Woodruff P, Camargo CJ. Acute asthma among pregnant women presenting to the emergency department. *Am J Respir Crit Care Med.* 1999;160:887–892.

26. Bonner S, Zimmerman B, Evans D, Irigoyen M, Resnick D, Mellins R. An individualized intervention to improve asthma management among urban Latino and African American families. *J Asthma.* 2002;39:167–179.

27. Markham A, Wilkinson J. Complementary/alternative medicine in the treatment of asthma. *Annal Allergy Asthma Immunol.* 2000;85:438–449.

28. York S, Brattice M. Complementary and alternative medicine for bronchial asthma: Is there new evidence? *Curr Opin Pulmonary Med.* 2004;10:37–43.

29. Hartert T, Peebles RS. Dietary antioxidants and adult asthma. *Curr Opin Allergy Clin Immunol.* 2001;1:421–429.

30. Fuhlbrigge A, Adams R. The effect of treatment of allergic rhinitis on asthma morbidity, including emergency department visits. *Curr Opin Allergy Clin Immunol.* 2003;3:29–32.

31. Koh YY, Kim CK. The development of asthma in patients with allergic rhinitis. *Curr Opin Allergy Clin Immunol.* 2003;3:159–164.

32. Finegold I. Is immunotherapy effective in allergic disease? *Curr Opin Allergy Clin Immunol.* 2002;2: 537–540.

33. Fineman S. The burden of allergic rhinitis: Beyond dollars and cents. *Ann Allergy Asthma Immunol.* 2002;88 Suppl 1:2–7.

34. Bousquet J, van Cauwenberge P, Khaltaev N, World Health Organization. *Allergic Rhinitis and Its Impact on Asthma.* In collaboration with the World Health Organization. Executive summary of the workshop report. 7–10 December 1999, Geneva, Switzerland. *Allergy* 2002;57:841–855.

35. Skoner D. Allergic rhinitis: Definition, epidemiology, pathophysiology, detection, and diagnosis. *J Allergy Clin Immunol.* 2001;108:S2–8.

36. de Shazo R, Kemp S. Clinical manifestations and evaluation of allergic rhinitis (rhinosinusitis); 2004. In: [Monograph on the Internet] 2005 UpToDate® [subscriber Web site] Waltham, MA. Available from: http://www.uptodate.com.

37. Li J. Allergy testing. *Am Fam Physician.* 2002;66: 621–624.

38. Custovic A, Simpson A, Chapman M, Woodcock A. Allergen avoidance in the treatment of asthma and atopic disorders. *Thorax.* 1998;53:63–72.

39. Corren J. Allergic rhinitis: Treating the adult. *J Allergy Clin Immunol.* 2000;105(6 Part 2 Suppl): S610–S615.

40. Salib R, Howarth P. Safety and tolerability profiles of intranasal antihistamines and intranasal corticosteroids in the treatment of allergic rhinitis. *Drug Safety.* 2003;26:863–893.

41. Abramson M, Puy R, Weiner J. Allergen immunotherapy for asthma. *Cochrane Rev.* 2004;2:CD001186.

42. Dinakar C, Portnoy J. Allergen immunotherapy in the prevention of asthma. *Curr Opin Allergy Clin Immunol.* 2004;4:131–136.

43. Crespo J, Rodriquez J. Food allergy in adulthood. *Allergy.* 2003;58:98–113.

44. Tang A. A practical guide to anaphylaxis. *Am Fam Physician.* 2003;68:1325–1332.

45. Belsito D. The diagnostic evaluation, treatment, and prevention of allergic contact dermatitis in the new millennium. *J Allergy Clin Immunol.* 2000;105:409–420.

Chapter 13

Respiratory Conditions

Karen A. Stemler

Illnesses of the respiratory system, whether the etiological source is viral, bacterial, or allergic, present with myriad symptoms. Symptoms affecting the upper and lower airway, cardiac, integumentary, and muscular systems are often reported in patients with upper and lower respiratory problems. Similar symptoms can occur in many different conditions, making it difficult for the practitioner to determine the underlying cause(s). This chapter sorts the possibilities and discusses the presentation, evaluation, and management of common respiratory illnesses in pregnant and nonpregnant women.

Common Symptoms

Upper and/or lower respiratory infections present with a number of symptoms (**Table 13-1**). Some of the most common complaints reported by patients with respiratory illnesses include nasal congestion, fever, and cough. In pregnancy, rhinorrhea, nasal congestion, sinus congestion, and postnasal drip are particularly common because of the underlying hormonal changes. Some of these same symptoms are seen with a viral or bacterial infection, or as part of an allergic response, making the diagnosis of

respiratory conditions more difficult in pregnancy. Selective symptoms are often grouped together and suggest a specific diagnosis, but more often a practitioner must consider several etiologies in order to arrive at a diagnosis. In addition, the patient may have underlying problems or comorbid conditions, which require a different or more aggressive management plan. A thorough history and physical exam are usually enough to make the appropriate diagnosis.

Nasal Congestion

The nose and the paranasal sinuses provide essential functions that help maintain a healthy respiratory tract by conditioning and purifying inspired air.[1] The coarse hairs line the distal nasal cavity and filter particles from the air. Mucous membranes cover the proximal nasal cavity and provide moisture to inspired air. If the secretions become thick or sticky, the mucous membranes may release mast cell mediators, resulting in mucosal inflammation. Nasal congestion can be caused by changes in the linings of the nose and sinuses as a result of infection.

Pregnancy-related changes make women more prone to nasal congestion, even without infection. Estrogen, progesterone, and placental

---

Table 13-1 **COMMON SYMPTOMS SEEN WITH A RESPIRATORY INFECTION**

General malaise, fever, chills
Loss of appetite
Difficulty sleeping
Ear pain or discomfort
Nasal congestion and/or rhinorrhea
Sore throat
Itchy eyes/ears/nose/throat and sneezing
Shortness of breath, wheezing, chest tightness, and/or cough
Enlarged lymph nodes
Myalgia

---

growth hormone as well as non-hormonal factors such as inflammatory changes, immunologic changes, and parasympathetic upregulation contribute to the development of nasal congestion in pregnancy.

Fever

Microorganisms such as bacteria or viruses and exotoxins induce macrophages and endothelial cells to produce fever-producing mediators or cytokines (i.e., interleukin-1, interleukin-6, and tumor necrosis factor). These chemical mediators or cytokines induce the release of prostaglandin E from the hypothalamus, which increases the set point of the thermoregulatory center. Once the set point has increased, the hypothalamus responds with vasoconstriction and shivering to increase the core body temperature to this new set point, and this action results in fever.[2]

Noninfectious disorders can also stimulate the production of cytokines. Tissue injury from trauma or surgery can induce a fever, as can neo-plasms such as leukemia or Hodgkin's disease. Fever also may occur if the hypothalamus is damaged, which can be seen with intracerebral bleeding, increased intracranial pressure, or trauma to the central nervous system. A fever due to hypothalamic damage will be unresponsive to antipyretic treatment.[2]

Several signs and symptoms occur as a result of fever alone. Because of the inflammatory properties of interleukin-1, leukocytosis, anorexia, and malaise are often noted. A person's heart rate will increase as the body's temperature increases. For every rise of 1°F, the heart rate will increase by 10 beats per minutes (BPM) (15 BPM for every increase of 1°C). Other conditions, such as inflammatory bowel disease, tuberculosis (TB), and Kawasaki disease, need to be considered if the heart rate does not rise as expected or is out of proportion to the degree of fever.[3] Other common manifestations due to fever are myalgia, arthralgia, fatigue, and headache. An alteration in mental status (e.g., confusion, delirium, agitation, uncoordination) can occur in the older adult with temperature elevations above 104°F (40°C), or with concurrent cerebral hypoxemia.[2]

Cough

Pathogens can enter the lungs through inhalation, aspiration from the oropharynx, direct spread from the upper to lower respiratory tract via the mucosal membrane, or through the blood. The cough reflex helps prevent bacteria from reaching the lower respiratory tract. Other defense mechanisms also help remove bacteria and other microorganisms.[4]

Each epithelial cell of the trachea and bronchus is lined with approximately 200 cilia, fluctuating several hundred times per minute, preventing stagnation of bacteria and keeping the flow upward toward the larynx. The mucosal membrane that lines the cilia has antimicrobial compounds (i.e., lysozyme and secretory immunoglobulin A antibodies) that target bacteria trapped by the cilia. If larger particles, secretions, or foreign bodies are aspirated, then the cough reflex is stimulated, forcing these substances upward.[4]

In smokers, the cilia become damaged or paralyzed. As a result, smokers have difficulty clearing respiratory secretions and have to rely on the cough reflex. If these mechanisms fail, the bacteria may still be inhibited by the macrophages and neutrophils that are present in the alveoli.[4] However, if microorganisms remain in the lower respiratory tract, infection may occur.

Cough can be a presenting symptom in many conditions. Relatively benign and self-limiting to serious complicated conditions can cause an acute or chronic cough. Acute cough is defined as a cough lasting for less than three weeks and is often caused by infections, allergies, or an acute exacerbation of asthma or bronchitis. Chronic cough persists for longer than three weeks and generally reflects a more persistent condition.

The presentation may provide clues pointing to a specific etiology or etiologies. In some situations a chest x-ray may be needed to rule out an underlying mass or tumor, or when the patient is acutely distressed, the diagnosis is unclear, or the condition is persistent. If the patient is a nonsmoker and has a normal chest radiograph, postnasal drip syndrome (PNDS), asthma, and/ or gastroesophageal reflux disease (GERD) are more likely considerations. The quality of cough in these cases, whether it is dry or productive, does not help to distinguish between the possibilities.[5] Another possible cause is the use of medications such as angiotensin-converting enzyme inhibitors (ACEIs).[5] **Table 13-2** and **Table 13-3** list common differential diagnoses to be considered when evaluating acute and chronic cough.

COUGH AND POSTNASAL DRIP SYNDROME

With PNDS, patients usually complain of drainage in the back of the throat that results in a constant need to clear the throat. Nasal discharge, cobblestone appearance of the oropharyngeal mucosa, or mucus in the oropharynx may also be noted, but are not specific to PNDS. Some patients will not have any upper respiratory signs or symptoms commonly found with PNDS, except for cough. These patients often respond well to first-generation antihistamine/ decongestant therapy. A good response to therapy indicates that PNDS was the likely cause of

---

Table 13-2 **DIFFERENTIAL DIAGNOSES OF ACUTE COUGH**[6,7]

Acute Cough (<3weeks duration)
Common cold (most common), leading to postnasal drip syndrome (PNDS)
Acute bacterial sinusitis, leading to PNDS
Allergic or environmental rhinitis
Acute bronchitis
Pertussis, leading to PNDS (suspect if exposed to a close contact with pertussis or if patient presents with a post-tussive emesis)
Chronic obstructive pulmonary disease exacerbation
Pneumonia
Pulmonary embolism
Congestive heart failure
Aspiration

Table 13-3 DIFFERENTIAL DIAGNOSES OF CHRONIC COUGH[5,6,7]

Chronic Cough (3–≥8 Weeks Duration)	Comments
Postnasal drip syndrome (most common)	
• Seasonal allergic rhinitis	• Allergy testing may be useful; consider pollen or animal dander
• Perennial allergic rhinitis	• Allergy testing may be useful; consider house dust mite or indoor mold
• Vasomotor rhinitis	• Excessive rhinorrhea/nasal congestion may be aggravated by temperature changes; Ipratropium bromide nasal spray may control vasomotor symptoms
• Postinfectious or postviral rhinitis	• Often present after a recent URI
• Chronic bacterial sinusitis	• Four-view sinus radiograph with >6mm of mucosal thickening, sinus opacity, or air fluid levels
• Allergic fungal sinusitis	• Consider skin testing for *Aspergillus* or other fungi
• Nonallergic rhinitis	• From medication overuse/rhinitis medicamentosa (from nasal oxymetazoline HCl) or substance use (e.g., snorting cocaine) or environmental/occupational triggers
• Nonallergic rhinitis associated with pregnancy	• Symptoms resolve postpartum
Asthma	• Consider with cough induced by cold/exercise and/or signs of wheezing/rhonchi and responsive to β_2-agonists
GERD	• Often without GI symptoms
Chronic bronchitis	• Relatively rare condition accounting for only 5% of chronic cough • Consider smoking cessation if appropriate and institute environmental controls
Pertussis	• Suspect and treat in patients who have an persistent cough and have been exposed to a close contact with pertussis or if patient presents with a post-tussive emesis
Related to medications	• Such as angiotensin converting enzyme inhibitors (ACEI)
Bronchiectasis	
Cystic fibrosis	
Chronic interstitial pulmonary disease	
Bronchogenic carcinoma	• Uncommon; seen more often in smokers or patients with occupational exposure
Postinfectious cough	• Diagnosis of exclusion
Psychogenic cough	• Diagnosis of exclusion

Abbreviations are: URI, upper respiratory condition; GI, gastrointestinal; GERD, gastrointestinal-esophageal reflux disease.

the cough.[5] Second generation, non-sedating antihistamines are not effective in treating an acute cough associated with the common cold. These agents also are not as effective as first-generation antihistamines in treating chronic nonallergic coughs due to PNDS.[5]

COUGH AND GERD

Patients with GERD may not exhibit typical symptoms (e.g., reflux or heartburn) or have other gastrointestinal (GI) symptoms, but can present only with a chronic cough.[5] The most specific and sensitive test to assess GERD is a 24-hour esophageal pH monitoring test. However, if esophageal pH testing is not available, a trial of antireflux medication can be used for the following situations: 1) if GI symptoms are consistent with GERD, or 2) if a chronic cough without GI symptoms is present and there is no underlying cause, such as pulmonary infiltrate, effusion, or mass (rule out with a normal chest radiograph), medication (e.g., ACEI), asthma, PNDS, or smoke inhalation.[5] Diet and lifestyle modifications should always be instituted concurrently with treatment. If the treatment fails, it may mean that the treatment was not sufficient to suppress the GERD or that another etiology should be considered. Further details on the management of GERD are in Chapter 17.

Physiologic Changes in Pregnancy

Many of the physiologic changes that occur in pregnancy affect the presentation and course of infections. The pregnant woman's chest expands, the subcostal angle increases, and the diaphragm rises by approximately 4 centimeters. However, these changes do not affect inhalation and exhalation during pregnancy.[8] Progester-

one, derived from the placenta, stimulates the brain's respiratory center producing a hyperventilatory state. Hyperventilation decreases the alveolar CO_2 tension and the arterial PCO_2. The body compensates by decreasing the plasma bicarbonate level, resulting in a minimal change in pH.[8] Given these natural changes, compensated respiratory alkalosis is noted in normal pregnancy. Some pregnant women have subjective symptoms from these changes and report breathlessness. **Table 13-4** describes common respiratory changes seen in pregnant women.

During pregnancy, the T helper cells decrease in number and cellular immunity is impaired, leading to a mildly immunocompromised state,[10,11] making pregnant women more prone to infection. Infections such as community-acquired pneumonia (CAP), Type A influenza, measles, TB, pneumocystis, and varicella pneumonia are more common and are often associated with more morbidity in pregnant than non-pregnant women. The compensatory respiratory mechanisms triggered by pregnancy reduce the respiratory system's capacity to compensate further if additional insults, such as those caused by infection, occur.

Management of Specific Respiratory Conditions

To differentiate between the most commonly found acute and chronic respiratory diagnoses, refer to **Table 13-5**.

Common Cold

The human rhinoviruses (HRVs), which include over 100 serotypes,[14,15] are most commonly associated with upper respiratory infections. HRV have been identified in 80% of the

Table 13-4 NORMAL PULMONARY VALUES IN NON-PREGNANT AND PREGNANT WOMEN

Term	Definition	Values		Clinical Significance in Pregnancy
		Non-pregnant	Pregnant	
Respiratory rate (RR)	Number of respirations per minute	16/min	Changes very little	
Tidal volume (V_T)	The amount of air moved in one normal respiratory cycle	450 mL	600 mL (increases up to 40%)	
Residual volume (RV)	The amount of air that remains in the lung at the end of a maximal expiration	1,000 mL	Decreases by approximately 200–800 mL	Improves gas transfer from alveoli to blood
Minute ventilation	The volume of air moved per minute; product of RR and V_T	7.2 L	9.6 L (increases up to 40% because of the increase in V_T)	Increases oxygen available for the fetus; complaints of shortness of breath, and mild compensated respiratory alkalosis noted (see text above)
Forced vital capacity (FVC)	The maximum amount of air that can be moved from maximum inspiration to maximum expiration	3.5 L	Unchanged	If over 1 L, pregnancy is usually well tolerated
FEV1	Forced expiratory volume in one second	Approximately 80%–85% of the vital capacity	Unchanged	Valuable to measure because there is no change due to pregnancy
PEFR	Peak expiratory flow rate	Calculation depends on height, age, sex, and co-existent pulmonary condition	Unchanged	Valuable to measure because there is no change due to pregnancy

Source: Reprinted with permission.[8]

Table 13-5 DIFFERENTIATING BETWEEN COMMON ACUTE AND CHRONIC RESPIRATORY DIAGNOSES[12,13]

Diagnosis	Key History	Key Physical Findings	Diagnostic Testing Considered Useful	Additional Comments
Common cold	Mild symptoms: rhinorrhea, sneezing, nasal congestion, post-nasal drip (PND)	Chest examination is normal	None	Antibiotics are not needed
Influenza	Moderate to severe symptoms: non-productive dry cough, fever 100°–104°F, fatigue		None	Influenza vaccine recommended yearly. Antiviral medications need to be taken within 2 days of symptom onset.
Acute sinusitis	Rhinorrhea, nasal discharge, unilateral maxillary, facial, or tooth pain, headache, fever	Decreased transillumination of sinus, mucopurulent nasal discharge, sinus tenderness with palpation or percussion	If needed, choose a limited CT scan (coronal plane)	Antibiotics reserved for persistent symptoms >7 days, which persist despite treatment with decongestants and analgesics. Reserve radiographs or CT scan for patients with >3 sinus infections/year or persistent sinus infections
Chronic sinusitis	Symptoms persistent for >12 weeks due to chronic inflammation and	Similar to acute sinusitis	Limited CT scan of the sinus (coronal plane) or if surgery planned, complete series of sinus films	Antibiotics are usually not effective; however, if acute/recurrent exacerbation,

(continues)

Table 13-5 DIFFERENTIATING BETWEEN COMMON ACUTE AND CHRONIC RESPIRATORY DIAGNOSES *(continued)*

Diagnosis	Key History	Key Physical Findings	Diagnostic Testing Considered Useful	Additional Comments
Chronic sinusitis (cont'd)	polyp development; allergies are often a trigger; key symptoms: nasal congestion, PND, purulent nasal discharge, headache, cough, and facial pressure			treatment same as acute sinusitis,[13] consider a referral to ENT/otolaryngology consult
Acute bronchitis	Symptoms present for <3 weeks; cough, chest discomfort, low-grade fever, rhinorrhea, throat pain, fatigue, headache, PND	Wheezing or rhonchi are commonly noted.	Peak expiratory flow readings (PEFRs); chest radiography (CXR) rarely needed	>90% are viral, antibiotics not needed. Cough may last 2 weeks
Chronic bronchitis	Persistent cough with an overproduction of sputum for 3 or more consecutive months in 2 consecutive years; symptoms: increased sputum, shortness of breath, cough	Lowered FEV1 — hospitalize, if FEV1 <40%; If O_2 saturation less than 90% and febrile, obtain CXR.	Possibly CXR or spirometry. Consider alpha, antitripsin if genetic disorder suspected	Subjective worsening in 1 or more chronic symptoms such as sputum production/purulence/viscosity, shortness of breath, dyspnea, or cough

Table 13-5 DIFFERENTIATING BETWEEN COMMON ACUTE AND CHRONIC RESPIRATORY DIAGNOSES *(continued)*

Diagnosis	Key History	Key Physical Findings	Diagnostic Testing Considered Useful	Additional Comments
Pneumonia	Persistent, acute cough, pleuritic chest pain, dyspnea, fever, fatigue, night sweats, malaise, myalgia, anorexia	Tachycardia, tachypnea, fever, diminished breath sounds, and inspiratory crackles; positive tactile fremitus, dullness to percussion, positive bronchophony, egophony, or whispered pectoriloquy		If needed in pregnancy, obtain posteroanterior CXR (not lateral)
Tuberculosis (latent)	Asymptomatic	Positive PPD, normal chest exam	CXR—negative	Positive exposure to TB, but not contagious
Tuberculosis (active)	Malaise, fatigue, night sweats, weight loss, fever, decreased appetite, cough >2 weeks, productive sputum with or without hemoptysis	Positive PPD; adventitious breath sounds may be auscultated	CXR—upper lobe infiltrates and unilateral hilar node enlargement; AFB, sputum culture	Isolate patient and immediately transfer in hospital to negative pressure room

Abbreviations are: CT, computed axial tomography; ENT, ear, nose, throat; FEV1, forced expiratory volume in 1 second; PPD, purified protein derivative tuberculin test; TB, tuberculosis; AFB, acid fast bacillus.

adult population who presented with the common cold during the fall and spring season.[15–17] Infections due to HRV have also been noted at other times during the year.[15] Other viruses associated with the common cold include the parainfluenza virus, adenovirus, respiratory syncytial virus, certain enteroviruses,[16] and the influenza A virus.[17]

The incubation period of the common cold is one to three days.[15] The duration of cold symptoms varies from less than 7 days to a maximum of 14 days,[14] with a mean duration of 9.5 to 11 days.[16] Rhinorrhea, sneezing, nasal obstructions, and postnasal drip are commonly reported.[6] In adults, nasal symptoms usually peak within 48 to 72 hours and then gradually subside.[15] Other symptoms such as headache, facial pressure, sneezing, irritated throat, hoarseness, and cough may also be reported.[6,14,16] Fever and malaise are less common.[15] If a rhinovirus is the causative agent, a sore throat is often the initial symptom.

ESSENTIAL HISTORY, AND PHYSICAL AND LABORATORY EVALUATION

Generally, a patient with the common cold will present with mild symptoms. On examination, the conjunctiva will be clear, but there may be increased lacrimation. There may be clear fluid behind the tympanic membrane indicating a serous otitis. There should be no erythema, bulging, or displacement of the bony landmarks. The nasal turbinates usually are erythematous and edematous with clear discharge noted bilaterally. The sinuses may be tender, but transillumination is normal. The posterior pharynx may be erythematous with minimal edema. If edema is present, it will be symmetrical. The tonsils should not exceed 1+ bilaterally (i.e., visible, but each tonsil is not encompassing more than 25% of posterior pharynx). The oral pharynx is usually free of exudates. Lymphadenopathy is uncommon. If lymph nodes are palpable, they will be small in size (i.e., ~0.5 cm) and located only in the anterior and/or posterior cervical chain. The heart rate and rhythm will be normal. Minor increases in heart rate may be due to a mild temperature elevation or insufficient fluid intake. The lungs will be clear, without any rales, rhonchi, or wheezing.

No laboratory tests are helpful in evaluating the common cold. Rapid antigen detection or serological tests have no clinical utility and are not cost effective or practical. Viral cultures can take up to seven days to obtain results. For these reasons, diagnostic testing is not recommended.[15]

MANAGEMENT

Lifestyle Regular health maintenance is important in maintaining proper immune function. Key points to focus on in patient education are regular and thorough hand washing, adequate sleep, sufficient fluid with balanced nutrition, and the use of appropriate measures to manage stress.

Medication Viral organisms are the most common cause of colds. In general, antibiotics are not needed. Bacterial co-infections are rare,[17] and the overuse of antibiotics can result in side effects, allergic reactions, and the development of antibiotic resistance.[18] Thus, antibiotic therapy is not recommended for the treatment of the common cold and should only be given if a secondary bacterial infection is strongly suspected.[15] Other treatments such as pseudoephedrine, intranasal ipratropium, and oral naproxen provide significant clinical benefits.

Complementary or Alternative Choices Herbal and homeopathic treatments have been tested in vitro and in controlled studies; however, due to small sample sizes, study limitations, and variable outcome results, the effectiveness and safety of these treatments remain uncertain,[15] especially in pregnant and lactating women. Some of the alternative choices that have been recommended for the common cold are zinc, echinacea, and vitamin C.[14]

PATIENT INSTRUCTIONS

Transmission occurs with hand-to-nose or hand-to-eye contact after exposure to the nasal secretions of the infected individual.[15] Good hand washing is the key to the prevention and control of the common cold. Adequate sleep and nutrition are essential in boosting the immune system's ability to combat and prevent further illness.

The following techniques may provide some relief from nasal or sinus congestion: 1) using a saline nasal solution two to four times per day; 2) steam treatments (e.g., breathing in steam from boiled water, steamy bath, or shower); and 3) drinking plenty of fluids. If a woman's symptoms worsen or no relief is noted in one to two weeks, she should return for re-evaluation.

MANAGEMENT DURING PREGNANCY AND LACTATION

Management of the common cold does not change in pregnancy or lactation. Medication use should be minimized but may be necessary to afford relief from moderate to severe symptoms. **Table 13-6** describes appropriate treatments for the common cold, as well as other respiratory conditions.

Influenza

Influenza viruses are responsible for approximately 200,000 hospitalizations and 36,000 deaths per year.[19] Pandemics due to influenza occur at regular intervals: the Spanish Flu in 1918–1919 (500,000 U.S. deaths), Asian Flu in 1957–1958 (69,800 U.S. deaths), and the Hong Kong Flu in 1968–1969 (33,800 U.S. deaths).[20] While deaths are higher during pandemics, influenza causes significant morbidity and mortality every year. The patients at highest risk include newborns, older adults, immunosuppressed patients, and the chronically ill.[21] Between October 2003 and January 2004, 93 influenza-associated deaths among children younger than 18 years old

were reported to the Centers for Disease Control and Prevention (CDC).[22]

ESSENTIAL HISTORY, AND PHYSICAL AND LABORATORY EVALUATION

Symptoms are acute, often affecting the sinus, pharyngeal, and lower airway. These same symptoms are found with other viral illnesses such as the common cold, except with influenza the symptoms are more severe. Myalgia and fatigue are commonly present. Cough and fever are often seen in patients with influenza.[23] **Table 13-7** compares the presentation for the common cold and influenza.

The approach to a patient suspected of having influenza is similar to that used in evaluating a cold. Complications are more frequent with influenza infections than with other upper respiratory infections, and patients may need to be evaluated for otitis media, dehydration, or other problems outlined in **Table 13-8**. High-risk individuals such as the very young and the elderly are particularly at risk for serious illness and worsening symptoms (**Table 13-9**). A thorough history and physical exam are essential in order to confirm the diagnosis and to identify complications.

Laboratory testing is of limited value in the evaluation of influenza. Viral cultures, such as Directigen, Flu A+B, Flu OIA, ZstatFlu, and QuickVue rapid-assays, are diagnostic tests used in office settings[21]; but these are generally used in practices that are part of the CDC monitoring system put in place to detect the types of circulating viruses and the level of infection present within a community in any given year. This information is used to determine what viral subtypes should be included in the influenza vaccine for the following year.[25] Some practices will collect nasal swab specimens on

Table 13-6 CHOOSING THE APPROPRIATE TREATMENT[12]

Diagnosis	Common Etiology	Preferred Rx	Alternative	Comments
Common cold	Rhinovirus, parainfluenza, adenovirus, RSV, enterovirus, influenza A	Supportive measures: saline nasal spray, steam, fluids, rest	Sudafed, Atrovent nasal spray	Antibiotics not recommended
Influenza	Influenza A and B	Supportive measures: saline nasal spray, steam, fluids, rest	Antiviral medications—need to be taken within 2 days of onset of symptoms	Antibiotics not recommended
Acute sinusitis	*Streptococcus pneumoniae* 31%, *Haemophilus influenza* 21%, viruses 15%, anaerobes 6%, *Staph. aureus* 4%, %, *M. catarrhalis* 2%, Group A strep 2%, fungal infections in immunosuppressed patients	Supportive therapy unless persistent symptoms (e.g., >7 days). If persistent, then treat: amoxicillin 500 mg tid, amoxicillin/clavulanic acid 875/125 mg bid, cefdinir 300 mg q12h or 600 mg qd, cefpodoxime 200 mg bid, or cefuroxime axetil 250 mg bid, or telithromycin 800 mg qd *If antibiotic used in past month*, treat with Augmentin or fluoroquinolone	*For penicillin/cephalosporin allergy, use:* clarithromycin 500 mg bid, TMP/SMX 1 double strength bid, qatifloxacin 400 mg qd, Levofloxacin 500 mg qd, moxifloxacin 400 mg qd, azithromycin, telithromycin, or doxycycline	Reserve antibiotics if symptoms continue × 7 days or more despite the use of decongestants/analgesics. May give antibiotics sooner if purulent nasal discharge, severe illness, facial pain, and fever noted. If antibiotics are needed, treat for 10–14 days
Sinusitis (chronic)	Most prominent: *Staphylococci* and respiratory anaerobes. Other pathogens are:	Topical nasal decongestant (Afrin) Oxymetazoline HCl (0.05%) × 3–5 days max,	Adequate fluids, steam inhalation, warm compresses to sinuses, and analgesics	ENT consult is recommended; Antibiotics are usually not effective

Table 13-6 **CHOOSING THE APPROPRIATE TREATMENT** *(continued)*

Diagnosis	Common Etiology	Preferred Rx	Alternative	Comments
	H. influenza, M. catarrhalis, Pseudomonas aeruginosa, group A *Streptococcus*, and *S. pneumoniae*	oral decongestants (pseudoephedrine), nasal corticosteroids, saline nasal spray, 2nd-generation antihistamines (fexofenadine/ loratadine) with known allergic rhinitis and mucolytics (Mucinex)		
Bronchitis (acute)	90% = viral 5%–10% = related *to Mycoplasma pneumoniae, C. pneumoniae*, bordetella pertussis; *S. pneumoniae, H. influenzae, M. catarrhalis* noted in underlying lung disease	Bronchodilator (albuterol), antihistamine, antitussive agents		Antibiotics generally not recommended, but patients with comorbidities often need treatment
Bronchitis (chronic)	*H. influenza, S. pneumoniae, Moraxella catarrhalis* (50%–60%)	Oxygen supplementation, β-adrenergic agonists (albuterol) and anticholinergic agents (ipratropium bromide), antibiotics (doxycycline), oral corticosteroids	Expectorants (Mucinex)	Referral to a pulmonologist is often recommended

(continues)

Table 13-6 CHOOSING THE APPROPRIATE TREATMENT *(continued)*

Diagnosis	Common Etiology	Preferred Rx	Alternative	Comments
Pneumonia	*S. pneumoniae* (most common)	Macrolides (azithromycin, clarithromycin), Fluoroquinolones (levofloxacin)	Penicillins (Augmentin), and cephalosporins	Avoid ciprofloxacin
Tuberculosis (latent)	*Mycobacterium tuberculosis*	Isoniazid 300 mg daily for 9 months (preferred)	300 mg daily for 6 months (see Table 13-23)	Need to identify if person is in certain risk groups

the first few patients who present with influenza symptoms during the flu season. Once influenza has been identified in the community, antiviral treatment may be an option for patients with severe underlying medical conditions. Other laboratory or diagnostic testing, such as chest x-rays, may be needed if complications are suspected.

Table 13-7 DIFFERENTIAL DIAGNOSIS: COMMON COLD AND INFLUENZA[21,23]

Common Cold	Influenza
Overall symptoms: mild	Overall symptoms: moderate-to-severe
Symptoms: gradual onset	Symptoms: abrupt onset
Cough: mild	Nonproductive, dry cough
Fever: not noted or low-grade 99°F (37.2°C)	Fever >100°–104°F (37.7°C)
Energy: normal or fatigue mild-to-moderate	Extreme fatigue or weakness
Headache: mild	Headache
Sore throat	Sore throat
Nasal congestion	Nasal congestion
Rhinitis	Rhinitis
Sneezing	Chills
	Myalgia
	Malaise: constant
	Photophobia

Abbreviations are: RSV, respiratory syncytial virus; tid, three times daily; bid, twice daily; q, every; h, hour; qd, daily; max, maximum.

- Otitis media
- Sinusitis
- Bronchitis
- Pneumonia
- Dehydration
- Exacerbation of current medical problem (e.g., asthma, diabetes, congestive heart failure)

MANAGEMENT

Lifestyle   Adequate hydration is important. Those infected with influenza should be encouraged to consume two or more liters of water or other fluids. Caffeine and alcohol intake should be decreased or eliminated to prevent further fluid loss. Thorough, frequent hand washing should also be encouraged.

Medication   Antiviral medications (i.e., amantadine hydrochloride, rimantadine hydrochloride, oseltamivir, zanamavir) are adjunctive therapies to the influenza vaccine. These medications should not be used as a substitute for the vaccine.[25] Amantadine, rimantadine, and oseltamivir are used both for the prevention and treatment of influenza, whereas Zanamavir is used only for the treatment of influenza. Amantadine and rimantadine are older antiviral drugs effective against influenza type A, not influenza type B.[25] Zanamavir and Oseltamivir are newer antiviral agents that are active against influenza type A and B.[25–27] Both work against the influenza virus enzyme neuroaminidase and are found to be safe. With Osteltamivir, mild transient symptoms of nausea, vomiting, and diarrhea have been reported.[26] When an antiviral

medication is used for prevention, the medication is 70% to 90% effective in healthy adults. If influenza-like symptoms have begun, the antiviral drugs can decrease symptoms and shorten the duration of illness by one to two days.[27] In order for the medication to be effective, the antiviral medication needs to be taken within two days of symptom onset. **Table 13-10** presents common antiviral medications, and **Table 13-11** details the use of antiviral medication for treatment and prophylaxis.

Complementary or Alternative Choices   Research on the use of complementary and alternative medications (CAMs) in the treatment of influenza is sparse and provides no guidance on the effectiveness or safety of these products for individuals infected with influenza.

PATIENT INSTRUCTIONS

Patient education regarding transmission and prevention should be given. Since adults can shed the influenza virus from one day before symptoms begin until five days later,[28] individuals who have had close contact in this time period with someone with influenza may become infected. Infected individuals should be instructed to avoid contact with pregnant women, children, older adults, and others who are immunocompromised or have a chronic illness.[28] Frequent hand washing, adequate rest, and adequate fluid and nutrition intake are the most important factors in preventing influenza. High-risk individuals should receive the influenza vaccine annually.

MANAGEMENT DURING PREGNANCY AND LACTATION

Complications relating to influenza have marked effects on the pregnant women and her

---

Table 13-9   HIGH-RISK FOR DEVELOPING INFLUENZA OR COMPLICATIONS RELATED TO INFLUENZA[21,23,24]

- People aged 65+
- Children younger than 2 years old
- Residents of a chronic care facility
- People with chronic medical disorders (e.g., cardiovascular disorders, diabetes, asthma, or other respiratory disorders)
- HIV-affected patients
- Pregnant women who will be in the second or third trimester of pregnancy during influenza season (November–March, sometimes extending to April) or earlier if the patient is at high risk for influenza secondary to chronic medical problem
- Health care workers
- Household contacts (including children) or caretakers of persons at high risk

---

growing baby. If a pregnant woman has influenza, the physiologic changes of pregnancy, such as heart rate acceleration, increased stroke volume, higher oxygen consumption, loss of lung capacity, and alterations in immunologic function, put the pregnant woman at increased risk for major medical complications.[28] Because of the increased risk of complications and hospitalizations related to influenza, pregnant women should be offered the influenza vaccine. If a pregnant woman has a medical condition that will increase her risk for complications from influenza (e.g., cardiopulmonary, including asthma), she should be vaccinated regardless of the stage of pregnancy.

Influenza Vaccine   The influenza vaccination can prevent illness from influenza virus Type A and B. If an individual becomes infected despite having received the vaccine, the clinical course tends to be milder and is associated with less morbidity. High-risk individuals, such as those listed in Table 13-9, should be offered the influenza vaccine annually. Chapter 2 provides more information about the indications,

---

Table 13-10   ANTIVIRAL MEDICATIONS FOR INFLUENZA[24]

Drug	Amantadine	Rimantadine	Oseltamivir	Zanamivir
Indication	Prevention and treatment	Prevention and treatment	Prevention and treatment	Treatment
Effective against subtype	Type A	Type A	Types A and B	Types A and B

Table 13-11 RECOMMENDED DAILY DOSAGE OF INFLUENZA ANTIVIRAL MEDICATIONS FOR TREATMENT AND PROPHYLAXIS[28]

	Age Group, years	
Antiviral Agent	**13–64**	**≥65**
Amantadine*		
Treatment, Influenza A	100 mg twice daily	≤100 mg/day
Prophylaxis, influenza A	100 mg twice daily	≤100 mg/day
Rimantadine[¶]		
Treatment,** influenza A	100 mg twice daily,[§§]	100 mg/day
Prophylaxis, influenza A	100 mg twice daily	100 mg/day[¶¶]
Zanamivir***[†††]		
Treatment, influenza A and B	10 mg twice daily	10 mg twice daily
Oseltamivir		
Treatment,[§§§] influenza A and B	75 mg twice daily	75 mg twice daily
Prophylaxis, influenza A and B	75 mg/day	75 mg/day

Note: Amantadine manufacturers include: Endo Pharmaceuticals (Symmetrel®, tablet and syrup); Geneva Pharms Tech and Rosemont (Amantadine HCL, capsule); USL Pharma (Amantadine HCL, capsule and tablet); and Alpharma, Copley Pharmaceutical, HiTech Pharma, Mikart, Morton Grove, Carolina Medical, and Pharmaceutical Associates (Amantadine HCL, syrup). Rimantadine is manufactured by Forest Laboratories (Flumadine®, tablet and syrup) and Corepharma, Impax Labs (Rimantadine HCL, tablet), and Amide Pharmaceuticals (Rimantadine ACL, tablet). Zanamivir is manufactured by GlaxoSmithKline (Relenza®, inhaled powder). Oseltamivir is manufactured by Hoffman-LaRoche, Inc. (Tamiflu®, tablet). This information is based on data published by the U.S. Food and Drug Administration (FDA), which is available at http://www.fda.gov.

* The drug package insert should be consulted for dosage recommendations for administering amantadine to persons with creatinine clearance ≤50 mL/min/1.73 m².

¶ A reduction in dosage to 100 mg/day of rimantadine is recommended for persons who have severe hepatic dysfunction or those with creatinine clearance ≤10 mL/min. Other persons with less severe hepatic or renal dysfunction taking 100 mg/day of rimantadine should be observed closely, and the dosage should be reduced or the drug discontinued, if necessary.

** Only approved by the FDA for treatment in adults.

§§ Rimantadine is approved by the FDA for treatment among adults. However, certain specialists in the management of influenza consider rimantadine appropriate for treatment in children (see American Academy of Pediatrics, *2000 Red Book: Report of the Committee on Infectious Diseases.* 25th ed. Elk Grove Village, IL: American Academy of Pediatrics; 2000.)

¶¶ Older nursing-home residents should be administered only 100 mg/day of rimantadine. A reduction in dosage to 100 mg/day should be considered for all persons aged ≥65 years, if they experience possible side effects when taking 200 mg/day.

*** Zanamivir is administered through inhalation by using a plastic device included in the medication package. Patients will benefit from instruction and demonstration of correct use of the device.

††† Zanamivir is not approved for prophylaxis.

§§§ A reduction in the dose of oseltamivir is recommended for persons with creatinine clearance, 30 mL/min.

Source: Adapted from Table 7, "Recommended Daily Dosage of Influenza Antiviral Medications for Treatment and Prophylaxis.[28]

effectiveness, and risks associated with the influenza vaccine.

Pneumonia

Persons affected by CAP face significant illness and possibly death. In the United States, approximately 500,000 individuals develop CAP each year.[29] It is estimated that approximately 175,000 cases of pneumococcal infection require hospitalization each year. Case fatality rates are estimated to be 5 to 7% but can be higher in more vulnerable populations.[30] The severity and prognosis are dependent upon the patient's age, immune status, and the presence of comorbid conditions. *Streptococcus pneumoniae* is the most common cause of CAP.[29] Other organisms such as *Staphylococcus aureas*, *Chlamydia pneumoniae*, *Haemophilus influenzae*, *Mycoplasma pneumoniae*, *Klebsiella pneumoniae*, *Legionella sp*, and *Staphylococcus aureus* are less common causes of CAP. Viral infections, such as those due to the influenza A virus or varicella, can also lead to pneumonia. Fungal infections (e.g., histoplasmosis, coccidiomycosis, and blastomycosis) are very rare causes of pneumonia.[31]

ESSENTIAL HISTORY AND PHYSICAL AND LABORATORY EVALUATION

In pneumonia, the following symptoms are most common: cough, pleuritic chest pain, shortness of breath, fever, fatigue, chills, night sweats, malaise, myalgia, and anorexia. The cough can be productive or nonproductive. Occasionally, an individual with pneumonia may report abdominal pain caused by an infiltrate of the right lower lobe that stimulates the tenth and eleventh thoracic nerves, thereby causing right lower quadrant pain.[32] The presentation of pneumonia is the same in both pregnant and nonpregnant women. Other diagnostic possibilities need to be excluded. The differential diagnosis includes asthma exacerbation or reactive airway disease, congestive heart failure, chronic obstructive pulmonary disease (COPD), pulmonary embolism, lung cancer, empyemia, lung abscess, pleurisy, and aspiration pneumonitis. If the patient is pregnant, amniotic fluid embolism and air embolism are also possibilities.[31]

If pneumonia is present, the main objective findings are tachycardia greater than 100 BPM, tachypnea greater than 25 breaths per minute, fever of more than 100°F, diminished breath sounds, and rales on inspiration. In the elderly, fever is often absent. A provider may suspect pneumonia in an older adult if she has an acute cough, shortness of breath, and mental status changes.[33] Tactile fremitus may be found on examination in individuals with pneumonia. Other causes for increased tactile fremitus include the presence of a compressed lung or solid mass.[32] Signs of consolidation may also be present with pneumonia. If consolidation is present, dullness will be heard over the affected lobe during percussion, and bronchophony, vocal resonance, and whispered pectoriloquy may be noted on auscultation.

Most providers will prefer to obtain a chest radiograph with anterior-posterior and lateral views to confirm the diagnosis. If pneumonia is present, the chest x-ray will commonly show infiltrates consistent with interstitial disease. In pregnancy, the chest radiograph may not be ordered unless the results will change patient management. During pregnancy, if a chest x-ray is needed, a postero-anterior view is preferred as this view exposes the mother and fetus to lower levels of radiation.[31] If a lateral chest x-ray is needed, the woman is exposed to 150 to 250 mRad, compared to only 5 to 30 mRad for a postero-anterior view.

MANAGEMENT

Medication   Antibiotics are needed for the treatment of most cases of pneumonia. Several choices are available. Macrolides (e.g., azithromycin, clarithromycin, erythromycin) are well-tolerated and effective in the treatment of pneumonia, making them the most commonly used agents. However, other good options are also available. Fluroquinolones (e.g., levofloxacin, gatifloxacin, moxifloxacin) are effective against *S. pneumoniae*, *M. pneumoniae*, *C. pneumoniae*, and *Legionella* species[34] and are the preferred treatment for older patients or those with comorbid illness (e.g., COPD). They are contraindicated in pregnancy or with patients under the age of 18.[35] Doxycycline is both inexpensive and effective, but it is contraindicated in pregnancy[36] as are the other tetracyclines and chloramphenicol.[31] Penicillins and cephalosporins are considered to be alternative treatments. Acyclovir has been shown to be efficacious in pneumonia caused by varicella zoster virus or herpes simplex virus.[37]

PREVENTION

Individuals at higher risk for acquiring pneumonia or who have underlying conditions that make it more likely that they will experience more severe infections should receive the pneumococcal and influenza vaccines. **Table 13-12** lists the high risk individuals who should be considered for vaccination with the pneumococcal vaccine (see the section on influenza above as well as Chapter 2 for further details on the influenza and pneumococcal vaccines).

Management during Pregnancy and Lactation
During pregnancy, CAP is more severe and more difficult to treat due to the anatomical and physiological changes that occur in normal pregnancy.[31] Most cases of pneumonia are seen in the second and third trimester, when these changes become more pronounced. Only an estimated 0% to 16% of pneumonia cases occur during the first trimester.[31]

REFERRAL

Most individuals can be managed on an outpatient basis and treated with oral antibiotics. **Table 13-13** lists factors that increase the risk of mortality. In the absence of these high risk factors, outpatient treatment with oral antibiotics can be initiated with close follow-up. Patients who have underlying medical conditions, more severe presentations, or who are older must be evaluated for inpatient admission. Depending on the severity of symptoms, the patient may either be observed for 24 hours or admitted.

Acute Sinusitis

Sinusitis is an inflammation of the paranasal mucosal sinuses. Usually the nasal cavity is also inflamed, and the term *rhinosinusitis* may be used. Sinusitis can either be acute, subacute, or chronic. Acute bacterial sinusitis presents with signs and symptoms of less than one month duration.[38] Viral, bacterial, and fungal infections as well as allergy or environmental irritants can cause acute sinus inflammatory reactions.[39] The maxillary and ethmoid sinuses are predominantly affected. Rarely, bacterial pathogens invade the frontal or sphenoid sinuses resulting in higher morbidity. Complications involving the orbit, the central nervous system,

Table 13-12 PNEUMOCCAL VACCINE: CONDITIONS PLACING INDIVIDUALS AT HIGH RISK[29]

Diabetes
Cardiovascular disease (including congestive heart failure and cardiomyopathy)
Pulmonary disease (including chronic obstructive pulmonary disease and emphysema; excluding asthma)
Alcohol abuse
Liver disease (including cirrhosis)
Cerebrospinal fluid leaks
Immune system disorders (i.e., anatomic or functional asplenia [splenectomy, sickle cell disease], nephrotic syndrome, HIV infection, leukemia, lymphoma, Hodgkin's disease, multiple myeloma, generalized malignancy)
Renal disease (including chronic renal failure and nephrotic syndrome)
Organ or bone marrow transplant
Chronic immunosuppressive treatment (e.g., chemotherapy or corticosteroids)
Certain living situations (i.e., nursing homes, long-term care facilities, incarceration facility)
Pregnant woman (only if high-risk condition is present)

or both can occur with untreated acute bacterial sinusitis. These include meningitis, subperiosteal abscess, orbital abscess, intraorbital or periorbital cellulitis, and cavernous sinus thrombosis.[39,40]

Most cases of acute rhinosinusitis are viral.[41] The two most common bacteria isolated from infected maxillary sinuses are *Streptococcus pneumoniae* and *Haemophilus influenzae*.[5,39,42,43] *Streptococcus pyogenes*, *Moraxella catarrhalis*, and anaerobic bacteria are rarely responsible for bacterial sinusitis but should be considered if symptoms persist despite treatment.[39] Fungal infections are rare and are mainly seen in immunocompromised patients (e.g., transplant recipients and those with diabetes, acquired immune deficiency syndrome (AIDS), or malignancies)[38,39,41] or in patients living in a geographic location with high humidity.[38]

ESSENTIAL HISTORY AND PHYSICAL AND LABORATORY EVALUATION

Aspiration of purulent secretions via a sinus puncture is considered the most accurate method of diagnosing sinusitis. Diagnosis is confirmed if the culture detects a minimum of 10^5 organisms per milliliter of a suspected pathogen. However, since this method is not commonly used, providers rely on the imperfect but more practical method of symptom review and clinical observations to diagnose acute rhinosinusitis. Unfortunately, it may be difficult for providers to distinguish between an acute bacterial sinusitis and a viral sinusitis. Hickner et al. reviewed seven studies published between 1976 and 1996 to determine predictors of acute bacterial rhinosinusitis.[39] Their study found the following symptoms were associated with sinusitis: unilateral or bilateral purulent rhinorrhea, mucopuru-

---

Table 13-13 INCREASED MORTALITY RISK WITH COMMUNITY-ACQUIRED PNEUMONIA

Age >50
Co-existing conditions
- Cancer (i.e., active/diagnosed within 1 year, excluding basal or squamous cell carcinoma)
- Chronic liver disease (i.e., cirrhosis, hepatitis)
- Congestive heart failure
- Stroke or transient ischemic attack
- Renal impairment (i.e., chronic renal disease or blood urea nitrogen >30 mg per dL or elevated creatinine)

Altered mental status (i.e., new onset)
Abnormal vital signs
- Temperature <95°F (35°C) or >104°F (40°C)
- Systolic blood pressure <90 mm Hg
- Pulse >124 beats per minute
- Respiratory rate >29 beats per minute

Other diagnostic data
- Radiographic finding: pleural effusion
- Random glucose >249 mg/dL
- Hematocrit <30%
- Sodium <130 mEq/L
- Arterial pH <7.35
- Arterial partial pressure of oxygen <60 mm Hg

---

lent nasal discharge on examination, unilateral maxillary, facial, or tooth pain. The more symptoms present, the higher the probability of an infectious sinusitis. Headache, fever, postnasal drip, and cough were often noted with an upper respiratory infection, and these symptoms were not highly predictive of a bacterial sinusitis.[39] Determining whether a patient has severe symptoms of acute sinusitis is important to determine if an urgent Ear-Nose-Throat (ENT) or surgical consult is necessary. **Table 13-14** describes signs and symptoms of bacterial and/or viral sinusitis, and **Table 13-15** provides those symptoms that necessitate an urgent ENT or surgical referral.

When evaluating a possible sinus infection, a thorough ENT, chest, and skin exam is recommended. The ears should be assessed for serous otitis or otitis media; the nose should be examined for a deviated septum, nasal polyps, foreign bodies, and tumors.[38] The provider should also check for purulent nasal discharge, erythema and edema of the sinuses (e.g., possible bacterial sinusitis), or pale, boggy turbinates (i.e., allergic rhinitis). The face, particularly over the maxillary sinuses, should be checked for any swelling or redness. The sinuses should be palpated for tenderness. **Figure 13-1** illustrates the normal landmarks for the sinuses. The sinuses

Table 13-14 SYMPTOMS OF SINUSITIS[13,38,39]

Signs and Symptoms Consistent with Bacterial Sinusitis	Nonspecific Symptoms Found in Both Viral or Bacterial Sinusitis
Mucopurulent nasal discharge	Fever
Unilateral maxillary pain/tooth pain	Headache
Unilateral facial pain	Generalized facial pain or tenderness
Unilateral sinus tenderness	Bilateral maxillary pain
Symptoms that initially improve and then worsen	Bilateral toothache/pain
No improvement with decongestants	Postnasal drip
Symptoms longer than 7 days	Cough

can be transilluminated to assess for blockage. Transillumination of the sinuses must be performed in a blackened room with an extremely bright source of light; otherwise, the exam will be inaccurate.[13] The throat should be examined for postnasal drip, erythema, swelling, or exudate. The chest and skin should be checked for signs of asthma or allergy. A neurologic exam, including a thorough eye examination, should be done if the patient complains of visual problems. If periorbital swelling, exophthalmos, abnormal extraocular movements, or decreased visual acuity are noted, urgent evaluation with an ENT specialist is necessary. Since radiographs and computed tomography (CT) scans are usually abnormal with both viral and bacterial rhinosinusitis, experts discourage the use of these tests for diagnosing sinusitis. These tests are reserved for use in patients with recurrent (>3 sinus infections per year) or persistent sinus infections.[13] (Refer to the section on "Chronic Sinusitis" below for further details regarding imaging.) If persistent symptoms are noted in a pregnant woman, consultation with an ENT specialist is warranted before further diagnostic testing or treatment is ordered.

Table 13-15 SYMPTOMS REQUIRING IMMEDIATE REFERRAL TO ENT SPECIALIST OR SURGEON[13,38,39]

High fever
Severe headaches
Facial swelling over one or more sinuses
Periorbital edema
Exophthalmos (seen with cavernous sinus disease)
Abnormal extraocular movements
Visual changes
Changes in mental status or other central nervous system symptoms (may be seen with periorbital abscess, brain abscess, or meningitis)

Figure 13-1 Illustration of the normal landmarks of the sinuses.

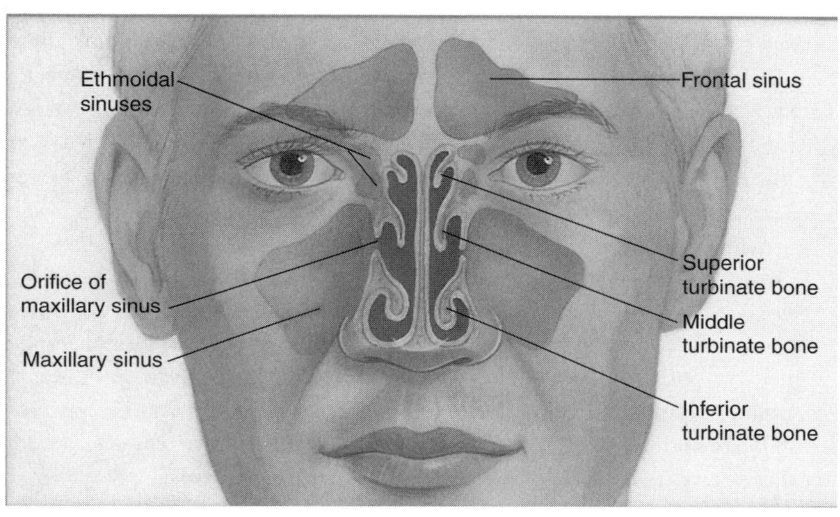

Source: Used with permission from Ghorayeb BY. Anatomy of the sinuses. Available at: http://www.ghorayeb.com/anatomy/sinuses.html.2004.

MANAGEMENT

Lifestyle In some situations, acute sinusitis can be exacerbated by allergies. If allergies are a potential trigger of acute sinusitis, environmental measures should be implemented to help control symptoms.

MEDICATION AND COMPLEMENTARY AND ALTERNATIVE CHOICES

Streptococcus pneumoniae is becoming increasingly resistant to antibiotics. In the United States, this pathogen is predominantly responsible for illnesses associated with bacterial sinusitis, community-acquired bacterial pneumonia, otitis media, and bacterial meningitis.[43] Bacterial pathogens are not as common a cause of acute sinusitis as providers may believe, and therefore, providers should be cautious before prescribing antibiotics.[6,39] In general, antibiotics are avoided unless symptoms have persisted for more than seven days and a bacterial infection is strongly suspected. If the patient has moderate-to-severe symptoms, fever, unilateral swelling and/or erythema isolated to one sinus, and sinus pain, then treatment should be initiated regardless of duration of symptoms.[39]

If mild symptoms have been present for fewer than seven days, then symptomatic treatment with oral and topical decongestants is usually effective. Other therapies include topical anticholinergics, nasal corticosteroids, zinc gluconate lozenges, vitamin C, and echinacea extract.[13] The use of steam, saline nasal spray, saline irrigation, and warm facial compresses may also be helpful and should routinely be recommended.

If symptoms are present for more than seven days or moderate to severe symptoms are present, supportive treatments should be continued and an antibiotic may be prescribed. Amoxicillin and trimethoprim/sulfamethoxazole are first-line antibiotics that are less costly and are equally as effective as the newer antibiotics (i.e., amoxicillin/clavulanate potassium, levofloxacin, cefuroxime axetil, clarithromycin, loracarbef, and ciprofloxacin). The management guidelines for the treatment of sinusitis are essentially the same for pregnant patients as for nonpregnant patients.[44] However, providers need to be aware that some of the medications used in the management of sinusitis are not recommended during pregnancy or lactation (**Table 13-16**). Amoxicillin and other penicillin derivative medications as well as the macrolides are safe to use in pregnancy.

PATIENT INSTRUCTIONS

Instructions include an explanation of the causes and treatment(s) for acute sinusitis. Proper adherence to non-prescriptive supportive treatments (steam treatments, normal saline nasal spray, and warm facial compresses) should be encouraged. Patients should also be instructed to return if their symptoms worsen or they develop swelling, facial redness, vision changes, severe headaches, or high fever.

Chronic Sinusitis

Sinusitis is defined by duration of symptoms: acute (<4 weeks), subacute (4–12 weeks) or chronic (>12 weeks).[38,43] *Chronic sinusitis* (CS) is commonly seen in primary care, allergy and immunology, and ENT specialty offices, since it affects over 30 million Americans.[47] CS results from chronic inflammatory mucosal changes with or without the development of polyps in the paranasal sinuses.[47] CS is caused by noninfectious (i.e., eosinophilia and mononuclear cells) and infectious (i.e., bacterial or viral) etiologies.[42] Noninfectious causes are more commonly reported than infectious causes. Noninfectious CS is strongly associated with allergy-related illness and chronic hyperplastic sinusitis with nasal polyposis.[42] The most common bacteria associated with the development of CS are *Staphylococci* and respiratory anaerobes; however, *H. influenzae*, *M. catarrhalis*, *Pseudomonas aeruginosa*, group A *Streptococcus*, and *S. pneumoniae* have also been detected.[38,42] It is believed that anaerobes develop after an initial bacterial infection as a result of mucus stasis, sinus obstruction, and hypoxia. CS can also develop from the same bacteria that caused an acute sinusitis.[41]

Several factors can worsen CS, with one of the main contributors being ostial blockage. The mucosa becomes thickened from inflammation despite antibiotic treatment. Mucosal inflammation inhibits normal mucociliary clearance, which may further obstruct sinus ostia.[42,47] Mucus immobility, sinus ostial obstruction, and hypoxia all contribute to the growth of anaerobic bacteria.[42] Allergy and eosinophilia also contribute to CS. Patients with allergies have a higher risk for extensive sinus disease.[48]

Nasal congestion and sinus complaints are common in pregnancy. However, as the fetus grows and the mother reaches her third trimester, her nasal symptomatology should decrease. During the later stages of pregnancy, blood shunts to the enlarging gravid uterus and away from the peripheral vascular system. Consequently, the nasal passages are less engorged, and there is less osteomeatal obstruction and a lower incidence of recurrent or chronic sinusitis.[44]

Table 13-16 Use of Medications in Pregnancy and Lactation[45,46]

Medication	Use	Mechanism of Action	Pregnancy Category	Lactation Effects	Possible Side Effects	Pregnancy (yes or no)
Acetylcysteine (Mucomyst)	Mucolytic purposes		B	Safety unknown	Bronchospasm, anaphylaxis, nausea, vomiting, rhinorrhea	Unknown
Albuterol	Asthma or bronchitis	Stimulates β_2-adrenergic receptors	C	Probably safe	Tremor, nervousness, nausea, tachycardia, palpitations, insomnia	Yes
Amantadine	Influenza A	Antiviral	C	Safety unknown	Nausea, dizziness, anxiety, irritability, dry mouth, headache, diarrhea, cardiac arrhythmias	No
Amoxicillin (Amoxil)	Bacterial infections	Bactericidal	B	Safe	Contraindicated in penicillin allergy or use with caution in cephalosporin allergy; nausea, vomiting, diarrhea, rash	Yes
Amoxicillin/ clavulanate potassium (Augmentin)	Bacterial infections	Bactericidal, inhibits β-lactamases	B	Safe—nursing infant may be at risk for diarrhea and candidiasis (rare)	Contraindicated with penicillin allergies; caution with liver/renal dysfunction; SE: diarrhea, nausea, vomiting, rash, mucocutaneous candidiasis	Yes
Azithromycin	Bacterial infections	Bactericidal	B	Probably safe	Diarrhea, nausea, abdominal pain, dizziness, rash	Yes
Budesonide nasal spray (Rhinocort aqua)	Allergic rhinitis	Corticosteroid	C	Probably safe	Epistaxis, pharyngitis, nasal irritation	Yes
Cefuroxime axetil (Ceftin)	Bacterial infections	Bactericidal	B	Safe	Caution with penicillin allergy, seizure disorder, renal dysfunction; SE: diarrhea, nausea, rash, abdominal cramps, elevated labs: BUN, creatinine, eosinophils, liver transaminases	Yes
Cetirizine (Zyrtec)	Allergic rhinitis	Antihistamine	B	Unknown	Drowsiness, fatigue, dry mouth, pharyngitis, dizziness	Yes

(continues)

Table 13-16 USE OF MEDICATIONS IN PREGNANCY AND LACTATION *(continued)*

Medication	Use	Mechanism of Action	Pregnancy Category	Lactation Effects	Possible Side Effects	Pregnancy (yes or no)
Chlorpheniramine (Chlor-Trimeton)	Allergic rhinitis	First generation non-selective antihistamine	B	Unknown	Drowsiness, dry mouth, constipation, dizziness, tachycardia	Yes
Ciprofloxacin (Cipro)	Bacterial infections	Bactericidal	C	Potential for significant effects on nursing infant (i.e., arthropathy in infant)	Contraindicated in patients under 18 years old and in pregnancy. Caution in seizure disorder, renal or liver dysfunction, sun exposure; Need to drink with plenty of water; SE: phototoxicity, nausea, diarrhea, vomiting, abdominal pain, headache, rash	No in pregnancy.
Clarithromycin (Biaxin)	Bacterial infections	Binds to P site of 50S ribosomal subunit, interfering with protein synthesis	C	Safety unknown, limited data available	Caution with liver or renal dysfunction; SE: QT prolongation, pseudomembranous colitis, diarrhea, abdominal pain, taste changes, nausea, rash	Not recommended when lactating.
Diphenhydramine (Benadryl)	Allergic rhinitis	First generation non-selective antihistamine	B	Probably Safe	Sedation, dry mouth, constipation, dizziness, tachycardia, wheezing, coordination problems, urinary retention, tinnitus	No
Doxycycline	Bacterial infections	Bacteriostatic	D	Unsafe	Headache, nausea, dyspepsia, diarrhea, rash, photosensitivity	No
Erythromycin	Bacterial infections	Bactericidal	B	Safe	Abdominal pain, abdominal cramps, stomatitis	Yes
Fexofenadine (Allegra)	Allergic rhinitis	Second generation selective antihistamine	C	Safe	Headache, dizziness, drowsiness	Yes, after second trimester
Fluticasone (Flonase)	Allergic rhinitis	Corticosteroid	C	Unknown	Pharyngitis, epistaxis, nasal burning, taste changes, sore throat, throat irritation, voice changes	Yes
Guaifenesin	Mucolytic uses	Increases volume and decreases viscosity of respiratory secretions	C	Unknown	Nausea, vomiting, GI irritation, headaches	Yes

Guaifenesin/ Pseudoephedrine (Entex)	Antitussive/ decongestant		C	Possibly unsafe based on small and limited studies	Nervousness, insomnia, headache, urinary retention, nausea, tachycardia, palpitations, tremor	No
Ipratropium nasal spray (Atrovent)	For rhinorrhea or rhinitis	Antagonizes aceylcholine receptors (anticholingergic); can decrease sputum production and cough	B	Sufficient literature not available	Anaphylaxis, bronchospasm, headache, URI, epistaxis, pharyngitis, nasal dryness/irritation	Yes, confined to severe asthma
Isoniazid	Antituberculosis	Bactericidal	C	Unknown	Hepatotoxicity, agranulocytosis, thrombocytopenia, peripheral neuropathy, leucopenia, optic neuritis, nausea, vomiting, diarrhea, rash	Yes
Levofloxacin (levaquin)	Bacterial infections	Bactericidal	C	Not safe	Contraindicated in patients under 18 years old (SE: arthropathy in children), in pregnancy, or if prolonged QT or arrhythmia noted; caution with seizure disorder and renal dysfunction; photosensitivity; SE: nausea, diarrhea, vomiting, abdominal pain, headache, rash	No in pregnancy. Must stop breastfeeding if medication used
Loracarbef (Lorabid)	Bacterial infections	Bactericidal	B	Safety unknown; limited literature available	Caution in pregnancy and lactation; SE: pseudomembranous colitis, low platelets, leukopenia, diarrhea, headache, nausea, vomiting, abdominal pain, rash	Yes
Loratadine (Claritin)	Allergic rhinitis	Selected antihistamine	B	Safe	Headache, fatigue, dry mouth	Yes
Naproxen	For pain and inflammation	Reduces prostaglandin synthesis	B—not for use in third trimester	Safe if used only in first and second trimesters, use with caution	Anaphylaxis, GI bleed, bronchospasm, abdominal pain, constipation, headache, rash, drowsiness, tinnitus	Avoided, especially in third trimester
NasalCrom	Allergic rhinitis	Mast cell stabilizer	B	Unknown	Sneezing, nasal burning, epistaxis, bad taste in mouth	Yes

(continues)

Table 13-16 Use of Medications in Pregnancy and Lactation *(continued)*

Medication	Use	Mechanism of Action	Pregnancy Category	Lactation Effects	Possible Side Effects	Pregnancy (yes or no)
Oseltamivir (Tamiflu)	Influenza A and B	Antiviral	C	Unknown	Nausea, vomiting, diarrhea, abdominal pain, headache	No
Oxymetazoline 0.05% (Afrin nasal spray)	For nasal congestion	Stimulates smooth muscle α-adrenergic receptors	C	Safety unknown, limited data available	Contraindicated: angle closure glaucoma; SE: nasal irritation, burning, dryness, rebound rhinitis if used for >5 days; hypertension (HTN)	Yes
Pseudoephridrine (Sudafed)	To decongest	Stimulates smooth muscle (sympathomimetic)	C	Safe	Arrhythmia, severe HTN, insomnia, headache, dizziness, nervousness, excitability, agitation, anxiety, palpitations, tachycardia, tremor	With caution; not to use with HTN, tachycardia, h/o palpitations, or glaucoma
Pyrazinamide	Anti-tuberculosis	Unknown	C	Unknown	Anorexia, rash, arthralgia, photosensitivity, gout, hepatotoxicity, thrombocytopenia, interstitial nephritis	No
Rifampin	Anti-tuberculosis		C	Probably safe	Renal failure, hepatotoxicity, thrombocytopenia, hemolytic anemia, leucopenia, interstitial nephritis, dizziness, abdominal pain, diarrhea, rash, stained contact lenses	Yes
Rimantadine	Influenza A	Inhibits viral replication	C	Unsafe	Hallucinations, insomnia, nervousness, dizziness	No
Trimethoprim/ sulfamethoxazole (Bactrim-DS/ Septra-DS)	Bacterial infections	Bactericidal	C	Unknown	Contraindicated with allergy to Sulfa, G6PD-deficiency, folate deficiency, liver or renal dysfunction. Serious SE are: Stevens-Johnson syndrome, agranulocytosis, blood dyscrasias, rash, nausea, vomiting, diarrhea, dizziness, headache, GI upset	No in lactating women. Avoid in pregnancy; do not use in third term.
Zanamavir (Relenza)	Influenza A and B	Antiviral	C	Unknown	Bronchospasm, nausea, dizziness, headache	No

Abbreviations: SE, side effects; GI, gastrointestinal; BUN, blood urea nitrogen; Cr, creatinine; HTN, hypertension; G6PD, glucose 6 phosphate dehydrogenase; URI, upper respiratory tract infection; h/o, history of.
Sources: Murphy JL. *Nurse Practitioners' Prescribing Reference.* 2nd ed: Prescribing Reference; 2004.[45]
Niebyl JR. Antibiotics and other anti-infective agents in pregnancy and lactation. *Am J Perinatol.* 2003;20:405–414.[46]

ESSENTIAL HISTORY AND PHYSICAL AND LABORATORY EVALUATION

The most common symptoms of CS are nasal congestion, postnasal drip, purulent nasal discharge, headache, cough, facial pressure, decrease or loss of the sense of smell, decreased ability to taste, and throat clearing.[42] Chronic or recurrent sinusitis often is related to allergic or environmental factors. If allergies are a triggering factor, symptoms such as itching of the nasal passages and sneezing are commonly reported.[39]

A thorough history should include questions about the initial presentation, how symptoms have changed over time, and whether the patient has symptoms suggestive of allergy or asthma. Common allergy symptoms include rhinorrhea; nasal congestion; itchiness of the eyes, ears, nose, mouth, and/or throat; repetitive sneezing; postnasal drip; and cough. Common asthma symptoms include chest tightness, shortness of breath, and/or wheezing.

A thorough eyes-ears-nose-throat, neck, cardiopulmonary, and skin assessment is necessary. The practitioner should note any eye discharge or darkening under the eyes. If both eyes have watery secretions with scant erythema to the conjunctiva, this suggests an allergic source. Allergic shiners, or darkening of the skin under the eyes, are also commonly seen in individuals with allergies. The ears should be examined for clear fluid behind the tympanic membrane (indicating possible serious otitis), or erythema, bulging of the tympanic membranes, and abnormal bony landmarkings (which can be seen with otitis media). The nasal turbinates should be assessed for color and texture. Pallor and bogginess are seen with allergies; erythema and edema in viral or bacterial infections. Also, the nasal passages should be checked for nasal discharge and polyps. The sinuses should be palpated. However, unlike an acute sinusitis, marked discomfort is not usually elicited upon palpation of the sinuses in individuals with CS. The throat should be checked for postnasal drip, which can be clear or purulent, as well as posterior pharyngeal erythema, or edema, any uvular deviation, pharyngeal exudate, and inflammation of the gums. The neck should be examined for any cervical lymphadenopathy, which may indicate an inflammatory or infectious source in the head, eyes, sinuses, ear, or throat. The jaw should be palpated for any tenderness or malalignment. Gums should be inspected for any swelling or erythema. The cardiac exam should include an evaluation of heart sounds, and the presence of tachycardia should be noted. Lungs should be assessed with particular attention for any wheezing or rhonchi. The skin should be inspected for patches of dryness or rashes that might indicate eczema.

A CT scan of the sinuses may be needed in the following circumstances: 1) to evaluate persistent symptoms despite appropriate treatment; 2) to determine anatomic abnormalities; or 3) to evaluate whether the patient is a candidate for endoscopic sinus surgery. The preferred diagnostic test in assessing obstruction to the sinus ostia is a limited CT scan of the sinus (coronal plane), as it provides a high-definition result. A full axial and coronal sinus CT scan, which is a more extensive and costly test, does not generally provide any additional clinical data that would be helpful in managing a patient with CS.[13] However, if sinus surgery is needed, a complete series is the preferred test. Magnetic resonance imaging is rarely used to diagnose sinusitis because it cannot distinguish between air and bone, but it may be helpful if a fungal infection or tumor is suspected.[38]

MANAGEMENT

Lifestyle Because the majority of patients with CS have an underlying allergy component, potential triggers need to be investigated and suggestions for eliminating allergens need to be offered.

Medication Initially, a topical nasal decongestant may be prescribed. Decongestants are useful because these agents can decrease nasal swelling and edema, thereby improving ostial patency, but this medication should be discontinued after three to five days to prevent rebound congestion. Long-term use of nasal corticosteroids has been approved to treat allergic, as well as perennial nonallergic rhinitis, although its use in CS is controversial.[49] Saline nasal sprays can also be used to help to liquefy secretions. Second-generation antihistamines (i.e., loratadine, fexofenadine, cetirizine) are often recommended; however, these medications should be reserved for patients with known allergic rhinitis. First-generation antihistamines (i.e., diphenhydramine) should be avoided; their anticholinergic effects may be too drying and actually prevent mucus drainage and clearance. If respiratory secretions are thickened, a guaifenesin tablet (600–1200 mg 2 ×/day) has been found to be beneficial in thinning the mucus and promoting drainage from the sinuses.[38] Guaifenesin 600 mg/pseudoephedrine 120 mg, one tablet every 12 hours, provides both systemic and mucolytic properties, and is often used in chronic rhinosinusitis.

Individuals with CS can develop superimposed acute infections. If there is a sudden exacerbation of symptoms, treatment would be the same as for acute sinusitis. However, if the symptoms are prolonged or persistent despite prior treatment(s) and/or the patient has a known history of CS, antibiotics probably will not be effective.[12] Mucosal thickening from chronic inflammation impedes normal mucociliary clearance, which can directly obstruct the ostiomeatal unit, and this process will continue despite antibiotic coverage.[12,42] Consultation with an otolaryngologist or ENT specialist is recommended when there is any suspicion of superimposed infection.

Complementary or Alternative Choices There are few choices of CAMs for the treatment of CS. Some that have been investigated include dietary and vitamin supplements, herbs, acupuncture, and homeopathic remedies. Some dietary supplements, such as Ma Huang or Bromelains have been used. Ma Huang contains ephedra alkaloids that have been used as a nasal decongestant; cardiovascular and neurologic side effects have been reported.[50] Bromelains, found in pineapple, exhibit proteolytic and anti-inflammatory effects that modify tissue permeability and reduce edema. In older studies, bromelains have been given to reduce nasal inflammation, nasal discharge, and headache. Unfortunately, the studies were few and the sample sizes were small. Therefore, the safety of the complementary or alternative choices is often uncertain or unknown, especially in pregnancy and during lactation.

PATIENT INSTRUCTIONS

Patients should be educated about a comprehensive treatment plan that involves adequate fluids, steam inhalation, warm compresses to sinuses, analgesics, decongestants, corticosteroid nasal inhalants, and saline nasal spray.

MANAGEMENT DURING PREGNANCY AND LACTATION

Management in pregnancy is individualized and depends on the underlying cause and severity of CS and the stage of pregnancy. Particular care must be taken during the first trimester (the period of organogenesis). If allergy is a precipitating factor of CS, then cromolyn sodium (Nasal Crom nasal spray) may be tried. NasalCrom is a mast-cell stabilizer that blocks allergens from releasing histamine. Mild symptoms of nasal irritation, flushing, or sneezing have been reported with its use. This medication is safe to use in pregnancy and can be used daily.[51] If this treatment is found to be ineffective or the woman's symptoms are intermittent, then an antihistamine may be tried. Chlorpheniramine (i.e., Chlor-Trimeton, a first-generation antihistamine) is considered safe and is the preferred antihistamine to use during pregnancy.[51] The prominent side effects are drowsiness and dry mouth. If Chlor-Trimeton is causing intolerable adverse effects or the medication is ineffective, a second-generation antihistamine such as loratadine (Claritin) or cetirizine (Zyrtec) may be tried. Loratadine and cetirizine were found to be safe in animal studies; the data regarding safety in pregnancy are incomplete. Pseudoepinephrine, an oral decongestant, is also relatively safe in pregnancy; in rare cases, fetal gastroschisis has been reported with its use during the first trimester.[44]

CONSULTATION

A referral to an ENT specialist is warranted when the patient is not responding to antibiotic treatment, symptoms have worsened, or the patient is experiencing recurrent sinusitis.[38] Table 13-15 defines the symptoms that require immediate referral. If the patient has nasal polyps, copious nasal secretions, chronic otitis media, immunodeficiency, allergies to several antibiotics, antibiotic resistance, or other circumstances that complicate the course of treatment, then a referral to an ENT specialist is also necessary. The specialist will determine whether sinus surgery is warranted. Chronic hyperplastic sinusitis with nasal polyposis often requires surgical intervention.[42] If an allergy is suspected and environmental controls and treatment have failed to prevent or improve the patient's outcome, a referral to an allergist is appropriate.

Acute Uncomplicated Bronchitis

Acute bronchitis is most frequently triggered by a viral infection because more than 90% of uncomplicated acute bronchitis cases are viral in origin.[52,53] Most of the other cases are due to atypical bacteria such as *Mycoplasma pneumoniae*, *Chlamydia pneumoniae* (TWAR strain), and *Bordetella pertussis*. *Streptococcus pneumoniae*, *Haemophilus influenzae*, and *Moraxella catarrhalis* can also cause acute bronchitis in adults but tend to be more common in individuals who have underlying lung disease.[53] Detecting the actual organism is not necessary in uncomplicated cases.[12,54] Rather, the diagnosis and management are based on clinical findings.

Acute bronchitis results from an inflammation or infection of the bronchial epithelium of the tracheobronchial tree. The alveoli are not affected. Inflammation results in airway hyperresponsiveness and production of mucus.[52] Acute bronchitis often presents with wheezing, rhonchi, and low peak flow readings. These findings make it difficult for providers to distinguish whether the "reactive airway" is simply from bronchitis or from undiagnosed asthma. If the diagnosis of asthma has not already been established, it is generally recommended to forgo diagnosis in patients with a cough until the symptoms have lasted longer than three weeks. Cough-variant asthma should be suspected in patients with nocturnal symptoms, or if symptoms are triggered by exposure to cold or exercise.[53]

With acute bronchitis, symptoms are usually present for less than three weeks duration, and the dominant symptom is a cough.[5,55] Patients may also report chest discomfort, low-grade fever,[52] and upper respiratory symptoms such as phlegm, rhinorrhea, throat pain, fatigue, headache, and postnasal drip.[52,55] These signs and symptoms are common and can be present with other respiratory problems. Other causes of cough such as postnasal drip, sinusitis, allergic rhinitis, GERD, asthma, and pneumonia should be ruled out.

ESSENTIAL HISTORY AND PHYSICAL AND LABORATORY EVALUATION

The diagnosis of bronchitis is primarily made from the history and physical examination findings. As when evaluating any respiratory condition, a history focusing on the evolution of symptoms and the length of time that symptoms have been present is essential. Eliciting a history of persistent cough, particularly with an onset after an upper respiratory infection, is highly suggestive of bronchitis. A physical examination can help confirm the diagnosis and exclude other possibilities. Fever, tachycardia, or tachypnea suggests more serious infection such as pneumonia, particularly if areas of focal consolidation are found during auscultation and percussion of the lung fields. Wheezing, rales, and rhonchi may be indicative of asthma or other obstructive lung conditions.

In general, laboratory and diagnostic testing is of little value. Chest radiography is not usually needed. However, if the patient has underlying cardiac or pulmonary disease (e.g., congestive heart failure, prior myocardial infarction, COPD/emphysema, chronic cough) or smokes, then further diagnostic testing may be warranted. In these cases, a chest x-ray and peak flow measurements may be helpful. Cultures are rarely taken because most cases are due to viral infections or inflammation. Consequently, antibiotics are not commonly used in the treatment of acute bronchitis except in selected cases, such as when bacterial infections are present.

MANAGEMENT

Many of the same measures discussed above that provide symptomatic relief from the common cold will also help individuals with acute bronchitis. Rest and hydration are particularly helpful.

MEDICATION

In uncomplicated acute bronchitis, management should be directed to the relief of cough. Different medication choices are available; the decision regarding which drug to use will depend on the underlying cause of the cough. For example, if a reactive airway or wheezing is noted, then a bronchodilator usually is helpful and can decrease the cough by as much as one week. If the cough is due to allergic rhinitis, an antihistamine may be beneficial. Antitussive agents are used to help suppress or control coughing when chest discomfort is noted from coughing. This is often helpful for a cough induced by cigarette smoking or postnasal drip. Coughing is one of the body's defense mechanisms and, therefore, antitussives may be used if suppressing the cough will not delay the patient's recovery. If a more productive cough would be beneficial to help clear the airways of mucus, then a protussive agent or expectorant is recommended.

Antibiotics have historically been prescribed for the treatment of uncomplicated acute bronchitis, but their use is no longer recommended. Providers have been most likely to prescribe antibiotics in the presence of purulent sputum or nasal discharge, wheezing, or rhonchi. However, purulent nasal or pharyngeal secretions do not necessarily indicate that the infection is due to bacteria. The use of antibiotics in the treatment of acute uncomplicated bronchitis does not improve clinical outcomes.[54,56,57] A 1988 literature review evaluated eight randomized controlled trials to determine whether the use of antibiotics for the treatment of acute bronchitis improved clinical outcomes. Antibiotics used in these studies were erythromycin, doxycycline, and trimethoprim/sulfamethoxazole. The meta-analysis found that the potential risk of adverse effects outweighed the benefits. The benefits of antibiotic use included decreased sputum production, decreased cough, and reduced work absenteeism by less than one day.[57] Risks included the development of side effects, the cost of antibiotics, and increased likelihood of encouraging antibiotic resistance. A 2004 Cochrane review had similar findings.[58] Therefore, antibiotics are generally not recommended in patients with acute bronchitis who have no other underlying pulmonary disease.[8,56,59]

PATIENT INSTRUCTIONS

Providers may feel pressure from patients to prescribe an antibiotic. According to Knutson and Braun,[54] patient satisfaction is related to the quality of the interaction between the patient and her provider, and not from the number of prescriptions received. Therefore, patient education is vital. Patients need to be informed of the diagnosis, treatment, and clinical course of acute bronchitis. They need to know why antibiotics are not needed and the risks associated with their use. For some patients, describing uncomplicated acute bronchitis as a "chest cold" makes it easier to accept the idea that an antibiotic is not necessary.[54]

MANAGEMENT DURING PREGNANCY AND LACTATION

The evaluation of acute bronchitis is the same during pregnancy and lactation. The treatment is also the same, although the practitioner must verify that a particular medication is safe in pregnancy. Table 13-16 lists medications mentioned in this chapter as well as pregnancy categories, lactation safety profiles, and whether the medication is used in pregnancy.

Chronic Bronchitis

Chronic bronchitis presents with a persistent cough and an overproduction of sputum for three or more consecutive months in two consecutive years. Chronic bronchitis is the fourth leading cause of death in the United States.[60] Symptoms are due to chronic inflammation, which results in erythema, edema, increased secretions, and mucosal friability of the bronchial airway.[61] In advanced stages, airway obstruction develops and leads to COPD. Certain factors have been found to contribute to the pathogenesis of COPD, including cigarette smoking, infections, and inhalation of dust.[12,62] Once COPD has developed, a patient can have periods of *acute exacerbations of chronic bronchitis (AECB)*. AECB is characterized as a subjective worsening in one or more chronic symptoms (e.g., sputum production/purulence/viscosity, shortness of breath, dyspnea, or cough).[63]

Up to 60% of AECB are caused by bacterial pathogens such as *Haemophilus influenza*, *Streptococcus pneumoniae*, and *Moraxella catarrhalis*.[62–64] *H. influenza* adheres to mucosal, oropharyngeal, and bronchial cells, causing an inflammatory response and damage of the lower respiratory mucosa. This process inhibits the immune system, allowing increased bacterial replication and worsening inflammation.[61] Other bacteria can also cause AECB but are less common. Atypical bacterial such as *Chlamydia pneumoniae*, *Enterobacteriaceae*, and *Pseudomonas* cause approximately 5 to 10% of cases of AECB. *Enterobacteriaceae* and *Pseudomonas*, which are Gram-negative pathogens, are more common in patients with advanced lung disease and decreased lung function.[62] Viral sources such as influenza, parainfluenza, respiratory syncytial virus, rhinovirus, and coronavirus[65] have been found in an estimated 20% to 50% of cases.[12,63]

ESSENTIAL HISTORY AND PHYSICAL AND LABORATORY EVALUATION

A thorough history and physical examination will help confirm the diagnosis of chronic bronchitis. Hallmark findings of chronic bronchitis include the persistence of symptoms and the presence of cough. However, other conditions may have similar presentations (**Table 13-17**), and individuals with chronic bronchitis can also develop other respiratory problems. Compare the subtle differences among **Figure 13-2** (normal radiographic findings of the female chest), **Figure 13-3** (radiograph showing an infiltrate), and **Figure 13-4** (radiograph showing congestive heart failure).

Individuals with AECB usually report an increase in cough, a change in the color, quantity, and consistency of sputum, or worsening dyspnea.[68] Forced expiratory volume in one second (FEV1) will decrease with acute infective exacerbations. The degree of severity can help determine the stage of COPD and direct management.[62] (Chapter 12 provides a description of pulmonary function testing.) If the FEV1 is less than 40%, the patient will often need to be hospitalized.[69] Patients with severe COPD usually have low O_2 saturation levels of 90% to 92%.[68] If the patient is febrile and/or the O_2 saturation is less than 92%, a chest x-ray should be obtained. Hyperventilation is usually seen on a chest x-ray in patients with chronic bronchitis; however, the finding of an infiltrate or effusion indicates that an infection is also present. Mental status changes and respiratory distress are signs of a severe exacerbation, and these patients should be transferred to the emergency room promptly via ambulance for further evaluation.

MANAGEMENT

Individuals with chronic bronchitis need to be under the care of a specialist skilled in the management of serious respiratory conditions. Oxygen supplementation, bronchodilators, antibiotics, and corticosteroids are commonly used in the management of chronic bronchitis and AECB. Beta-adrenergic agonists (i.e., albuterol, metaproterenol) and anticholinergic agents (i.e., ipratropium bromide) are recommended to improve airflow during an acute exacerbation. Antibiotics may be needed, especially in severe exacerbations.[68] A 1995 meta-analysis showed a small but statistically significant improvement in symptoms and peak expiratory flow readings following antibiotic treatment in patients with

Table 13-17 DIFFERENTIAL DIAGNOSIS FOR BRONCHITIS[53,66,67]

Possible Diagnosis	History	Physical Exam	Laboratory Findings
Pneumonia	Fever >101°F Cough Shortness of breath Malaise	Rales/crackles Focal fremitus Positive egophony Lowered peak flow readings	Infiltrate on chest x-ray (Refer to Figure 13-3)
Congestive heart failure	Shortness of breath Cough	Rales or crackles on auscultation Lowered O_2 saturation	Chest x-ray findings: • increased cardiothoracic ratio >0.5 • pulmonary venous congestion • pulmonary venous hypertension and interstitial edema (superior pulmonary venous distention, large hila with indistinct borders, Kerley's B lines) Severe pressure (i.e., pulmonary capillary wedge pressure >25 mm Hg): • alveolar edema • pleural effusions (biventricular failure). (Refer to Figure 13-4.)
Pulmonary embolism	Cough Shortness of breath Chest pain with inspiration Malaise	Tachycardia Hypotension Wheezing on auscultation	• Chest x-ray: normal • EKG (80% = nonspecific changes; 20% = S wave in Lead I, Q wave in Lead III, T wave inversion in Lead II, positive • D-Dimer positive • Doppler ultrasound (deep vein thrombosis) • VQ scan (intermediate to high probability) • Helical/spiral CT (abnormal) Pulmonary angiogram (confirmation).

(continues)

Table 13-17 DIFFERENTIAL DIAGNOSIS FOR BRONCHITIS *(continued)*

Possible Diagnosis	History	Physical Exam	Laboratory Findings
Myocardial infarction	Midsternal, exertional chest pain Shortness of breath Dizziness Diaphoresis Nausea/vomiting Weakness Radiation to arm/chest/back/shoulder	Diaphoresis, cool, moist skin, anxious affect; tachycardia and hypertension (bradycardia and hypotension with inferior wall MI); jugular vein distention, rales/crackles, and S3 heart sound if left ventricular heart failure present	ST wave elevation/inversion on EKG Positive exercise perfusion stress test
Upper respiratory tract infection	Milder symptoms of rhinorrhea Nasal congestion Postnasal drip Afebrile or low-grade fever <101°F	See section on Common Cold	Not helpful
Noncompliance to medications	Non-applicable	Exacerbations of usual symptoms	Patient's report of missed medication and lack of support for other diagnosis
Cough-variant asthma	Cough lasting longer than 3 weeks Allergy symptoms Chest tightness Shortness of breath and/or wheezing	Diminished breath sounds or wheezing Decreased peak flow readings Possible lowered O_2 saturation	Pulmonary function test or methacholine challenge test

Abbreviations are:: EKG, electrocardiogram; VQ, ventilation perfusion imaging; CT, computed axial tomography; MI, myocardial infarction.

COPD.[70] Oxygen supplementation may be required with severe hypoxia. If respiratory failure occurs, noninvasive positive-pressure ventilation is used to increase ventilation.

Because individuals with chronic bronchitis are at risk of developing COPD, encouraging smokers to stop may slow the progression of chronic bronchitis and prevent the development of severe COPD. All smokers should be counseled to stop smoking, especially those with underlying respiratory conditions, and smoking cessation medications prescribed as needed. Assessing the patient's home environment is also critical, as second-hand smoke, occupational and home inhalants or pollutants, and social contact with an illness can all cause a relapse or recurrence of symptoms. To prevent exacerbations, all individuals with chronic bronchitis should receive the influenza vaccine annually.

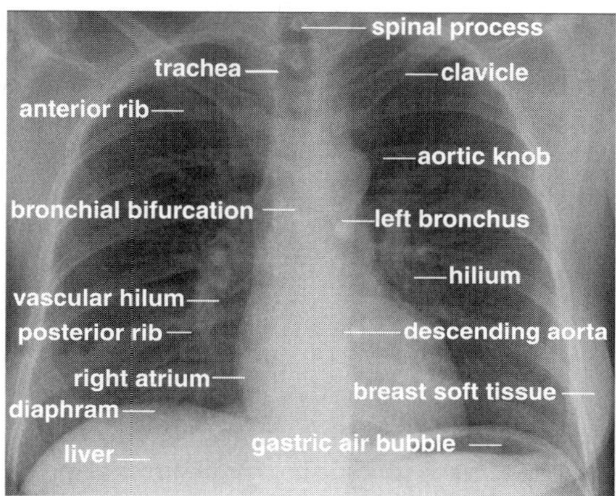

Figure 13-2 Normal chest radiograph of a female.

Source: Used with permission from Yale University. Available from: http://info.med.yale.edu/intmed/cardio/imaging/contents. html.

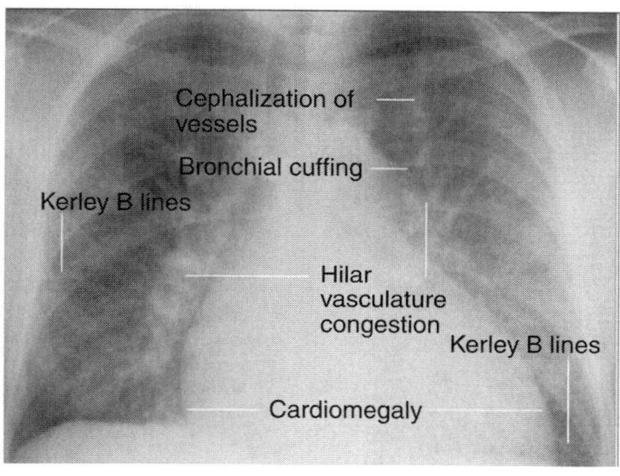

Figure 13-3 Chest radiograph of a female who has chronic bronchitis. Note infiltrate.

Source: Used with permission from Yale University. Available from: http://info.med.yale.edu/intmed/cardio/imaging/contents.html.

Expectorants, mucolytics, mucokinetics, antiproteases, and antioxidants are alternative therapies that have shown some benefit.[71] Expectorants (e.g., Mucinex) are only effective if given in higher doses (i.e., 600–1200 mg 2 x/day). Mucolytics (e.g., Acetylcysteine) help to decrease the viscosity of sputum; however, these medications often do not reach the distal airways where mucus plugging often is noted. Mucokinetic agents decrease mucus adhesiveness and increase airway patency. These agents have been shown to be beneficial in patients with COPD; however, further research is needed to assess the efficacy of mucokinetics. Antiprotease (e.g., α-1 antiprotease) is costly and has a high risk for adverse effects. Other alternative antiproteases are still being developed. Since cigarette smoking is a heavy oxidant and smoking is known to be correlated with chronic bronchitis, the use of antioxidants has been considered.

Latent Tuberculosis Infection

Mycobacterium tuberculosis is a bacterium that is spread from person to person through respiratory droplets. Bacteria are expelled from a person with active pulmonary or laryngeal TB either through sneezing, coughing, talking, or singing. Bacteria can also be released into the environment during medical procedures or sputum/tissue collection or analyses such as sputum induction, aerosolization during bronchoscopy, handling of tissue or bodily secretions.[72] The bacteria can remain in the air for several hours, so if a susceptible individual inhales the bacteria, infection may result.

Figure 13-4 Congestive Heart Failure.

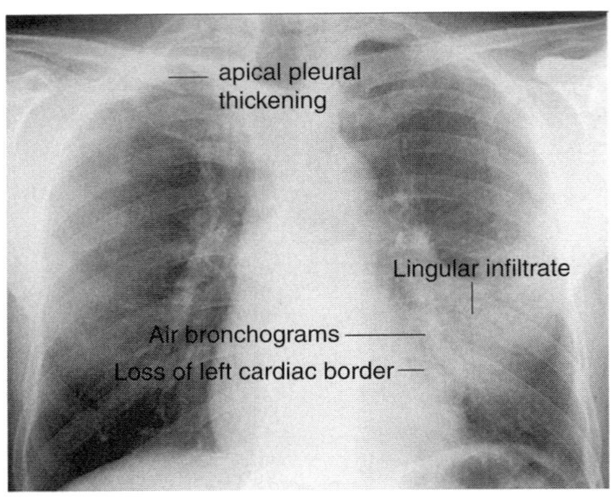

Source: Used with permission from Yale University. Available from: http://info.med.yale.edu/intmed/cardio/imaging/contents.html.

Four main factors increase the chance of infection with *M. tuberculosis*: 1) the number of organisms released in the air; 2) the concentration of bacteria in relation to the space and the amount of ventilation (e.g., bedroom vs. non-enclosed backyard); 3) immune status of the exposed person; and 4) length of exposure to the infected environment.[72] Infection is most likely to occur if the exposed individual has close contact with a contagious individual over a prolonged period of time.[73] Household contacts are generally more at risk.

Once a person is exposed to the bacteria, local inflammation and consolidation can occur. The tubercle bacilli enter the lymphatic system and reach the paratracheal lymph nodes, which surround the trachea, and the hilar lymph nodes, which are located near the mediastinum. This process forms the initial pulmonary lesion, or the *Ghon focus*. Some bacilli also enter the bloodstream and are transported to various organs, where they may later become activated.[72,73] The organs that are mainly affected are the lung (particularly the upper lobes), brain, kidneys, and bones. The bacilli can also be found in the bone marrow, liver, and spleen; however, *M. tuberculosis* is rarely detected in these locations because they do not favor replication of the bacilli.

Within several days after the exposure, *granulomata* are formed. A granuloma is a nodule of inflammatory tissue formed when macrophages and T cells surround the TB bacterium. The formation of granulomata prevents further replication and dissemination of disease. Once cell-mediated immunity develops between 2 and 12 weeks after infection, replication of *M. tuberculosis* ceases; however, a small amount of viable bacilli remains in the granuloma.[72] The granulomata and the Ghon focus may fibrose and calcify, leaving the TB infection dormant for several years; however, viable bacilli can be reactivated. Clusters of granulomata form tubercles, the nodular lesion of TB.[73]

The risk of developing active infection depends on the patient's age, immune status, and the presence of comorbid medical conditions. Some conditions that place the individual at a higher risk of progressing to active tuberculosis are listed, from highest to lowest risk: 1) untreated advanced human immunodeficiency virus (HIV) infection; 2) old healed TB; 3) chronic renal failure; 4) poorly controlled diabetes; 5) silicosis; 6) low body weight (10% below normal); and 7) gastrectomy.[74] The relative risk of an HIV-infected individual with a positive *purified protein derivative* (PPD) having active TB is 35 to 162 times higher than it is in the general population.[74] HIV positive individuals are also at high risk of reactivation of old infection. There is a twofold risk of tuberculosis conversion in individuals on antiretroviral therapy for HIV.[74] Given these statistics, it is imperative that all HIV-infected individuals be tested and if the results are positive receive treatment for latent TB infection.[74] In most individuals, for every 10 years postinfection, the lifetime risk of reactivation TB decreases by 10%.[75]

ESSENTIAL HISTORY AND PHYSICAL AND LABORATORY EVALUATION

Latent tuberculosis infection (LTBI) is an inactive form of TB that indicates the individual has been exposed to TB. If a person is diagnosed with latent TB, there is no lung damage, the person is asymptomatic, and is not contagious to others; however, she is at risk for developing the active form of TB.[74] Overall, there is a 10% chance of the active form developing; this percentage increases dramatically in certain high-risk groups.[72,74] **Table 13-18** lists groups who should be tested for TB.

While most LTBIs are asymptomatic, some will present with unusual findings such as erythema nodosum or phylectenular conjunctivitis.[73] In erythema nodosum, mildly erythematous subcutaneous nodules are noted, usually on the lower extremities. Phylectenular conjunctivitis produces small grey or yellow nodules in the conjunctiva that result in discomfort, pain, and increased tearing in the affected eye. These findings are the result of hypersensitivity reactions to the TB bacterium. Providers need to be aware that patients presenting with these symptoms may be infected and should be tested for TB.

Tuberculin Skin Testing   TB is detected with a Mantoux tuberculin skin test. Tuberculin skin testing is recommended for two groups of individuals who are at higher risk for TB compared to the general U.S. population: 1) those with a greater risk of exposure to *M. tuberculosis* and 2) those who have a current medical condition that increases their risk for conversion from LTBI to active TB.[74] Once infected, individuals are at an increased risk for developing active disease within the first two years.[74]

It is essential to screen selected individuals and treat persons with LTBI to eliminate the progression to active TB disease. According to the CDC, a decision to screen is also a decision to treat.[74] Therefore, all individuals with positive screening tests require treatment for either latent or active TB. However, not all patients will want to comply with these recommendations. While all patients with active disease require treatment, some patients with latent infection may refuse prophylactic medication. They may not be willing or able to comply with medication regimes requiring daily long-term dosing or they may refuse because of the possible adverse effects associated with the medication. In this situation, a careful assessment of the risks is important. Patients at lower risk of progression, such as those who have tested positive years ago or who are at higher risk of developing hepatotoxicity, may be less likely to benefit from prophylactic treatment.

The initial screening done to determine whether an individual has been exposed to TB is the PPD. Exposed individuals who have developed latent or active infection will develop an indurated area at the site of the PPD placement. The amount of induration determines whether

---

Table 13-18 TUBERCULOSIS SCREENING[72,76]

Those at Higher Risk of Exposure

Persons born in countries with high incidence or prevalence of TB (e.g., Africa, Asia, Latin America, Caribbean)

Persons who had contact with a known or suspected case of TB

Persons who visit regularly (e.g., daily) or reside in residential facilities or group settings (e.g., nursing homes or other long-term care facilities, correctional facilities, homeless shelters, in-patient psychiatric institutions, hospitals)

Persons who will be involved in "high-risk" residential facilities or group settings; may be screened at college entrance/work clearance/routine physical examinations

Health care workers or employees of a "high-risk facility or group setting" (annual testing)

Those at High Risk for Converting from Latent TB Infection to Active TB Disease

HIV+ or at risk for HIV

Alcohol abuser

Intravenous drug user and other illegal substance user (e.g., cocaine or crack user)

Low socioeconomic or impoverished settings (e.g., homeless, malnourished, large number of family members in small space).[72]

Recent infection with *M. tuberculosis* in the past 2 years and not treated.[72]

Pulmonary fibrotic lesions on chest x-ray (evidence of TB without adequate treatment)

Immunosuppressive risk factors:

- Chronic corticosteroid use
- Immunosuppressive therapy
- Organ transplant recipient (i.e., particularly renal or cardiac)
- Diabetes mellitus
- Silicosis
- Head and neck cancers
- Hematologic and reticuloendothelial diseases (e.g., leukemia, Hodgkin's disease)
- Gastrointestinal concerns (e.g., intestinal bypass, gastrectomy, jejunoileal bypass, chronic malabsorption syndromes)
- End-stage renal disease
- Malnutrition, low body weight (<10% below ideal body weight)

---

a test is considered positive or negative. Low-risk individuals must have more induration than higher risk individuals in order for their tests to be considered positive. All PPD readings, whether they are positive or negative, should be recorded in millimeters and entered into the patient's chart.

Placing the PPD using an incorrect technique can result in false-negative results. The Mantoux tuberculin skin test is administered by using 0.1 mL of PPD, which contains five tuberculin units (TUs). A one-quarter to one-half inch, 27-gauge needle on a tuberculin syringe is used to place an intradermal injection in the anterior or volar surface of the forearm, which will form a pale wheal approximately 6 millimeters (mm) to 10 mm in diameter.[77] This wheal subsides approximately 20 minutes after placement. If a wheal does not develop from the injection, then the test was administered incorrectly and should be repeated. If administered correctly, the results of the test should be read by a trained health care provider in 48 to 72 hours. The reading is based on the size of the induration (semifirm to firm swelling), not erythema, at the site of skin testing. **Table 13-19** describes how to correctly plant a PPD, and **Table 13-20** explains how to correctly interpret the PPD result.

There are only a few contraindications to PPD placement. The PPD is contraindicated if a person has had an allergic or necrotic skin reaction from prior skin testing. In addition, a false-negative result can occur if the tuberculin skin testing is done near the time a live vaccine (i.e., measles, mumps, rubella, varicella, oral polio, yellow fever, oral typhoid, and bacilli Calmette–Guérin (BCG)) was administered. Therefore, the test should be done on either the same day as a live-virus vaccine is given or four to six weeks later to prevent suppression of the PPD response.[72]

Infants, children, pregnant women, HIV infected individuals, other immunosuppressed individuals, and persons who had the bacilli Calmette-Guérin (BCG) vaccine may receive the tuberculin skin test. BCG vaccine is administered in many underdeveloped countries as a preventive measure against TB. Unfortunately, the effectiveness of BCG ranges from 0% to

80%.[79] BCG has failed to control TB because it does not consistently prevent infection or active disease.[72,79] In addition, the protection induced by the BCG vaccine wears off over time. Therefore, because most adults received BCG in childhood, a positive PPD cannot be assumed to be due to the BCG vaccine. False-positive results usually result only if the BCG was given in recent months; otherwise, a positive tuberculin skin test should be considered positive, regardless of whether the patient had been vaccinated with BCG.[72,74]

Practitioners should ask about the timing and results of prior PPD tests. Individuals who test positive and have a history of a prior negative test

---

Table 13-19 CORRECT PURIFIED PROTEIN DERIVATIVE OF TUBERCULIN (PPD) PLACEMENT

Dose: PPD 0.1 mL (5 TU)
Needle size: 27-gauge 1/4 to 1/2 inch tuberculin syringe
Type of injection: intradermal
Site: Anterior or volar surface of forearm
Results: Pale wheal approximately 6–10 mm in diameter. If wheal does not develop, repeat test in opposite arm.

Table 13-20 CORRECT INTERPRETATION OF PPD RESULTS

Read: 48–72 hours after placement by trained health care provider
Measure: Induration (i.e., semifirm to firm swelling) from left to right (i.e., perpendicular to long axis of arm)
Record: Chart all results (negative or positive). If no induration, indicate 0 mm

within the last two years have a higher risk of developing active TB[72,74]; therefore, initiating treatment should be highly encouraged. Midwives should also ask about possible exposure to individuals with TB, even if the PPD is negative. If exposure occurred within two weeks of placement of the PPD, individuals may have false-negative PPD results. In this situation, the PPD should be planted but also repeated later. The tubercle bacillus grows slowly over a period of 2 to 12 weeks.[72] Therefore, exposed individuals should be retested in 10 to 12 weeks after the initial PPD to ensure adequate time has elapsed for the PPD to detect an immune response if infection developed after exposure. If the test remains negative on the follow-up test, the person does not have LTBI. **Table 13-21** lists the criteria needed for a PPD to be considered positive.

If the PPD is positive, the health care practitioner needs to rule out active TB. Symptoms related to active TB include malaise, fatigue, nocturnal sweating, weight loss, fever and chills, decreased appetite, and cough for longer than two weeks. Other symptoms may include chest pain, productive sputum with or without hemoptysis, lymphadenopathy, and diarrhea. Some patients have atypical presentations.[80] These patients may report fatigue or other vague symptoms that may be attributed to another health concern or psychological stress. Physical findings can also be minimal in atypical presentations. Fever may not be present. Cough may be mild, nonproductive, and intermittent. Therefore, it is essential to obtain a chest x-ray irrespective of whether the patient has symptoms. If radiographic evidence of upper lobe granulomatous or fibronodular infiltrates are noted, immediate evaluation is needed to rule out active TB.[76,81]

MANAGEMENT

Medication Treatment of LTBI is critical for the occurrence of TB disease to decrease in the United States. With successful treatment, the chance for conversion to active disease will significantly decrease. If untreated, there is a risk for active disease and transmission of *M. tuberculosis* to other individuals. The preferred medication is isoniazid (INH) 300 mg, once a day for nine months.[74] An alternative medication is rifampin given daily. One of the major side effects from all the antituberculosis medications is hepatitis or hepatotoxicity. Other serious side effects include: blood dyscrasia[44] (i.e., agranulocytosis, leukopenia, aplastic anemia, thrombocytopenia), seizures, optic neuritis, peripheral neuropathy, and parethesias. Common reactions with INH include: GI complaints (i.e., nausea, vomiting, diarrhea, epigastric discomfort), dizziness, tinnitus, agitation, and rash.

Rifampin is a common treatment for LTBI. The side effects are similar to INH with two additional potentially serious complications: renal failure and interstitial nephritis. Other side effects related to rifampin include headache, fatigue, pruritis, and a reddish-orange discoloration of body fluids. Rifampin interacts with oral contraceptive agents, so an alternative non-hormonal contraceptive method needs to be offered. If a patient is HIV-positive and taking protease inhibitors or non-nucleoside reverse transcriptase inhibitors, rifampin must be used with extreme caution. Other medications offered for LTBI are rifabutin and pyrazinamide. **Table 13-22** lists medications used to treat latent TB.

If a person has a history of liver disease, alcohol overuse, continues to use alcohol or other

Table 13-21 PPD TESTING: AMOUNT OF INDURATION NEEDED FOR A TEST TO BE CONSIDERED POSITIVE[72,74]

≥5 mL	≥10 mL	≥15 mL
HIV+ Recent contacts of TB case CXR with granulomatous (fibrosis) changes consistent with history of TB Organ transplant patients or other immunocompromised patients (receiving prednisone 15 mg/day or more for at least 1 month)	Foreign-born individuals, living in United States for less than 5 years Injection drug users Residents and employees of high-risk settings (prisons, in-patient psychiatric institutions, homeless shelters, long-term care facilities, nursing homes, other residential facilities, and hospitals Microbacteriology laboratory personnel Children younger than 4 years of age (risk of developing TB is high during the first 2 years of life)[72] Infants, children, and adolescents exposed to adults in high-risk categories Recipient of BCG vaccine	No known risk factors for TB (should have met criteria to initiate testing)

Abbreviations are: TB, tuberculosis; CXR, chest x-ray; BCG, Bacillus Calamette-Guerin

hepatotoxic agents (e.g., acetaminophen) while on antituberculosis medication, then the person is more at risk for hepatotoxicity. The risk of hepatotoxicity also increases with age and is most likely to occur in individuals older than 35.[82] A thorough clinical evaluation is needed to screen for other problems or concerns that may put the patient at risk for hepatic dysfunction. Given the potential risks involved with treatment, close clinical monitoring and follow-up is essential. Baseline laboratory work is recommended for certain patients but is not necessary for the general population.[81] If the patient is HIV-positive, pregnant, postpartum (i.e., under 3 months), has a history of liver disease (chronic hepatitis B or C, alcoholic hepatitis, cirrhosis), drinks alcohol regularly, taking other medications for chronic medical conditions, or if there

Table 13-22 MEDICATIONS USED TO TREAT TUBERCULOSIS INFECTION: DOSES, TOXICITIES, AND MONITORING REQUIREMENTS[74]

Recommended Treatment Regimens for Treatment of Latent Tuberculosis Infections in Adults

Drug	Interval	Comments
Isoniazid	Daily for 9 months	Preferred treatment
Isoniazid	Twice weekly for 9 months	Acceptable alternative treatment, but must be delivered via directly observed therapy
Isoniazid	Daily for 6 months	Not indicated for HIV-infected individuals, children, and those with fibrotic lesions on chest x-ray Acceptable alternative but offer only if Option 1 or Option 2 cannot be given
Rifampin plus pyrazinamide	Daily for 2 months	Acceptable alternative, refer to guidelines before using with HIV-positive individuals
Rifampin plus pyrazinamide	Twice weekly for two to three months	Use only if other alternatives can not be given.
Rifampin	Daily for four months	For use in those who cannot tolerate pyrazinamide. Acceptable alternative

is a concern for liver involvement, then baseline laboratory tests are needed. Depending on the history and which antituberculosis medication is being considered, the following may be ordered: liver function tests, complete blood count with platelet count (CBC/PLT), and kidney function tests (blood urea nitrogen [BUN] and creatinine [Cr]).[82] If there is a risk of hepatitis or if there is an elevation of the aspartate aminotransferase (AST) or alanine aminotransferase (ALT), then hepatitis serologies (i.e., hepatitis A IgG/IgM, hepatitis B [HBsAg, HBsAb, HBcAb], and hepatitis C [HCV Ab]) may also be ordered to rule out other causes of abnormal laboratory results and to detect conditions that may increase the likelihood of drug-induced hepatoxicity. **Table 13-23** lists the conditions that

place the patient at risk for hepatotoxicity while on antituberculosis medication.

During treatment, the frequency of laboratory testing is dependent on the medication chosen and the patient's current health status. If the patient has abnormal baseline liver function tests or if the patient develops symptoms while on treatment, strict follow-up with clinical evaluation and laboratory correlation is an absolute necessity. Antituberculosis medication should be withheld if the transaminase levels are three times the upper limit of normal; further consultation is necessary. Some specialists may recommend continued treatment as long as the patient remains asymptomatic, unless the transaminase levels exceed five times the upper limit of normal.[79] Fre-

Table 13-23 INCREASED RISK OF HEPATOTOXICITY ON ANTITUBERCULOSIS MEDICATIONS

HIV-positive

Pregnant women

Postpartum period (less than 3 months)

Hepatitis B

Hepatitis C

Alcoholic hepatitis

Cirrhosis

Regular alcohol consumption

Multiple medication use for other medical problems

General risk for chronic liver disease

quency of follow-up testing will depend on the patient's symptoms and the level of the test result (e.g., slightly abnormal vs. critical reading). If antituberculosis medications are discontinued, the signs and symptoms of hepatotoxicity should resolve.[82] The following tests may be ordered periodically throughout treatment: AST, ALT, bilirubin, BUN, Cr, CBC/PLT count. Depending on whether the patient has any comorbidities, weekly to monthly visits are recommended to ensure tolerance of the prescribed therapy. Patients should be informed about the side effects associated with treatment and advised to stop their medication and return for re-evaluation if symptoms occur.[81] The use of INH or pyrazinamide is contraindicated in patients with active hepatitis and end-stage liver disease.[81] If moderate-to-severe liver disease is noted in the presence of LTBI, consultation with an infectious disease specialist, TB expert, or pulmonologist is recommended.

PATIENT INSTRUCTIONS

Patients must be educated about latent TB, their risk for developing active TB, treatment options, benefits related to the medication (e.g., cure of TB infection and prevention of active TB), risks associated with treatment, and major symptoms or side effects of the medication. They should be instructed to discontinue the medication and contact their health care provider for further evaluation if they develop symptoms of drug-induced hepatitis, which may include anorexia, nausea, vomiting, jaundice, myalgia, fatigue, or excessive itching to the skin.[81,82]

MANAGEMENT DURING PREGNANCY AND LACTATION

The decision to test should follow the same guidelines as for non-pregnant women. Only high-risk individuals need to be tested in pregnancy. Individuals who test positive usually require treatment in pregnancy. According to Smith,[78] the most effective way to prevent congenital TB in newborn infants is to treat and prevent the disease in pregnancy. Although the risk of congenital TB is rare,[83] if the mother has or develops active TB during pregnancy, the risk of neonatal complications (i.e., prematurity, fetal growth retardation) increases twofold. Other complications include low birth weight and fetal mortality. Maternal complications associated with active TB include hypertension, respiratory failure, oligohydramnios, premature labor, and premature rupture of membranes.[83]

Initiation of therapy in pregnancy can be a dilemma for health care providers. Potential risks and side effects as well as the known benefits should be carefully considered. Careful screening for evidence of liver dysfunction is necessary. Women with liver impairment, alcohol use, or chronic, heavy use of agents that can be hepatotoxic (i.e., acetaminophen), should be excluded from antituberculosis treatment during the antepartum period.[84] If a person has emigrated from a high-prevalence country (e.g., Africa, Asia, Latin America, Carribean), uses intravenous drugs, is HIV positive, has another immunocompromised condition, or recently has been infected, then the initiation of therapy should not be delayed on the basis of pregnancy,[81] but strict laboratory and clinical monitoring is necessary.[84] Treatment of LTBI can be started as early as the first trimester.[74] Regular visits are scheduled on a monthly to weekly basis during pregnancy. Incorporating the surveillance needed for those on TB prophylaxis into routine prenatal care makes follow-up easier, because patients may be more compliant with appointments scheduled during pregnancy than in the postpartum period.[84]

INH for 9 months is the preferred medication for the treatment of LTBI in pregnant women,[81] although rifampin is considered safe and can be an alternative treatment.[74] Some research has shown that INH and rifampin both cross the placenta, but teratogenic effects have not been reported.[74] Pyridoxine 25 to 50 mg (vitamin B_6) needs to be given concurrently with INH to help prevent peripheral neuropathy.[74] Breastfeeding may be continued while on antituberculosis agents such as INH and rifampin.[74]

Active Tuberculosis

In 2004, there were 14,511 cases of active TB reported to the CDC in the United States.[85]

Active TB infection can occur anywhere in the body. The most common site is the lung, but infection also occurs in the kidneys, bone, soft tissue, lymph nodes, and brain. **Table 13-24** describes the presentation of common extrapulmonary infections. Extrapulmonary TB is more common in immunocompromised HIV-positive patients. The impaired immune response to *M. tuberculosis* allows the bacilli to spread to one or multiple non-pulmonary sites. Invasive procedures are needed to establish a diagnosis.[72]

Patients may present with fever, fatigue, malaise, persistent cough longer than two weeks, chest pain, productive sputum with or without hemoptysis, night sweats, weight loss, fever, chills, and decreased appetite. Symptoms can be few and nonspecific. The specific symptoms reported by patients as well as associated PPD and radiographic findings vary according to whether infection is present, its type, and location. **Table 13-25** describes PPD and chest x-ray findings associated with latent and active TB. Certain chest x-ray findings are indicative of active TB. Calcified nodules can be detected (**Figure 13-5**).[72] Upper lobe infiltrates and unilateral hilar node enlargement[73,79] may be noted in individuals with active infection; however, abnormalities occur in fewer than 30% of those with primary infection.[72] These radiographic findings are highly specific for active TB and, if found as an incidental finding on chest x-rays done for other indications, warrant further investigation. All individuals with radiographic findings suggestive of TB require PPD testing if it has not been performed recently.

Individuals suspected or known to have active TB require the use of measures to pre-

Table 13-24 **TYPES OF TUBERCULOSIS (TB)**[72]

Types of TB	Key Diagnostic Findings
Pulmonary tuberculosis	• *Reactivation of latent infection*: Infiltrate in upper lobes of one or both lungs, with cavitation. • *Primary TB from recent infection*: Middle or lower lung zone infiltration usually with ipsilateral hilar adenopathy. • *Old tuberculosis*: Nodular or fibrotic lesions (if PPD+, treat). • *Negative CXR*: Normal in HIV+ or other cause for immune suppression.
Extrapulmonary tuberculosis	
• Tuberculosis lymphadenitis	• Painless enlargement of one or more lymph nodes (e.g., posterior-anterior cervical chain or supraclavicular fossa). Biopsy needed for diagnosis.
• Genitourinary tuberculosis	• Symptoms of dysuria, frequency, hematuria, flank pain; urinalysis with hematuria and pyuria. Urine culture will be negative. Culture urine for mycobacterium, fully evaluate for TB.
• Skeletal tuberculosis	• Swelling and decreased range of motion of affected site. Symptoms are subtle and, therefore, diagnosis often delayed. CT, MRI, or bone biopsy may be needed when TB is suspected. Vertebral TB can lead to spinal cord compression and irreversible neurological symptoms, including paraplegia.
• Central nervous system tuberculosis –TB meningitis	• Symptoms of headache, neck stiffness, and loss of consciousness. CT of the head and lumbar puncture needed for diagnosis.
• Abdominal tuberculosis	• Clinical signs and symptoms depend on the site involved. Lesions can be found throughout GI tract (mouth to anus). Most common sites are terminal ileum and cecum. Laparoscopy or colonoscopy (with biopsy) is recommended for diagnosis.
• Pericardial tuberculosis	• Symptoms of chest pain (dull, aching, affected by position and inspiration), cough, dyspnea, orthopnea, edema; possible cardiac tamponade and hemodynamic changes.
Disseminated tuberculosis	• Due to immunosuppression, the bacterium proliferates and disseminates to multiple organs.

vent the spread of infection to others. These measures include: having the patient wear a specially designed face mask when being transported within a medical facility, being evaluated or cared for in a health care facility only in negative pressure rooms, and following standard respiratory precautions. Once the patient is hospitalized, sputum samples are collected

Table 13-25 CATEGORIES OF FINDINGS RELATING TO TB DIAGNOSIS[72]

Classification	Exposure	PPD reading	Chest X-Ray Findings	Symptoms
No potential infection	No	Negative	Not needed	None
Positive exposure, no infection	Yes	Negative	Not needed	None
LTBI—no disease	Yes	Positive	Negative	None
TB—active disease	Yes	Positive	Positive	Yes

Figure 13-5 Calcified Nodules in TB

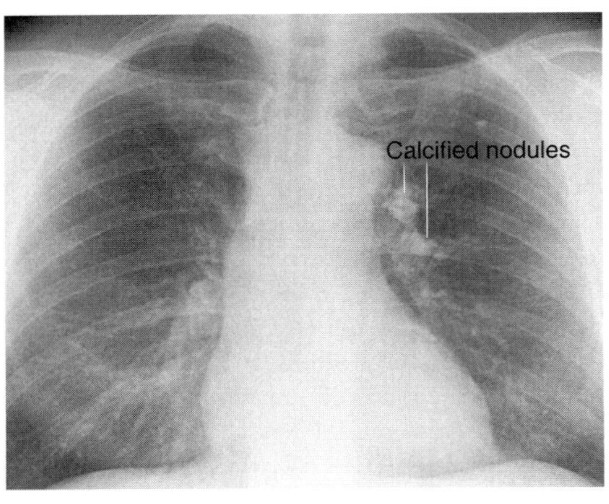

Chest radiograph showing patient with active tuberculosis. Note the calcified nodules.
Source: Used with permission from Yale University. Available from: http://info.med.yale.edu/intmed/cardio/imaging/contents.html

and sent for an acid-fast bacilli sputum smear and sputum culture.[72] If the sputum cultures are negative and the chest x-ray findings on multiple x-rays remain stable, the management guidelines are the same as those for LTBI.[81] Individuals diagnosed with active infection usually require treatment for 6 and 18 months, length of treatment depends on which regimen is used.[86] Most patients will have culture-negative sputum within two months of initiation of treatment. If cultures remain positive for longer than three months, the patient should be evaluated for nonadherence, malabsorption, or drug resistance.[86] Cure is achieved through comprehensive treatment that includes monitoring to ensure compliance and prevention of drug-resistant organisms, evaluation of contacts, and patient education.

References

1. Porth CM. Control of respiratory function. In: Porth CM. *Pathophysiology: Concepts of Altered Health States.* 7th ed. Philadelphia: Williams & Wilkins; 2005.

2. Kunert MP. Alterations in temperature regulation. In: Porth CM. *Pathophysiology: Concepts of Altered Health States.* 7th ed. Philadelphia: Williams & Wilkins; 2005.

3. Majeed HA. Differential diagnosis of fever of unknown origin in children. *Curr Opin Rheumatol.* 2000; 12:439–444.

4. Bloch KC. Infectious diseases. In: Ganong WF, editor. *Pathophysiology of Disease.* New York: Lange/ McGraw-Hill; 2003. pp. 58–90.

5. Irwin RS, Boulet LP, Cloutier MM, Fuller R, Gold PM, Hoffstein V, et al. Managing cough as a defense mechanism and as a symptom: A consensus panel report of the American College of Chest Physicians. *Chest.* 1998;114 Suppl 2:133S–181S.

6. Irwin RS, Madison JM. Primary care: The diagnosis and treatment of cough. *N Engl J Med.* 2000;343: 1715–1721.

7. Brashers VL, Hayden K. Differential diagnosis of cough: Focus on lung malignancy. *Lippincott's Prim Care Pract.* 2000;4:374–389.

8. ACOG technical bulletin. Pulmonary disease in pregnancy. *Int J Gynecol Obstet.* 1996;54:187–196.

9. Magriples U, Copel JA. Obstetrics. In: Noble J, editor. *Textbook of Primary Care Medicine.* 3rd ed. St. Louis: Mosby; 2001. pp. 350–359.

10. Moses RL, Paige T, Cavalli G, Broker B, Malhotra R, Shrager D, et al. Laryngotracheobronchitis in pregnancy and its clinical implications. *Otolaryngol Head Neck Surg.* 1997;116:401–403.

11. Ie S, Rubio ER, Alper B, Szerlip HM. Respiratory complications of pregnancy. *Obstetric and Gynecological Survey.* 2001;57:39–46.

12. Gilbert DN, Moellering RC, Sande MA. *The Sanford Guide to Antimicrobial Therapy.* 33rd ed. Hyde Park, VT: Sanford; 2003.

13. Rhinosinusitis Guideline Team. University of Michigan Health System. Acute Rhinosinusitis in Adults. Ann Arbor, MI: University of Michigan Health System; 2005 Feb. Available on the Internet: http://cme.med.umich.edu/pdf/guideline/rhino05.pdf.

14. Fendrick AM. Viral respiratory infections due to rhinoviruses: Current knowledge, new developments. *Am J Ther.* 2003;10:193–202.

15. Rotbart HA, Hayden FG. Picornavirus infections: A primer for the practitioner. *Arch Fam Med.* 2000; 9:913–920.

16. Arruda E, Pitkaranta A, Witek TJ Jr, Doyle CA, Hayden FG. Frequency and natural history of rhinovirus infections in adults during autumn. *J Clin Microbiol.* 1997;35:2864–2868.

17. Makela MJ, Puhakka T, Ruuskanen O, Leinonen M, Saikku P, Kimpimaki M, et al. Viruses and bacteria in the etiology of the common cold. *J Clin Microbiol.* 1998;36:539–542.

18. Kaiser L, Lew D, Hirschel B, Auckenthaler R, Morabia A, Heald A, et al. Effects of antibiotic treatment in the subset of common-cold patients who have bacteria in nasopharyngeal secretions. *Lancet.* 1996; 347:1507–1510.

19. Centers for Disease Control and Prevention. *Key Facts about the Flu: Overview.* Atlanta: CDC. Available on the Internet: http://www.cdc.gov/flu/keyfacts.htm

20. National Vaccine Program Office. *Pandemics and Pandemic Scares in the 20th Century.* Washington, DC: United States Department of Health and Human Services; 2004 February 12. [Monograph on the Internet.] Available at http://www.hhs.gov/nvpo/pandemics/flu3.htm.

21. Singh S. Preparing your practice for the influenza season. *Patient Care for the Nurse Practitioner.* 2001:24–37. Internet based publication available at http://www.patientcarenp.com.

22. Centers for Disease Control and Prevention. Update: influenza activity-United States, 2003–2004 season. *MMWR.* 2004;53:284–287.

23. Monto AS, Gravenstein S, Elliott M, Colopy M, Schweinle J. Clinical signs and symptoms predicting influenza infection. *Arch Intern Med.* 2000;160: 3243–3247.

24. Centers for Disease Control and Prevention. Influenza. In: Atkinson W, Hamborski J, Wolfe C, editors. *Epidemiology and Prevention of Vaccine-Preventable Diseases: The Pink Book.* 8th ed. Waldorf, MD: Public Health Foundation; 2004. pp. 213–231.

25. Centers for Disease Control and Prevention. Neuraminidase inhibitors for treatment of influenza A and B infections. *MMWR.* 1999;48(RR-14):1–9.

26. Hayden FG, Treanor JJ, Fritz RS, Lobo M, Betts RF, Miller M, et al. Use of the oral neuraminidase inhibitor Oseltamivir in experimental human influenza: Randomized controlled trials for prevention and treatment. *JAMA.* 1999;282:1240–1246.

27. Hayden FG, Osterhaus ADME, Treanor JJ, Fleming DM, Aoki FY, Nicholson KG, et al. Efficacy and safety of the neuraminidase inhibitor Zanamivir in the treatment of influenza virus infections. *N Engl J Med.* 1997;337:874–880.

28. Centers for Disease Control and Prevention. Prevention and Control of influenza: Recommendations of the Advisory Committee on Immunization Practices (ACIP). *MMWR Recommendations and Reports.* 2005, 54(early release):1–40.

29. Centers for Disease Control and Prevention. Prevention of pneumococcal disease: Recommendations of the Advisory Committee on Immunization Practices (ACIP). *MMWR.* 1997;46 (RR-08):1–24.

30. Centers for Disease Control and Prevention. Pneumococcal disease. In: Atkinson W, Hamborski J, Wolfe C, editors. *Epidemiology and Prevention of Vaccine-Preventable Diseases: The Pink Book.* 8th ed. Waldorf, MD: Public Health Foundation; 2004. pp. 233–245.

31. Lim WS, Macfarlane JT, Colthorpe CL. Pneumonia in pregnancy. *Thorax.* 2001;56:398–405.

32. Seidel HM, Ball JW, Dains JE, Benedict GW. *Mosby's Guide to Physical Examination.* 5th ed. St. Louis: Mosby; 2003.

33. Roof SK. Common problems of the cardiovascular and respiratory systems. In: Dains JE, Baumann LC, Scheibel P, editors. *Advanced Health Assessment and Clinical Diagnosis in Primary Care.* St. Louis: Mosby; 1998. pp. 85–146.

34. Thibodeau K, Viera AJ. Atypical pathogens and challenges in community-acquired pneumonia. *Am Fam Physician.* 2004;69:1699–1706.

35. Abramowicz M. Treatment guidelines: Drugs for pneumonia. *Med Lett.* 2003;1:83–88.

36. Leiner S, Mays M. Pharmacologic management of common lower respiratory tract disorders in women. *J Midwifery Women's Health.* 2002;47:167–181.

37. Mandell LA, Bartlett JG, Dowell SF, File TM Jr, Musher DM. Update of practice guidelines for the management of community-acquired pneumonia in immunocompetent adults. *Clin Infect Dis.* 2003;37: 1405–1433.

38. Dykewicz MS. Rhinitis and sinusitis. *J Allergy Clin Immunol.* 2003;111:S520–S529.

39. Hickner JM, Bartlett JG, Besser RE, Gonzales R, Hoffman JR, Sande MA. Principles of appropriate antibiotic use for acute rhinosinusitis in adults: Background. *Ann Intern Med.* 2001;134:498–505.

40. American Academy of Pediatrics. Clinical practice guidelines: Management of sinusitis. *Pediatrics.* 2001; 108:798–808. *Erratum Pediatrics.* 2001;1085: A24 and 2002;109:40.

41. Wald ER. Microbiology of acute and chronic sinusitis in children and adults. *Am J Med Sci.* 1998;316: 13–20.

42. Hamilos DL. Chronic sinusitis. *J Allergy Clin Immunol.* 2000;106:213–227.

43. Snow V, Mottur-Pilson C, Hickner JM. Principles of appropriate antibiotic use for acute sinusitis in adults. *Ann Intern Med.* 2001;134:495–497.

44. Sobol SE, Frenkiel S, Nachtigal D, Wiener D, Teblum C. Clinical manifestations of sinonasal pathology during pregnancy. *J Otolaryngol.* 2001;30:24–28.

45. Murphy JL. *Nurse Practitioners' Prescribing Reference,* 2nd ed. Prescribing Reference; 2004.

46. Niebyl JR. Antibiotics and other anti-infective agents in pregnancy and lactation. *Am J Perinatol.* 2003;20: 405–414.

47. Hoover GE, Newman LJ, Platts-Mills TAE, Phillips CD, Gross CW, Wheatley LM. Chronic sinusitis: Risk factors for extensive disease. *J Allergy Clin Immunol.* 1997;100:185–191.

48. Newman LJ, Platts-Mills TAE, Phillips D, Hazen K, Gross CW. Chronic sinusitis: Relationship of computed tomographic findings to allergy, asthma, and eosinophilia. *JAMA.* 1994;271:363–367.

49. Starke PR, Chowdhury BA. Efficacy of intranasal corticosteroids for acute sinusitis. *JAMA.* 2002;287: 1261–1262.

50. Asher BF, Seidman M, Snyderman C. Complementary and alternative medicine in otolaryngology. *Laryngoscope.* 2001;111:1383–1389.

51. Schatz M, Petitti D. Antihistamines and pregnancy. *Ann Allergy Asthma Immunol.* 1997;78:157–159.

52. Oeffinger KC, Snell LM, Foster BM, Panico KG, Archer RK. Diagnosis of acute bronchitis in adults: A national survey of family physicians. *J Fam Pract.* 1997;45:402–409.

53. Gonzales R, Bartlett JG, Besser RE, Cooper RJ, Hickner JM, Hoffman JR, et al. Principles of appropriate antibiotic use for treatment of uncomplicated acute bronchitis: Background. *Ann Intern Med.* 2001; 134:521–529.

54. Knutson D, Braun C. Diagnosis and management of acute bronchitis. *Am Fam Physician.* 2002;65: 2039–2044.

55. Gonzales R, Barrett PH, Crane LA, Steiner JF. Factors associated with antibiotic use for acute bronchitis. *J Gen Intern Med.* 1998;13:541–548.

56. Lindbaek M, Hjortdahl P. Resistance to antibiotics: Restricted prescribing resulted in reduction of resistant strains. *BMJ.* 1998;317:1521–1522.

57. Fahey T, Stocks N, Thomas T. Quantitative systematic review of randomised controlled trials comparing antibiotic with placebo for acute cough in adults. *BMJ.* 1998;316:906–910.

58. Smucny J, Fahey T, Becker L, Glazier R. Antibiotics for acute bronchitis. [update of Cochrane Database Syst Rev. 2000;(4):CD000245; PMID: 11034678]. *Cochrane Database of Systematic Reviews.* 2004;(4):CD000245.

59. Bent S, Saint S, Vittinghoff E, Grady D. Antibiotics in acute bronchitis: A meta-analysis. *Am J Med.* 1999; 107:62–67.

60. Grossman RF. Guidelines for the treatment of acute exacerbations of chronic bronchitis. *Chest.* 1997;112 Suppl 6:S10–S13.

61. Nelson S, Mason CM. The inflammatory response in chronic bronchitis. *Semin Respir Crit Care Med.* 2000; 21:79–86.

62. Eller J, Ede A, Schaberg T, Niederman MS, Mauch H, Lode H. Infective exacerbations of chronic bronchitis:

Relation between bacteriologic etiology and lung function. *Chest.* 1998;113:1542–1548.

63. Sethi S. Infectious etiology of acute exacerbations of chronic bronchitis. *Chest.* 2000;117 Suppl 2:S380–S385.

64. Ball P. Epidemiology and treatment of chronic bronchitis and its exacerbations. *Chest.* 1995;108 Suppl 2:43S–52S.

65. Baughman RP, Pina E. Infections in acute exacerbation of chronic bronchitis: What are they and how do we know? *Semin Respir Crit Care Med.* 2000;21:87–96.

66. Givertz MM, Colucci WS. Heart failure. In: Noble J, editor. *Primary Care Medicine.* 3rd ed. St. Louis: Mosby; 2001. pp. 578–596.

67. Lipchik RJ, Presberg KW. Venous thromboembolism and pulmonary hypertensive diseases. In: Noble J, editor. *Primary Care Medicine.* St. Louis: Mosby; 2001. pp. 728–739.

68. Stoller JK. Acute exacerbations of chronic obstructive pulmonary disease. *N Engl J Med.* 2002;346:988–994.

69. Emerman CL, Effron D, Lukens TW. Spirometric criteria for hospital admission of patients with acute exacerbations of COPD. *Chest.* 1991;99:595–599.

70. Saint S, Bent S, Vittinghoff E, Grady D. Antibiotics in chronic obstructive pulmonary disease exacerbations: A meta-analysis. *JAMA.* 1995;273:957–960.

71. Jones KL, Robbins RA. Alternative therapies for chronic bronchitis. *Am J Med Sci.* 1999;318:96–100.

72. American Thoracic Society/Centers for Disease Control and Prevention. Diagnostic standards and classification of tuberculosis in adults and children. *Am J Respir Crit Care Med.* 2000;161:1376–1395.

73. Milburn HJ. Primary tuberculosis. *Curr Opin Pulm Med.* 2001;7:133–141.

74. Centers for Disease Control and Prevention. Targeted tuberculin testing and treatment of latent tuberculosis infection. ATS/CDC Committee on Latent Tuberculosis Infection, June 2000; *MMWR Recommendations and Report.* 2000;49 (RR06):1–54.

75. Horsburgh CRJ. Priorities for the treatment of latent tuberculosis infection in the United States. *N Engl J Med.* 2004;350:2060–2067.

76. Ozuah PO, Ozuah TP, Stein REK, Burton W, Mulvihill M. Evaluation of a risk assessment questionnaire used to target tuberculin skin testing in children. *JAMA.* 2001;285:451–453.

77. Brinton K, Rybin A. Interpreting the PPD: TB skin-testing of patients with previous BCG vaccination. *Nurse Pract.* 2000;25:18–20, 22.

78. Smith KC. Congenital tuberculosis: A rare manifestation of a common infection. *Curr Opin Infect Dis.* 2002;15:269–274.

79. American Thoracic Society/Centers for Disease Control and Prevention. Targeted tuberculin testing and treatment of latent tuberculosis infection. *Am J Respir Crit Care Med.* 2000;161:S221–S247.

80. Miller LG, Asch SM, Yu EI, Knowles L, Gelberg L, Davidson P. A population-based survey of tuberculosis symptoms: How atypical are atypical presentations? *Clin Infect Dis.* 2000;30:293–299.

81. American Thoracic Society/Centers for Disease Control and Prevention. Treatment of tuberculosis. *MMWR.* 2003;52(RR 11): 1–77.

82. Nolan CM, Goldberg SV, Buskin SE. Hepatotoxicity associated with isoniazid preventative therapy: A 7-year survey from a public health tuberculosis clinic. *JAMA.* 1999;281:1014–1018.

83. Figueroa-Damian R, Luis Arredondo-Garcia JL. Neonatal outcome of children born to women with tuberculosis. *Arch Med Res.* 2001;32:66–69.

84. Boggess KA, Myers ER, Hamilton CD. Antepartum and postpartum isoniazid treatment of latent tuberculosis infection. *Obstet Gynecol.* 2000;96:757–762.

85. Centers for Disease Control and Prevention. Trends in tuberculosis rates—United States, 2004. *MMWR Weekly.* 2005;54(10):245–249.

86. Small PM, Fujiwara PI. *Medical Progress: Management of Tuberculosis in the United States.* 2001;345:189–200.

Cardiovascular Disease in Women

Eileen Wyner

Julie Marfell

Deborah Karsnitz

Mary Ellen Rousseau

Cardiovascular disease (CVD) is the leading killer of women in the United States, accounting for more than one-half million deaths annually. This exceeds the number of male deaths from CVD and of the next seven causes of death in women combined. It translates into approximately one death every minute. Coronary heart disease (CHD) accounts for the majority of CVD deaths in women, with nearly two-thirds of these women dying suddenly without any previously recognized symptoms.[1]

Two of the major risk factors for CHD are hypertension and dyslipidemia. Both are modifiable and can be prevented by lifestyle changes and, if needed, controlled by medications. It is for this reason that prevention is essential. Hypertension is the most potent and modifiable risk factor in more than 500,000 cases of stroke and 1 million heart attacks in the United States annually.[2] The National Cholesterol Education Program (NCEP) guidelines clearly document the importance of elevated low-density lipoprotein (LDL) levels and their link to the development of CHD.[3] Appropriate management of women with elevated blood pressure and/or elevated cholesterol can prevent CVD. Mortality has increased over the last 20 years because of the increased prevalence of risk factors such as smoking, obesity, and sedentary lifestyle, as well as diabetes and the disease processes mentioned above.

Women also are less likely to be counseled about control of risk factors, because CHD is still perceived to be a man's disease. Providers must be aware that multiple risk factors are associated with a substantial increase in the risk of subsequent cardiac events.[4,5] Women's health providers must also take into account newly identified risk factors that adversely affect women's risk of CHD. These include menstrual irregularity due to polycystic ovarian syndrome (PCOS), pregnancy losses, and age at menopause. In addition to other risks (e.g., endometrial cancer), women with PCOS are more at risk for metabolic syndrome and diabetes, which puts them at risk for CHD in later years.[6] Women who experience early menopause lose the protection afforded by endogenous estrogen to the cardiac system and are at greater risk for more extensive atherosclerosis.[7]

Risk Identification

Screening for heart disease in women should begin before middle age. This is why midwives and women's health providers need to take an active role in identification, screening, and treatment or referral of at-risk women. The U.S. Preventive Services Task Force (USPSTF)[8] strongly recommends that clinicians routinely screen men aged 35 years and older and women aged 45 years and older for lipid disorders, and treat abnormal lipids in people who are at increased risk of CHD. The USPSTF recommends that clinicians routinely screen younger adults (men aged 20–35 and women aged 20–45) for lipid disorders if they have a higher than average risk of CHD. These risks include diabetes, a family history of CVD before age 50 years in male relatives or age 60 years in female relatives, a family history suggestive of familial hyperlipidemia, and the presence of multiple personal risk factors for CHD (e.g., tobacco use, hypertension). The NCEP ATP III Guidelines suggest the first fasting lipid profile be drawn at age 20 and repeated every five years, again making women in the reproductive years optimal candidates for intervention.[3] During pregnancy, women are particularly motivated toward a healthier lifestyle, including smoking cessation. Prenatal care provides an opportunity to discuss limiting weight gain, screen for diabetes and hypertension, and provide counseling on healthy behavior change that can benefit the fetus and long-term health of the mother. Menopause provides another opportunity to provide patient education and screening for chronic illnesses, especially heart disease and diabetes. The optimal interval for screening is uncertain but on the basis of other guidelines and expert opinion, reasonable options include every five years, with shorter intervals for those who have lipid levels close to those warranting therapy, and longer intervals for low-risk people who have had low or repeatedly normal lipid levels.[8] The USPSTF found

good evidence that lipid measurement in low-risk young adults can detect individuals at increased long-term risk of heart disease, but the absolute reduction in risk as a result of treating dyslipidemia in most people is small before middle age. Fair evidence suggests that a substantial proportion of the benefits of treatment may be realized within five years of initiating therapy. The USPSTF concludes that the net benefits of screening for lipid disorders in low-risk young people are not sufficient to make a general recommendation. No upper age limit for screening has been established.

Another risk factor for CHD is arterial inflammation, which is essential to development and progression of atherosclerosis. An elevated C-reactive protein is closely associated with increased risk in women.[9] This inflammation leads to plaque formation, erosion, and rupture. The 2002 Women's Health Initiative demonstrated that C-reactive protein and lipids were significantly ($P < .001$) better at predicting risk than lipids alone.[10]

Because women throughout their reproductive years can benefit from lipid and blood pressure screening, midwives and women's health providers sit in an essential position as gatekeepers for cardiovascular risk reduction. They also can provide a pivotal role in implementing new screening guidelines as new recommendations are issued. Obstetric and gynecologic visits are an ongoing opportunity for risk assessment, encouraging healthful lifestyle strategies and health interventions for women. Given that obesity rates have reached epidemic proportions, early interventions such as diet, exercise, and smoking cessation are of great importance even in very young women, particularly before diseases such as hypertension and diabetes have emerged.

Hypertension

Hypertension, a condition of elevated blood pressure, affects approximately 50 million Americans and is the leading reason for office visits to health care providers in the United States today. Nearly 60% of those affected are women. The prevalence of hypertension increases in women across the lifespan at a higher rate and with greater associated morbidity and mortality than in men.[11] There is also a high prevalence of hypertension and of resultant end organ damage in African Americans relative to whites. Only 53% of patients with identified hypertension are presently being treated with prescription medications; 29% of these patients have their blood pressure under control.[12] The control and prevention of morbidity and mortality from hypertension is an important challenge for health care providers, especially as the population ages.

Physiology

The underlying pathology that leads to the development of hypertension is not completely understood, although several mechanisms have been proposed. The circulatory system provides for the delivery and removal of products to the cells throughout the body. The flow of blood occurs because of the pressure differential established by the pumping action of the heart. An elevation in blood pressure comes about in one of two ways or both: an increase in *cardiac output (CO)* or an increase in total *peripheral vascular resistance (PVR)*. CO is a result of left ventricular pump function, which depends on several factors. These include venous return, the contractile state of the ventricular muscle, and aortic input impedance, which is the complex relation between unsteady flow and pressure throughout the cardiac cycle.[13]

PVR occurs mainly in small muscular arteries and arterioles. Small changes in arterial diameter have a profound effect on flow (resistance). The diameter of small arteries and arterioles is controlled by the contractile state of their smooth muscle.

The above definitions assume that pressure and flow in circulation are steady, which of course they are not. CO depends on the interaction between the mechanics of ejection and the properties of the vessels. Pressure and flow respond to cyclical changes at all sites in the system, although the effect is somewhat dampened in the capillaries. This damping is due to the elastic properties of the large arteries, and is called the *Windkessel or cushioning function*. The pressure energy generated by the left ventricle is converted to elastic energy by distending the large arteries. When the pressure falls as the ejection is complete, the large vessels compress and the energy is converted once more to pressure. This pressure accounts, in large part, for the diastolic blood pressure. Thus, arterial compliance (stiffness being the reciprocal of compliance) is an important factor in damping pressure oscillation; pulse pressure will increase when arteries stiffen, for example, with age.[13]

Women with several years of hypertension but without target organ damage have increased PVR in all vascular areas. PVR is the hallmark of established hypertension. Altered cardiac function may also contribute to the hypertension. Additionally, hypertension itself causes cardiac and vascular remodeling and hypertrophy. Cardiac index and stroke volume are generally normal or reduced, but heart rate may be increased compared to women without hypertension. In established hypertension, there is also a reduction in arterial compliance and a central shift in blood volume, which may be related to reduced venous compliance. Blood volume and extracellular fluid volume are generally normal.[13]

Target organ damage associated with hypertension results primarily from events occurring at the microvascular level.[14] Examples include myocardial ischemia, renal damage, retinopathy, or slowly advancing dementia. Another central and early effect of CVD is chronic inflammation.

For many years, diastolic and *mean arterial pressures*, the steady component of the flow, were considered the best guides for hypertension-related risk. However, epidemiologic studies in the past decade have demonstrated that systolic blood pressure and pulse pressure are independent markers of cardiovascular risk.[15,16] The Framingham study showed that systolic blood pressure, diastolic blood pressure, and pulse pressure were positively related to outcome when entered into correlation analysis individually; when these variables were entered in combination, the association was negative for diastolic blood pressure, whereas pulse pressure was a good indicator for outcome in middle aged and elderly individuals.[4,17] In an analysis of the Framingham Heart Study published in 2003, researchers found that while each component of blood pressure was associated with risk for congestive heart failure, a rise in pulse and systolic pressure conferred greater risk than diastolic pressure.[18]

Risk Factors

Several associated factors play key roles in the prediction of risk for hypertension. If there is a positive family history of hypertension, or of stroke in women under the age of 65 or men under the age of 55, the individual is at risk for developing hypertension. African Americans and the elderly, those who are inactive physi-cally, smoke, and/or have an elevated *body mass index (BMI)* are also at greater risk. Finally, those individuals who have diabetes or dyslipidemia are at an increased risk of becoming hypertensive. In turn, hypertension has been identified as a risk factor for stroke, myocardial infarction, renal failure, congestive heart failure, progressive atherosclerosis, retinopathy, and dementia.[19]

Definition of Hypertension and Recommendations

The Fifth Report of the Joint National Committee on Prevention, Detection, Evaluation, and Treatment of High Blood Pressure (JNC 5) defined hypertension as a systolic blood pressure greater than or equal to 140 mm Hg and a diastolic blood pressure of 90 mm Hg or more.[19] The JNC 7 Guidelines incorporate evidence from hypertension outcome studies that were published between January 1997 and April 2003.[20] One study that was central to the development of the management guidelines of JNC 7 was the Antihypertensive and Lipid-Lowering Treatment to Prevent Heart Attacks (ALLHAT) Trial.[21] This was a randomized, double blind, multicenter clinical trial sponsored by the National Heart, Lung and Blood Institute (NHLBI). The purpose of this trial was to determine the effectiveness of diuretic therapy in a head-to-head comparison with other commonly prescribed medications used to treat hypertension and prevent cardiovascular complications. The results demonstrated that thiazide-type diuretics were superior to calcium channel blockers (CCBs), angiotensin converting enzyme inhibitors (ACEIs), and alpha-adrenergic blockers in the treatment of high blood pressure and in the prevention of some forms of heart disease. The alpha-adrenergic blocker category was dropped from the trial early in 2000 because there was a 25% increase in cardiovascular events. ALLHAT determined that thiazide-type diuretics should be the first drugs initiated in the medication management of hypertension.[21] The Second Australian National Blood Pressure Trial (2003) was a prospective, randomized, open-label study that was comprised of predominantly older subjects. Its purpose was to compare the treatment of hypertension with diuretics versus ACEI. Initiating treatment with ACEIs in older subjects, particularly men, led to better outcomes than if treatment was initiated with diuretics. Both drugs demonstrated reductions in blood pressure; however, it is noteworthy that this study did not involve a comparison of all drug classes.[22]

The JNC 7 Guidelines, which are the latest in a series of guidelines issued by the National High Blood Pressure Education Program, identify several key concepts in the prevention and management of hypertension.[23] Perhaps the most significant feature is the identification of a new hypertensive class: prehypertension. This class identifies individuals with a systolic blood pressure between 120–139 mm Hg and a diastolic blood pressure of 80–89 mm Hg as being prehypertensive. Each incremental increase of 20/10 mm Hg from a blood pressure reading of 115/75 mm/hg doubles the risk for CVD. Patients with prehypertension are thus at risk for CVD and are advised to adopt lifestyle modifications to lower their blood pressure. The introduction of this classification impresses upon health care providers the need for intervention at the earliest possible sign of blood pressure elevation to prevent future complications. JNC 7 identifies adults over the age of 50 with a systolic blood pressure greater than 140 mm Hg as being at more risk for CVD than if they had an elevated diastolic pressure. Thiazide-type diuretics are recommended as the preferred initial drug therapy for most patients with uncomplicated hypertension; more than one drug may be necessary to reach the blood pressure goal. The goal for treated blood pressure has been defined as <140/90 mm Hg in the general population and <130/80 mm Hg for patients with diabetes or chronic kidney disease.[23] JNC 7 also emphasizes the importance of motivation on the patient's part in order for the treatment to be effective.[22,23]

Lifestyle modification is encouraged in those with normal readings to prevent the development of hypertension and is an intrinsic part of the management of all classifications of hypertension, whether or not medications are required.[23] JNC 7 has classified blood pressure readings as normal (<120 mm Hg systolic and <80 mm Hg diastolic), prehypertension (120–139 mm Hg systolic and 80–89 mm Hg diastolic), Stage 1 hypertension (140–159 mm Hg systolic and 90–99 mm Hg diastolic), and Stage 2 hypertension (systolic ≥160 mm Hg and diastolic ≥100 mm Hg) (**Table 14-1**).[23]

Evaluation

The assessment of an individual with hypertension is based on the following objectives: identify cardiovascular risk factors or concomitant disorders that may affect prognosis and guide treatment, reveal identifiable causes of hypertension, and determine whether target organ damage and cardiovascular disease are present. These factors will help structure the management plan. Because hypertension is an asymptomatic disease until there is end organ damage, a thorough history is important. Pertinent family history includes hypertension or CVD. Pertinent personal

Table 14-1 HYPERTENSIVE STAGES ACCORDING TO JNC 7[23]

Blood Pressure	Diagnosis	Treatment Recommendations
<120/<80	Normal BP	None
120–139/80–89	Prehypertensive	Therapeutic lifestyle changes (TLC)
140–159/90–99	Stage I	TLC plus pharmacologic treatment
≥160/≥100	Stage II	TLC plus pharmacologic treatment

history includes whether the patient already has documented hypertension, CVD, diabetes, or renal disease. The provider should assess risk factors such as an elevated BMI, whether the lifestyle is active or sedentary, high fat and sodium levels in the diet, tobacco use, and alcohol and substance abuse, and evaluate previous blood pressure readings.[24]

The course of hypertension involves insidious damage that can be clinically silent for a decade or more. It typically presents in the fourth decade of life and is often preceded by a period of lability. Ninety-five percent of patients with hypertension have primary or essential hypertension. This means that there is no specific cause for the elevated blood pressure. Secondary hypertension occurs rarely and is attributed to illnesses such as Cushing's syndrome, pheochromocytoma, primary aldosteronism, or substance use (Table 14-2).[25–27]

Measurement of blood pressure is the only way to screen for hypertension; it should be measured at every office visit, regardless of the reason for the visit. It takes more than one elevated reading to label a patient as hypertensive. An accurate diagnosis requires three elevated readings over several office visits using accurate equipment and measurement technique.[28]

An accurate measurement requires the appropriate equipment. The sphygmomanometer must be appropriately calibrated. The inflatable portion of the cuff needs to surround at least 80% of the circumference of the arm. The lower edge of the cuff should be 2 to 3 cm above the antecubital fossa. A false elevation in pressure will result from a cuff that is too small. The woman should be advised to avoid caffeine and tobacco for at least 30 minutes prior to the office visit. She should sit quietly without talking in a chair with back and arm support and her feet on the ground for approximately five minutes. These are significant—not trivial—points necessary to obtain valid blood pressure measurements. An increase of 5 mm Hg or less can significantly increase the number of patients classified as prehypertensive or hypertensive, leading to a change in the management plan. Two or more readings, separated by at least two minutes, are averaged together and documented at each visit. Blood pressure should be checked in both arms.[25]

The term *white coat hypertension (WCH)* is used to identify patients who have elevated blood pressure readings in a medical provider's office, but not in their own environment. It is now well understood that this is not a benign condition and that these patients may also be at risk for cardiovascular events. WCH can occur at any age, but primarily it affects people over the age of 65, with women more commonly affected than men. There is a lower incidence of end organ damage in patients with WCH in comparison to patients with similar levels of sustained hypertension.[29]

Table 14-2 **DIFFERENTIAL DIAGNOSES FOR SECONDARY HYPERTENSION**[25,26,27]

Causes of Secondary Hypertension	History or Physical Findings	Diagnostic Studies
Hyperparathyroidism	Kidney stones	Protein in urine
	Osteoporosis	
	Depression	PTH
	Lethargy	
	Muscle weakness	Elevated creatinine
	Renal dysfunction	
	Abdominal bruits	
	Nocturia	
	Diabetes	
	Hematuria	
Renovascular disease	Edema	Creatinine clearance
	Elevated BUN & Creatinine	
Chronic kidney disease	Proteinuria	Renal ultrasound
		Estimated glomerular filtration rate
Pheochromocytoma	Labile hypertension	Elevated urine vanillyl-mandelic acid
	Family history of endocrine disorders	
	Hypertension after abdominal palpation	
	Headaches	
	Diaphoresis	
	Palpitations	
Hyperaldosteronism	Hypokalemia	Low potassium level
	Hypernatremia	
	Headache	
	Weakness	
	Fatigue	
	Muscle cramps	
	Polyuria	
	Polydipsia	
	Nocturia	
	Paresthesias	
Cushing's syndrome	Weight gain	Dexamethasone-suppression test
	Fatigue	
	Weakness	
	Hirsutism	
	Amenorrhea	
	Moon facies	
	Dorsal hump	

(continues)

Table 14-2 DIFFERENTIAL DIAGNOSES FOR SECONDARY HYPERTENSION *(continued)*

Causes of Secondary Hypertension	History or Physical Findings	Diagnostic Studies
Coarctation of the aorta	Arm blood pressure > leg blood pressure Late systolic murmur Decreased or delayed femoral pulses	Abnormal chest x-ray
Hypothyroid	Fatigue, weight loss, hair loss, diastolic hypertension, muscle weakness	Elevated TSH
Hyperthyroid	Heat intolerance, weight loss, palpitations, systolic hypertension, exophthalmos, tremor, tachycardia	TSH Levels
Sleep apnea	Snoring Daytime sleepiness	Sleep studies with oxygen saturation
Drugs and substances associated with hypertension	Immunosuppressants including corticosteroids NSAIDs Cox-2 Inhibitors Estrogens Weight loss agents Stimulants—nicotine, amphetamines Bromocriptine Nardil Testosterone Pseudoephedrine Licorice Antidepressants, especially venlafaxine Buspirone Clozapine Ergotamine St. John's Wort Anabolic steroids Cocaine Ecstasy	

Abbreviations are: PTH, parathyroid hormone; NSAID, non-steroid anti-inflammatory drug; TSH, thyroid stimulating hormone.

The presence of WCH makes it more difficult to establish a diagnosis. Two methods may be helpful in clarifying the actual readings: *ambulatory blood pressure monitors (ABPMs)* and *home monitoring*. ABPMs provides information about a patient's blood pressure during her daily activities as well as at rest. These readings are usually lower than the readings obtained in the provider's office. ABPM readings have been found to correlate better than office measurements with the likelihood of identifying patients at risk for a cardiovascular event. The readings are recorded while the patient is sleeping, when it is expected that blood pressure will be lower. Patients who have sustained blood pressure elevation while sleeping are at increased risk for experiencing a cardiovascular event.[23] An ABPM is not informative or cost effective enough to use in the routine evaluation of elevated blood pressure. It is best used in patients with clinic readings that the provider suspects may not be representative of the patient's true blood pressure. Home monitoring is not only helpful in differentiating WCH versus true hypertension, but it is also beneficial in monitoring response to the treatment plan. It is imperative that the provider checks the device for accuracy and is confident that the patient is using the device correctly. Studies have shown that it is best to avoid wrist and finger monitors because the brachial artery-based monitors are more accurate. It is important to explain to women that they need to take the same steps at home when checking their blood pressure that are taken in the office to ensure accuracy. Blood pressure readings are usually lower at home than in the office, so any values above 135/85 mm/Hg at home are considered elevated.[28]

Physical Examination

The goal of the physical examination is to assess whether there is evidence of end organ damage. The examination includes accurate blood pressure measurements; height, weight, and waist circumference (>35 inches in women is considered to be abdominal obesity). The BMI should be calculated. A full evaluation of the optic fundi can be performed to assess for arteriolar narrowing, increased vascular tortuosity, or A-V nicking, hemorrhages, exudates, and disc edema. The thyroid is palpated to evaluate for any nodules or enlargements. The carotid pulses are assessed for the presence of bruits. The cardiac and lung exams evaluate for symptoms of congestive heart failure and the presence of S_3 and S_4 heart sounds. The peripheral vasculature is assessed for the presence of bruits, and abnormalities in bilateral arm pressures. The abdomen is palpated for masses and bruits. The neurologic exam targets any focal deficits.[24]

Laboratory Tests

Laboratory evaluation of women with hypertension requires diagnostic tests that will assess for the level of end organ damage, identify patients who are at high risk for developing CVD, and screen for secondary causes of hypertension. Tests that are commonly performed include a complete blood count (CBC), urinalysis for the presence of albumin, serum electrolytes (potassium), thyroid-stimulating hormone, and chemistry for creatinine, fasting glucose, and lipid profiles. An electrocardiogram (ECG) is done to identify patients who have already developed complications such as left atrial enlargement and ventricular hypertrophy. When a secondary cause of hypertension is identified, it is necessary to refer the patient to the appropriate medical specialist for further evaluation; in this case, treatment is out of the scope of primary care.[19,23,24]

Management

LIFESTYLE MODIFICATION

Once the diagnosis of hypertension has been determined, the appropriate treatment needs to be implemented. The absolute goal of hypertensive treatment is to decrease CVD and renal disease, as well as morbidity and mortality. Morbidity includes target organ damage, the effect that sustained elevated blood pressure has on specific organ systems. Damage to these systems can include: left ventricular hypertrophy, coronary artery disease (CAD), heart failure, stroke, transient ischemic attack, chronic kidney disease, peripheral arterial disease, and retinopathy. Treatment options for the management of hypertension start with lifestyle modifications; in many cases the use of medications will also be necessary.

Lifestyle modifications refer to behaviors that individuals adopt with the goal of preventing disease. When disease is already present, these behavioral changes can still help manage the course of disease. Patients who have hypertension and who have implemented major lifestyle modifications have been found to decrease their blood pressure, which in turn decreases their cardiovascular risk.[20] There is also evidence that these modifications enhance the efficiency of antihypertensive drug therapy. Lifestyle modifications are indicated for the treatment of hypertension at all stages.[20] Some women may be unable to maintain these modifications long-term, but they are well proven as safe and cost-effective treatment modalities.[12]

With a weight reduction of 10 to 12 pounds, women who have an elevated BMI have a demonstrated systolic blood pressure reduction of 5 to 20 mm Hg.[30] A reduction in the systolic blood pressure of 8 to 14 mm Hg has been documented in patients who have adopted the Dietary Approaches to Stop Hypertension (DASH) eating plan.[31] This diet is rich in foods high in potassium such as fruits, vegetables, and low-fat dairy products (**Table 14-3**).

A systolic blood pressure reduction of 2 to 8 mm Hg has been documented in patients who reduce their sodium intake.[33] The adoption of 30 minutes of daily exercise has been found to decrease systolic blood pressure by 4 to 9 mm Hg. Daily alcohol intake is an important factor that is often not fully evaluated when the patient is first assessed. The daily alcohol intake should consist of no more than 1 ounce of ethanol alcohol. This translates into 2 ounces of 100-proof whiskey, 10 ounces of wine, or 24 ounces of beer. A decrease in the systolic blood pressure of 2 to 4 mm Hg will correlate with decreased alcohol intake.[20] Although caffeine does acutely raise blood pressure, there are no studies to support a direct relationship between sustained caffeine intake and hypertension. However, the same cannot be said of tobacco use. Each smoked cigarette causes significant elevations in blood pressure. In fact, patients who continue to smoke while they are on antihypertensive medications may not be as protected from CVD as patients who don't smoke.[19] **Table 14-4** describes strategies to manage hypertension.[30]

Many patients in the United States use dietary or nutritional supplements to control their blood pressure. These preparations are not under the strict regulations of the Food and Drug

Table 14-3 DIETARY APPROACHES TO STOP HYPERTENSION (DASH) EATING PLAN, BASED ON 2,000 CALORIES PER DAY[32]

Food Group	Daily Servings (Except as Noted)
Grains and grain products	7–8
Vegetables	4–5
Fruits	4–5
Low-fat or fat-free dairy foods	2–3
Meats, poultry, and fish	≤2
Nuts, seeds, and dry beans	4–5 per week
Fats and oils	2–3
Sweets	5 per week
Sodium intake	1,500–2,400 mg (start at 2,400 mg with the goal of reducing to 1,500 mg per day)

Administration (FDA) and, therefore, there is no standardization of their ingredients. Their safety and efficacy are in question. Few clinical trials support the use of these herbal and botanical supplements for the treatment of hypertension. There is particular concern about the potential for serious herb–drug interactions. However, since 1980, evidence has been accumulating in randomized controlled studies and cohort studies that the "Mediterranean Diet," rich in fresh fruits and vegetables, offers protection against hypertension.[34,35]

PHARMACOTHERAPEUTICS

Pharmacologic treatment of hypertension is indicated to achieve blood pressure values of less than 140/90 mm Hg in the general population and less than 130/80 mm Hg in patients with diabetes and renal disease. Patients who already have evidence of CVD, end organ damage, or blood pressure values in Stage 1 at diagnosis should begin lifestyle modifications and drug therapy simultaneously. Patients who have Stage 2 hypertension should begin lifestyle modifica-

tions and usually require treatment with a two-drug combination.[23] **Table 14-5** lists classes of antihypertensive medications with their mechanism of action and side effects.[23,36,37]

The most common classes of medications in use for hypertensive treatment are identified below:

- *Thiazide diuretics* block the re-absorption of sodium, thereby decreasing intravascular volume, intracellular sodium, and peripheral resistance. They block the excretion of calcium in the distal tubule, which has been shown to be somewhat protective against development of osteoporosis in elderly women. The primary side effects include hypokalemia (low potassium), hypomagnesemia, hyponatremia (low sodium), and gout.[23,36,37]
- *Beta Blockers (BB)* have been used for blood pressure reduction for decades. The exact mechanism of their action is not clear, but the beta blockers decrease

Table 14-4 MANAGEMENT OF BLOOD PRESSURE FOR ADULTS[30]

BP Classification	SBP mm Hg	DBP mm Hg	Lifestyle Modification	Initial Drug Therapy Without Compelling Indication	Initial Drug Therapy With Compelling Indications
Normal	<120	And <80	Encourage		Drug(s) for compelling indications.
Prehypertension	120-139	or 80-89	Yes	No antihypertensive drug indicated.	
Stage 1 Hypertension	140-159	or 90-99	Yes	Thiazide-type diuretics for most. May consider ACEI, ARB, BB, CCB, or combination.	Drug(s) for the compelling indications. Other anti-hypertensive drugs (diuretics, ACEI, ARB, BB, CCB) as needed.
Stage 2 Hypertension	≥160	or ≥100	Yes	Two-drug combination for most (usually thiazide-type diuretic and ACEI or ARB or BB or CCB)	

Abbreviations are: BP, blood pressure; SBP, systolic blood pressure; DBP, diastolic blood pressure; ACEI, angiotensin converting enzyme inhibitor; ARB, angiotensin receptor blocker; BB, beta blocker; CCB, calcium channel blocker.

cardiac output, renin release, catecholamine release, and peripheral resistance. Side effects include bronchospasm, decreased libido, and fatigue.[23,36,37]

- *Angistems in Converting Enzyme Inhibitors (ACEIs)* block the conversion of angiotensin I to angiotensin II by inhibiting angiotensin converting enzyme. Nearly 20% of patients develop a cough when using this category of drug. Hyperkalemia is also a possible side effect. These medications should not be prescribed to patients who have had an episode of angioedema in the past because of the risk of recurrence while on ACEIs.[23,36,37]

- *Angiotensin Receptor Blockers (ARBs)* block the action of angiotensin at the receptor site. They are a good alternative to ACEIs in patients who complain of cough.[23,36,37]

- *Calcium Channel Blockers (CCBs)* block the calcium-dependent contraction of

Table 14-5 CLASSIFICATION OF ANTIHYPERTENSIVES[23,36,37]

Classification	Mechanism of Action	Common Side Effects	Serious Side Effects
Angiotensin converting enzyme inhibitors (ACEI)	Blocks angiotensin converting enzyme and prevents the formation of angiotensin II. This results in arteriolar and venous dilation, and decreased peripheral resistance and arterial blood pressure. Renal blood flow is also increased.	Cough Taste disturbances Rash	Contraindicated in pregnancy during second and third trimesters. Orthostatic hypotension with concurrent use of diuretics.
Angiotensin II receptor blockers	Blocks the effects of angiotensin II on specific tissue. Produces the same hemodynamic effects as ACEI but has fewer side effects (SE).	Same as ACEI but not as severe and SE do not occur as often.	Hypotension in patients who are volume depleted.
Beta blockers (BB)	Antihypertensive effect is not fully understood. Beta$_2$ blockers inhibit receptors in the peripheral vasculature, bronchi, pancreas, and liver. Heart rate is decreased as well as contraction force and cardiac output.	Reduced exercise tolerance. Cool extremities.	Bronchospasm Exacerbates congestive heart failure Elevates triglycerides Decreases high density lipoprotein
Calcium channel blockers (CCB)	Relaxes arteriolar smooth muscle and decreases peripheral vascular resistance.	Headache Flushing Palpitations Ankle edema	Bradycardia Sinoatrial dysfunction 2nd and 3rd degree heart blocks
Alpha$_1$ antagonists	Lowers blood pressure by arteriolar dilation.	Fatigue Weakness Nasal congestion Headache	First dose syncope and orthostatic hypotension
Central alpha agonists	Reduces sympathetic vasoconstriction and decreases total peripheral vascular resistance.	Sedation Drowsiness	Orthostatic hypotension Hyperkalemia
Thiazide diuretics	Arteriolar vasodilation.	Rash Fatigue Impotence Photosensitivity Acute gout	Hypercalcemia Glucose intolerance Hypercholesterolemia Hypertriglyceridemia

vascular smooth muscle. Common side effects include constipation and peripheral edema. Use of short-acting CCBs in the treatment of hypertension is controversial, because they have been shown to increase cardiovascular mortality.[37,38] On the other hand, agents such as verapamil are considered effective, well tolerated, and as safe as diuretics, ACEIs, or BBs in the long-term treatment of hypertension.[38] Long-acting CCBs are very effective antihypertensive agents.

- *Alpha Blockers.* According to the ALLHAT Study, there is no indication for these medications in the treatment of hypertension because of the increased number of reports of cardiovascular events.[21]

Table 14-6 lists commonly prescribed oral antihypertensive medications.[23,36,37]

The JNC 7 recommends the use of thiazide-type diuretics as the initial therapy for most patients with hypertension. These drugs can be used either alone or in combination with BBs, CCBs, ACEIs, and ARBs.[23] When initiating drug therapy in younger patients, the lowest recommended dose should be utilized. Older patients should be started at one-half of the normal dose. The dose then can be gradually adjusted upwards until the blood pressure goal is achieved or the maximum dose is reached. When the maximum dose has been reached, a second drug from another class and dose is added as needed to reach goal blood pressure.[19] Patients with Stage 1 hypertension should be treated with a thiazide-type diuretic, but any of the other medication classes, alone or in combination, could also be considered. Patients with Stage 2 hypertension should be treated with a minimum two-drug combination, one of which should be a thiazide-type diuretic.[23]

Women diagnosed with hypertension need close surveillance. This is true regardless of the treatment plan. The success of any chosen therapy is dependent not only upon the actual therapy but also upon the level of motivation and compliance that the patient demonstrates. Because hypertension is asymptomatic, some patients have difficulty accepting their diagnosis. It is hard to commit to treatment for a condition that is not perceived as a health issue. Denial makes it difficult to take medications correctly and to follow diet and exercise recommendations. Frequent office visits are helpful because they allow the opportunity for patients and providers to identify any barriers to care and to adjust the plan in order to achieve goal blood pressure.[23]

Women should have an office visit scheduled for one month after treatment has begun. Further follow-up should be scheduled at monthly intervals until the goal blood pressure has been reached. At that point office visits can be scheduled every three to six months with biannual renal function monitoring. More frequent office visits may be required if the blood pressure is difficult to control or if there are other medical conditions present. The office visit is an opportunity for the provider to evaluate the success of lifestyle modifications such as diet and exercise. It is also the time to identify any issues the patient may be having with compliance. Many patients appear to be failing medication therapy when in fact medication cost or side effects may be discouraging them from taking the medication as prescribed.[23] The success of treatment is not only the improved blood pressure measurement, but also the woman's ability to maintain healthy changes.

Table 14-6 ORAL ANTIHYPERTENSIVES[23,36,37]

Class	Drug Name (Trade Name)	Usual Dose Range, mg/d (daily frequency)
Angiotensin converting enzyme inhibitors	benazepril (Lotensin[†])	10–40 (1–2)
	captopril (Capoten[†])	25–100 (2)
	enalapril (Vasotec[†])	2.5–40 (1–2)
	fosinopril (Monopril)	10–40 (1)
	lisinopril (Prinivil, Zestril[†])	10–40 (1)
	moexipril (Univasc)	7.5–30 (1)
	perindopril (Aceon)	4–8 (1–2)
	quinapril (Accupril)	10–40 (1)
	ramipril (Altace)	2.5–20 (1)
	trandolapril (Mavik)	1–4 (1)
Angiotensin II antagonists	candesartan (Atacand)	8–32 (1)
	eprosartan (Tevetan)	400–800 (1–2)
	irbesartan (Avapro)	150–300 (1)
	losartan (Cozaar)	25–100 (1–2)
	olmesartan (Benicar)	20–40 (1)
	telmisartan (Micardis)	20–80 (1)
	valsartan (Diovan)	80–320 (1)
Calcium channel blockers (CCB) non-dihydropyridines	diltiazem extended release (Cardizem CD, Dilacor XR, Tiazac[†])	180–420 (1)
	diltiazem extended release (Cardizem LA)	120–540 (1)
	verapamil immediate relesase (Calan, Isoptin[†])	80–320 (2)
	verapamil long acting (Calan SR, Isoptin SR[†])	120–360 (1–2)
	verapamil–Coer (Covera HS, Verelan PM)	120–360 (1)
Calcium channel blockers (CCB) dihydropyridines	amlodipine (Norvasc)	2.5–10 (1)
	fetodipine (Plendil)	2.5–20 (1)
	isradipine (Dynacirc CR)	2.5–10 (2)
	nicardipine sustained release (Cardine SR)	60–120 (2)
	nicardipine long-acting (Adalat CC, Procardia XL)	30–60 (1)
	nisoldipine (Sular)	10–40 (1)
Alpha$_1$ blockers	doxazosin (Cardura)	1–16 (1)
Central alpha$_2$ agonists and other centrally acting drugs	prazosin (Minipress[†])	2–20 (2–3)
	terazosin (Hytrin)	1–20 (1–2)
	clonidine (Catapres[†])	0.1–0.8 (2)
	clonidine patch (Catapres-TTS)	0.1–0.3 (1 weekly)
	methyldopa (Aldomet[†])	250–1,000 (2)
	reserpine (generic)	0.05[‡]–0.25 (1)
	guanfacine (generic)	0.5–2 (1)
Direct vasodilators	hydralazine (Apresoline[†])	25–100 (2)
	minoxidil (Loniten[†])	2.5–80 (1–2)

*These dosages may vary from those listed in the *Physician's Desk Reference.* Stamford, CT: Thompson Healthcare; 2006.

[†] Are now or will soon become available in generic preparations.

[‡] A 0.1 mg dose may be given every other day to achieve this dosage.

The JNC 7 includes the category of "compelling indications." Individuals with hypertension who have co-morbidities have a "compelling indication" and require more aggressive management. They may also respond better to a particular class of antihypertensive medication. For example, JNC 7 recommends that individuals with chronic renal disease and hypertension receive a mutliple-drug regimen; three drugs may be needed to achieve blood pressures less than 130/80. Treatment with an ACEI or ARB is preferred because these medications have been shown to slow the progression of renal disease.[23]

Ischemic heart disease (IHD) is the most common form of end organ damage. The most frequently used medications for the management of IHD include BBs, CCBs, or ACEIs. Heart failure may directly result from IHD but can also be due to systolic hypertension. It is often treated with the same medications as well as aldosterone blockers and loop diuretics in the end stages of disease. Women with diabetes and renal disease usually will require more intensive therapy to achieve blood pressure control. There are compelling data to support the use of ACEIs and ARBs to reduce diabetic nephropathy, albuminuria, and coronary events.[23] However, all classifications of drugs are suitable for treatment.

Midwives and other women's health providers may begin medications in conjunction with a consulting physician and can monitor women on medications who have stable blood pressures. All individuals with blood pressures that remain elevated on medications, or have abnormal ECG findings or cardiac symptoms should be referred to a cardiologist for an evaluation as soon as possible.

Special Populations

AFRICAN AMERICANS

There is an increased prevalence and severity of hypertension and its complications in the African-American population.[40] This population possesses physiologic characteristics that contribute to this risk, such as low circulating renin and excessive levels of angiotensin. African Americans are also more likely to have the salt-sensitive gene, higher levels of intracellular calcium stores, and a higher incidence of obesity. Research has shown that this population experiences a significant decline in systolic blood pressure when sodium intake is restricted. Thiazide-type diuretics and CCBs are usually the first drugs of choice for blood pressure control. ACEIs are commonly indicated in the setting of other comorbid conditions, but they should be used with caution. There is as much as a fourfold increased risk of angioedema in African Americans with the use of ACEIs.[21]

WOMEN

Reproductive-aged women with hypertension are more limited in their contraceptive choices than normotensive women, particularly if they have end-organ damage. Pregnancy also poses risks for the mother as well as the fetus. Selecting a contraceptive product that balances the need for safety with the need to find a product that is easy to use and effective can be especially difficult. In order to provide guidance, the World Health Organization (WHO) has established guidelines to help provide women with underlying medical conditions with the broadest array of options. Contraceptive options are rated for their safety in women with many different underlying conditions such as migraine headaches, human immunodeficiency virus infection, and diabetes, as well as hypertension. Ratings range from 1 (safest) to 4 (least safe). The WHO criteria are defined as follows:[41]

1. use method in any circumstances
2. generally use the method
3. use of method not usually recommended unless other more appropriate methods are not available or acceptable
4. method not to be used

Contraceptive choices for hypertensive women are affected by the degree of hypertension, the extent to which it is well controlled, and the presence of comorbidities. Of the hormonal options, progestin-only options are deemed safer than estrogen-containing products and can be used in most situations. Progestin-only pills and Depo Provera are rated as Category 1 and Category 2 respectively unless the blood pressure is >160/90 or other conditions are present. Estrogen-containing products (combined oral contraceptives, ring, patch) are generally placed in Category 3, but their safety rating is lowered to Category 4 when blood pressure levels exceed >160/90 or comorbidities are present. A full description of all these recommendations is available on the Web.[41]

Older women are at higher risk for adverse outcomes than reproductive-aged women. The risk of CVD increases in women after menopause, but with the treatment of hypertension the stroke mortality rate will decrease in women over 50 years of age.[11]

For many years, reports of hypertension with the use of menopause hormone therapy (MHT) were rare. However, since the release of the results of the Women's Health Initiative[10] in 2002, hypertension has concerned both providers and researchers because of the correlation between exogenous estrogen and heart disease. If a woman has hypertension and chooses to use MHT, she should be monitored closely, even though elevations in blood pressure are rare.[42]

PREGNANCY AND PRECONCEPTION

Chronic hypertension occurs in 1% to 5% of pregnant women.[43] Chronic hypertension is a serious medical complication in pregnancy with increased maternal and perinatal morbidity and mortality.[43] The diagnosis of chronic hypertension in pregnancy is made on the basis of a prior diagnosis or persistent elevation of blood pressure of at least 140/90 mm Hg on two occasions more than 24 hours apart, before the 20th week of gestation.

The NHLBI issued a revised report in 2000 on high blood pressure in pregnancy.[43] Ideally, preconception counseling is provided to select a drug regimen that will minimize any fetal effects. Frequent prenatal visits are recommended, although the number and spacing of visits is individualized depending on maternal and fetal status. Blood pressure and urine protein should be assessed at each visit. Laboratory tests including CBC, platelet count, uric acid, 24-hour urine for protein, and liver enzymes are obtained to establish a baseline and repeated as necessary. Consultation with and/or referral to a physician for management of women with hypertension during pregnancy is essential. Pregnant women with chronic hypertension are at risk for both superimposed pre-eclampsia and fetal growth restriction.[43,44] Close monitoring for these complications is important. Baseline sonographic evaluation is recommended at 18 to 20 weeks gestation. A follow-up sonogram can be obtained at 28 to 32 weeks and can be repeated monthly until term if adequate fetal growth is uncertain to ensure appropriate fetal growth. Serial sonography is not necessary if adequate fetal growth is found on the clinical exam.[43] Serial non-stress tests and biophysical profiles may be used if there is evidence of growth restriction or pre-eclampsia or if these conditions cannot be excluded. Non-stress tests and biophysical profiles are not essential in women with mild chronic hypertension as long as there is normal fetal growth and no evidence of pre-eclampsia.[44] Lifestyle modifications during pregnancy for women with hypertension should also be recommended; however, weight loss and vigorous exercise during pregnancy are not advised. Nutrition counseling can provide the woman with information needed to choose an appropriate diet. Restricting work and home activities may be necessary.

Medication regimens used prior to pregnancy may be altered depending on the risk-benefit analysis for an individual woman. Whether continuing the use of a thiazide diuretic during pregnancy is beneficial or not is unclear. A benefit has been suggested based on theoretical grounds,[44] and it is thought to be "probably safe".[23] Initiating diuretic therapy during pregnancy is controversial because it may affect maternal and fetal electrolyte balance and fluid volume.[23,43] These same effects may be seen in women who become pregnant while taking diuretics, so maternal and fetal monitoring are crucial if diuretic use is continued.

Women who are diagnosed with hypertension before conception and are on medication present a challenge to the provider. While they are not considered teratogenic in the first trimester, use of anti-hypertensives in the second and third trimester has resulted in severe intrauterine growth retardation (IUGR) and

fatal neonatal renal insufficiency. Anti-hypertensive medications (listed in the general order of preference) used in pregnancy include methyldopa, labetalol, and the BBs.

Hypertension in pregnancy is classified into four categories according to the National High Blood Pressure Education Program's Working Group Report on High Blood Pressure in Pregnancy:[43]

1. *Chronic Hypertension* is that which has been diagnosed before pregnancy or before the 20th week of pregnancy. Most pre-pregnancy medications, including diuretics, can be continued. Evaluation by an obstetrician skilled in the management of hypertension should be obtained at the earliest possible date. ACEIs and ARBs should be discontinued and another medication regime substituted if needed. Some women may be suspected of having pre-existing chronic hypertension but not meet the definition due to late entry to care or the lack of recent pre-pregnancy blood pressure measurements. These women can be considered to have developed chronic hypertension if blood pressure elevations persist longer than 6 to 12 weeks postpartum.

2. *Preeclampsia* is defined as the presence of hypertension in conjunction with proteinuria ($\geq$300 mg in a 24-hour collection or $\geq$1+ in a random urine sample) after 20 weeks gestation. Abnormal coagulation studies and liver function tests (LFTs), symptoms such as headache, visual changes, and epigastric pain, and higher levels of proteinuria make the diagnosis more certain.

Eclampsia indicates the presence of seizure activity not due to other causes.

3. Preeclampsia superimposed on chronic hypertension has the features of both disorders. Markers of concern depend on a woman's baseline status. In women who are well controlled, a sudden rise in blood pressure or the development of new-onset proteinuria may indicate the presence of superimposed preeclampsia. The diagnosis in women with preexisting proteinuria or poorer control will be harder to make. In these women, sudden increases in proteinuria or blood pressure levels indicate that superimposed preeclampsia is developing.

4. Transient hypertension or gestational hypertension occurs late in pregnancy without proteinuria and usually disappears with delivery. Women who are overweight or who have a history of elevated blood pressures are at risk for this condition.[45,46]

An accurate diagnosis and treatment plan for hypertension in pregnancy depends on distinguishing hypertension that originates during pregnancy from hypertension that was present but unrecognized before the pregnancy. The key diagnostic feature is the presence or absence of protein in a 24-hour urine collection. Several medication classes are available that are effective and considered safe for the fetus. Methyldopa is the drug of choice for oral administration; hydralazine is the drug of choice for parenteral administration. The chief side effects of dry mouth, sedation, and elevated LFTs may make methyldopa difficult for some women to tolerate. BBs are also very well tolerated. Although preliminary data suggested that IUGR was associated with the use of BBs, a retrospective review has demonstrated that hundreds of women have used these medications without any fetal complications.[47] Labetalol, which is a combination of alpha and BBs, is frequently prescribed from preconception through pregnancy, delivery, and lactation. Women who are already well controlled with thiazide-type diuretics may continue on these medications; they require close monitoring for IUGR, which may be related to volume depletion. Nitroprusside should also be avoided because cyanide, a by-product of the drug's metabolism, accumulates to toxic levels in the fetal compartment.[48]

The foregoing discussion of the management of hypertensive disorders during pregnancy is not comprehensive. As a general rule, midwives who care for women with hypertensive disorders during pregnancy do so in close consultation with a physician skilled in the management of these problems. Resources for adequate and ongoing fetal assessment are essential.

Alternative Therapies

Consumption of fish may be protective against CVD. A prospective cohort study of women enrolled in the Nurse's Health Study found a significantly lower risk of thrombotic stroke among women who ate fish two or more times per week.[49] Fish containing higher levels of omega-3 fatty acids seem to be the most protective. These include sardines, trout, salmon, tuna, halibut, crab, mackerel, shrimp, and scallops. Pregnant women are advised by the FDA to avoid shark, swordfish, king mackerel, and tilefish because these fish contain high levels of mercury. Up to 12 ounces of fish with lower levels of mercury (such as shrimp, canned light tuna, salmon, pollock, and catfish) may be consumed by pregnant women each week.[50]

Other alternative therapies are less extensively researched. Vitamin C intake has been associated with decreased risk of CHD in women.[51] The recommendations found to be most effective, especially in prehypertensive women, are the lifestyle modifications described earlier in this chapter. These modifications have been shown to affect blood pressure and help individuals reach their target blood pressure goals and maintain those levels.

Hyperlipidemia

Although CHD is the single largest cause of death in both men and women, and is two to three times more common in women after menopause, many women are unaware of these facts. When women are queried about potential causes of death, the majority assume that they have a greater risk of dying from breast cancer than heart disease. The American Heart Association estimates that direct and indirect costs of CHD were approximately $368.4 billion dollars in 2002.[52]

The NCEP has released a series of guidelines for the treatment and management of high cholesterol since 1988. The most recent guideline, the Adult Treatment Panel III (ATP III), was released in 2001.[31] The ATP III recommendations focus on lowering LDL levels, because high LDL levels are thought to have a strong causal relationship to CVD. It also identifies what levels of total cholesterol, LDL, high-density lipoprotein (HDL), and triglycerides are thought to be optimal, acceptable, or elevated (**Table 14-7**). These categories vary depending on the individual's risk status and are used to determine whether lifestyle modifications or medication is needed and whether the response to therapy is

acceptable. ATP III promotes the use of a scoring system to predict the risk of developing CVD over the next 10 years. Individual attributes such as age, gender, and smoking status are entered into an algorithm and a score is generated. The higher the score, the higher the risk. Those at highest risk are those who require treatment for hyperlipidemia.

Definitions

Cholesterol is a fat-like substance used by the body to form hormones and cell membranes. Cholesterol is carried through the bloodstream in molecules called *lipoproteins*. Excess cholesterol deposits in the interior of blood vessels cause an inflammatory process that contributes to heart disease. This inflammatory process begins a chain of events in the blood vessels that leads to plaque rupture, thrombus formation, and embolization of clots into the blood vessels, causing occlusion and ischemia in surrounding tissue.

Lipoproteins are classified according to their size, specifically their density. LDL cholesterol has been shown to be the major cause of CHD. A 1% reduction in LDL levels has been associated with a 1% reduction in the risk of developing cardiovascular disease.[31] Women with elevated cholesterol levels have twice the risk of developing heart disease than do women with lower cholesterol levels.[53]

HDL cholesterol is often referred to as the "good cholesterol" and the goal of therapy is to increase the HDL levels. HDL participates in reverse cholesterol transport. HDL attracts free cholesterol in the blood and transports it to the liver for secretion as bile.[54] Triglycerides are another form of fat in the bloodstream that is utilized for energy. A high triglyceride level can cause the

Table 14-7 LIPOPROTEIN PROFILES[3]

Type of Lipoprotein	Serum levels (mg/dL)	Classification by ATP III
Low-density lipoprotein cholesterol	<70	Therapeutic goal for those at highest risk
	<100	Optimal
	100–129	Near optimal/above optimal
	130–159	Borderline high
	160–189	High
	≥190	Very high
Total cholesterol	<200	Desirable
	200–239	Borderline high
	≥240	High
High-density lipoprotein cholesterol	<40	Low
	≥60	High
Triglycerides	<150	Normal
	150–199	Borderline high
	200–499	High
	≥500	Very High

blood to appear creamy or milky; higher levels of triglycerides are associated with an increased risk of heart disease. All of these serum levels are measured in a lipoprotein profile.

Evaluation

Identification and management of risk factors is essential in preventing CHD. The first step is to determine the individual's total cholesterol profile. The National Cholesterol Program ATP III recommends a fasting lipoprotein panel every five years for patients over the age of 20.[31] The USPSTF recommends that clinicians routinely screen younger adults (men aged 20–35 and women aged 20–45) for lipid disorders if they have other risk factors for CHD.[8] Screening can be done with a fasting lipid panel measuring total cholesterol (TC), LDL, HDL, and triglyc-

erides. Non-fasting TC and HDL values can also be used but are less accurate. If a nonfasting TC is >200 mg/dL or nonfasting HDL is <40 mg/dL, the patient should be reevaluated using a fasting sample.[55]

The presence of risk factors should also be evaluated; categories include: major independent risk factors, life-habit risk factors, and emerging risk factors. Major risk factors are used to determine whether treatment is needed and include factors such as diabetes, tobacco use, hypertension, HDL <40 mg/dL, age ≥55 in women, and a family history of premature CHD (in a first-degree male relative at age ≤55 years or a first-degree female <65 years). Life-habit risk factors are defined as obesity (BMI >30), physical inactivity, and an atherogenic diet. Life-habit risk factors do not change the cholesterol goal, but are targeted to increase the likelihood of achieving normal lipid values. Emerging risk factors include: changes in lipoprotein (a), homocysteine, prothrombotic factors, or proinflammatory factors, impaired fasting glucose, and subclinical atherosclerosis.

Once the fasting lipoprotein panel has been obtained, the number of major risk factors present is determined. If two or more risk factors are present, the Framingham Risk Assessment can be used to determine the individual's risk that CVD will develop over the next 10 years.[18] Scores fall into one of three categories: 1) high risk (>20% chance of developing CVD over 10 years), 2) intermediate risk (between 10% and 20%), and 3) low risk (<10%).[3] See **Table 14-8** for a copy of the tool, which is also posted on the National Institute of Health Web site: http://hin.nhlbi.nih.gov/atpiii/calculator.asp.

The Framingham Risk Score and the LDL level are used to determine if drug therapy is needed. In order to be accurate, LDL levels should be drawn after a 9- to 12-hour fast. Accuracy is also affected by acute episodic events such as myocardial infarction, surgery, trauma, or infection; by the presence of conditions such as pregnancy; and by lifestyle factors such as weight loss and dietary changes. A waiting time of eight weeks after these conditions resolve or stabilize is recommended before LDL levels are repeated. This will allow the level to equilibrate; and the sample will then be a true representation of LDL status.[31]

LDL levels are also used to monitor therapy. A lipoprotein profile should be obtained six weeks after initiation or change in medication(s). Once the target LDL level has been reached, a lipoprotein profile should be repeated at least every four to six months.[32]

Management

LIFESTYLE CHANGES

All patients with an elevated LDL are treated with lifestyle changes. These measures have been identified as the most cost-effective means to reduce the risk for CHD. Lifestyle changes alone may not be sufficient to reach goal LDL, but they should still be maintained when pharmacological treatment is added.[56]

The major principles of therapeutic lifestyle changes (TLCs) include healthy diet, increased activity, exercise, smoking cessation, and decreased alcohol intake. The diet should include foods that are low in saturated fats and cholesterol, high in fiber, and contain plant stanols and sterols. Margarines and olive oil-based salad dressings are excellent sources for plant stanols and sterols. Good sources of soluble fiber foods include cereal grains, legumes, and fruits. Referral to a registered dietician may be very beneficial for patients to fully understand the principles of the diet. Patients should be advised to maintain or attain a normal weight, to stop smoking, and to exercise daily. After six weeks of TLC, the fasting lipoprotein panel should be rechecked. If the goal LDL still has not been reached, dietary changes and activity levels are reviewed and changes recommended. If no improvement is seen in LDL six weeks after intensifying lifestyle strategies, then the clinician should consider adding a lipid lowering agent.

The role of vitamins and antioxidants in the metabolism of homocysteine for those at increased cardiovascular risk is controversial. Supplementation with folic acid and other B vitamins (B_6 and B_{12}) has been found to lower homocysteine levels. However, the prevalence of

Table 14-8 RISK ASSESSMENT TOOL FOR ESTIMATING 10-YEAR RISK OF DEVELOPING HEART DISEASE[32]

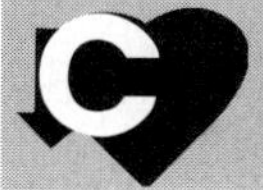

The risk assessment tool below uses recent data from the Framingham Heart Study to estimate 10-year risk for "hard" coronary heart disease outcomes (myocardial infarction and coronary death). This tool is designed to estimate risk in adults aged 20 and older who do not have heart disease or diabetes. Use the calculator below to estimate 10-year risk.

Age:	☐ years
Gender:	○ Female ○ Male
Total Cholesterol:	☐ mg/dL
HDL Cholesterol:	☐ mg/dL
Smoker:	○ No ○ Yes
Systolic Blood Pressure:	☐ mm/Hg
Currently on any medication to treat high blood pressure.	○ No ○ Yes

Calculate 10-Year Risk

Total cholesterol - Total cholesterol values should be the average of at least two measurements obtained from lipoprotein analysis.

HDL cholesterol - HDL cholesterol values should be the average of at least two measurements obtained from lipoprotein analysis.

Smoker - The designation "smoker" means any cigarette smoking in the past month.

Systolic blood pressure - The blood pressure value used is that obtained at the time of assessment, regardless of whether the person is on antihypertensive therapy (treated hypertension carries residual risk).

More Information - Determining 10-year (short term) risk for developing CHD is carried out using Framingham risk scoring. The risk factors included in the Framingham calculation are age, total cholesterol, HDL cholesterol, systolic blood pressure, treatment for hypertension, and cigarette smoking. Because of a larger database, Framingham estimates are more robust for total cholesterol than for LDL cholesterol. Note, however, that LDL cholesterol remains the primary target of therapy. The Framingham risk score gives estimates for "hard CHD," which includes myocardial infarction and coronary death.

elevated homocysteine levels appears to be low in the general U.S. population. Nor has the exact relationship between homocysteine levels and CVD, as well as the strength of this relationship if it exists, been determined. Those thought most likely to benefit from monitoring and supplementation are those with a strong family history of CVD. Therefore the ATP III concludes that it is premature to recommend routine supplementation, particularly in nutrient-replete individuals, and recommends following the Institute of Medicine's (IOM) recommended daily allowance for dietary folate of 400 μg per day until further data are available from ongoing clinical trials. The one exception is for those with a strong family history who may benefit from drawing a homocysteine level and supplementation if it is elevated.[31]

Oxidative stress and the oxidation of LDL have been shown to be important steps in the progression of CHD. However, clinical trials on the impact of antioxidant supplementation on the prevention or progression of CVD have had conflicting results. Consequently, the ATP III does not recommend antioxidant supplementation to reduce LDL levels; rather they recommend following the dietary standards set by the IOM. The IOM has increased its recommendations for dietary antioxidants for women to 90 mg/d for Vitamin C and to 15 mg/d of Vitamin E.[31] While the use of herbal and botanical dietary supplements for the prevention of CVD is not supported by ATP III, it does stress the need to query patients about their use in order to identify any potential drug interaction.

Moderate alcohol consumption of no more than two drinks per day for men and not more than one drink per day for women also appears to be cardioprotective. However, because alcohol has the potential of being abused, a thorough discussion of the risks and benefits of alcohol consumption, including the importance of moderation, is warranted.

Weight Reduction Weight reduction is an important part of TLC. A reduction in LDL cholesterol of 5% to 8% has been documented with a 10-lb weight loss. A client's weight, BMI, and waist circumference should be obtained at regular intervals. A decrease in total caloric intake to maintain desirable body weight or to prevent weight gain is recommended. The ATP III recommends that the provider first discuss dietary changes with the patient and then discuss weight loss if needed, once dietary improvements have been implemented. This stepped approach is recommended in order to prevent overwhelming the patient by asking for too many changes at one time. A loss of 10% body weight over six months has been associated with reduced cardiovascular risks.

Weight loss can be achieved by reducing caloric consumption. Teaching women to read food labels to identify and reduce hidden fat is helpful. Women should be advised to reduce the intake of saturated fats in their diets to less than 7% of total calories and dietary cholesterol to less than 200 mg/day. Patients who adhere to these recommendations can reduce their LDL levels by 8% to 10% and their total cholesterol by 3% to 5%. Lowering the intake of saturated fatty acids has been reported to decrease the incidence of CHD by 24%. High protein, high fat, low carbohydrate diets are not recommended by ATP III, but a decrease in excess carbohydrates found in fat-free products is recommended.[31]

A complete dietary assessment should be performed. One easy tool is the dietary "CAGE" assessment, which evaluates whether a woman is consuming foods thought to raise LDL-cholesterol

(Table 14-9). These include cheese, animal fats, meals eaten outside the home, and high fat commercial products like candy and cakes.

Exercise is the other key to successful weight loss and improves cardiovascular health. Women should be encouraged to obtain 30 minutes of moderate intensity activity on most days of the week and to incorporate physical activities into daily routines. Wearing a pedometer can make it easier to achieve a goal of 10,000 steps a day (Table 14-10).[31]

Tables 14-11 through 14-14 summarize dietary and lifestyle modifications that will help women achieve and maintain a healthy lifestyle.

PHARMACOTHERAPEUTICS

Pharmacologic therapy is often required to lower LDL levels to an acceptable level, especially in high-risk individuals. There are four major classes of medications available for cholesterol control on the market today.

Table 14-9 DIETARY CAGE FOR ASSESSMENT OF INTAKES OF SATURATED FAT AND CHOLESTEROL[32]

CAGE	Description
C	Cheese and other sources of dairy fats: whole milk, 2% milk, ice cream, cream, whole fat yogurt
A	Animal fats: hamburger, ground meat, frankfurters, bologna, salami, sausage, fried foods, fatty cuts of meats
G	Got it away from home: high fat meals either purchased and brought home or eaten in a restaurant
E	Eat (extra) high-fat commercial products: candy, pastries, doughnuts, cookies

---

HMG CoA Reductase Inhibitors (Statins)   Statins are considered the gold standard of cholesterol management. Recent studies have shown that statins are highly effective in lowering LDL and therefore the risk for CHD.[55] They inhibit the β-hydroxy-β-methylglutaryl–coenzyme A reductase enzyme, which is essential for the synthesis of cholesterol. They also increase the uptake of LDL by the liver. They have been shown to affect platelet aggregation and deposition, fibrinogen, and endothelial vasodilation and blood viscosity, which may be the reason for their effectiveness in stroke prevention. Side effects include but are not limited to fatigue, abdominal pain, myalgias, constipation, and, in rare incidences, rhabdomyolysis (by-products of skeletal muscle destruction accumulate in the renal tubules and produce acute renal failure). It is important to monitor LFTs before initiating treatment, after the first six weeks of therapy, and every three months for a year. After a year, biannual LFT measurements are adequate with the caveat that LFTs should be repeated after each dosage adjustment. Statins can cause elevations in liver enzymes. If transaminase levels persistently exceed three or more times the normal limit, the FDA recommends discontinuation of the medication.[31] These medications are contraindicated in patients with liver disease and in women who are pregnant and lactating.[24]

While statin use has been associated with myopathy and hepatic injury, statins can also lead to myalgias, muscle aches, and weakness without elevations in creatine kinase (CK). Serious myopathy is rare, but all patients on statins should be instructed to report any muscle aches or weakness after a statin is started. Baseline CK levels are suggested for individuals prescribed dual therapy, but are not generally necessary if on monotherapy. However, CK

Table 14-10 EXAMPLES OF MODERATE PHYSICAL ACTIVITY IN HEALTHY ADULTS[32,57]

- Brisk walking: 3 to 4 mph for 30 to 40 minutes
- Swimming: laps for 20 minutes
- Bicycling (for pleasure or transportation): 5 miles in 30 minutes
- Raking leaves: for 30 minutes
- Moderate lawn mowing: push a powered mower for 30 minutes
- Home care: heavy cleaning
- Basketball: 15–20 minutes
- Golf: pulling a cart or carrying clubs
- Social dancing: 30 minutes

Moderate intensity is defined as 4 to 7 kcal/min or 3 to 6 METS. METS (work metabolic rate/resting metabolic rate) are multiples of the resting rates of oxygen consumption during physical activity. One MET represents the approximate rate of oxygen consumption of a seated adult at rest, or about 3.5 mL/min/kg.

levels should be obtained in all individuals who develop symptoms of muscle weakness or pain. If myopathy is suspected or confirmed, statin drug therapy should be discontinued immediately.[31]

Nicotinic Acid (Niacin) This medication is particularly beneficial in lowering triglycerides and increasing HDL. It impairs the hepatic synthesis of very low density lipoproteins (VLDL), which is essential for the production of LDL. It is unclear what the mechanism is by which HDL is increased, but it is the best available agent for that purpose. The most commonly reported side effect is that of flushing, which can be a severe enough side effect to cause patients to stop taking it. Patients can take an aspirin or ibuprofen one-half hour prior to each dose to relieve the flushing if the symptoms are severe, provided neither is contraindicated.[58] Titrating the dose up slowly, avoiding caffeine and alcohol, and taking niacin with meals may help reduce the flushing. It is available in three formulations: immediate release, sustained release, and extended release. The latter two formulations reduce the incidence and severity of flushing. Niacin may cause elevated LFTs and is contraindicated in patients with liver disease, peptic ulcer, and in pregnant and lactating women.[24]

Bile Acid Sequestrants These are the oldest available agents and are particularly beneficial in lowering the LDL levels when combined with other lipid-lowering medications. They inhibit the return of bile acids from the bowel to the liver, which decreases the production of cholesterol and increases its excretion in the feces. Their chief side effects are gastrointestinal (GI) symptoms. They also may affect absorption of other medications and can raise triglyceride levels.[31]

Fibric Acid Derivatives These medications are excellent for rapidly lowering dangerously elevated triglycerides. They work by increasing the clearance of VLDL from the plasma and increase

Table 14-11 FOUR COMPONENTS OF THERAPEUTIC LIFESTYLE CHANGE (TLC)[32]

Component	Recommendation
LDL-raising nutrients	
Saturated fats*	<7% of total calories
Dietary cholesterol	<200 mg/d
Therapeutic options to lower LDL	
Plant stanols/sterols	2 g/d
Increased viscous (soluble) fiber	10–25 g/d
Total calories (energy)	Adjust total caloric intake to maintain desirable body weight/ prevent weight gain.
Physical activity	Include enough moderate exercise to expend at least 200 kcal/d.

* Trans-fatty acids are another LDL-raising fat that should be minimized.

the secretion of cholesterol into bile. The most commonly reported side effects are GI in nature as well as rash and elevated LFTs. Fibric acid derivatives are known to induce rhabdomyolysis.[59] These medications are contraindicated in patients with liver or renal disease and in pregnant and lactating women.[24] **Table 14-15** lists classes of medications used to manage hyperlipidemia, with mechanisms of action and side effects.[60,61]

PRESCRIBING LIPID-LOWERING MEDICATIONS

Medications are indicated when three to six months of TLC have failed to lower LDL to the desired goal. In individuals with extremely elevated levels, the interval can be shortened. The class of drug chosen depends on which component(s) of the cholesterol panel need adjustment, as well as on whether comorbidities are present. In general, the NCEP concludes that a statin is the drug of choice for most individuals with hyperlipidemia.[31] They have been found to reduce LDL levels by 30% to 40%.[58] Therapy is begun

at the usual starting dose but may need to be adjusted upward in order to achieve the goal LDL level. If LDL levels do not respond to higher statin doses, a second agent should be added. Zetia (ezetimise) is a cholesterol absorption inhibitor that can be added to a statin for greater effectiveness. It can also be used as single agent therapy, or in combination with a bile acid sequestant. Bile acid sequestants are often given in combination with statins to lower LDL levels. Nicotinic acid can also be used to enhance the effectiveness of statins and may be particularly useful in individuals who are unable to tolerate the sequestrants or have high triglyceride levels. In contrast, the fibrates do not seem to enhance LDL lowering when combined with statins. They are used in selected situations if patients are unable to tolerate other products or have very specific forms of dyslipidemia.[31]

Goal levels have consistently been lowered over the years and vary by risk status. For *high risk individuals*, the ATP III recommended that the LDL goal be <100 mg/dL; a 2004 update

Table 14-12 THE THERAPEUTIC LIFESTYLE CHANGE DIET[32]

Component	Recommendation
Polyunsaturated fat	Up to 10% of total calories
Monounsaturated fat	Up to 20% of total calories
Total fat	25%–35% of total calorie*
Carbohydrate[†]	50%–60% of total calories*
Dietary fiber	20–30 grams per day
Protein	~ 15% of total calories

* ATP III allows an increase of total fat to 35% of total calories and a reduction in carbohydrate to 50% for persons with metabolic syndrome. Any increase in fat intake should be in the form of other polyunsaturated or mono-unsaturated fat.
[†]Carbohydrate should derive predominantly from foods rich in complex carbohydrates, including grains (especially whole grains), fruits, and vegetables.

lowered this recommendation to an optional goal of <70 mg/dL. Drug therapy should be considered at an LDL level of ≥100 mg/dL, with the goal of therapy to be <70 mg/dL. Based on information from clinical trials released after ATP III, some experts are beginning to recommend lipid-lowering therapy in all high-risk individuals, even those with LDL levels <100 mg/dL, with a goal of reducing LDL levels by 30% to 40%.[58] High-risk individuals are considered to be those with already established cardiac disease (history of myocardial infarction, unstable angina, coronary artery procedures), those who have conditions considered to be CHD risk equivalent (peripheral artery disease, abdominal aortic aneurysm, carotid artery disease, diabetes), or those with 2 or more risk factors with a 10-year risk for CHD >20%.[58]

Moderate high-risk individuals have a goal LDL level <130 mg/dL according to ATP III, but newer guidelines suggest an optional lower goal of <100 mg/dL. ATP III recommended initiating therapy at levels >130 mg/dL; updated guidelines give an option to begin drug therapy at LDL levels of 100 to 129 mg/dL with the goal of reducing LDL to <100 mg/dL.[58] Moderate high-risk individuals are defined as those with two or more risk factors (smoking, hypertension, low HDL levels, family history of premature CHD, and age) resulting in a 10-year risk of 10% to 20%. *Moderate risk individuals*, defined as those with 2 or more risk factors resulting in a ten-year risk of <10%, have a target LDL goal of <130 mg/dL. Drug therapy should be initiated with these individuals with an LDL level of greater than or equal to 160 mg/dL. Individuals at *low risk* (with 0 to 1 risk factor) have a goal of <160 mg/dL. Drug therapy should be considered when the LDL is above or equal to 190 mg/dL,[31] but can be considered at levels between 160 to 189 mg/dL according to the newest guidelines.[58]

As stated earlier, the LDL level should be checked after the first six weeks of therapy. If the LDL goal has not been reached, the medication dose can be increased, or another agent can be added. The LDL should be reevaluated six weeks after changes are made in the medication regime to monitor the response to treatment. Once the LDL goal is reached, the patient should have laboratory tests every four to six months. These tests should include LFTs as well as the fasting lipid profile. If LDL goals are not met, the treatment plan needs to be carefully reviewed with the patient to ensure compliance. If the patient has been consistent and compliant with both TLC and medication therapy, the patient should be referred to a lipid specialist for a more

Table 14-13 DIETARY REDUCTION OF LOW DENSITY LIPOPROTEIN CHOLESTEROL[32]

Dietary Component	Dietary Change	Approximate LDL Reduction
Major		
Saturated fat	<7% of calories	8%–10%
Dietary cholesterol	<200 mg/d	3%–5%
Weight reduction	Lose 10 lb	5%–8%
Other Options		
Viscous fiber	5–10 g/d	3%–5%
Plant sterol/stanol esters	2 g/d	20%–30%
Cumulative estimate		20%–30%

intensive evaluation and consultation regarding medication management.[3]

METABOLIC SYNDROME

The ATP III has identified metabolic syndrome as a new secondary target for cardiovascular risk reduction therapy.[23,62] *Metabolic syndrome* is a constellation of atherosclerotic risk factors including dyslipidemia (triglycerides ≥150 mg/dL, HDL <50 mg/dL in women), insulin resistance (fasting glucose >110 mcg/dL), obesity (specifically central obesity—waist circumference >35 inches in women; with a BMI >30), and hypertension (>130/85).[31] The diagnosis is made when three or more of these risk factors are present. Patients with this syndrome have a threefold risk of developing CAD and stroke. African-American and Hispanic-American women have a significantly higher prevalence. The major treatment options for managing this syndrome include weight loss, increased physical activity, and treatment of dyslipidemia.[61] **Table 14-16** lists drugs commonly used to lower lipid levels.

Compliance with TLC and medications for a lifetime is challenging. It is imperative that women being treated for hyperlipidemia, whether with TLC alone or with medications, understand the need for long-term intervention and lifelong lifestyle changes. The greatest likelihood of success occurs when there is a close working relationship between the patient and provider. Frequent follow-up visits will allow for the patient and the provider to discuss and evaluate how the treatment is progressing and identify at an early stage any obstacles to treatment.

Reproductive Issues

The identification and management of hyperlipidemia in women of reproductive age deserves special attention. While hyperlipidemia is a chronic problem, suspension or delaying of treatment due to pregnancy or lactation has not been found to increase maternal mortality. The normal changes that occur during pregnancy cause a significant rise in all the sub-fractions of the total cholesterol profile. These elevations may persist for more than one year postpartum. It is helpful

Table 14-14 LIFESTYLE RECOMMENDATIONS FOR A HEALTHY HEART[32]

Food Items to Choose More Often	Food Items to Choose Less Often	Recommendations for Weight Reduction	Recommendations for Increased Physical Activity
Breads and Cereals ≥6 servings/day, adjusted to caloric needs Breads, cereals, especially whole grain; pasta; rice; potatoes; dry beans and peas; low-fat crackers and cookies **Vegetables** 3–5 servings/day of fresh, frozen, or canned without added fat, salt, or sauce **Fruit** 2–4 servings/day of fresh, frozen, canned, or dried **Diary Products** 2–3 servings/day of fat-free, $\frac{1}{2}$%, 1% milk, buttermilk, yogurt, cottage cheese **Eggs** ≤2 egg yolks/week egg whites or egg substitute **Meat, Poultry, Fish** ≤5 oz/day Lean cuts of loin, leg, round; extra lean hamburger; cold cuts made from lean meat or soy protein; skinless poultry; fish **Fats and Oils** Amount adjusted to caloric level; unsaturated oils, soft or liquid margarines and vegetable oil spreads, salad dressings, seeds, and nuts	**Breads and Cereals** Many bakery products (i.e., doughnuts, biscuits, butter rolls, muffins, croissants, sweet rolls, Danish, cakes, pies, cookies, coffee cakes) Many grain-based snacks including chips, cheese puffs snack mix, regular crackers, buttered popcorn **Vegetables** Fried or prepared with butter, cheese, or cream sauce **Fruits** Fried or served with butter or cream **Dairy Products** Whole milk/2% milk, whole-milk yogurt, ice cream, cream, cheese **Eggs** Egg yolks, whole eggs **Meat, Poultry, Fish** Higher fat meat cuts; ribs, T-bone steak, regular hamburger, bacon, sausage cold cuts, salami, bologna, hot dogs; organ meats; liver, brains, sweetbreads, poultry with skin, fried meat; fried poultry; fried fish **Fats and Oils** Butter, shortening, stick margarine, chocolate, cocoanut	**Weigh Regularly** Record weight, BMI, and waist circumference **Lose weight gradually** Goal: lose 10% of body weight in 6 months; lose $\frac{1}{2}$–1 lb/week. **Develop Healthy Eating Patterns** • Choose healthy foods (see column 1) • Reduce intake of foods in column 2 • Limit the number of eating occasions • Select sensible portion size • Avoid second helpings • Identify and reduce hidden fat by reading food labels to choose products lower in saturated fat and calories • Identify and reduce sources of excess carbohydrates such as fat-free and regular crackers; cookies and other desserts; snacks; and sugar-containing beverages	**Make Physical Activity Part of Daily Routine** • Reduce sedentary time • Walk, wheel, or bike ride more; drive less; take the stairs instead of elevator; and get off the bus a few stops early and walk the remaining distance; mow the lawn with a push mower; clean the house; rake the leaves; garden; push a stroller; do exercises or pedal a stationary bike while watching TV; play actively with children; take a brisk 10-minute walk or wheel before work, during work breaks, and after dinner **Make Physical Activity Part of Exercise or Recreational Activities** • Walk, wheel, or jog; bicycle or use an arm pedal bicycle; swim or perform water aerobics; play basketball; join a sports team; play wheelchair sports; golf, pull cart or carry clubs; canoe; cross-country ski; dance; take part in exercise program at work, home, school, or gym

Table 14-14 LIFESTYLE RECOMMENDATIONS FOR A HEALTHY HEART *(continued)*

Food Items to Choose More Often	Food Items to Choose Less Often	Recommendations for Weight Reduction	Recommendations for Increased Physical Activity
TLC Diet Options Stanol/sterol- containing margarines, Viscous fiber food sources: barley, oats, psyllium, apples, bananas, berries, citrus fruits, nectarines, peaches, pears, plums, prunes, broccoli, brussels sprouts, carrots, dry beans, peas, soy products (tofu, miso)			

to have a fasting lipoprotein profile in women with risk factors prior to pregnancy to properly evaluate the presence of hyperlipidemia. Fatty streak formulation begins very early in fetal life, and it is greatly increased by maternal hypercholesterolemia during pregnancy. It is beneficial to the fetus to have maternal lipid levels as close to normal as possible prior to conception.[63] The only recommended treatment for hyperlipidemia during pregnancy and lactation is TLC. Pharmacologic management during pregnancy and lactation is contraindicated. No well-controlled studies of these medications in pregnancy exist, nor are they likely to be done in the future. Cholesterol and other products of cholesterol biosynthesis are essential components for fetal development. The studies that have been done show that statins, usually the preferred drug, also inhibit prolactin release in rats and theoretically could interfere with the initiation of lactation.[64]

Chest Pain

Office visits for the evaluation of chest pain are most commonly attributed to non-life–threatening events; however, life-threatening etiologies such as cardiac and pulmonary causes must be identified as quickly as possible. A careful and detailed history focused upon the patient's presentation must be obtained to best direct treatment. The history and physical examination have been shown to correctly differentiate non-organic chest pain from organic chest pain in most cases. The differential diagnosis for chest pain includes cardiac conditions, pulmonary pathology, GI disease, musculoskeletal causes, and psychological distress.

Differential Diagnosis

CARDIAC

CAD is the most important cardiac source of chest pain. CAD impairs blood supply to the heart and can present with a variety of symptoms. A classic presentation of *angina pectoris* may be characterized by complaints of a sudden onset of pain that is described as heavy or squeezing. It may radiate to the jaw, neck, shoulder, arm, or upper abdomen. There may also be complaints of dyspnea, diaphoresis, and nausea. Women

Table 14-15 CLASSIFICATIONS OF MEDICATIONS FOR MANAGEMENT OF HYPERLIPIDEMIA[32,36,37,60,61]

Classification	Mechanism of Action	Common Side Effects	Serious Side Effects
HMG-CoA reductase inhibitors (statins)	Reduces synthesis and secretion of lipoproteins in the liver	Myopathy Increased liver enzymes	Uncommon Relative contraindication concomitant use of cyclosporine, macrolide antibiotic, various antifungal agents and cytochrome P-450 inhibitors
Bile acid sequestrants	Bind bile acids in the intestine promote the conversion of cholesterol in the liver into bile acids	Constipation Bloating Flatulence Indigestion Decreased absorption of other drugs	Uncommon Contraindications triglycerides >200 mg/dL
Nicotinic acid	Increases the lipolysis, which increases the shift in cholesterol to HDL and decreases triglyceride production	Flushing Hyperglycemia Gout Nausea Dyspepsia Vomiting Diarrhea Abdominal pain	Hepatotoxicity
Fibric acid derivatives	Affects fatty acid oxidation and reduces the formation of very low density lipoproteins and triglycerides and raises HDL cholesterol	Dyspepsia, myalgia, flatulence	Gallstones, myopathy

Abbreviations are: HMG-CoA, hydroxymethyl glutaryl-coenzyme A.

often do not experience this traditional constellation of symptoms, but will report chest discomfort, nausea, dyspnea, and exertional fatigue. Many women report fatigue, without associated chest pain.

Atypical angina (atypical chest pain) is a term that denotes angina-like chest pain. Atypical angina differs in the location, quality, or other characteristics from more typical angina, yet is still suggestive of cardiac chest pain. Fifty percent of these patients will be diagnosed with CAD when evaluated by angiography, and the remaining 50% may have other non-cardiac causes of chest pain.[24] A diagnosis of *microvas-*

Table 14-16 PHARMACOTHERAPY FOR LIPID REDUCTION[32,37]

Trade Name	Generic Name	Dose
HMG CoA reductase inhibitors		
Mevacor	lovastatin	10–80 mg qhs
Zocor	simvastatin	20–80 mg qhs
Pravachol	pravastatin	10–40 mg qhs
Lescol	fluvastatin	20–80 mg qd
Lipitor	atorvastatin	10–80 mg qd
Crestor	rosuvastatin	10–40 mg qhs
Nicotinic acid		
Niacin	crystalline nicotinic acid	1.5 to 4.5 g
Niaspan	extended release nicotinic acid	1 to 2 g
Bile acid sequestrants		
Questran	cholestyramine	4 to 24 g qd
Colestid	colestipol	5 to 30 g qd
Welchol	colesevelam HCl	2.6 to 4.4 g qd
Fibric acid derivatives		
Lopid	gemfibrozil	600 mg bid
Tricor	fenofibrate	mg qd

Abbreviations are: HMG-CoA reductase inhibitors, Hydroxymethyl glutaryl-coenzyme A; QHS, every night; QD, daily; BID twice daily.

cular angina is given to a small group of patients who complain of either typical or atypical chest pain. Women are affected more frequently than men. The most common symptom is long-lasting pain at rest. Patients with microvascular angina usually have normal arteries at angiography despite having ECG changes at rest and exercise. The prognosis is excellent.

Mitral valve prolapse (MVP) is a cardiac valvular abnormality. It results from the systolic displacement of an abnormally thickened, redundant mitral leaflet into the left atrium during systole. Patients are usually asymptomatic but may present with atypical chest pain. Patients may present with symptoms of chest discomfort described as prolonged pain. Two-dimensional echocardiography is the diagnostic test of choice because cardiac auscultation has a low sensitivity. Symptomatic patients, including those with syncope, anxiety, or palpitations, require further evaluation. Antibiotic prophylaxis for delivery is required only if regurgitation is present.

Aortic dissection is a life-threatening medical emergency found more commonly in older men than women and in individuals with a history of hypertension. It commonly presents with an acute onset of severe chest or interscapular pain that is described as "ripping" or "tearing," but the presentation may be subtler if the patient experiences a slow leak through the intima (the innermost layer of the wall of an artery or vein). The pain may radiate to the extremities and abdomen. Neurologic deficits may be noted on the physical exam due to diminished blood supply to the central nervous system.

PULMONARY

Causes of pleuritic chest pain include pericarditis, pulmonary embolism, spontaneous pneumothorax, and other conditions that lead to inflammation or distention of the pleura. Pleuritic pain is usually worsened by deep inspiration and coughing, but not affected by movement or palpation. The severity of pain is related to the degree of inflammation and is typically worse in infectious conditions. A *pulmonary embolism (PE)* is characterized by the acute onset of dyspnea with pleuritic chest pain. PE should always be considered in women who present with these symptoms if they are taking oral contraceptives or hormonal therapy; are currently pregnant or have recently given birth; have any past history of thrombolitic events; have an underlying connective tissue disorder; or have been diagnosed as having antiphospholipid syndrome. A *spontaneous pneumothorax* is characterized by a sudden onset of stabbing pleuritic chest pain. It occurs in younger people and patients with known emphysema. See Chapter 13 for further details.

GASTROINTESTINAL

Approximately 60% of patients who complain of chest pain have normal coronary arteries and may actually be experiencing pain due to an esophageal disorder. Esophageal pain does share similar qualities with anginal chest pain, so the latter must be completely ruled out before the diagnosis of esophageal pathology can be made. Esophageal pain usually has a dull, persistent quality to it and may be associated with dysphagia (difficulty in swallowing). The pain may radiate to the interscapular region and be aggravated by bending forward. Patients may report that their symptoms develop after meals.

Gastroesophageal reflux disease (GERD) is the most common cause of non-cardiac chest pain in women. It is described as a squeezing or burning sensation that may last from one minute to several hours. Conditions that decrease lower esophageal sphincter pressure, such as pregnancy, can predispose women to GERD. Other GI diseases such as cholecystitis, pancreatitis, and peptic ulcer disease are also sources of complaints of chest pain. The pain is intermittent, long-lasting, and localized to the right upper quadrant. More information on these conditions can be found in Chapter 17.

MUSCULOSKELETAL

Musculoskeletal chest pain is a frequent reason for ambulatory office visits; it may be attributed to overexertion or trauma. *Costochondritis* is an inflammatory condition causing localized swelling, erythema, warmth, and tenderness at the costochondral or chondrosternal junction. It is more common in women than men. The pain may be sharp and localized to a specific area or diffuse and poorly localized. Movement, palpitation, and deep breathing aggravate the pain. The symptoms may last for a variable amount of time with the intensity sharp to dull.

PSYCHOLOGICAL

Palpitations associated with atypical chest pain can be a prominent component of panic disorder and are more common in women than men. Patients usually complain of chest tightness or heaviness in association with palpitations as well as dizziness from hyperventilation and dyspnea. The symptoms may last for hours and occur over several days. Rest does not relieve the symptoms. Refer to Chapter 9 for further details.

Evaluation

The first step in evaluating chest pain is to determine whether the patient's complaints warrant emergent hospitalization. Delays in receiving health care are a major predictor of poor outcome and are particularly prevalent among women, especially post-menopausal women.[65] A detailed history includes a complete pain description in the history of present illness. The pain severity can range from mild, described as a low, dull ache, to severe, described as a heavy substernal weight. Other words frequently used to describe the quality of pain include: squeezing, tight, constricting, or burning. It is also important to verify whether or not the pain radiates to the arms, jaw, or back, as well as to clarify whether or not the onset of pain was abrupt, gradual, or vague. Patients should be screened for the presence of any co-existing cardiac risk factors. Younger patients who present with ischemic quality chest pain need to be questioned about cocaine use. When a patient reports chest pain and has known cardiac risk factors, an affirmative answer to any of the following questions requires urgent medical evaluation:

- Has the pain lasted longer than 20 seconds?
- Is it getting worse? Does it occur at rest or at night?
- Does it occur with exertion? Is this a new complaint?
- Is there shortness of breath with this pain?

The physical examination can be completely normal in a woman with CAD. When the patient presents urgently, the examination is deferred in favor of immediate transport of the patient to the emergency department.

The complete assessment for chest pain begins with general appearance and vital signs. The presence or absence of certain signs may help rule in or rule out various clinical entities. The skin is evaluated for the presence of pallor or cyanosis to assess perfusion. Bilateral measurements of blood pressure and peripheral pulses are obtained. Discrepancies may indicate the presence of a dissecting aneurysm. New focal deficits found on evaluation of cranial nerves can also suggest an aortic dissection. Tachypnea and tachycardia accompanied by pleuritic chest pain may be indicative of PE. The chest wall should be examined and palpated for pain, particularly at the costochondral junctions, to help rule out pain of musculoskeletal origin. The heart and lungs should be auscultated for consolidation, murmurs, clicks, or murmurs indicating underlying cardiac disorders or pulmonary conditions. The abdomen is evaluated via auscultation, percussion, and palpation for the presence of pain or masses. For example, epigastric and right upper quadrant tenderness suggest cholecystitis, while a pulsating abdominal mass found on palpation could indicate an abdominal aneurysm.

The results of the history and physical examination guide decisions regarding further testing. An ECG will be normal in as many as one-third of patients who present with angina and is not sufficient evidence of lack of disease in a high-risk patient. Ambulatory ECG recordings may be useful in detecting ST segment depression associated with ischemia. Exercise electrocardiography (ETT) is a sensitive, specific, and low-cost test to detect high-risk coronary disease. The test cannot be interpreted unless the resting ECG is normal. Women are more likely to have changes suggestive of ischemia but are less likely to have significant CAD on ETT. The high false-negative rate in women may be due to the fact that some women simply cannot complete the full exercise protocol. Stress echocardiography is a more expensive test than the ETT, but it is more sensitive and specific in detecting regional changes in contractility during stress either introduced with exercise or pharmacologically.[48]

Management

Management of chest pain is dependent on the exact diagnosis. Specific treatment for many of these conditions begins with referral to a cardiologist. Treatment of cardiac chest pain may include medications and surgical intervention. Musculoskeletal chest pain can be treated with heat and ice therapy, nonsteroidal anti-inflammatory drugs, and physical therapy. Many GI causes of pain can be treated with dietary changes or antacids; others require referral to a gastroenterologist. Patients with symptoms of a panic disorder should be referred for psychotherapy.

Special Issues

Chest pain that is attributed to CAD is uncommon in women during pregnancy. However, women do frequently complain of symptoms that could be anginal in nature, such as dyspnea and fatigue. These symptoms are generally a response to the hemodynamic changes of pregnancy. Chest pain during pregnancy is commonly secondary to the thoracic distortion caused by elevation of the diaphragm and flaring of the ribs to accommodate the growing fetus. A rare cause of abrupt, tearing chest pain and interscapular pain in pregnancy is aortic dissection. This type of pain requires urgent medical evaluation.

Heart Sounds

Heart sounds are normally low in pitch except in the presence of significant disease. There are four basic heart sounds: S_1, S_2, S_3, and S_4. S_1 and S_2 are the most distinct sounds. S_3 and S_4 may or may not be present and both are difficult to hear. Their absence is not unusual but the presence of a loud S_4 does indicate an abnormality.[66]

S_1 indicates the beginning of systole and results from the closure of the arterioventricular valves. It is best heard at the apex of the heart and is louder, lower in pitch, and longer than S_2. The S_1 sound is referred to as "lubb." S_2 indicates the end of systole and results from the closure of the semilunar valves. It is best heard at the base of the heart and has a higher pitch and shorter duration than S_1. The S_2 sound is referred to as "dubb." S_2 is actually two sounds. The closure of the aortic pulmonic valve contributes to most of the sound of S_2, masking the sound of the pulmonic valve closing. The pulmonic valve closure occurs slightly later, giving S_2 two distinct components. When audible, this is referred to as split S_2. S_3 is a low-pitched sound that resembles a gallop and occurs early in diastole. S_4 resembles the rhythm of "Tenn-es-see" and occurs late in diastole. S_4 can be heard in patients at any age; it is common in patients who have CHD. CHD can cause increased resistance to filling due to the loss of compliance of the ventricular walls. It also is heard in patients who are in high output states such as severe anemia, thyrotoxicosis, and pregnancy.[66]

Heart murmurs are prolonged extra sounds that can be heard during systole or diastole. Murmurs are caused by a disruption in the flow of blood into, through, or out of the heart. Many murmurs are benign; however, valvular disorders commonly produce murmurs.[66]

Evaluation

Evaluation and management of heart murmurs are affected by the presence or absence of symptoms. It is important to ascertain if the patient is experiencing dyspnea, cough, chest pain, or palpitations, and whether these symptoms are associated with rest or activity. The woman needs to be questioned about past medical history to screen for rheumatic heart disease or any congenital abnormalities. A careful physical examination of the heart is performed with the patient in the supine, sitting, and standing position. The examination may be hindered by body habitus, because obesity affects the transmission of heart sounds to the chest wall surface. Tests such as an ECG, echocardiogram, or Doppler flow studies may be necessary to assess the status of a murmur.

Murmurs are classified according to their timing and duration, pitch, intensity, pattern, quality, location, radiation, and respiratory phase variations. Murmurs are most commonly referred to by their intensity. They are graded between I to VI, with the intensity increasing as the grade gets higher.

While it is out of the scope of this chapter to review all types of murmurs, two conditions commonly seen in primary care are addressed: flow murmurs and mitral valve prolapse.

Flow murmurs are also referred to as ejection or innocent murmurs. They are systolic murmurs heard in the absence of any identifiable disease and are classified as benign. These murmurs are asymptomatic. They commonly occur in the setting of hyperdynamic or high output conditions such as fever, anemia, hyperthyroidism, and pregnancy. Flow murmurs are common in patients under the age of 35. It is not uncommon for these murmurs to come and go when followed in serial exams. They are usually best heard at the base of the heart with a crescendo-decrescendo pattern. Their intensity is usually Grade III or less. Echocardiograms are not indicated in the evaluation of flow murmurs because these murmurs are not pathologic and are considered to be normal variants.[24]

MVP is also referred to as the click-murmur syndrome. MVP should be suspected if a mid-systolic click is heard on examination. It may be accompanied by mitral valve regurgitation; the murmur of mitral valve regurgitation is best heard at the apex and is holosystolic. It is often described as having a high pitch blowing quality and may have a crescendo-decrescendo pattern. It is equally common in both men and women. Patients may complain of symptoms such as palpitations, atypical chest pain, cold extremities, migraine headache, and panic attacks. Women are more likely than men to present with symptoms. However, MVP is most frequently asymptomatic and is discovered during routine physical examination. The discovery of a clicking or snapping sound on examination is diagnostic for MVP.

Echocardiography is helpful in confirming the diagnosis of MVP. This test will show the degree of mitral regurgitation or thickening of the valvular leaves. Patients with thickened redundant valvular tissue have the highest risk for developing bacterial endocarditis; they should receive antibiotic prophylaxis for certain invasive medical procedures. Not all procedures place the patient at risk. In general, risky procedures are those that may produce bacteremia with organisms associated with endocarditis (**Table 14-17**). Women with MVP with regurgitation have somewhat lower risk of developing bacterial endocarditis but should receive antibiotics. It is important to clarify the diagnosis of MVP so that the appropriate patients receive antibiotics. Inappropriate antibiotic use is unnecessary and can lead to antibiotic resistance.[67,68]

Recommendations governing antibiotic coverage and appropriate medication(s) vary according to risk status (**Table 14-18**). High-risk individuals are those with prosthetic valves, a prior history of endocarditis, some types of congenital cardiac abnormalities, or required cardiac surgery. Moderate risk individuals are those with less significant congenital cardiac disease, acquired valvar dysfunction (such as rheumatic heart disease), hypertrophic cardiomyopathy, and MVP with valvar regurgitation and/or thickened leaflets. Individuals with MVP withour valvar regurgitation and those with physiologic, functional, or innocent heart murmurs are not at greater risk than the general public for bacterial endocarditis and do not require prophylaxis.[67]

In the event that MVP is suspected, the American Heart Association recommends that if:[67]

1) A distinctive murmur or click suggestive of mitral value regurgitation is

---

Table 14-17 PROCEDURES REQUIRING ANTIBIOTIC PROPHYLAXIS IN AT-RISK INDIVIDUALS WITH MITRAL VALVE PROLAPSE[67,68,69,71]

Indicated	Not Indicated
Tonsils, adenoids	Endotracheal intubation
Surgery involving respiratory mucosa	Flexible bronchoscopy with or without biopsy
Bronchoscopy with rigid scope	Tympanostomy tube insertion
Sclerotherapy for esophageal varices	Endoscopy with or without biopsy
Esophageal stricture dilation	Intrauterine device insertion and removal
Endoscopic retrograde cholangiography with biliary obstruction	Vaginal hysterectomy
Biliary tract surgery	Vaginal delivery
Surgery involving intestinal mucosa	Caesarian delivery
Cystoscopy	Incision of surgically scrubbed skin
Urethral dilation	Urethral catheterization
Dental extractions	Uterine dilation and curettage
Dental cleaning with expected bleeding	Therapeutic abortion
Periodontal procedures	Sterilization
Implants	Dental X-rays
Root canal	Fluoride treatment
	Restorative dentistry

heard, the patient should receive antibiotic prophylaxis.

2) Regurgitation is suspected or cannot be ruled out, prophylaxis should be given if the procedure is urgent, considered invasive, and time or resources are not available to obtain confirmatory testing.

3) Testing is completed and no regurgitation or echocardiographic features consistent with regurgitation or abnormal valves is found, prophylaxis is not needed and should not be given.

Special Considerations

During pregnancy there is an increase of 50% in the circulating blood volume producing the systolic flow murmur that is so common in pregnancy. Echocardiography also demonstrates a slight increase in the size of all four cardiac chambers. The chamber enlargement may persist for 6 months or more postpartum and may be reflective of the maternal weight gain. Late in pregnancy and while lactating, many women have a so-called mammary soufflé. This murmur is secondary to the increased blood flow in the breasts and can be heard in both systole and diastole anywhere in the breast. Women who have valvular lesions that restrict CO are referred to a cardiologist when pregnant.[45] **Table 14-19** lists the differential diagnoses for heart murmurs.

Varicose Veins

The venous circulation is comprised of a deep system, a superficial system, and a set of perforating veins that direct blood from the superficial system to the deep system within the calf. The deep system handles approximately 80% to 90% of venous return and is composed of the femoral, popliteal, and tibial veins. The superficial system is comprised of the greater and lesser saphenous veins and their branches; these veins drain into the deep system. The saphenous veins lie in the subcutaneous tissue where they are more susceptible to trauma. The perforating veins direct blood flow between the superficial system to the deep system within the calf. They are also referred to as the communicating veins.

Table 14-18 ANTIBIOTICS USED FOR ENDOCARDITIS PROPHYLAXIS IN AT-RISK INDIVIDUALS[39,67,68]

Clinical Procedure	Drug & Dose	Penicillin Allergy
Dental, oral, respiratory, esophageal	Amoxicillin 2 g	Clindamycin 600 mg Cephalexin 2 g Azithromycin 500 mg
Genitourinary, non–esophageal gastrointestinal procedures		
Moderate risk women	Amoxicillin 2 g	Vancomycin 1 g IV
High risk women	Add Gentomycin to Amoxicillin or vancomycin	

Table 14-19 DIFFERENTIAL DIAGNOSIS OF HEART MURMURS[24,70,71]

Systolic Murmurs
  Flow Murmurs: Ejection Murmurs, Innocent
    Murmurs
  Aortic Sclerosis
  Aortic Stenosis
  Mitral Valve Prolapse
  Pulmonic Stenosis
  Ventricular Septal Defect
Diastolic Murmurs
  Aortic Regurgitation
  Mitral Stenosis
Both Systolic and Diastolic Murmurs
  Pericardial Rub
  Patent Ductus Arteriosus
  Venous Hum

These veins have valves that prevent retrograde flow of the blood.

Varicose veins affect the superficial veins of the legs. The etiology of varicose veins is unclear, but both genetic and environmental factors seem to play a role. They may be the result of a venous abnormality such as a structural weakness of the vein wall or an incompetent venous valve. In some people, poorly functioning valves cause an abnormal flow toward the superficial system. Over time the veins widen, elongate, and become tortuous. Factors such as a history of trauma may make the patient more susceptible to varicose veins. Other conditions such as pregnancy and obesity often can cause varicose veins, secondary to a rise in the intraluminal venous pressure. The greater saphenous system is more commonly involved; thus, varicosities are often noted in the medial and anterior thigh, calf, and ankle region. Varicosities located in the posterior calf and the lateral ankle regions are attributed to the lesser saphenous system.

Evaluation

Varicose veins are the most common manifestation of chronic venous disease. Prevalence increases with age. Varicose veins affect both men and women; however, women more commonly seek medical advice because of cosmetic concerns. Many patients complain of a range of symptoms such as heaviness in the legs, aching, burning, swelling, leg cramps, or itching. Patients usually awaken without symptoms; however, their symptoms may become progressively worse through the day. These symptoms are usually worse with standing and improve with walking and elevation. Women complain of worsening symptoms premenstrually, suggesting a hormonal influence. In rare instances, the varicosities are so severe that ulcerations or superficial thrombophlebitis may occur.

An appropriate history includes age of onset, family history of varicose veins, any personal history of leg trauma, deep vein thrombosis (DVT) or lower extremity surgery, and prior pregnancies. It is also important to note any aggravating or alleviating factors in the patient's self-management. The physical examination includes the patient's height, weight, and BMI. The extremities are evaluated for the location and extent of the varicosities. Veins should be mapped, noting the size and exact location after the patient has been standing for five to ten minutes.

Management

Patients seek medical intervention for varicose veins for two reasons: symptom relief and better cosmetic appearance. Without intervention varicosities will worsen over time. Benefit can be derived from simple interventions, including leg elevation and compression stockings. Women should be advised to take frequent breaks during the day to elevate their legs, because this will help to decrease swelling and improve circulation.

Compression stockings are graduated stockings with a higher pressure at the ankle and less pressure proximally to the knee and the thigh. These specially fitted stockings can be obtained at a medical supply pharmacy. Compression stockings work by decreasing the venous pressure, reflux, and residual venous volume of varicosities. However, their benefit only lasts while they are worn. Compression stockings should be put on first thing in the morning when the legs are at their thinnest because the veins are at their lowest pressure. They should be removed each evening. Leg elevation following removal is recommended. The use of regular stockings is not recommended simply because they do not have any extra compression value. Ace bandages wrapped around the legs do not provide any extra support and the level of compression may actually make the varicosities worse; in rare instances they may cause DVT.

In obese women, weight reduction is a significant aspect of the plan of care and should be incorporated at the beginning. Increasing activity as well as changing nutritional habits should be encouraged.

Invasive treatments such as sclerotherapy and surgery are available, but a full course of conservative treatment should be attempted before seeking surgical intervention. Veins should also be evaluated by Doppler ultrasound of the affected extremity. Sclerotherapy has been used with variable success. There is a 65% recurrence rate within five years. The best success occurs in cases where the primary varicose veins

are small and there is no evidence of proximal venous incompetence. Sclerotherapy is contraindicated in women who are obese, pregnant, have large veins, or reflux. The technique involves injecting hypertonic saline into the lumen of the vein. Pressure dressings are then applied and need to be left in place for several weeks. The solution causes an inflammatory reaction that produces fibrosis and obliteration of the vein lumen. Surgery is indicated in cases when the varicosities are large, symptomatic, and cosmetically troubling. The recurrence rate is approximately 20%.[48]

Deep Vein Thrombosis

Untreated, DVT may progress to pulmonary embolus, which is life threatening. Nearly a half a million people are diagnosed with DVT annually. The cause of acute thrombosis formation in the venous system is unclear but, in most instances, factors contributing to the three basic elements of Virchow's triad (intimal damage, stasis, and hypercoagulability) can be identified. Vessel wall injury contributes to DVT after trauma or surgery that damages the vascular lining. Venous stasis occurs when there is immobility, such as with paralysis or an orthopedic injury. Stasis may also occur when there is slow venous flow from proximal obstruction occurring with slow growing tumors or pregnancy. Less common are hypercoagulopathies such as the lupus anticoagulant/antiphospholipid antibody syndrome.

Evaluation

Because the clinical presentation of a DVT may be subtle, the physical examination may not be sufficient to diagnose DVT. The patient may complain of lower extremity tightness or aching with activity that is relieved with rest and elevation. The differential diagnosis includes Baker's cyst, osteoarthritis, muscle injury, or cellulitis. Risk factors for developing a DVT include obesity, tobacco use, hypertension, varicose veins, pregnancy, and oral contraceptive use. The presence of unilateral leg edema is a sensitive indicator of DVT. Edema may be noted distal to the level of the DVT. The involved area may be warm and tender to the touch and erythematous in color; a thrombosed vein may be palpable as a superficial cord. Pain may be elicited with compression of the knee. Homan's sign, that is, the presence of calf pain with dorsiflexion of the foot, may be positive.

Duplex scanning and contrast venography are commonly used to make the diagnosis. The duplex scan is a two-dimensional ultrasound and Doppler ultrasound that compresses the vein to assess for any changes in venous flow. The lack of compressibility of the thigh vein and abnormal Doppler color flow are highly specific for a DVT. Serial studies may be needed in cases where the ultrasound is negative but the physical examination is clinically consistent with DVT. Contrast venography is the definitive technique for diagnosing DVT and is considered the gold standard. However, this invasive test is so uncomfortable for the patient that it is difficult to obtain a quality study. There is also a small risk of phlebitis. It is technically unsuccessful in up to 20% of patients and requires considerable expertise for both its performance and interpretation.[48]

Special Considerations

Pregnancy and the postpartum period are well-established risk factors for DVT. The risk of DVT is present throughout pregnancy and increases in the third trimester. One possibility for this is that during this time all three of Virchow's triad may be present. The stasis is due to the compression of the large veins because of the gravid uterus. Endothelial injury may occur with the delivery itself and can be associated with vascular injury and changes at the uteroplacental surface. This might exaggerate the vascular intimal injury and increase the risk of DVT postpartum. Hypercoagulability is also associated with pregnancy. Any woman with prior DVT has increased risk. There are more reports of DVT during pregnancy in the left leg as opposed to the right leg. This may be due to increased venous stasis in the left leg because of the disproportionate pressure on the left iliac vein by the gravid uterus. The rate is higher after a Cesarean section than with a vaginal birth. DVT is also seen more frequently with advanced maternal age.

Diagnosis during pregnancy is generally confined to physical examination findings and the duplex ultrasound. The ultrasound results can be difficult to interpret because of the venous compression of the uterus. Treatment during pregnancy is complicated by risks to the mother and fetus. Oral anticoagulants, such as warfarin, cross the placenta and are contraindicated because they enter the fetal circulation. Parenteral medications such as heparin do not cross the placenta and do not appear to pose any added risk to the mother unless administrated within 24 hours prior to delivery. Then there may be an increased risk of maternal hemorrhage.

Women who use combined hormonal contraceptives are at risk for developing DVT; the risk is highest during the first year of use. First-generation oral contraceptive pills (OCPs), which were removed from the market in 1989, had more than 50 µg of estrogen and posed a significant risk for DVT and PE. Second-generation OCPs introduced in 1967 have less than 50 μg of estrogen. The third-generation OCPs contain the new progestins, desogestrel and gestodene, which have been shown to double or triple the risk of thromboembolic disease when compared with the second-generation oral contraceptives. The possible explanation for this is that third-generation oral contraceptives lead to acquired resistance to activated protein C, the most potent endogenous anticoagulant. This being said, the overall risk is still low. Healthy women are still excellent candidates for using OCPs but consideration should be given to starting on a second-generation preparation. Third generation agents, which are less androgenic, should be used only in women who also have acne or hirsutism. Women with a prior history of DVT or any other thrombophilia should not use oral contraceptives or other combined hormonal contraceptive (CHC) methods. Women with underlying medical conditions that increase their risk, such as obesity, hypertension, or tobacco use, should be carefully screened before prescribing CHC methods. Originally it was thought that women on MHT were not at risk for DVT because the dose of estrogen was so much lower than with OCPs. After the 2002 Women's Health Initiative,[10] it became apparent that even at the lower doses of estrogen, women were at significant risk for thromboembolic events including DVT, stroke, and myocardial infarction. Women on MHT need to have a full explanation of the risks of estrogen use that must be balanced against the severity of symptoms of menopause.[7,70] Women must be assessed for DVT with the same vigilance as women on CHC.

Conclusion

Raising awareness of heart disease in women is an essential role for midwives and women's health providers. Lifestyle interventions are effective in preventing CVD in all individuals regardless of their underlying risk(s). They have been deemed Class I Recommendations (useful and effective) by the American Heart Association's Evidence-Based Guidelines for Cardiovascular Disease Prevention in Women.[1] Raising women's awareness of the power of lifestyle modifications must begin as early as childhood and should be stressed as much as prenatal care, safer sex, and consistent contraception use from the very beginning of a young woman's reproductive years. Minority and elderly women have the least information about heart disease and need better access to care, risk assessment, and education.[1] Women's health providers are in an ideal position to teach the importance of good nutrition, healthy weight, and daily exercise before chronic diseases arise in middle adulthood. Evaluation of a woman's risks and encouragement for her to adopt or maintain healthy behaviors must be a routine part of every health care visit.

References

1. Mosca L, Appel L, Benjamin E, et al. Evidence-based guidelines for cardiovascular disease prevention in women. *Circulation.* 2004;109:672–693.
2. Diehl Y. Unclear and present danger. *Adv Nurse Pract.* 2002;10(10):73–78.
3. United States Department of Health and Human Services, National Heart, Lung and Blood Institute. *Third Report of the National Cholesterol Education Program (NCEP) Expert Panel on Detection, Evaluation, and Treatment of High Blood Cholesterol in Adults (Adult*

Treatment Plan III) Executive Summary. NIH Publication no. 01-3670. Washington, DC: NIH; May 2001.

4. Franklin SS, Khan SA, Wong ND, Larson MG, Levy D. Is pulse pressure useful in predicting risk for coronary heart disease? The Framingham Heart Study. *Circulation.* 1999;100:354–360.

5. Domanski M, Mitchell G, Pfeffer M, Neaton JD, Norman J, Svendsen K, et al. Pulse pressure and cardiovascular disease-related mortality: Follow-up study of the Multiple Risk Factor Intervention Trial (MRFIT). *JAMA.* 2002;287:2677–2683.

6. Ehrmann DA. Polycystic ovary syndrome. *N Engl J Med.* 2005;352:1223–1236.

7. Rousseau M. Hormone replacement therapy: Short-term versus long-term use. *J Midwifery Women's Health.* 2002;47:461–470.

8. Agency for Healthcare Research and Quality. United States Preventive Services Task Force. *Screening for Lipid Disorders in Adults.* [release date 2001] Available from: http://www.ahrq.gov/clinic/uspstf/uspschol.htm.

9. Venugopal SK, Devaraj S, Jialal I. Effect of C-reactive protein on vascular cells: Evidence for a proinflammatory, proatherogenic role. *Curr Opin Nephrol Hypertens.* 2005;14:33–37.

10. Rossouw JE, Anderson GL, Prentice RL, LaCroix AZ, Kooperberg C, Stefanick ML, et al. Risks and benefits of estrogen plus progestin in healthy postmenopausal women: Principal results from the Women's Health Initiative randomized controlled trial. *JAMA.* 2002;288:321–333.

11. Hirao-Try Y. Hypertension and women: Gender specific differences. *Clin Excell Nurse Pract.* 2003;7:4–8.

12. August P. Initial treatment of hypertension. *N Engl J Med.* 2003;348:610–617.

13. Mayet J, Hughes A. Cardiac and vascular pathophysiology in hypertension. *Heart.* 2003;89:1104–1109.

14. Struijker Boudier HAJ, Cohuet GMS, Baumann M, Safar ME. The heart, macrocirculation and microcirculation in hypertension: A unifying hypothesis. *J Hypertens.* 2003;21 suppl 3:S19–23.

15. Darne B, Girerd X, Safar M, Cambien F, Guize L. Pulsatile versus steady component of blood pressure: A cross-sectional analysis and a prospective analysis on cardiovascular mortality. *Hypertension.* 1989;13:392–400.

16. Dart AM, Kingwell BA. Pulse pressure—a review of mechanisms and clinical relevance. *J Am Coll Cardiol.* 2001;37:975–984.

17. Franklin SS. Cardiovascular risks related to increased diastolic, systolic and pulse pressure. An epidemiologist's point of view. *Pathol Biol* (Paris). 1999;47:594–603.

18. Haider AW, Larson MG, Franklin SS, Levy D. Framingham Heart Study. Systolic blood pressure, diastolic blood pressure, and pulse pressure as predictors of risk for congestive heart failure in the Framingham Heart Study. *Ann Intern Med.* 2003;138:10–16.

19. Lookinland S, Beckstrand L. Evidence-based treatment of hypertension. *Adv Nurse Pract.* 2003;11:32–39.

20. Chobanian A, Bakris G, Black HR, Cushman WC, Green LA, Izzo JLJ, et al. The Seventh Report of the Joint National Committee on Prevention, Detection, Evaluation, and Treatment of High Blood Pressure: The JNC 7 Report. *JAMA.* 2003;289:2560–2572.

21. The ALLHAT Officers and Coordinators for the ALLHAT Collaborative Research Group. Major outcomes in high-risk hypertensive patients randomized to angiotensin-converting enzyme inhibitor or calcium channel blocker vs. diuretic. *JAMA.* 2002;288:2981–2997.

22. Wing L, Reid C, Ryan P, et al. A comparison of outcomes with angiotensin-converting-enzyme inhibitors and diuretics for hypertension in the elderly. *N Engl J Med.* 2003;348:583–592.

23. National Heart Lung and Blood Institute. Seventh Report of the Joint National Committee on Prevention, Detection, Evaluation, and Treatment of High Blood Pressure (JNC 7). [monograph on the Internet]. Available from: http://www.nhlbi.nih.gov/guidelines/hypertension/jnc7full.htm.

24. Goroll A, Mulley A, May L. Cardiovascular problems. In: *Primary Care Medicine: Office Evaluation and Management of the Adult Patient.* Philadelphia: Lippincott Williams and Wilkins; 2000. pp. 69–211.

25. Mayet J, Coats AJ. Diagnosis and investigation of essential and secondary hypertension. *European Heart Journal.* 1998;19(3):372–377.

26. Onusko E. Diagnosing secondary hypertension. *American Family Physician.* 2003;67(1):67–74.

27. Schapera CH. Potential causes of secondary hypertension. *American Family Physician.* 2003;68(1):42.

28. McFadden C, Townsend R. Blood pressure measurement: Common pitfalls and how to avoid them. *Consultant.* 2003;43:161–165.

29. Pickering T. Recommendations for the use of home (self) and ambulatory blood pressure monitoring.

American Society of Hypertension Ad Hoc Panel. *Am J Hypertens*. 1996;9:1–11.

30. Karanja N, Erlinger TP, Pao-Hwa L, Miller ER, Bray GA. The DASH diet for high blood pressure: From clinical trial to dinner table. *Cleve Clin J Med*. 2004; 71:745–753.

31. National Heart, Lung and Blood Institute, National High Blood Pressure Education Program. JNC 7 Express. *The Seventh Report of Joint National Committee on the Prevention, Detection, Evaluation and Treatment of High Blood Pressure*. NIH Publication No. 03-5233, December 2003.

32. National Heart, Lung and Blood Institute, National Cholesterol Education Program. *Third Report of the National Cholesterol Education Program Expert Panel on Detection, Evaluation, and Treatment of High Blood Cholesterol in Adults (Adult Treatment Panel III) Final Report*. NIH Publication No. 02-5215. Washington, DC: NIH; 2002. Accessible on the Internet. http://www.nhlbi.nih.gov/guidelines/cholesterol/atp_iii.htm.

33. Harsha DW, Sacks FM, Obarzanek E, Svetkey LP, Lin PH, Bray GA, et al. Effect of dietary sodium intake on blood lipids: Results from the DASH-sodium trial. *Hypertension*. 2004;43:393–398.

34. Rimm EB. Stampfer MJ. Diet, lifestyle, and longevity—the next steps? *JAMA* 2004;292:1490–1492.

35. Panagiotakos DB, Pitsavos CH, Chrysohoou C, Skoumas J, Papadimitriou L, Stefanadis C, et al. Status and management of hypertension in Greece: Role of the adoption of a Mediterranean diet: The Attica study. *J Hypertens*. 2003;21(8):1483–1489.

36. Murphy J. Nurse practitioners prescribing reference. *Prescribing Reference*. 2004;11(1):3–5.

37. PDR staff. 2004 Physician's Desk Reference with PDR electronic library on CD-ROM. Washington, DC: Thompson PDR; 2003.

38. Hernandez RH, Armas-Hernandez MJ, Velasco M, Israili ZH, Armas-Padilla MC. Calcium antagonists and atherosclerosis protection in hypertension. *Am J Therap*. 2003;10:409–414.

39. Hayek E. Griffin B. Mitral valve prolapse: Old beliefs yield to new knowledge. *Cleve Clin J Med*. 2002;69:889–896.

40. Martins D, Norris K. Hypertension treatment in African Americans: Physiology is less important than sociology. *Cleve Clin J Med*. 2004;71:735–743.

41. World Health Organization (WHO) *Medical Eligibility Criteria for Contraceptive Use*, 3rd ed. 2004. Available from: http://www.who.int/reproductive health/publications/mec/mec.pdf.

42. Mueck AO, Seeger H. Effect of hormone therapy on BP in normotensive and hypertensive postmenopausal women. *Maturitas*. 2004;49:189–203.

43. National Institutes of Health, National Heart, Lung and Blood Institute, National High Blood Pressure Education Program. *Working group report on high blood pressure in pregnancy*. NIH Publication No. 00-3029. Washington, DC: NIH; 2000.

44. Gabbe S, Niebyl J, Simpson J. Hypertension. In: *Obstetrics: Normal and Problem Pregnancies*. New York: Churchill Livingstone; 2002.

45. Setaro JF, Caulin-Glaser T. Pregnancy and cardiovascular disease. In: Burrow GN, Duffy TP, Copel JA, editors. *Medical Complications during Pregnancy*. 6th ed. Philadelphia: Elsevier Saunders, 2004. pp. 103–129.

46. James PR, Nelson-Piercy C. Management of hypertension before, during, and after pregnancy. *Heart*. 2004;90:1499–1504.

47. Lindheimer M, Roberts J, Cunningham F, Chesley L. Introduction, history, controversies, and definitions. In: Lindheimer M, Cunningham F, Roberts J, editors. *Chesley's Hypertensive Disorders in Pregnancy*. 2nd ed. Saddle River, NJ: Prentice Hall; 1999. pp. 3–41.

48. Leppert P, Peipert J. Cardiovascular system. In: *Primary Care for Women*. Philadelphia: Lippincott Williams and Wilkins; 2004. pp. 267–337.

49. Rexrode K, Iso H, Stampfer M, Manson J, Colditz G, Speizer F, et al. Intake of fish and omega-3 fatty acids and risk of stroke in women. *JAMA*. 2001;285:304–312.

50. Environmental Protection Agency. Fish Advisories: What you need to know about mercury in fish and shellfish, 2004. EPA and FDA advice for women who might become pregnant, women who are pregnant, nursing mothers, young children. [Monogram found on the Internet]. Available from: http://epa.gov/waterscience/fishadvice/advice.html.

51. Osganian S, Stampfer M, Rimm E, Spiegelman D, Hu F, et al. Vitamin C and risk of coronary heart disease in women. *Am Coll Cardiol*. 2003;42:246–252.

52. American Heart Association. American Heart Association leaders testify on Hill. *Advocacy News*. June 6, 2002. Available from: http://www.americanheart.org/presenter.jhtml?identifier=3002938.

53. Endoy M. CVD in women: Risk factors and clinical presentation. *J Am Acad Nurse Pract*. 2004;8:33–39.

54. Hansen M. *Pathophysiology: Foundations of Disease and Clinical Intervention*. Philadelphia: WB Saunders; 1998.

55. Leake N. The heart of the matter: National guidelines urge more aggressive cholesterol treatment. *Adv Nurse Pract*. 2002;10:42–47.

56. Grundy S, Leeman J, Bairey Merz C, Brewer H, Clark L, Hunninghake D, et al. Implications of recent clinical trials for the national cholesterol education program adult treatment panel III guidelines. *Circulation*. 2004;110:227–239.

57. U.S. Department of Health and Human Services. *Physical Activity and Health: A Report of the Surgeon General*. Atlanta, GA: U.S. Department of Health and Human Services, Centers for Disease Control and Prevention, National Center for Chronic Disease Prevention and Health Promotion, 1996.

58. Meagher EA. Addressing cardiovascular disease in women: Focus on dyslipidemia. *J Am Board Fam Pract*. 2004;17:424–437.

59. Morimoto S, Fujioka Y, Tsutsumi C, Masai M, Okumra T, Yuba M, et al. Mizoribine-induced rhabdomyloysis in rheumatoid arthritis patient receiving bezafibrate treatment. *Am J Med Sci*. 2005;329:211–213.

60. Mody F. Combining mechanisms of action of drugs used in the management of dyslipidemia to achieve treatment goals. *Lipid Management Today*. 2004 September.

61. Berra K. Clinical update on the use of niacin for the treatment of dyslipidemia. *J Am Acad Nurse Pract*. 2004;14:526–534.

62. Scott C. Diagnosis, prevention, and intervention for the metabolic syndrome. *Am J Cardiol*. 2003;92(1a):35–42.

63. Napoli C, Glass C, Witztum J, et al. Influence of maternal hypercholesterolaemia during pregnancy on progression of early atherosclerotic lesions in childhood: Fate of early lesions in children (FELIC) study. *Lancet*. 1999;354:1234–1240.

64. Weiner C, Buhimschi C. *Drugs for Pregnant and Lactating Women*. London: Churchill Livingston; 2003.

65. Beery TA. Gender bias in the diagnosis and treatment of coronary artery disease. *Heart Lung*. 1995;24:427–435.

66. Seidel H, Ball J, Dains J, Benedict G. *Mosby's Guide to Physical Examination*. St. Louis: Mosby; 2003.

67. Dajani AS, Taubert KA, Wilson W, Bolger AF, Bayer A, Ferrieri P, et al. Prevention of bacterial endocarditis: Recommendations by the American Heart Association. *Clin Infect Dis*. 1997;25:1448–1458.

68. Triezenberg D, Helmen J, Pearson M, Bercaw DM. Clinical inquiries. When should patients with mitral valve prolapse get endocarditis prophylaxis? *J Fam Pract*. 2004;53:223–228.

69. Grimes DA. Schulz KF. Antibiotic prophylaxis for intrauterine contraceptive device insertion. *Cochrane Database of Systematic Reviews*. (2):CD001327, 2001.

70. Hackley B, Rousseau ME. Managing menopausal symptoms after the women's health initiative. *J Midwifery Women's Health*. 2004;49(2):87–95.

71. Swartz, M, editor. The heart. In: *Textbook of Physical Diagnosis*. WB Saunders Company: Philadelphia; 2002. pp. 345–390.

Chapter 15

Anemias

Kimberly
Updegrove

Anemia is defined as a lower than normal number of red blood cells (RBCs) in the blood, usually measured as a decrease in the concentration of hemoglobin (Hb), the iron-rich protein in the blood that carries oxygen to all cells, and hematocrit (Hct), the relative concentration of the solid constituents of the blood. Anemia is not a diagnosis in and of itself, but a symptom of an underlying condition. The finding of lower than expected Hb or Hct should lead the health care provider to explore the possible diagnoses that lead to abnormal laboratory values.

Anemia is common in the United States, with the highest rates seen among young women (4.5%) and elderly men (4.8%).[1] The Centers for Disease Control and Prevention (CDC) estimates that 10% of nonpregnant women of childbearing age have iron deficiency, and 3% have iron deficiency anemia.[2] 6.3% of pregnant women are iron deficient in the first trimester, a number that rises to 30% during the third trimester.[3] Risks to the fetus increase with maternal iron deficiency anemia; a study by Scholl and colleagues demonstrated an adjusted odds ratio of 3.1 (CI 1.16-4.39) for preterm delivery and an AOR of 2.66 (CI 1.15-6.17) for low birth weight as a result of iron deficiency anemia.[4]

Although anemia is found in all populations, the underlying etiologies vary by race. Certain inherited red cell disorders occur more frequently in specific populations, such as sickle cell disease in persons of African descent, beta thalassemia in those of Mediterranean heritage, and alpha thalassemia in Asians and African Americans. In the United States, anemia is more common among African Americans, Native Americans, natives of Alaska, immigrants from developing countries, and people of lower socioeconomic status.[5,6] While genetics accounts for some of these differences, it does not completely explain why rates of anemia vary so dramatically between different populations. Untangling how genetics, nutrition, and the environment interact and lead to anemia is a focus of ongoing research, as is attempting to understand the specific health consequences of anemia in different populations.[2,7]

Primary care practitioners need to be comfortable identifying and treating anemias and hemoglobinopathies, especially those that occur most frequently. This chapter provides midwives and women's health providers the background needed to understand the pathophysiology, clinical presentation, diagnostic methods, and management of the most common anemias.

Physiology

The erythrocyte, or red blood cell (RBC), carries oxygen to tissues. Each RBC is a biconcave disk. RBCs are manufactured in the bone marrow; *erythropoiesis*, the term for RBC formation, is controlled by a complex set of feedback loops. In general, an increased supply of RBCs in circulating body fluids inhibits erythropoesis and anemia stimulates it.[8] *Erythropoietin*, which is produced in the fetal liver as well as in the adult kidneys and liver in response to hypoxia, stimulates the bone marrow to manufacture RBCs. Bone marrow stem cells go through a series of transformations that ultimately lead to the release of *reticulocytes*, the youngest mature form of RBCs. RBCs continue to mature for one to two days after their release into the blood circulation.

RBCs contain Hb, which is the portion of the RBC that binds with oxygen. Hb is formed only during the early stages of RBC maturation. Mature RBCs are incapable of producing Hb because they lack the necessary protein-synthesizers found only in reticulocytes. Because of this, if Hb is damaged during the production or maturation of an RBC, then it cannot be repaired later. Mature RBCs lack a nucleus; they are incapable of repairing damage from aging or trauma. Consequently, RBCs have a limited lifespan. Certain elements, such as iron and vitamin B_{12}, are necessary for the production and maturation of RBCs. Inadequate dietary intake, depleted physiologic stores, or inflammation (which blocks the release of iron from the reticuloendothelial system) can lead to inadequate levels of critical RBC building materials and result in anemia. Normal RBC production depends on having a functioning bone marrow, adequate erythropoietin level (which is dependent on functioning liver and kidneys in the adult), and the availability of all essential substrates. **Figure 15-1** is a flowchart of the life cycle of RBCs.

Hb is composed of two sections: the *heme* and the *globin*. The heme portion is made up of an iron atom in the center of a protoporphyrin ring. Each section of hemoglobin contains four heme groups, and these are responsible for giving the blood its red color and for carrying oxygen within the blood cell. The globin portion is composed of protein and contains four polypeptide chains. **Figure 15-2** illustrates the hemoglobin molecule. Differences among types of hemoglobin lie in the sequencing and kinds of amino acids that make up the chains. Normal adult RBCs contain approximately 97.5% hemoglobin A1, which is composed of two alpha and two beta chains. The remainder of the hemoglobin in normal adult erythrocytes is hemoglobin A2, which has two alpha and two delta chains. The alpha chains remain the same as in hemoglobin A1, but delta chains are substituted for beta chains. A normal variant, fetal hemoglobin, or Hb F, is found in large amounts in the human fetus. Its structure is similar to hemoglobin A1, except that gamma chains replace the beta chains. It has a higher affinity for oxygen, thus facilitating the movement of oxygen from the mother's circulation to her fetus. Hb F is normally replaced by Hb A soon after birth of the infant. **Table 15-1** describes the normal Hb variants.

RBCs live an average of 120 days. At the end of their life span, macrophages of the reticuloendothelial system in the liver, spleen, and lymph nodes destroy the aging RBCs by cleaving the globin and heme portions of the hemoglobin molecule. Globin is further digested down to

Figure 15-1 Life cycle of red blood cells (RBCs).

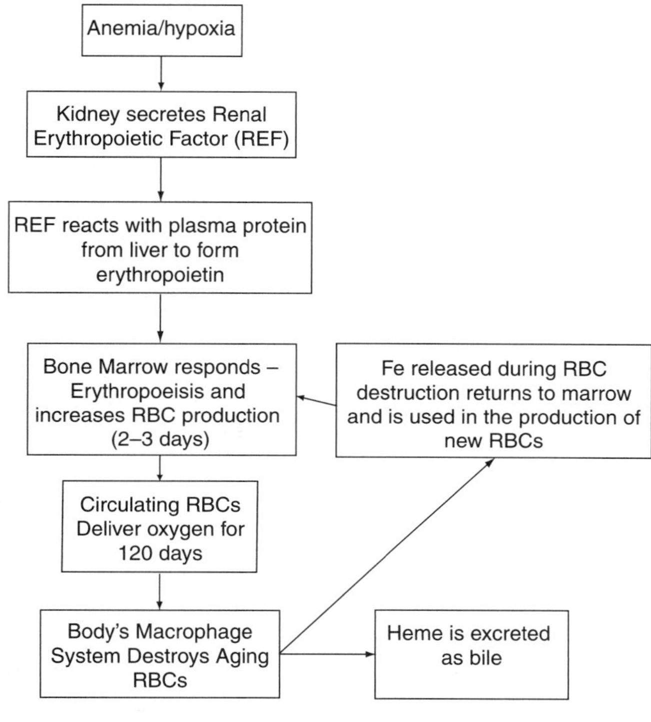

Abbreviation is: fe, iron

amino acids, which then are utilized by the phagocytes for protein synthesis or released into the blood. The heme is first converted to biliverdin (green pigment) and then to bilirubin (yellow pigment), which is then excreted in bile. Iron from the heme is returned to the bone marrow and reused in the production of new RBCs. Recycled iron from Hb catabolism is essential to Hb synthesis.

Hemoglobinopathies

Inherited disorders can affect either the globin portion of the Hb, as in the hemoglobinopathies, or the heme portion of the Hb, as in the sideroblastic anemias and porphyrias. *Porphyrias*, such as erythropoietic protoporphyria, are a group of disorders in which abnormal genetic pathways lead to deficiencies in the production of essential enzymes needed for the synthesis of heme. Excessive levels of metabolic intermediates are produced and build up in the skin, urine, serum, or other tissues, causing symptoms such as abdominal pain, neurologic changes, hyperbilirubinemia, photosensitivity, and other complications. Many sideroblastic anemias are caused by unknown genetic abnormalities that affect heme production. These

Figure 15-2 Hemoglobin molecule and red blood cells (RBCs).

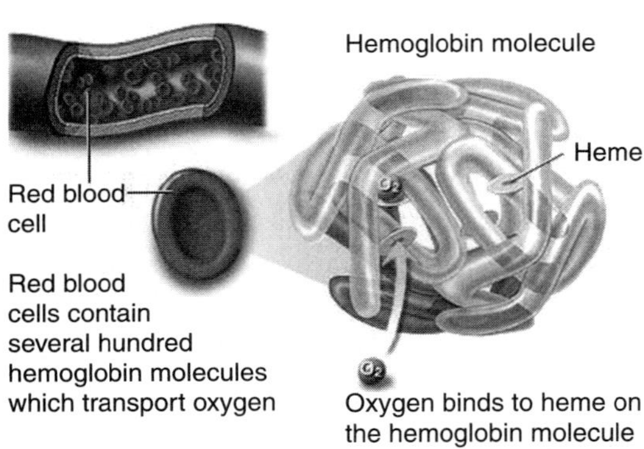

Source: Reprinted from the National Library of Medicine, National Institutes of Health (http://www.nlm.nih. govmedlineplus/ency/imagepages/19510.htm).

conditions are relatively rare compared to the hemoglobinopathies.

Hemoglobinopathies are caused by genetic defects that result in an abnormal hemoglobin structure. These structural flaws fall into three categories:

- Structural defects can be present in the Hb molecule. Alterations in the gene for one of the two Hb subunit chains— alpha or beta—are called mutations. Often, mutations change a single amino acid building block in the subunit, and are innocuous. Sometimes, as with sickle cell anemia, this single change produces a disease state.

- Diminished production of one of the two Hb subunit chains can occur. In normal Hb, equal numbers of alpha and beta chains are necessary for normal function. Imbalances damage RBCs, making them vulnerable to destruction and causing anemia.

- Abnormal associations of otherwise normal subunits can occur. Normally, one alpha subunit and one beta subunit combine to produce a normal Hb dimer. With severe alpha thalassemia, for instance, the beta globin subunits begin to associate into groups of four (called *tetramers*) because of diminished alpha chain partners. These tetramers are functionally inactive and are incapable of binding with oxygen. In severe beta-thalassemia, alpha globin subunits rapidly degrade because of a lack of a partner from the beta globin gene cluster.

In combination, these abnormalities lead to increased destruction of more fragile RBCs, and to a lesser extent they impair RBC production, resulting in significant anemia.

Table 15-1 NORMAL HEMOGLOBIN

Hb A1	Normal adult	2 alpha chains; 2 beta chains	Up to 98% in adults
Hb A2	Normal adult	2 alpha chains; 2 delta chains	Up to 3% in adults
Hb F	Normal fetus and early infancy	2 alpha chains; 2 gamma chains	May continue in small amounts throughout life

Abnormal Hb chains and the resulting hemoglobinopathies are differentiated by letter. If an offspring inherits an abnormal gene for Hb from only one parent, the individual is *heterozygous*, meaning that one-half of the circulating hemoglobin is normal and one-half is abnormal. Individuals with the sickle cell trait have inherited normal Hb A from one parent and Hb S from the other. Sickle cell trait is an example of a heterozygous presentation. When identical abnormal genes are inherited from both parents, the offspring is *homozygous* and all of the Hb is abnormal; this is the case, for example, in those with sickle cell disease.

Not all Hb abnormalities are harmful, and some may cause only mild-to-moderate anemia. However, some mutations can be so harmful that individuals cannot survive long enough to pass on these mutations to future generations. Consequently, harmful mutations tend to die out, but those that confer survival value persist and can become widespread in the population.[8] The sickle cell gene is an example. Hb S, which is found in those with sickle trait or disease, is insoluble at low oxygen tensions. Hypoxia changes the shape of the normally biconcave RBC to a sickle shape. These abnormal cells hemolyze, which produces anemia and causes stasis in the microcirculation, leading to significant end-organ damage. The sickle gene originated in African populations and confers resistance to malaria in those with heterozygous presentations. While many individuals with sickle disease historically died before reaching reproductive age, those with the trait are commonly unaffected, live normal healthy lives, and pass on the gene to their offspring. Offspring who inherit the trait benefit from the protective effect this gene carries against malaria and, at

the same time, avoid the devastating consequences of sickle disease, which is the result of the homozygous expression of Hb S. In some areas of Africa, 40% of the population carries the trait; among African Americans, its incidence is about 10%.[8] **Table 15-2** provides other examples of clinically significant variant homozygous Hb.

It is possible to inherit two different abnormal Hb genes: one each from the mother and father. The resulting anemia is known as a *compound heterozygous variant anemia*. Among the more common of these are Hb SC disease, sickle/beta thalassemia, Hb E/beta thalassemia, and alpha thalassemia/Hb constant spring. Some of these anemias have mild presentations; others are disabling. The severity of the presentations of these conditions depends on which amino acid(s) are altered. **Table 15-3** describes the most common heterozygous conditions.

Classification of Anemia

There are two classification systems used to describe anemia. One is based on the underlying cause of the anemia such as acute or chronic blood loss, RBC destruction, or malfunction in RBC production or maturation. The other system describes anemia by the size, shape, and color of the RBC. Both approaches help focus the investigation of the cause of anemia for the individual patient.

Etiology

Three categories are used to describe the functional causes of anemia: proliferative disorders, maturational disorders, and hemolytic disorders.

Table 15-2 CLINICALLY SIGNIFICANT VARIANT HOMOZYGOUS HEMOGLOBINS

Type of Hb	Diagnosis	Clinical Implications	Notes
Hb C	Hb C disease	Mild hemolytic anemia/splenomegaly	Trait is benign. Target cells are seen on peripheral smear.
Hb S	Sickle cell disease	Potentially life-threatening disease	Trait is benign.
Hb E	Hb E disease	Mild microcytic anemia/splenomegaly	Trait is benign. Common in southeast Asia. Target cells are seen on peripheral smear.
Hb Constant Spring (Hb CS)	Thalassemia disease	Decreased Hb because of unstable alpha chain protein. Mild anemia.	Named for area of identification: Constant Spring, Jamaica.
Hb H	Hb H disease	Moderately severe hemolytic anemia.	Seen in people with three-gene alpha thalassemia deletion and those with Hb CS. See Hb H and Hb Barts on electrophoresis.
Hb Bart	Hb Bart disease or alpha thalassemia major	Hydrops fetalis—fetal death in utero likely	All four alpha chains are deleted; only gamma chains exist.

Proliferative disorders include those in which production of RBCs is decreased. Examples of proliferative disorders include anemias due to bone marrow failure; reduced levels of hormones such as erythropoietin, thyroid, or androgens needed for RBC production; or insufficient levels of essential nutrients such as iron, folate, and vitamin B_{12}. Bone marrow failure can be the result of exposure to myelotoxic drugs, malignancies of the bone marrow, or chronic diseases. Erythropoietin production is reduced in the presence of renal disease and certain endocrine disorders. Iron may not be available because of the presence of inflammation (which blocks the release of recycled iron removed by the reticuloendothelial system) or from inadequate dietary intake. Iron deficiency, the most common proliferative disorder found in women, is discussed later in this chapter.

Maturational disorders can also lead to anemia. In maturational disorders, the bone marrow functions normally and has all of the essential ingredients needed to produce RBCs, but problems occur in the pathways that allow RBCs to develop normally. Two different processes can lead to maturational disorders: either an essential element (such as vitamin B_{12} or folate) needed for the maturation but not for initial production of

Table 15-3 CLINICALLY SIGNIFICANT VARIANT HETEROZYGOUS HEMOGLOBINS

Type Hemoglobin	Diagnosis	Clinical Implications	Notes
Hb SC	Hb SC disease	Similar to sickle cell disease, but milder	A gene for Hb S is inherited from one parent and the gene for Hb C from the other; ex. 60% Hb C and 40% Hb S.
Hb S; some normal Hb with varying amounts of normal/abnormal beta globin.	Sickle/beta thalassemia. (If there is no normal beta globin, this is sickle/beta0 thalassemia. If there are some normal beta globins, it is sickle/beta+thalassemia.)	Dependent on the quantity of normal Hb produced by the beta-thalassemia gene. If none, symptoms are identical to those of sickle cell anemia. If there are some normal beta globins, symptoms are much milder.	Most common in persons of Mediterranean descent (Italian, Greek, Turkish).
Hb E/beta thalassemia	Thalassemia intermedia	Severe anemia probable.	Most often seen in persons with southeast Asian background.
Hb H/alpha thalassemia	Alpha thalassemia/Hb CS	Anemia	Mutation of alpha globin where both alpha gene clusters are deleted and replaced by Constant Spring and Hb H (formed by beta globin).

RBCs is lacking; or there is a structural defect in the Hb itself (i.e., in the thalassemias) that adversely affects maturation. Anemias that result from genetic or acquired defects in iron metabolism, such as the sideroblastic anemias, also adversely affect RBC maturation.

Hemolytic disorders, or increased RBC breakdown, may occur because of abnormal phagocytic activity or an increased fragmentation, such as warm or cold antibody hemolysis. In warm antibody hemolysis (also called immunoglobulin G [IgG] mediated hemolysis), IgG binds RBCs and macrophages ingest the IgG-bound membrane. This type of hemolysis is seen in patients with diseases such as non-Hodgkin lymphoma, systemic lupus erythematosus, and chronic lymphocytic leukemia. Hemolysis can also result from enzymatic deficiencies on the cellular level such as in glucose-6-phosphate dehydrogenase (G6PD). Severe hemolysis can be accompanied by symptoms such as hepatomegaly, splenomegaly, hematuria, and jaundice.

Anemia can also result from acute or chronic blood loss. Chronic blood loss leads to the loss of recycled iron, depletion of iron stores, and anemia. Usually symptoms are mild until anemia is severe. Acute blood loss is more obvious: frank bleeding, jaundice, and tarry stools may be noted depending on the origin and cause of the blood loss.

Morphology

Anemias are also classified according to size of the RBCs. *Macrocytic anemias* are those in which the mean corpuscular volume (MCV) is larger than normal. Conditions such as hypothyroidism, alcohol abuse, and liver disease, anemias resulting in increased production of reticulocytes (which are normally bigger than fully mature RBCs), and the megaloblastic anemias caused by vitamin B_{12} and folic acid deficiencies can all lead to macrocytosis (the condition in which unusually large number of macrocytes, i.e., large erythrocytes, are in the circulating blood). *Microcytic anemias*, those with smaller than normal RBCs, include iron deficiency anemia, the thalassemias, Hb E disorders, sideroblastic anemia, and lead toxicity. *Normocytic anemias* are those in which the cell size is normal; they are caused by acute blood loss or by hemolytic disorders such as Hb S disease, glucose-6-phosphate dehydrogenase (G6PD) deficiency, aplastic anemia, chronic diseases, and acquired hemolytic anemias.

RBCs also can be described by their color and shape. *Hypochromic anemia*, of which iron deficiency anemia is the most common, results from a reduction in red cell Hb and makes the RBCs appear pale in color. Thalassemia and sickle cell disease, like iron deficiency anemia, are both hypochromic and microcytic. *Normochromic anemias* are those in which the amount of hemoglobin in the cell is normal and, therefore, the color of the RBCs is also normal. Normochromic anemias are most common in conditions where there is acute blood loss or in the early stages of anemia before deficiencies are so low that RBC production is impaired. However, *normochromic normocytic anemias* can herald more significant problems, albeit rarely. If a low white blood cell (WBC) count or if a low platelet count is noted, or if nucleated RBCs or immature WBCs are seen on the peripheral smear, more serious causes such as cancer should be considered and immediate referral for a bone marrow biopsy is warranted. The shape of the RBC also can be quite distinctive in certain anemias and can indicate potential etiologies that should be considered. For example, spherocytes seen on a peripheral smear can indicate an autoimmune hemolytic anemia or an inherited condition called spherocytosis (also hemolytic in nature). The Laboratory section later in this chapter discusses tests that describe the morphological characteristics of anemia.

Routine Screening

Routine screening for anemia is controversial, and authorities differ in their recommendations. Because most anemia in women of childbearing age is related to iron deficiency,[9] the main purpose of anemia screening in this population is to detect those specifically at risk for iron deficiency. The American College of Obstetricians and Gynecologists (ACOG) recommends that Hb levels be measured as part of routine care of the woman with excessive menstrual flow, and for those women over the age of 65 years at high risk for anemia due to chronic diseases or poor nutritional intake.[1] In addition, ACOG recommends that women of certain ethnicities be screened for hemoglobinopathies. Individuals at higher risk include those whose ancestors originated from parts of the world where the abnormal hemoglobins are more common, such as the Mediterranean, Africa, East India, the Middle East, and Asia. Those of Hispanic descent and those who have family members with a hemoglobinopathy are also at risk. The U.S. Preventive Services Task Force, in direct contrast, states that there is insufficient evidence to call for routine screening of asymptomatic, nonpregnant adults.[1] The CDC recommends screening low-risk nonpregnant women every 5 to 10 years beginning in adolescence. However, if a woman has a history of risk factors such as heavy menses, blood loss, low iron intake, or a previous diagnosis of iron-deficiency anemia, the CDC recommends annual screening. No routine screening for iron deficiency is recommended for postmenopausal women.[10] A clinician should consider screening for anemia when a patient's symptoms, physical findings, or risk profile suggest the presence of anemia. Women with poor nutrition or whose ethnic heritage puts them at risk for nutritionally based anemia or a hemoglobinopathy should also be considered candidates for screening.

Anemia screening requires the use of standard ranges for normal Hb and/or Hct that are specific for age, sex, and stage of pregnancy (**Table 15-4**). The CDC defines these values based on data obtained from the third National Health and Nutrition Examination Survey. Lifestyle must be considered also when determining normal levels of Hb and Hct. Smokers and those living in high altitudes (>3000 feet) have a higher limit of normal Hb levels because they need a greater red cell mass in order to maintain tissue oxygen levels.[11] According to the CDC, the normal upper limit for smokers is 0.3 g/dL higher for Hb and 1.0% higher for Hct than nonsmokers.[10]

The U.S. Congress first called for a national sickle cell anemia screening program in 1972 to identify women of childbearing age and children under the age of seven at high risk. Screening of neonates was adopted in the United States after it became apparent that prophylactic administration of long-term antibiotics to well infants with sickle cell anemia could prevent or decrease incidences of sepsis.[1,12,13] Successful clinical trials using prophylactic penicillin in the United States and Jamaica in the 1980s led to widespread adoption of newborn hemoglobinopathy screening programs.[14] Although not universally implemented, newborn screening programs are recommended by the CDC and the American

Table 15-4 NORMAL HEMOGLOBIN AND HEMATOCRIT LEVELS

Patient Profile	Hemoglobin Level (g/dL)	Hematocrit Level (%)
Nonpregnant, ≥18	≥12.0	35.7%
Pregnant, first trimester	11.0	33.0
Pregnant, second trimester	10.5	32.0
Pregnant, third trimester	11.0	33.0

Academy of Pediatrics.[15] Newborn screening allows for enrollment in comprehensive specialty care programs and parental education to recognize serious complications.

Whether screening for hemoglobinopathies should be universal or targeted to specific populations continues to be a subject of debate. Current recommendations are based on prevalence. Populations with higher prevalence rates should be screened, whereas those with low prevalence may not need screening. Screening in pregnancy is recommended in particular for women of African or Mediterranean descent. The preferred screening test is Hb electrophoresis.[16]

Clinical Presentation

Symptoms associated with anemia may result from: cellular hypoxia due to low Hb and Hct levels; the compensatory mechanisms triggered by anemia; and/or the underlying cause of anemia. Hypoxia is caused by either a reduction in the amount of Hb secondary to decreased production or increased destruction of RBCs, or by a decrease in the overall volume of blood available for oxygen transport.[17] A woman with anemic hypoxia may report a range of symptoms depending on the cause and severity of the anemia. These symptoms can include: pallor and fatigue from low Hb levels associated with chronic anemia; a racing heart rate and dizziness with hypovolemia from acute blood loss; or symptoms such as peripheral neuropathy because of vitamin B deficiency. Symptoms will be most pronounced in those with lower Hb and Hct levels, in anemias of acute onset, and in those with severe underlying disease.

Women associate fatigue with anemia. However, fatigue is an uncommon symptom unless anemia is severe or sudden. When anemia occurs suddenly, the presentation can be dramatic and may include symptoms of congestive heart failure or hypovolemia. With acute anemia, the body does not have time for compensatory protective mechanisms to develop. Consequently, patients may report symptoms such as fainting from orthostatic changes due to hypovolemia. On physical examination, the midwife may note pulse rates over 120 beats per minute (BPM) and significant flow murmurs. However, chronic anemia develops slowly and is often well tolerated until the red cell mass reaches critically low levels. With chronic anemia the human body has time to respond and compensates by:

- Increasing cardiac output
- Shunting blood to vital organs
- Decreasing the oxygen affinity of RBCs so that more oxygen is delivered to tissues
- Increasing erythropoietin levels in order to stimulate RBC production

Although these symptoms are more commonly a result of other conditions, subjective symptoms that may alert the clinician to the possibility of anemia include fatigue, lethargy, dizziness, and anorexia. Decreased tolerance for exercise, dyspnea, and palpitations are all associated with moderate-to-severe anemia. Women with moderate anemia may have pasty or sallow skin, colorless creases of the palms, pale gums, nail beds, and eyelids. As anemia worsens and compensatory mechanisms fail, more severe symptoms develop, such as breathlessness, dizziness, angina pectoris, headache, memory loss, inability to concentrate, insomnia, irregular heartbeat, anorexia, tachypnea, excessive sweating, swelling of hands or feet, thirst, tinnitus, and unexplained bleeding or bruising.

Other factors that influence whether a particular woman experiences symptoms from anemia are her normal baseline Hb and Hct levels. Patients with low but stable Hb levels may be able to better tolerate a level of anemia that a woman with a higher baseline could not. For example, a woman with iron deficiency anemia whose Hct drops slowly to 28 may remain asymptomatic, but a woman whose Hct falls suddenly to this same level because of a postpartum hemorrhage may experience significant symptoms and require a blood transfusion.

Some anemias cause specific symptoms that suggest a particular underlying etiology. For instance, pernicious anemia is often diagnosed because of the onset of neurologic symptoms such as numbness or tingling in the extremities. Patients with sickle cell disease may report pain and swelling of the hands and feet, painful joints, or jaundiced eyes and skin due to the rapid breakdown of RBCs.

Essential History, Physical Examination, and Laboratory Data

Once anemia has been diagnosed by laboratory testing, further history, physical, and targeted laboratory evaluation can discern the underlying cause(s).

History

Because there are many different causes of anemia, the initial history will need to elicit all possible etiologies. Midwives should ask questions about dietary intake in order to uncover iron, folate, and vitamin B_{12} deficiencies. They should ask about environment exposures to lead or other toxins as well as drugs that can trigger hemolysis. They should query about symptoms that may indicate a specific cause such as the presence of tarry stools seen in gastrointestinal (GI) bleeding. Personal characteristics such as age, ethnic heritage, or pregnancy status may also help pinpoint a specific etiology. A positive family history for anemia may raise the possibility of an inherited disorder.

Physical Examination

Beginning with the head, the physical examination should include: careful inspection of the skin and eyes for jaundice; scrutiny of the mouth and throat for sores; and examination of the tongue for redness, swelling, and shine (glossitis). Facial deformities such as bony prominences should be noted, because these findings are associated with chronic severe hemolytic anemias and thalassemia. Other physical indications of anemia include: skin changes such as pallor, dryness, edema; signs of bleeding such as petechiae or bruising; and brittle, ridged, or spoon-shaped nails. Patients with acute or severe anemia will appear in distress with tachycardia, a gallop rhythm, and tachypnea. Cardiomegaly and hepatomegaly may be present in very severe presentations.

Vital signs can help gauge the severity of the anemia. Orthostatic blood pressures are particularly helpful because they can provide objective measurements of the degree of hypovolemia commonly seen in anemias of acute onset. Orthostatic hypotension is defined as a decrease of at least 20 mm Hg in systolic blood pressure when an individual moves from a supine to a standing position. To perform this assessment, blood pressure and heart rate should be measured with the patient in a supine, sitting, and standing position, following a few general principles:

- Obtain the initial blood pressure in the supine position ensuring that the brachial artery is at the level of the heart.
- Allow patient to rest supine for at least five minutes before obtaining baseline measurements.
- Allow patient to sit for two to three minutes before obtaining vital signs in the sitting position.
- Have the patient stand for two to three minutes and obtain the last measurement in the standing position.

Many systems must work in concert in order to maintain a stable blood pressure during position change. When a person moves, muscle contractions in the legs compress the veins forcing blood upward toward the heart; one-way valves in the veins prevent stasis. In addition, signals sent by baroreceptors located in the carotid arteries and the aorta stimulate the sympathetic nervous system. The sympathetic nervous system responds by coordinating changes in peripheral resistance, heart rate, and cardiac contractility in order to maintain a stable blood pressure. An array of etiologies such as spinal cord problems, brain tumors, multiple sclerosis, medications, cardiac conditions, and hypovolemia can disrupt normal autonomic function. In patients with intact autonomic nervous systems, the pulse will increase by 5 to 12 BPM when standing after lying supine, and the blood pressure will remain stable. Sympathetic autonomic failure should be suspected if the pulse rate fails to rise in the presence of a fall in blood pressure when standing. A substantial increase in the standing pulse rate suggests a contracted intravascular volume. A drop in systolic blood pressure of 20 mm Hg or more, a drop in diastolic blood pressure of 10 mm Hg or more, or a rise in the pulse rate of 20 beats or more is considered an abnormal response.

Laboratory Data

Laboratory data are required in order to make the diagnosis of anemia and to determine the type of anemia. The most commonly used tests for screening for iron deficiency are Hb concentration and Hct.[10] These tests are also commonly used in the diagnosis of other suspected causes of anemia and to determine if already identified anemias are responding appropriately to treatment. Table 15-1 charts normal Hb levels. **Figures 15-3** and **15-4** are decision trees for screening children and women of childbearing age, respectively. **Figure 15-5** depicts how pregnant women are screened for anemia.

COMPLETE BLOOD COUNT

Second to Hb and Hct, a differential, complete blood count (CBC) and reticulocyte count are most commonly used as screening tools. These tests generally are more available and less expensive than biochemical tests for iron status (e.g., erythrocyte protoporphyrin concentration, serum ferritin concentration, and transferrin saturation) although they are later indicators of changes in iron status.

The CBC yields a morphological view of the RBC and describes the anemia by cell size, color, and shape. The size of an RBC determines the classification of the anemia as microcytic, normocytic, or macrocytic, and is measured by MCV. The MCV is the average volume of RBCs as measured in femtoliters (fL). Low in cost and easily obtained, this is a particularly useful test to classify anemia. A low MCV (<80) indicates *microcytic anemia*. An

Figure 15-3 Screening of high-risk infants and preschool children for anemia.

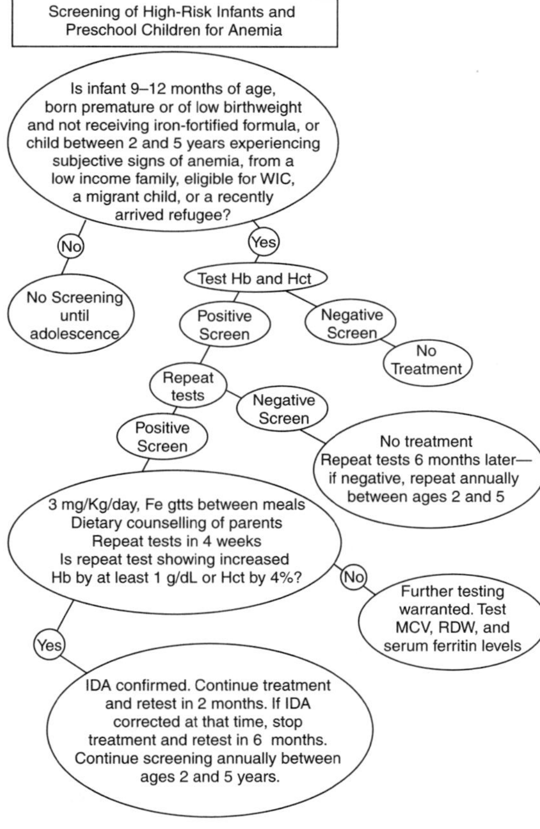

Abbreviations are: IDA, iron deficiency anemia; WIC, women, infant and children program; RDW, red blood cell distribution width.

Figure 15-4 Screening of nonpregnant women of childbearing ages for anemia.

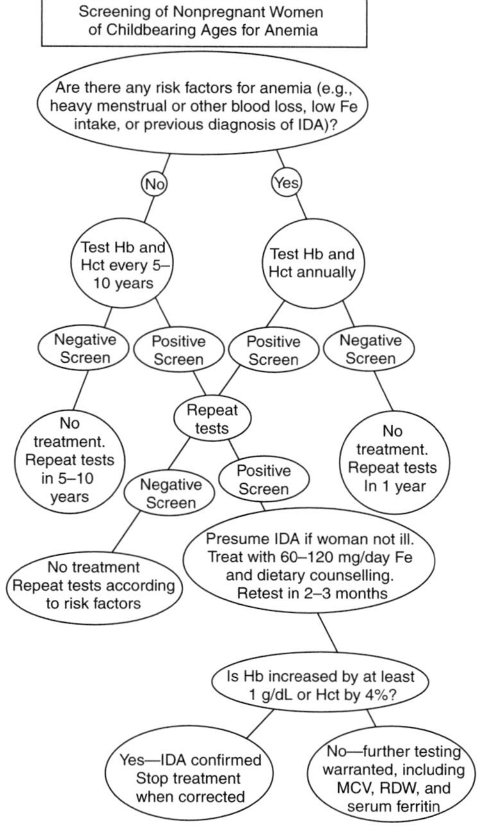

Abbreviations are: IDA, iron deficiency anemia; WIC, women, infant and children program; RDW, red blood cell distribution width.

elevated MCV (>100) suggests that *macrocytic anemia* such as folate/vitamin B_{12} deficiency or reactive reticulocytosis is present. Color and shape of the RBC provide further clues to the underlying cause of anemia. Normal MCV results show 80 to 100 fL.

PERIPHERAL SMEAR

A peripheral smear examines the shape of RBCs and is helpful in suggesting specific etiologies that should be considered. Examples of abnormal findings found on the peripheral smear are in **Table 15-5**.

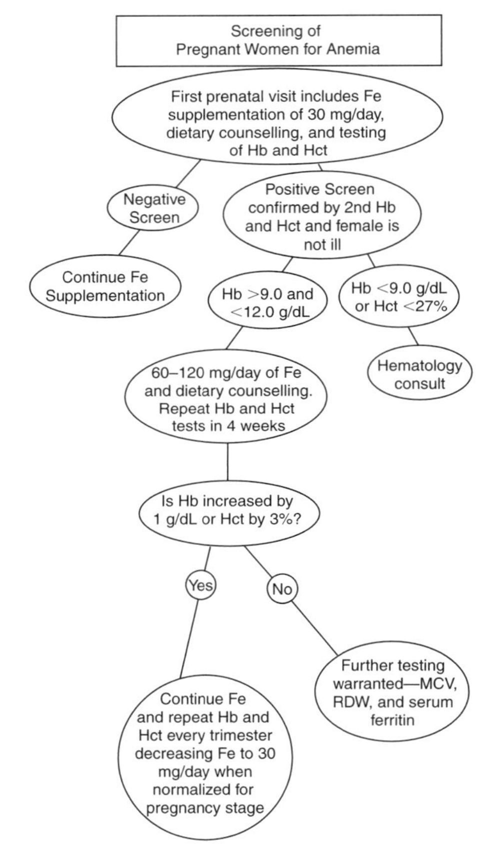

Figure 15-5 Screening of pregnant women for anemia.

RETICULOCYTE COUNT

A reticulocyte count is helpful in two situations. First, it can help discern the underlying cause of anemia and second, once the etiology is identified, it can help reassure the clinician that the prescribed treatment is effective. A reticulocyte count measures how rapidly immature RBCs are made by the bone marrow and released into the bloodstream. Reticulocytes circulate in the blood for about two days before reaching maturity. Normally, about 1% to 2% of circulating RBCs are reticulocytes. The reticulocyte count increases in response to rapid blood loss or in the presence of diseases in which RBCs are prematurely destroyed, as the body attempts to rapidly replace lost RBCs. If the count is higher than normal, it suggests acute blood loss or hemolytic anemia and responsive bone marrow. If the count is low or normal in the presence of anemia, it suggests that the bone marrow is unable to respond to the body's feedback system.[18] For example, a reticulocyte count can be low in anemias due to hypoproliferation because of insufficient levels of critical elements, such as iron, which are necessary for the production of RBCs. Once iron supplementation begins, the bone marrow will respond and the production of reticulocytes will increase. Therefore, a reticulocyte count is often ordered to monitor the effectiveness of treatment.

RED BLOOD CELL DISTRIBUTION WIDTH

A red blood cell distribution width (RDW) measures the uniformity of the RBCs' size. The normal RDW level is 10.2% to 14.5%. A high RDW means that the RBCs vary significantly in size. Evaluating the RDW in conjunction with the MCV can help narrow down possible causes of anemia. If both the RDW and MCV are increased, then conditions such as liver disease, hemolytic anemia, vitamin B_{12} deficiency, or folic acid deficiency must be considered. Iron deficiency anemia is the most common cause of a high RDW and low MCV, but thalassemia intermedia must also be considered. A high RDW reading found in combination with a low

Table 15-5 DIFFERENTIAL DIAGNOSIS OF ANEMIA BASED ON PERIPHERAL SMEAR FINDINGS

Findings on Peripheral Smear	Associated Anemia
Schistocytes or fragmented cells	Microangiopathic hemolytic anemia
Spherocytes	Hereditary spherocytosis or autoimmune hemolytic anemia
Ghost or bite cells	G6PD deficiency
Sickle-shaped cells	Sickle cell disease
Target cells	Hemoglobin C
Stippled RBCs	Lead poisoning
Teardrop cells	Thalassemia major; severe iron deficiency
Howell-Jolly bodies	Sickle cell anemia
Heinz bodies	G6PD; alpha thalassemia; unstable form of hemoglobin; congenital hemolytic anemia

MCV can also be seen after a hemorrhage because of the release of immature RBCs from the bone marrow (leading to an increased variation in size) and a loss of recycled iron. A high RDW level but normal MCV level can be seen early in the course of iron deficiency anemia, vitamin B_{12} deficiency, or folic acid deficiency.

ERYTHROCYTE PROTOPORPHYRIN, OR FREE ERYTHROCYTE PROTOPORPHYRIN

Erythrocyte protoporphyrin is the immediate precursor of Hb. It increases when sufficient iron is not available for the production of Hb. Without an adequate amount of iron, the body is unable to synthesize heme, and protoporphyrin accumulates. A normal reading for this test is between 16 and 65 mcg/dL in adults. A concentration of ≥ 70 mcg/dL of RBCs in adults often indicates iron deficiency. Other reasons for it to be elevated include infection, inflammation, and lead poisoning. The level of protoporphyrin can be used to estimate the blood lead level. This test can be used instead of Hb, because they have similar sensitivity and specificity for predicting iron deficiency in nonpregnant women, and both are inexpensive tests.[19]

FERRITIN LEVELS

Ferritin is a protein that stores iron in the body. Serum ferritin concentration in the blood is directly proportional to the amount of stored iron in the body. Most of the iron that is not already bound by the heme portion of Hb is stored as ferritin in the liver, bone marrow, and spleen; the remaining iron is found in transferrin in myoglobin, and a small amount in the enzyme systems active in energy metabolism. The average value in U.S. women is 43 mcg/L. It is an early indicator of the compromised status of iron in the body because the body will deplete its stores of ferritin before iron deficiency becomes a problem. If a woman has a low Hb or Hct, a serum ferritin concentration of ≤ 15 mcg/L confirms iron deficiency. Levels of ferritin > 15 mcg/L suggest that iron deficiency is not the cause of anemia and other etiologies should be considered. Although a good early indicator of iron status, this test is costly and only available through limited laboratories. Serum ferritin levels are also affected by chronic infections, inflammation, and liver damage, all of which cause elevations of the levels that mask diminishing iron stores. A high serum ferritin level can be seen in the presence of other conditions such as renal disease, iron overload, or other anemias (megaloblastic, hemolytic, the thalassemias).

TRANSFERRIN

Transferrin saturation indicates how much transferrin has vacant iron-binding sites. Transferrin is manufactured by the liver and can be used to monitor liver function as well as nutrition. This value is dependent on two laboratory measures: serum iron concentration and *total iron-binding capacity (TIBC)*. It is calculated by dividing serum iron concentration by TIBC and multiplying by 100 to express as a percentage. If the result is <16% in adults, it confirms iron deficiency. The TIBC is considered to be less sensitive than serum ferritin for reflecting iron stores in the body.

SERUM IRON

Serum iron concentration is a measure of the total amount of iron in the blood bound to the protein transferrin. Many factors alter this amount, including eating recently (increased level), infections and inflammations (decreased level), and time of day the sample was drawn. As such, this test is not an accurate indicator of iron status alone, but together with serum ferritin and transferrin levels, it can help determine what type of anemia is present.

TOTAL IRON BINDING CAPACITY

The TIBC is a measure of the iron-binding capacity within the serum, or how much iron the blood would carry if the transferrin were fully saturated. It increases when the serum iron concentration is low and decreases when it is high. The level can also be increased because of medications such as fluorides and birth control pills.

HEMOGLOBIN ELECTROPHORESIS

Hb electrophoresis measures the different types of Hb in the blood. It is a test conducted when familial or ethnic history suggests an increased risk for an inherited abnormality such as sickle cell trait. As indicated in Table 15-1, normal adult Hb consists mainly of Hb A1, a small amount of Hb A2, and a minor amount of Hb F.

OTHER TESTS

Other tests can be conducted to confirm suspicions about specific types of anemia. For example, abnormal GI blood loss can be tested by a chemical hemoccult test of a rectal smear. Folate and vitamin B_{12} levels should be checked in the presence of macrocytic anemia.

Treatment

Treatment of anemia is dependent upon the underlying cause of the anemia as well as the severity of symptoms. For purposes of describing specific, selected anemias and their recommended treatments, they are classified here according to the MCV as microcytic, macrocytic or normocytic anemias.

Microcytic Anemias

IRON DEFICIENCY ANEMIA

Iron deficiency anemia is the most common anemia in the world. In developed countries such as the United States, anemia is often seen when the person has insufficient iron because of increased requirements seen in infancy, adolescence, or pregnancy; inadequate iron intake; decreased iron absorption; or increased blood loss from heavy menses, bleeding of the GI tract, and other conditions.[18] It is especially common in toddlers between the ages of 1 and 2, and women in their childbearing years; however, it is rarely seen in teenage boys and young men, or older children and adults over the age of 50. Causes of decreased iron absorption also include gastrectomy, achlorhydria, or chronic diarrhea. In developing countries located in tropical climates, the most common cause is an infestation of hookworm, which causes intestinal blood loss.

Iron absorption is regulated by receptors located predominantly in the duodenum and upper jejunum. Regulation of absorption is not completely understood, but it is clear that dietary factors, gastric acid, and medications are among the potential influences on the rate of absorption. An imbalance can be caused by failure to absorb enough iron (usually due to insufficient intake of absorbable dietary iron) or excessive loss of iron (e.g., hemorrhagic event). The onset of iron deficiency anemia is gradual. RBC production falls in response to declining iron reserves. Initially, the anemia is normochromic and normocytic, but as iron stores become further depleted, hypochromic microcytic anemia develops. Laboratory evaluation of iron deficiency anemia will show lower than normal Hb, Hct, and reticulocyte levels as well as abnormal values of serum ferritin, erythrocyte protoporphyrin, and transferrin saturation.[20] Hb levels fall before Hct in iron deficiency, but both are late indicators. A positive screening test should be confirmed by repeat Hb and Hct. If the tests agree and the girl or woman is not ill, a presumptive diagnosis of iron-deficiency anemia can be made.

These laboratory findings are similar to those found in individuals with thalassemia trait, sideroblastic anemia, or lead poisoning, which also cause microcytic anemias. However, unlike individuals with iron deficiency anemia, these individuals will have abnormal cells (i.e., target cells, anisocytes, and poikilocytes) on the peripheral smear. Low serum iron and ferritin levels in combination with an elevated TIBC are diagnostic of iron deficiency in well individuals. Fever, cancer, or other inflammatory processes will raise the serum ferritin, causing an inaccurate clinical picture and masking iron deficiency anemia.[18] A bone marrow biopsy may be necessary in selected complicated cases to determine the status of iron stores.

Management of iron deficiency anemia includes iron supplementation. While there are many forms of iron supplements, some are absorbed more efficiently than others (**Table 15-6**). All supplements are better absorbed if taken between meals, but the GI side effects can be a deterrent. Side effects include GI upset, such as nausea, diarrhea, heartburn or constipation, and black or tarry stools. Starting supplements with daily dosing and slowly increasing to three times per day may be helpful in avoiding severe side effects. Taking smaller doses several times per day may also help alleviate these effects. Tolerance of iron supplementation is related to the level of elemental iron concentration. Ferrous gluconate, although more expensive than ferrous sulfate, has a lower elemental iron concentration and is therefore easier for patients to tolerate. Supplementation is more effective if enteric-coated and time-release products are avoided. Calcium, tannins present in many teas, and phytic acid in legumes, cereals, and nuts can impair absorption and should not be consumed at the same time as iron

Table 15-6 COMMON TYPES OF IRON SUPPLEMENTATION

Iron Supplement	Absorption Rate	Usual Dosage	Common Trade Names
Ferrous sulfate	high	325 mg PO qd, bid, or tid	Slow Fe, Feratab, Fer-iron
Ferrous gluconate	high	325 mg PO	Fergon
Ferrous fumarate	high	200 mg PO qd or bid	FemIron, Feostat
Carbonyl iron	low	45 mg PO tid	Feosol

supplements if possible. Absorption of both iron and folic acid is increased if taken with vitamin C, so patients can be encouraged to take the supplement with citrus juice.

Hb and Hct should be retested after two to three months of therapy. If the anemia does not respond to iron treatment despite compliance after four weeks (indicated by an increase in Hb concentration of at least 1 g/dL or in Hct of at least 4%), additional laboratory tests such as a MCV, RDW, and serum ferritin concentration are needed.[10] If these tests confirm iron deficiency anemia, treatment should continue for an additional two months before rechecking Hct and Hb.

THALASSEMIAS

The thalassemias are inherited hemolytic anemias in which the body produces defective Hb. The RBCs in persons with thalassemias are unusually fragile and microcytic in appearance. The cause of these disorders is not fully understood, but one theory is that a mutation of an operon gene, which regulates the production of hemoglobin chains, alters the rate of chain synthesis.[21] There are many variants of the thalassemias; however, they are categorized into two basic classifications, alpha or beta, depending on which Hb chain is affected.

Alpha Thalassemia   The *alpha thalassemias* include several variants depending on the number of genes involved in the production of Hb. Only alpha chains are affected. Four genes regulate alpha globin synthesis. In homozygous alpha thalassemia, also known as Hb Bart's, a condition incompatable with life, all four genes are missing. Fetuses affected by this condition often die late in pregnancy or at birth. The loss of three genes causes Hb H disease, which is a moderately severe form of thalassemia. The loss of two genes leads to the development of alpha thalassemia minor and causes mild anemia resembling iron deficiency anemia. Loss of one gene leads to a silent carrier state, or alpha+thalassemia trait; there are no symptoms, but the person may still have a small amount of Hb Bart's that can be seen on electrophoresis.

Alpha thalassemias are more common in certain populations. All of the alpha thalassemia disorders are relatively common among those from Southeast Asia and China; up to 25% of Black individuals carry at least one gene responsible for the development of alpha thalassemia and the thalassemia missing one or two genes are more common in Blacks than are those with all genes absent.

Table 15-7 shows the classification of alpha thalassemia by genotype.

Table 15-7 CLASSIFICATION OF ALPHA THALASSEMIA BY GENOTYPE

Genotype	Description
$--/--$	Hemoglobin Bart's; homozygous alpha thalassemia
$\alpha -/--$	Hemoglobin H disease
$\alpha -/\alpha -$	May be homozygous alpha+thalassemia (or alpha0 thalassemia trait if $--/\alpha\alpha$)
$\alpha -/\alpha\,\alpha$	Silent carrier state, or alpha+thalassemia trait

Beta Thalassemia Beta thalassemias are inherited disorders of beta globin synthesis. Abnormal hemoglobin synthesis causes microcytosis, ineffective erythropoiesis, and hemolysis. In the homozygous state, beta globin is completely absent (beta0 thalassemia) or markedly reduced (beta+ thalassemia). Disease severity is dependent on the degree of abnormal beta chain synthesis and the amount of beta globins that are present. Beta0 thalassemia, also known as beta thalassemia major or Cooley anemia, can be fatal in children. Individuals with beta0 thalassemia may have characteristic mongoloid faces due to cranial and facial bone abnormalities. Beta+ thalassemia, also known as beta thalassemia intermedia, causes severe anemia. However, the anemia is not severe enough to require blood transfusions. Growth failure, bone deformities, and enlarged liver and spleen are common problems for patients afflicted with beta thalassemia intermedia. On electrophoresis, Hb F is more prevalent than usual, and Hb A2 is increased. Hb A levels vary depending on which type of beta thalassemia is present; it is absent in beta0 thalassemia and markedly reduced in beta+ thalassemia. **Table 15-8** shows the classification of beta thalassemia by genotype.

The heterozygous state is known as beta thalassemia minor and typically presents with mild symptoms. Mild anemia, microcytic erythrocytes, and splenomegaly are seen. Hemoglobin electrophoresis shows Hb A with slightly increased Hb A2, and normal or slightly increased Hb F.

Beta thalassemia is more commonly found in people from countries surrounding the Mediterranean or from Southeast Asia. Individuals of Black, Mediterranean, or Southeast Asian descent should be screened, as should anyone whose family members have been diagnosed with thalassemia. Laboratory evaluation includes CBC, MCV, and Hb electrophoresis. **Table 15-9** describes the Hb electrophoresis findings commonly seen in the various thalassemias. The MCV is always low in beta thalassemia. Genetic counseling should be offered to couples if both are carriers. Prenatal diagnosis is possible through DNA analysis of amniocytes obtained through amniocentesis or chorionic villus sampling.

LEAD POISONING

Lead poisoning should be suspected in children who are anemic, although it can also affect adults. Lead levels should be drawn if lead exposure is suspected as the cause of anemia. Women who engage in pica behavior, particularly of soil or paint chips or who are from countries such as Mexico, Jamaica, and the Balkan states where lead levels are known to be high, are at increased risk of having elevated lead levels. Supplementation with calcium and iron may be particularly helpful in these individuals and may prevent further absorption of iron from the environment or release of stored lead in the bones. Chapter 3 provides further details about screening, prevention, and management of lead poisoning.

Table 15-8 CLASSIFICATION OF BETA THALASSEMIA BY GENOTYPE

Genotype*	Description
B0/B0 or B0/B+ or B+/B+	Beta thalassemia major, or beta0 thalassemia, or Cooley's anemia
B0/B+ or B+/B+	Beta + thalassemia, or beta thalassemia intermedia
B/B+ or B/B0	Beta thalassemia minor, beta thalassemia trait, or silent carrier trait

*B0 = no beta chains; B+ = reduced production.

Macrocytic Anemias

The most common causes of macrocytic anemia are vitamin B_{12} deficiency and folic acid deficiency. Other causes include leukemia, myelofibrosis, and multiple myeloma; drugs that affect DNA synthesis such as chemotherapeutic agents; alcohol; arsenic; and endocrine diseases such as hypothyroidism. Laboratory findings commonly seen with macrocytic anemias include an increased MCV, a low reticulocyte count, and hyper-segmented polymorphonuclear leukocytes on the peripheral smear.[22]

FOLIC ACID DEFICIENCY ANEMIA

Folic acid deficiency anemia is the most common of the megaloblastic anemias. Folic acid is a B vitamin needed for the production of RBCs. When the folic acid level is deficient, too few RBCs will be produced, and they will be macrocytic. It is found most commonly in infants and teenagers as a result of insufficient intake, but can also result from an inability to absorb the vitamin. Folic acid is found in foods such as cheese, eggs, green vegetables, meats, milk, mushrooms, and yeast. Most breads are now fortified with folic acid. Foods high in folic acid should be eaten raw or cooked as little as possible; light and heat destroy it. Folic acid is dependent on the presence of vitamin C for absorption. For this reason, a smoker is at increased risk for folic acid anemia. Deficiency may be seen in pregnancy, because the need is increased by a factor of eight. This disorder can be corrected in three to six weeks with supplementary treatment of 1 mg folic acid per day, but treatment should be continued for six months with periodic blood tests to make certain that the deficiency is corrected.

PERNICIOUS ANEMIA

Pernicious anemia is a type of megaloblastic anemia that is caused by lack of intrinsic factor, a protein needed to absorb vitamin B_{12} from the GI tract. Intrinsic factor is normally produced by cells within the stomach. Its absence may result from chronic gastritis or surgery to remove or reduce the size of the stomach. Vitamin B_{12} is necessary for the formation of RBCs and the maintenance of healthy nerve cells. B_{12} deficiency can lead to fatigue, shortness of breath, tingling sensations in hands and feet, difficulty walking, and diarrhea. Neurologic symptoms are likely to be the primary complaint that suggests this diagnosis, because they tend to be difficult to ignore.

Pernicious anemia is the most common type of *vitamin B12 deficiency anemia*. The onset of this disease tends to be slow, spanning decades.[23] The average age of diagnosis is 60 years. Women, especially those of Scandinavian or

Table 15-9 Hemoglobin Electrophoresis Findings Seen with Different Causes of Anemia

Type of Hb	Normal Adult	Alpha Thalassemia Minor	Alpha Thalassemia Major	Beta Thalassemia Minor	Beta 0 Thalassemia Major	Beta + Thalassemia Major	Sickle Cell Trait	Sickle Cell Disease	Hg H Dis.
Hb A1	95%–98%	90%	—	>90%	0%	1%–3%	60%	—	Up to 90%
Hb A2	2%–3%	4%–5.8%	—	Slight increase	Up to 10%	Up to 9%	<3.5%	<3.5%	<2%
Hb F	0.8%–2%	—	—	Up to 2.5%	Up to 90%	Up to 90%	<2%	Up to 15%	<5%
Hb S	—	—	—	—	—	—	20%–40%	70%–98%	—
Hb Bart	—	5%–10%	15%–20%	—	—	—	—	—	2%–10%
Hb H	—	—	—	—	—	—	—	—	5–40%

*There are slight variations in references across labs—always check with the lab conducting the test.

Northern European descent, are at higher risk of developing this condition. It occurs more commonly in individuals with autoimmune endocrine diseases such as type 1 diabetes, hypoparathyroidism, Addison's disease, hypopituitarism, Graves disease, chronic thyroiditis, myasthesia gravis, secondary amenorrhea, and vitiligo.[23] It is also more commonly found in individuals who have family members with the disease. Rarely, infants and children are born lacking the ability to produce effective intrinsic factor. Congenital pernicious anemia is an inherited autosomal recessive disorder.

Laboratory findings seen in pernicious anemia include an elevated MCV, low Hct and Hb levels, reduced amounts of serum B_{12}, and decreased WBCs, platelets, and reticulocytes.

Adequate treatment of pernicious anemia requires monthly vitamin B_{12} injections beginning with 1000 mcg per week for six weeks and then 1000 mcg intramuscularly every month for life. This therapy corrects the anemia. It may also reverse any neurologic damage caused by vitamin B_{12} deficiency, if therapy is instituted early in the course of the disease. Neurologic defects may persist if treatment is delayed. Only about 1% of vitamin B_{12} is absorbed, so some health care providers recommend that elderly patients with gastric atrophy take oral vitamin B_{12} supplements in addition to monthly injections. A well-balanced diet is essential to providing other elements necessary for healthy blood cell development, such as folic acid, iron, and vitamin C.

Normocytic Anemias

ACUTE BLOOD LOSS

Acute anemia is caused by hemolysis or acute hemorrhage and leads to a precipitous drop in the number of RBCs. Hypoxia results from a reduction in the oxygen-carrying capacity of the blood caused by the loss of RBCs. Decreased intravascular volume leads to hypovolemia and the development of hypotension. Symptoms progress from mild tachycardia and normal blood pressure to tachycardia, tachypnea, and decreased pulse pressure. Marked tachycardia and significantly decreased blood pressure are seen when 40% or more of the normal blood volume is lost.

Midwives will most often see acute blood loss as a result of postpartum hemorrhage (PPH), a potentially life-threatening complication of both vaginal and cesarean section deliveries. Although traditionally defined as a blood loss of greater than 500 mL, recognition that the normal blood loss from vaginal and cesarean delivery often exceeds this level has led to a broader definition of PPH. Any bleeding that results in signs and symptoms of hemodynamic instability, or bleeding that could result in hemodynamic instability if left untreated, is considered PPH. Any bleeding resulting in a decrease in postpartum Hct of 10% from the prenatal Hct is also considered PPH.[24] The initial evaluation of PPH involves identification of the cause of bleeding. Treatment will vary according to the underlying etiology and may include appropriate management of uterine atony, diagnosis and repair of cervical or vaginal lacerations, and removal of retained placental tissue.

HEMOLYTIC ANEMIA

Hemolytic anemias are a result of premature destruction of RBCs. As a group, these anemias occur with less frequency than those caused by excessive blood loss or decreased production. Whether inherited or acquired, hemolytic anemia occurs when the bone marrow is unable to compensate for the premature loss of RBCs by increasing their production, resulting in anemia. There are many types of hemolytic anemias, including sickle cell anemia, paroxysmal nocturnal hemoglobinuria, Hb SC disease, hemolytic anemia due to G6PD deficiency, idiopathic autoimmune hemolytic anemia, non-immune hemolytic anemia caused by chemical or physical agents, secondary immune hemolytic anemia, and alpha and beta thalassemia.

Hemolytic anemias can be classified as intrinsic or extrinsic. *Intrinsic hemolytic anemias* are inherited disorders and include the thalassemias and sickle cell disease. Destruction of the RBC is due to a defect in the cell itself, causing the RBC to be more vulnerable and have a shortened life span. *Extrinsic hemolytic anemias*, also called autoimmune hemolytic anemia, are acquired. The RBCs are healthy and are produced normally. However, hemolysis occurs from exposure to drugs or infections that destroy RBCs or from entrapment of RBCs in the spleen. Specific causes include infections such as hepatitis, cytomegalovirus, Epstein Barr virus, typhoid fever, *E. coli*, or streptococcus; medications such as penicillin, antimalaria medications, sulfa medications, or acetaminophen; leukemia or lymphoma; autoimmune disorders such as systemic lupus erythematosus, rheumatoid arthritis, Wiskott Aldrich syndrome, or ulcerative colitis; or various tumors. Some types of extrinsic hemolytic anemia are temporary, resolving spontaneously over several months. Others become chronic with periods of remissions and recurrence.

General symptoms of hemolytic anemia include classic signs of anemia, such as fatigue, pallor, shortness of breath, tachypnea, jaundice, dark urine, and enlarged spleen (which leads to further hemolysis when the spleen fails to filter out spherocytes and other abnormal red cells). A hemolytic crisis, which is rare, presents with fever, chills, tachycardia, and hemoglobinuria (a potential cause of renal failure).

Specific laboratory findings are indicative of hemolysis. The Hb and Hct levels will be low. Usually the RBCs will be normochromic-normocytic, but may also be macrocytic (as in megaloblastic anemia) or microcytic (as in chronic intravascular hemolysis). The Coomb test will be positive. Additional tests will be necessary in order to identify the specific cause of hemolysis. **Table 15-10** shows typical laboratory results seen in hemolytic anemias.

Treatment, complications, and outcome depends on the specific type and cause of hemolytic anemia as well as the patient's age, overall health, medical history, extent of disease, and tolerance for specific medications, procedures, or therapies. Treatment may include vitamin and mineral supplements, dietary changes, pharmacologic management, the avoidance of medications known to trigger hemolysis, or splenectomy. There is no known prevention for hemolytic anemias.

Hereditary Hemolytic Anemia   Inherited forms, or hereditary hemolytic anemia, are most often caused by hereditary spherocytosis, a congenital hemolytic icterus in which the RBCs are spherical in shape and drop their Hb.[8] The spherical shape is caused by abnormalities in the protein network that maintains shape and flexibility of cell membrane. Other RBC defects causing hereditary hemolytic anemia include hereditary elliptocytosis and hereditary stomatocytosis.

Glucose-6-Phosphate Dehydrogenase   G6PD is an X-linked genetic disease that affects the G6PD enzyme, rendering it useless. Without active G6PD, normal Hb will undergo changes that

Table 15-10 LABORATORY FINDINGS SEEN IN HEMOLYTIC ANEMIA

Type of Blood Test	Expected Result
Hemoglobin/hematocrit	Low
Indirect bilirubin	High
Serum haptoglobin	Low
Urinalysis	Possible Hb, hemosiderin, urobilinogen
Reticulocyte count	High
RBC	Low
Serum LDH	High

Abbreviation: LDH, lactate dehydrogenase.

make it incapable of carrying oxygen. In addition, the G6PD enzyme is normally responsible for blocking effects of oxidizing agents on RBCs. Without the protection provided by the G6PD enzyme, hemolysis occurs in response to illness, stress, and exposure to oxidant medications such as sulfa or macrodantin. Consuming fava beans may also trigger hemolysis in some individuals, especially those of Mediterranean descent, who are more likely to have a particular variant of G6PD deficiency. G6PD is also common among African Americans.[25] Individuals with mild symptoms may not be diagnosed in childhood. A triggering event such as those listed above may occur at any time and lead to testing and diagnosis. Management includes avoidance of precipitants, prompt diagnosis and treatment of all infections, genetic counseling, and prenatal diagnostic testing if a woman is G6PD deficient. Individuals with G6PD deficiency who require surgery need to make sure that their physician is aware that they have this condition. Travelers to countries such as Haiti and certain areas in the Dominican Republic and Mexico, where malaria is prevalent, are urged by the CDC to take antimalarial medications prophylactically. However, Primaquine, which is one of several available prophylactic regimens, can cause a fatal hemolysis in G6PD deficient persons, and should not be prescribed unless the woman's G6PD status is known.[26]

Autoimmune Hemolytic Anemias Autoimmune hemolytic anemias can be classified as cold-antibody hemolytic anemias or warm-antibody hemolytic anemias. *Warm antibody hemolytic anemias* are most common and cause 70% of all cases of autoimmune hemolytic anemias. They occur when the body produces autoantibodies that coat RBCs at normal body temperatures, causing them to be destroyed by the spleen, liver, or bone marrow. Warm antibody hemolytic anemias are more common in women than men; 30% of these anemias are associated with lymphoma, leukemia, lupus, or connective tissue disease. Treatment generally consists of large doses of intravenous or oral corticosteroids. If medication is unsuccessful, the spleen is surgically removed. As a last resort, immune system suppressants are used. Warm-antibody hemolytic anemias are often severe, with Hb levels of 7.0 or less, and can be fatal.[18] A hematology consult is warranted for these patients.

Cold-antibody hemolytic anemias are often mild, short-lived, and resolve without treatment. They may develop acutely in people with pneumonia, mononucleosis, or other acute infections. Cold-antibody anemias also can be chronic, sometimes lifelong, and these occur most commonly in women over 40 and in the presence of arthritis. Individuals with cold-antibody hemolytic anemia often have few symptoms. As with warm antibody anemias, autoantibodies cause RBC destruction. The triggering episode leading to hemolysis in this anemia is often exposure to cold temperatures that results in fatigue, joint aches, and acrocyanosis of the arms and hands.

SICKLE CELL ANEMIA

The sickle cell anemias are hereditary conditions occurring when a sickle gene mutation on the beta chain of hemoglobin is inherited from one or both parents. Sickle cell disease occurs when the offspring receives sickle cell mutations from both parents; sickle cell trait occurs if only one parent passes on the mutation. Hb S polymerizes, or increases its molecular weight under low oxygen tension, forcing the hemoglobin carrying RBCs to assume an abnormal crescent or sickle shape. While a normal RBC lives for approximately 120 days, the sickled RBC lives only for 10 to 12 days. RBC production can not keep up and chronic anemia develops.

Symptoms of sickle cell disease are proportionate to the percentage of affected RBCs. Individuals with sickle trait have fewer affected RBCs and minimal symptoms. Those with sickle cell disease can develop significant complications that include chronic anemia, arthralgia, and episodes of acute pain. In sickle cell anemia, the deformed RBCs easily adhere to vascular endothelium, increasing the potential for decreased blood flow and vascular obstruction. Sickled blood cells also cannot carry enough oxygen to nourish the body's tissues. As

a result, patients experience organ damage as well as hemolytic anemia and vasculopathy. Organ damage is often silent until well advanced. Individuals with sickle cell disease can have acute exacerbations and experience a sickle cell crisis. During a sickle cell crisis, capillary blood flow diminishes, leading to stasis and vascular occlusion within capillaries, decreasing oxygen and nutrition to the involved tissue, and causing severe anoxic pain. The most commonly affected sites are the limbs and abdomen. If circulating blood volume is severely reduced by the crisis, shock and death may ensue. Sickle cell crises often occur without any identifiable precipitating cause.

Sickle cell anemia is seen predominately in Blacks and those of Mediterranean descent. There are currently approximately 50,000 Americans with sickle cell disease. Population rates vary: 1 in every 375 African Americans; 1 in every 3,000 Native Americans; 1 in every 20,000 Hispanics; and, 1 in every 60,000 Caucasian Americans have sickle cell disease.[27] Life expectancy for those affected is decreased, on average by 25 to 30 years.[28] The average age at death is 50 years.[29] The mortality rate in children peaks between ages one and three because of sepsis caused by *Streptococcus pneumoniae*.

Persons with sickle cell anemia experience a number of symptoms specific to this particular disease. Included is hand-foot syndrome where symptoms include pain and swelling of the hands and feet and possibly fever, representing vascular occlusion of blood vessels in the extremities. Fatigue, paleness, shortness of breath, delayed growth and puberty in children, and slight build in adults all result from the anemia. Pain in joints or organs of the body can last for hours to weeks, sometimes requiring hospitalization for management. Jaundice of the eyes and skin can be present due to excessive rapid breakdown of RBCs. Damage to the spleen is associated with frequent infections, particularly pneumonia. Damage to the retina causes vision problems, and damage to the vessels in the brain can result in stroke. Persistent ulcers on the legs can develop due to impaired circulation. Renal disease results from blockages in the vasculature of the kidney and urinary tract, sometimes requiring kidney transplant. One of the most ominous sequelae of sickle cell disease is acute chest syndrome, which is caused by impaired circulation in the lungs from vascular blockages and can be life-threatening. Acute chest syndrome is characterized by chest pain and fever.

The diagnosis of sickle cell anemia is typically made during newborn screening. Hb S is the most common abnormal hemoglobin detected by newborn screening programs in the United States.[14]

Management of the patient with sickle cell disease is age- and case-dependent, collaborative in nature, and often involves health care providers from several specialties. Treatment plans are mainly focused on specific symptoms. Folic acid supplementation is essential because of the rapid RBC turnover in patients. Pain is treated with analgesics and may include narcotics. Dialysis is used in the presence of kidney disease. Bone marrow transplant can be curative, but is used rarely; stem cell transplants (from bone marrow or cord blood) are also rarely performed. The risks of this procedure and the difficulty of finding a genetic match are the limiting factors. New medications stimulate the production of Hb F because Hb F inhibits sickling of cells. Other drugs are used to increase oxygen binding to sickle cells.[30,31] Careful documentation of all complications is critical to

lifetime care, as childhood health markers can be used to predict the number and severity of complications, or crises, in later years.[32]

Care of the adolescent with sickle cell disease requires acknowledgment of the difficult developmental tasks of this age, and the need to stress compliance with medication regimens and clinic visits. Peer support groups and one-on-one guidance counseling can be helpful. Self image and self-esteem issues will manifest themselves particularly during the teen years, warranting close observation and intervention when necessary.

Health care providers seeing the adolescent or adult patient with sickle cell anemia for the first time should order a CBC, reticulocyte count, and hemoglobin electrophoreses if a recent test is unavailable. Other baseline tests include urinalysis, liver function tests, urea, creatinine, and electrolytes levels, and a chest x-ray. Additional testing may be necessary in the presence of complications. The patient's immunization record should be reviewed, and vaccinations provided if missing.

A review of the patient's ophthalmologist exams should be obtained, and the patient's understanding of the disease and its complications should be reviewed. Family planning and genetic counseling services should be discussed, and the availability of prenatal diagnosis should be mentioned when appropriate.

Adult patients with sickle cell disease should have regular medical evaluations approximately every three to six months[33] if stable and more frequently if complications are experienced. A blood count and reticulocyte count should be obtained at each of these visits. Urinalysis and chemistry tests should be obtained at minimum once a year. With advancing age, complications such as chronic organ failure often require more frequent visits and more extensive laboratory evaluations. Patients should be counseled about seeking immediate treatment for high fever, productive cough, and acute symptoms such as dyspnea, weakness, or dizziness. Painful episodes are often managed at home with rest, fluids, and analgesics. Persistent pain requires further evaluation. Cigarette smoking and excessive alcohol intake should be avoided. A well-balanced, moderate exercise program is often possible with supervision.[33]

All contraceptive options are suitable for those with sickle cell disease. Although sickle cell disease can cause major complications during pregnancy and has implications for the health of the fetus, pregnancy is not prohibited.[33] Women should seek care early in pregnancy and should receive expert consultation by professionals experienced in the management of sickle cell disease. Biweekly visits prior to 28 weeks, and weekly visits thereafter, are appropriate. All pregnant patients with sickle cell disease should receive 1 mg of folic acid daily in addition to the usual prenatal vitamins, minerals, and iron supplements, unless iron stores are known to be increased. They should be screened for the presence of red cell alloantibodies, regardless of their transfusion history. The woman should be told if antibodies are present and given written information in case she delivers at a hospital other than the one planned for delivery.[33] The father should also have his Hb type identified through Hb electrophoresis. If he carries the sickle cell trait or is a carrier of another hemoglobinopathy (including thalassemia), the possibility of amniocentesis to identify sickle cell disease in the fetus should be raised early in pregnancy.

Pregnancies of women with sickle cell disease have increased rates of intrauterine growth retardation, preterm labor, and premature delivery; rates are higher among women with Hb SS than with SC or S beta thalassemia.[29] Eclampsia, thrombophlebitis, phyelonephritis, and spontaneous abortions all may occur with increased frequency as well. These complications should be treated the same as in patients without sickle cell disease.[33]

Aplastic Anemia

Aplastic anemia was first described in 1888 when Dr. Paul Ehrlich, a German pathologist, studied the case of a pregnant woman who died of bone marrow failure.[34] The autopsy revealed a near absence of all hematopoietic cells (hence, the name aplastic). Whether inherited, acquired, or idiopathic, aplastic anemia is characterized by a markedly decreased production of all three types of blood cells by the bone marrow: RBCs, WBCs, and platelets. It reflects a primary defect in, or damage to, stem cells or the marrow micro environment.

Aplastic anemia has no affinity for one gender over another, but is seen more often in people of Asian origin.[35] It is primarily found in young adults (15–30 years of age) and the elderly ($\geq$60 years). The incidence of aplastic anemia is estimated to be 5 to 10 cases per 1,000,000 each year.[34] Aplastic anemia is most often acquired[35] as a result of severe illness such as human immunodeficiency virus, hepatitis, or Epstein Barr virus, long-term exposure to industrial chemicals, or use of anticancer drugs and other medications. Although not completely understood, there is some evidence that the body's autoimmune responses are responsible for acquired aplastic anemia. Hereditary aplastic anemia is rare but can be seen with Fanconi's anemia, Shwachman-Diamond syndrome, and dyskeratosis congenita. *Idiopathic aplastic anemia* refers to those cases where the cause is unknown.

Symptoms that should raise the health care provider's suspicion of aplastic anemia include unexplained bleeding (nosebleeds or easy bruising), frequent infections, or fatigue that is unusually severe. Physical findings include general signs of anemia, such as pallor and tachycardia, and signs of thrombocytopenia, such as petechiae, purpura, or ecchymoses. Short stature, microcephaly, hypogonadism, mental retardation, and skeletal anomalies may be seen in cases of inherited aplastic anemia such as Fanconi's anemia. The diagnosis can be made when a CBC reveals abnormally low counts of at least two of the three types of blood cells and a bone marrow biopsy confirms these low counts in the marrow itself. Laboratory results will reveal RBCs that appear normal in size and coloration, but with a very low number of reticulocytes. Platelets and WBCs will also be normal in structure, but decreased in number.

Treatment of this anemia first requires discontinuing exposure to any substance that may be causing the disorder. RBC transfusions are sometimes used as temporary relief for mild or moderate disease while the underlying cause is managed. Severe disease is frequently fatal, but may respond to a bone marrow or stem cell transplant. Infections are seen frequently as a result of reduced white cell production and require antibiotic therapy.[34,36] Current clinical trials include exploring the use of immunosuppressive agents such as antithymocyte globulin,[36] which appear to improve marrow functioning in about 70% of study patients.[35] Bone marrow transplants resolve some cases, but appear to be more effective in younger patients (80% survival rate) than older patients (40%–70% survival). Left untreated, death is likely.

ANEMIA OF CHRONIC DISEASE

Anemia of chronic disease is associated with a wide range of chronic malignant, autoimmune, leukemic, inflammatory, and infectious disease conditions.[37] It is a disorder with multiple names, and sometimes is called hypoferremia of inflammatory disease, anemia of inflammation, or iron-reutilization anemia (reflecting the bone marrow's inability to use stored iron in developing RBCs). The elderly are most at risk for this anemia, although anyone with a chronic disease may develop it. Developing slowly over time, this anemia reflects the suppressed production of RBCs in the bone marrow. Symptoms depend on the underlying cause, but will be mild in most cases. A transfusion is sometimes necessary.[38] Chronic liver failure tends to produce the most severe symptoms. Laboratory evaluation will show low hemoglobin with an increased ferritin level. It is sometimes microcytic, but often normocytic in nature. Other laboratory data may include:

- Low transferrin iron saturation percentage
- Low TIBC
- Low transferrin
- Normal serum transferring receptors

Anemia due to chronic disease may coexist with other anemias. For example, an individual with rheumatoid arthritis, in addition to an anemia of chronic disease, also may develop iron deficiency from chronic GI bleeding secondary to medication therapy. Treatment involves identification and eradication or treatment of the underlying cause. Supplementing with iron is not helpful until the underlying cause is addressed, and, can be harmful since some pathogens and cancer cells can proliferate in an iron-rich environment.

Physiology of Pregnancy and Anemia

Pregnancy is a time of remarkable yet natural and expected changes in blood volume. Blood volume increases beginning in the first trimester, primarily due to an increase in plasma rather than RBCs. Because plasma increases more than the solids in the circulating body fluids, pregnancy is a state of relative hemodilution, meaning that there is an expected decrease in Hb, Hct, and RBC count, but no change in MCV and in mean cell hemoglobin concentration (MCHC). This disproportion peaks in the second trimester, which can disguise the presence or severity of other anemias.[18] Diagnosis of iron deficiency anemia in pregnancy requires serial evaluation of the indices in order to differentiate between dilutional anemia and progressive iron deficiency anemia.[22] In pregnancy, the expanded blood volume, growth of the fetus, placenta, and other maternal tissues increases the demand for iron threefold in the second and third trimesters to approximately 5 mg iron/day.[39]

The CDC recommends routine iron supplementation of pregnant women at a low dose of 30 mg/day beginning at the first prenatal visit. Dietary counseling should be given at this time, and screening for anemia should occur at this first visit. Presumptive diagnosis of iron deficiency anemia is made if a positive screening (of Hb and Hct) is confirmed by a second test, and the woman is not ill. If the Hb is less than 9 g/dL or Hct is less than 27%, a hematology consult should be considered. Treatment of anemia should be an oral dose of 60 to 120 mg/day of iron, and dietary counseling. If repeat testing at four weeks shows no response (the Hb does not increase by 1 g/dL or Hct by 3%) despite compliance, further evaluation is recommended, with MCV, RDW, and serum ferritin concentration. When the Hb normalizes for the stage of pregnancy, the dose of iron can be decreased to 30 mg/day.[10]

Pregnant women who are at higher risk of hemoglobinopathies should be screened. If a woman tests positive for any of these conditions, her partner should also be tested to more completely evaluate the risks to the fetus and neonate. The baby has a 25% chance of having sickle cell anemia if both parents are carriers of the trait. A carrier usually shows no signs of disease other than mild anemia and can be identified by electrophoresis. However, during pregnancy, women who carry sickle cell trait are more likely to experience a higher incidence of asymptomatic bacteriuria and possibly pyelonephritis.[25] Women with compound anemias with two abnormal variant Hbs such as sickle cell anemia, Hb S/Hb C disease, and Hb S/beta thalassemia may experience more frequent and severe sickle cell crises during the pregnancy.[40] In addition, persons with Hb S-beta thalassemia experience higher rates of splenomegaly than those with homozygous sickle cell disease.[32]

Postpartum evaluation to confirm resolution of anemia should be performed in women at risk for persistent anemia. All women whose anemia continued throughout the third trimester, who experienced excessive blood loss during delivery, or who were pregnant with twins or multiples should be screened at their six-week postpartum visit. Treatment and follow-up during the postpartum period is the same for nonpregnant women.[1]

Conclusion

Anemias and hemoglobinopathies present a fairly predictable picture once the basic pathophysiology is understood. Primary care providers need to understand how to screen for, diagnose, and treat anemia, as well as how to determine when consultation is warranted. The most common types of anemia are manageable by the primary care provider who is committed to working with women to maximize quality of life.

References

1. U.S. Preventive Services Task Force. Screening for iron deficiency anemia—including iron prophylaxis. Chapter 22. In: *Guide to Clinical Preventive Services.* 2nd ed. Washington, DC: U.S. Department of Health and Human Services; 1996 [Monograph on the Internet; cited Jan 2004.] Retrieved November 29, 2005, from http://www.text.nlm.nih.gov/cps/www/cps.28.html.

2. Centers for Disease Control and Prevention. Iron deficiency–United States, 1999–2000. *MMWR.* 2002; 51:897–899. [Monograph available on the Internet.] Retrieved November 27, 2005, from: http://www.cdc.gov/mmwr/preview/mmwrhtml/mm5140a1.htm.

3. Centers for Disease Control and Prevention. Pediatric and Pregnancy Nutrition Surveillance System. Maternal Health Indicators available on the Internet. Retrieved November 29, 2005, from: http://www.cdc.gov/pednss/pnss_tables/pdf/.

4. Scholl TO, Hediger ML, Fischer RL, Shearer JW. Anemia vs. iron deficiency: Increased risk of preterm delivery in a prospective study. *Am J Clin Nutr.* 1992; 55:985–988.

5. Pilch SM, Senti FR, editors. Assessment of the Iron Nutritional Status of the U.S. Population Based on Data Collected in the *Second National Health and Nutrition Examination Survey, 1976–1980.* Rockville, MD: Life Sciences Research Office, Federation of American Societies for Experimental Biology; 1984.

6. Centers for Disease Control and Prevention. Pediatric Nutrition Surveillance System—United States, 1980–1991. *MMWR.* 1992;41(SS-7):1–24.

7. Ramakrishnan U, Frith-Terhune A, Cogswell M, Khan L. Dietary intake does not account for differences in low iron stores among Mexican American and non-Hispanic white women. *Third National Health and Nutrition Examination Survey, 1988–1994.* The American Society for Nutritional Sciences. *J Nutr.* 2002;132:996–1001.

8. Ganong W. Circulating body fluids. In: *Review of Medical Physiology.* 16th ed. Norwalk, CT: Appleton and Lange; 1993. pp. 469–493.

9. Dallman PR, Siimes MA, Stekel A. Iron deficiency in infancy and childhood. *Am J Clin Nutr.* 1980;33: 86–118.

10. Centers for Disease Control and Prevention (CDC). Recommendations to prevent and control iron deficiency in the U.S. *MMWR.* 1998;47(RR-3):1–36.

11. Engstrom J, Sittler C. Nurse-midwifery management of iron-deficiency anemia during pregnancy. *J Nurse Midwifery.* 1994;39(2):20S–34S.

12. Norris CF, Mahannah SR, et al. Pneumococcal colonization in children with sickle cell disease. *J Pediatr.* 1996;129:821–827.

13. Hord J, Byrd R, et al. *Streptococcus pneumoniae* sepsis and meningitis during the penicillin prophylaxis era in children with sickle cell disease. *J Pediatr Hematol Oncol.* 2002;24:470–472.

14. Centers for Disease Control and Prevention. Newborn screening for sickle cell disease: Public health impact and evaluation. In: *Developing, Implementing, and Evaluating Population Interventions. Part IV, in Genetics and Public Health in the 21st Century 2000.* [Monograph on the Internet; cited Jan. 20, 2004.] Available from:http://www.cdc.gov/genomics/info/books/21stcent4a.html.

15. Newborn Screening Committee of The Council of Regional Networks for Genetic Services (CORN). *National Newborn Screening Report—1993.* Atlanta: CORN; 1998. pp. 16,156–160, 169.

16. Agency for Health Care Policy and Research. Laboratory screening for sickle cell disease. Chapter 6. Sickle Cell Disease: Screening, Diagnosis, Management, and Counseling in Newborns and Infants. In *AHCPR Archived Clinical Practice Guidelines.* [Monograph on the

Internet; cited Jan 21 2005.] Available from: http://www.ncbi.nlm.nih.gov/books/bv.fcgi?rid=hstat6.section.17035.

17. Groer M, Shekleton M. Oxygenation and cellular metabolism. In: *Basic Pathophysiology. A Conceptual Approach.* St. Louis: C.V. Mosby Company; 1979. pp.179–194.

18. Schlichtmann J, Graber M. Anemia. In: *University of Iowa Family Practice Handbook 1999.* Chapter 5. [Monograph on the Internet; cited Jan 2004.] Available from:www.vh.org/Providers/ClinRef/FP Handbook/Chapter05/02-5.html.

19. Family Practice Notebook.com. Erythrocyte Protoporphyrin. [Monograph on the Internet; cited Jan. 21 2005.] Available from:www.fpnotebook.com/HEM67.html.

20. U.S. Dept. of Health and Human Services. *Healthy People 2010.* [Monograph on the Internet; cited Dec. 2003.] Available from: http://www.healthypeople.gov/.

21. Groer M, Shekleton M. Genetic teratogenic disease mechanisms. In: *Basic Pathophysiology. A Conceptual Approach.* St. Louis: C.V. Mosby Company; 1979. pp. 19–46.

22. Laros R. Maternal hematologic disorders. In: Creasy R, Resnik R. *Maternal-Fetal Medicine.* 3rd ed. Philadelphia: WB Saunders Company; 1994. pp. 905–933.

23. MEDLINE. *Medical encyclopedia: Pernicious anemia* [cited Dec. 2003.] Available from: http://www.nlm.nih.gov/medlineplus/ency/article/000569.html.

24. Wainscott M. Pregnancy, Postpartum Hemorrhage. In: *emedicine.com.* [Monograph on the Internet; cited Sept. 14, 2004.] Available from: http://www.emedicine.com/emerg/topic481.html.

25. Varney H, Kriebs JM, Gegor CL. Screening for and collaborative management of antepartal complications. In: *Varney's Midwifery.* 4th ed. Sudbury, MA: Jones and Bartlett; 2004.

26. Centers for Disease Control and Prevention. Prescription drugs for malaria. [Monograph on the Internet; cited Nov. 11, 2004.] Available from: http://www.cdc.gov/travel/malariadrugs.html.

27. Agency for Health Care Policy and Research. Sickle cell disease: Screening, diagnosis, management, and counseling in newborns and infants. In: *Clinical Practice Guideline No. 8. Publication No. 93-0562.* Rockville, MD: Agency for Health Care Policy and Research; 1993.

28. Platt, OS, Brambilla, DJ, Rosse WF, et al. Mortality in sickle cell disease: Life expectancy and risk factors for early death. *N Engl J Med.* 1994;330:1639–1644.

29. Claster S, Vichinsky E. Managing sickle cell disease. *BMJ.* 2003;327:1151–1155.

30. Bunn HF. Pathogenesis and treatment of sickle cell disease. *N Engl J Med.* 1997;337:762–769.

31. National Institutes of Health. Sickle Cell Anemia. Found in Medline Plus, Medical Encyclopedia. [Monograph on the Internet; cited Nov. 10, 2004.] Available from: http://www.nlm.gov/medlineplus/ency/article/000527.html.

32. Tyagi S, Chaoudhry VP, Saxena R. Subclassification of HbS syndrome: Is it necessary? *Clin Lab Haematol.* 2003;25:377–381.

33. National Institutes of Health. *Management and Therapy of Sickle Cell Disease.* NIH Publication No. 95-2117. Revised Dec 1995. 3rd ed. Washington, DC: National Institutes of Health, National Heart, Lung, and Blood Institute.

34. Segel G, Lichtman M. Aplastic anemia. In: Lichtman M, Beutler E, Kipps T, Seligsohn U, Kaushansky K, Prehal S, editors. *Williams Hematology.* 7th ed. New York: McGraw-Hill; 2006. pp. 419–436.

35. Bakhshi S. Aplastic Anemia. In: eMedicine. [Monograph on the Internet; updated Nov. 2005.] Available from: http://www.emedicine.com/med/topic162.htm.

36. National Marrow Donor Program. Aplastic anemia (severe)—basic. [Monograph on the Internet; cited Nov. 2005.] Available from: http://www.marrow.org/PATIENT/aplastic_anemia.html.

37. Iron Disorders Institute. Anemia. [Monograph on the Internet; cited Nov. 2005.] Available from: http://www.irondisorders.org.

38. Merck Manual. Anemia [cited Dec. 2003]. Available from: http://www.merck.com/mrkshared/mmanual_home2/sec14/ch172/ch172e.jsp.

39. National Research Council. *Recommended Dietary Allowances.* 10th ed. Washington, DC: National Academy Press; 1989.

40. Miller S, Sleeper LA, Pegelow CH, Enos LE, Wang WC, Weiner S, et al. Prediction of adverse outcomes in children with sickle cell disease. *N Engl J Med.* 2000;342:1612–1613.

Chapter 16

Endocrine

Melissa D. Avery

Karyn D. Baum

Diabetes and thyroid disorders are the most commonly seen endocrine diseases in the primary care setting. All health care providers must be aware of the symptoms, diagnostic tests, and common treatments for these conditions. Thyroid disorders, particularly hypothyroidism, are more common in women and must be considered during the childbearing period and as women age. Untreated thyroid disorders have been linked to serious medical consequences including infertility, miscarriage, pre-eclampsia, low birth weight, and neuropsychological sequelae in children. Thyroid disorders are more prevalent in the elderly; as the population ages over the next several decades, caregivers will be diagnosing and treating more and more patients with these conditions.

The United States is facing an epidemic of obesity and, consequently, diabetes. A 2002 study of U.S. adults utilizing National Health and Nutrition Examination Survey (NHANES) data documented the prevalence of obesity in U.S. adults in 1999 to 2000 at 30.5%, an increase from 22.9% in 1988 to 1994.[1] A 2004 study suggested that poor diet and physical inactivity, known risk factors for type 2 diabetes, may soon overtake cigarette smoking as the most common cause of death in the United States.[2] Recognizing and counseling women at risk for diabetes should be a major focus of preventive education in the primary care setting.

As primary care providers, midwives must be prepared to appropriately screen, diagnose, and consult or refer new cases of thyroid disease or diabetes to physicians for management as appropriate. Continuing collaborative care of women with thyroid disease or diabetes may be appropriate depending on the setting, wishes of the patient, and the interests and expertise of the provider.

Thyroid Disorders

Thyroid disorders are the second most common endocrine disorder affecting women of reproductive age, behind diabetes mellitus.[3] Untreated thyroid disorders are present in up to 10% of the adult population, are commonly found in women of all age groups,[4] and have been associated with outcomes such as miscarriage in 60% of overtly hypothyroid patients.[5] Although most midwives, having made a diagnosis of thyroid disease, will refer the patient for care, in some cases the midwife may monitor and manage stable hypothyroid patients on an ongoing basis, depending on her expertise and practice setting.

The thyroid gland produces three hormones: calcitonin, thyroxine (T_4), and triiodothyronine (T_3). Calcitonin regulates calcium metabolism. T_3 and T_4 are generally considered to be the "thyroid hormones"; T_3 is more potent although T_4 is more plentiful. T_3 and T_4 are produced by the thyroid as part of a negative feedback control mechanism. The hypothalamus, in response to circulating levels of free T_3 and free T_4, produces thyroxine-binding globulin (TBG). TBG signals the anterior pituitary gland to synthesize thyroid stimulating hormone (TSH). TSH controls the production of T_3 and T_4. Finally, rising T_3 and T_4 levels signal the hypothalamus to decrease production of TBG (**Figure 16-1**).

Hypothyroidism

EPIDEMIOLOGY

The exact prevalence of hypothyroidism has been difficult to quantify for several reasons. First, rates vary significantly among populations. For example, in one study carried out in Colorado (n = 25,862), 9.5% of subjects at a State Fair were found to have elevated serum thyrotropin (TSH) levels.[6] A longitudinal study in England found that 7.5% of women and 2.8% of men had TSH levels greater than 6 mIU/L.[7] Rate variations may be partially due to differences in iodine intake, although this cannot fully explain the wide range in results. For instance, one area of endemic iodine deficiency reported rates of hypothyroidism as high as 17%,[8] while another noted a rate of only 2.1%.[9] Additionally, there is evidence that average TSH values are higher in whites than blacks.[10,11]

Secondly, the exact definition of the disease state has changed with both the sensitivity of

the assays used and the definition of normal ranges for TSH results. Various studies have used upper limits ranging from 4.1 mIU/L[12,13] to 4.5 mIU/L,[10] 5.1 mIU/L,[6,14] and 6 mIU/L.[7] In general, the rate of abnormally elevated TSH levels is likely close to the 5% postulated by Vanderpump and Tunbridge,[15] the 4.7% found in a population in Milan, Italy,[16] and the 4.6% noted in a stratified sample from multiple ethnic and geographic distributions in the NHANES III.[10]

Hypothyroidism affects women to a much greater degree than men, with a prevalence of 4% to 10% in women.[17] A study of over 94,000 Norwegians noted a prevalence of hypothyroidism in 4.8% of women as compared to 0.9% of men.[13] Hypothyroidism is often undiagnosed as well. This Norwegian study noted that 6% of women had TSH values above normal (4.1 mIU/I).[13] Another study found that 2.2% of 9403 women randomly tested during their second trimester of pregnancy were hypothyroid (TSH 6 mIU/L or greater).[18]

Hypothyroidism consists of overt and subclinical hypothyroidism, each of which should be considered separately. *Overt hypothyroidism*, which is less common and more obvious to the clinician, is diagnosed by laboratory findings of a low serum free T_4 concentration with elevated serum TSH concentration.[19] Rates for overt hypothyroidism among the general population are approximately 0.3% to 0.4%.[6,10]

Subclinical hypothyroidism is defined as "a serum TSH concentration above the statistically defined upper limit of the reference range when serum free T_4 concentration is within normal range."[19] Subclinical hypothyroidism is much more common than overt hypothyroidism. It occurs in 4% to 8.5% of the U.S. adult population without known thyroid disease.[6,10,20] As

Figure 16-1 Thyroid physiology.

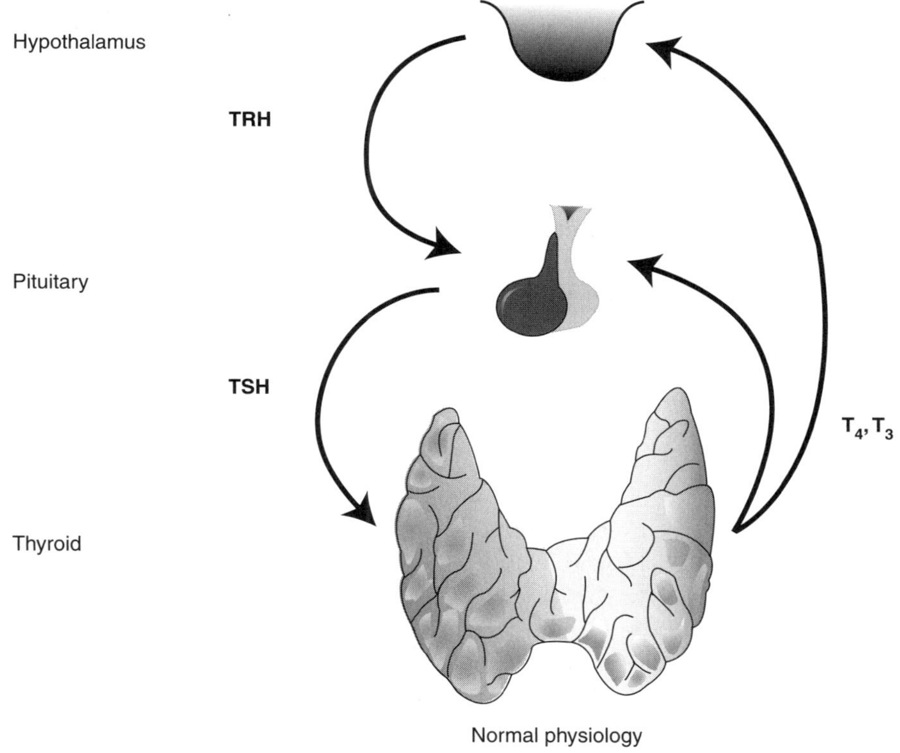

Abbreviations are: TRH, thyroid; TSH, thyroid stimulating hormone.
Source: Reprinted with permission from Current Science Group. Atlas of Clinical Endocrinology, 1999.

with most thyroid disease, subclinical hypothyroidism is more common in women than men. In one community in England, 8% of women and 3% of men had the disorder based on laboratory findings.[21] Subclinical hypothyroidism may progress to overt hypothyroidism over time, but rates of progression are debated. Rates of progression reportedly vary from 3% to 20% per year, with risks being greater in those with thyroid antibodies.[19,22] Patients with higher TSH values (above 9 mIU/L) [14] and positive antithyroid antibodies are more likely to

progress to overt hypothyroidism over a five-year period.

Clearly, both types of hypothyroidism are relatively common and underdiagnosed medical conditions. In one screening study, 103 of 114 hypothyroid patients were not taking medication.[6] Both conditions are more common in women, especially as they age. A small but significant percentage of pregnant women therefore are likely to have undiagnosed hypothyroidism.

By its nature, subclinical hypothyroidism is a laboratory diagnosis only. Although people with subclinical hypothyroidism can report any of the symptoms discussed below, usually patients are clinically well.

SYMPTOMS

Symptoms of thyroid disease vary widely among patients and correspond with the acuity of the loss of thyroid function, thus leading to a delay in diagnosis in some cases. Symptoms are less obvious when the loss of thyroid hormone occurs gradually rather than abruptly, such as after thyroidectomy or radioiodine therapy.[23]

Most symptoms are believed to reflect one of two changes that occur after the loss of thyroid hormones:[24] a generalized slowing of the metabolic process, and an accumulation of matrix glycosaminoglycans in the interstitial spaces of many tissues.

The classical symptoms of overt hypothyroidism are listed in **Table 16-1**[24] and include drier skin, poorer memory, weight gain, edema, constipation, and feeling colder. Sensitivities for these symptoms are low and range from 2.9% to 28.3%, meaning that the absence of any given symptom would not rule out the disorder. Specificities fare slightly better, with rates of 74.7% to 97.6%.[6] However, positive predictive values are only 8% to 12%[6] for any given symptom, so the diagnosis should not be based upon the presence or absence of any given complaint.

A less common but important complaint is infertility.[12] One case series of hypothyroid women found that incompletely treated hypothyroidism was associated with preterm labor as well as miscarriage and fetal death.[5,18] Additionally, one case series by Haddow and colleagues suggested a link between untreated hypothyroidism during pregnancy and subsequent delays in neuropsychological development of the child.[25]

Table 16-1 COMMON SYMPTOMS OF HYPOTHYROIDISM*

Drier skin, thin hair
Poorer memory
Slower thinking
Weaker muscles
More tired
More muscle cramps
Feeling colder
Puffier eyes
Deep voice (current)
Hoarse voice (current)
More constipation
Depression

*Symptoms are listed in order of discriminatory ability.
Source: Data are adapted from Canaris et al.[6] and Surks.[24]

The difficulty of diagnosing hypothyroidism in pregnancy is that many of the classic symptoms, such as fatigue, are common in pregnancy as well. Parasthesias and weight gains are symptoms frequent in both conditions, so clinicians must have a high index of suspicion in order to make a diagnosis of new-onset hypothyroidism in these women.

SIGNS

Clinical manifestations of hypothyroidism can be found in almost every organ system, owing to the wide variety of impacts that thyroid hormones have upon the body.

Cardiovascular   Both overt and subclinical hypothyroidism appear to affect the cardiovascular system, most commonly by bradycardia, mild hypertension, and a narrowed pulse pressure.[26] Subclinical hypothyroidism has been associated with impaired left ventricular diastolic dysfunction at rest, systolic dysfunction at effort, and enhanced risk for myocardial infarction.[27]

Hypothyroidism also prolongs the QT interval and may dispose patients to torsade de pointes[26] (a distinctive type of ventricular tachycardia), although data are conflicting.[28] In one large cross-sectional study in The Netherlands, subclinical hypothyroidism was found to be a strong indicator of risk for aortic atherosclerosis (odds ratio 1.7; CI 1.1-6) and myocardial infarction (odds ratio 2.3; 1.3-4) in women with a mean age of 69.[29] However, in an analysis of the literature for the U.S. Preventive Services Task Force (USPSTF), Helfand concluded that the evidence on whether subclinical hypothyroidism increases the risk of hyperlipidemia, artherosclerosis, and other adverse outcomes associated with overt hypothyroidism is inconsistent.[14]

Endocrinologic   The thyroid gland itself should always be examined in cases of suspected hypothyroidism. Examination findings can vary from a tender, slightly enlarged thyroid to an entirely normal exam to a nonpalpable atrophic gland. It is helpful to exclude obvious nodules.

Gastrointestinal   Scattered reports link celiac disease[30] and malabsorption[31,32] with hypothyroidism. Two cases of intestinal obstruction have been reported in the literature as well as pseudo-obstruction and acute abdomen.[33]

Hematologic   Patients with hypothyroidism and diabetes mellitus type 1 have a relatively high incidence of pernicious anemia (6.3% in one series of 63 patients), with a higher rate in women (8.5% in the same study). Anemia also is associated with hypothyroidism.[34]

Metabolic   A generalized slowing of the metabolic rate causes a variety of metabolic changes, including weight gain (although weight loss is not unheard of). Laboratory alterations associated with hypothyroidism include elevated creatinine kinase, serum oxaloacetic transaminase, lactate dehydrogenase, serum cholesterol, and serum carotene. Hypothyroid patients also have high cholesterol levels, most specifically low-density lipoprotein.

Neuromuscular   There are a wide variety of signs and symptoms linked to overt hypothyroidism, from general intelligence decline to memory impairment to perceptual and visuospatial function impairment.[35] Treatment will often lead to improvement. Overt hypothyroidism has been associated with carpal tunnel syndrome. Several small series suggest that subclinical hypothyroidism causes similar, if less pronounced, changes.[36,37] Individuals with this condition have also been reported to have higher scores on scales of anxiety and depression, although this finding has not been consistent.[38]

Overt hypothyroidism has long been associated with dementia, although the evidence that treatment reverses the dementia is lacking.[39] Subclinical hypothyroidism has also been linked to dementia;[40] however, high-quality studies have not been performed to establish a causal link.

Myxedema coma is a rare but potentially fatal consequence of untreated hypothyroidism. It is usually precipitated by an acute illness or trauma in a patient with underlying hypothyroidism.[41] A high index of suspicion is crucial in patients presenting with unexplained coma.

Respiratory   Overt hypothyroidism is a recognized cause of obstructive sleep apnea syndrome,[42] and the current recommendation is to treat those with subclinical hypothyroidism and sleep apnea with hormone replacement.

Reproductive   Hypothyroidism is considered by some to be a potential cause of infertility.[12] Data are lacking as to whether treatment will reverse this problem, which usually manifests as ovulatory dysfunction. Two small case series recommend screening infertile women for hypothyroidism,[12,43] but no studies have been reported on whether fertility is improved by L-thyroxine treatment.

Skin The skin is cool due to decreased blood flow.[24,44] Dryness results from atrophy of the cellular layer and hyperkeratosis. Hair may be coarse, and hair loss is common. Patients may also complain of thin, brittle nails.[45] Skin discoloration may occur; a yellowish hue, the result of carotemia, may be imparted on the skin, particularly on the palms, soles, and nasolabial folds. Generalized myxedema is likely the most characteristic dermatologic sign of hypothyroidism, with skin appearing swollen, pale, dry, waxy, and firm to the touch.

SCREENING FOR THYROID DISEASE

Table 16-2 lists the recommendations from several major organizations about screening for thyroid disease, including during pregnancy.[46–50] Notably, false positives are a significant concern in the screening for thyroid disease. In one study, 8 of 19 mildly elevated TSH levels reverted to normal with treatment by placebo.[51] Therefore, a reasonable first step if confronted by an abnormal TSH is to repeat the test.

DIAGNOSIS

Accompanied by a thorough history and physical examination addressing the signs and symptoms discussed above, appropriate laboratory testing is crucial in the diagnosis of hypothyroidism (**Table 16-3**). A sensitive TSH assay (with a functional sensitivity of at least 0.02 mIU/L[19]) is recommended as the primary

---

Table 16-2 RECOMMENDED GUIDELINES FROM LEADING HEALTH CARE ORGANIZATIONS ABOUT SCREENING FOR THYROID DISEASE

Organization	Screening Recommendation
American College of Physicians[50]	Reasonable to screen women >50 years old
American College of Obstetricians and Gynecologists[1,45]	Insufficient data to recommend routine screening for asymptomatic women
American Association of Clinical Endocrinologists[51]	Screening TSH should be routine before pregnancy or during first trimester
U.S. Preventive Services Task Force[12]	Insufficient evidence for or against screening in nonpregnant adults. Pregnant adults are not addressed.
American Thyroid Association, American Association of Clinical Endocrinologists and the Endocrine Society[15]	Obtain a TSH prior to or during pregnancy if a woman has a family or personal history of thyroid disease, diabetes mellitus type 1, signs or symptoms suggestive of hypothyroidism, or personal history of autoimmune disorders
American Thyroid Association[48]	All adults >35 years should be screened every 5 years
American Academy of Family Physicians	Recommend against screening patients ≤60 years and non-neonates

Table 16-3 EXPECTED LABORATORY FINDINGS WITH THE MAJOR CATEGORIES OF THYROID DISEASE

Diagnosis	TSH	Free T_4	Free T_3
Pituitary insufficiency	Normal/Low	Low	Low/Normal
Overt Hypothyroidism	Elevated	Low	Low to High
Subclinical Hypothyroidism	Elevated	Normal	Normal
Euthyroid	Normal	Normal	Normal
Subclinical Hyperthyroidism	Low	Normal	Normal
Overt Hyperthyroidism	Low	High/Normal	High

preliminary test used to evaluate suspected subclinical or overt hypothyroidism.[47]

Other available tests should be ordered judiciously because they may not change the treatment plan and can increase costs. These tests include[47,52]:

- Serum Free T_4 (FT_4)
- Thyroid antibodies: anti-thyroid peroxidase (elevated in Hashimoto's thyroiditis)
- Free T_3
- Antithyroglobulin autoantibodies
- Thyroid scan or ultrasound (needed if suspect structural abnormality)

It is important to note that during pregnancy, serum TSH and free T_4 values should remain unchanged, unlike total T_3 and T_4 levels, which increase due to the increase in TBG.[4,34] Even hormone replacement therapy and oral contraceptive use can increase total T_4 levels above the reference range.[17]

There are three settings in which TSH may not be a useful tool:[23]

1. Known or suspected pituitary or hypothalamic disease.
2. Hospitalized patients receiving dopaminergic or glucocorticoid medications, or with *euthyroid sick syndrome* (defined as abnormal thyroid function tests associated with acute non-thyroid, non-pituitary illness).[53]
3. Use of drugs that affect TSH secretion. Drugs that decrease secretion include dopamine, phenytoin, and octreotide. Drugs that increase TSH secretion include dopamine antagonists and amiodarone.

Table 16-4 outlines the findings seen in overt and subclinical hypothyroidism.

TREATMENT

Overt Hypothyroidism On the whole, treatment for overt hypothyroidism is quite effective and safe; the mainstay of treatment remains levothyroxine sodium (Synthroid). Adverse effects of replacement with levothyroxine include nervousness, atrial fibrillation, and, in about one-fifth of patients with angina pectoris, exacerbation of chest pain. Treatment with thyroid replacement is usually lifelong[17] and requires periodic monitoring of TSH levels.

There is no single agreement as to the ideal method for initiating treatment. Some specialists have advocated that women with newly diagnosed hypothyroidism should be started on a daily dose

Table 16-4 DIFFERENTIAL DIAGNOSIS OF HYPOTHYROIDISM

Primary Hypothyroidism

Chronic autoimmune thyroiditis
  Goitrous
  Atrophic
Transient hypothyroidism
  Subacute lymphocytic thyroiditis
  Subacute granulomatous thyroiditis
  Postpartum thyroiditis
  Subtotal thyroidectomy
  Post-radiation therapy for Graves disease
  Post-viral subacute thyroiditis
Iatrogenic
  Post-thyroidectomy
  Radioiodine therapy or external radiation
Iodine deficiency or excess
Infiltrative diseases
  Fibrous thyroiditis
  Hemachromatosis
  Sarcoidosis
Drugs
  Lithium
  Amiodarone
  Interferon-alpha
  Perchlorate
Highly active antiretroviral therapy (HAART)

Secondary Hypothyroidism

Pituitary disease
Hypothalamic disease
Other causes
  Generalized thyroid hormone resistance
  Recovery from severe illness
  Untreated primary adrenal insufficiency
  Depression
  Amyloidosis
  Assay error due to interfering substances
  Over-treatment of overt hyperthyroidism

of 25 mcg to 50 mcg of levothyroxine,[34,54] while others have recommended that a higher replacement dose be initiated, especially if the patient is young and without heart disease. Doses should then be slowly increased until the patient is euthyroid by clinical and laboratory standards. TSH levels take about four weeks to adjust after a dose change, so in general it is not useful to test more frequently than every four to six weeks.

Subclinical Hypothyroidism The advisability of treating subclinical hypothyroidism has been debated over the past several years. Many authorities have concluded that treatment for all patients with asymptomatic subclinical hypothyroidism is not warranted,[55] while others believe that treatment is safe and may prevent the subsequent development of overt hypothyroidism. Other experts feel that subclinical hypothyroidism is mild thyroid failure and deserves medical treatment.[56] The debate over the advisability of treating subclinical hypothyroidism is fueled by poor quality research; small randomized trials have produced inconsistent results.[14]

Several large reviews have advocated treatment for those with a TSH greater than 10 mIU/L in nonpregnant adults.[19,20,22,55] These patients are more likely to have symptoms attributable to thyroid disease and progress to overt hypothyroidism.[14] Treatment at levels between 5 and 10 mIU/L is more controversial because it is not clear that early treatment leads to improvement in long-term outcomes.[14,47] The American Association of Clinical Endocrinologists recommends treatment for those with lower abnormal TSH levels only if they also have a goiter, certain medical conditions, or test positive for antithyroid perioxidase antibodies.[47] If treatment is initiated for subclinical hypothyroidism, the American Association of Clinical Endocrinologists recommends starting levothyroxine at at 25 to 50 mcg daily and rechecking TSH levels in six to eight weeks. Dosages should be adjusted until the TSH level is between 0.3 and 3 mIU/L.[47] One 2004 review advocated a focused approach (**Figure 16-2**).[20]

Figure 16-2 Suggested approach to diagnosis and management of subclinical hypothyroidism.

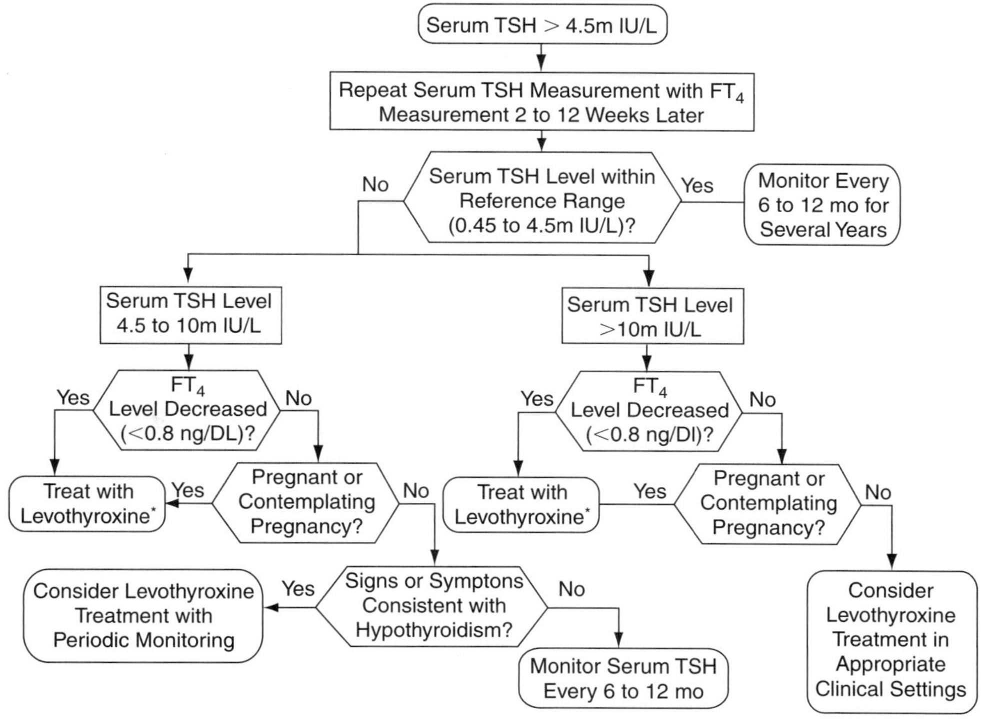

The normal range of free T_4 (FT_4) is 0.8 to 2.0 ng/dL (10-25 pmol/L); the normal range of thyroid-stimulating hormone (TSH) is 0.45–4.5 mIU/L.

*In rare instances a slightly elevated serum TSH represents hypothalamic/pituitary disease. In these situations the FT_4 is extremely low when the TSH is only slightly elevated, in contrast to primary hypothyroidism in which the TSH increases exponentially with small decreases in serum FT_4 concentration.

Source: Reprinted with permission from the Journal of the American Medical Association 2004; 291 (2).

TREATMENT AND MANAGEMENT DURING PREGNANCY

Hypothyroidism is not a common occurrence during pregnancy but must be recognized by health care practitioners to ensure optimal maternal and fetal health. Estimates of the incidence of new hypothyroidism (subclinical and overt) in pregnant women have been reported to range from 0.2% to 2.5%.[34] Rates are significantly higher in patients with insulin-dependent diabetes. Hypothyroidism has also been associated with a greater risk of preterm delivery and pre-ecclampsia as well as miscarriage, although causal links have not been clearly established.[57]

Authorities are unclear as to whether treating pregnant women with subclinical hypothyroidism is appropriate. Certainly, treating women with a

TSH greater than 10m IU/L would be consistent with the reviews discussed in the previous section of this chapter. While for ethical reasons there have not been randomized-control trials, there is some retrospective case review evidence showing a higher rate of fetal loss and abnormalities in women with untreated subclinical hypothyroidism during pregnancy.[5] The American Association of Clinical Endocrinologists recommend routine screening and treatment of subclinical hypothyroidism in pregnancy,[47] whereas American College of Obstetricians and Gynecologists (ACOG) does not, even for those with hyperemesis or mildly enlarged thyroid glands.[58] These different interpretations result from the lack of good evidence to determine the best approach. Therefore, the decision to treat during pregnancy should be individualized and consultation obtained as appropriate.

The goals of treatment during pregnancy are to maintain a normal free T_4 value and a normal TSH. These goals are based upon data associating elevated TSH levels in the mother with undesired outcomes, including fetal death.[18] It should be noted that there are no trials, especially randomized trials, that assess whether treating pregnant mothers who have elevated TSH levels prevents these outcomes.

Monitoring hormone levels is crucial. During pregnancy, TBG levels increase, as do total T_4 and T_3 levels. Many women with pre-existing hypothyroidism will require a dose increase during pregnancy; one study found that 69.5% of pregnant women required a dose increase during pregnancy.[5] Women may require as much as a 50% dose increase in order to remain euthyroid.[4] TSH levels should be checked in pregnant women with known hypothyroidism at 22 weeks and 28 weeks gestation.[34] After delivery, dose requirements will decrease to preconception levels.[59]

For those pregnant women with newly diagnosed hypothyroidism, monitoring will be the same as for their nonpregnant counterparts. TSH levels should be measured monthly until they are clinically and numerically euthyroid.

Hyperthyroidism

EPIDEMIOLOGY

In general, hyperthyroidism is less commonly found than hypothyroidism, with approximately 1% to 2.5% of the overall population having an abnormally low serum TSH level.[6,10,13,60] Once again, women are twice as likely as men to have a TSH below normal.[13] Only about 0.2% of pregnancies are complicated by hyperthyroidism[61] compared with 10 times that incidence in hypothyroidism. Graves disease accounts for 95% of those cases.[61]

Hyperthyroidism also is divided into two types: overt and subclinical hyperthyroidism. Subclinical hyperthyroidism is the more common condition, with approximately 0.7% of the U.S. population having the condition.[10] *Overt hyperthyroidism* is defined as having a low TSH as well as an elevated serum free T_4 level, and is usually caused by Graves disease.

Unlike hypothyroidism, untreated overt hyperthyroidism in pregnancy has been convincingly shown to lead to poor fetal outcomes, and must be promptly recognized and carefully treated. Controversy remains as to the necessity for treatment of subclinical hyperthyroidism. In general, pregnant women with asymptomatic subclinical hyperthyroidism and an uneventful pregnancy should not be treated.[62] While there may be some evidence that untreated hyperthyroidism may lead to complications, there is enough clear evidence of unintended side effects from antithyroid drugs that treatment in these cases is generally unwarranted.

OVERT HYPERTHYROIDISM

Symptoms A variety of symptoms are associated with hyperthyroidism, at times making the diagnosis challenging (**Table 16-5**). Notably, the elderly can have a very different presentation for hyperthyroidism. They may present with an altered or even decreased set of symptoms that may include constipation, apathy, and angina or congestive heart failure.[63] One case series in France noted that the most common presenting symptoms were tachycardia, fatigue, and weight loss.[64] A second case series of 65 elderly hyperthyroid patients confirmed the difference in presentation and found that the incidence was approximately equal for men and women at this age (age range 50–78 years).[65] The etiology of hyperthyroidism also changes with age; one study of patients aged 20 to 78 years of age found that toxic multinodular goiter was the etiology for 43.1% of cases, whereas Graves disease accounted for only 21.4% of cases.[66]

SIGNS

Cardiovascular Tachycardia is common in hyperthyroidism, even subclinical hyperthyroidism, as is widened pulse pressure. Hyperthyroidism has been associated with several types of cardiac dysfunction. Atrial fibrillation has long been linked to hyperthyroidism, and several experts have advocated routine TSH testing in all patients presenting with new-onset atrial fibrillation. However, several studies, including a large Canadian study, have refuted the utility of screening for hyperthyroidism in patients with atrial fibrillation.

A 2002 review concluded that subclinical hyperthyroidism was associated with increased heart rate and atrial arrhythmias.[27] A small retrospective study in women reported that both

Table 16-5 SYMPTOMS OF HYPERTHYROIDISM

More Common Symptoms
Weight loss
Tachycardia/palpitations
Anxiety/nervousness
Heat intolerance
Increased perspiration
Tremor
Weakness
Increased appetite (decreased appetite in the elderly)
Frequent defecation

Less Frequent Symptoms
Urinary frequency
Oligomenorrhea or amenorrhea
Gynecomastia in men
Erectile dysfunction
Dysphagia
Hypokalemia periodic paralysis
Angina (elderly patients)
Insomnia

Symptoms Specific to Graves Disease
Exophthalmos
Diplopia
Dry eyes (from lid retraction)

Source: Watts RS. Hyperthyroidism. In: *Saunders Manual of Medical Practice.* St. Louis: WB Saunders; 1996. pp. 638–641.

subclinical and overt hyperthyroidism were associated with diastolic dysfunction.[67] Pulmonary hypertension has been associated with hyperthyroidism.[68]

Hyperthyroidism increases the overall cardiac output and may occasionally lead to a blunted ability to respond to exercise demands, leading to anginal symptoms. For this reason, some experts have advocated screening all patients with new-onset angina with a TSH.[26]

Endocrinologic   Once again, the thyroid gland should always be examined when a clinician is concerned about hyperthyroidism. In one study, over 60% of patients with hyperthyroidism had a diffusely palpable thyroid, and 19% had a nodular thyroid. Patients over 40 years of age, however, were more likely to have a normal exam.[69] A palpable thrill or bruit may also be found on exam. A solitary nodule should lead to an immediate referral to an endocrinologist.

Gastrointestinal   Many texts note that hyperthyroidism can lead to secretory diarrhea; however, the primary literature is mostly comprised of case reports. There have also been case reports of severe dysphagia.[70,71]

Hematologic   Thyroid hormones generally stimulate erythropoiesis, but there have been associations proposed between hyperthyroidism and anemia. There are case reports of several types of anemia, including autoimmune hemolytic anemia[72] and Evans syndrome[73,74] that resolve upon re-establishment of the euthyroid state. The best evidence for a link between hyperthyroidism and anemia comes from the National Thyrotoxicosis Therapy Follow-Up Study, which reported that 10–15% of over 20,000 women were found to be anemic, demonstrating an association but not necessarily a causal link.[75]

Metabolic   Weight loss has long been associated with uncontrolled hyperthyroidism, especially in the elderly.[64] Osteoporosis has also been linked to hyperthyroidism.[76] Rarely, hypokalemic paralysis has been associated with hyperthyroidism.[77]

Neuromuscular   Hyper-reflexia has been linked to hyperthyroidism for decades.[78,79] In fact, for years the "Achilles reflex time" was used to help

screen for and diagnose thyrotoxicosis.[80,81] Hyperthyroidism also may cause muscle weakness and even paralysis, with or without hypokalemia.[72,77,82,83] Depression and anxiety also have been associated with hyperthyroidism.[84] In one small study, insomnia was a discriminating feature of hyperthyroidism in patients in Turkey.

Ophthalmologic   Opthalmopathy is apparent in 20% to 40% of patients with Graves disease. Signs include proptosis, lid retraction, and conjunctivitis. In more severe cases, exopthalmos may develop. Rarely, compression of the optic nerve or entrapment of extraocular muscles may occur.[85] Unfortunately, exopthalmos is often irreversible even after treatment.

Reproductive   Graves disease in pregnancy carries an approximately 1% risk of fetal thyrotoxicosis from the transplacental transfer of thyroid-stimulating antibodies or fetal hypothyroidism from transplacental transfer of antithyroid drugs and thyroid-blocking antibodies.[86] It is not clear how best to monitor the fetal thyroid status, but one study suggested that serial ultrasonographic measurement of the fetal thyroid can help to identify cases of fetal hypothyroidism.[87] Additionally, a fetal heart rate baseline above 160 may suggest its development, and in these cases measuring TSH receptor antibody levels may be helpful.[88] Prompt treatment in these cases with oral propylthiouracil (PTU) can help alleviate the consequences. If neonatal hyperthyroidism does develop, it is generally self-limited and resolves by three to four months of age because the maternal antibodies are no longer being transmitted. Women with uncontrolled hyperthyroidism also have an increased risk for low-birth weight babies as well as pre-eclampsia in several studies.[89,90]

Respiratory Hyperthyroidism has been linked to asthma exacerbations.[91,92] In addition, the symptoms of hyperthyroidism may mimic the side effects of bronchodilators,[93] making it more difficult to diagnose these patients.

Skin Thyroid hormones affect the growth and formation of hair. Skin in patients with hyperthyroidism is warm, moist, and smooth. Hyperpigmentation in crease areas, similar to that seen in Addison's disease, may also be noted. Scleromyxedema has also been reported rarely.[44] Approximately 5% of patients have Plummer's nail, a concave contour and distal onycholysis.[94]

Graves disease has some specific skin manifestations. Approximately 0.5% to 4% of patients have pre-tibial myxedema and 1% have acropachy, a triad consisting of digital clubbing, soft tissue swelling, and periosteal new bone formation.[44]

SUBCLINICAL HYPERTHYROIDISM

Table 16-2 reviews the screening recommendations of major medical groups. Screening for hyperthyroidism is largely predicated upon data suggesting a higher risk of cardiovascular complications, mainly atrial fibrillation, in individuals with asymptomatic subclinical hyperthyroidism. However, a well-respected Canadian study that evaluated thyroid function in patients with recent-onset atrial fibrillation concluded that routine TSH screening of patients with new-onset atrial fibrillation has a low yield.[95] In addition, there is little evidence that treating subclinical hyperthyroidism leads to conversion to normal sinus rhythm.[19]

DIAGNOSIS

A history and physical directed toward assessing for signs, symptoms, and secondary etiologies of hyperthyroidism should be performed before any laboratory work is ordered. When hyperthyroidism is suspected, an appropriate laboratory workup should be performed. All patients with overt hyperthyroidism will have elevated serum concentrations of free T_4 and/or free T_3.

The best initial test to evaluate hyperthyroidism is the serum TSH. Other laboratory tests that may be used include:[96]

- Serum free T_3 and/or T_4 levels
- Twenty-four-hour thyroid radioiodine uptake and scan in patients with high free T_3 and/or T_4. Note that routine thyroid scans of patients with newly diagnosed hyperthyroidism are controversial. Some experts recommend this testing only in patients without opthalmopathy (because the etiology of the hyperthyroidism is still in doubt);[54] however, a 2002 study noted that thyroid nodules associated with Graves were more likely to be malignant.[97] Because of the results of that study, other experts are recommending routine thyroid scans in all patients.[88]
- Consider pituitary magnetic resonance imaging if serum free T_3 and T_4 levels are elevated but TSH is normal or high. These values may indicate thyrotropin-secreting pituitary tumor.

Circulating TSH receptor levels are often ordered. However, if the patient presents with opthalmopathy, she can be diagnosed with Graves disease without ordering the additional test.

Table 16-3 reviews the expected laboratory results for the most common types of hyperthyroidism. As noted in the hypothyroidism diagnostics section, keep in mind the three situations that may affect TSH levels: pituitary or hypothalamic disease; hospitalized patients with certain medications or euthyroid sick syndrome; and medications affecting TSH secretion.

The full workup for a newly diagnosed individual with hyperthyroidism is beyond the scope of this chapter. Prompt referral to an endocrinologist is warranted in these cases, especially if she is pregnant.

Subclinical hyperthyroidism, like subclinical hypothyroidism, can be difficult to diagnose given its lack of symptoms. In addition, several other causes of low serum TSH and normal serum free T_3 and T_4 exist, including central hypothyroidism, dopamine and glucocorticoid therapy, and recovery from hyperthyroidism.[96]

Differential Diagnosis   The most common etiology of hyperthyroidism is Graves disease, with 60% to 80% of patients with hyperthyroidism having Graves, depending upon regional factors.[98] Other causes are listed in **Table 16-6**. The differential can essentially be broken down into three main categories: primary hyperthyroidism, secondary hyperthyroidism, and additional causes.

Transient hyperthyroidism of hyperemesis gravidarum (THHG) should be considered in any woman in the early stages of pregnancy who presents with new hyperthyroidism. THHG is a self-limiting hyperthyroid condition in the setting of hyperemesis gravidarum and has been postulated to be responsible for 40% to 70% of the thyroid function abnormalities in pregnancy.[99] No treatment is required, and it generally resolves by 18 weeks of gestation.[100]

Postpartum women with pre-existing diabetes mellitus type 1 are at a significant risk for developing postpartum hyperthyroidism. One

Table 16-6 DIFFERENTIAL DIAGNOSIS OF HYPERTHYROIDISM

Primary Hyperthyroidism

Hyperthyroid goiter (Graves disease)
Multinodular hyperthyroid goiter (toxic multinodular goiter)
Autonomous hyperfunctioning nodule (Plummers disease)

Secondary Hyperthyroidism

Transient hyperthyroidism (e.g., critical illness)
Pregnancy
    High HCG levels (first 4 months pregnancy)
    Molar pregnancy
    Transient hyperthyroidism of hyperemesis gravidarum
Postpartum thyroiditis (particularly in patients with diabetes mellitus)
Struma ovarii (thyroid tissue within dermoid tumors and teratomas)
TSH-induced hyperthyroidism
    TSH-secreting pituitary ademonas
    Partial resistance to feedback (defect in T_3 receptor)

Other Causes

Medications inhibiting T_4 to T_3 conversion (i.e., amiodarone)
Iodine-induced hyperthyroidism
Recovery from hyperthyroidism
Drugs
    Dopamine and glucocorticoids
Thyrotoxicosis facitia
    Over-replacement/overuse of thyroid hormone
    Consumption of beef contaminated with bovine thyroid gland (rare)

cohort study found that 25% of women with diabetes mellitus type 1 developed postpartum thyroid dysfunction, in almost all cases of thyroiditis.[101] The hyperthyroidism is usually mild and transient, but patients are at an increased risk to develop subsequent hypothyroidism.

TREATMENT

Overt Hyperthyroidism   Treatment for tumors or secondary hyperthyroidism are not considered here, because these topics are beyond the scope of this text. Should the clinician suspect either of these etiologies, prompt referral to a specialist is warranted.

The goal of treatment is to control symptoms and restore euthyroidism. In general, treatment is somewhat more complex than for hypothyroidism. Hyperthyroidism treatment is very dependent upon the etiology of the disease. In addition, more options are available to the patient and optimal recommendations are still being investigated.

The treatment options for Graves disease include medications, usually propylthiouracil (PTU) or methimazole (Tapazole); surgery (either partial or total thyroidectomy [TT]); or radioablation.[102] Both PTU and methimazole inhibit the production of T_4 and T_3. PTU inhibits iodine and peroxidase from interacting with thyroglobulin and forming T_4 and T_3. Methimazole blocks oxidation of iodine in the thyroid and blocks iodine incorporation into tyrosine to form T_4 and T_3.

Although the antithyroid drugs PTU and methimazole have similar efficacy, there are situations when one agent is preferred. Methimazole has a longer half-life than PTU, allowing a once-daily dosing that can improve patient adherence to treatment. PTU historically has been the drug of choice for treating pregnant and breastfeeding women because of its limited transfer into the placenta and breast milk,[102] but both may be used. One 2003 evidence-based re-view noted that, in general, methimazole is preferred over PTU because it appears to be slightly more efficacious and may have lower rates of some minor and severe side effects, particularly hepatitis and vasculitis.[103] However, the studies included in this review varied in size and quality and excluded pregnant women. ACOG Guidelines recommend the use of either PTU or methimazole, but not iodine 131, in pregnancy.[58] Therefore, the treatment needs to be tailored to the individual.

Unfortunately, antithyroid drugs achieve remission in only 30% to 40% of cases. Some experts believe that, over time, relapse is quite likely.[88] Radioiodine, administered as oral 131I, usually results in euthyroidism in 6 to 18 weeks. Hypothyroidism is an inevitable result.[102] Radioiodine treatment is contraindicated during pregnancy.

Surgery should be reserved for the rare patient who is allergic to both PTU and methimazole, is poorly compliant with medications, or who has large goiters causing difficulty swallowing.[88,104] There are two general options, subtotal thyroidectomy (ST) and TT. One randomized controlled trial did not find any convincing evidence for improved outcomes with more radical approaches and recommended subtotal resection.[105] A large meta-analysis reported that TT and ST had similar complication rates; 8% of patients undergoing ST had persistent or recurring hyperthyroidism as compared to none of the TT patients (all of whom became hypothyroid).[106]

Adjuvant therapies for Graves disease include beta-blockers, inorganic iodide, and lithium. Beta-blockers are used to decrease the adrenergic symptoms of hyperthyroidism, including palpitations, tachycardia, anxiety, tremor, and heat intolerance. Atenolol, metoprolol, and propranolol are all commonly used for this purpose.[88] There is no consensus as to when to start beta-blocker therapy, but most clinicians prescribe it when the patient is experiencing adrenergic symptoms. A common starting dose of propranolol is 40 mg per day. Higher doses may be needed initially and then titrated downward as euthyroidism is achieved.[88] Lithium has been found to minimize the transient increase of thyrotoxicosis often seen after antithyroid therapy is withdrawn and to enhance the effectiveness of radio-iodine therapy,[107] although the effect of lithium on cure rates may not be significant.[108]

SUBCLINICAL HYPERTHYROIDISM

In general, treatment is not recommended for individuals with subclinical hyperthyroidism unless TSH values fall below 0.1 mIU/L.[19] Some experts do believe that clinicians should consider treatment in the elderly, because of the association with increased cardiovascular mortality.[27] If persistent TSH suppression below 0.1 mIU/L is confirmed, the American Association of Clinical Endocrinologists recommends that treatment be considered, particularly in the presence of other conditions such as atrial fibrillation, unexplained weight loss, osteopenia, cardiovascular disease, and mutinodular goiter.[47] **Figure 16-3** summarizes the recommendations from a review of subclinical thyroid disease and its clinical implications.

TREATMENT AND MANAGEMENT DURING PREGNANCY

Overt hyperthyroidism in pregnancy can lead to serious consequences for both the mother and the child; these patients should be referred for physician management. In one study, women with uncontrolled hyperthyroidism were nine times more likely to have low birth weight babies than women who had always been euthyroid. The same study noted that women with controlled hyperthyroidism had only a twofold increased risk of delivering a low birth weight baby. There was also an increased risk of pre-eclampsia for women with undertreated hyperthyroidism.[109]

Hyperthyroidism in pregnancy is treated with thioamides, usually PTU and methimazole.[3,100] When used during pregnancy, both PTU and methimazole expose the fetus to a 5% to 10% risk of hypothyroidism.[110] Less common but more potentially serious is the development of fetal thyroid enlargement secondary to PTU-induced hypothyroidism. In rare cases the thyroid can be large enough to induce respiratory distress in the newborn.[111] In order to minimize these complications, the lowest dose of antithyroid medications needed to maintain a woman's TSH in the upper limits of normal is prescribed in pregnancy.[47]

In the past, PTU has generally been the drug of choice because experimental data seemed to indicate that placental transport of PTU may be less than that with methimazole. However, other studies indicate that placental transport is similar with both drugs.[102] In addition, a study of 77 mothers with Graves disease found no differences in measures of fetal thyroid status at birth between fetuses exposed to PTU compared to those exposed to methimazole.[110] PTU is recommended by some authorities as the drug of first choice because of a small but real chance of fetal anomalies such as aplasia cutis with methimazole,[62] although ACOG considers the use of either drug to be acceptable in pregnancy.[61] Even less clear is whether long-term outcomes of the mother and child are any different after PTU and methimazole use. Both PTU and methimazole seem to be safe for use during breastfeeding.[62]

Figure 16-3 Suggested approach to diagnosis and management of subclinical hyperthyroidism.

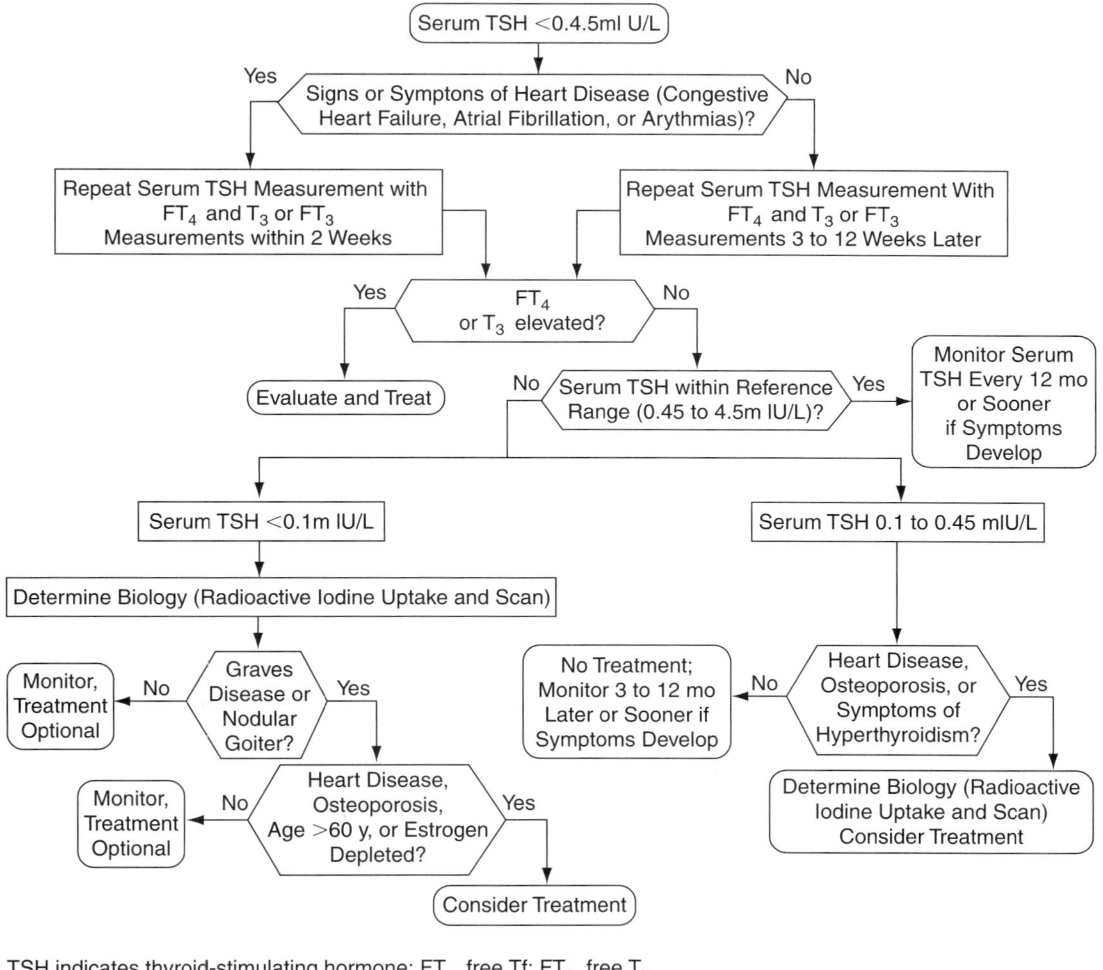

TSH indicates thyroid-stimulating hormone; FT4, free Tf; FT3, free T3.

Source: Reprinted with permission from the Journal of the American Medical Association. 2204; 291 (2).

Iodine is contraindicated in pregnancy because of the risk of fetal thyroid ablation. ACOG recommends that women avoid pregnancy for at least four months after 131I treatment.[3]

Thyroid function tests should be monitored monthly during pregnancy, and doses of PTU or methimazole should be liberally adjusted in order to maintain the euthyroid state. Pregnant women may also require dose decreases if the TSH rises into the normal range.[62,100]

WHEN TO REFER TO A SPECIALIST

Most authorities agree that all patients with a new diagnosis of hyperthyroidism should be referred to an endocrinologist for the initial evaluation and institution of a treatment plan. Pregnant women with hyperthyroidism should be managed by a physician, although a midwife may be part of the health care team. The diagnosis and management of hypothyroidism is relatively straightforward; consequently these individuals may not require referral to an endocrinologist. However, referral to an endocrinologist should be considered if a patient with hypothyroidism is unresponsive to treatment, has other concurrent endocrine disorders, or is found to have a thyroid nodule or other structural changes in the thyroid gland.[47]

Diabetes

Epidemiology

It has been estimated that at least 20.8 million individuals in the United States have diabetes, including approximately 6.2 million undiagnosed cases.[112] These statistics include the 2.2% of individuals under age 20 and the approximately 1 in 400 to 600 children and adolescents with type 1 diabetes. The prevalence is approximately the same for men and women. Diabetes occurs more frequently in African American, American Indian, Latino, and Asian populations than in non-Hispanic whites, as well as in those with a family history of diabetes, dyslipidemia, hypertension, previously recognized pre-diabetes, and in women with previous gestational diabetes mellitus (GDM) and polycystic ovarian syndrome.[112,113]

Diabetes, broadly defined as a group of heterogeneous metabolic disorders resulting in hyperglycemia, is a consequence of either inadequate insulin production, inadequate insulin secretion, or a combination of the two.[114] There are four main categories of diabetes. This chapter focuses on the two primary types of diabetes: type 1 and type 2. The prevalence of diabetes in adults is approximately 9.6%[112] of individuals and may be higher when cases of undiagnosed diabetes are included. If current trends continue, it has been estimated that the number of U.S. adults with diabetes will increase from 11 million to 29 million by 2050.[115] Approximately 90% to 95% of cases of diabetes are type 2, and only 5% to 10% represent type 1.[112]

The third category of diabetes includes such causes as a variety of genetic disorders including genetic defects of the pancreatic beta cell and genetic abnormalities of the insulin receptor, pancreatic diseases, drug and chemical induced diabetes, infections, and genetic syndromes associated with diabetes.[114] A fourth category, GDM, is defined as the onset or first recognition of diabetes during pregnancy. Women with GDM should be retested after six weeks postpartum to determine whether the condition has resolved or if diabetes has persisted. Women who develop GDM are at significant risk of developing overt diabetes later in life and should be screened at one- to three-year intervals depending on postpartum blood glucose testing results.[113,116]

Pathophysiology

The development of diabetes results from complicated interactions among genetics, lifestyle choices, and environmental factors.[117] Types 1 and 2 diabetes represent different pathophysiologic mechanisms that result in a similar phenotypic picture of hyperglycemia. In normal physiology, insulin is synthesized in and secreted by the pancreatic beta cells. Insulin is secreted in response to a meal and is important is the metabolism of carbohydrate, fat, and protein. However, the ability of insulin to enable glucose utilization by the target tissues of skeletal muscle, the liver, and adipose tissue is its primary postmeal function. Insulin allows energy use by the target tissues by binding to receptors on cell membranes in target tissues and allowing glucose transport into the cells. Excess energy is stored as glycogen in muscle and as fat in adipose tissue.[118]

Type 1 diabetes is characterized by autoimmune destruction of the pancreatic beta cells resulting in an inability to produce and secrete insulin.[114,117,118] Some individuals have a genetic tendency toward autoimmune cell destruction, and this may also be triggered by a viral infection. Although many individuals with type 1 diabetes may not have a first degree relative with diabetes, relatives of those with diabetes are at increased risk for the disease.[117] Other individuals may have a genetic tendency toward beta cell destruction in the absence of an autoimmune process.[118] The process can occur slowly over months or years, or very quickly over several weeks.[117,118] Symptoms of hyperglycemia typically appear when 80% of the beta cells have been destroyed.[118] Type 1 diabetes occurs more commonly in children and adolescents but is also diagnosed in adults of all ages.[117]

Type 2 diabetes is believed to represent insulin resistance, but may include a relative insulin deficiency or an insulin secretory defect combined with insulin resistance.[114] In type 2 diabetes, the target tissues (muscle, liver, adipose) gradually lose their sensitivity to insulin over time, thus preventing efficient use of glucose in most tissues with the exception of the brain, which does not require insulin for glucose utilization. This loss of tissue sensitivity is referred to as *insulin resistance*.[118] As insulin tissue sensitivity declines, insulin secretion increases, initially resulting in a mild hyperinsulinemic state. Over time, the pancreas loses its ability to secrete enough insulin to maintain euglycemia and the result is *hyperglycemia*. Abnormalities in carbohydrate, protein, and fat metabolism occur that are related to the inability of insulin to act at the target tissue level in many body systems.

Genetics and lifestyle both play a larger role in type 2 diabetes,[113,117] and many individuals with type 2 diabetes have a positive family history of diabetes; factors such as obesity and lack of physical activity are also common.[117] Type 2 diabetes is a progressive disease with increasing loss of function of the pancreatic beta cells over time and decreasing effectiveness of oral medications.[118,119] Therefore, achieving treatment goals becomes more difficult the longer an individual has type 2 diabetes.[117,120]

Signs and Symptoms

The classic symptoms of significant hyperglycemia are polydypsia, polyuria, and unexplained weight loss. These symptoms are seen more often in type 1 diabetes when acute pancreatic beta cell destruction occurs; in type 2 diabetes where insulin resistance leads to hyperinsulinemia and then hyperglycemia, symptoms may not be as evident at the onset of the disease.[117,118] Polyphagia, blurred vision, and increased susceptibility to infections may also occur. When diabetes control is less than ideal, ketoacidosis and nonketotic hyperosmolar syndrome (cellular dehydration that results from the effects of hyperglycemia and resulting increased osmotic pressure in the extracellular fluid) may occur.[117] Often, particularly in type 2 diabetes, there may be no symptoms for a number of years before diagnosis.[117,118,121]

The chronic hyperglycemia that accompanies poorly controlled diabetes affects many organ systems. Complications of diabetes include cardiovascular disease, peripheral vascular disease, retinopathy, neuropathy, and nephropathy. Diabetes represents the leading cause of end-stage renal disease, nontraumatic amputation of the lower extremities, and adult blindness.[117] Cardiovascular disease is the major cause of death in individuals with diabetes.[118] It has been estimated that the direct costs of providing medical care to individuals with diabetes are approximately $92 billion and when indirect costs, such as loss of work time, disability, premature death, are included, the cost is $132 billion.[112]

Essential History and Physical Exam

The patient should have a complete history including full exploration of the chief complaint and a thorough review of systems. The midwife is most likely to be seeing a woman for reasons other than diabetes, so paying attention to risk factors is important. Careful screening permits prevention counseling and increases the likelihood of early diagnosis. The physical examination should be appropriate to the purpose of the visit and to any findings from the history.

Once a diagnosis of diabetes has been made, a thorough examination and laboratory workup are required to evaluate the diagnosis and possible complications, and to develop a plan for immediate and ongoing treatment.

This evaluation should begin with a complete medical history including past medical and family medical history; current review of systems particularly related to complications of diabetes; patterns of dietary intake and physical activity; risk factors for cardiovascular disease (CVD); contraceptive and reproductive history; use of tobacco, alcohol, or other substances; current medication use including over-the-counter medications and herbal or other supplements; and any cultural or other lifestyle factors that might influence the management of diabetes. Physical examination includes: height, weight, and blood pressure; fundoscopic examination; examination of the oral cavity; palpation of the thyroid gland; cardiac and abdominal examination; assessment of pulses; and foot, skin, and neurologic examinations. Accompanying laboratory evaluations include hemoglobin A1c (HgA1c), fasting lipids, urinalysis for microalbuminuria, ketones, protein and sediment, TSH, serum creatinine, and electrocardiogram as indicated.[122] A technical report from the Agency for Healthcare Research and Quality summarizes the available literature recommending the use of glycated hemoglobin and microalbuminuria (measured in a 24-hour urine collection) in the management of diabetes.[123]

LABORATORY TESTING

Three recommended methods exist for blood glucose testing to diagnose diabetes. Each must be confirmed by a repeat test on a different day unless there is unequivocal hyperglycemia. Testing can include a random blood glucose level when accompanied by classic symptoms of hyperglycemia (polydypsia, polyuria, and weight loss); fasting blood glucose following an eight hour fast, or testing two hours after consumption of 75 grams of a standard glucose solution.[114]

Table 16-7 describes the diagnostic criteria for each test. Individuals with impaired fasting glucose (IFG) or impaired glucose tolerance (IGT) (fasting plasma glucose ≥100 and <126 mg/dL; 2-hour post-glucola ≥140 and <200 mg/dL) are now referred to as having pre-diabetes, reflecting their increased level of risk for developing overt diabetes in the future.[114]

A large number of individuals are believed to have undiagnosed type 2 diabetes. Using data from NHANES III in the United States, a recent study estimated that nearly 12 million U.S. overweight adults have pre-diabetes and may benefit from programs designed to prevent the development of type 2 diabetes.[124] Type 2 diabetes has been estimated to be present for at least four to seven years in a study of the United States and Australian populations, and may be present for as long as nine to twelve years before diagnosis. As many as 50% or more of individuals may have developed a complication by the time of diagnosis.[121]

Although there are no randomized controlled trials demonstrating benefits of earlier diagnosis and treatment of diabetes, the American Diabetes Association (ADA) has made recommendations based on expert opinion for screening for type 2 diabetes. Clinicians should consider screening (testing in the absence of symptoms) of all individuals who are age 45 and older as well as those with hypertension or a body mass index of >25 kg/m^2 at three-year intervals.[113] **Table 16-8** presents the ADA criteria for testing for diabetes in asymptomatic adults. In addition, those who have a first degree relative with diabetes, belong to a high risk ethnic population (African American, Hispanic, American Indian, Asian, Pacific Islander), have a high density lipoprotein (HDL) cholesterol level of ≤35 or triglycerides ≥250, or IFG or IGT on previous testing should be screened for diabetes. Women with previous GDM, who have given birth to an infant weighing over nine pounds or who have polycystic ovarian syndrome (PCOS), are also at increased risk. The USPSTF recommends screening only adults with hypertension or hyperlipidemia.[125]

Table 16-7 **CRITERIA FOR THE DIAGNOSIS OF DIABETES MELLITUS**

1. Symptoms of diabetes plus casual plasma glucose concentration ≥200 mg/dL (11.1 mmol/L). Casual is defined as any time of day without regard to time since last meal. The classic symptoms of diabetes include polyuria, polydipsia, and unexplained weight loss.

or

2. FPG ≥126 mg/dL (7.0 mmol/L). Fasting is defined as no caloric intake for at least 8 h.

or

3. Two-hour post-load glucose ≥200 mg/dL (11.1 mmol/L) during an OGTT. The test should be performed as described by WHO, using a glucose load containing the equivalent of 75 g anhydrous glucose dissolved in water.

Abbreviations are: FPG, Fasting plasma glucose; OGTT, oral glucose tolerance test.

In the absence of unequivocal hyperglycemia, these criteria should be confirmed by repeat testing on a different day. The third measure (OGTT) is not recommended for routine clinical use.

Source: Reprinted with permission from The American Diabetes Association. © 2005. American Diabetes Association; Standards of Medical Care in Diabetes (Position Statement). *Diabetes Care.* 2005;28(S1):S43-49.

Table 16-8 TESTING CRITERIA FOR DIABETES IN ASYMPTOMATIC ADULTS

1. Testing for diabetes should be considered in all individuals at age ≥45 years, particularly in those with a BMI 25 kg/m2,* and, if normal, should be repeated at 3-year intervals.
2. Testing should be considered at a younger age or be carried out more frequently in individuals who are overweight (BMI 25 kg/m2)* and have additional risk factors:
   - Are habitually physically inactive
   - Have a first-degree relative with diabetes
   - Are members of a high-risk ethnic population (e.g., African American, Latino, Native American, Asian American, Pacific Islander)
   - Have delivered a baby weighing >9 lb or have been diagnosed with GDM
   - Are hypertensive (140/90 mm Hg)
   - Have an HDL cholesterol level 35 mg/dl (0.90 mmol/L) and/or a triglyceride level 250 mg/dL (2.82 mmol/L)
   - Have PCOS
   - On previous testing, had IGT or IFG
   - Have other clinical conditions associated with insulin resistance (e.g., PCOS or acanthosis nigricans)
   - Have a history of vascular disease

Abbreviations are: IGT, impaired glucose tolerance; IFG, impaired fasting glucose.
*May not be correct for all ethnic groups. Abbreviation: PCOS, polycystic ovarian syndrome.
Source: Used with permission from the American Diabetes Association: Standards of Medical Care in Diabetes, ©2004. *Diabetes Care.* 2005;28(Suppl 1):S15-S35.

Differential Diagnosis

Individuals presenting with classic symptoms of diabetes should be carefully screened for diabetes and other possible conditions. Classic symptoms are much more likely to present in individuals with type 1 diabetes than type 2.[122] Because type 2 diabetes is much more prevalent and likely exists for several years prior to diagnosis, the clinician should be alert to risk factors for diabetes related to age, obesity, and ethnicity as well as symptoms of diabetes complications (**Table 16-9**).

Diabetes should be managed by a physician who is experienced in the management of diabetes. A multidisciplinary team approach to diabetes treatment, including nurses, registered dieticians, and behavioral health professionals as well as the primary physician has been associ-ated with improved outcomes and is preferred. If laboratory values can not be brought into the range of recommended ADA guidelines, then referral to an endocrinologist for more intensive management is warranted.[122]

Management

Because the management of type 1 and type 2 diabetes varies significantly, they will be discussed separately. The primary objectives of diabetes treatment are to bring blood glucose within or close to normal limits and to prevent or delay the development of complications. The Diabetes Control and Complications Trial (DCCT)[126] demonstrated a reduction in microvascular complications with tight control of type 1 diabetes, although tight control of blood glucose was shown to increase the risk of hypoglycemia and weight gain. Similarly, the

Table 16-9 DIFFERENTIAL DIAGNOSIS FOR DIABETES BY SIGNS AND SYMPTOMS

Polydypsia/polyuria
  Diabetes mellitus type 1
  Diabetes mellitus type 2
  Diabetes insipidus
Obesity
  Excessive caloric intake
  Diabetes type 2
  Hypothyroidism
  Cushing disease
  Fluid retention
  Smoking cessation
  Drug effects
    Steroids
    NSAIDs
    Oral contraceptives
    Some antidepressants
Weight loss
  Diabetes type 1
  Hyperthyroidism
  Cancer
  Depression
  Anorexia
  Drug effects
    Sedatives
    Antidepressants
    NSAIDs
    Antibiotics
  Idiopathic
  Gastrointestinal causes (malabsorption and
    sprue)

United Kingdom Prospective Diabetes Study (UKPDS) demonstrated that tight control (goal of fasting plasma glucose <6 mmol/L, equivalent to approximately 108 mg/dL, and pre-meal blood glucose of 4 to 7 mmol/L, equivalent to approximately 72 to 126 mg/dL, for those on insulin) reduced microvascular complications in individuals with type 2 diabetes.[127,128]

For individuals with either type 1 or type 2 diabetes, based on the results of the DCCT and UKPDS trials, the ADA recommends a goal for nonpregnant adults of HbA1c below 7%, which represents a value approximately 1% above the normal limits of 4% to 6%.[122] This measurement allows an assessment of blood glucose levels over the previous two- to three-month period. HbA1c levels should be checked at least twice annually for individuals meeting the target goals, and quarterly for those outside the target. Because CVD is a major cause of death for individuals with diabetes, and because diabetes, hypertension, and dyslipidemia are all independent risk factors for CVD, management of blood pressure and lipids is essential in the treatment of diabetes. **Table 16-10** shows ADA-recommended blood glucose treatment goals as well as accompanying recommendations for blood pressure and lipid treatment goals. Information included in ADA publications and other sources provides data for clinicians on the management of lipids and blood pressure that is beyond the scope of this chapter. See also Chapter 14.[122,129–131]

TYPE 1 DIABETES

Individuals with type 1 diabetes are managed with insulin therapy to replace what the pancreatic beta cells can no longer produce in sufficient quantity, and a dietary plan of meals and snacks spaced throughout the day, so that euglycemia is maintained. To minimize the formation of antibodies, human insulin is used. Insulin is manufactured in rapid, short, intermediate, and long-acting forms. It can be given by multiple subcutaneous injections or constant infusion via an insulin pump.[132,133] Since the DCCT trial, intensive therapy is preferred to minimize the risk of microvascular complications.[126] However, these benefits

Table 16-10 SUMMARY OF RECOMMENDATIONS FOR ADULTS WITH DIABETES

Factor	Parameter
Glycemic control	
AIC	<7.0%*
Preprandial plasma glucose	90–130 mg/dL (5.0–7.2 mmol/L)
Postprandial plasma glucose†	<180 mg/dL (<10.0 mmol/L)
Blood pressure	<130/80 mm Hg
Lipids‡	
LDL	<100 mg/dL (<2.6 mmol/L)
Triglycerides	<150 mg/dL (<1.7 mmol/L)
HDL	>40 mg/dL (>1.1 mmol/L)

*Referenced to a nondiabetic range of 4.0–6.6% using a DCCT-based assay. †Postprandial glucose measurements should be made 1–2 h after the beginning of the meal, generally peak levels in patients with diabetes. ‡Current NCEP/ATP III guidelines suggest that in patients with triglycerides 200 mg/dl, "non-HDL cholesterol" (total cholesterol minus HDL) be utilized. The goal is 130 mg/dl. For women it has been suggested that the HDL goal be increased by 10 mg/dl.
Source: Reprinted with permission from The American Diabetes Association: Standards of Medical Care (Position Statement), ©2004. *Diabetes Care.* 2004;27:S15–S35.

must be balanced with the increased risks of weight gain and hypoglycemia observed in the DCCT trial.[122] **Table 16-11** outlines the major types of insulin and their duration of action and peak effect.

Consideration is given to using both short and longer acting insulins together to control fasting blood glucose levels and to minimize *postprandial excursions* (increase and subsequent decrease) in blood glucose. Pre-prandial insulin needs are determined based on carbohydrate intake.[134] Most individuals with type 1 diabetes require at least three insulin injections daily or they use an insulin pump that provides a basal level of insulin infusion along with boluses taken before each meal. Determination of the exact dosing regimen is based on individual parameters that include diet, physical activity level, blood glucose levels, and types of insulin used.[132,133]

Regular exercise is important for those with type 1 diabetes and is one of the variables con-sidered when calculating dietary and insulin needs. Several well-known professional athletes have competed successfully while managing type 1 diabetes. Important considerations are monitoring blood glucose before and after exercise, using carbohydrates as needed to prevent hypoglycemia, and avoiding exercise if fasting blood glucose is >250 with ketosis or >300 without ketosis.[135]

TYPE 2 DIABETES

Dietary management, also referred to as *medical nutrition therapy (MNT)*, and exercise are important cornerstones of both the initial and ongoing management of type 2 diabetes. The goals are weight reduction and an improvement in insulin sensitivity (reduction in insulin resistance) as well as reduction of cardiovascular risk factors by controlling lipids and blood pressure. MNT should be provided by a registered dietician who works as a part of the diabetes care team. Goals include: prevention of large excursions in blood

Table 16-11 TYPES OF INSULIN AND PHARMACODYNAMICS*

Type of Insulin (manufacturer)	Onset (h)	Peak (h)	Duration (h)
Rapid Acting			
Insulin lispro (Humalog)	0.25	0.5–1.5	4–5
Insulin aspart (Novolog)	5–10 min	1–3	3–5
Short Acting			
Regular human (Humulin R, Novolin R, Velosulin BR)	0.5–1	2–4	5–7
Intermediate Acting			
NPH human (Humulin N, Novolin N)	1–2	6–14	18–24
Lente Human (Humulin L, Novolin L)	1–3	6–14	18–24
Long Acting			
Ultralente human (Humulin U)	6	18–24	24–48
Insulin glargine (Lantus) Insulin analog	1.5	Flat	24

*These times may vary widely in individuals

glucose level; encouraging carbohydrate intake that incorporates dietary fiber from whole grains, fruit, and vegetables; obtaining 15% to 20% of calories from protein, and reducing the proportion of saturated fat, *trans*-fatty acids, and cholesterol in the diet. Diets should be individualized to accommodate individual preferences and lifestyle and should be culturally appropriate.[134] A 2004 study comparing low carbohydrate (<30 g/d) and conventional (500 calorie/day reduction) diets among a group of obese adults after one year, over 80% of whom had diabetes or metabolic syndrome, found similar weight loss but improved triglyceride and HDL cholesterol levels for those on the low carbohydrate diet.[136] HbA1c levels were lower for a sub-group of individuals with diabetes who were on the low carbohydrate diet.[136] More research is needed to confirm these findings.

Including regular exercise to improve cardiovascular fitness is important to management. A minimum of 30 minutes of exercise three times weekly is suggested. Studies have demonstrated improvements in carbohydrate metabolism and insulin sensitivity using regimens of 30 to 60 minutes of aerobic activity three to four times weekly. Results are more impressive in individuals with milder diabetes and those with greater degrees of insulin resistance. Initial monitoring of exercise sessions and regular follow-up with diabetes team members is likely to improve adherence to the exercise program.[135] Depending on the age of the individual, length of time since diagnosis of diabetes, and possible diabetes complications, careful evaluation of cardiovascular status may be warranted prior to initiating an exercise program.

When MNT and exercise do not result in meeting the desired blood glucose goals, medication is added to the therapeutic regimen. **Table 16-12** describes the major classes of oral hypoglycemic medications, their mechanism of action, side effects, and dosing schedules. Sulfonylureas or metformin (Glucophage) are often the first drug of choice when adding medication to the MNT and exercise plan. Sulfonylureas are less expensive than other medications; first-generation drugs are less expensive than the newer second-generation preparations, but second-generation preparations are more potent, have a shorter half life, and fewer side effects.[137] A recent study of first line drug costs with newly diagnosed type 2 diabetes demonstrated that short-term cost savings may be obtained when sulfonylureas are used as the first choice medication if diet and exercise alone are not sufficient to achieve the ADA recommended blood glucose levels.[138]

Metformin is commonly used and may also have a positive effect on blood lipids, which can result in less weight gain or even weight loss when compared to other medications. It may be useful in obese individuals but should be avoided in those with kidney disease. Metformin is also contraindicated for individuals with alcoholism or binge drinking behavior as

well as hepatic dysfunction. Thiazolidendiones are newer medications that may also be used as an initial choice of medication or as adjunct therapy with other medications. The first drug developed in that class, troglitazone (Rezulin), was removed from the market because of hepatocellular injury; individuals taking this class of medication should be observed for hepatic changes.[137,139]

Alpha glucosidase inhibitors help reduce post-prandial hyperglycemia by delaying glucose absorption in the intestinal tract, but may have gastrointestinal side effects such as flatulence, abdominal pain, and diarrhea that make it unacceptable to some individuals. They are usually used as an adjunct to other medications. Meglitinides are another class of medication and may be used in combination with other oral hypoglycemics.[137]

Acarbose (Precose) helps to reduce post-prandial hyperglycemia, but may have gastrointestinal side effects that make it unacceptable to some individuals. It is usually used as an adjunct to other medications. Glitinides are another newer class of medication and may be used in combination with other oral hypoglycemics.

Insulin therapy may be used initially in type 2 diabetes, but is often reserved until blood glucose goals cannot be met with other medications. Often patients prefer to start oral medications initially and reserve insulin, which must be taken by injection, until later. Nearly half of individuals with type 2 diabetes in the UKPDS study required insulin within six years of their diagnosis.[140] Monotherapy, whether it is diet and exercise, oral medication, or insulin, will not be sufficient for the majority of patients with type 2 diabetes over time. A study examining diet, sulfonylureas, metformin, and insulin as individual therapies in those newly

Table 16-12 ORAL MEDICATIONS FOR THE TREATMENT OF TYPE 2 DIABETES

Medication Class (examples)	Mechanism of Action	Common Side effects	Dosing
Sulfonylureas First generation – chlorpropramide (Diabenese), tolbutamide (Orinase), tolazimide (Tolinase) Second generation – glyburide (Micronase), glipizide (Glucotrol), glimepiride (Amaryl)	• Stimulate insulin secretion, increase sensitivity of beta pancreatic cells, reduce hepatic glucose production • Decrease appetite (tolbutamide, toloyamide)	• Weight gain • Hypoglycemia	• Duration of action 12–24 hours • Dose varies by drug. • Initiate low dose and increase every 1–2 weeks until desired objective reached.
Biguinides (metformin)	• Decrease hepatic glucose output • Enhance tissue responsiveness to insulin	• GI upset • Lactic acidosis	• 500 mg once or twice daily with meals • Increase by 500 mg every 1–2 weeks to meet goals, 2500 mg max dose
Alpha-glucosidase inhibitors (alpha-carbose, miglitol)	• Interfere with carbohydrate metabolism, thus slowing absorption Used along with other medication.	• GI cramping, distension, flatulence, impaired Fe absorption • Hypoglycemia when used with other drugs.	• Start with 25 mg tid with meals • Maximum dose 50–100 mg tid
Meglitinides (repaglinide, nateglinide)	• Stimulate beta cell secretion of insulin	• Hypoglycemia • Weight gain	• Taken before meals • Start 0.5 mg with each meal if A1c $<$8, 102 mg if A1c $>$8
Thiazolidinediones (pioglitazone, rosiglitazone)	• Increase insulin sensitivity in muscle and fat	• Weight gain • Monitor hepatocellular enzymes (1 drug removed from market due to hepatocelluar injury.	• Dosage varies by drug. • Begin with low dose. • Increase monthly until goals or maximum dose reached.

diagnosed with type 2 diabetes found that only 50% of participants could maintain blood glucose goals with any kind of monotherapy at three years, but by nine years that number was 25%.[119] Initiation of insulin therapy should be overseen by a physician skilled in the management of diabetes. Referral to a diabetologist may be helpful at any point but is required if good control cannot be achieved or maintained.

Because of the epidemic of type 2 diabetes and the diagnosis of diabetes in younger individuals who will require therapy for many years, experts in the field have recommended that the progression from diet and exercise, to drug monotherapy, to combined therapy and insulin use, including consideration of earlier insulin use in some cases, should be more rapid in order to achieve blood glucose goals more quickly and slow the development of diabetes complications.[141,142] Intensive treatment using metformin as the initial medication has been shown to reduce costs in the long term by reducing the costs of hospitalization associated with the development of diabetes complications.[143]

PATIENT EDUCATION

Patient education is critical for effective management of both type 1 and type 2 diabetes, including before and during pregnancy, because the patient is considered to be a key part of the diabetes care team. Goals for blood glucose, lipids, and blood pressure can be met only if the individual with diabetes is educated about all aspects of diabetes management and understands how to work with other members of the diabetes care team to maximize desired outcomes. The ADA believes education is so important that the organization has developed national standards for diabetes self-management education[144] for use by health care entities in developing their local diabetes education programs. The task force that recently revised these standards included diabetes care professionals and representatives from a number of organizations and federal agencies involved in diabetes care.

Self-obtained blood-glucose monitoring (SBGM) is a key component of diabetes management, so all individuals with diabetes need to be educated in this method. SBGM and regular HbA1c measurements are used to adjust diet, activity, and medication regimens. In addition, MNT is crucial for an individual to be able to manage her diabetes. A good understanding of general dietary principles as well as ways to adapt dietary recommendations to accommodate individual food preferences, changing activity levels, and the presence of illness is critical. Nutrition education should ideally be provided by a registered dietician who is experienced in working with individuals with diabetes.[134]

Ongoing access to a dietician is also helpful. In particular, individuals with type 1 diabetes need to be educated in principles related to insulin adjustment in order to compensate for variations in diet and activity. Use of an intensive management regimen assumes that the individual will be educated to make adjustments in insulin dosages according to daily blood glucose levels as well. ADA standards include the recommendation that diabetes education be provided by a team representing various professions, and that this team be comprised of experts in providing diabetes education.[144]

PREVENTION OF TYPE 2 DIABETES

Several recent studies have demonstrated that type 2 diabetes can be prevented or at least delayed.[145–147] The most impressive was a randomized controlled trial of lifestyle intervention, metformin, and placebo.[145] The Diabetes

Prevention Program Research Group randomized over 3000 nondiabetic individuals at 27 centers into each of the three treatment groups. The sample included obese individuals age 25 and older; 68% were women, and 45% represented minority groups. The lifestyle group received an intensive intervention program with goals of a 7% reduction in initial body weight through a healthy low fat diet and moderate intensity exercise of 150 minutes per week. The metformin group was prescribed 850 mg twice daily; both metformin and placebo groups received written information and a single visit recommending standard healthy lifestyle advice. After an average follow-up period of nearly three years, the lifestyle group had a reduced incidence of diabetes of 59% and the metformin group of 31% compared to controls. Both interventions were significantly more effective than placebo, and lifestyle was more effective than metformin.[145]

The ADA has established recommendations for the delay or prevention of type 2 diabetes.[148] The argument includes the following points: diabetes is known to be a serious health problem with significant public burden; the early course of the disease and significant risk factors are known; tests to detect the pre-disease state exist; and there are safe methods to delay or prevent the disease. However, it is not yet known if there are cost-effective ways to implement preventive interventions for those at high risk. At a minimum, ADA suggested that some interventions, particularly lifestyle modification, are probably worthwhile, even in the absence of good cost-effectiveness data. The ADA recommendations include: awareness among individuals at high risk for type 2 diabetes of the benefits of weight loss and exercise; screening for diabetes among individuals at high risk; counseling those with pre-

diabetes; monitoring of lipids and other cardiovascular risk factors; and follow-up counseling for those identified at risk for diabetes.[148] Underscoring the magnitude of the public health burden of type 2 diabetes is a recent estimate of the number of adults over 45 years of age with impaired glucose tolerance, impaired fasting glucose, or pre-diabetes. Researchers estimated that in the year 2000 there were over 9 million overweight adults with one of these conditions that could potentially benefit from preventive strategies.[124]

In addition to pre-diabetes, another area of concern for preventive strategies is that group of individuals with a constellation of physical and laboratory measurements known as the *metabolic syndrome*. This condition was defined in the Third Report of the National Cholesterol Education Program Expert Panel on Detection, Evaluation and Treatment of High Blood Cholesterol in Adults (Adult Treatment Panel III).[129] These measures include abdominal obesity, hypertriglyceridemia, low HDL cholesterol, hypertension, and high fasting blood glucose. Using these diagnostic criteria and data from NHANES III and the 2000 U.S. Census, an estimated 47 million individuals (22%–24% of U.S. adults) have the metabolic syndrome.[149,150] At risk for diabetes and coronary heart disease, these individuals represent a tremendous opportunity for intervention and prevention. Studies of cost-effective means to deal with this increasing problem are needed.[149] **Table 16-13** lists Internet resources related to diabetes.

IMPACT OF PREGNANCY AND BREASTFEEDING

A preconception care program is essential for women with type 1 or type 2 diabetes who wish to become pregnant.[151,152] Preconception care may be difficult because over half of pregnancies

---

Table 16-13 RESOURCES FOR OBESITY AND DIABETES INFORMATION AND GUIDELINES

Resource Description	Resource location
Centers for Disease Control and Prevention (CDC) Data on prevalence of diabetes	http://cdc.gov/diabetes/pubs/.estimates.htm#incidence
U.S. Preventive Services Task Force Recommendations on screening for type 2 diabetes	http://www.ahrq.gov/clinic/erduspstf/diabscr/diabetrr.htm
Agency for Healthcare Research and Quality Recommendations on the use of glycated Hg and microalbuminuria to monitor diabetes	http://www.ahrq.gov/clinic/epcsums/glycasum.htm
National Heart, Lung Blood Institute Aim for a healthy weight; information for professionals	http://nhlbi.nih.gov/guidelines/obesity/ob_gdlns.htm

---

in the United States are unplanned or unintended. However, as part of overall diabetes management, women of childbearing age should be counseled on appropriate contraceptive methods, and the importance of preconception care should be stressed at all health care visits. Despite the fairly well documented benefits, only about 30% of women with diabetes receive preconception care.[152,155]

Preconception care should be provided by an interdisciplinary team[151] with an overall goal to bring HbA1c levels to under 1% above the normal limits (<7%) in order to reduce the occurrence of anomalies and other complications.[153,154] Major malformations in the fetus, such as cardiovascular, central nervous system, skeletal, and genitourinary anomalies, are known to occur more frequently in diabetic women.[152] Malformations are believed to be the result of maternal hyperglycemia during the

sensitive period of organogenesis. Near-normal blood glucose control prior to conception is essential in the prevention of these abnormalities.[153,154] Higher rates of malformations are observed with increasing levels of HbA1c.[155] Additional risks for women with pre-existing diabetes include spontaneous abortion, stillbirth, and preterm labor as well as macrosomia.[151,154] Because of the association between diabetes and autoimmune thyroid disease, women with diabetes should undergo thyroid testing prior to pregnancy.[156] Initiation of 1-mg folic acid daily is recommended for three months prior to conception to reduce the incidence of neural tube defects.[156]

Once a woman with type 1 or 2 diabetes has become pregnant, care should be coordinated by a physician skilled in the management of diabetes in pregnancy. Midwives may certainly be involved as a member of the care team. Care of a diabetic patient will be similar to care provided during the preconception period: the focus is on keeping blood glucose levels close to the normal range in order to provide a healthy environment for fetal growth and development.[151,152,155] It is also important to quickly recognize and treat hypoglycemia that may occur early in pregnancy. Hypoglycemia is common during pregnancy in women with pre-existing diabetes following overnight fasting, and this may occur even before a pregnancy diagnosis is confirmed. Although the major focus of care is preventing hyperglycemia,[152,155] strict control of blood glucose is associated with episodes of severe hypoglycemia (requiring assistance from another person and possibly including coma). Human clinical studies have not demonstrated an association between maternal hypoglycemia and fetal anomalies; but the evidence is too scanty to be able to dismiss any association with certainty. The safest course is to reduce both hyper- and hypoglycemia, particularly severe episodes.[157]

Reviews provide information and parameters for the management of the antenatal care for women with pre-gestational diabetes.[152,155,156] Evaluations for retinopathy and nephropathy should occur early in pregnancy. Diabetic nephropathy occurs in 5% to 10% of pregnancies and contributes to increased risk for hypertensive complications and preterm labor. An ultrasound to evaluate for the presence of anomalies should occur at about 18 to 20 weeks gestation.[152] Nutrition and exercise continue to be important in the management of diabetes during pregnancy. Women of normal pre-pregnant weight are prescribed a diet of 30 to 35 kcal/kg of body weight. Recommendations include 40% to 50% of calories form good quality complex carbohydrates, 20% from protein, and 30% to 40% from unsaturated fats.[152] Griffith and Conway recommended a slightly different composition using fewer carbohydrates to improve glycemia and reduce the incidence of macrosomia. That formula is 40% carbohydrate, 35% protein, and 25% fat.[155,156]

Insulin, which does not cross the placenta, historically has been the medication of choice for treating hyperglycemia in pregnancy. Recent reviews have examined the use of oral hypoglycemic medications in pregnancy, including pre-gestational diabetes and GDM. Several studies recommend the use of glyburide for GDM, a condition diagnosed after organogenesis has occurred.[152,155,158,159] Metformin, a Category B drug, has been studied during pregnancy in the treatment of women with PCOS (but not diabetes). A lower incidence of GDM (3% vs. 31%) was observed in those treated with metformin throughout their pregnancy.[160] Although not all studies concur,[158] some experts have recommended not using metformin in pregnancy, but instead using insulin until further research confirms safety.[152,156,161,162]

In general, insulin dosages are reduced in the first trimester to prevent hypoglycemia resulting from increased insulin sensitivity in the first trimester as well as nausea and vomiting. Insulin levels are generally the highest between 28 and 32 weeks gestation.[152] Newer short-acting insulins such as lispro (Humalog) and aspart (Novolog) may help reduce postprandial hyperglycemia, episodes of hypoglycemia between meals, and Hgb A1c.[156] Because of a higher rate of thyroid disease during pregnancy and the postpartum period for women with diabetes, thyroid function testing is recommended. A plan for continuing dietary and blood glucose monitoring, increased fetal surveillance, and timing of delivery should be developed among members of the care team, including the pregnant woman and her family.

Care during the third trimester focuses on preventing stillbirth, promoting intrauterine fetal growth and oxygenation, and planning the appropriate time for the birth. Planning is important in order to maximize fetal/neonatal health and minimize maternal morbidity related to birth. Continued blood glucose monitoring and fetal surveillance will provide the information for developing this plan. Twice weekly fetal assessment using the biophysical profile and/or non-stress test has been recommended beginning at 32 weeks gestation. If test results remain normal and blood glucose control is good, the woman may be allowed to progress to her due date. Cesarean section is recommended for those with an estimated fetal weight that is more than 4250 to 4500 grams.[152,155,159]

If labor and a vaginal birth are planned, the goal is to maintain the blood glucose approximately 80 to 110 mg/dL during labor.[152,156] Intravenous insulin is typically used. Controlling hyperglycemia during labor will reduce the likelihood of neonatal hypoglycemia.[152,156] The physician will manage blood glucose and insulin levels, and make other medical decisions in the plan of care. Midwives may be involved in labor management and delivery; although the exact role of the midwife will vary depending on the wishes of the pregnant woman and the particular health care facility.

The postpartum care of women with diabetes is similar to that for women without diabetes. Women with type 1 or 2 diabetes should continue to be managed by a physician-directed team with the goal of continued glycemic control. Insulin needs decrease rapidly after the birth and may be reduced by approximately half of the antepartum dose as meals are initiated.[153,157] Recovery status should be determined as for any other woman and should include appropriate recommendations for family planning methods. Provision of an appropriate and effective contraceptive is an important step in preconception care for a possible next pregnancy. Because of evidence that the incidence of childhood diabetes is lower among those who were breastfed, breastfeeding should be encouraged and supported. Breastfeeding may also promote improved glycemic and lipid profiles in women with diabetes.[157,163] Goals for care during pregnancy, in addition to improving pregnancy outcomes, include establishing a healthy lifestyle that can be maintained.[153]

References

1. Flegal KM, Carroll MD, Ogden DL, Johnson CL. Prevalence and trends in obesity among US adults, 1999–2000. *JAMA*. 2002;288(14):1723–1727.

2. Mokdad AH, Marks JS, Stroup DF, Gerberding JL. Actual causes of death in the United States, 2000. *JAMA*. 2004;291(10):1238–1245.

3. American College of Obstetricians and Gynecologists. ACOG Practice Bulletin. Clinical management guidelines for obstetrician-gynecologists. Number 37, August 2002. Thyroid disease in pregnancy. *Obstetr Gynecol*. 2002;100(2):387–396.

4. Adlersberg MA, Burrow GN. Focus on primary care. Thyroid function and dysfunction in women. *Obstet Gynecol Surv*. 2002;57; Suppl 3:S1–7.

5. Abalovich M, Gutierrez S, Alcaraz G, Maccallini G, Garcia A, Levalle O. Overt and subclinical hypothyroidism complicating pregnancy. *Thyroid*. 2002; 12(1):63–68.

6. Canaris GJ, Manowitz NR, Mayor G, Ridgway EC. The Colorado thyroid disease prevalence study. *Arch Intern Med.* 2000;160(4):526–534.

7. Tunbridge WM, Evered DC, Hall R, et al. The spectrum of thyroid disease in a community: The Whickham survey. *Clin Endocrinol* (Oxford). 1977;7: 481–493.

8. Baral N, Lamsal M, Koner BC, Koirala S. Thyroid dysfunction in eastern Nepal. *Southeast Asian J Trop Med Public Health.* 2002;33(3):638–641.

9. Knudsen N, Jorgensen T, Rasmussen S, Christiansen E, Perrild H. The prevalence of thyroid dysfunction in a population with borderline iodine deficiency. *Clin Endocrinol.* 1999;51(3):361–367.

10. Hollowell JG, Staehling NW, Flanders WD, Hannon WH, Gunter EW, Spencer CA, et al. Serum TSH, T_4, and thyroid antibodies in the United States population (1988 to 1994): National Health and Nutrition Examination Survey (NHANES III). *J Clin Endocrinol Metab.* 2002;87(2):489–499.

11. Schectman JM, Kallenberg GA, Hirsch RP, Shumacher RJ. Report of an association between race and thyroid stimulating hormone level. *Am J Public Health.* 1991;81:505–506.

12. Lincoln SR, Ke RW, Kutteh WH. Screening for hypothyroidism in infertile women. *J Reprod Med.* 1999;44(5):455–457.

13. Bjoro T, Holmen J, Kruger O, Midthjell K, Hunstad K, Schreiner T, et al. Prevalence of thyroid disease, thyroid dysfunction and thyroid peroxidase antibodies in a large, unselected population. The Health Study of Nord-Trondelag (HUNT). *Eur J Endocrinol.* 2000;143(5):639–647.

14. Helfand M. Screening for subclinical thyroid dysfunction in nonpregnant adults: A summary of the evidence for the U.S. Preventive Services Task Force. *Ann Intern Med.* 2004;140(2): 128–141.

15. Vanderpump M, Tunbridge W. The epidemiology of thyroid disease in a community. In: Braverman LE, Utiger RD, editors. *The Thyroid.* 9th ed. Philadelphia: Lippincott-Raven; 1996. pp. 474–482.

16. Rivolta G, Cerutti R, Colombo R, Miano G, Dionisio P, Grossi E. Prevalence of subclinical hypothyroidism in a population living in the Milan metropolitan area. *J Endocrinol Invest.* 1999;22(9): 693–697.

17. Redmond GP. Hypothyroidism and women's health. *Int J Fertil Womens Med.* 2002;47(3):123–127.

18. Allan WC, Haddow JE, Palomaki GE, Williams JR, Mitchell ML, Hermos RJ, et al. Maternal thyroid deficiency and pregnancy complications: Implications for population screening. *J Med Screen.* 2000;7(3): 127–130.

19. Surks MI, Ortiz E, Daniels GH, Sawin CT, Col NF, Cobin RH, et al. Subclinical thyroid disease: Scientific review and guidelines for diagnosis and management. *JAMA.* 2004;291(2):228–238.

20. Col NF, Surks MI, Daniels GH. Subclinical thyroid disease: Clinical applications. *JAMA.* 2004;291(2): 239–243.

21. Vanderpump MP, Tunbridge WM. Epidemiology and prevention of clinical and subclinical hypothyroidism. *Thyroid.* 2002;12(10):839–847.

22. Fatourechi V. Subclinical thyroid disease. *Mayo Clin Proc.* 2001;76(4):413–416.

23. Ross DS. Diagnosis of and screening for hypothyroidism. In: Rose BD, Rush J, editors. UpToDate. Edition 12.1; 2004. [Homepage on the Internet; subscription service.] Available from: http://www.uptodate.com.

24. Surks M. Clinical manifestations of hypothyroidism. In: Rose BD, Rush J, editors. UpToDate 12.1; 2004. [Homepage on the Internet; subscription service.] Available from: http://www.uptodate.com.

25. Haddow J, Palmieri EA, Lombardi G, Fazio S. Maternal thyroid deficiency during pregnancy and subsequent neuropsychological development of the child. *N Engl J Med.* 1999;341:549–555.

26. Klein I, Ojamaa K. Thyroid hormone and the cardiovascular system. *N Engl J Med.* 2001;344(7): 501–509.

27. Biondi B, Palmieri EA, Lombardi G, Fazio S. Effects of subclinical thyroid dysfunction on the heart. *Ann Intern Med.* 2002;137(11):904–914.

28. Lehmann MH, Frankovich D, Baga JJ, Pires LA, Schuger CD, Steinman RT, et al. Does subclinical hypothyroidism explain the increased susceptibility of women to torsades de pointes? *Am J Cardiol.* 1997;79(7):963–965.

29. Hak AE, Pols HA, Visser TJ, Drexhage HA, Hofman A, Witteman JC. Subclinical hypothyroidism is an independent risk factor for atherosclerosis and myocardial infarction in elderly women: The Rotterdam Study. *Ann Intern Med.* 2000;132(4): 270–278.

30. Alaswad B, Brosnan P. The association of celiac disease, diabetes mellitus type 1, hypothyroidism, chronic liver disease, and selective IgA deficiency. *Clin Pediatr.* 2000;39(4):229–231.

31. Jauk B, Mikosch P, Gallowitsch HJ, Kresnik E, Molnar M, Gomez I, et al. Unusual malabsorption of levothyroxine. *Thyroid.* 2000;10(1):93–95.

32. Kubota S, Fukata S, Matsuzuka F, Kuma K, Miyauchi A. Successful management of a patient with pseudomalabsorption of levothyroxine. *Int J Psychiatry Med.* 2003;33(2):183–188.

33. Kumar N, Wheeler MH. Hypothyroidism presenting as acute abdomen. *Postgrad Med J.* 1997;73(860): 373–374.

34. Mooney CJ, James DA, Kessenich CR. Diagnosis and management of hypothyroidism in pregnancy. [Erratum appears in JOGNN. 1998;27(2):531]. *JOGNN Nurs.* 1998;27(4):374–380.

35. Dugbartey AT. Neurocognitive aspects of hypothyroidism. *Arch Intern Med.* 1998;158(13):1413–1418.

36. Monzani F, Caraccio N, Del Guerra P, Casolaro A, Ferrannini E. Neuromuscular symptoms and dysfunction in subclinical hypothyroid patients: Beneficial effect of L-T4 replacement therapy. *Clin Endocrinol.* 1999;51(2):237–242.

37. Misiunas A, Niepomniszcze H, Ravera B, Faraj G, Faure E. Peripheral neuropathy in subclinical hypothyroidism. *Thyroid.* 1995;5(4):283–286.

38. Cooper DS. Clinical practice. Subclinical hypothyroidism. *N Engl J Med.* 2001;345(4): 260–265.

39. Clarnette RM, Patterson CJ. Hypothyroidism: Does treatment cure dementia? *J Geriatr Psychiatry Neurol.* 1994;7(1):23–27.

40. Davis JD, Stern RA, Flashman LA. Cognitive and neuropsychiatric aspects of subclinical hypothyroidism: Significance in the elderly. *Curr Psychiatry Rep.* 2003;5(5):384–390.

41. Mazzaferri EL. Adult hypothyroidism. 1. Manifestations and clinical presentation. *Postgrad Med.* 1986; 79(7):64–72.

42. Kittle WM, Chaudhary BA. Sleep apnea and hypothyroidism. *South Med J.* 1988;81(11):1421–1425.

43. Arojoki M, Jokimaa V, Juuti A, Koskinen P, Irjala K, Anttila L. Hypothyroidism among infertile women in Finland. *Gynecol Endocrinol.* 2000;14(2): 127–131.

44. Leonhardt JM, Heymann WR. Thyroid disease and the skin. *Dermatol Clin.* 2002;20(3):473–481, vii.

45. Fitzgerald PA. Diseases of the thyroid gland. In: Tierney LM, McPhee SJ, Papadakin MA, editors. *Current Medical Diagnois and Treatment.* New York: McGraw-Hill; 2003. pp. 1081–1107.

46. American College of Obstetricians and Gynecologists. Committee Opinion. Screening for hypothyroidism. Number 241, September 2000. *Int J Gynaecol Obstet.* 2001;75(3):342–343.

47. AACE Thyroid Task Force. American Association of Clinical Endocrinologists medical guidelines for clinical practice and treatment of hyperthyroidism and hypothyroidism. *Endocr Pract.* 2002;8:457–469.

48. Ladenson PW, Singer PA, Ain KB, Bagchi N, Bigos ST, Levy EG, et al. American Thyroid Association guidelines for detection of thyroid dysfunction. [Erratum appears in Arch Intern Med 2001 Jan 22; 161(2):284.] *Arch Intern Med.* 2000;160(11): 1573–1575.

49. American Academy of Family Physicians. Summary of policy recommendations for periodic health examinations Revision 5.7. Leawood (KS): American Academy of Family Physicians (AAFP); 2005 Apr. 15 p. Accessed at National Guidelines Clearinghouse http://www.guideline.gov/summary/summary.aspx?doc_id=7292&nbr=004340&string=american+AND+academy+AND+family+AND+physicians.

50. American College of Physicians. Screening for thyroid disease. Clinical guideline, part 1. *Ann Intern Med.* 1998;129(2):141–143.

51. Jaeschke R, Guyatt G, Gerstein H, Patterson CJ, Molloy W, Cook D, et al. Does treatment with L-thyroxine influence health status in middle-aged and older adults with subclinical hypothyroidism? *J Gen Intern Med.* 1996;11:744–749.

52. Brent GA. Maternal thyroid function: Interpretation of thyroid function tests in pregnancy. *Clin Obstet Gynecol.* 1997;40(1):3–15.

53. Spencer CA. Clinical utility and cost-effectiveness of sensitive thyrotropin assays in ambulatory and hospitalized patients. *Mayo Clin Proc.* 1988;63(12): 1214–1222.

54. Woeber KA. Update on the management of hyperthyroidism and hypothyroidism. *Arch Intern Med.* 2000;160(8):1067–1071.

55. Chu JW, Crapo LM. The treatment of subclinical hypothyroidism is seldom necessary. *J Clin Endocrinol Metab.* 2001;86(10):4591–4599.

56. McDermott MT, Ridgway EC. Subclinical hypothyroidism is mild thyroid failure and should be treated. *J Clin Endocrinol Metab.* 2001;86(10):4585–4590.

57. Poppe K, Glinoer D. Thyroid autoimmunity and hypothyroidism before and during pregnancy. *Hum Reprod Update.* 2003;9(2):149–161.

58. American College of Obstetrics and Gynecology. ACOG practice bulletin. Clinical Management Guidelines for Obstetrician-Gynecologists. Thyroid

disease in pregnancy. Number 37, August 2002. *Obstet Gynecol.* 2002;100:387–396.

59. Montoro MN. Management of hypothyroidism during pregnancy. *Clin Obstet Gynecol.* 1997;40(1):65–80.

60. Wiersinga WM. Subclinical hypothyroidism and hyperthyroidism. Prevalence and clinical relevance. *Neth J Med.* 1995;46(4):197–204.

61. Masiukiewicz US, Burrow GN. Hyperthyroidism in pregnancy: Diagnosis and treatment. *Thyroid.* 1999;9(7):647–652.

62. Mandel SJ, Cooper DS. The use of antithyroid drugs in pregnancy and lactation. *J Clin Endocrinol Metab.* 2001;86(6):2354–2359.

63. Bailes BK. Hyperthyroidism in elderly patients. *AORN J.* 1999;69(1):254–258.

64. Trivalle C, Doucet J, Chassagne P, Landrin I, Kadri N, Menard JF, et al. Differences in the signs and symptoms of hyperthyroidism in older and younger patients. *J Am Geriatr Soc.* 1996;44(1):50–53.

65. Kawabe T, Komiya I, Endo T, Koizumi Y, Yamada T. Hyperthyroidism in the elderly. *J Am Geriatr Soc.* 1979;27(4):152–155.

66. Diez JJ. Hyperthyroidism in patients older than 55 years: An analysis of the etiology and management. *Gerontology.* 2003;49(5):316–323.

67. Donatelli M, Assennato P, Abbadi V, Bucalo ML, Compagno V, Lo Vecchio S, et al. Cardiac changes in subclinical and overt hyperthyroid women: Retrospective study. *Int J Cardiol.* 2003;90(2–3):159–164.

68. Marvisi M, Brianti M, Marani G, Del Borello R, Bortesi ML, Guariglia A. Hyperthyroidism and pulmonary hypertension. *Respir Med.* 2002;96(4):215–220.

69. Greenwood RM, Daly JG, Himsworth RL. Hyperthyroidism and the impalpable thyroid gland. *Clin Endocrinol.* 1985;22(5):583–587.

70. Branski D, Levy J, Globus M, Aviad I, Keren A, Chowers I. Dysphagia as a primary manifestation of hyperthyroidism. *J Clin Gastroenterol.* 1984;6(5):437–540.

71. Ming RH, Dreosti LM, Tim LO, Segal I. Thyrotoxicosis presenting as dysphagia. A case report. *S Afr Med J.* 1982;61(15):554.

72. Ogihara T, Katoh H, Yoshitake H, Iyori S, Saito I. Hyperthyroidism associated with autoimmune hemolytic anemia and periodic paralysis: A report of a case in which antihyperthyroid therapy alone was effective against hemolysis. *Jpn J Med.* 1987;26(3):401–403.

73. Lee FY, Ho CH, Chong LL. Hyperthyroidism and Evans syndrome. A case report. Taiwan i Hsueh Hui Tsa Chih. *J Formos Med Assoc.* 1985;84(2):256–260.

74. Yashiro M, Nagoshi H, Kasuga Y, Isobe H, Kitajima S, Nakagawa T, et al. Evans syndrome associated with Graves disease. *Intern Med.* 1996;35(12):987–990.

75. Perlman JA, Sternthal PM. Effect of 131I on the anemia of hyperthyroidism. *J Chronic Dis.* 1983;36(5):405–412.

76. Ben-Shlomo A, Hagag P, Evans S, Weiss M. Early postmenopausal bone loss in hyperthyroidism. *Maturitas.* 2001;39(1):19–27.

77. Wu CC, Chau T, Chang CJ, Lin SH. An unrecognized cause of paralysis in ED: Thyrotoxic normokalemic periodic paralysis. *Am J Emerg Med.* 2003;21(1):71–73.

78. Evered D. Diseases of the thyroid gland. *Clin Endocrinol Metab.* 1974;3(3):425–450.

79. Gross MA. Achilles-reflex timing in diagnosis of thyroid status. *NY State J Med.* 1971;71(19):2283–2291.

80. North KA. The Achilles reflex in thyrotoxicosis. *N Z Med J.* 1967;66(413):16–18.

81. Nordyke RA. Screening for thyrotoxicosis by the achilles reflex time. *Pac Med Surg.* 1966;74(1):8–12.

82. Bazzani M, Benati L, Bosi M, Iorini M, Panizza M. Hypokalemic thyrotoxic paralysis: A rare cause of tetraparesis with acute onset in Europeans. *Ital J Neurol Sci.* 1998;19(5):307–309.

83. Reisin RC, Martinez O, Moran M, Rovira M, Roccatagliata G, Pardal A, et al. Thyrotoxic periodic paralysis in caucasians. Report of 8 cases. *Neurologia.* 2000;15(6):222–225.

84. Demet MM, Ozmen B, Deveci A, Boyvada S, Adiguzel H, Aydemir O. Depression and anxiety in hyperthyroidism. *Arch Med Res.* 2002;33(6):552–556.

85. Scott IU, Siatkowski MR. Thyroid eye disease. *Semin Ophthalmol.* 1999;14(2):52–61.

86. Nachum Z, Rakover Y, Weiner E, Shalev E. Graves disease in pregnancy: Prospective evaluation of a selective invasive treatment protocol. *Am J Obstet Gynecol.* 2003;189(1):159–165.

87. Cohen O, Pinhas-Hamiel O, Sivan E, Dolitski M, Lipitz S, Achiron R. Serial in utero ultrasonographic measurements of the fetal thyroid: A new complementary tool in the management of maternal hyperthyroidism in pregnancy. *Pren Diagn.* 2003;23(9):740–742.

88. Ginsberg J. Diagnosis and management of Graves disease. *CMAJ.* 2003;168(5):575–585.

89. Millar LK, Wing DA, Leung AS, Koonings PP, Montoro MN, Mestman JH. Low birth weight and preeclampsia in pregnancies complicated by hyperthyroidism. *Obstet Gynecol.* 1994;84(6):946–949.

90. Phoojaroenchanachai M, Sriussadaporn S, Peerapatdit T, Vannasaeng S, Nitiyanant W, Boonnamsiri V, et al. Effect of maternal hyperthyroidism during late pregnancy on the risk of neonatal low birth weight. *Clin Endocrinol.* 2001;54(3):365–370.

91. Luong KV, Nguyen LT. Hyperthyroidism and asthma. *J Asthma.* 2000;37(2):125–130.

92. White NW, Raine RI, Bateman ED. Asthma and hyperthyroidism. A report of 4 cases. *S Afr Med J.* 1990;78(12):750–752.

93. Zacharisen MC, Fink JN. Hyperthyroidism complicating asthma treatment. *Allergy Asthma Proc.* 2000; 21(2):71–74.

94. Ai J, Leonhardt JM, Heymann WR. Autoimmune thyroid diseases: Etiology, pathogenesis, and dermatologic manifestations. *J Am Acad Dermatol.* 2003; 48(5):641–659; quiz 660–662.

95. Krahn AD, Klein GJ, Kerr CR, Boone J, Sheldon R, Green M, et al. How useful is thyroid function testing in patients with recent-onset atrial fibrillation? The Canadian Registry of Atrial Fibrillation Investigators. *Arch Intern Med.* 1996;156(19): 2221–2224.

96. Ross DS. Diagnosis of hyperthyroidism. In: Rose BD, Rush J, editors. UpToDate. Edition 12.1; 2004. [Homepage on the Internet; subscription service.] Available from: http://www.uptodate.com.

97. Stocker DJ, Foster SS, Solomon BL, Shriver CD, Burch HB. Thyroid cancer yield in patients with Graves disease selected for surgery based on the basis of cold scintiscan defects. *Thyroid.* 2002;12:305–311.

98. Weetman AP. Graves disease. *N Engl J Med.* 2000; 343(17):1236–1248.

99. Caffrey TJ. Transient hyperthyroidism of hyperemesis gravidarum: A sheep in wolf's clothing. *J Am Board Fam Pract.* 2000;13(1):35–38.

100. Mestman JH. Hyperthyroidism in pregnancy. *Endocrinol Metab Clin N Am.* 1998;27(1):127–149.

101. Gerstein HC. Incidence of postpartum thyroid dysfunction in patients with type I diabetes mellitus. *Ann Intern Med.* 1993;118(6):419–423.

102. Streetman DD, Khanderia U. Diagnosis and treatment of Graves disease. *Ann Pharmacother.* 2003; 37(7-8):1100–1109.

103. Cooper DS. Antithyroid drugs in the management of patients with Graves disease: An evidence-based approach to therapeutic controversies. *J Clin Endocrinol Metab.* 2003;88(8):3474–3481.

104. Mestman JH. Hyperthyroidism in pregnancy. *Clin Obstetr Gynecol.* 1997;40(1):45–64.

105. Witte J, Goretzki PE, Dotzenrath C, Simon D, Felis P, Neubauer M, et al. Surgery for Graves disease: Total versus subtotal thyroidectomy—results of a prospective randomized trial. *World J Surg.* 2000; 24(11):1303–1311.

106. Palit TK, Miller CC, 3rd, Miltenburg DM. The efficacy of thyroidectomy for Graves disease: A meta-analysis. *J Surg Res.* 2000;90(2):161–165.

107. Bogazzi F, Bartalena L, Campomori A, Brogioni S, Traino C, De Martino F, et al. Treatment with lithium prevents serum thyroid hormone increase after thionamide withdrawal and radioiodine therapy in patients with Graves disease. *J Clin Endocrinol Metab.* 2002;87(10):4490–4495.

108. Bal CS, Kumar A, Pandey RM. A randomized controlled trial to evaluate the adjuvant effect of lithium on radioiodine treatment of hyperthyroidism. *Thyroid.* 2002;12(5):399–405.

109. Millar LK, Wing DA, Leung AS, Koonings PP, Montoro MN, Mestman JH. Low birth weight and preeclampsia in pregnancies complicated by hyperthyroidism. *Obstet Gynecol.* 1994;84(6):946–949.

110. Momotani N, Noh JY, Ishikawa N, Ito K. Effects of propylthiouracil and methimazole on fetal thyroid status in mothers with Graves hyperthyroidism. *J Clin Endocrinol Metab.* 1997;82(11):3633–3636.

111. Gallagher MP, Schachner HC, Levine LS, Fisher DA, Berdon WE, Oberfield SE. Neonatal thyroid enlargement associated with propylthiouracil therapy of Graves disease during pregnancy: A problem revisited. *J Pediatr.* 2001;139(6):896–900.

112. Centers for Disease Control and Prevention. National Diabetes Fact Sheet: General information and national estimates on diabetes in the United States, 2005. Atlanta: U.S. Department of Health and Human Services, Centers for Disease Control and Prevention, 2005.

113. American Diabetes Association. Screening for type 2 diabetes. *Diabetes Care.* 2004;27; Suppl 1:S11–14.

114. American Diabetes Association. Diagnosis and classification of diabetes mellitus. *Diabetes Care.* 2005;28 Suppl 1:S43–49.

115. Boyle JP, Honeycutt AA, Venkat Narayan KM, Hoerger TJ, Geiss LS, Chen H, et al. Projection of diabetes burden through 2050. *Diabetes Care.* 2001;24(11):1936–1940.

116. American Diabetes Association. Gestational diabetes mellitus. *Diabetes Care*. 2004;27:S88–90.

117. Powers A. Diabetes. In: Braunwald E, Fauci, A, Kasper, D Eds. *Harrison's Principles of Internal Medicine*. 16th ed. New York: McGraw Hill; 2005.

118. Guyton AH, Hall JE. *Textbook of Medical Physiology*. 10th ed. Philadelphia: W.B. Saunders; 2000.

119. Turner RC, Cull CA, Frighi V, Holman RR. Glycemic control with diet, sulfonylurea, metformin, or insulin in patients with type 2 diabetes mellitus: Progressive requirement for multiple therapies (UKPDS 49). UK Prospective Diabetes Study (UKPDS) Group. *JAMA*. 1999;281(21):2005–2012.

120. Liebl A. Challenges in optimal metabolic control of diabetes. *Diabetes Metab Res Rev*. 2002;18 Suppl 3:S36–41.

121. Harris MI, Klein R, Welborn TA, Knuiman MW. Onset of NIDDM occurs at least 4–7 yr before clinical diagnosis. *Diabetes Care*. 1992;15(7):815–819.

122. American Diabetes Association. Standards of medical care in diabetes. *Diabetes Care*. 2005;28 Suppl 1: S4–36.

123. Golden S, Boulware LE, Berkenblit G, Brancati F, Chandler G, Marinopolous S, et al. Use of glycated hemoglobin and microalbuminuria in the monitoring of diabetes mellitus. Evidence Report/ Technology Assessment No. 84 (Prepared by Johns Hopkins Evidence-based Practice Center under contract No. 290-97-0006). AHRQ Publication No. 04-E0001. Rockville, MD: Agency for Healthcare Research and Quality, U.S. Department of Health and Human Services, October 2003.

124. Benjamin SM, Valdez R, Geiss LS, Rolka DB, Narayan KM. Estimated number of adults with prediabetes in the US in 2000: Opportunities for prevention. *Diabetes Care*. 2003;26(3):645–649.

125. U.S. Preventive Services Task Force. Screening for Type 2 Diabetes Mellitus in Adults: Recommendations and Rationale. Rockville, MD: Agency for Healthcare Research and Quality, U.S. Department of Health and Human Services, February 2003. http://www.ahrq.gov/clinic/3rduspstf/diabscr/ diabetrr.htm.

126. The effect of intensive treatment of diabetes on the development and progression of long-term complications in insulin-dependent diabetes mellitus. The Diabetes Control and Complications Trial Research Group. *N Engl J Med*. 1993;329(1993):977–986.

127. UK Prospective Diabetes Study (UKPDS) Group. Effect of intensive blood-glucose control with metformin on complications in overweight patients with type 2 diabetes (UKPDS 34). *Lancet*. 1998; 352(9131):854–865.

128. UK Prospective Diabetes Study (UKPDS) Group. Intensive blood-glucose control with sulphonylureas or insulin compared with conventional treatment and risk of complications in patients with type 2 diabetes (UKPDS 33). *Lancet*. 1998;352(9131): 837–853.

129. National Cholesterol Education Program. Third Report of the National Cholesterol Education Program (NCEP) Expert Panel on Detection, Evaluation, and Treatment of High Blood Cholesterol in Adults. Executive Summary. National Institutes of Health, National Heart, Lung and Blood Institute, NIH Publication No. 01-3670, 2001.

130. Arauz-Pacheco C, Parrott MA, Raskin P. Hypertension management in adults with diabetes. *Diabetes Care*. 2004;27 Suppl 1:S65–67.

131. Haffner SM. Dyslipidemia management in adults with diabetes. *Diabetes Care*. 2004;27; Suppl 1:S68–71.

132. American Diabetes Association. Insulin administration. *Diabetes Care*. 2004;27(1):S106–109.

133. American Diabetes Association. Continuous subcutaneous insulin infusion. *Diabetes Care*. 2004;27(1): S110.

134. Franz MJ, Bantle JP, Beebe CA, Brunzell JD, Chiasson JL, Garg A, et al. Nutrition principles and recommendations in diabetes. *Diabetes Care*. 2004; 27; Suppl 1:S36–46.

135. Zinman B, Ruderman N, Campaigne BN, Devlin JT, Schneider SH. Physical activity/exercise and diabetes. *Diabetes Care*. 2004;27; Suppl 1:S58–62.

136. Stern L, Iqbal N, Seshadri P, Chicano KL, Daily DA, McGrory J, et al. The effects of low-carbohydrate versus conventional weight loss diets in severely obese adults: One-year follow-up of a randomized trial. *Ann Intern Med*. 2004;140(10):778–785.

137. Buttaro TM, Bailey PP, Sandberg-Cook J. *Primary Care: A Collaborative Practice*. 2nd ed. St. Louis: Mosby; 2003.

138. Ramsdell JW, Braunstein SN, Stephens JM, Bell CF, Botteman MF, Devine ST. Economic model of first-line drug strategies to achieve recommended glycaemic control in newly diagnosed type 2 diabetes mellitus. *Pharmacoeconomics*. 2003;21(11): 819–837.

139. Koda-Kimble M, Young LY, Dradjan WA, Guglielmo BJ, Alldredge BK, Corelli RL. *Applied Therapeutics: The Clinical Use of Drugs*. 8th ed. Philadelphia: Lippincott Williams & Wilkins; 2005.

140. Wright A, Burden ACF, Paisey RB, Cull CA, Holman RR. Sulfonylurea Inadequacy: Efficacy of addition of insulin over 6 years in patients with type 2 diabetes in the U.K. Prospective Diabetes Study (UKPDS 57). *Diabetes Care.* 2002;25(2):330–336.

141. Nathan DM. Clinical practice. Initial management of glycemia in type 2 diabetes mellitus. *N Engl J Med.* 2002;347(17):1342–1349.

142. Rosenstock J. Basal insulin supplementation in type 2 diabetes; refining the tactics. *Am J Med.* 2004;116 Suppl 3A:10S–16S.

143. Clarke P, Gray A, Adler A, Stevens R, Raikou M, Cull C, et al. Cost-effectiveness analysis of intensive blood-glucose control with metformin in overweight patients with type II diabetes (UKPDS No. 51). *Diabetologia.* 2001;44(3):298–304.

144. Mensing C, Boucher J, Cypress M, Weinger K, Mulcahy K, Barta P, et al. National standards for diabetes self-management education. *Diabetes Care.* 2004;27; Suppl 1:S143–S150.

145. Knowler WC, Barrett-Connor E, Fowler SE, Hamman RF, Lachin JM, Walker EA, et al. Reduction in the incidence of type 2 diabetes with lifestyle intervention or metformin. *N Engl J Med.* 2002;346(6):393–403.

146. Tuomilehto J, Lindstrom J, Eriksson JC, et al. Prevention of type 2 diabetes mellitus by changes in lifestyle among subjects with impaired glucose tolerance. *N Engl J Med.* 2001;344:1343–1350.

147. Tataranni PA, Bogardus C. Changing habits to delay diabetes. *N Engl J Med.* 2001;344(18):1390–1392.

148. Sherwin RS, Anderson RM, Buse JB, Chin MH, Eddy D, Fradkin J, et al. Prevention or delay of type 2 diabetes. *Diabetes Care.* 2004;27; Suppl 1:S47–54.

149. Ford ES, Giles WH, Dietz WH. Prevalence of the metabolic syndrome among US adults: Findings from the third National Health and Nutrition Examination Survey. *JAMA.* 2002;287(3): 356–359.

150. Park YW, Zhu S, Palaniappan L, Heshka S, Carnethon MR, Heymsfield SB. The metabolic syndrome: Prevalence and associated risk factor findings in the US population from the Third National Health and Nutrition Examination Survey, 1988–1994. *Arch Intern Med.* 2003;163(4): 427–436.

151. American Diabetes Association. Preconception care of women with diabetes. *Diabetes Care.* 2004;27; Suppl 1:S76–78.

152. Gabbe SG, Graves CR. Management of diabetes mellitus complicating pregnancy. *Obstet Gynecol.* 2003;102(4):857–868.

153. Ray JG, O'Brien TE, Chan WS. Preconception care and the risk of congenital anomalies in the offspring of women with diabetes mellitus: A meta-analysis. *QJM.* 2001;94(8):435–444.

154. Kendrick JM. Preconception care of women with diabetes. *J Perinat Neonatal Nurs.* 2004;18(1):14–25; quiz 26–27.

155. Griffith J, Conway DL. Care of diabetes in pregnancy. *Obstet Gynecol Clin North Am.* 2004;31(2): 243–256.

156. Moore T. *Diabetes in Pregnancy.* 5th ed. Philadelphia: WB Saunders; 2004.

157. ter Braak EW, Evers IM, Willem Erkelens D, Visser GH. Maternal hypoglycemia during pregnancy in type 1 diabetes: Maternal and fetal consequences. *Diabetes Metab Res Rev.* 2002;18(2):96–105.

158. Langer O. Oral hypoglycemic agents in pregnancy: Their time has come. *J Matern Fetal Neonatal Med.* 2002;12(6):376–383.

159. Reece EA, Homko C, Miodovnik M, Langer O. A consensus report of the Diabetes in Pregnancy Study Group of North America Conference, Little Rock, Arkansas, May 2002. *J Matern Fetal Neonatal Med.* 2002;12(6):362–364.

160. Glueck C, Wang P, Kobayashi S, Phillips H, Sieve-Smith L. Metformin therapy throughout pregnancy reduces the development of gestational diabetes in women with polycystic ovary syndrome. *Fertil Steril.* 2002;77(3):520–525.

161. Preece R, Jovanovic L. New and future diabetes therapies: Are they safe during pregnancy? *J Matern Fetal Neonatal Med.* 2002;12:365–375.

162. McCarthy EA, Walker SP, McLachlan K, Boyle J, Permezel M. Metformin in obstetric and gynecologic practice: A review. *Obstet Gynecol Surv.* 2004;59(2): 118–127.

163. Kjos SL, Henry O, Lee RM, Buchanan TA, Mishell DR, Jr. The effect of lactation on glucose and lipid metabolism in women with recent gestational diabetes. *Obstet Gynecol.* 1993;82(3):451–455.

Chapter 17

Gastrointestinal

Diane Angelini

Diane Hodgman

Edie McConaughey

In 2001, the National Center for Health Statistics estimated that hospital emergency department (ED) visits neared 107.5 million. The top reasons cited for these visits were stomach pain and abdominal cramps. A review of adult ED visits categorized cases in which abdominal pain was the primary presenting symptom as follows: 18% admitted; 25% undifferentiated; 12% female pelvic-related; 12% urinary tract; and 9.3% surgical gastrointestinal (GI).[1] Women of reproductive age present to the ED with abdominal pain in two-thirds to three quarters of cases annually in the United States.[2] Additionally, 13 to 44 of every 10,000 pregnant women require nonobstetric, usually abdominal, surgery during pregnancy.[3] Thus, abdominal assessment and management therapies are salient components of primary care for midwives and women's health providers.

Introductory sections of this chapter include history-taking and physical assessment skills specific to the abdomen, and generic sections on nausea, vomiting, diarrhea, and constipation. The remaining sections are divided by location of complaint within the abdomen. The upper abdomen includes gastroesophageal reflux disease (GERD), cholecystitis, gastritis, and pancreatitis.

Mid abdomen encompasses peptic ulcer disease (PUD), bowel obstruction, aneurysm, inflammatory bowel disease (IBD), and irritable bowel syndrome (IBS). The last section on the lower abdomen focuses on GI issues, including appendicitis, diverticulitis, parasites, and rectal bleeding. Urinary and gynecologic conditions are addressed in Chapter 18.

Health History and Physical Assessment

Both common and life-threatening conditions can precipitate abdominal pain. The clinician must assess several organs to identify the source of the problem, determine its severity, and treat or make a referral for treatment.[4] A list of common conditions producing abdominal pain by location, radiation, and symptoms is presented in **Table 17-1**.

The acuity of the problem determines whether immediate hospitalization and surgery are warranted.[5] The sudden onset of severe pain may signify acute and progressive deterioration such as a ruptured appendix or a ruptured ectopic or aortic aneurysm. Any movement usually exacerbates the

"

Table 17-1 ABDOMINAL PAIN BY MAIN LOCATION WITH SIGNS AND SYMPTOMS[5,6]

Diagnosis	Pain Location	Visual Pain Radiates	Symptoms	Signs
Hepatitis	RUQ	Right shoulder	• Fatigue • Malaise • Anorexia	• Hepatic tenderness • Hepatomegaly • Increased bilirubin • Jaundice • Increased liver enzymes
Cholecystitis Cholelithiasis	RUQ Epigastric pain	Back, right scapula, mid-epigastric, sudden onset with associated nausea	• Anorexia • Nausea • Severe pain • Prolonged episodes	• RUQ tenderness • Jaundice • Vomiting • Increased WBC • Peritoneal irritation
Pancreatitis	Mid-epigastric region LUQ	Radiates to back, left shoulder, may have peritonitis, knife-like pain	• Pain radiating to back or chest	• Fever • Rigidity • Rebound tenderness • Nausea • Vomiting • Jaundice • Abdominal distention • Diminished bowel sounds
Gastric Ulcer Duodenal Ulcer	Mid-epigastric LLQ pain	Radiation to back, if posterior ulcer, peritonitis with perforation, may awaken patient from sleep	• Abrupt pain if perforated • Burning pain	• Tenderness in epigastric and/or RUQ
Aortic Aneurysm	Periumbilical – especially into back flanks	Epigastric or back pain, flank, hip pain May be colicky	• Abdominal, back or flank	• Vague to severe GI symptoms
Appendicitis	Early – periumbilical	May present with peritoneal signs	• Anorexia • Nausea	• Vomiting • Localized RLQ

Table 17-1 ABDOMINAL PAIN BY MAIN LOCATION WITH SIGNS AND SYMPTOMS
(continued)

Diagnosis	Pain Location	Visual Pain Radiates	Symptoms	Signs
	Late – RLQ at McBurney point		• Pain	guarding and tenderness late • Rovsing sign • Iliopsoas sign • Obturator sign • WBC increased • Left shift • Low grade fever
Crohn's disease or ulcerative colitis	RLQ Central pain	May radiate to back	• Chronic, watery diarrhea with blood, mucus • Anorexia • Weight loss • Fatigue	• Fever • Cachexia • Anemia • Leukocytosis
Diverticulitis	LLQ Rare RLQ	Generalized	• Recurrent LLQ pain	• Fever • Vomiting • Diarrhea • Chills • Tenderness over descending colon
GYN – ovarian cyst, ovarian torsion, ectopic, PID	RLQ, LLQ, suprapubic	Radiation to groin or right shoulder	• Symptoms of pregnancy • Lower abdominal pain • Nausea • Dyspareunia	• Tenderness • Mass • Fever • Cervical motion tenderness • Cervical discharge
Urolithiasis or nephrolithiasis	Flank	Radiates to labia	• Hematuria dysuria	• Flank pain • CVAT
Cystitis	Suprapubic pain		• Urgency • Dysuria • Frequency • Hematuria	• Flank pain

Abbreviations are: RUQ, right upper quadrant; LUQ, left upper quadrant; RLQ, right lower quadrant; LLQ, left lower quadrant; CVAT, costovertebral angle tenderness; PID, pelvic inflammatory disease.

degree of pain. Additional warning signs include rebound, rigidity, tachycardia, postural hypotension, and absence of bowel sounds.[5,6] Consideration of any abnormalities in stool and urine characteristics should also be included.

An accurate and detailed history and physical exam are the basic tools needed for diagnosing abdominal pain.[7] The initial interview will alert the clinician to specific parts of the physical examination that need further investigation and laboratory testing. Key elements of the initial interview are presented in **Table 17-2**.

A general health assessment includes information from the woman's past medical and surgical history that will identify chronic or recurrent conditions that might affect the diagnosis. A complete menstrual/sexual/obstetric/gynecologic history and determination of the possibility of pregnancy in any woman of childbearing age are required.[8] Evidence of eating disorders, sexual/physical abuse, or substance abuse is elicited. Finally, a complete list of medications (prescription or nonprescription), as well as any use of complementary or alternative therapies, should be obtained.[4] **Table 17-3** lists causes of abdominal pain by quadrant.

The physical examination follows the history. A systematic approach is used when performing the exam.[4,9,10] An initial observation of physical appearance includes alertness, comfort level, and movement without distress. Components of the examination are discussed in the order in which they should be performed. Having an empty bladder will lessen the woman's discomfort.[4,9]

Inspection

The abdomen is initially inspected, observing for shape, symmetry, pulsations, and any visible scars.

Auscultation

Both the frequency and character of bowel sounds aid in the assessment of motility. Sounds are generally increased in diarrhea and early intestinal obstruction, and decreased in peritonitis and ileus.[5] Vascular sounds are assessed for bruits; the liver and spleen are assessed for rubs

---

Table 17-2 **KEY ELEMENTS OF PATIENT HISTORY**[4,5,7]

Location	Where is the pain located? Specific point of pain? Does pain radiate? Change in location over time? Superficial or deep?
Onset	When did it begin? Gradual or rapid onset. Intermittent onset.
Duration	Continuous, recurrent, chronic, or intermittent? Pain steadily intensifying?
Description	What does the pain feel like—sharp, dull, burning, stabbing, cramping, colic-like? How severe is it? Differentiate between visceral pain, deep somatic pain, and referred pain.
Associated Symptoms	Is the pain accompanied by other symptoms—vomiting, diarrhea, constipation, flatus, belching, jaundice, change in menstrual pattern, vaginal discharge, weight loss, heartburn, presence of melena, mucus or pus in the stool, urinary symptoms?
Exacerbating or Alleviating Factors	What makes the pain better or worse—position, breathing, drinking, medications, menstrual cycle, bowel movements, stress?

Table 17-3 ABDOMINAL PAIN BY QUADRANT[5,9]

RUQ	LUQ
Acute cholecystitis	Diverticulitis
Biliary colic/stones	Gastric ulcer
Duodenal ulcer	Gastritis
Hepatitis	Herpes zoster
Herpes zoster	Lower lobe pneumonia (left-sided)
Lower lobe pneumonia (right-sided)	Myocardial ischemia
Myocardial ischemia	Nephrolithiasis (left-sided)
Nephrolithiasis (right-sided)	Pancreatitis
Pancreatitis	Pericarditis
Retrocecal appendicitis	Pulmonary embolism
Subphrenic abscess	Splenic rupture
Perforated peptic ulcer	Pyloric obstruction

RLQ	LLQ
Appendicitis	Colon perforation
Cecal perforation	Constipation
Constipation	Early appendicitis
Crohn's disease	Ectopic pregnancy
Diverticulosis	Endometriosis
Ectopic pregnancy	Kidney or ureteral stone
Endometriosis	Ovarian cyst
Intestinal obstruction	Salpingitis
Kidney or ureteral stone	Sigmoid diverticulitis
Ovarian cyst	Sigmoid perforation
Regional enteritis	Strangulated hernia
Salpingitis	Ulcerative colitis
Strangulated hernia	
Perforated duodenal ulcer	
Pelvic inflammatory disease	

Abbreviations: RUQ, right upper quadrant; LUQ, left upper quadrant; RLQ, right lower quadrant; LLQ, left lower quadrant.

if a mass or infection in these areas is suspected.[5,10] Auscultation of cardiac and pulmonary systems is included.

PERCUSSION

Percussion of the abdomen in all four quadrants follows. This technique is useful for determining the size and location of liver and spleen and identifying ascites and masses.[4,5,10]

PALPATION

Palpation is the most critical physical assessment technique, especially when the chief complaint is abdominal pain. All four quadrants are palpated using light palpation and then deep palpation, *examining the most painful area last.* This technique is useful for identifying abdominal tenderness, masses and organs, and muscular resistance.[5,10] Observation of involuntary tenderness, rigidity, or rebound tenderness and the type of pain response elicited are additional assessment parameters. **Table 17-4** describes common maneuvers used in abdominal evaluation. Bimanual pelvic and rectal exams to rule out gynecologic causes of abdominal pain complete the physical examination.

The history and physical examination are supplemented by a number of diagnostic tests that can be ordered in the primary care setting. The laboratory tests and imaging for specific conditions will be presented as the topics are covered. If the woman presents with symptoms of a chronic nature that have not responded to initial treatment regimens, a referral is made to an internist or a gastroenterologist for further evaluation, depending on the suspected condition as well as the severity and complexity of the presentation.

Nausea and Vomiting

Definition

Nausea and vomiting (NV) are common distressing symptoms with a number of underlying causes, including pregnancy. They may represent a physiologic homeostatic response to an ingested toxin or indicate a disease process of the GI tract, adjacent organs, or the central nervous system (CNS).[1] They can be secondary symptoms of many different primary diseases of the GI tract or the CNS. Careful attention to the principal causes of NV while performing the history and physical will assist the clinician in making a diagnosis. Most acute cases of NV, whether caused by infection, toxins, or pregnancy, can be remedied. Chronic NV persisting for greater than one month is not within the scope of this chapter.

Nausea can be defined as an unpleasant sensation of sickness with the imminent need to vomit.[11–13] This queasiness may or may not be followed by vomiting. Vomiting is defined as the forceful oral expulsion of gastric contents associated with the contraction of the abdominal and chest wall musculature.[12,14] Three components are present in this process: nausea; retching (spasmodic respiratory and abdominal movements, "dry heaves"); and vomiting. Vomiting is usually preceded by nausea although nausea and retching can occur without vomiting. Vomiting includes both voluntary and involuntary processes. Vomiting should be distinguished from regurgitation, a passive process where there is retrograde flow of esophageal contents into the mouth, which is common in GERD.[12,13]

Associated phenomena accompanying the vomiting episode include: mouth opening; hypersalivation; inhibition of gastric motility; retroperistaltic contraction in the small bowel, duodenum, and stomach; tachycardia; breath holding; posturing; contraction of abdominal muscles; and ejection of gastric contents through the open mouth.[15]

Pathophysiology

Vomiting is the reflex that allows the body to rid itself of toxins. The act of vomiting is under the control of two medullary centers: the vomiting center in the dorsal portion of the lateral reticular formation including the dorsal vagal complex ("vomiting center"), and the chemoreceptor trigger zone (CTZ) in the area of the floor

Table 17-4 MANEUVERS IN EVALUATING THE ABDOMEN[5,11]

Sign	How Elicited	Differential Diagnosis
Rebound	Gentle deep pressure over abdomen with quick release produces severe pain on release	Local or general peritonitis
Guarding	Patient resistance to gentle pressure on abdominal wall	Voluntary or involuntary response to palpation related to perforated viscera (internal organs) or internal bleeding
Iliopsoas sign	Pain or resistance on extension of thigh	Retroperitoneal irritation—endometriosis, hemorrhage
Murphy sign	Pause in inspiration as examiner palpates under liver	Cholecystitis
Rovsing sign	Palpation of LLQ causes pain in RLQ	Appendicitis
McBurney point	Point at which palpation of RLQ two-thirds distance between umbilicus and right iliac crest causes pain	Appendicitis
Obdurator sign	Pain on rotation of flexed thigh especially with internal rotation	Perforated appendix

of the fourth ventricle.[16,17] The vomiting center receives input via the vagus and sympathetic nerves; it is activated directly by signals from the cerebral cortex, signals from sensory organs, or from the vestibular apparatus of the inner ear (motion sickness, Ménière's disease, benign positional paroxysmal vertigo).[14,17,18] Individuals vary considerably in the response threshold of their vomiting centers to different stimuli.[17]

The CTZ can be activated by toxic substances in the blood (e.g., drugs, chemotherapeutic agents, hypoxia, uremia, radiation therapy), or it can be affected by signals in the stomach and small intestines via the vagal efferent nerves.[13,17,18] Activation of either pathway can lead to emesis. Specific neurotransmitters in the CTZ identify substances as harmful and relay impulses to the vomiting center to initiate the vomiting cycle, which will expel the toxins. The responsible neuro-

transmitters include serotonin, dopamine, acetylcholine, histamine, and neurokinin-1 neuropeptide. Because stimulation of neurotransmitters induces vomiting, interference with transmission of these neurotransmitters will prevent the vomiting center from being activated. Antiemetics act in this fashion by blocking at least one of the neurotransmitters.[18] Examples include: Zofran as a serotonin antagonist; Phenergan and Compazine as a dopamine antagonist; Scopolamine as an anticholinergic; and Antivert or Dramamine as antihistamines.

Diagnosis

Acute symptoms are usually caused by medications, obstructions in the GI tract, infectious gastroenteritis, endocrine and metabolic causes, inflammatory processes within the peritoneal cavity, post-anesthesia and CNS disease.[12,15,19,20] The differential diagnosis of NV includes, but is not limited to, causes displayed in **Table 17-5**.

DRUG-INDUCED ETIOLOGIES

Ingesting almost any drug can cause vomiting. Adverse reactions to medications are among the most common causes of NV. Many drugs act on the CTZ to cause NV, including opiates, dopamine agonists, nicotine, digoxin anesthetics, and chemotherapy agents. Other commonly used agents such as aspirin, nonsteroidal anti-inflammatory drugs (NSAIDs), and antibiotics cause damage to the gastric mucosa and activate the vomiting center.[12,14]

Table 17-5 DIFFERENTIAL DIAGNOSIS FOR NAUSEA AND VOMITING[12,19]

Drug Induced Etiologies	**Disorders of the Gut and Peritoneum**
Cancer Chemotherapy Agents	Mechanical Obstruction
Analgesics	Small intestinal obstruction
Aspirin	Functional Gastrointestinal (GI) Disorders
Nonsteroidal anti-inflammatory drugs	Gastroparesis (Weakness of gastric peristalsis)
Anti-gout medications	Irritable bowel syndrome
Cardiovascular Medications	Organic GI Disorders
Anti-arrhythmics	Peptic ulcer disease
Anti-hypertensives	Cholecystitis
Beta blockers	Pancreatitis
Calcium channel blockers	Crohn's disease
Diuretics	Hepatitis
Hormonal Medications	
Oral contraceptives	**Infectious Etiologies**
Antibiotics	Viral/bacterial gastroenteritis
Macrolides	
Tetracycline	**Endocrine Etiologies**
Sulfonamides	Pregnancy
Acyclovir	Uremia
Nicotine	Diabetic ketoacidosis
Narcotics	Hyperthyroidism
Radiation Therapy	
Alcohol Abuse	**Central Nervous System**
	Increased intracranial pressure
	Emotional/psychiatric
	Migraine
	Seizure disorder
	Labyrinthine disorders
	Motion sickness
	Labyrinthitis
	Ménière's disease

Medications usually produce acute rather than chronic NV, because the symptoms tend to present soon after use. Radiation treatment for cancer can also cause NV, especially when the abdomen is in the radiation field. Other substances such as alcohol cause vomiting by local action on the GI tract along with central action on the brainstem.[12]

DISORDERS OF THE GUT AND PERITONEUM

Mechanical obstruction of the stomach and small bowel can produce significant nausea, vomiting, and abdominal pain that can be chronic, intermittent, or acute.[12] Gastroparesis, a disorder of motility, along with other organic and inflammatory GI disorders (e.g., PUD, cholecystitis, pancreatitis, appendicitis) will also cause varying degrees of NV.[12,14]

INFECTIOUS ETIOLOGY

Acute infections with bacterial, viral, and parasitic pathogens are characterized by sudden and explosive outbreaks of profuse vomiting, frequently in the morning.[14,15] Acute illness resulting in vomiting is most prevalent in children under three years old and in young adults 20 to 30 years of age.[12] Gastroenteritis occurs at a rate of 1.2 infections per person per year, and many episodes occur in the fall and winter seasons.[12,19] Infections with Norwalk virus or other enteral viruses are often associated with symptoms of headache, chills, muscular pain, sweating, diarrhea, and fever, all of which suggest a viral syndrome.[20]

Food poisoning by bacteria such as *Staphylococcus aureus*, *Salmonella*, *Shigella*, or *Clostridium perfringens* present with diarrhea but are also associated with NV via toxins that act on the area postrema.[19] The area postrema is on the dorsal surface of the medulla oblongata at the caudal end of the fourth ventricle. A careful history will help to define the source of the contamination.

CENTRAL NERVOUS SYSTEM ETIOLOGY

Acute meningitis, migraine, and increased intracranial pressure from hemorrhage or infection may produce vomiting with or without nausea. Labyrinthine disorders such as labyrinthitis and Ménière's disease produce NV with associated vertigo. Motion sickness caused by repetitive movements activates the vestibular nuclei causing pallor, diaphoresis, salivation, and NV.[15,19]

ENDOCRINE ETIOLOGY

Endocrine and metabolic causes of NV include diabetic ketoacidosis, uremia, and hyperthyroidism.[19] These conditions activate the area postrema and may disrupt the normal GI motor activity.

Nausea and vomiting in pregnancy (NVP) is the most common endocrine cause of vomiting. NVP is usually mild and self-limiting, typically beginning in the early first trimester and resolving 90% of the time by 20 weeks gestation.[21] There are usually no adverse outcomes.

Hyperemesis gravidarum, a severe form of NVP, affects 0.5% to 1% of pregnant women.[21] Persistent vomiting leads to dehydration, ketosis, electrolyte imbalance, and more than 5% loss of body weight. Risk factors for hyperemesis include previous history, multiple gestation, gestational trophoblastic disease, and a family history of this condition.[22]

Clinical Findings

The history focuses on detailing the location, description, pattern of radiation, associated symptoms, and the exacerbating or alleviating factors.[15,23] The onset and duration of symptoms will assist in differentiating between acute and chronic NV. Acute NV is usually quickly diagnosed, whereas chronic NV presents a greater challenge in determining the underlying cause and providing satisfactory treatment.[12,15,20] Referral to a gastroenterologist is warranted when the primary care clinician diagnoses or suspects a serious chronic disease such as Crohn's disease.

The physical examination includes vital signs to assess for tachycardia or orthostatic hypotension, which are common in dehydration caused by vomiting. Decreased skin turgor and dry mucous membranes are also seen with dehydration. Assessment of bowel sounds and observation of abdominal distention are critical to rule out intestinal obstruction. Abdominal palpation may reveal tenderness or guarding that could signify an inflammatory or infectious disease such as ulcer, cholecystitis, or peritonitis.[19]

Most individuals with acute NV will be diagnosed by history and physical. However, laboratory tests and imaging may assist with the diagnosis of long-standing NV. Frequently ordered tests include complete blood count (CBC), serum electrolytes, serum pregnancy testing, urinalysis, thyroid function testing, amylase, lipase, and liver and kidney function tests. Abdominal radiographs, barium contrast radiography, upper GI endoscopy, or contrast radiography are several diagnostic tools ordered to exclude serious organic causes.

Management

Whether hospitalization is necessary to replenish fluids and electrolytes must be decided. When treatment can be accomplished at home, clear liquids are introduced followed by a high-protein, low-fat diet as tolerated. The diet is gradually increased to include bland solid foods. Supportive therapy can be used when dehydration and electrolyte imbalances are not present. Pharmacologic management with antiemetic drugs can be utilized to prevent or minimize NV (**Table 17-6**).

The anticholinergic/antimuscarinic agent scopolamine comes as a transdermal patch; it is used primarily for prophylaxis and treatment of motion sickness.[12,15,19] Antihistamine agents (e.g., meclizine, diphenhydramine) are available over the counter (OTC) and by prescription. These drugs are useful for disorders of labyrinthine origin such as motion sickness, vertigo, and migraine.[12,19] Dopamine antagonists (e.g., phenothiazines, butyrophenones, benzamides) block dopamine receptors in the area postrema and are used for more severe episodes of NV including those caused by motion sickness, vertigo, and migraine.[10,12] Finally, serotonin receptor antagonists (e.g., ondansetron [Zofran], granisetron [Kytril], or dolasetron [Anzemet]) act on both central and peripheral locations with their primary site of action at the CTZ.[12] These drugs are well tolerated and have less likelihood of GI upset and headaches. However, they are expensive, and many insurance plans require prior authorization. Prescription marijuana (dronabinol) has been used as an appetite stimulant and antiemetic, and is most useful for treating nausea from chemotherapy.[10] No drugs are without side effects; they are individualized to the patient's needs. Combination therapy with two or more classes of drugs with different mechanisms of action is also utilized.

Midwives will most frequently encounter this problem in women coming for prenatal care because NV is a common occurrence in early pregnancy. While NV will be a relatively minor

Table 17-6 COMMONLY USED ANTIEMETIC MEDICATIONS[12,18,19]

Action	Medications	Clinical Use	Side Effects
Muscarinic/ cholinergic antagonists	Scopolamine (TransdermScop)	Motion sickness	Drowsiness Sedation Dry mouth/eyes
Histamine agonists	Meclizine (Antivert) Dimenhydrinate (Dramamine) Diphenhydramine (Benadryl)	Motion sickness Vertigo	Sedation Dry mouth Hypotension
Dopamine agonists	Phenothiazines Promethazine (Phenergan) Prochlorperazine (Compazine)	Post-operative nausea/ vomiting (NV) Opioid-induced NV Toxins	Sedation Anxiety Mood disturbance
Dopamine agonists	Butyrophenones Droperidol (Inapsine)	Post-operative NV Chemotherapy-induced NV	Sedation Hypotension Tachycardia
Dopamine agonists	Benzamides Metaclopramine hydrochloride (Reglan)	Opioid induced Effective for gastric stasis First-line therapy	Extra-pyramidal symptoms
Serotonin antagonists	Ondansetron (Zofran) Granisetron (Kytril)	Chemotherapy or post- operative NV Hyperemesis	Constipation Headache

and short-lived reaction for most women, others will experience significant distress and can benefit from more aggressive management. The American College of Obstetricians and Gynecologists (ACOG) recommends a stepped approach to this problem, beginning with simpler regimens and adding on medications if the woman does not see improvement. Once other possible causes of NV have been ruled out, ACOG[22] recommends to:

1. Start with Vitamin B_6 10 to 25 mg three to four times daily.

2. Add on Doxylamine 12.5 mg three or four times daily if monotherapy with Vitamin B_6 does not provide relief. Doxylamine is available as the OTC sleep aid, Unisom. Each Unisom tablet contains 25 mg; breaking the scored tablet in half will provide the recommended dosage.

3. Add other antiemetic medications, in particular Promethazine 12.5 to 25 mg every four hours or Dimenhydrinate 50 to 100 mg every four to six hours.

If these measures do not provide relief, a woman may require another prespective anti-emetic medication, intravenous hydration, or even parental nutritional therapy if symptoms are severe and persistent.[22]

Nonpharmacologic therapy is also considered as an adjunct treatment for NV. Acupuncture, acupressure, and ginger have been utilized with perioperative vomiting, NVP, postoperative nausea, motion sickness, and chemotherapy-induced vomiting.[23,24] Ginger can be used as grated fresh ginger steeped in tea, or eaten as candied ginger. Hypnosis has also been proposed for prevention of anticipatory chemotherapy-induced NV.[20]

Diarrhea

Diarrhea is defined as passage of frequent or unformed stools. It is characterized by an increase in water content, volume or frequency of stools, and a decrease in consistency of stools. Diarrhea can be attributed to a number of causes including infectious agents such as bacteria, viruses, parasites; bacterial and chemical toxins; diet; medications; and functional causes.[5] Acute episodes of diarrhea last less than 14 days, while persistent and chronic diarrhea continues for longer than 14 days.

Most cases of acute diarrhea are attributed to viral infections, with viral gastroenteritis as the most common cause. Other GI and systemic symptoms may occur concurrently including nausea, vomiting, abdominal pain, fever, anorexia, or myalgias.[25] This disease can range from a mild, self-limited 24-hour syndrome to a more fulminate illness requiring hospitalization.

In the United States, over 200 million episodes of acute diarrhea occur each year (1.4 episodes/person/year). These episodes result in more than 900,000 hospitalizations and 6000 deaths annually.[26]

Details learned from the clinical history help to establish the cause of the illness, especially specifics about recent travel, living situation, occupation, and sexual preference. Indications for medical evaluation include: profuse watery diarrhea; dysentery (passage of many stools containing blood and mucus); fever greater than 101.3°F; passage of greater than six unformed stools in 24 hours; diarrhea with severe abdominal pain in adults $\geq$50 years; and diarrhea in the elderly or the immunocompromised.[27]

Diarrhea is considered mild when there is no change in activities of daily living. Moderate diarrhea results in forced changes of activities, and severe diarrhea can result in confinement to bed.[27] Assessment of the severity of the illness, examination of the stool, presence of fever, vomiting, and dysentery all help determine the course of treatment. Dehydration is common with diarrhea and should be promptly treated.

Diagnosis

The patient history includes stool character; timing of bowel movements; symptom duration; pain; fever; weight loss; medications; medical history; travel history; and relationship of diarrhea to food consumption.[10] The physical exam focuses on abdominal tenderness and hyperactive bowel sounds as well as assessment of vital signs, orthostatic changes, temperature, weight loss, and skin turgor.

Viral diarrhea is characterized by the destruction of villus mucosa, which decreases the intestinal surface area available for absorption and ion secretion. Norwalk virus and rotavirus are the agents responsible for greater than 50% of these viral infections.[28] Bacterial diarrhea causes inflammation of the colon, resulting in red and white blood cells in the stool. Common etiologies are *Salmonella*, *Shigella*, *Escherichia coli*, *Yersinia*, and *Campylobacter*.[28] Characteristic features of bacterial diarrhea include elevated temperature and multiple stools per day that are bloody and explosive. Normal feces should have few or no red or white blood cells.[28]

Food poisoning occurs when an enterotoxin is ingested from contaminated food or when infectious agents within the stomach produce enterotoxins. Nausea and vomiting may present along with diarrhea. The suggestion of a suspicious food is important, especially if similar symptoms are present in other persons exposed to the same food. Traveler's diarrhea is most commonly found in travelers visiting developing semitropical or tropical countries. Symptoms can include nausea, vomiting, abdominal pain, and increased bowel movements. The most common sources of traveler's diarrhea are contaminated food and water.

Escherichia coli O157:H7, a common cause of diarrhea, is estimated to cause more than 20,000 infections each year, often from ingestion of contaminated beef or water.[28] Symptoms include abdominal pain, bloody stool, and the absence of fever. Protozoan diarrhea, such as *Giardia lamblia*, is characterized by complaints of chronic diarrhea, bloating, and excessive flatulence. The typical stool specimen is noninflammatory and does not contain blood, pus, or eosinophils.[28]

Antibiotic therapy contributes to the development of diarrhea. When normal bowel flora are destroyed by antibiotic use, an overgrowth of *Clostridium difficile* can produce a pseudo-membranous colitis causing infectious diarrhea.[28] Individuals who have Crohn's disease or ulcerative colitis along with those who have acquired immune deficiency syndrome (AIDS) can also present with acute diarrhea; when these complications are present, they warrant referral to a gastroenterologist.

Because most diarrheal illnesses are self-limited or viral and last less than one day, microbiologic investigation (i.e., stool examination for white blood cells, ova and parasites or blood; stool culture) is unnecessary but can be considered if the patient is dehydrated, febrile, or presents with blood or pus in the stool.[5,26] Referral to an ED is indicated when the individual presents with diarrhea-induced dehydration accompanied by an inability to tolerate oral fluid replacement.

Management

The most important intervention in acute diarrhea is repletion of fluids and electrolytes. Boiled starches, cereals with salt, saltine crackers, bananas, yogurt, broths, steamed vegetables, and fruits are ideal foods during acute diarrhea episodes. Avoidance of dairy products is recommended. In cases of mild diarrhea, patients may avoid high fiber foods, fats, alcohol, and caffeine to rest the bowel.

Antimotility agents, such as codeine, diphenoxylate with atropine (Lomotil), and loperamide (Imodium), reduce urgency and frequency of bowel movements. Loperamide is the first-line treatment because of efficacy and safety. Bismuth subsalicylate (Pepto-Bismol) reduces bowel movements, helps to relieve vomiting, and has antibacterial properties that help with prevention of traveler's diarrhea.[28] These agents should be avoided in patients with bloody diarrhea or suspected inflammatory diarrhea to avoid masking more serious conditions.[26]

Antibiotic therapy should be considered for patients with symptoms of acute dysentery and/or traveler's diarrhea. A quinolone antibiotic (e.g., ciprofloxacin [Cipro]) is recommended for three to five days, unless stool culture results dictate otherwise. Metronidazole is effective for *Giardia*, *Clostridium difficile*, colitis, and intestinal amebiasis. Antibiotic treatment should not begin until stool culture results are obtained.[10,28]

Constipation

Constipation is defined as infrequent or difficult evacuation of feces with bowel movements less frequently than every three to four days. When asked to identify symptoms, individuals also include straining or hard stools as part of the definition. An international expert panel developed consensus criteria for defining constipation as symptoms persisting for at least 12 weeks in the preceding year (**Table 17-7**).[29]

It is estimated that constipation affects 4 million people in the United States, with increased numbers occurring in children, women, and those of advancing age; this corresponds to a prevalence of approximately 2% in the general population.[30] Constipation is the most common chronic digestive complaint in the United States, but it rarely leads to hospitalization. It is usually diagnosed by the patient's history and exclusion of other diseases. Constipation, as a symptom, is associated with a number of diseases such as colonic inertia, megacolon, pelvic outlet obstruction, and IBS.[30] A systematic approach in the primary care setting will help to provide symptomatic relief, exclude serious disease, and minimize unnecessary testing. If initial assessment reveals GI tract dysfunction, referral to a gastroenterologist is indicated.

The majority of individuals diagnosed with constipation complain of mild symptoms that are not associated with structural abnormalities, intestinal motility disorders, or systemic disease. Dietary review reveals inadequate consumption of dietary fiber and fluids. Structural abnormalities, such as obstructive lesions, must be excluded. Systemic diseases, such as neurologic gut dysfunctions, endocrine disorders, and electrolyte abnormalities (e.g., hypercalcemia or hypokalemia), may also cause constipation. Finally, medications such as anticholinergics, diuretics, narcotics, and calcium and iron supplements may contribute to the condition. Severe or refractory constipation occurs with slow colonic transit times, disorders of the rectum or pelvic floor, and IBS.[31,32]

Table 17-7 **DEFINITION OF CONSTIPATION**[29]

Within the last 12 months, at least 12 weeks (not necessarily consecutive) of at least two of the following, at least 25% of total defecations:

- Straining
- Lumpy or hard stool
- Feeling of incomplete evacuation
- Feeling of anorectal obstruction
- Manual maneuvers to assist defecation (e.g., digital evacuation) **OR** fewer than three defecations per week

In addition:

- Absence of loose stools
- Insufficient criteria for irritable bowel syndrome

Constipation in women may be associated with alterations in sex hormones during the phases of the menstrual cycle. A small number of women experience constipation as a consequence of hysterectomy, although the exact mechanism (e.g., decreased hormone levels, sphincter relaxation, nerve injury, or psychologic) is unclear.[31–34] A history of physical or sexual abuse can also result in increased GI complaints.[31]

Clinical examination begins with a detailed history that includes symptoms from the individual's own point of view. It is essential to elicit typical bowel habits including timing, frequency, and result. Completion of a symptom diary can assist this process. A comprehensive list of prescription and nonprescription medications is obtained including medication regimens utilized to relieve symptoms. A systematic systems review can assist with excluding metabolic or neurologic diseases for which constipation is a symptom.

The physical examination includes complete abdominal examination, noting the type of bowel sounds and the presence of masses or hernias. The examination of the anus, rectum, and perineum is performed in the left lateral position initially, observing the descent and elevation of the perineum during simulated evacuation and retention.[29] The anal reflex "wink" test can be elicited by light touch. Digital examination evaluates tone of the anal sphincter during squeezing and expulsive forces. Additionally, a rectovaginal exam is included to assess for the presence of a rectocele.

Laboratory studies include a CBC, serum electrolytes, calcium, and thyroid stimulating hormone to exclude other metabolic disorders. Stool guiac testing for occult blood is also in-cluded. Healthy individuals less than 50 years old with mild symptoms and no evidence of other disease processes can be started with a trial of fiber supplements and or laxatives. Structural evaluation of the GI tract is indicated for all adults with new onset of unexpected and prolonged symptoms, with the presence of occult blood, and with individuals who have risk factors for colon cancer.[32] Flexible sigmoidoscopy or colonoscopy allows visualization and the ability to perform tissue biopsy. Barium enema allows visualization but is limited by the inability to gather tissue sampling. Individuals who do not respond to conservative management require further investigation by a gastroenterologist to evaluate the functional assessment of colonic motility and pelvic floor function.

Treatment measures consist of dietary alterations and medications and laxatives. The addition of fiber in the diet and adequate fluid intake are emphasized as the first line in efforts to increase colonic transit time and increase GI motility.[29,32,33] Treatment is started for at least 7 to 10 days beginning with twice-daily doses of an appropriate laxative. Individuals are counseled that response is not immediate and adjustments can occur after the initial treatment. Side effects include increased gaseousness and distention that diminishes after several days.[29,33,34] Pharmacologic treatments include stool softeners, osmotic, and saline laxatives, nonabsorbable carbohydrates, polyethylene glycol solutions, and stimulant agents. **Table 17-8** lists common laxative agents used for constipation.

In summary, because constipation is the most frequent GI complaint in the general population, clinicians must obtain the patient's own perceptions of the actual disturbance in bowel

Table 17-8 COMMONLY USED MEDICATIONS FOR CONSTIPATION[29,32,33]

Type	Generic/Trade Name	Dose	Side Effects and Comments
Fiber	Bran	1 cup/day	Bloating, flatulence
	Psyllium (Metamucil)	1 tsp up to tid	Bloating, flatulence
	Methylcelluose (Citrucel)	1 tsp up to tid	Minimal bloating
	Calcium Polycarbophil (Fibercom)	2–4 tablets qd	Bloating, less gas
Stool surfactant	Docusate Sodium (Colace)	100 mg bid	
	Mineral oil	15–45 mL qd or bid Stool lubricated	May cause pneumonia, if aspirated
Stimulants	Bisacodyl (Ducolax)	10 mg suppositories up to 3 times/wk Rectal burning	Abdominal cramps
	Pericolace	1-2 tabs qd Dehydration	Abdominal cramps
	Senna (Senokot, ExLax)	2 tabs qd to 4 tabs bid	Possible cramping; avoid daily use
Osmotic laxative	Magnesium (Milk of Magnesia, Epsom salt)	15–30 ml PO qd – bid	Abdominal cramps
Enemas	Tap water	500 mL/rectum	Mechanical lavage
	Phosphate enema (Fleet)	1 U/rectum	For acute constipation
	Soap suds enema	Up to 1500 mL/rectum	Impaction
Hyperosmolars	Sorbitol	15–30 mL qd – bid	Cramps, bloating, flatulence
	PEG (Golytely, Miralax)	4 L PO over 2–4 h	Used before colonoscopy
	Magnesium citrate	10 oz	Lemon flavored

function to determine whether true constipation exists. Some women will need to be informed about normal bowel patterns and reassured; others will begin treatment. Medications that cause constipation can be adjusted; a trial of fiber and pharmacologic agents can be instituted. The infrequent metabolic, neurologic, or obstructive diseases for which constipation is a symptom must be excluded prior to treatment; if any of these conditions are suspected, referral is necessary. Finally, referral is also indicated when constipation is refractory to treatment after an adequate trial.

Gastroesophageal Reflux Disease

GERD is defined as tissue damage that results from abnormal chronic excessive backflow of gastric contents into the esophagus leading to symptoms, mucosal inflammation, and injury.[35–37] This is a motility disorder that is primarily characterized by heartburn and regurgitation.

Epidemiology

GERD is one of the most common GI disorders. Heartburn or regurgitation symptoms occur in approximately 20% to 60% of the population in a given year with nearly 1% of all visits to a family physician being for GERD or GERD-related symptoms.[38–42] More than 60 million Americans experience symptoms at least once per month, and more than 15 million Americans experience daily symptoms.[43] Pregnant women have the highest incidence of daily heartburn, and older adults are the most likely to seek treatment.[43,44] Eighteen million adults in the United States use medications for indigestion at least 2 times weekly.[43] Long-term consequences of untreated GERD are the potential for erosive esophagitis, stricture, and ulcer, Barrett's metaplasia, and rarely, the occurrence of esophageal cancer.[39] Barrett's esophagus occurs when chronic acid exposure causes squamous epithelial cells to be replaced by metaplastic columnar epithelium, a precursor to adenocarcinoma of the esophagus.[37]

Pathophysiology

The pathophysiology of GERD is multifactorial and is believed to involve lower than normal esophageal sphincter pressures. It is believed that the lower esophageal sphincter fails to close, allowing reflux of acid into the unprotected lining of the esophagus.[39] The disease state is not always from acid overproduction; it occurs from the length of time and frequency of esophageal acid exposure. Normally, the mucus-secreting glands of the normal esophagus are able to neutralize gastric acid and protect the mucosal integrity.[37] Individuals with GERD may exhibit alterations in this protective mechanism. Peristalsis, salivary pH, esophageal epithelium, and the characteristics and quantity of gastric fluids are thought to play a significant role in tissue ulceration.[43] Risk factors that predispose to reflux include esophageal motility disorder, hiatal hernia, and obesity. Additional external factors may include diet, medications, and smoking.

Diagnosis

Because of the potential complications of GERD and the negative effect it has on quality of life, early and accurate diagnosis is essential. Clinical signs and symptoms along with thorough medical history are the most useful diagnostic tools in primary care assessment.

The most common symptoms of GERD include heartburn (retrosternal burning possibly radiating to the neck) and acid regurgitation (the return of gastric contents into the pharynx or esophagus). **Table 17-9** lists the signs and symptoms of GERD.

These symptoms commonly occur after eating, especially after large fatty meals, and are frequently noticed at night. They are exacerbated by recumbency, straining, or bending over and are usually relieved with antacids.[46] When these symptoms occur in a typical pattern, the clinician can establish the diagnosis of GERD and begin treatment empirically without further diagnostic testing. GERD symptoms should be differentiated from those related to cardiac, gastric, infectious, and biliary diseases. **Table 17-10** presents the differential diagnosis for GERD.

Diagnostic testing by endoscopy is usually reserved for those who are refractory to empiric antireflux therapy in the initial two weeks or for those who present with atypical "alarm" symptoms.[37] Endoscopy has the advantage over barium studies of providing direct visualization and availability to obtain biopsy samples.

Management

The goals of treatment are to relieve symptoms and prevent further complications, in addition

Table 17-9 SIGNS AND SYMPTOMS OF GERD[36–38,40,42–45]

Uncomplicated esophageal
Heartburn (pyrosis)
Regurgitation
Water brash
Frequent hiccups
Globus (ball in your throat)
Mild epigastric pain
Dyspepsia
Nausea and/or vomiting

Atypical extra-esophageal symptoms
Chronic throat clearing
Chronic hoarseness and/or sore throat
Chronic cough
Dental erosions
Asthma
Sleep apnea

Alarm symptoms*
Dysphagia (difficulty swallowing)
Weight loss
Atypical noncardiac chest pain
Shortness of breath
Gastrointestinal bleeding

*Refer immediately to a physician.

Table 17-10 DIFFERENTIAL DIAGNOSIS FOR GERD[36,42,47]

Peptic ulcer disease
Nonulcer dyspepsia
Biliary disease
Obstruction
Gastroparesis
Nonsteroidal anti-inflammatory drug gastritis
Malignancy
Complications of reflux including stricture or
    ulceration
Cholelithiasis
Myocardial ischemia, unstable angina
Esophagitis
Esophageal spasm

to healing any esophageal erosions. Primary care clinicians can play an active role by assisting patients in initiating treatment and helping with lifelong management of this chronic disease. Treatment includes the following lifestyle modifications: adjustments in diet (avoiding peppermint, coffee, chocolate, fried or fatty foods); sleep position with elevated shoulders and head; and smoking cessation. These lifestyle adjustments are usually begun prior to and continue concurrently with medication as recommended by the American Gastroenterology Association as first-line treatment.[44]

Pharmacologic management, the primary approach to treatment, can help control GERD symptoms by increasing gastric pH (antacids), decreasing acid production (histamine-2 receptor antagonists [H$_2$RAs]), suppressing acid secretion (proton pump inibitors [PPIs]), or enhancing esophageal clearance, thus promoting gastric emptying (promotility agents). Sucralfate (Carafate) provides a protection layer over the mucosa to reduce direct exposure of tissue to acids.[37,48] **Table 17-11** lists the commonly used medications for GERD.

The American Gastroenterology Association recommends initial self-treatment with antacids and OTC H$_2$RAs. OTC medications can provide rapid relief, reduce the frequency and severity of symptoms, and provide the primary treatment regimen for short-term treatment of GERD.[43] If resolution of symptoms does not occur with OTC medications, further evaluation is necessary for diagnosis. PPIs or higher doses of H$_2$RAs are usually initiated next. A two-week trial of treatment with a PPI is recommended as a cost-effective and quick

Table 17-11 MEDICATIONS USED FOR GERD AND PUD[36–38,45,48]

Antacids/Alginic Acids – Treatment of mild heartburn, reflux

Drug	Mechanism	Comments
Aluminum or magnesium formulations (e.g., Maalox, Mylanta, Rolaids) Bicarbonate	• Increase pH • Neutralize acidic gastric contents	• Frequent dosing needed • Potential medication interactions • Bicarbonate can cause sodium retention—avoid in pregnancy

Histamine H_2 receptor antagonists (H_2RA) – Treatment of duodenal ulcers, uncomplicated GERD, stress ulcers

Drug	Mechanism	Comments
Cimetedine (Tagamet) 400 mg bid for 6–8 wks 400 mg/day maintenance pregnancy category B Ranitidine (Zantac) 150 mg bid for 6–8 wks 150 mg/day maintenance pregnancy category B Famotidine (Pepcid) 20 mg bid for 6–8 wks 20 mg/day maintenance pregnancy category B Nizatidine (Axid) 150 mg bid for 6–8 wks 150 mg/day maintenance pregnancy category B	• Inhibit acid production • Compete with histamine • Bind to H_2 receptors of parietal cells	• Side effects include: diarrhea, headache, drowsiness, fatigue, muscle pain, constipation • Decrease dose in persons with decreased creatinine clearance

Proton pump inhibitors (PPI) – Treatment of gastric and duodenal ulcers and GERD that are not responsive to H_2 antagonists

Drug	Mechanism	Comments
Omeprazole (Prilosec) 20 mg/day for 4 wks 10 mg/day maintenance pregnancy category C	• Suppress gastric acid production • Require acid environment for activation—take dose 30–60 min before meal	• Caution for use in severe hepatic disease and chronic renal failure • Do not take with H_2 antagonists

(continues)

Table 17-11 MEDICATIONS USED FOR GERD AND PUD *(continued)*

Proton pump inhibitors (PPI) – Treatment of gastric and duodenal ulcers and GERD that are not responsive to H2 antagonists

Drug	Mechanism	Comments

Lansoprazole (Prevacid)
    30 mg/day for 4 wks
    15 mg/day maintenance
    pregnancy category B
Rabeprazole (Aciphex)
    20 mg/day
    pregnancy category B
Pantoprazole (Protonix)
    40 mg/day
    pregnancy category B		

Prostaglandin analogs – Prevention of NSAID-induced gastric ulcers

Drug	Mechanism	Comments

Misoprostol (Cytotec)
    200 mcg qid—taken for
    duration of NSAID therapy
    *Pregnancy category X
 	
*Absolute contraindication in pregnancy
	• Acid suppression
	• Increase mucosal blood flow—decreased basal and food stimulated acid secretion
		• Care for use in persons <18 years old and renal failure
		• Side effects: diarrhea, abdominal pain, cramping, exacerbation of inflammatory bowel disease

Sulfated polysaccharides – Short-term and maintenance treatment of duodenal ulcers

Drug	Mechanism	Comments

Sucralfate (Carafate)
    1 g qid for 6-8 wks
    1 g bid maintenance
    pregnancy category B
	• Viscous gel that adheres to epithelial cells and erosions
	• Increase mucosal resistance	

Prokinetics – Improve acid clearance from the esophagus

Drug	Mechanism	Comments

Metoclopramid (Reglan)
    5–10 mg 30 min before
    meals and qhs
    pregnancy category B
Cisapride (Propulsid) (withdrawn in 2002 because of fatal cardiac arrythmias)
	• Strengthen the LES
	• Improve muscle action and emptying of stomach
	• Increase GI motility
		• CNS side effects—drowsiness, irritability, extra pyramidal effects

Abbreviation: LES, lower esophageal sphincter.

method for diagnosing uncomplicated GERD.[49] In instances with the presence of "alarm" symptoms, referral to a gastroenterologist for further evaluation and endoscopy is indicated.

Once referral is initiated, additional testing and/or surgery may be indicated. Endoscopy, barium esophagram, Bernstein testing, and ambulatory 24-hour pH monitoring are additional tools to aid in completing the diagnosis.[50] Endoscopy is the gold standard because it provides direct visualization. The Bernstein test alternates an infusion of saline with hydrochloric acid. GERD is diagnosed by the rapid amelioration of symptoms once the acid is withdrawn.[43] The 24-hour intraesophageal pH-monitoring test identifies excessive reflux with or without symptoms as well as the duration and pattern of the reflux.[42] Anti-reflux surgery is an option for a carefully selected population.[50] Once surgery is complete, long-term GERD therapy with PPIs will continue.[37]

Once acid-suppressing medications have been initiated, follow-up occurs at two weeks and at six to eight weeks. Evaluation consists of the patient's subjective response regarding symptom abatement. Therapy continues for eight weeks if symptoms are controlled, and then a downward titration of medication dosage begins.[37] Because of the chronic nature of this disease, long-term treatment is often necessary to prevent symptoms and relapsing illness.[43] Both continuous and intermittent symptom-directed treatments offer good control for chronic GERD symptoms.

Pregnancy Considerations

Heartburn, one of the major symptoms of GERD, affects 30% to 50% of all pregnant women, and up to 80% in some populations.[51] The occurrence of heartburn increases as gestation progresses. A relaxed esophageal sphincter from increases in estrogen and progesterone has a role in the pathophysiology, along with the mechanical effects of the gravid uterus increasing intraabdominal pressure.[48,51] Clinical history is usually sufficient to make the diagnosis of reflux. Additional testing is needed if GERD symptoms are complicated by suspicion of stricture or ulcer.[37] Antacids are considered safe and, along with lifestyle changes, should be first-line treatment. Antacids containing bicarbonate should be avoided in pregnancy due to electrolyte alterations. If additional treatment is needed to control symptoms, H_2RAs and PPIs can safely be utilized. Table 17-11 contains pregnancy safety categories of common medications used for GERD. The major goal of treatment is to relieve symptoms, which will alter quality of life.

Gallbladder Disease

Gallstones are the most common reason for admission to hospitals for abdominal pain in developed countries.[49] While most gallstones do not cause severe symptoms, complications of gallbladder disease include cholecystitis and pancreatitis. Gallstones can obstruct the billiary duct and the gallbladder, and its capsule can become inflamed. When symptoms become severe, surgical intervention is required. Laparoscopic surgery is most common. Ductal stones can be treated with endoscopic retrograde pancreatography and sphincterotomy with extraction of stones. Oral dissolution and lithotripsy are reserve treatments for those at high-risk for other medically related conditions or those who fail surgical options.

Incidence of Gallbladder Disease

More than 20 million persons have gallbladder disease in the United States.[52] The multicenter Italian study of cholelithiasis examined nearly 33,000 subjects aged 30 to 69 in 18 cohorts in 10 regions throughout Italy.[53] The overall rate of gallstone disease was 18.8% in women and 9.5% in men. Gallstones are reportedly seen most frequently between ages 60 and 74[52]; others quote 40 to 69 as being the critical cutoff for higher incidences of gallstone-related surgeries.[54]

Risk Factors

The incidence of cholelithiasis is greater in women than men and increases with age. Risk factors include obesity, genetic predisposition, rapid weight loss, sedentary lifestyle, diet rich in animal and refined sugars, diabetes, and use of oral contraceptives and other drug therapies.

Gallstones are most prevalent among Native Americans, especially the Pima Indians, and Hispanic Americans when compared to other groups.[52] Pregnancy can also increase the risk of gallstone formation[55]; sludge within the gallbladder is commonly seen on ultrasound in pregnant women.[56] Elevated progesterone levels in pregnancy also contribute to biliary stasis and slower emptying times.

Estrogen and progesterone alter the biliary system among those using oral contraceptives and other hormonal replacement therapies. Most studies show that estrogen is associated with higher rates of gallstones.[57,58] Women under the age of 40 and those taking high-dose estrogens (i.e., 50 mcg) have been noted to have the greatest risk.[59] There is a minor increase in the rate of gallstone formation after initiating oral contraceptives.[60]

Obese and morbidly obese patients who have undergone gastric bypass surgery have a high incidence of developing gallstones.[61,62] Another factor is rapid weight loss, secondary to what is believed to be fluctuations in gallbladder bile mucin increase. Ursodeoxycholic acid may be recommended in patients going through rapid weight loss to decrease this effect.[63]

Other related risk factors for gallstones include diabetes mellitus, serum hypertriglycerides, cirrhosis, gallbladder stasis, and selected drugs, such as ceftriaxone. Physical activity is an effective preventive measure.[64] Moderate coffee usage is associated with a reduced risk of gallstones in a large cohort study of women.[65] Risk factors associated with gallbladder disease are listed in **Table 17-12**.

Pathophysiology and Gallstone Formation

The gallbladder is a pear-shaped organ lying beneath the liver on the right side of the abdomen.

Table 17-12 RISK FACTORS ASSOCIATED WITH GALLBLADDER DISEASE IN WOMEN[50,52,55–58,61,62]

- Female gender
- Advancing age
- Estrogen
  - Pregnancy
  - Postpartum
  - Exogenous estrogen
- Rapid weight loss
- Hypertriglyceridemia
- Obesity
- Native Americans
- Genetic predisposition
- Diabetes mellitus

It functions as a storage reservoir for bile produced by the liver to aid in digestion. There is a high concentration of bile salts, pigments, and cholesterol within the bile storage pool. When foods high in fat content are eaten, the gallbladder contracts and bile salts are ejected into the intestine. These bile salts and bile acid aid in the absorption of lipids and help to eliminate them.

Gallstones are composed of a mixture of cholesterol, calcium bilirubinate, proteins, and mucin. They can be classified by presence or absence of cholesterol in origin and either black-pigmented or brown-pigmented in color. Most stones are thought to have a mixed composition. In industrialized countries, cholesterol-based stones account for the majority of gallstones.

Black-pigmented stones are formed in the gallbladder and result from hemolysis. They are associated with sickle cell disease and liver cirrhosis. Brown-pigmented stones are associated with bacterial or parasitic infections of the biliary tract and are more commonly seen in Asians.[56] Brown stones usually form in the intrahepatic bile duct.[65] In very severe cases of cholecystitis, there is accompanying inflammation of the gallbladder along with occlusion of the cystic duct. *Choledocholithiasis* is defined as stones obstructing the common duct; *cholangitis* is an infectious complication related to bile obstruction.

Acute cholangitis occurs when an obstructed common bile duct becomes contaminated with bacteria. Treatment is with broad-spectrum antibiotics along with the use of other techniques such as endoscopy decompression of the biliary tract. Delay in treatment can result in liver abscesses or septicemia. Gallbladder stasis contributes to gallstone formation because it allows sludge (muddy sediment, which is a precursor to stones) and crystals to build up in the gallbladder longer than necessary and adds to delay in normal emptying times. Sludge can be detected by ultrasound and is composed of cholesterol and calcium bilirubinate in a thick mucin gel. Although sludge can lead to gallstones, it can also disappear spontaneously. Sludge is primarily seen in pregnancy.

Symptoms

Gallstone disease can be symptomatic. However, it should be noted that 70% of stones in the gallbladder do not cause symptoms.[67] Gallstone disease can be evidenced as colicky, stabbing, spasmodic pain in the epigastric area or specifically in the right upper quadrant (RUQ) of the abdomen, often radiating to the right scapular area, and lasting from two to four hours per episode. This colicky pain is caused primarily from the impaction of gallstones in the cystic duct leading to gallbladder distention.

NV may or may not be seen; the emesis may be bile stained. Diaphoresis and low-grade fever may be noted. The gallbladder is rarely palpable. Patients may have localized tenderness or guarding in the RUQ area, often following a fatty or heavy meal. Murphy sign may be noted, that is, tenderness on deep palpation under the right costal margin upon inspiration, bringing the inflamed gallbladder into contact with the examiner's hand. Murphy sign is usually seen in conjunction with acute cholecystitis. Anorexia, dyspepsia, and tachycardia may be noted.

Leukocytosis with left shift and fever can be noted with acute cholecystitis. Laboratory testing includes assessing the white blood count and liver function tests for elevation in enzymes that can signal potential biliary obstruction and liver disease. Elevations of serum bilirubin and alkaline phosphatase, in particular, can signal potential gallbladder disease and are often noted during biliary obstruction.[56] High elevations can be seen with a common duct stone. Serum amylase and lipase may be ordered additionally if pancreatitis is suspected. Pancreatitis develops in 5% of all patients with gallstones. Small stones can obstruct the pancreatic duct or allow reflux of bile into the duct.

Differential Diagnosis

The differential diagnosis of common causes of severe acute epigastric pain include: biliary colic, PUD, worsening esophagitis and GERD, esophageal spasm, acute pancreatitis-related gallstone disease, myocardial infarction, and pneumonia (**Table 7-13**).

Imaging

Ultrasound is the imaging method of choice for diagnosing gallstones. It detects gallstones with a specificity and sensitivity of more than 95% but is less helpful for biliary sludge. Ultrasound is also less sensitive for bile duct stones because the lower bile duct is inaccessible due to surrounding structures and bowel gas.[56] Confirmation of gallbladder disease on ultrasound includes gallbladder wall thickening or edema and a sonographic Murphy sign, where a positive Murphy sign is seen during palpation with

Table 17-13 COMMON CAUSES OF SEVERE ACUTE EPIGASTRIC PAIN

- Acute pancreatitis
- Myocardial infarction
- Peptic ulcer disease/severe GERD
- Esophagitis/esophageal spasm
- Biliary colic
- Pneumonia

Source: Reprinted with permission.[49]

the ultrasound transducer. In one study that compared ultrasound with direct percutaneous miniendoscopy, endoscopy did show better evidence for smaller stones of 1 to 3 mm.[69]

If the diagnosis is unclear, a *cholescintigraphy*, a nuclear medicine scan, can also be performed; it has a sensitivity and specificity of approximately 95%.[69] Magnetic resonance cholangiography is another noninvasive technique for evaluating the bile ducts. It has been found to be superior to ultrasound for detecting stones in the cystic duct but less sensitive to diagnosing thickening of the gallbladder wall.[70]

Endoscopic retrograde cholangiopancreatography (ERCP) involves injecting contrast dye directly into the biliary tree. Its primary use in gallstone- or gallbladder-related disease is in diagnosing choledocholithiasis (common duct stones) and cholangitis.[71] Since ultrasound is not sensitive enough for detecting and identifying common duct stones, ERCP is more helpful in making this diagnosis. ERCP was developed in the 1970s, and its sensitivity and specificity for stone disease exceed 90%.[56] With ERCP, the pancreatic duct is gently filled with contrast material under fluoroscopy. Visualization of the common bile duct is seen as well as the whole biliary tract, including the gallbladder. With ERCP, *sphincterotomy*, the actual removal of stones and the placement of stents, can be performed. The goal is to eliminate the barrier preventing passage of the stones and assist with stone extraction.

Small stones may pass spontaneously or can be pulled into the duodenum with a balloon catheter or basket. Larger stones may need to be broken up and fragmented. There have been a number of studies documenting the successful use of ERCP in pregnancy.[72–75] Magnetic resonance cholangiopancreatography (MRCP) is a newer diagnostic technique that uses magnetic resonance imaging and is an alternative to ERCP, but is more costly to operate and is currently limited to large medical centers.[76]

Endoscopy ultrasound is a technique in which an ultrasound transducer is attached to the tip of an endoscope, similar to routine endoscopy. Detection for bile duct stones is about 95%. This also affords fewer complications (i.e., slight pancreatitis) than ERCP.

Treatment Options

Initial therapies include intravenous fluids, antiemetics, surgical consultation, pain relief, and possibly broad spectrum antibiotics. Laparoscopic cholecystectomy has rapidly replaced open cholecystectomy for surgical treatment because it allows for a shorter hospitalization and length of stay. Laparoscopic cholecystectomy has a 5% rate of conversion to open cholecystectomy.[56] Common bile duct injuries are more frequent with laparoscopy than with open cholecystectomy. Acute cholecystitis and previous gastroduodenal surgery are no longer contraindications to laparoscopic procedures but do have a higher conversion rate. **Figure 17-1** describes an approach to the management of uncomplicated gallstones.

The main disadvantage of laparoscopy has been a higher incidence of injury to the common hepatic or bile ducts, approximately 0.2%.[49] The technique requires more skill on the surgeon's part than open laparotomy, and consequently the learning curve for this technique may be responsible for the higher rate of injury.

Nonsurgical treatment options include oral dissolution therapy, contact dissolution, and lithotripsy for shattering the stones with shock waves (**Table 17-14**). Less than 10% of

---

Figure 17-1 Approach to uncomplicated gallstones.[56]

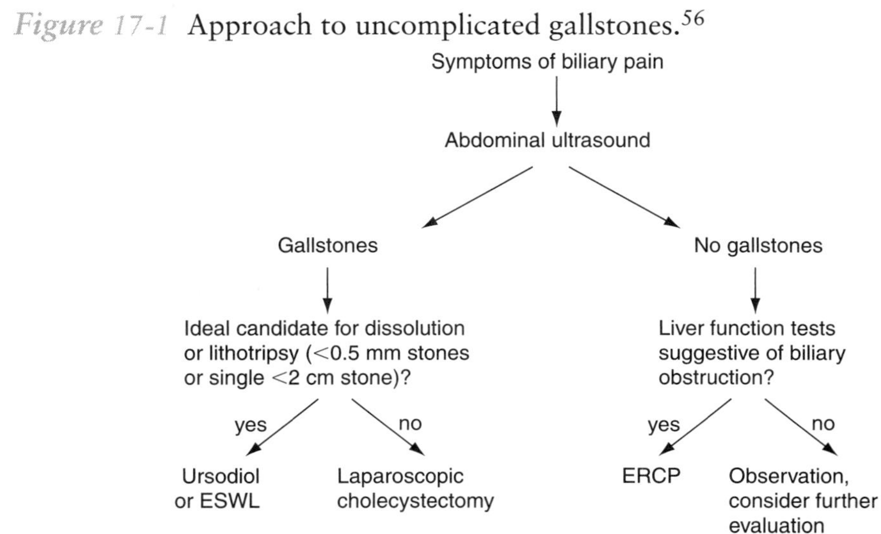

Abbreviations: ESWL, extracorporeal shock-wave lithotripsy; ERCP, endoscopic retrograde cholangiopancreatography.
Source: Reprinted with permission.[56]

gallstones are thought to be suitable for non-surgical treatment, and success rates vary.[49] Stones can also re-form. In general, these treatments should be used only in patients in whom surgery is not an option. Urodeoxycholic acid is a naturally developed bile acid, which dissolves cholesterol gallstones at doses of 8 mg/kg/day. The criteria for identifying appropriate candidates include:

- Stones must be cholesterol in composition.

- No calcification is seen on scan.
- A patent cystic duct must be evident.
- Gallstones should be less than 1 cm diameter.
- There should be no evidence of acute cholecystitis.

The success of oral therapy is dependent on both the bile to dissolve the cholesterol and the ability of the gallbladder to clear the debris of materials from the disintegrating stones. Treatment may be required for two years or more.

Table 17-14 NONOPERATIVE THERAPIES FOR SYMPTOMATIC GALLSTONES

Agent	Advantages	Disadvantages
Oral bile acid dissolution: ursodeoxycholic acid (Actigall), at 8–10 mg/d	Stone clearance 30%–90% with zero percent mortality	50% recurrence of stones; dissolves noncalcified cholesterol stones; optimal for stones <5 mm; symptom relief does not start for 3–5 wks; may take 6–24 months for results
Contact solvents methyl-*tert*-butyl ether/*n*-propyl acetate	Stone clearance 50%–90%	70% recurrence of stones; experimental—insufficient data; duodenitits; hemolysis; nephrotoxicity; mild sedation
Extracorporeal shock-wave lithotripsy electrohydraulic	Stone clearance 70%–90%	70% recurrence; not FDA approved; performed only at centers with electromagnetic expertise; selection criteria require no more than one radiolucent stone (<20 mm in diameter), patent cystic duct, functioning gallbladder in a patient with symptomatic gallstones without complications

Source: Reprinted with permission from Ahmed A, Cheung R, Keefe E. Management of gallstones and their complications. *Am Fam Physician.* 2001;61:1673–1680.

Dose-related diarrhea has been noted in these patients. Some combined therapies may be more beneficial and have fewer side effects.[77] Dissolution rates vary, and the best results occur in patients with small buoyant stones. Incomplete dissolution and stone recurrence are possible complications. Results can be monitored with abdominal ultrasound.

Contact dissolution involves using specific solvents that are available in only a few medical centers. These agents include methyl-tert-butyl ether (MTBE) and n-propyl acetate.[77] The ideal patient selection criteria are the same as for oral methods. A direct needle puncture of the gallbladder is performed, using a transhepatic approach. The success of this method depends on the solubility of the stone in the chosen solvent and adequate mixing within the gallbladder itself. Success is measured by monitoring tube cholecystograms. Oral agents can be used concomitantly. The most experience with dissolution agents has been with MTBE. Major complications relate to toxicity of the agents and procedural techniques.

Lithotripsy is the third nonsurgical method for treatment of gallstones. Lithotripsy uses high-energy shock waves to break up stones so they can pass spontaneously or dissolve with the use of oral agents. Various types of lithotriptors or wave generators are used commercially. This technique is most effective in patients with a single large gallstone or fewer than three stones. Additional criteria for successful lithotripsy include adequate gallbladder functioning, low body mass, mild symptoms and solitary radiolucent stones with diameters of 20 mm or less. Very small stones are difficult to target and treat effectively. Pregnancy is an obvious contraindication to lithotripsy usage.

Fewer than 20% of patients are considered eligible for this type of therapy. The complication rate is less than 5% but can include biliary colic, common bile duct obstruction, or pancreatitis.[56] Stone recurrence rates range from 3% to 12% at one year and are higher with multiple stones. These rates can fluctuate depending on the use of oral agents to reduce the rate of symptom recurrence.[78,79]

Gastritis

Gastritis is defined as an inflammation of the stomach (gastric mucosa) resulting in mucosal injury, cell damage, and regeneration.[80] When viewed endoscopically, abnormal features include erythema, erosions, and subepithelial hemorrhages.[47,80–83] Gastritis is not a single disease, but rather a group of disorders that all cause inflammation, but differ in their clinical features, histology, or causative mechanisms.[84] The classification of gastritis includes acute gastritis from *Helicobacter pylori* (*H. pylori*) or other infectious agents, and chronic atrophic gastritis.[84,85] Infection with *H. pylori,* a Gram negative flagellate, is the major cause of nonautoimmune chronic gastritis.[86] However, not all damage is accompanied by inflammation. In contrast, the term that describes epithelial damage and regeneration without inflammation is referred to as *gastropathy*.[82] This damage is caused mainly by drugs, such as NSAIDs, aspirin, and alcohol.[80]

Epidemiology

Gastritis is more common in men than women and has an overall prevalence of 5% to 10% of the population.[5] The rate of gastritis among persons diagnosed with *H. pylori* is 30% to 40%, but many individuals are asymptomatic, especially in the initial acute phase.[80,86] The exact epidemiology of *H. pylori* and its mode of transmission remain unclear.[80] Diagnosis is made by gastroscopic biopsy. Greater than 90% of the population affected with chronic gastritis have detectable levels of *H. pylori* on biopsy. The remaining 10% originate from causes such as chemical injury from drugs, gastroduodenal reflux, Crohn's disease, or infections with other agents.[85] The prevalence of gastritis increases as the population ages, with more than 50% of the cases occurring in those over 50 years of age.[87] *H. pylori* infection is a major cause of PUD and also increases the risk for gastric adenocarcinoma.[87] A list of differential diagnoses for PUD is in **Table 17-15**.

Etiology

In addition to the presence of *H. pylori*, there are other co-factors for gastritis: spicy and salty foods (in susceptible individuals); alcohol; NSAIDs; stress; infections; bile reflux; pancreatic reflux; and irradiation.[47,83,86] Onset of *H. pylori* infection may result in acute gastritis with an associated transient increase in gastric acid secretion.[84] Progression often leads to the more chronic form.

Table 17-15 DIFFERENTIAL DIAGNOSIS FOR PEPTIC ULCER DISEASE[47,88]

Gastroesophageal reflux disease
Cholelithiasis
Pancreatitis
Gastritis
Nonulcer dyspepsia
Neoplasm
Cardiac (i.e., angina, myocardial infarction, pericarditis, dissecting aneurysm)
Early appendicitis

Gastritis develops with inflammatory changes occurring in the superficial mucosa only. The disease can then progress to atrophic gastritis, where the inflammation extends to the deep portions of the mucosa with distortion and destruction of the glands; frequently, this begins in the antrum of the stomach and then continues into the body and fundus of the stomach. Chronic gastritis initially involves the superficial and glandular areas of the gastric mucosa, progresses to glandular destruction, and may ultimately lead to gland metaplasia and atrophy.[84] Finally, a loss of glandular structures with thinning of the mucosa becomes evident as gastric atrophy ensues. Changes to the morphology of gastric cells can occur as gastritis progresses. This intestinal metaplasia is an important predisposing factor for gastric cancer.[84] The etiology of gastric cancer is multifactorial.

Diagnosis

Patients with gastritis often present with nonspecific clinical symptoms and epigastric pain. Such symptoms include bloating, anorexia, weight loss, and NV, which may be exacerbated by eating.[7] The clinician must be able to differentiate the symptoms of gastritis from several other conditions such as PUD, GERD, nonulcer dyspepsia, gastric adenocarcinoma, pancreatitis, and gastroparesis.[47] Laboratory testing and imaging will help to clarify the diagnosis.

Imaging

Endoscopy with biopsy is the gold standard diagnostic tool for detecting gastritis and *H. pylori*.[47,84] Several biopsy samples are obtained to determine the presence of urease, which is a product of *H. pylori*. Alternately, serum immunoglobulin G antibody testing is an inexpensive and convenient test. It is less accurate than biopsy and is associated with a high false-positive rate because the antibodies remain present following treatment.[47,89] An upper GI series is not sensitive for the detection of *H. pylori*,[81] and stool antigen testing also has only limited value.

The C-urea breath test is a sensitive, noninvasive method of detecting active *H. pylori* gastritis and is useful in the primary care setting. This test detects urease and is more specific than serology testing.[5,89] However, the presence of *H. pylori* does not correlate with disease severity, but only with the presence or absence of the disease.[90] The C-urea breath test is most useful when there is not an additional indication for an endoscopic exam. It is most accurate at diagnosing the eradication of the disease once treatment is complete.[90,91]

Laboratory testing includes a CBC and vitamin B_{12} level for those who have chronic gastritis and those with active bleeding. Stool cultures also help to identify bleeding by the presence of melena (tarry stools).

Treatment

The primary treatment objective is to decrease pain, initiate healing, and avoid recurrences. Initially, nonpharmacologic treatments such as avoiding foods that worsen symptoms are recommended. Alcohol, tobacco, aspirin, and NSAIDs, which irritate the mucosa, should be avoided.[47] When medication is instituted, treatment for 10 to 14 days is indicated. A list of commonly used medications is in **Table 17-16**. Because of increasing resistance to antibiotics among these patients, newer formulations of drugs that target the stomach more specifically are being investigated.[92]

With new onset dyspepsia for those under 50 years of age, *H. pylori* screening is performed by serology antibody IgG. If positive, the clinician should begin eradication therapy to decrease the chance of active ulcer disease. Oral clarithromycin is used in combination with amoxicillin and lansoprazole or omeprazole (triple therapy) for the treatment of *H. pylori* infection and duodenal ulcer disease. Clarithromycin also is used orally in combination with omeprazole (dual therapy) or ranitidine bismuth citrate in patients with an active duodenal ulcer. Other multiple-drug regimens including clarithromycin (with or without amoxicillin, lansoproprazole, omeprazole, or ranitidine bismuth citrate) are used for the treatment of *H. pylori* infection associated with PUD.[95] If the patient presents with serious symptoms or is older than 50 years, then referral for further evaluation with endoscopy is indicated.

Pancreatitis

The pancreas is an elongated organ that lies in the back of the mid-abdomen. Its functions include production of digestive juices and certain hormones, including insulin responsible for regulating blood glucose. The pancreas is 20% endocine (secretes to systemic circulation) and 80% exocrine (secretes outwardly through excretory ducts).[96] The islets of Langerhans produce insulin, glucagons, and somatostatin, all of which are involved in food production. The acinar cells compose the exocrine portion of the pancreas that secretes pancreatic juices. These include bicarbonate and digestive enzymes that flow into the duodenum from the main pancreatic duct. The pancreas sits outside the posterior curve of the stomach, behind the duodenum and the spleen. It has three entities: the head, body, and tail. The point where it joins the common bile duct is the ampulla of Vater, which empties into the duodenum.

Table 17-16 SUGGESTED TREATMENTS FOR *HELICOBACTER PYLORI*[45,47,88,92–94]

Pharmacology	Dose	Regimen	Pharmacology	Dose	Regimen
Bismuth subsalicylate +	525 mg qid	14 days	Bismuth subsalicylate +	525 mg qid	14 days
Metronidazole +	250 mg qid	14 days	Metronidazole +	500 mg tid	14 days
Tetracycline +	500 mg qid	14 days	Tetracycline +	500 mg qid	14 days
H$_2$RA	bid	28 days	PPI (omeprazole 20 mg bid or lansoprazole 30 mg bid)	bid	14 days
PPI (Omeprazole 20 mg bid or Lansoprazole 30 mg bid) +		14 days	PPI (Omeprazole 20 mg bid or Lansoprazole 30 mg bid +)		14 days
Clarithromycin +	500 mg bid	14 days	Clarithromycin +	500 mg bid	14 days
Amoxicillin	1000 mg bid	14 days	Metronidazole	500 mg bid	14 days
Ranitidine bismuth citrate +	400 mg bid	14 days			
Clarithromycin +	500 mg bid	14 days			
Amoxicillin or	1000 mg bid	14 days			
Metronidazole or	500 mg bid				
Tetracycline	500 mg bid				

Acute pancreatitis is defined as inflammation of the pancreas and is associated with sudden onset of severe abdominal pain. Most problems related to acute pancreatitis do not lead to complications. However, some patients may progress to a more serious episode warranting intensive medical care. It is critical to uncover the underlying cause of pancreatitis because it affects which specific treatment will be implemented. *Chronic pancreatitis* is the result of repeated episodes of acute pancreatitis, often due to chronic alcoholism. The reported incidence of acute pancreatitis in the United States is as high as 79.8 per 100,000.[97]

Causes of Acute Pancreatitis

GALLSTONE PANCREATITIS

Because the gallbladder and pancreas share a common drainage duct, gallstones blocking this duct will backup pancreatic enzymes. Possible explanations include reflux of bile into the pancreatic duct secondary to obstruction of the ampulla during passage of gallstones, or obstruction at the ampulla due to stones or edema. Only about 3% to 7% of patients with gallstones will develop pancreatitis. Gallstones occur more frequently in women and, therefore, more women develop this disorder.[98] In developed countries, gallstone pancreatitis is the most common variety[99,100] accounting for 45% of the cases.[96] Pancreatic and periampullary tumors are also responsible for obstructive causes.

ALCOHOL-RELATED PANCREATITIS

More commonly seen in men, this occurs in individuals with long-standing alcohol-related issues and accounts for approximately 35% of all cases. Recurrent attacks suggest an alcoholic origin. The diagnosis can often only be made after definite signs of chronic pancreatitis appear. In a study of 1,068 cases of acute pancreatitis in pooled data from five European countries, the majority of the 288 who had recurrent pancreatitis were men.[101] Alcohol was the most frequent factor in 57% of those studied.

DRUG-RELATED PANCREATITIS

Many medications can induce pancreatitis.[96] These drugs include: HIV therapy such as didanosine; antimicrobial drugs such as sulfonamides and tetracycline; diuretics; drugs used in treating IBD; immunosuppressive agents; neuropsychiatric agents such as valproic acid; and anti-inflammatory drugs. Others like estrogen and tamoxifen may act by inducing hypertriglyceridemia. Toxins from certain spiders, scorpions, the Gila monster lizard, and certain insects can also be culprits.[102,103]

HEREDITARY CONDITIONS

Serum triglyceride levels above 1000 mg/dL can initiate attacks of acute pancreatitis, but the eti-

ology of this action is unclear.[104] Hypertriglyceridemia accounts for a small number of acute pancreatitis cases. The genetic basis for hereditary pancreatitis now includes mutations in at least one allele of the cystic fibrosis transmembrane conductance regulator.[105,106] Genetic testing may be helpful in the future to identify and manage other patients with hereditary causes of pancreatitis.

Other causes of hypertriglyceridemia include alcohol, obesity, diabetes mellitus, hypothyroidism, pregnancy, estrogen or tamoxifen therapy, nephrotic syndrome, and beta blockers.[107]

POST-ENDOSCOPIC RETROGRADE CHOLANGIOPANCREATOGRAPHY PANCREATITIS

ERCP is an endoscopic procedure used to diagnose and/or remove gallstones blocking the main duct. ERCP-induced pancreatitis is often mild. Post-ERCP patients often may have elevated amylase levels with possible complaints of upper abdominal pain, nausea, and/or vomiting following the procedure (**Table 17-17**).[108]

INFECTIONS

Cases of pancreatitis have also been associated with the following organisms: viruses including mumps, Coxsackie virus, varicella zoster, viral hepatitis, and mononucleosis; bacterial infections including *Mycoplasma* and *Legionella*; fungal infections such as *Aspergillus*; and parasitic infections such as *Toxoplasma gondii*, *Cryptosporidium*, and *Ascaris*.[97]

HYPERCALCEMIA

Hypercalcemia can lead to pancreatitis. This is thought to be due to calcium deposits within the pancreatic duct and the activation of trypsinogen. Hyperparathyroidism is also

Table 17-17 PRIMARY CAUSES OF ACUTE PANCREATITIS[96,98,101,102,104,106,107]

- Gallstones
- Alcohol-induced
- Drug-related
- Hereditary conditions
- Post ERCP-induced
- Infections (viral, mumps, mononucleosis)
- Hyperlipidemia
- Hypercalcemia
- Pregnancy
- Idiopathic
- Trauma
- Venom (spider, scorpion, reptile bites)
- Hypertriglyceridemia

Abbreviation: ERCP, endoscopic retrograde cholangiopancreatography

believed to be associated with pancreatitis; however, the incidence is low.

PREGNANCY

The most common cause of pancreatitis during pregnancy is gallstones. However, hyperlipidemia still needs to be considered. Pregnancy causes metabolic and hormonal changes that add to the risk of developing gallstones. For certain women with a genetic predisposition to hypertriglyceridemia, this level will most likely become elevated during pregnancy.

IDIOPATHIC

No obvious cause is responsible for approximately 10% of all cases of pancreatitis.[96] Additional testing may be necessary including an abdominal computed tomography (CT) scan. As mentioned earlier, other causes can include trauma and pancreatitis related to venoms from scorpions and spider bites. Two uncommon causes include pancreatic tumors and penetrating PUD.

Symptoms

Patients often present following ingestion of a fatty meal or following an episode of drinking. The primary symptoms are dull epigastric pain radiating to the back that often is associated with NV. Epigastric tenderness or pain is constant for most. Others will complain of sudden, constant pain in the upper part of the abdomen. The pain may wrap around the trunk and involve the left flank. Rebound is generally absent, but guarding may be seen. Some people will have limited abdominal tenderness. In those with gallstone-related pancreatitis, gallbladder and RUQ pain may occur initially. This pain can extend to the right flank and shoulder. In severe cases, shock or coma may present. If alcohol is the main cause, patients may present as malnourished, and may complain of *steatorrhea* (offensive, foul-smelling stools that are pale in color). For these patients, symptoms can worsen when eating, lying down, or drinking alcohol.

DIAGNOSTIC TESTING

Systemic signs of acute pancreatitis include hyperglycemia, hypocalcemia, elevated white count, and an elevated serum amylase ($>$200) during the first 24 to 72 hours. In more severe cases, patients can present with a distended and tender abdomen, hypotension, tachypnea, tachycardia, fever, and jaundice.[109] **Figure 17-2** illustrates the rates of systemic signs of acute pancreatitis.

During cases of acute pancreatitis, enzymes that usually flow from the pancreas into the digestive tract can be detected in the bloodstream. Two commonly used enzyme tests for pancreatitis are amylase and lipase.

Increases in serum amylase levels suggest acute pancreatitis. This is one of the first values to rise

Figure 17-2 Systemic signs of acute pancreatitis.

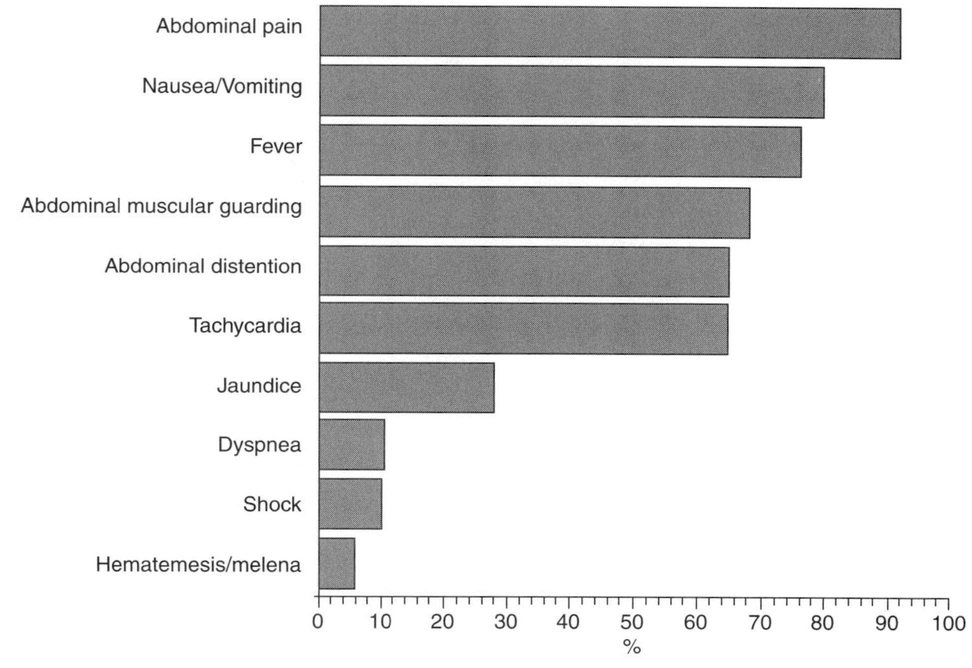

Source: Reprinted with permission.[109]

and is the most commonly used diagnostic test when evaluating acute pancreatitis. It appears within 2 to 12 hours of onset, peaks within 24 hours, and often returns to normal within 72 hours. Amylase can rise with other disorders such as cholecystitis, bowel obstruction, and ectopic pregnancy. However, during episodes of acute pancreatitis, serum amylase often rises threefold. Normal amylase levels are 25 to 125 U/L. Amylase levels do not correlate with disease severity. Very high amylase levels are usually seen when gallstones are the underlying cause.

Elevated levels of serum lipase confirm the pancreatic origin of elevated serum amylase lev-els. Lipase levels begin to rise within four to eight hours of an acute episode, peak at 24 hours, and return to normal after 8 to 14 days. The sensitivity of serum lipase ranges from 85% to 100%, and it has close to 100% specificity. Normal serum lipase levels are 20 to 180 IU/L. Serum lipase is helpful in those patients who present late with acute pancreatitis and is more sensitive than amylase in alcohol-induced pancreatitis. Elevated amylase and lipase levels can also be found in other diseases. Combining enzyme tests does not improve diagnostic accuracy; daily measurement of enzymes has no utility.[110] A CBC, serum glucose, calcium, blood urea nitrogen (BUN), creatinine, bilirubin, and alkaline phosphatase levels should be drawn as part of the evaluation. Transaminase levels and triglycerides will need to be obtained in selected cases.

Imaging

Abdominal films can show the scattered calcifications that are seen in chronic pancreatitis. However, ultrasound, CT, and ERCP are also useful in evaluation and management.[111] They provide different types of information to the clinician.

ERCP is still the gold standard for diagnosis and staging of pancreatitis because sensitivity for ERCP is approximately 75% to 95% and specificity is 90% or more. It is invasive and does carry some morbidity and mortality (0.1%–1.0%).[112] The main role of ERCP in pancreatitis is to identify or confirm common duct stones and provide access for sphincterotomy, stone removal, or stent placement.

MRCP is providing a useful alternative to ERCP. With MRCP, the pancreatic ducts and fluid collections can be visualized. However, quality, sensitivity, and specificity of MRCP vary across centers and with the skill of the operator.[113] For chronic pancreatitis, MRCP is now being considered the primary imaging technique.[113]

Ultrasound and CT are capable of depicting ductal and other pancreatic changes and eliminating disorders in the differential diagnosis (such as gallstones). With helical or other CT scanners and the use of contrast, the pancreas can be visualized in detail. In 1985, Balthazar et al.[114] classified the scope and severity of pancreatic inflammation seen on CT into five categories that correlate with clinical course. According to Balthazar, patients with a low severity index have very little morbidity; those with a severity index of 7 to 10 have a higher morbidity rate.[114]

Treatment

Treatment options follow the primary etiology for pancreatic disease. Treatment of gallstone pancreatitis would include treating nausea and vomiting, correcting fluid and electrolyte imbalance, and treating any local complications. Complete bowel rest (to decrease pancreatic secretions and intrapancreatic pressure), use of narcotics for pain relief, antiemetics, H_2RAs, PPIs, intravenous nutrition, and supportive care are all treatment options. About 30% of patients with severe acute pancreatitis will develop an infection in the pancreatic tissues. Antibiotics can be useful to reduce the infection rate in those patients with severe necrotizing pancreatitis.

Fentanyl or toradol are often the drugs of choice for pain control. Morphine is used less frequently for pain because it is thought to increase pressure in the sphincter of Oddi. Repeated doses of meperidine can be problematic because accumulation of the metabolite normeperidine may cause neuromuscular irritation and potential seizures.

Scoring Systems

Most acute attacks of pancreatitis are mild, with recovery occurring in five to seven days. In patients with either chronic episodes or severe necrotizing pancreatitis, the morbidity and mortality increase. Within 48 hours of an admission for pancreatitis, the severity of the disease should be rated using a multifactor scoring system to improve the accuracy of diagnosis and to predict disease severity.

The Apache II score is believed to be the most accurate predictor of disease severity and can be updated continuously.[115] Apache II appears to be as accurate at 24 hours as other scoring systems are at 48 hours. Other providers use Ranson's criteria at both the time of admission and at 48 hours.[116] During the initial 48 hours, the criteria include: a drop in hematocrit; a rise in BUN; arterial PO_2; base deficit; serum calcium levels; and estimated fluid sequestration. If three or fewer of these signs are present, the mortality rate approaches 1% and indicates the patient is less seriously ill. If four or more signs are present, the mortality rate can reach 25%, and about 50% of the patients are seriously ill (**Table 17-18**).

Peptic Ulcer

PUD comprises ulcerations occurring in the stomach (gastric ulcers) and those occurring in the duodenum (peptic ulcers). Essentially, ulcers are the result of an imbalance between mucosal protective factors and various mucosal damaging mechanisms. *Ulcers* are circumscribed mucosal damage extending through the muscularis submucosa; they are distinct from gastritis erosions that are superficial and confined to the mucosa. Any portion of the GI tract exposed to aggressive action by acid or pepsin may be involved.

Epidemiology

The yearly incidence of PUD is estimated at 15 to 30 cases per 1000 individuals.[88] An estimated 250,000 to 500,000 individuals are diagnosed yearly with 75% of ulcers considered duodenal ulcers and 25% considered gastric ulcers.[87,117] There is a 10% lifetime risk of PUD in the United States.[88] The incidence of gastric ulcers is continuing to rise with the widespread use of

Table 17-18 RANSON'S CRITERIA FOR PREDICTING PANCREATIC DISEASE SEVERITY[116]

At admission
  Age >55 years
  White count >16,000/mm^3
  Blood glucose >200 mg/dL (>11 mmol/L)
  Serum LDH >350 IU/L
  AST (SGOT) >250/L

After 48 hours
  Hematocrit drop >10 percentage points
  BUN rise >5 mg/dL (>1.8 mmol/L)
  Arterial PO_2 >60 mm Hg
  Base deficit >4 mEq/L
  Serum calcium >8 mg/dL (>2 mmol/L)
  Estimated fluid sequestration >6 L

If 3 or fewer of these signs are present, the mortality rate approaches 1%, and few patients are seriously ill. If 4 or more signs are present, the mortality rate can reach 25%, and about 50% of patients are seriously ill.

both OTC NSAIDs and smoking.[88] At one time, gastric ulcers were more prevalent in men, but the gender gap has almost disappeared.[88] The economic burden accounts for an estimated $5.65 billion each year from direct patient care and indirect loss of productivity costs.[93]

Etiology

The etiology of ulcer formation remains unclear. Acid must reach the mucosa for PUD to occur. The GI tract normally has protective mechanisms that assist in preventing PUD: the gastric mucosal barrier; cytoprotection; and the secretion of protective mucus and bicarbonate.[88,117] However, any disruption can cause an ulceration to form.

Damage to mucosa from secretion of urease and other enzymes by *H. pylori* causes most peptic ulcers.[88,93] The prevalence of *H. pylori* is 20% to 50% in Western countries; it is more prevalent in developing countries and in poor sanitary conditions. It occurs more commonly in the elderly, in African Americans, Hispanics, and immigrants from Asia and Africa. *H. pylori* is associated with 65% of gastric ulcers and 90% of duodenal ulcers[88,117]; it is seen in up to 50% of the general population by age 50 and continues to increase thereafter.[88] Eradication leads to long-term remission of chronic PUD in the absence of NSAID use.[118]

Smoking causes an altered blood flow that results in hypoxic damage to the mucosa, and it also interferes with mucosal protective factors. Smoking cigarettes will delay healing and increase the risk of bleeding.[88,117]

NSAID use, the most common cause of ulcers in *H. pylori*-negative individuals, is mainly associated with gastric ulcers. NSAIDs damage the gastric mucosa by decreasing mucosal prostaglandin production, which in turn interferes with mucus secretion and mucosal blood flow via inhibition of the cyclooxygenase-1 (COX-1) enzyme. NSAIDs cause analgesia and anti-inflammatory effects by inhibiting the COX-2 enzyme. Most recently, the use of selective COX-2–inhibiting NSAIDs such as celecoxib (Celebrex) was recommended because of decreased risks of gastroduodenal ulcers.[88,117] In 2004, Merck & Co. withdrew its drug rofecoxib (Vioxx) from the worldwide market. While the coxibs have been proven to be effective for reducing arthritis symptoms, their safety has been controversial. The early clinical studies of the coxibs raised concern about their cardiovascular safety. The Vioxx Gastrointestinal Outcomes Research study was not designed to address the issue of cardiovascular side effects, but it did show an increased risk of myocardial infarction in patients treated with rofecoxib ($P < .01$)[119] A meta-analysis of large clinical trials of celecoxib (including the CLASS study)[120] did not show any increased risk of cardiovascular events.[121] Two pharmacoepidemiologic analyses demonstrated that rofecoxib was associated with an increase in the risk of myocardial infarction.[122,123] There is concern about patients using any NSAIDs for the same reason. Moreover, many individuals over the age of 50 are advised to take low dose aspirin, which may negate the proposed benefit of COX-2 inhibitors compared to NSAIDs.

Diagnosis

Presenting symptoms may include varying degrees of mild symptoms to severe abdominal pain. It is impossible to distinguish gastric from duodenal ulcers based on symptoms alone because both typically present with epigastric tenderness and a burning or gnawing pain.[87,88,117] Tachycardia, hypotension, anorexia, hematemesis, melena, or NV may also present. Often an exacerbation during the night or early morning hours is related to circadian changes in acid secretion. The influence of food may vary with the disease: eating can alleviate symptoms of duodenal ulcers but may precipitate pain with gastric ulcers.[87,88,95,117] The health history should provide information about exacerbating factors such as use of alcohol, NSAIDs, and smoking.

The physical examination focuses on identifying complications of PUD. Vital signs and orthostatic blood pressures are obtained to identify any blood loss from bleeding ulcers. A thorough abdominal examination is necessary to note any masses or evidence of an acute abdomen. A rectal examination should be included to identify any GI bleeding.

Other than a CBC to determine anemia or stool test for occult blood, routine laboratory test results may be unremarkable. *H. pylori* testing with the C urea breath test, stool antigen test, serologic antibody testing, or endoscopic biopsy is performed.[45,118] Conventional upper GI radiologic studies are not always accurate in diagnosing PUD. Endoscopy should be obtained on individuals who present with alarm symptoms as well as those who older than 45 years who present with dyspeptic symptoms.[88]

Treatment

Initially, counseling to quit smoking, avoid alcohol, and stop the intake of NSAIDs is crucial. Diet has not been shown to relate to ulcer development or healing, but avoiding foods that aggravate dyspeptic symptoms is recommended. Empiric pharmacologic therapy consists of a H_2RA or PPI for six to eight weeks to decrease acid secretion; efficacy is greater with PPIs. Refer to Table 17-11 for pharmacologic agents used for antisecretory therapy. If no response occurs in 10 to 14 days, a diagnostic study—preferably endoscopy—is indicated. Antibiotics are prescribed to treat *H. pylori* when bacteria are present.[45] Table 17-16 presents the treatment regimen commonly used with PUD.

Immediate investigation with endoscopy is indicated if the patient presents with dyspepsia and "alarm" symptoms: anemia; GI bleeding; anorexia; early satiety; weight loss; or new onset for those age 50 or more.[45,88] Cure of *H. pylori* decreases ulcer recurrence and promotes healing; therefore, antibiotics are indicated for all *H. pylori*-positive patients. Confirmation of eradication of *H. pylori* is necessary when there are complicated ulcers associated with bleeding, perforation, or obstruction or when symptoms persist.[88]

Pregnancy Considerations

PUD is uncommon in all women of childbearing age and rare during pregnancy. Often the woman will present with nonspecific abdominal tenderness. The signs and symptoms are often attributed to reflux and may improve with antacids. Dyspepsia is a typical occurrence in pregnancy, with many women complaining of NV in early gestation as well as heartburn symptoms in later pregnancy. The occurrence of *H. pylori* in patients with ulcers is well documented; however, the incidence has not been investigated during pregnancy.[94]

If the woman has known PUD, exacerbations occur more commonly as pregnancy reaches late third trimester in response to the increase in serum gastrin. Pregnancy provides a beneficial effect on the course of the disease through several factors that include decreased gastric acid output and increased gastric mucus secondary to progesterone.[124] Complications are rare but may include perforation, hemorrhage, and obstruction. Treatment consists of antacids and H_2RAs as the first line of therapy, with avoidance of symptom-producing foods and adverse factors such as smoking, caffeine, alcohol, and NSAIDs.[125] Misoprostol is indicated for ulcer prevention but is contraindicated in pregnancy (class X) because of its abortifacient effects. Endoscopy is reserved for those cases where confirmatory diagnosis is necessary.

Bowel Obstruction

Bowel obstruction occurs when a blockage exists in either the large bowel or the small bowel.

The exact location of the obstruction is key because the differential diagnosis will vary with symptomatology. This section on bowel obstruction focuses on small bowel obstruction (SBO) because 60% to 80% of all intestinal obstructions are in the small bowel.[126,127]

Epidemiology

The incidence of SBO varies but is thought to represent 20% of all surgical admissions for acute abdominal pain.[127,128] Fifty to 70% of patients admitted with SBO require surgery, and the overall mortality is close to 5%.

Etiology

Three common causes of SBO are adhesions, Crohn's disease, and neoplasms.[129] In the past, hernias were a major cause of SBO, but in the United States, improvements in health care and in elective hernia repair make hernias a less common cause of SBO.[130,131]

Adhesions are a result of previous surgery and may form soon after surgery or take years to develop. Adhesions account for 70% of SBO, primarily because of the increased frequency of abdominal surgeries.[131] With adhesions, bowel loops become wrapped around or between adhesions, and bowel ischemia and tissue necrosis ensue. In pregnancy, the frequency of SBO from adhesions is highest in the third trimester.[132]

Other, less commonly seen causes of SBO include: gallstone ileus' parasitic disease; phytobezoar (intragastric concretion of vegetable fibers); IBD; diverticulitis; malignancies; hematomas; intussusception; and volvulus.[128,133,134] With *intussusception*, one portion of the bowel "telescopes" over the next, resulting in edema and obstruction and eventually to bowel is-

chemia.[135] *Volvulus* refers to torsion of a segment of the alimentary tract. The most common sites for volvulus are the sigmoid colon and the cecum.

Symptoms and History/Physical Findings

The most common symptoms are abdominal distention; cramp-like abdominal pain; nausea; vomiting; inability to or difficulty in passing flatus; and obstipation (extreme constipation). The inability to pass flatus and obstipation may or may not be seen because the colon needs 12 to 24 hours to empty after the onset of bowel obstruction. The presence of constant abdominal pain or a change in pain status to that of "constant pain" can be signs of impending strangulation. Because adhesions account for the majority of bowel obstructions, all patients with abdominal pain should be asked whether they have had previous abdominal surgery.

Physical findings on presentation may include fever, tachycardia, hypotension, oliguria, and dehydration. Abdominal inspection may reveal surgical scars, distention, and tympany (to percussion). Gross or occult blood may be present in the stool depending on the cause. Bowel sounds may be exaggerated. Laboratory tests including a CBC, electrolytes, renal studies, and urinalysis are commonly ordered to assess degree of dehydration. An elevated white blood count with left shift may be evident. Amylase and liver enzymes may also be elevated.

Imaging

The supine abdominal x-ray is the primary imaging test when SBO is suspected, although the use of CT is increasing. Both modalities are equally sensitive in diagnosing SBO. CT is valuable in defining the cause of the obstruction and its severity, thus influencing clinical management decisions.[132] CT sensitivity for high-grade obstruction is 81% to 94%, and for low grade obstruction is 48% to 50%.[131] CT correctly identifies the obstructive cause in 73–95% of cases but can be limited in differentiating adhesions from small tumor recurrences.[132] There are a number of types and degrees of obstruction (**Table 17-19**).

While a CT scan may demonstrate changes in ischemic bowel segments accurately and assists in determining the primary cause of ischemia, the findings in bowel ischemia are not always specific.[135] A combination of clinical symptoms, laboratory findings, and imaging studies is needed to determine a clinical diagnosis.

Treatment

The primary goals in the treatment of SBO include assessing the degree of hydration, metabolic status, and need for/timing of surgical intervention. Although treatment will depend on the specific cause, in the case of suspected, imminent, or occurring strangulation, immediate surgical intervention is necessary as soon as the patient is stable, or following resuscitative measures (i.e., hydration and electrolyte balance) in an intensive care setting. If there is suspicion of lower bowel strangulation, a period of close observation prior to surgery may be warranted. Conservative management is confined to patients with partial obstruction, because they can be managed with nasogastric suction and intravenous fluids.

Regardless of degree, suspicion of SBO is reason for immediate referral to a physician. It is recommended that potentially obstructed patients be observed for no longer than 12 to 24 hours prior to intervention. In one retrospective study of patients with SBO secondary to adhesions, the period of observation in patients managed medically was 2 to 12 days (average 6.9 days); while for those who underwent surgery, the range was 1 to 14 days (average 5.4 days).[136]

Table 17-19 **TERMINOLOGY IN BOWEL OBSTRUCTION**[8]

Term	Definition
Simple obstruction	Bowel obstruction with an intact blood supply
Strangulating obstruction	Bowel obstruction with resultant ischemia
Closed-loop obstruction	A segment of bowel occluded at two points along its course with the sites of obstruction adjacent to each other
Partial obstruction	Luminal narrowing, permitting the passage of some gas and intestinal contents
Complete obstruction	Total luminal occlusion
Obturation obstruction	Bowel obstruction caused by an intraluminal mass
Functional obstruction (pseudo-obstruction)	Symptoms of mechanical obstruction in the absence of luminal occlusion or compression

Abdominal Aortic Aneurysm

The overall incidence of abdominal aortic aneurysm (AAA) is approximately 15 to 37 per 100,000 patients a year.[137] Risk increases with age; AAA is rarely seen in women under the age of 55. It presents four to five times more commonly in men.[138,139] AAA is responsible for substantial morbidity and mortality. Surgical repair of AAA is expensive. In the United States, each procedure costs an estimated $25,000.[140]

Risk Factors

Age and male gender are key risk factors for AAA. Smoking is also believed to be a major risk factor and promotes the rate of aneurysm growth. In one study of veterans, the excess prevalence associated with smoking accounted for 78% of all aneurysms greater than or equal to 4 cm in diameter.[139] The number of years someone has smoked is significant. White race and connective tissue disorders (Marfan and Ehlers-Danlos syndromes) are other risk factors for AAA.

AAA is more common in patients who have atherosclerosis, and hypertension also has a small effect. A family history of abdominal aneurysm increases the risk of developing the disease.

Clinical Symptoms

Most aneurysms remain quiescent until they rupture. They are often detected during a workup for unrelated acute or chronic abdominal pain because the primary finding with AAA is abdominal or back pain. Physical examination may identify a pulsatile aneurysm at or above the umbilicus (the aorta bifurcates at the umbilicus), and a bruit may be detectable. Suspicion of this diagnosis leads the midwife to request an immediate physician evaluation.

Patients who present with a ruptured abdominal aneurysm (if they survive long enough to get to an ED) often present with abdominal or back pain, hypotension, and possibly a pulsing abdominal mass. Rupture produces hemorrhage and severe hypotension. The survival rate for someone who suffers a ruptured AAA is less than 50%.

AAA presents with abdominal and back pain. Thus the differential includes renal colic; pancreatitis; diverticulitis; coronary disease; mesenteric ischemia; and biliary tract disease. Cardiogram changes may be consistent with acute coronary syndrome disease or pulmonary embolism. For any patient presenting with chest pain, the provider needs to consider AAA.[141] The treatment for AAA is completely different than for acute coronary syndrome, and that makes early and accurate diagnosis critical.

Incidental identification during imaging has led to an increased number of AAAs being discovered over the last decade. CT of the abdomen and use of magnetic resonance imaging, cardiac catherizations, and imaging prior to preoperative workups have all contributed to the higher rates of diagnosis.

Imaging

Ultrasound is an extremely sensitive and specific test for diagnosing and monitoring AAA. Potential problems with ultrasound are that it is dependent on the technician's skill, and is technically difficult when overlying gas or obesity is present. Contrast spiral CT scan can image the abdomen in detail; however, it is more costly. CT angiography is very sensitive and also very accurate. Magnetic resonance angiography may be more accurate, but again is more expensive.[142]

Clinical Management

Aneurysms that are less than 4 cm are at a low risk of rupture. As they increase to 5 to 7 cm, the risk of rupture increases. Aneurysms that change quickly also pose significant risk for rupture. "Watchful waiting" is the management policy for aneurysms ≤4.0 cm, and ultrasound surveillance is usually performed on a regular basis for such aneurysms. Controlling high blood pressure is essential during this period.[143]

Surgery is indicated when aneurysms are ≥5.5 cm, painful, expanding rapidly, or become evident while diagnosing other problems. Surgery involves resection of the aorta using a synthetic graft prosthesis for replacement.

AAA and Pregnancy

Although aortic aneurysms are not common in women under 40 years of age, they can be an incidental finding. If discovered incidentally, clinical management must be geared toward avoiding a fatal rupture because that risk increases as the pregnancy progresses.[144] There is one case report of a woman who delivered vaginally with a known aneurysm of small diameter (incidental thoracic aortic aneurysm).[145]

Inflammatory Bowel Disease

IBD includes two primary entities: ulcerative colitis and Crohn's disease.[146] Both diseases are characterized by chronic intestinal inflammation. In Crohn's disease, any part of the digestive tract from mouth to anus can be involved with the inflammatory process. In ulcerative colitis, the inflammation is limited to the colon and rectum. IBD can also be associated with extra-intestinal manifestations involving liver, skin, eyes, and joints.[147] IBD potentially causes lifelong medical problems often leading to disability and can be associated with an increased risk of colorectal cancer. However, each disease has distinct features. These disorders commonly occur early in life; 15% to 20% present before age 16.[147]

If symptoms lead to a suspicion of inflammatory bowel disease, prompt referral to a GI specialist is required.

Epidemiology

For ulcerative colitis, the incidence and prevalence rates range from 3 to 15 per 100,000 and 50 to 80 per 100,000, respectively.[147] For Crohn's disease, the incidence in the United States is 6 to 7 per 100,000 and the prevalence rate is 28 to 104 per 100,000.[148] The incidence of Crohn's disease has been increasing over the last half century; whereas the rate of ulcerative colitis has remained stable.[149] There also appears to be a geographic relationship to IBD prevalence; in the United States, the prevalence is highest in the North and lowest in the South.[150]

Both diseases appear in young people and usually peak in those between ages 15 and 30. A second peak for Crohn's disease occurs in patients between 50 and 80 years old. These diseases are not gender-specific.[151] IBD has a higher incidence in patients of Jewish background and lower incidence in Black and Hispanic populations as compared to Caucasians.[152] Disease incidence is highest in developed, urbanized countries.

Genetic and Immunological Basis for IBD

Using both animal and human models, it has been shown that Crohn's disease is driven by the production of interleukin-12 (IL-12) and interferon-γ.[153] Ulcerative colitis is likely driven by the production of IL-9. Mutations in the gene that encodes nucleotide-binding oligomerization domain 2 (NOD2) protein have been found in one subgroup of patients with Crohn's disease. The present working hypothesis is that IBD is the result of exaggerated and unusual mucosal immune response to the microflora present in the intestinal mucosa,[153] and this is partially genetically induced. It is thought that effector-cell responses to mucosal antigens induce the inflammatory response in IBD.

The best evidence for the role of genetic factors in determining susceptibility comes from studies that are conducted with twins. The rate for Crohn's disease is as high as 58% in identical twins.[154,155] It is thought that IBD is not inherited as a Mendelian trait but as a more complex entity with contributing genes; the identification of NOD2/ CARD 15 mutations on chromosome 16 have now been linked to susceptibility to Crohn's disease.[156]

Evidence shows that smoking lessens the risk of developing ulcerative colitis but may increase the risk for Crohn's disease.[157,158]

Crohn's Disease

Crohn's disease is characterized by transmural mucosal inflammation. Any part of the GI tract can be affected, but the most common sites are the terminal ileum, cecum, perianal area, and colon. Segments of normal bowel between affected areas are commonly referred to as *skip lesions*. The intersection of these areas produces a mucosal "cobblestone" appearance on endoscopy. The inflammatory characteristics of Crohn's disease often lead to fibrosis and obstruction. Sinus tracts within the serosa secondary to inflammation often precede the development of fistulae.

Approximately 80% of patients have small bowel involvement, most commonly the distal ileum, with some patients having exclusive ileitis. 50% of patients have both ileum and colonic involvement. Fewer patients have mouth or esophageal involvement, but approximately one-third may have perianal disease.[159] Patients may complain of nonspecific GI symptoms for many years prior to being diagnosed. Diarrhea, abdominal pain, weight loss, malaise, fever, and night sweats [160] are typical clinical symptoms. Crampy abdominal pain is a common complaint regardless of where the inflammation lies. Weight loss is common because patients often state that they feel better when they are not eating. Weight loss can also be attributed to malabsorption. Fever may be part of the overall inflammatory response. Bacterial overgrowth may lead to *steatorrhea* (passage of fat in large amounts in the feces because of the failure to digest and absorb it) in some patients. Crohn's disease may mimic appendicitis clinically with anorexia, diarrhea, vomiting, fever, and elevated white blood cell counts. Other patients may not present with any symptoms until narrowing of the bowel lumen causes symptoms. Diagnostic signs include narrowing of the gut lumen that will lead to strictures and bowel obstruction, abscess formation, and fistulae. Gross rectal bleeding is much less frequent than in ulcerative colitis, although in some patients the stools will be hemoccult-positive. A history of prolonged diarrhea without bleeding and with other symptoms of IBD or extra-inflammatory presentation or with a family history of IBD warrants an evaluation for Crohn's disease. In patients who have developed bowel wall perforation, signs of peritonitis may be seen, such as fever, abdominal pain, and tenderness.

The diagnosis of ileitis or ileal Crohn's disease is often made by a barium study of the small bowel. Colonoscopy may be performed to rule out involvement of the colon. Intestinal biopsy can be performed to confirm the diagnosis; it will show focal ulcerations, both acute and chronic. Patients with Crohn's disease may have symptoms mimicking IBS and lactose intolerance; diagnosis may be delayed in these individuals.

The diagnosis includes involvement of the small bowel, absence of gross bleeding, bothersome perianal disease, and the development of granulomas and fistulae. The provider will need to exclude other infections such as *Campylobacter*, *Shigella*, amebic disease, lymphoma, or other diseases such as appendicitis or diverticulitis.

Crohn's disease can be assessed based on severity: mild-to-moderate in patients who are ambulatory and are not yet dehydrated or obstructed; moderate-to-severe in patients who have failed treatment for mild disease and present with fulminating and more severe symptomatology; severe (fulminant disease) when despite treatment (i.e., with steroids) symptoms persist; and patients in remission who are asymptomatic following treatment (no steroids).[161]

A typical course for Crohn's disease is that of intermittent exacerbations of symptoms with periods of remission. The remission period is lengthened with the use of medications including immunomodulators.

Treatment Regimes

Patients with mild symptoms are often started on oral sulfasalazine or 5-aminosalicylic acid (5-ASA) compounds, one of which is Mesalamine. These are thought to have some advantages over sulfasalazine because of their controlled release in the bowel and fewer side effects. These drugs are the main treatments for outpatient management. They possess both anti-inflammatory and antibacterial properties.

They are partially absorbed in the jejunum. Sulfa is best in colonic disease. Antibiotics may also be initiated prior to beginning any corticosteroid therapy. Prednisone is the treatment for those patients failing the above drug therapies or in those with severe or worsening symptoms.[162] Initial dosing is 40 to 60 mg/day. Most patients will respond to this dosing regime with a gradual tapering to 5 mg/wk. Long-term therapy is maintained with sulfa or oral 5-ASA agents. **Figure** 17-3 illustrates a proposed treatment algorithm for mild-to-moderate Crohn's disease.

In refractory disease after prednisone fails, immunomodular agents such as azathioprine or 6-mercaptopurine are initiated. These immunomodulators have a steroid sparing effect and reduce symptoms significantly.[163] Methotrexate also has been shown to be an effective alternative for the patient who is unresponsive to immunomodulators. The provider needs to monitor hepatotoxicity closely in these patients. Antibodies specific for tumor necrosis factor[162] and surgical removal of the segments of the intestines that are obstructive are other treatment options. A number of options, including monoclonal antibodies, peptide recombinant proteins, oligonucleotides, and modulators of specific pathways, present new treatment options for the future.[163] Cytokine-specific immunomodulators, modulators of cell adhesion, modulators of intracellular signaling cascades, modulators of growth factors, probiotics, and hematopoietic stem cell renewal are also included as potentially effective future therapies.[163]

COMPLICATIONS

Extraintestinal complications may include eye involvement with uveitis, skin disorders such as erythema nodosum, peripheral arthritis, and

Figure 17-3 Suggested treatment algorithm for mild-to-moderate Crohn's disease that uses the latest evidence-based approach to induction[162]

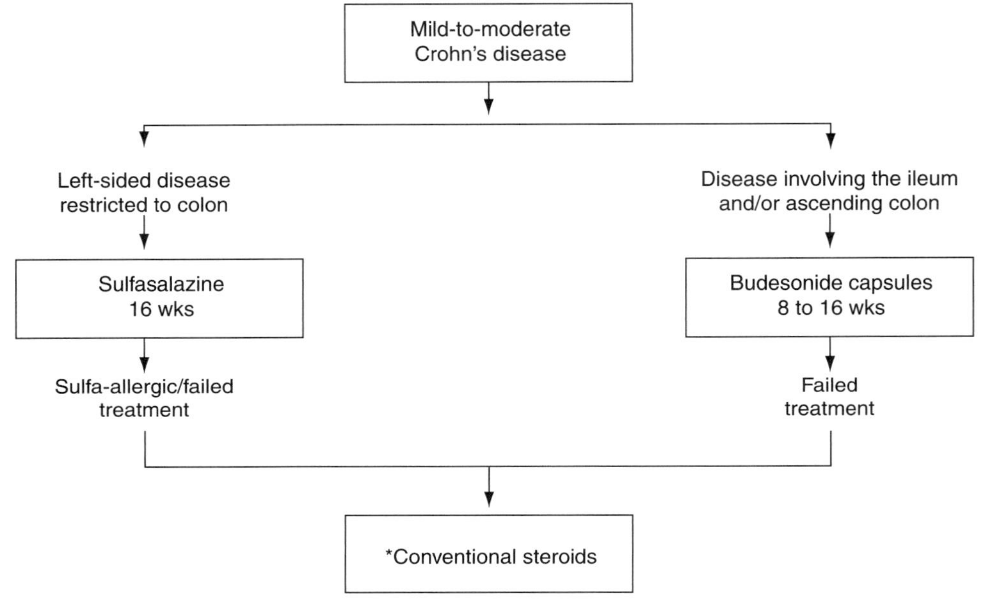

*If the patient is not improving, need to reclassify patient as having moderate-to-severe disease and evaluate for treatment with infliximab, immunomodulators, or surgery.

sclerosing cholangitis. Specific complications related to malabsorption have been seen. There is an increased risk of colon cancer, and the incidence of small bowel cancer in Crohn's disease is also higher than in the general population. Surgery for intestinal resection and later re-anastomosis still has a 10% to 15%/year clinical recurrence rate.[164] Other GI complications include fulminant colitis, toxic megacolon, and abscess.

Ulcerative Colitis

Ulcerative colititis is defined by recurring episodes of chronic inflammation that specifically involve the mucosa layer of the colon; it invariably involves the rectum. Sometimes it is limited to the rectum as *ulcerative proctitis*. With ulcerative colitis, the histology involves the presence of ulcerations and chronic inflammation leading to *crypt abscesses*, defined as the presence of acute inflammatory cells in crypts. Unlike the skip lesions associated with Crohn's disease, the mucosal involvement is continuous and uniform.

Patients usually present with mild, moderate, or severe disease. In mild disease, the inflammation is confined to the rectum or rectosigmoid. There may be intermittent rectal bleeding, the passage of mucus, mild and often bloody diarrhea with loose stools. Mild abdominal cramping pain and periods of constipation with bloody mucus are commonly seen, but the passage of gross blood is the main feature.[160] In moderate disease, the inflammatory process extends to the splenic flexure. Patients complain of frequent bloody stools, abdominal pain that is crampy, low-grade fever, and diarrhea. In severe disease, patients have more extensive colonic involvement. There is an increase in the number of loose stools per day, severe cramping, fever, and bleeding that often necessitates blood transfusions. There may be rapid weight loss leading to a poor nutritional state. Physical exam findings may include pallor, weight loss, abdominal tenderness, and positive stool guiac. The differential diagnosis includes infectious disease, other cancers, and use of NSAIDs.

The diagnosis is confirmed by flexible sigmoidoscopy at the onset of symptoms. The presence of crypt abscesses on biopsy is diagnostic for ulcerative colitis. Colonoscopy is useful when the diagnosis is in question, symptoms are in remission, or if only routine surveillance is necessary. Performing a colonoscopy or barium enema in a patient with severe disease may trigger megacolon and possible perforation.

The course of ulcerative colitis involves intermittent exacerbations alternating with periods of complete remission. A small percentage of patients continue to be symptomatic and do not achieve remission. In those with proctitis only, 20% resolve spontaneously and many others do well following drug therapy. For those patients who have disease limited to the distal colon, surgery is rarely required. Surgical intervention with colectomy is limited to those patients who are refractory to medical therapy or have massive hemorrhage, colonic perforation, extenuating toxic megacolon, or carcinoma. Approximately 30% of patients undergo colectomy after 15 to 25 years of living with the disease.[165]

TREATMENT REGIMENS

Lactose intolerance is frequently noted in patients with ulcerative colitis, and patients should undergo breath analysis to confirm this diagnosis. Nutritional counseling may also include restricting fresh fruit and vegetables, caffeine, and carbonated beverages. Nicotine therapy may benefit some patients with ulcerative colitis.[166]

The first-line treatment for ulcerative proctitis is topical 5-ASA suppositories or steroid foams. High remission rates can be achieved with suppositories and oral sulfa and 5-ASA agents also may be used if needed. Systemic steroids are rarely indicated with this section of colon.[167]

Therapy for mild-to-moderate disease can be started with 5-ASA or hydrocortisone enemas. 5-ASA drugs are a first-line therapy but steroids may be necessary; when the patient reports chronic steroid use, the midwife should include the possible systemic steroid side effects in the assessment. Oral agents of sulfasalazine (azyfidine), mesalamine (pentasa, asacol), and balsalazide (colazal) have been proven to be effective in active ulcerative colitis. As in Crohn's disease, prednisone should be used for patients who have more severe symptoms or who are refractory to treatment. Therapy is similar to that for Crohn's disease. Budesonide is a glucocorticoid with first-pass metabolism in the liver and produces less steroid toxicity.

In the severely ill patient who is at risk of megacolon and bowel perforation, hospitalization is crucial. Bowel rest, nutrition, and parenteral steroids may be necessary. Broad-spectrum antibiotics are often used, and total parenteral nutrition may be indicated. Immunomodular therapy with azathioprine or 6-mercaptopurine may be considered. Adjunctive treatment with psychotropic agents may be beneficial for some patients.

Patients with toxic megacolon (colon dilated to ≥6 cm) who do not respond to therapy may need a colectomy. Toxic megacolon occurs more commonly with ulcerative colitis than with Crohn's disease.

Complications

As with Crohn's disease, extra-intestinal complications are seen. Local complications include hemorrhage, fulminant colitis, intestinal perforation or stricture, and the development of colon cancer. The risk of developing colon cancer is related to both duration and extent of disease. There is an increased risk of colon cancer seven to eight years after disease onset, and if the GI tract above the splenic flexure is affected. The risk also increases in patients with a family history of colon cancer.[168] Yearly surveillance colonoscopy is indicated.

Irritable Bowel Syndrome

IBS involves complex symptoms that include abdominal pain and alterations in bowel functioning. IBS has no structural or biochemical markers and no pathophysiological mechanism has been discovered.[169] It is primarily a symptom-based syndrome and a diagnosis of exclusion. It is classified into three types: IBS-C (constipation); IBS-D (diarrhea); and IBS-A (alternating). IBS is believed to be the most common functional disorder of the GI tract.[170,171] It accounts for 36% to 50% of all GI consultations, which translates to approximately 3.5 million medical visits in the United States annually.[171] IBS has a clear impact on health costs—8 million dollars annually—as well as being the cause of significant time away from the workplace.[172,173]

Epidemiology

The prevalence of IBS ranges from 14% to 24% for women and 5% to 19% for men.[174,175] Population-based studies have found a 2:1 female predominance of IBS in North America. There appear to be equal numbers of IBS patients who experience primarily constipation, primarily diarrhea, or who alternate between the two conditions. Half of new IBS patients are under 35 years of age.[176]

Neurophysiology and Psychosocial Factors

The intestinal tract is controlled by the *enteric nervous system (ENS)*, which is sometimes called the "brain-in-the-gut" because it regulates patterns of intestinal behavior.[177] Early stages of enteric neuropathy may be expressed as IBS-like symptoms when there is dysregulation of the brain–gut axis. Peripheral enteric neuropathology or visceral hyperalgesia may be the underlying cause of increased sensitivity to distention at least in a subset of patients. Contractions of the intestinal muscle (altered gut reactivity) underlie the sensations often referred to as cramping-abdominal pain. This pattern occurs more frequently and with stronger muscular contractions in IBS patients.[178] Intestinal mast cells, which act as immune/inflammatory cells, are also known to proliferate during any exposure to GI threats such as parasites. This parallel pattern supports the premise of increased visceral hypersensitivity with IBS.[179] The interactions of the ENS and the bowel are paving the way for future research and treatment strategies as well as helping biomedical scientists to understand the nature of overall pain in IBS.[180] **Figure** 17-4 is a neurophysiologic model of IBS.

Psychosocial factors also play a key role in IBS and may be the most critical component of symptom severity.[181] Up to 50% of patients suffer from paranoia, anxiety, depression, somatization, and phobias. There is also a two- to threefold increase in a history of physical sexual abuse.[182] **Figure** 17-5 is a conceptual model of IBS.

Symptomatology

A thorough history includes both physiologic symptoms and psychosocial factors such as stress, social support, and lifestyle. The provider must be alert to significant symptoms, which include rectal bleeding; severe weight loss; fever; and anorexia that might indicate more

---

Figure 17-4 The neurophysiologic model for the enteric nervous system (ENS) is the same as for the central nervous system (CNS). Sensory neurons, interneurons, and motor neurons are connected synaptically for information transfer from the sensory neurons to interneuronal integrative circuits to motor neurons to gastrointestinal effector systems. Gastrointestinal effector systems are the musculature, secretory epithelium, and blood vascular system. The ENS organizes and coordinates the activity of the musculature, secretory glands, and blood vessels to generate the moment-to-moment behavior of the whole organ. Bidirectional flow of neural signals is continuous between the CNS and the ENS.

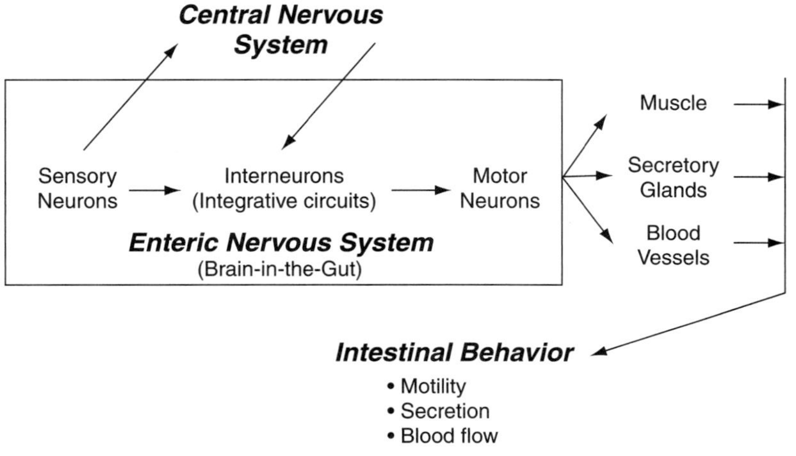

Source: Reprinted with permission.[177]

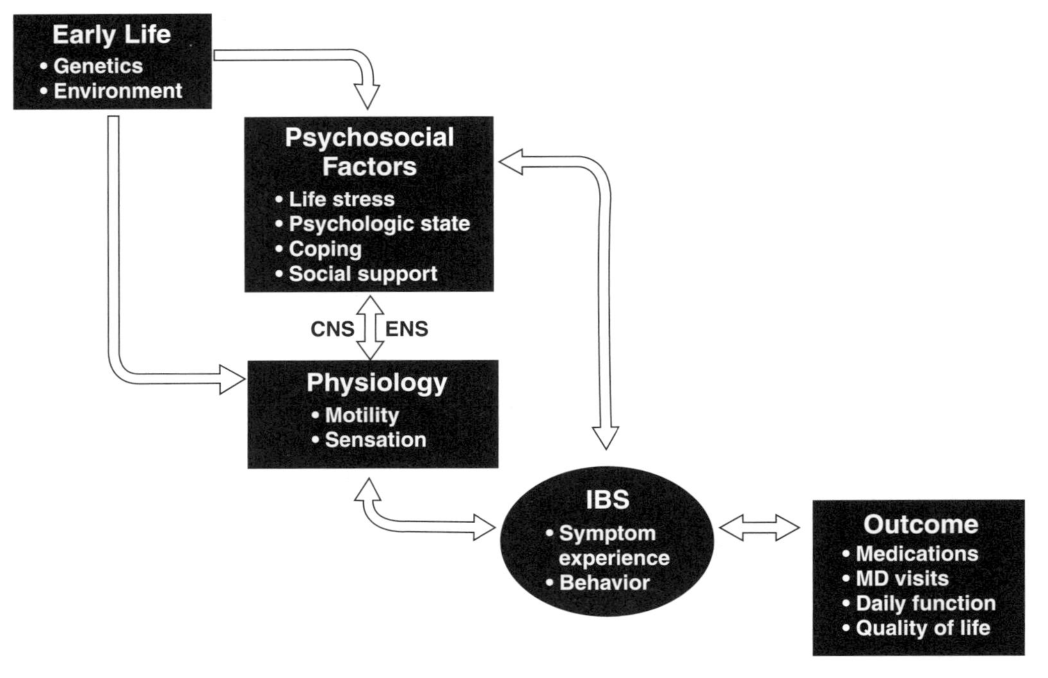

Figure 17-5 Conceptual model of irritable bowel syndrome (IBS) depicting the relationship between early life, psychosocial factors, physiology, symptom experience, and behavior and outcome.

Source: Reprinted with permission.[183]

significant pathology than IBS. Other symptoms that may indicate IBS include: constipation; diarrhea; abdominal cramping; abdominal pain relieved by defecation; pain associated with looser or more frequent stools; alternating diarrhea and constipation; mucus stools; dyspepsia; bloating; and gas. Symptoms are worse at times of increased stress in IBS patients.[170] Patients may only complain of altered bowel habits, which is why a detailed history becomes critical. They may also complain of symptoms unrelated to intestinal disease that include sexual dysfunction; dysmenorrhea; dyspareunia; urinary symptoms; and rheumatologic symptoms including fibromyalgia.[184,185] Any medication history and a dietary assessment may offer additional clues to the diagnosis.

Criteria for Diagnosis of IBS

In the absence of any set markers for IBS, symptoms alone are used to define the syndrome (**Table 17-20**). Multinational teams have worked on developing consensus-based criteria using the Delphi method of consensus approach;

Table 17-20 DIAGNOSTIC CRITERIA FOR IRRITABLE BOWEL SYNDROME*

Twelve weeks† or more in the past 12 months of abdominal discomfort or pain that has two of three features:

- Relieved with defecation
- Onset associated with a change in frequency of stool
- Onset associated with a change in form (appearance) of stool

The following symptoms are not essential for the diagnosis, but when/if present, they increase the confidence in the diagnosis and may be used to identify subgroups of IBS:

- Abnormal stool frequency ($>$3/day or $<$3/week)
- Abnormal stool form (lumpy/hard or loose/watery stool) $>$1/4 of defecations
- Abnormal stool passage (straining, urgency, or feeling of incomplete evacuation) $>$1/4 defecations
- Passage of mucus $>$1/4 of defecations
- Bloating or feeling of abdominal distention $>$1/4 of day

*In the absence of structural or metabolic abnormalities to explain the symptoms.
†The 12 weeks need not be consecutive.
Source: Reprinted with permission.[183]

these are known as the Rome criteria.[183] Rome I was published in 1994 and revised in 1999 and 2000 (Rome II).

Laboratory testing may be needed to rule out other diagnostic possibilities. Occult stool analysis and CBC are recommended. A sedimentation rate may be ordered as well as serum chemistries, and stool for ova and parasites based on travel, geographic history, and symptom history. A 24-hour stool collection may be ordered depending on the degree of diarrhea. Thyroid testing may be ordered to rule out hyper/hypothyroid disease. In those patients over 50 years of age, a colonoscopy will be included to rule out more serious diseases such as neoplastic and serious inflammatory diseases of the bowel. A flexible sigmoidoscopy may be ordered, but usually it has a low yield. It is sometimes used in younger patients with persistent diarrhea to exclude other diseases of the GI tract.

Treatment Options

There are a number of different approaches to treatment, as dictated by the wide variance in symptoms. Dual therapies are used to manage multiple symptoms. Treatment is usually a long-term process of seeing what works best for the individual. Within this process, establishing a solid patient–provider relationship is key.

Dietary Modifications

A thorough dietary history is needed. The patient will need to keep a food diary to determine if there is a relationship between certain foods and symptoms. Lactose intolerance is commonly seen.[186] Caffeine can also be problematic because it is a gut stimulant. Many food intolerances can affect the bowel pattern and cause increased gas production, diarrhea, or abdominal pain. Hypersensitivity and allergies to certain foods can also create an immunologic response. Foods most commonly associated with IBS symptoms include: milk, eggs, fish, nuts, shellfish, soybeans, and wheat.[187] Celiac disease and gluten enteropathy are found with intolerance of wheat-based products.

Constipation should be treated initially with an increase in dietary fiber to 20 to 30 gm of dietary fiber/day. Patients should start with breakfast fiber cereal and then add portions of fruits and green leafy vegetables daily; fiber supplements can also be used. For patients with diarrhea, pain, gas, or bloating, adding fiber and increasing water consumption may be helpful. There are no current recommendations on dietary modifications if pain and bloating are the major symptoms, other than keeping a diary to see which foods are problematic.

The use of prebiotics and probiotics in the treatment strategy is increasing as intestinal microflora have been found to ameliorae the severity of IBS. *Probiotics* are live bacteria food supplements that benefit the host animal by improving the intestinal microbial balance.[188] *Prebiotics* are nondigestible food substances or supplements that are fermented by host bacteria, alter intestinal flora, and stimulate the growth of healthy bacteria. Both enhance the growth of healthy bacteria such as *Lactobacillus*.

Pharmacologic Therapies

The 5HT4 agonists have been used to treat constipation or pain with constipation, especially if fiber or bulking agents and laxatives are ineffective. Tegaserod (Zelnorm) is one of these drugs. 5HT4 receptors are located in the GI tract and affect neurons. Tegaserod stimulates the release of certain neurotransmitters that in turn stimulate the peristaltic reflex and increase small and large bowel fluid secretion.[188] In large, multicenter, randomized controlled trials, this drug was found to be effective, with diarrhea the most frequently reported side effect.[189,190] Originally approved by the Food and Drug Administration (FDA) for women only, it is now approved for men as well. Dosage is 6 mg twice a day prior to meals.

For patients whose primary symptom is diarrhea, loperamide (Imodium) decreases intestinal transit, increases water absorption, and may be helpful for resting the anal sphincter tone. However, it is not more effective than placebo for treating global IBS symptoms or abdominal pain.[169]

Alosetron (Lotronex) has been studied[190,192] as a treatment option for patients with IBS. The most common adverse event was constipation that affected up to 28% of patients. Acute ischemic colitis has been associated with the drug. Because of these potentially serious side effects, it was removed from the U.S. market in November 2000, just months after its approval. It was re-approved in June 2002. The recommended starting dose is 1 mg/day, which is half the dose used in clinical trials. Dosage may be increased slowly. Providers who prescribe alosetron must agree to participate in a prescribing program that requires them to attest to their qualifications to diagnose and treat IBS, and to also report serious adverse affects to the manufacturer or the FDA. Both provider and patient must sign a consent form that becomes part of the medical record. It is appropriate only for women with severe diarrhea-predominant IBS who have failed conventional therapy.[170]

Antispasmodic agents, which induce smooth muscle relaxation, are commonly used to treat IBS. A meta-analysis of 23 randomized clinical trials involving 1880 patients found five drugs to be more effective than placebo.[193] Most of these drugs are not available in the United States. The two most used antispasmodics in the United States are hyoscyamine (Levsin) and dicyclomine, neither of which has been found to be more effective than placebo. **Table 17-21** summarizes the common medications used in IBS management.

The use of antidepressants to treat pain is supported by several randomized controlled trials involving tricyclic antidepressants (TCAs).[194,195] Antidepressants must be used on a continual basis and not on an "as needed" regimen; it takes two

Table 17-21 MEDICATIONS USED TO MANAGE IRRITABLE BOWEL SYNDROME

Predominent Symptom	Medication	Dose	AFP Level of Evidence	Comment
Diarrhea	loperamide (Imodium)	2–4 mg up to 4x/d	Level A	Use as needed or prophylactically in times of anticipated stress
	cholestyramine (Questran)	4 g 1–6x/d	Level C	Second-line agent
	alosetron (Lotronex)	1 mg/d titrated to 2x/d if tolerated	Level A	Restricted use to female patients only
Constipation	Fiber	Start low and titrate up to 20–30 g/d	Level A	May worsen bloating
	Osmotic laxative	Magnesium citrate, lactulose, or polyethylene glycol dosed as appropriate	Level C	
Abdominal pain	Antispasmodics and anticholinergics (e.g., dicyclomine [Bentyl], hyoscyamine [Levsin])	Dicyclomine 10–20 mg, 2–4 x/d	Level B	Use as needed only
	Tricyclic antidepressants (e.g., amitriptyline [Elavil])	Start amitriptyline, 10–25 mg at bedtime or 2x/d, or desipramine (Norpramin) 50 mg 3 x/d	Level A	Needs to be given daily, not as needed and, therefore, generally reserved for patients with more severe pain. FDA approved for short-term treatment of women
Gas or bloating	tegaserod (Zelnorm) simethicone (Mylanta)	40–125 mg up to 4x/day as needed		Anecdotal evidence only
Comorbid depression or anxiety	Antidepressants or anxiolytics	Dose as appropriate		Treating depression has been shown to improve bowel symptoms

Source: Reprinted with permission.[170]

to four weeks to see symptom improvement. TCAs, which include amitriptyline (Elavil), slow the movement of contents through the GI tract and may be helpful in patients with predominantly IBS diarrhea. TCAs are used to control pain and not for treatment of depression. Selective serotonin reuptake inhibitors, such as paroxetine (Paxil), fluoxetine (Prozac), and sertraline (Zoloft) are usually prescribed for patients with IBS and depression. Behavioral therapy can be used as adjunctive therapy.

It is reasonable for the midwife to begin dietary modifications and initiate treatment for symptoms of diarrhea or constipation. When symptoms persist, referral to a physician is essential.

Appendicitis

Appendicitis should always be considered as a diagnostic possibility in cases where lower abdomen pain, particularly right sided, is the primary presenting problem. Appendicitis was first described in 1886.[196] The lifetime risk of appendectomy is 12% for men and 25% for women, making it the most commonly performed operation in the world.[197,198] More than 250,000 appendectomies are performed in the United States each year, making it the most common abdominal operation performed on an emergency basis as well.[199] The incidence is highest among 10- to 19-year-olds.

In more than 15% of appendectomies performed, there is no pathologic evidence of appendicitis.[200] One small study attempted to investigate the morbidity, mortality, and costs of removing a normal appendix in patients with suspected appendicitis.[201] Complications occurred in 16 patients and in 5, a re-operation was needed. The mean hospital stay was 4.4 days and in cases of complication, 7.4 days stay.

An organized approach to the investigation of suspected appendicitis can minimize costs without compromising care. Midwives who suspect a diagnosis of appendicitis are responsible for arranging for physician care promptly.

Pathophysiology

The primary pathophysiology in appendicitis is acute obstruction of the appendiceal lumen. The most common cause is a *fecalith*, which is a hard mass consisting of inspissated feces; they are found in 40% of all acute appendicitis cases and 90% of ruptured appendices.[202]

Appendiceal obstruction leads to further abdominal distention and impaired outflow, which eventually causes an enlargement and engorgement of the appendix. Ischemic changes are seen. There is an increase in intestinal bacteria within the obstructed appendix. As the appendix becomes inflamed, adjacent organs and the omentum begin to wall off further contents. Once significant inflammatory changes occur, necrosis sets in, and the appendix may form a localized abscess or perforate and cause generalized peritonitis. In one study of patients in whom the appendix had perforated, 65% showed inflammatory changes that had been in existence for greater than 48 hours.[203]

The goal is to promptly diagnose appendicitis and minimize complications such as perforations. The rate of normal findings at surgery for appendicitis can be as high as 15% to 30% [201] in the non-pregnant woman and even higher in pregnant women, where the need to prevent perforation is critical, especially during the second and third trimesters.

The majority of women with acute appendicitis complain of right lower quadrant (RLQ) pain. The appendix most often lies in the retrocecal or pelvic position relative to the cecum in the RLQ. It averages 9 to 10 cm in length. The diameter ranges from 0.5 to 1 cm. On abdominal exam, an inflamed appendix produces tenderness and discomfort at what is commonly referred to as the McBurney point.

Differential Diagnosis

For obvious reasons, assessing for appendicitis in premenopausal women can be more difficult because of the potential for pregnancy. Gynecologic disorders, such as ectopic pregnancy, simple and complex right ovarian masses, right ovarian torsion, endometriosis, urinary tract disease, mittelschmerz pain, and pelvic inflammatory disease, can produce appendicitis-like symptoms. Obtaining an accurate last menstrual period date and ordering a pregnancy test will assist in establishing the diagnosis. The Manchester Trial Group in the United Kingdom proposed that until proven otherwise, any female who has reached puberty, who is amenorrheic, irregular, has delayed menses, or is having unprotected sex, should be considered potentially pregnant.[204]

The differential diagnosis for appendicitis includes constipation, Crohn's disease, diverticulosis, intestinal obstruction, Meckel diverticulum, pyelonephritis and strangulated hernia, and any other RLQ disorders. Age, medical history, and related factors need to be considered as well. Misdiagnosis occurs more commonly in the very young and very old, among women more than men, and in patients with higher levels of comorbid illnesses.[200] **Table 17-22** specifies conditions that mimic appendicitis.

Symptoms and Findings on Examination

The first symptoms of appendicitis may be mild in intensity, with minor cramping and gradual onset of pain or slight nausea, feelings of indigestion, bowel changes, or anorexia. These symptoms worsen to include loss of appetite, periumbilical pain, nausea, vomiting, and/or diarrhea in young adolescents. Not all patients have vomiting. The signs and symptoms that are most predictive of acute appendicitis are RLQ pain, abdominal rigidity, and migration of pain from the periumbilical region to the RLQ.[205] Coughing or walking can aggravate the pain. Some patients may have voluntary guarding to avoid any motion tenderness in the area. Fever and rebound tenderness may present as well as leukocytosis. Some patients will have only a mild elevated white count. An elevated neutrophil ratio or left shift appears to be a good predictor of acute appendicitis.[206] A urinalysis is often performed to rule out renal calculi and pyelonephriti. **Figure** 17-6 is an algorithm describing how to evaluate pain in the right lower quadrant RLQ.

A helpful mnemonic to assess abdominal pain is the mnemonic PQRST,[208,209] where P = what provokes the pain; Q = quality (what does it feel like?); R = radiation (where does it radiate?); S = severity (rate the pain on a scale of 1 to 10); T = time and treatment (how long have you had it and what has been done already?).

In addition, some patients may have a positive psoas sign, which is RLQ pain on passive extension of the right hip. With the patient supine, the clinician raises the patient's right leg while providing counter-resistance. The resulting increase in RLQ pain may indicate appendicitis. Other physical exam findings associated with appendicitis include obturator sign (RLQ pain on passive internal rotation of the flexed right hip), Rosving sign (RLQ pain upon palpation of the left lower quadrant), and RLQ pain on rectal exam.

Table 17-22 CONDITIONS THAT MIMIC APPENDICITIS[197,200,204–207]

Non-OB/Gyn Conditions	OB/Gyn Conditions
Constipation	Ectopic pregnancy
Pyelonephritis	Right ovarian masses
Urinary calculi	Endometriosis
Bowel obstruction	Mittelschmerz
Gastroenteritis	Ovarian torsion
Acute mesenteric adenitis	Pelvic inflammatory disease
Diverticulosis	
External and strangulated hernia	
Perforated duodenal ulcer	
Meckel diverticulum	

When history and physical findings are consistent with a diagnosis of acute appendicitis, appendectomy is often performed without further evaluation. If the symptomatology is less acute, then a period of observation reasonable. The patient should have nothing by mouth, an intravenous line should be established, early surgical consultation obtained, and prophylactic antibiotics ordered if surgery is pending.

Imaging

Ultrasound has only 40% to 90% sensitivity, 86% to 100% specificity, and a positive predictive value of 89% to 93% for appendicitis.[210–212] Ultrasound also has poor sensitivity for perforation. However, it can be helpful for identifying alternative diagnoses in the differential list. A normal-appearing appendix is seen in fewer than 5% of patients.[210] Ultrasound is often reserved for pregnant women, those with high suspicion of gynecologic-related diseases, or in cases where radiation exposure from CT needs to be minimized. Findings on ultrasound suggesting appendicitis include a noncompressible appendix with a thickened wall, distention of the lumen, and free fluid in the pelvis. The

use of transvaginal ultrasound in conjunction with transabdominal ultrasound imaging seems to improve the overall detection rate for appendicitis [212] and is sensitive for evaluation of gynecologic disorders.

For patients with suspected appendicitis, spiral computed tomography has a sensitivity of 90 to 100%, a specificity of 91% to 99%, a positive predictive value of 95% to 97% and an accuracy of 94% to 100%.[208,213] With improvements in CT imaging, including spiral CT, the entire abdomen can be effectively scanned at high resolution in thin slices during a single period. High-resolution pictures of the appendix and localized tissue surrounding it can be visualized, so alternative causes of abdominal pain can be discovered as well. CT is far more accurate than ultrasound and is being used with greater frequency despite radiation exposure.[209]

CT findings diagnostic of appendicitis include distended appendix, thickened appendiceal wall, and peri-appendiceal inflammation.

Another indication of appendicitis is the CT arrowhead sign, which is an arrowhead-shaped collection of contrast medium that localizes to the upper part of the cecum near the appendix

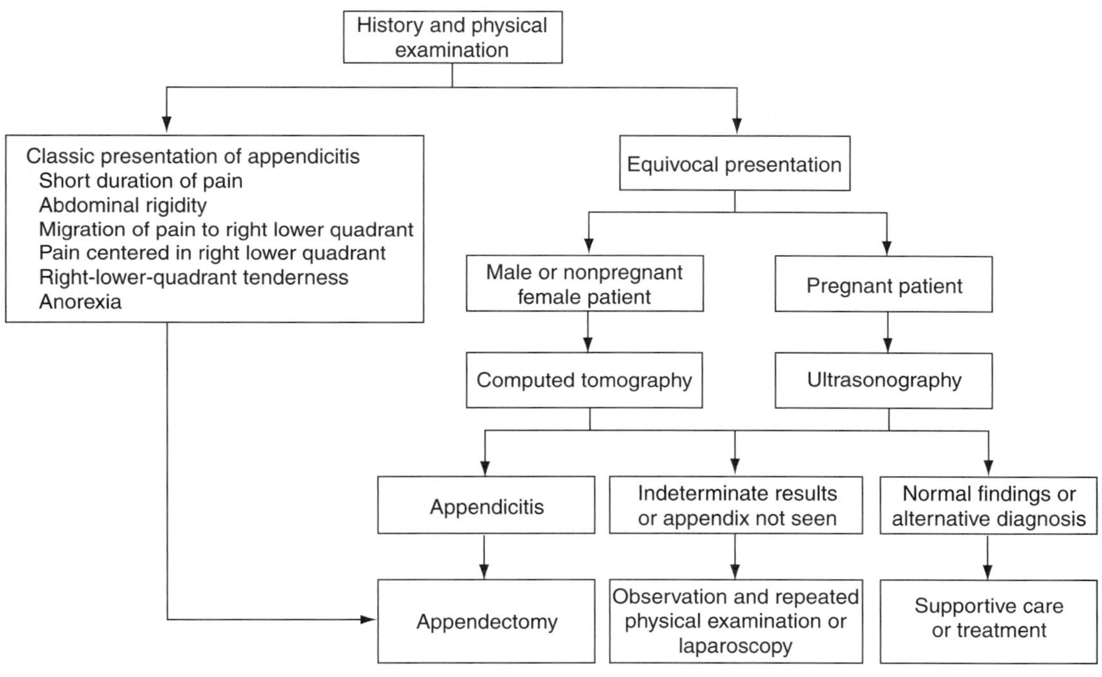

Figure 17-6 Clinical algorithm to evaluate pain in the right lower quadrant when appendicitis is suspected. If gynecologic disease is suspected, a pelvic and endovaginal ultrasonographic examination should be considered.[205]

(**Figure 17-7**). Some authors suggest scanning solely in the appendix area[216] and others scan the entire abdomen.[217] However, spiral CT is critical for obtaining adequate slices and thereby accurate imaging.

Although CT has been shown to be effective for the diagnosis of acute appendicitis, retrospective studies found that its effect on management decisions and rates of unnecessary appendectomy varies.[218,219] Many, but not all, prospective studies have found that the use of CT is helpful in diagnosing appendicitis. Comparison of initial evaluation with actual post-case outcomes has shown a 98% positive predictive value in diagnosing appendicitis.[220] In this study, CT led to a change in management in 59 patients and prevented unnecessary appendectomy (n = 13), unnecessary hospitalization (n = 39), and treatment delay.[220] A cost analysis of the impact of avoiding unnecessary observation and appendectomy, versus the cost of CT scan, demonstrated an average cost savings of $447.00 per patient with the use of CT.

Another study involved 99 patients suspected of having appendicitis who were evaluated by CT and ultrasound after the initial

Figure 17-7 Arrowhead sign in appendix with appendicitis. (a) Transverse computed tomographic (CT) image shows focal symmetric thickening of the upper portion of the cecum with an associated arrowhead-shaped collection of contrast medium (arrow) formed as contrast material funnels into the partially coapted cecal wall adjacent to the occluded appendiceal orifice. (b) Transverse CT image shows the inflamed appendix (arrows) with stranding of the adjacent mesenteric fat.

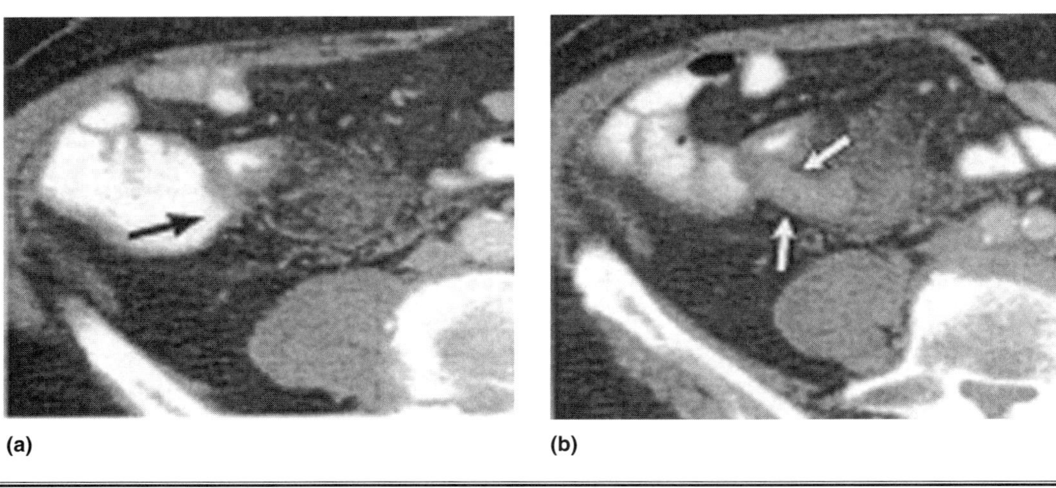

(a)   (b)

Source: Reprinted with permission of Radiological Society of North America.[214]

management had been completed.[221] Two hours later, each patient was re-evaluated clinically and the imaging results reported. A final management plan was then developed. CT led to cancellation of planned surgery for six patients, none of whom were found to have appendicitis; all six were female. The rate of unnecessary appendectomy was reduced from 50% to 17%, a statistically significant difference. Only 50% of the women initially scheduled to have surgery actually had appendicitis. Raman et al.[222] looked at gender-related performance of non-focused helical CT and found it to be highly accurate in both men and women for acute appendicitis, although there was a slight but significant decrease in sensitivity in thin women.

Rosen et al.[223] studied the value of abdominal CT in the ED for patients with nontraumatic abdominal pain and found that CT reduced the hospital admission rate by 28% of patients and changed the surgical management in 40%.

Perez et al.[224] found that the use of preoperative abdominal CT scanning has not improved the accuracy of the diagnosis of appendicitis at their institution. CT resulted in a significant increase in ED preoperative length of stay and the finding of a normal appendix at surgery. Earlier input by surgeons increased the rate of accurate clinical diagnosis and decreased the number of CT scans ordered.[225] Others report that CT is useful, but high accuracy rates have not been reproducible. The test may be beneficial only in selected patients with equivocal findings.[215]

Wise et al.,[226] in a comparative assessment of CT and sonographic techniques for appendiceal imaging, found that a standard abdominal-pelvic CT scan was a better initial exam for adult patients. Focused appendiceal CT with colonic contrast material should be used in diagnosing difficult cases.

Another study indicated that intravenous contrast material improves the delineation of a thickened appendix as well as improved detection of surrounding inflammation.[216] Using enteric contrast material (either orally or rectally) permits views of the terminal ileum and cecum.

CT does involve exposure to significant doses of radiation. Estimates are that helical CT gives a dose of about 3 mSv, which is four times the dose used in plain abdominal radiography.[227]

Operative Choices

Diagnostic laparoscopy is not usually needed in men or children with suspected appendicitis symptoms. However, among women of childbearing age, laparoscopy can be useful because multiple reproductive tract complications can exist that may require surgical intervention. Cervini et al. [207] noted that the surgeon on call at the time of patient admission is a critical factor in determining whether a patient will receive a laparoscopy or open appendectomy. In general, the approach to surgery, whether open or by laparoscopy, depends on the confirmation of appendicitis after considering history of prior surgery, age, gender, and body weight. Laparoscopy may offer an advantage when the diagnosis is not confirmed, because this technique allows for inspection of other abdominal organs.

Infection is the most common complication following appendectomy, occurring more commonly in cases in which the appendix has perforated.

Pregnancy and Appendicitis

Appendicitis is the most common cause of an acute abdomen in pregnancy.[228] It has been postulated that the appendix rises higher in the abdomen as gestation advances. However, a recent study has shown that in all three trimesters, affected women complained of RLQ pain.[229] Fever and leukocytosis are not clear indicators of appendicitis in pregnancy, but a left shift may be more suggestive. Preterm labor is a known complication; preterm delivery is rare.

Imaging in pregnancy had been previously limited to ultrasound, but other options such as helical or spiral CT may also be used.[230] CT imaging can be safely used in the second and third trimesters. This test takes approximately 15 minutes. Radiation exposure is approximately 300 mrad, one-third of the radiation exposure in an average abdominal/pelvic CT scan, and well below the accepted safe level of fetal exposure of 5 rads. On CT, an enlarged appendix greater than 6 mm, inflammatory changes, and a positive arrowhead sign can be seen.

Diverticular Disease

Diverticular disease primarily involves the colon and is a commonly seen entity that increases in frequency with age.[231] There are two forms of diverticular disease: *diverticulosis* is an asymptomatic diverticular disease; *diverticulitis* has associated inflammation. Many patients have diverticulosis, but diverticulitis is seen in only one in five people.[232] Diverticulosis can cause massive lower GI bleeding, although the majority of patients are asymptomatic.[231] An estimated 20% of patients manifest clinical symptoms. The disease is common in developed countries, with the highest rates seen in the United States, Europe, and Australia.[233] The incidence seems to rise within societies or countries when there is a reduction in dietary fiber uptake.[234] Men and women are affected equally by diverticular disease.

Anatomical Description

Diverticula are formed when colonic mucosa and submucosa herniate through the muscle layers of the colon. The hypothesis for the formation of diverticula is the following. Hard stools caused in part by low fiber diets exert increased pressure on the lumen of the colon. Because less frequent, small volume, firm stools are commonly seen in low fiber diets, the colon must increase the number of muscle contractions needed to pass the stool. Small arteries, called *vasa recta*, supply the rectum. The sites where they enter the colon are relatively weak areas, and it is at these areas where diverticula are formed in response to the increased pressure. The bleeding that ensues is from the neck of the vessels at the base of the diverticula.[235] Diverticula can vary in number from a few to several hundred. They are typically 5 to 10 mm in diameter but can exceed 2 cms. Most are single lesions located in the sigmoid and arising from the antimesenteric border of the colon.[231] Most cases requiring surgery involve the sigmoid. Diverticulitis is an uncommon complication of pregnancy.[236]

The signs and symptoms of diverticular bleeding are usually painless *hematochezia* (passage of bloody stools, in contradistinction to *melena*, or tarry stools) and occasionally mild lower left quadrant abdominal pain. Rarely is the bleeding severe.

Diverticular bleeding occurs in about 3% of patients who have diverticulosis.[2] It presents as acute bright red or maroon colored bleeding that is painless. Spontaneous resolution of this bleeding occurs in 75% to 85% of patients, and greater than 50% of the time there will be no recurrence.[237,238]

Etiology

Low dietary fiber predisposes to the development of diverticular disease.[239,240] Increasing dietary fiber may be preventive by causing large bulky stools that result in a wider colon. Dietary fiber also aids in preventing constipation. Lack of vigorous exercise may also be a risk factor for diverticular disease. In one prospective study of approximately 48,000 men in the United States who were free of known disease, the risk of developing diverticular symptoms was inversely related to overall physical activity.[241] Other mechanisms thought to underlie diverticular disease include inter-related processes such as muscular dysfunction, visceral hypersensitivity, and inflammation.[242]

Symptoms

Most patients with diverticulosis are either asymptomatic or have minor symptoms. In these patients, diverticulosis is often diagnosed on a routine colonoscopy. Some patients complain of intermittent abdominal pain, bloating, excessive gas, and irregular bowel movements. Nausea, anorexia, passage of small hard stools, or diarrhea may present in some patients. **Table 17-23** lists the differential diagnosis for acute diverticulitis.

On physical exam, fullness or mild tenderness in the left lower quadrant can be elicited, and rebound or guarding is often absent. A CBC is warranted to evaluate for anemia. If a hemoccult test is positive, it is necessary to rule out colon cancer. The presence of bleeding is a significant risk for an unrelated lesion.[234]

If the physical exam excludes the presence of hemorrhoids as the source of the bleeding or in

Table 17-23 **DIAGNOSIS OF ACUTE DIVERTICULITIS**[231]

Differential Diagnosis	Clinical Scenarios and Diagnostic Considerations
Acute appendicitis	Suspect if RLQ symptoms exist or it does not resolve with medical therapy.
Crohn's disease	Suspect if apthous ulcers ("mouth sores") are present, there is perianal involvement, or chronic diarrhea.
Colonic carcinoma	Suspect if the patient has lost weight, or is bleeding. Diagnose with colonic evaluation after acute inflammation resolved.
Ischemic colitis	Suspect in a high-risk patient, or if bloody diarrhea or thumbprinting is present. Diagnose with limited flexible sigmoidoscopy.
Pseudomembranous colitis	Suspect with antibiotic use or if patient has diarrhea. Diagnose with stool toxin or limited flexible sigmoidoscopy.
Complicated ulcer disease	Suspect if patient has pneumoperitoneum or peritonitis, or with clinical history, NSAID use, or dyspepsia.
Ovarian cyst, abscess, torsion	Suspect if female patient with unilateral pain. Diagnose with pelvic or transvaginal ultrasound.
Ectopic pregnancy	Suspect in female patient of childbearing age. Diagnose with pregnancy test and ultrasound.

the presence of a prior history of diverticular bleeding, the patient should be referred to a gastroenterologist.

Imaging Techniques

Barium enema is the gold standard for diagnosing uncomplicated diverticular disease and noting its extent and severity. However, it is contraindicated when diverticular disease is complicated by abscess and peritonitis.[243] A gastroenterologist can perform colonoscopy after urgent bowel cleansing. Colonoscopy should be avoided in diverticular disease when the risk of perforation is high.

In acute diverticulosis or suspected perforation, water soluble contrast studies are preferred to barium. CT is helpful for cross-sectional imaging for complicated diverticular disease. CT has a reported sensitivity ranging from 85% to 97%[243] and also assists in diagnosing other complications or disease entities that may confuse the differential diagnosis. An alternate approach to diagnosis utilizes mesenteric angiography and radionuclide bleeding scans when there is active bleeding. Extravasation of contrast can be seen in the lumen of the colon.[235]

Treatment

Increasing the amount of dietary fiber uptake can be the first line of treatment for minimally problematic diverticular disease. Fiber combined with increased fluid intake causes stools to become softer and easier to pass. This decreases constipation and pressure on the bowel walls. However, rapidly increasing fiber intake can result in gas, bloating, and diarrhea. To eliminate this discomfort, patients should slowly increase their intake of fiber over six to eight weeks. Soluble fiber can be found in fruit, green leafy vegetables, and cereals; insoluble fiber is in fruits, vegetables, edible skins, whole grains, nuts, and commercial bulking agents.

Diverticulitis

Diverticulitis results from inflammation of herniated bowel pockets when food lodges in the diverticula and ferments. Diverticulitis can lead to subsequent perforation, with sequelae including infection, fever, abscess, and eventual peritonitis. The most common symptoms include left lower quadrant pain or tenderness, fever, and elevated white count with possible left shift. Signs of localized peritoneal inflammation may present with involuntary guarding. Patients with minimal symptoms can be treated on an outpatient basis. A clear liquid diet and broad-spectrum antibiotics are continued for seven to ten days. Patients are often hospitalized for bowel rest, intravenous hydration, and broad-spectrum intravenous antibiotics.[234,244] Pain medication is administered, but because morphine is thought to increase intracolonic pressure, it is rarely used. Nasogastric suction may be required. Improvement is anticipated in 48 to 72 hours.

Following the first episode of diverticulitis, surgery is seldom warranted. Only 20% to 30% of patients will have recurrent episodes[232] that may warrant elective surgical treatment so that perforation and obstruction are avoided. Sigmoid resection and primary anastomosis is the most common operation. Complications include abscess, peritonitis, fistula formation, and hemorrhage.[244]

Intestinal Worms

Parasitic worms infect more than 25% of the world's population.[245] The most common parasitic worms include the roundworm, *Ascaris lumbricoides*; the hookworms, *Necator americanus* and *Ancylostoma duodenale*; and the whipworm, *Trichuris trichiura*.[245] Children of school age are particularly at risk for the clinical manifestations of the disease, but adults are also affected, particularly when they live in or visit areas with poor sanitary conditions. Clinical features caused by these worms include iron-deficiency anemia and malnutrition. Treatment with anthelmintics is inexpensive and can decrease morbidity associated with these infections.[245–247]

Roundworm

Roundworm (*Ascaris lumbricoides*) disease affects more than 1.4 billion people and occurs mostly in developing countries. Immigrants and travelers to these countries account for four million individuals infected in the United States.[248] Transmission is fecal-oral.[248,249] Adult worms inhabit the small intestine and, once fertilized, pass their eggs through feces to contaminate soil. The eggs mature into larvae that are the infectious stage. In poor sanitary conditions, larvae are spread from human via soil (fertilizer or poor hygiene) to another human host.[248,249] Once ingested, the larvae migrate through the lungs during their maturation process and settle in the small intestine where they develop into adults.

Clinical manifestations of infection are pulmonary (cough, dyspnea, chest discomfort) and intestinal (anorexia, nausea, vomiting). Many individuals do not have evidence of clinical disease unless there is a heavy worm infestation. These cases can be associated with bowel obstruction and with hepatobiliary and pancreatic ascariasis.[248,249] Diagnosis is based on identifying ova or mature worms in stool specimens. Treatment includes mebendazole (Vermox) 100 mg twice daily for three days, pyrantel pamoate 11 mg/kg once, or a single dose of albendazole 400 mg.[248,249] Iron therapy is also needed to correct any anemia.

Hookworm

Human hookworm disease (*Ancylostoma duodenale* and *Necator americanus*) is widely distributed in underdeveloped tropical and subtropical parts of the world and has sporadic distribution in the Southeastern United States.[250,251] Infections in developed countries are more common in immigrants and travelers returning from areas where infections are endemic.[252]

Hookworms are small (1 cm), long, creamy white nematodes that live in the upper small intestine attached to the mucosa. Most worms will live in a host from two to five years. Adult worms lay eggs that pass in feces to hatch in warm, moist topsoil. In this larval stage, they become infective to humans. Contact with contaminated soil for as few as 5 to 10 minutes can allow the skin to be penetrated by the larvae. These larvae are carried through venous circulation to the lungs, where they can make their way up to the pharynx and esophagus to be swallowed. They enter the small intestine where they mature into adults.[250,251]

The adult female, once fertilized, produces an estimated 10,000 to 20,000 eggs per day that pass in the feces. The eggs first appear in the stool five to six weeks after initial invasion by the larvae.[250] The spread of infection is most prevalent in areas with poor sanitary practices, that is, cultures where infected individuals defecate in areas frequented by others and those that use human excrement as fertilizer for crops.[250] The incidence decreases once adequate sanitation procedures are utilized.

Symptoms may begin early in the course of infection with intense pruritus, edema, and erythema at the site of larval penetration. Once in the lungs, larvae may produce mild coughing and wheezing. Additional symptoms include epigastric pain, diarrhea, and weight loss. The major clinical findings attributed to hookworm disease are iron deficiency anemia, eosinophilia, and chronic protein malnutrition.[250,251,253] Diagnosis is based upon fecal smear examination for hookworm ova. The drug of choice for treatment is mebendazole 100 mg twice a day for three days, with the second choice being single dose abendazole. Iron replacement is recommended for the anemia.[250,251,253]

Whipworm

Trichuris trichiura (whipworm) is the third most common nematode worldwide.[254] In the United States, this is seen mostly in immigrants from tropical areas and in rural areas of the Southeast. Infection is caused by ingestion of whipworm eggs from contaminated drinking water and food. The eggs hatch into larvae in the small intestine and migrate to the proximal colon as they mature into adults.[254] Many individuals are asymptomatic, but severe infestations can cause abdominal pain, diarrhea, weight loss, and anemia. Diagnosis is made by the presence of whipworm ova in the feces. Whipworm is effectively treated with Mebendazole, 100 mg for three days, or a single 400-mg dose of albendazole.[254]

Rectal Bleeding

Definitions

Rectal bleeding includes lower GI bleeding and is alternately described as colonic bleeding or small bowel bleeding. In this chapter, lower gastrointestinal bleeding refers to bleeding from below the ligament of Treitz. *Hematochezia* refers to bright red bleeding from the rectum. *Melena* is tarry colored, "sticky" malodorous stool. Degradation of hemoglobin from rectal bleeding over at least 14 hours causes the black color [235] and sticky texture. A minimum of 60 mL of blood will produce a black stool, and volume more than 60 mL can produce melena for up to seven days.[255] Other causative agents of black stool include bismuth (found in anti-diarrheal products), licorice, and iron preparations. Maroon-colored stools evolve from maroon-colored blood mixed with melena and are often seen as an indication of lower GI bleeding, but can also represent upper GI bleeding that had a rapid transit time through the GI tract. The American Gastroenterological Association has delineated guidelines for the standardization of the term *occult bleeding* in reference to chronic GI blood loss. It is defined as the initial presentation of a positive *fecal occult blood test (FOBT)* result and/or iron-deficiency anemia when there is no other obvious source of the bleeding.[256] *Obscure bleeding* refers to bleeding of unknown origin that is recurrent or persistent in nature, after a negative initial or primary endoscopy. Further delineation of terms includes the following: obscure occult bleeding is recurrent iron deficiency anemia and/or a recurrent positive FOBT. Obscure-overt is the recurrent passage of visible blood.[256]

Incidence

The incidence of lower GI bleeding is estimated to be between 20 and 27 per 100,000 adults.[237] It is less frequent than upper GI bleeding, but in all GI bleeding accounts for more than 300,000 hospitalizations annually in the United States.[257] The majority of patients who have lower GI bleeding (85%) have bleeding episodes that are self-limiting and remain hemodynamically stable.[235] Risk for GI bleeding is increased by ingestion of aspirin and calcium antagonists.[258–261] Excessive or long-term use of NSAIDs and COX inhibitors has been associated with GI bleeding. The risk of dying from lower GI bleeding has been reported as 3.6% in the United States.[261]

The most common etiology is from diverticulosis, followed by angiodysplasia, cancer, polyps, colitis, and anorectal sources.[256]

Angiodysplasia

Angiodysplasia, a degenerative structural abnormality of the normally distributed vasculature (also referred to as vascular ectasia), can cause either brisk bleeding or slow intermittent blood loss.[257] The incidence is 10% to 40% of cases of acute lower GI bleeding.[262,263] Most ectasia are degenerative lesions seen in an aging population. Those patients in whom this disease is diagnosed by either colonoscopy or helical CT can be treated with angiographic embolization or endoscopic techniques to achieve hemostasis.[264]

Neoplasms and Postpolypectomy Bleeding

Neoplastic lesions are seen in 2% to 26% of cases of lower GI bleeding.[265] The presenting complaint is often a history of a small amount of intermittent rectal bleeding.

Colonoscopy is the diagnostic tool of choice to further investigate the etiology of the bleeding. If the lesion(s) are small, they can be excised during the colonoscopy. If the lesions are large or extensive, a surgical approach is used for definitive treatment.

Polyps will need to be removed during colonoscopy as well. Post-polypectomy bleeding is seen anywhere from immediately to 17 days after the procedure.[266] Endoscopy can be utilized to resolve the bleeding in the majority of cases.

Hemorrhoids and Anal Fissures

Perianal disease encompasses both hemorrhoids and anal fissures. They are a common cause of minor rectal bleeding. Because the patient often does not seek treatment, the incidence is probably grossly under-reported. Hemorrhoids are seen with equal frequency in men and women, with a higher incidence in the fourth to sixth decades. They are rarely seen in women under age 20.

The *dentate line* is the demarcation line that distinguishes between external and internal hemorrhoids. Internal hemorrhoids arise from the superior hemorrhoidal vascular plexus; their primary locations correspond to the end branches of the middle and superior hemorrhoidal veins.[267,268] They are normal vascular tissue. As a consequence of aging or aggravating conditions, the muscle fibers that attach the vascular cushions to the anal sphincter become stretched and deteriorate.[267,268] Congestion, edema, and bleeding then ensue. Internal hemorrhoids, unlike external hemorrhoids, have a grading system (**Table 17-24**).

Aggravating conditions that predispose women to hemorrhoids include pregnancy, diarrhea, pelvic tumors, prolonged sitting, and straining with defecation. Chronic constipation, obesity, and low-fiber diets also predispose patients to hemorrhoids.

The symptoms of hemorrhoids are caused by the edema and displacement of the submucosal lining of the anal canal. The painless bleeding seen with this disease is usually from internal hemorrhoids. Women will often describe minimal bright red bleeding noted on the toilet tissue or around stools. Other symptoms of internal hemorrhoids include prolapse, itching, and a mucus discharge. The itching of the perianal

Table 17-24 INTERNAL HEMORRHOID CLASSIFICATION[267]

Grade	Description
Grade I	Visible with anoscope; may extend into anal canal
Grade I	Prolapses outside anal canal; may reduce spontaneously
Grade III	Same degree of prolapse; requires manual reduction
Grade IV	Unable to be reduced; may strangulate

skin is caused by exposure to leakage of rectal contents around the hemorrhoid. If harsh cleaning or scratching occurs, the skin may become more inflamed and a recurrent cycle develops. Severe pain may occur if the prolapsed internal hemorrhoid becomes strangulated.

External hemorrhoids are dilations of the inferior (external) hemorrhoidal plexus, below the dentate line, and are covered with squamous epithelium that contains many pain receptors.[267] External hemorrhoids may become thrombosed, and extreme pain usually is seen in the acute phase of this condition. Eventually, symptoms improve when the overlying anoderm sloughs; at this time bleeding may occur. Anal skin tags are the result of healing redundant skin. Their only significance is the potential impact on hygiene after defecation.

An examination of the anorectal anatomy begins with inspection for any obvious lesions, changes in color, and assessment of discomfort on palpation. Observation can be made of fistulae, perianal dermatitis, or condyloma. Digital examination is best performed with the patient in the left decubitus position. If the patient is able to strain during the exam, it will reduce the discomfort. The examining finger performs a 360° sweep around the anal canal. Anoscopic assessment is an office procedure to visualize the anal canal.

Referral to a primary care physician or gastroenterologist is indicated when the diagnosis of hemorrhoids is not confirmed with the digital exam. The diagnosis of internal hemorrhoids is accomplished with the use of anoscopy or sigmoidoscopy. If a fresh clot is seen at the site of the hemorrhoid, the diagnosis of the etiology of the bleeding is confirmed. Hemorrhoidal disease is not diagnosed definitively until all other sources of visible or occult bleeding have been excluded. The differential diagnosis of rectal bleeding includes external hemorrhoids, rectal varices, fissures, ulcers, polyps, and tumors.[235]

Nonsurgical therapy for hemorrhoids consists of increased dietary fiber, lubricant rectal suppositories with or without steroids, and warm sitz baths. See **Table 17-25** for dietary sources of fiber. Preparations made with psyllium seeds and methylcellulose add bulk to the stool. The increased bulk causes the stool to become softer and easier to pass.

Local anesthetics can be used for symptomatic relief from the discomfort of painful external hemorrhoids. Choices include 5% Lidocaine ointment, dibucaine ointment or cream (0.5%–1.0%), benzocaine, dyclonin, and pramoxine (**Table 17-26**). Witch hazel acts as an astringent. If it is kept cold, the amelioration of discomfort when applied may be improved. Use of a topical steroid may reduce inflammation. Topical steroids and analgesic creams or ointments should not be used for more than one week because of the potential for tissue inflammation or thinning of the skin.

Anoscopic therapy involves the following choices of treatment: injection sclerotherapy, rubber band ligation, cryosurgery, infrared photocoagulation, and electrocoagulation.[268] Surgical treatment is utilized when medical or anoscopic methods fail. It also may be used when the hemorrhoids no longer can be reduced man-

Table 17-25 **DIETARY SOURCES OF FIBER**

Fruits	Vegetables	Legumes	Grains
Apples (with skin)	Beans	Baked beans	Whole wheat breads
Peaches (with skin)	Cabbage	Cooked dried peas	Whole wheat cereals
Raspberries	Broccoli	Cooked kidney beans	Bran
Oranges	Carrots	Cooked or canned lima beans	Rye bread
Bananas	Brussels sprouts	Cooked lentils	Pumpernickel bread
Dried apricots	Peas	Cooked navy beans	
Dates	Potatoes		
Prunes	Parsnips		
Raisins			
Pear (with skin)			

ually. Signs and symptoms of thrombosis of an external hemorrhoid include acute perianal pain in association with a palpable mass. The pain often lasts two to three days, but may persist longer and gradually resolve. The appearance of a thrombosed hemorrhoid is that of an edematous,[268] exquisitely tender area, a portion of which appears much darker in color. If the hemorrhoid becomes thrombosed, excision will provide definitive treatment, but must be done within 48 to 72 hours of the onset of symptoms.

A meta-analysis of 18 studies compared the approaches to treatment. The following conclusions were delineated. Hemorrhoidectomy was more effective than sphincter dilation or rubber band ligation in preventing recurrent symptoms. Surgery was associated with more complications and pain. Rubber band ligation was more effective than sclerotherapy and was associated with the need for fewer further therapies.[269]

Anal Fissures

Anal fissures are tears or rents in the distal anal canal. They may be caused by trauma from the passage of firm stool and are seen in patients with Crohn's disease, tuberculosis, and leukemia. Fissures can be either acute or chronic in nature. Examination of the anal tissue is difficult to perform in many patients because of the severe discomfort at the site of the fissure. On inspection, a new fissure has the appearance of a recent laceration. If the fissure has become chronic, its appearance will include a slightly raised area around the defect, and white horizontal fibers of the internal anal sphincter are seen at the base of the defect.[270] The location where the fissures are most often seen is at the midline, primarily in the posterior aspect and secondarily in the anterior aspect of the anal

canal. Spasm occurs at the site of the exposed internal sphincter muscle. The spasm is painful and also causes the fissure to pull further apart, thus aggravating the condition and preventing healing from occurring. Elevated anal pressure is seen in patients with fissures. The mechanism has been hypothesized to be a result of increased tone of the internal anal sphincter. Blood perfusion is inversely related to pressure. Because the perfusion in the area of the fissures is reduced, it seems logical that medication to increase perfusion would be beneficial. Topical nitroglycerin increases the blood flow and thus decreases the pressure of the internal anal sphincter. The recommended dose is 0.2% topical glyceryl trinitrate, one half of a pea-size amount applied twice per day for six to eight weeks.[271] This concentration needs to be prepared by a pharmacist because it is not commercially available in the United States. A study performed to evaluate the effectiveness of this approach found that the success rate of this regimen was lower in patients who had concomitant hemorrhoids and duration of fissures more than six months.[271] A multicenter study designed to compare differing dosages concluded that the highest healing rate was found with a 0.4% concentration of gyceryl trinitrate ointment.[272]

Medical therapy of anal fissures is designed to promote healing and disrupt the cycle of spasm and resultant inadequate or failed healing of the defect. Relaxation of the anal sphincter, atraumatic passage of stool, and analgesia are the main goals of medical therapy. Sitz baths help to promote relaxation of the sphincter; stool softeners and bulking agents prevent firm stools; and topical anesthetic creams provide pain relief.

Varous modalities have been employed with variable success. Botulinum toxin has been used

Table 17-26 HEMORRHOIDAL THERAPEUTICS

Type	Generic/Trade Name	Form	Dosage	Side Effects/Comments
Bulk-forming agents				
	Psyllium			
	Metamucil	Powder	1–3 tsp, up to qid	Mix with at least 8 oz liquid
	Metamucil	Wafer	1–2 up to tid	Take with at least 8 oz liquid
	Fiberall	Powder	1 tsp up to tid	Take with at least 8 oz liquid
	Konsyl	Powder	1 full tsp or 6-g packet in 8 oz liquid	Increase PO fluids
	Konsyl	Tablets	625 mg/tab 2 tabs 1–4 x/d	Increase PO fluids
	Polycarbophil			
	Fibercon	Tablet	2 tabs /1–4 x/d	Not to exceed 6 g in 24 h
	Perdiem	Caplet	2 caplets up to qid	
	Mitrolan	Chewable tablets	500 mg 2 tabs qid	
	Methylcellulose			
	Citrucel	Caplets	2 caplets up to 6 x/d	Take with at least 8 oz liquid
	Citrucel	Powder	1 heaping tablespoon up to tid	Take with at least 8 oz liquid
	Malt soup extract			
	Maltsupex	Tablets	4 tabs 4 x/d then 2–4 tabs/h	
	Maltsupex	Powder	2 tsp for 3–4 d, then 1–2 tsp/h	
	Maltsupex	Liquid	2 tsp bid for 3–4 d, then 1–2 tsp/h	
Stool softeners				
	Docusate sodium/ Colace	Capsule	50 mg/1–6 daily	Take as single or divided doses
	Docusate sodium/ Colace	Capsule	100 mg/1–3 daily	
	Docusate sodium/ Colace	Syrup/ 20 mg	15–45 mL 1 or 2 x/d	

Table 17-26 HEMORRHOIDAL THERAPEUTICS *(continued)*

Type	Generic/Trade Name	Form	Dosage	Side Effects/Comments
	Modane Soft Capsules	Capsule	1–3 caps/d	
	Modane Bulk Powder	Powder	1 tsp in 8 oz liquid 1–3 x/d	
	Docusate calcium/ Surfak	50 mg capsule	2–3 caps/d	
	Docusate calcium/ Surfak	240 mg	1 cap/d	
Steroids				
	Hydrocortisone acetate	Suppositories,	25 mg	2–4 x/d p.r.n. after defecation. Pregnancy category C maximum use 2–3 weeks
	Hydrocortisone acetate/CaldeCORT light/Cortaid/ Lamacort	Cream/ ointment	1–2.5%	2–4 x/d after defecation. Pregnancy category C
	Hydrocortisone acetate/Anusol HC-1	Ointment`	1.12%	Apply not more than 3–4 x/d Pregnancy category C
Anesthetic/ steroid	Pramoxine HCL/ Anusol Hemorrhoidal Ointment	Ointment, cream, lotion, foam	1%/1%. Apply externally up to 5 x/d	May be applied partially into anus
	Pramoxine + Hydrocortisone/ Analpram HC	Cream	1%/1%	2–4 times daily Pregnancy category C
	Pramoxine + Hydrocortisone/ Analpram HC	Cream or Lotion	2.5%/1%	2–4 x/d Pregnancy category C
Topical Anesthetic				
	Dibucaine/ Nupercainal	Ointment	0.5% applied topically qid p.r.n.	Do not use if skin is broken
	Dibucaine/ Cinchocaine	Cream	1.0% applied topically qid p.r.n.	Do not use if skin is broken
	Lidocaine/Lignocaine/ Xylocaine	Ointment	5%	Prn/do not use if skin is broken

(continues)

Table 17-26 **HEMORRHOIDAL THERAPEUTICS** *(continued)*

Type	Generic/Trade Name	Form	Dosage	Side Effects/Comments
	Benzocaine/ Americaine Anesthetic Lubricant	Lotion, cream	6%	Apply topically p.r.n.
	Benzocaine	Aerosol/spray	5%–20%	Apply topically p.r.n.
	Benzocaine	Liquid	20%	Apply topically p.r.n.
	Benzocaine	Gel	15%–20%	Apply topically p.r.n.
	Benzocaine	Ointment	20%	Apply topically p.r.n.
	Dyclonine/ Dyclocaine	Solution	0.5%–1.0%	Apply topically p.r.n. Alleviates pain in 2–10 min. Pregnancy category C
	Pramoxine/ Pramocaine	Gel, cream, lotion, spray	1% 3–4 x/d	Alleviates pain in 2–5 min extended duration of action; apply topically Pregnancy category C
Antipruritic				
	Witch hazel/Tucks	Liquid or pads	50%/apply locally up to 6 x/d	May use as a wipe after defecation
	Hamamelis water	Liquid	Apply locally up to 6 x/d	

Sources: 1. Data from: Medical Economics Staff. Drug Information for the Health Care Professional: Micromedex: 21st ed.: 2001. 2. Lowy S. Hemorrhoids in Singleton JK, Sandowski SA, GreenHrnandez C, Horvath TV, DiGregorio RV, Holzemer SP. Philadelphia: Lippincott, Williams & Wilkins. 1999; pp 309–311. 3. Saver D, Soll AH, Targownik L. Hemorrhoids [Online]. 2004 [cited April 7]; Available from URL: http://www.firstconsult.com.

to treat chronic anal fissures. The mechanism of action is the inhibition of the release of acetylcholine from nerve endings, thereby affecting the spasm of the sphincter. Temporary fecal or flatus incontinence is a possible side effect. A small study devised to evaluate the long-term course of patients treated with botulinum has shown a recurrence rate as high as 42%.[273] The efficacy of botulinum toxin and nitroglycerin were compared in a study of 50 adult patients.[274] Analysis suggested a superior result with the use of botulinum; however, some of the patients improved

when the alternate medication was tried. However, pooled analysis does not support the efficacy of these approaches. A 2003 Cochrane review reporting the results of a metaanalysis of 31 randomized controlled studies that used various medical treatments (nitroglycerin ointment, isosorbide dinitrate, botulinum toxin (Botox), diltiazem, nifedipine (hydrocortisone, lignocaine, bran, placebo) concluded that medical treatment was only marginally better than placebo. Surgery was found to be significantly more effective.[275]

Surgical therapy for anal fissures is used when healing has not occurred with the use of medical approaches. The goal of the surgery is to achieve relaxation of the internal anal sphincter. Lateral internal sphincterotomy involves the division of the internal anal sphincter from its distal-most end for a distance equal to the length of the fissure, or up to the dentate line.[270] Risks of this surgery include infection, fistulas, and incontinence of flatus or stool, which are usually transient.[270] A long-term follow-up study of this method reported a 3% rate of deleterious effect on quality of life.[276]

Colon Cancer

Colon cancer is the third most common cancer found in women.[277] Presenting signs and symptoms in the majority of patients include, in order of frequency, abdominal pain, change in bowel habit, hematochezia or melena, weakness, anemia without other GI symptoms, and weight loss. The etiology of the abdominal pain can be because of a partial obstruction, peritoneal dissemination, or intestinal perforation. Hematochezia is more frequently seen in cancers of the rectum.[278] Iron deficiency anemia is a more common finding in advanced stages of colorectal cancer (CRC). The amount of bleeding reflects the site of the cancer more than the stage of the disease; cecal and ascending colon tumors have a fourfold higher amount of bleeding than that caused by cancers at other sites.[279] When hemorrhage is one of the presenting signs in CRC, it was initially thought that the disease process was in an earlier stage; however, this observation has not been born out in subsequent analysis.[280] Tumors in the right side of the colon tend to have lesions that are fungating or polypoid, whereas left-sided lesions are more often annular or encircling lesions that constrict and narrow the bowel lumen. This is the etiology of the symptoms of constipation, diarrhea, or bowel obstruction.[281,282] Abdominal distention and NV are other symptoms seen in CRC. Fifteen to twenty percent of patients will present initially with metastatic disease. Signs and symptoms of advanced disease include RUQ pain; abdominal distention; early satiety; supraclavicular adenopathy; or periumbilical nodules.[280] The most common sites of metastases are regional lymph nodes, liver, lung, and peritoneum.[280]

CRC is diagnosed either as a result of the clinical workup for the previous signs and symptoms or as a consequence of indicated routine screening. The use of FOBT in the absence of a positive family history of CRC or any other risk factor should be performed during annual health screening exams beginning at age 50. The rationale for this approach is that CRC is infrequently found in women under age 50. Studies have shown that colonoscopic detection of CRC is uncommon in asymptomatic patients who are younger than 50 years of age.[283] FOBT should be done by obtaining two samples from each of three consecutive stools. Sigmoidoscopy and colonoscopy are other choices for initial screening. The American College of Gastroenterology recommends colonoscopy as the first choice for a screening methodology.[284]

Women with increased risk for developing CRC should be offered screening and advised of various screening options. Twenty-five percent of patients who develop CRC will have had a positive family history.[285] Increased risks include the number of first degree relatives (parent, sibling, or child) with a history of CRC or adenomatous polyps, the age at diagnosis, and a history of familial adenomatous polyposis, or hereditary nonpolyposis colon cancer. These all increase the risk in the range of two- to sixfold.[286] Because the average risk of CRC in patients with a positive family history is the same at age 40 as the general population at age 50, routine screening is advised beginning at age 40 in this population. Additionally, many experts recommend that screening be initiated ten years before the age of occurrence of the index CRC. IBD in the form of either ulcerative colitis or Crohn's disease is associated with an increased risk of CRC, especially if the disease is extensive or has been present for a minimum of eight to ten years.[286]

The incidence of colon cancer in pregnancy has been described as 1 in 13,000.[287,288] Symptoms of colon cancer in pregnancy are similar to those in nonpregnant women. Rectal bleeding is not as frequent as abdominal pain, constipation, NV, and abdominal distention.[289,290] The size and location of the cancer will influence symptoms. Left colonic cancers tend to cause partial or complete intestinal obstruction; larger lesions are more likely to cause obstruc-tion.[290,291] Distal cancers are more often associated with rectal bleeding than are proximal cancers. Signs of CRC in pregnancy include anemia and associated fatigue and weakness. Hypoactive or high-pitched bowel sounds also may be heard in cases of obstruction. Colonic perforation is seen slightly more commonly in pregnant women than in the general population. Signs of perforation include abdominal tenderness, rebound discomfort, abdominal rigidity, and hypoactive bowel sounds.[290,291]

Women frequently present to a gynecology clinic with abdominal pain, believing that abdominal and pelvic complaints will be gynecologic in origin. Therefore, it is essential that the woman's health care provider understands the range of differential diagnoses. In this way, a thorough history and physical exam and appropriate laboratory studies can be obtained. If the results dictate, an appropriate and timely referral to a specialist should be achieved.

References

1. Kamin R, Nowicki T, Courtney D, Powers R. Pearls and pitfalls in the emergency department evaluation of abdominal pain. *Emerg Med Clin North Am.* 2003; 21:61–72.

2. Powers R, Gertler A. Abdominal pain in the ED: Stability and change over 20 years. *Am J Emerg Med.* 1995;13:301–303.

3. Visser B, Glasgow R, Mulvihill K, Mulvihill S. Safety and timing of nonobstetric abdominal surgery in pregnancy. *Dig Surg.* 2001;18:409–417.

4. Seidel HM, Ball JW, Dains JE, Benedict GW. Abdomen. In: *Mosby's Guide to Physical Examination.* 5th ed. St. Louis: Mosby; 2003.

5. Shaw B. Primary care for women: Comprehensive assessment of gastrointestinal disorders. *J Nurse Midwifery.* 1995;40:216–230.

6. Graber MA. General surgery. In: Graber MA, Toth PP, Herting RL, editors. University of Iowa. *The Family Practice Handbook.* 3rd ed. St. Louis: Mosby; 1997. pp. 380–411.

7. Charney P, Khaund R, Rucker LM, Sieldecki D. Gastroenterology. In: Rucker LM, editor. *Essentials of Adult Ambulatory Care.* Baltimore: Williams & Wilkins; 1997.

8. Varney H, Kriebs JM, Gegor, CL. Basics of management of care. In: Varney H, Kriebs JM, Gegor CL. *Varney's Midwifery.* 4th ed. Boston: Jones and Bartlett; 2004. pp 29–46.

9. Barkauskas VH, Baumann LC, Darling-Fisher CS. *Health and Physical Assessment.* 3rd ed. St. Louis: Mosby; 2002.

10. Shaw B. Primary care for women: Management and treatment of gastrointestinal disorders. *J Nurse Midwifery.* 1996;41:155–172.

11. Finkel MA. Abdominal pain. In: Scharder J, Hayden SR, Wolfe R, Barken RM, Rosen P, editors. *Rosen and*

Barkin's 5-Minute Emergency Medicine Consult. Baltimore: Lippincott Williams & Wilkins; 1999.

12. Quigley EMM, Hasler WL, Parkman HP. AGA technical review on nausea and vomiting. *Gastroenterology*. 2001;120:263–286.

13. McQuaid KR. Nausea and vomiting. In: Tierney LM, McPhee SJ, Papadakis MA, editors. *Current Medical Diagnosis and Treatment*. New York: McGraw-Hill Companies; 2003.

14. Lee M. Nausea and vomiting. In: Feldman M, Friedman LS, Sleisenger MH, editors. *Sleisenger and Fordtran's Gastrointestinal and Liver Disease: Pathophysiology, Diagnosis, Management*. 7th ed. Philadelphia: Saunders; 2002. pp. 119–130.

15. Koch KL. Approach to the patient with nausea and vomiting. In: Yamada T, Alpers DH, Owyang C, Powell DW, Silverstein FE, editors. *Textbook of Gastroenterology*. 2nd ed. Philadelphia: JB Lippincott; 1995. pp. 731–745.

16. Greenberg M. Nausea and vomiting. In: Rosen P, Barken R, Hayden S, Scharder J, Wolfe R. *The 5 Minute Emergency Medicine Consult*. Philadelphia: Lippincott Williams & Wilkins; 1999. pp. 1216–1217.

17. Friedman LS, Isselbacher KJ. Nausea, vomiting, and indigestion. In: Fauci AS, Brownwald E, Isselbacker KJ, Wilson JD, Martin JB, Kasper DL, et al., editors. *Harrison's Principles of Internal Medicine*. 14th ed. New York: McGraw-Hill Companies; 1998. pp. 230–236.

18. Garrett K, Tsuruta K, Walker S, Jackson S, Sweat M. Managing nausea and vomiting: Current strategies. *Crit Care Nurse*. 2003;23:31–50.

19. Hasler WL. Approach to the patient with nausea and vomiting. In: Yamada T, Alpers DH, Kaplowitz N, Laine L, Owyang C, Powell DW, editors. *Textbook of Gastroenterology*. 4th ed. Philadelphia: Lippincott Williams & Wilkins; 2003.

20. Parkman HP. New advances in the diagnosis and management of nausea and vomiting. *Case Manager*. 2002;13:83–87.

21. Quinlan JD, Hill DA. Nausea and vomiting of pregnancy. *Am Fam Physician*. 2003;68:121–128.

22. ACOG. Nausea and vomiting of pregnancy. ACOG Practice Bulletin, Clinical Management Guidelines for Obstetrician-Gynecologist, 2004; 52:803–815.

23. Koch KL, Frissora CL. Nausea and vomiting during pregnancy. *Gastroenterol Clin North Am*. 2003;32:201–234.

24. Jewell D. Nausea and vomiting in early pregnancy. *Am Fam Physician*. 2003;68:1561–1570.

25. Harris LA, Kim MK. Acute gastroenteritis. In: Leppert PC, Peipert JF, editors. *Primary Care for Women*. 2nd ed. Philadelphia: Lippincott Williams & Williams; 2004. pp. 451–458.

26. Thielman NM, Guerrant RL. Acute infectious diarrhea. *N Engl J Med*. 2004;350:38–47.

27. Dupont HL. The practice parameters committee of the American College of Gastroenterology: Guidelines on acute infectious diarrhea in adults. *Am J Gastroenterol*. 1997;92:1962–1975.

28. Salen PN, Heller MB. Diarrhea and proctitis. In: Harwood-Nuss A, editor. *The Clinical Practice of Emergency Medicine*. Philadelphia: Lippincott Williams & Wilkins; 2001.

29. Locke GR 3rd, Pemberton JH, Phillips SF. AGA technical review on constipation. *Gastroenterology*. 2000; 119:1761–1766.

30. Sonnenberg A, Koch TR. Physician visits in the United States for constipation: 1956–1986. *Dig Dis Sci*. 1989;34:606–611.

31. Rich HG. Constipation. In: Leppert PC, Peipert JF, editors. *Primary Care for Women*. 2nd ed. Philadelphia: Lippincott Williams & Wilkins; 2004. pp. 476–481.

32. McQuaid KR. Alimentary Tract. In: Tierney LM, McPhee SJ, Papadakis MA, editors. *Current Medical Diagnosis and Treatment*. 42nd ed. New York: McGraw-Hill; 2003.

33. Wolf JL. Bowel function. In: Carlson KJ, Eisenstat SA, Frigoletto FD, Schiff I, editors. *Primary Care of Women*. 2nd ed. St. Louis: Mosby; 2002. pp. 133–141.

34. Stollman N, Raskin J. Diverticular disease of the colon. *J Clin Gastroenterol*. 1999;29:241–252.

35. Schwizer W, Fox M. *Helicobacter pylori* and gastroesophageal reflux disease: A complex organism in a complex host. *J Pediatr Gastroenterol Nutr*. 2004;38: 12–15.

36. Ray SW, Secrest J, Ch'ien APY, Corey RS. Managing gastroesophageal reflux disease. *Nurse Pract*. 2002; 27: 36–53.

37. Flynn CA. The evaluation and treatment of adults with gastroesophageal reflux disease. *J Fam Pract*. 2001;50:57–58,61–63.

38. O'Malley P. Gastric ulcers and GERD: The new "plagues" of the 21st century update for the clinical nurse specialist. *Clin Nurse Spec*. 2003;17:286–289.

39. Williams JL. Gastroesophageal reflux disease: Clinical manifestations. *Gastroenterol Nurs*. 2003;26:195–200.

40. Tutuian R. Management of gastroesophageal reflux disease. *Am J Med Sci*. 2003;326:309–318.

41. DeVault KR, Castell DO. Guidelines for the diagnosis and treatment of gastroesophageal reflux disease. *Arch Intern Med.* 1995;155:2165–2173.

42. American Gastroenterology Association. Improving the management of GERD evidence based therapeutic strategies. 2002.

43. Cohen P. Gastroesophageal reflux disease. In: Singleton JK, Sandowski SA, Green-Hernandez C, Horvath TV, DiGregorio RV, Holzemer SP, editors. *Primary Care.* Philadelphia: Lippincott; 1999. pp. 273–276.

44. Szarka LA, DeVault KR, Murray JA. Diagnosing gastroesophageal reflux disease. *Mayo Clin Proc.* 2001; 76:97–101.

45. Howden CW, Hunt RH. Guidelines for the management of *Helicobacter pylori* infection. *Am J Gastroenterol.* 1998;93:2330–2338.

46. Spechler SJ. Clinical manifestations and esophageal complications of GERD. *Am J Med Sci.* 2003;326: 279–284.

47. Ferri FF. *Ferri's Clinical Advisor Instant Diagnosis and Treatment.* St. Louis: Mosby; 2003. p. 356.

48. Poneros JM, Friedman LS. Gastroesophageal reflux and peptic ulcer disease. In: Carlson KJ, Eisenstat SA, Frigoletto FD, Schiff I, editors. *Primary Care of Women.* 2nd ed. St. Louis: Mosby; 2002. pp. 119–125.

49. Beckingham IJ. ABC of diseases of liver, pancreas, and biliary system gallstone disease. *BMJ.* 2001;322: 91–94.

50. DeVault KR, Castell DO. Updated guidelines for the diagnosis and treatment of gastroesophageal reflux disease. *Am J Gastroenterol.* 1999;94:1434–1442.

51. Zimmermann EM, Christman GM. Approach to the female patient with gastrointestinal disease. In: Yamada T. editor. *Textbook of Gastroenterology.* 2nd ed. Philadelphia: JB Lippincott; 1995. pp. 1023–1039.

52. Everhart J, Khare M, Hill M, Maurer K. Prevalence and ethnic differences in gallbladder disease in the U.S. *Gastroenterology.* 1999;117:632–639.

53. Attili A, Carulli N, Roda E, Barbara B, Capocaccia L, Menotti A, et al. Epidemiology of gallstone disease in Italy: Prevalence data of the multicenter Italian study on cholelithiasis (MICOL). *Am J Epidemiol.* 1995;141:158–165.

54. Barbara L, Sama C, Morselli-Labate Taroni F, Rusticali A, Festi D, et al. A ten-year incidence of gallstone disease. The Sirmione Study. *J Hepatol.* 1993;18 Suppl 1:S43, Poster Abstract.

55. Valdivieso V, Covarrubias C, Siegel F, Cruz F. Pregnancy and cholelithiasis: Pathogenesis and natural course of gallstones diagnosed in early puerperium. *Hepatology.* 1993;17:1–4.

56. Kaufman J, Carr-Locke D. Gallstones. In: Carlson K and Eisenstat S, editors. *Primary Care of Women.* 2nd ed. St. Louis, MO: C.V. Mosby; 2002. pp. 111–118.

57. Hulley S, Grady D, Bush T, Furberg C, Herrington D, Riggs B, et al. Heart and Estrogen/progestin Replacement Study (HERS) Research Group. Randomized trial of estrogen plus progestin for secondary prevention of coronary heart disease in postmenopausal women. *JAMA.* 1998;280:605–613.

58. Grodstein F, Colditz G, Stampfer M. Postmenopausal hormone use and cholecystectomy in a large prospective study. *Obstet Gynecol.* 1994;83:5–11.

59. Strom B, Tamragouri R, Morse M, Lazar E, West S, Stolley P, et al. Oral contraceptives and other risk factors for gallbladder disease. *Clin Pharmacol Ther.* 1986; 39:335–341.

60. Thijs C, Knipschild P. Oral contraceptives and the risk of gallbladder disease: A meta analysis. *Am J Public Health.* 1993;83:1113–1120.

61. Stampfer M, Maclure K, Colditz G, Manson J, Willett W. Risk of symptomatic gallstones in women with severe obesity. *Am J Clin Nutr.* 1992;55:652–658.

62. Shiffman M, Sugarman H, Kellum J, Brewer W, Moore E. Gallstone formation after rapid weight loss: A prospective study in patients undergoing gastric surgery for treatment of morbid obesity. *Am J Gastroenterol.* 1991;86:1000–1005.

63. Shiffman M, Kaplan G, Brinkman-Kaplan V, Vickers F. Prophylaxis against gallstone formation with urodeoxycholic acid in patients in very low calorie diet program. *Ann Intern Med.* 1995;122:899–905.

64. Leitzmann M, Rimm F, Willett W, Spiegelman D, Grodstein F, Stampfer M, et al. Recreational physical activity and the risk of cholecystectomy in women. *N Engl J Med.* 1999;341:777–784.

65. Leitzmann M, Stampfer M, Willett N, Spiegelman D. Coffee intake is associated with lower risk of symptomatic gallstone disease in women. *Gastroenterology.* 2002;123:1823–1830.

66. Carey MC. Pathogenesis of gallstones. *Am J Surg.* 1993;165:410–419.

67. Bateson M. Fortnightly review: Gallbladder disease. *BMJ.* 1999;318:1745–1748.

68. Zakko S, Srb S, Ramsby G. Sensitivity of percutaneous endoscopy compared with ultrasonography in the detection of residue or mucosal lesions after topical gallbladder dissolution. *Gastrointest Endosc.* 1995;42: 434–438.

69. Fink-Bennett D, Freitas J, Ripley S, Bree R. The sensitivity of hepatobiliary imaging and real time ultrasonography in the detection of acute cholecystitis. *Arch Surg.* 1985;120:904–906.

70. Park M, Yu J, Kim Y, Kim M, Kim J, Lee S, et al. Acute cholecystitis: Comparison of MR cholangiography and ultrasound. *Radiology.* 1998;209:781–785.

71. Berk C. Gallbladder. In: Singleton J, Sandowski S, Green-Hernandez C, Horath T, DiGregorio R, Holzemer S, editors. *Primary Care.* Philadelphia: Lippincott; 1999. pp. 267–272.

72. Jamidar P, Beck G, Hoffman B, Lehman G, Hawes R, Agrawal R, et al. Endoscopy retrograde cholangiopancreatography in pregnancy. *Am J Gastroenterol.* 1995;90:1263–1267.

73. Barthel J, Chowdhury T, Miedema B. Endoscopic sphincterotomy for the treatment of gallstone pancreatitits during pregnancy. *Surg Endosc.* 1998;12: 394–399.

74. Nesbitt T, Kay H, McCoy MC, Herbert W. Endoscopic management of biliary disease during pregnancy. *Obstet Gynecol.* 1996;87:806–809.

75. Cappell M. The fetal safety and clinical efficacy of gastrointestinal endoscopy during pregnancy. *Gastroenterol Clin North Am.* 2003;32:123–179.

76. Kallou A, Kantsevoy S. Gallstones and biliary diseases. *Gastroenterology Clin Office Pract.* 2001;28: 1–19.

77. Ahmed A, Cheung R, Keeffe E. Management of gallstones and their complications. *Am Fam Physician.* 2000;61:1673–1680,1687–1688.

78. Cesmeli E, Elewaut A, Kerre M, DeBuyzere M, Afschrift M, Elewaut A. Gallstone recurrence after successful shock wave therapy. The magnitude of the problem and predictive factors. *Am J Gastroenterol.* 1999;94:474–479.

79. Tsumita R, Sugiura N, Abe A, Ebara M, Saisho H, Tsuchiya Y. Long-term evaluation of extracorporeal shock wave lithotripsy for cholesterol gallstones. *J Gastroenterol Hepatol.* 2001;16:93–99.

80. Yardley JH, Hendrix TR. Gastritis, duodenitis, and associated ulcerative lesions. In: Yamada T, Alpers DH, Owyang C, Powel DW, Silverstein, FE, editors. *Textbook of Gastroenterology.* 2nd ed. Philadelphia: Lippincott; 1995. pp. 1456.

81. Carrilho-Ribeiro L, Serra D, Pinto-Correia, Velosa J, Moura M. Quality of life after cholecystectomy and after successful lithotripsy for gallbladder stones: A matched pairs comparison. *European J Gastroenterol Hepatol.* 2002;14(7):741–744.

82. Dohil R, Hassall E, Jevon G, Dimmick J. Gastritis and gastropathy of childhood. *J Pediat Gastroenterol Nutr.* 1999;29:378–394.

83. Correa P. Chronic gastritis: A clinico-pathological classification. *Am J Gastroenterol.* 1988;83:504–509.

84. Friedman LS, Peterson WL. Peptic ulcer and related disorders. In: Fauci AS, Brownwald E, Isselbacker KJ, Wilson JD, Martin JB, Kasper DL, et al., editors. *Harrison's Principles of Internal Medicine.* 14th ed. New York: McGraw-Hill; 1988. pp. 1596–1616.

85. Genta RM. The gastritis connection: Prevention and early detection of gastric neoplasms. *J Clin Gastroenterol.* 2003;36 Suppl:S44–49.

86. Dixon MF, Genta RM, Yardly JH, Correa P. Classification and grading of gastritis—the updated Sydney system. *Am J Surg Pathol.* 1996;20:1161–1181.

87. Peterson WL, Fendrick AM, Cave DR, Peura DA, Garabedian-Ruffalo SM, Laine L. *Helicobacter pylori*-related disease: guidelines for testing and treatment. *Arch Intern Med.* 2000;160:1285–1291.

88. Cohen P. Peptic ulcer disease. In: Singleton JK, Sandowski SA, Green-Hernandez C, Horvath TV, DiGregorio RV, Holzemer SP, editors. *Primary Care.* Philadelphia: Lippincott; 1999. pp. 330–334.

89. Eltumi M, Brueton MJ, Francis N. Diagnosis of *Helicobacter pylori* gastritis in children using the urea breath test. *J Clin Gastroenterol.* 1999;28:238–240.

90. Lewis JD, Kroser J, Bevan J, Furth EE, Metz DC. Urease-based tests for helicobacter pylori gastritis: Accurate for diagnosis but poor correlation with disease severity. *J Clin Gastroenterol.* 1997;25:415–420.

91. Shetty AK, Correa H, Udall J, Schmidt-Sommerfeld E. Pathological case of the month: Helicobacter pylori gastritis. *Arch Ped Adol Med.* 1997;151: 855–856.

92. Peek RM. Optimizing *Helicobacter pylori* eradication therapies. Evidence-based. *Gastroent.* 2004;5:4–5.

93. American Society of Health-System Pharmacists, Inc. ASHP therapeutic position statement on the identification and treatment of *Helicobacter pylori*-associated peptic ulcer disease in adults. *Am J Health Syst Pharm.* 2001;58:31–37.

94. Scott LD, Abu-Hamda E. Gastrointestinal disease in pregnancy. In: Creasy RK, Resnik R, editors. *Maternal-Fetal Medicine*. 4th ed. Philadelphia: WB Saunders; 1999. pp. 1038–1053.

95. Chey W, Scheiman J. Peptic Ulcer Disease. In: Friedman S, McQuaid K, Grenndell J, editors. *Current Diagnosis and Treatment in Gastroenterology*, 2003. New York: McGraw Hill. pp. 323–340.

96. Nam J, Murthy S. Acute pancreatitis—the current status in management. *Expert Opin Pharmacother*. 2003;4:235–241.

97. Go V. Etiology and epidemiology of pancreatitis in the United States. In: Bradley E III, editor. *Acute Pancreatitis: Diagnosis and Therapy*. New York: Raven Press; 1994. pp. 235–239.

98. Riela A, Zinsmeister A, Melton L, DiMagno E. Etiology, incidence and survival of acute pancreatitis in Olmsted County, Minnesota [abstract]. *Gastroenterology*. 1991;100:A296.

99. Mitchell RM, Byrne MF, Baillie J. Pancreatitis. *Lancet*. 2003;361:1447–1455.

100. Godil A, Chen Y. Endoscopic management of benign pancreatic disease. *Pancreas*. 2000;20:1–13.

101. Gullo L, Migliori M, Pezzilli R, Olah A, Farkas G, Levy P, et al. An update on recurrent acute pancreatitis: Data from five European countries. *Am J Gastroenterol*. 2002;97:1959–1962.

102. Cole L. Unraveling the mystery of acute pancreatitis. *Nursing*. 2001;31:58–63.

103. Pinchbeck T. The treatment of pancreatitis. *Nurs Times*. 2003;99:26–27.

104. Toskes P. Hyperlipidemic pancreatitis. *Gastroenterol Clin North Am*. 1990:9:783–791.

105. Sharer N, Schwarz M, Malone G, Howarth A, Painter J, Super M. Mutations of the cystic fibrosis gene in patients with chronic pancreatitis. *N Engl J Med*. 1998;339:645–652.

106. Choudari CP, Yu A, Imperiale T, Fogel E, Sherman S, Lehman G. Significance of heterozygous cystic fibrosis gene in idiopathic pancreatitis [abstract]. *Gastroenterology*. 1998;114 G1818, Part 2, Suppl S:A447.

107. Hozumi Y, Kawang M, Saito T, Miyata M. Effect of tamoxifen on serum lipid metabolism. *J Clin Endocrinol Metab*. 1998;83:1633–1635.

108. Aliperti G. Complications related to diagnostic and therapeutic endoscopic retrograde cholangiopancreatography. *Gastrointest Endosc Clin N Am*. 1996;6: 379–407.

109. Kahl S, Zimmermann S, Malfertheiner P. Acute pancreatitis: Treatment strategies. *Dig Dis*. 2003;21: 30–37.

110. Yadav D, Agarwal N, Pitchumoni C. A critical evaluation of laboratory tests in acute pancreatitis. *Am J Gastroenterol*. 2002;97:1309–1318.

111. Turner MA. The role of US and CT in pancreatitis. *Gastrointest Endosc*. 2002;56:(6) Suppl):S241-S245.

112. Sharma S, Larson K, Adler Z, Goldfarb M. Role of endoscopic retrograde cholangiopancreatography in the management of suspected choledocholithiasis. *Surg Endosc*. 2003;17:868–871.

113. Kalra M, Maher M, Sahani D, Digmurthy S, Saini S. Current status of imaging in pancreatic diseases. *J Comput Assist Tomogr*. 2002;26:661–675.

114. Balthazar E, Ranson J, Naidich D, Megibow A, Caccavale R, Cooper M. Acute pancreatitis: Prognostic value of CT. *Radiology*. 1985;156: 767–772.

115. Larvin M, McMahon M. Apache II score for assessment and monitoring of acute pancreatitis. *Lancet*. 1989;2:201–205.

116. Ranson J, Rifkind K, Roses D, Fink S, Eng K, Spencer F. Prognostic signs and the role of operative management in acute pancreatitis. *Surg Gynecol Obstet*. 1974;139:69–81.

117. Ferri F. *Ferri's Clinical Advisor Instant Diagnosis and Treatment*. St. Louis: Mosby; 2003. pp. 617–618.

118. Moss SF, Sood S. *Helicobacter pylori*. *Curr Opin Infect Dis*. 2003;16:445–451.

119. Bombardier C, Laine L, Reicin A, Shapiro D, Burgos-Vargas R, Davis B, et al. Comparison of upper gastrointestinal toxicity of rofecoxib and naproxen in patients with rheumatoid arthritis. VIGOR Study Group. *N Engl J Med*. 2000;343: 1520–1530.

120. Silverstein FE, Faich G, Goldstein JL, Simon LS, Pincus T, Whelton A, Makuch R, et al. Gastrointestinal toxicity with celecoxib vs nonsteroidal anti-inflammatory drugs for osteoarthritis and rheumatoid arthritis: The CLASS study: A randomized controlled trial. Celecoxib Long-term Arthritis Safety Study. *JAMA*. 2000;284:1247–1255.

121. White WB, Faich G, Borer JS, Makuch RW. Cardiovascular thrombotic events in arthritis trials of the cyclooxygenase-2 inhibitor celecoxib. *Am J Cardiol*. 2003;92:411–421.

122. Ray WA, Stein CM, Daugherty JR, Hall K, Arbogast PG, Griffin MR. COX-2 selective non-

steroidal anti-inflammatory drugs and risk of serious coronary heart disease. *Lancet.* 2002;360:1071–1073.

123. Solomon DH, Schneeweiss S, Glynn RJ, Kiyota Y, Levin R, Mogun H, Avorn J. Relationship between selective cyclooxygenase-2 inhibitors and acute myocardial infarction in older adults. *Circulation.* 2004;109:2068–2073.

124. Zimmerman EM, Christman GM. Approach to the female patient with gastrointestinal disease. In: Yamada T editor. *Textbook of Gastroenterology.* 2nd ed. Philadelphia: JB Lippincott; 1995. pp. 1023–1039.

125. Landon MB. Gastrointestinal disease. In: Gabbe SG, Niebyl JR, Simpson JL, editors. *Obstetrics Normal and Problem Pregnancies.* 4th ed. New York: Churchill Livingstone; 2002. pp. 1124–1131.

126. Welch J. General consideration and mortality in bowel obstruction. In: Welch JP, editor. *Bowel Obstruction: Differential Diagnosis and Clinical Management.* Philadelphia: WB Saunders; 1990, pp. 59–95.

127. Delabrousse E, Destrumelle N, Brunelle S, Clair C, Mantion G, Kastler B. CT of small bowel obstruction in adults. *Abdom Imaging.* 2003;28:257–266.

128. Maglinte D, Heitkamp D, Howard T, Kelvin F, Lappas J. Current concepts in imaging of small bowel obstruction. *Radiol Clin North Am.* 2003;41: 263–283.

129. Miller G, Boman J, Shrier I, Gordon P. Etiology of small bowel obstruction. *Am J Surg.* 2000;180: 33–36.

130. Frager D. Intestinal obstruction: Role of CT. *Gastroenterol Clin North Am.* 2002;31:777–799.

131. Burkill G, Bell J, Healy J. Small bowel obstruction: The role of computed tomography in its diagnosis and management with reference to other imaging modalities. *Eur Radiol.* 2001;11:1405–1422.

132. Connolly M, Unti J, Nora P. Bowel obstruction in pregnancy. *Surg Clin North Am.* 1995;75:101–113.

133. Friedman J, Odland M, Bubrick M. Experience with colonic volvulus. *Dis Colon Rectum.* 1989;32:409–416.

134. Cohen P. Bowel obstruction. In: Singleton J, Sandowski S, Green-Hernandez C, Horwath T, DiGregono R, Holzemer S, editors. *Primary Care.* Philadelphia: Lippincott; 1999. pp. 258–261.

135. Wiesner W, Khurana B, Ji H, Ros P. CT of acute bowel ischemia. *Radiology.* 2003;226:635–650.

136. Shih S, Jeng K, Lin S, Kao C, Chou S, Wang H, et al. Adhesive small bowel obstruction: How long can patients tolerate conservative treatment? *World J Gastroenterol.* 2003;9:603–605.

137. Bickerstaff L, Hollier L, VanPeenen H, Melton L, Pairolero P, Cherry K. Abdominal aortic aneurysms: The changing natural history. *J Vasc Surg.* 1984;1: 6–12.

138. Singh K, Bonaa K, Jacobsen B, Bjork L, Solberg S. Prevalence of and risk factors for abdominal aortic aneurysms in a population-based study: The Tromso study. *Am J Epidemiol.* 2001;154:236–244.

139. Lederle F, Johnson G, Wilson S, Chute E, Littooy F, Bandyk D, et al. Prevalence and associations of abdominal aortic aneurysm detected through screening. *Ann Intern Med.* 1997;126:441–449.

140. Brox A, Filion K, Zhang X, Pilote L, Obrand D, Haider S, et al. In hospital cost of abdominal aortic aneurysm repair in Canada and the United States. *Arch Internal Med.* 2003;163:2500–2504.

141. Herkner H. Challenge for emergency physicians. *BMJ.* 2003;326:1134.

142. Ernst C. Abdominal aortic aneurysm. *N Engl J Med.* 1993;328:1167–1172.

143. Lederle F, Wilson S, Johnson G, Reinke D, Littooy F, Acher C, et al. Immediate repair compared with surveillance of small abdominal aortic aneurysms. *N Engl J Med.* 2002;346:1437–1444.

144. Lee M, Huang A, Gillen-Goldstein J, Funai E. Labor and vaginal delivery with maternal aortic aneurysm. *Obstet Gynecol.* 2001;98:935–938.

145. Williams G, Gott V, Brawley R, Schauble J, Labs J. Aortic disease associated with pregnancy. *J Vasc Surg.* 1988;8:470–475.

146. Cheung O, Regueiro M. Inflammatory bowel disease emergencies. *Gastroenterology Clin North Am.* 2003; 32:1269–1288.

147. Keighley M, Stockbrugger R. Inflammatory bowel disease. *Aliment Pharmacol Ther.* 2003;18 Suppl 3: 66–70.

148. Jewell D. Ulcerative colitis. In: Feldman M, Scharschmidt B, Sleisinger M, editors. *Gastrointestinal and Liver Disease: Pathophysiology/ Diagnosis/ Management.* Philadelphia: WB Saunders; 1998. p. 1735.

149. Whelan G. Epidemiology of inflammatory bowel disease. *Gastroenterol Clin North Am.* 1990:24: 101–109.

150. Sonnenberg A, McCarty D, Jacobsen S. Geographic variation of inflammatory bowel disease in the United States. *Gastroenterology.* 1991;100:143–149.

151. Trallori G, Palli D, Saieva C, Bardazzi G, Bonanomi A, d'Albasio G, et al. A population-based study of

inflammatory bowel disease in Florence over 15 years (78–92). *Scand J Gastroenterol.* 1996;31:892–899.

152. Roth M, Petersen G, McElree C, Feldman E, Rotter J. Geographic origins of Jewish patients with inflammatory bowel disease. *Gastroenterology.* 1989;97: 900–904.

153. Bouma G, Strober W. The immunological and genetic basis of inflammatory bowel disease. *Nat Rev Immunol.* 2003;3:521–533.

154. Bonen D, Cho J. The genetics of inflammatory bowel disease. *Gastroenterology.* 2003;124:521–536.

155. Orholm M, Binder V, Sorensen T, Rasmussen L, Kyvik K. Concordance of inflammatory bowel disease among Danish twins. Results of a nationwide study. *Scand J Gastroenerol.* 2000;35:1075–1081.

156. Tamboli C, Cortot A, Colombel JF. What are the major arguments in favor of the genetic susceptibility for inflammatory bowel disease? *Eur J Gastroenterol Hepatol.* 2003;15:587–592.

157. Boyko E, Koepsell T, Perera D, Inui T. Risk of ulcerative colitis among former and current cigarette smokers. *N Engl J Med.* 1987;316:707–710.

158. Silverstein M, Lashner B, Hanauer S, Evan A, Kirsner J. Cigarette smoking in Crohn's disease. *Am J Gastroenterol.* 1989;84:31–33.

159. Farmer R, Hawk W, Turnbull R, Jr. Clinical patterns in Crohn's disease: A statistical study of 615 cases. *Gastroenterology.* 1975;68:627–635.

160. Marion J, Concert C. Inflammatory bowel disease. In: Singleton S, Sandowski S, Green-Hernandez C, Howath T, DiGregorio, Holzemer S, editors. *Primary Care.* Philadelphia: Lippincott; 1999. pp. 319–325.

161. Hanauer S, Meyers S. Management of Crohn's disease in adults. *Am J Gastroenterol.* 1997;92:559–566.

162. Sandborn W, Feagan B. Mild to moderate Crohn's disease—defining the basis for a new treatment algorithm. *Aliment Pharmacol Ther.* 2003;18:263–277.

163. Katz S. Update in medical therapy of ulcerative colitis: Newer concepts and therapies. *J Clin Gastroenterol.* 2005; 39(7):557–569.

164. Rutgeerts P, Geboes K, Vantrappen G, Beyls J, Kerremans R, Hiele M. Predictability of the post operative course of Crohn's disease. *Gastroenterology.* 1990;99:956–963.

165. Langholz E, Munkholm P, Davidsen M, Binder V. Colorectal cancer risk and mortality in patients with ulcerative colitis. *Gastroenterology.* 1992;103: 1444–1451.

166. Sandborn W, Tremaine W, Offord K, Lawson G, Petersen B, Batts K, et al. Transdermal nicotine for mildly to moderately active ulcerative colitis: A randomized, double-blind, placebo-controlled trial. *Ann Intern Med.* 1997;126:364–371.

167. Marshall J, Irvine J. Rectal aminosalicylate therapy for distal ulcerative colitis: A metaanalysis. *Aliment Pharmacol Ther.* 1995;9:293–300.

168. Nuako K, Ahlquist D, Mahoney D, Schaid D, Siems D, Lindor N. Familial predisposition for colorectal cancer in chronic ulcerative colitis: A case control study. *Gastroenterology.* 1998;115:1079–1083.

169. Brandt L, Bjorkman D, Fennerty MB, Locke G, Olden K, Peterson W, et al. Systematic review on the management of irritable bowel syndrome in North America. *Am J Gastroenterol.* 2002;97 11 Suppl: S7–26.

170. Viera A, Hoag S, Shaughnessy J. Management of irritable bowel syndrome. *Am Fam Physician.* 2002;66: 1867–1874.

171. Gunn M, Cavin A, Mansfield J. Management of irritable bowel syndrome. *Postgrad Med J.* 2003;79: 154–158.

172. Talley N, Gabriel S, Harmsen W, Zinsmeister A, Evans R. Medical costs in community subjects with irritable bowel syndrome. *Gastroenterology.* 1995;109: 1735–1741.

173. Camilleri M, Williams D. Economic burden of irritable bowel syndrome reappraised with strategies to control expenditure. *Pharmacoeconomics.* 2000;17:331–338.

174. Talley N, Zinsmeister A, Melton L. Irritable bowel syndrome in a community: Symptom subgroups, risk factors and health care. *Am J Epidemiol.* 1995; 142:76–83.

175. Talley N, O'Keefe E, Zinsmeister A, Melton L. Prevalence of gastrointestinal symptoms in the elderly: A population based study. *Gastroenterology.* 1992; 102:895–901.

176. Maxwell P, Mendall M, Kumar D. Irritable bowel syndrome. *Lancet.* 1997;350:1691–1695.

177. Wood J. Neuropathophysiology of irritable bowel syndrome. *J Clin Gastroenterol.* 2002;35:S11–22.

178. Chey W, Jin H, Lee M, Sun S, Lee K. Colonic motility abnormality in patients with irritable bowel syndrome exhibiting abnormal pain and diarrhea. *Am J Gastroenterol.* 2001;96:1499–1506.

179. Hunt R. Evolving concepts in the pathophysiology of functional gastrointestinal disorder. *J Clin Gastroenterol.* 2002;35 Suppl 1:S2–6.

180. Tougas G. The nature of pain in irritable bowel syndrome. *J Clin Gastroenterol*. 2002;35 Suppl:S26–30.

181. Drossman D. Do psychosocial factors define symptom severity and patient status in irritable bowel syndrome? *Am J Med*. 1999;107:41S-50.

182. Delvaux M, Denis P, Allemand H. Sexual abuse is more frequently reported by IBS patients than by patients with organic digestive disease or controls: Results of a multicenter inquiry. *Eur J Gastroenterol Hepatol*. 1997;9:345–352.

183. Ringel Y, Drossman D. Irritable bowel syndrome: Classification and conceptualization. *J Clin Gastroenterol*. 2002;35:S7-S10.

184. Whorwell P, McCallum M, Creed F, Roberts C. Non-colonic features of irritable bowel syndrome. *Gut*. 1986;27:37–40.

185. Hudson J, Goldenberg D, Pope H, Keck P, Schlesinger L. Co-morbidity of fibromyalgia with medical and psychiatric disorders. *Am J Med*. 1992; 92:363–367.

186. Floch M, Naragan R. Diet in the irritable bowel syndrome. *J Clin Gastroenterol*. 2002;35 Suppl:S45–52.

187. Niec A, Frankum B, Talley N. Are adverse food reactions linked to irritable bowel syndrome? *Am J Gastroenterol*. 1998;93:2184–2190.

188. Berrada D, Canenguez K, Lembo T. New approaches to the medical treatment of irritable bowel syndrome. *Curr Gastroenterol Rep*. 2003;5:337–342.

189. Muller-Lissner S, Fumagalli I, Bardhan K, Pace F, Pecher E, Nault B, et al. Tegaserod, a5HT (4) receptor partial agonist, relieves symptoms in irritable bowel syndrome patients with abnormal pain, bloating and constipation. *Aliment Pharmacol Ther*. 2001; 15:1655–1666.

190. Whorwell P, Krumholz S, Muller-Lissner S, Schmitt C, Dunger-Baldauf C, Rueegg P. Tegaserod has a favorable safety and tolerability profile in patients with constipation—predominant and alternating forms of irritable bowel syndrome [abstract]. *Gastroenterology*. 2000;118:A1204.

191. Camilleri M, Northcutt A, Kong S, Dukes G, McSorley D, Mangel A. Efficacy and safety of alosetron in women with irritable bowel syndrome: A randomized placebo controlled trial. *Lancet*. 2000; 355:1035–1040.

192. Camilleri M, Chey W, Mayer E, Northcutt A, Heath A, Dukes G, et al. A randomized controlled trial of the serotonin type 3 receptor antagonist alosetron in women with diarrhea–predominant irritable bowel syndrome. *Arch Intern Med*. 2001;161:1733–1740.

193. Poynard T, Regimbeau C, Benhamou Y. Meta-analysis of smooth muscle relaxants in the treatment of irritable bowel syndrome. *Aliment Pharmacol Ther*. 2001;15:355–361.

194. Wald A. Psychotropic agents in irritable bowel syndrome. *J Clin Gastroenterol*. 2002;35 Suppl 1:S53–57.

195. Clouse R, Prakash C, Anderson R, Lustman P. Antidepressants for functional gastrointestinal symptoms and syndromes: A meta-analysis. [abstract] *Gastroenterology*. 2001;120 3252 Suppl 1:A642.

196. Fitz R. Perforating inflammation of the vermiform appendix with special reference to its early diagnosis and treatment. *Trans Assoc Am Physicians*. 1886;1: 106–144.

197. Addiss D. Shaffer N, Fowler B, Tauxe R. The epidemiology of appendicitis and appendectomy in the United States. *Am J Epidemiol*. 1990;132:910–925.

198. Korner H, Sondenaa K, Soreide J, Anderson E, Nysted A, Lende T, et al. Incidence of acute non-perforated and perforated appendicitis: Age-specific and sex specific analysis. *World J Surg*. 1997;21: 313–317.

199. Owings M, Kozak L. Ambulatory and inpatient procedures in the United States, 1996. Vital Health Stat. Series 13,139. Hyattsville, MD: National Center for Health Statistics; November 1998. p. 26.

200. Flum D, Morris A, Koepsell T, Dellinger E. Has misdiagnosis of appendicitis decreased over time? *JAMA*. 2001;286:1748–1753.

201. Bijnen C, Van Den Broek W, Bijnen A, DeRuiter P, Gouma D. Implications of removing a normal appendix. *Dig Surg*. 2003;20:115–121.

202. Mercer B, Witlin A. Appendicitis in pregnancy. In: Gleicher N, editor. *Principles and Practice of Medical Therapy in Pregnancy*. 3rd ed. Stamford, CT: Appleton & Lange; 1998. pp. 1512–1515.

203. Hale D, Jaques D, Molloy M, Pearl R, Schutt D, D'Avis J. Appendectomy: improving care through quality improvement. *Arch Surg*. 1997;132:153–157.

204. Mockway-Jones K. *Emergency Triage: Manchester Triage Group*. London: BMJ Publishing Group; 1997.

205. Paulson E, Kalady M, Pappas T. Suspected appendicitis. *N Engl J Med*. 2003;348:236–242.

206. Ng K, Lai S. Clinical analysis of the related factors in acute appendicitis. *Yale J Biol Med*. 2002;75:41–45.

207. Cervini P, Smith L, Urbach D. The surgeon on call is a strong factor determining the use of a laparoscopic approach for appendectomy. *Surg Endosc.* 2002;16:1774–1777.

208. Lane M, Liu D, Huynh M, Jeffrey R, Mindelzun R, Katz D. Suspected acute appendicitis: Nonenhanced helical CT in 300 consecutive patients. *Radiology.* 1999;213:341–346.

209. Neumayer L, Kennedy A. Imaging in appendicitis: A review with special emphasis on the treatment of women. *Obstet Gynecol.* 2003;162:1404–1409.

210. Birnbaum B, Wilson S. Appendicitis at the millennium. *Radiology.* 2000;215:337–348.

211. Jeffrey R Jr, Laing F, Townsend R. Acute appendicitis: Sonographic criteria based on 250 cases. *Radiology.* 1988;167:327–329.

212. Caspi B, Zbar A, Mavor E, Hagay Z, Appelman Z. The contribution of transvaginal ultrasound in the diagnosis of acute appendicitis: An observational study. *Ultrasound Obstet Gynecol.* 2003;21:273–276.

213. Kamel I, Goldberg S, Keogan M, Rosen M, Raptopoulos V. Right lower quadrant pain and suspected appendicitis: non-focused appendiceal: A review of 100 cases. *Radiology.* 2000;217:159–163.

214. Rexroad J. The CT arrowhead sign. *Radiology.* 2003; 227:44–45.

215. Ujiki M, Murayama K, Cribbins A, Angelos P, Dawes L, Prystowsky J, et al. CT scan in the management of acute appendicitis. *J Surg Res.* 2002;105:119–122.

216. Rao P, Rhea J, Novelline R, McCabe C, Lawrason J, Berger D, et al. Helical CT technique for the diagnosis of appendicitis: Prospective evaluation of a focused appendix CT examination. *Radiology.* 1997;202:139–144.

217. Jacobs J, Birnbaum B, Macari M. Megibow A, Isreal G, Maki D, et al. Acute appendicitis: Comparison of helical CT diagnosis focused technique with oral contrast material v. non-focused technique with oral and intravenous contrast material. *Radiology.* 2001;220:683–690.

218. Lee S, Walsh A, Ho H. Computed tomography and ultrasonography do not improve and may delay the diagnosis and treatment of acute appendicitis. *Arch Surg.* 2001;136;556–562.

219. Rao P, Rhea J, Rattner D, Venus L, Novelline R. Introduction of appendiceal CT: Impact on negative appendectomy and appendiceal perforation rates. *Ann Surg.* 1999;229:344–349.

220. Rao P, Rhea J, Novelline R, Mostafavi A, McCabe C. Effect of computed tomography of the appendix on treatment of patients and use of hospital resources. *N Engl J Med.* 1998;338:141–146.

221. Wilson E, Cole J, Nipper M, Cooney D, Smith R. Computed tomography and ultrasonography in the diagnosis of appendicitis: When are they indicated? *Arch Surg.* 2001;136:670–675.

222. Raman S, Kadell B, Vodopich D, Sayer J, Cryer H, Lu D. Patient gender-related performance of non focused helical computed tomography in the diagnosis of acute appendicitis. *J Comput Assist Tomogr.* 2003;27:583–589.

223. Rosen M, Siewert B, Sands D, Bromberg R, Edlow J, Raptopoulos V. Value of abdominal CT in the emergency department for patients with abdominal pain. *Eur Radiol.* 2003;13:418–424.

224. Perez J, Barone J, Wilbanks T, Jorgensson D, Corvo P. Liberal use of computed tomography scanning does not improve diagnostic accuracy in appendicitis. *Am J Surg.* 2003 185:194–197.

225. Safran D, Pilati D, Folz E, Oller D. Is appendiceal CT scan overused for evaluating patients with right lower quadrant pain? *Am J Emerg Med.* 2001;19:199–203.

226. Wise S, Labuski M, Kasales C, Blebea J, Meilstrup J, Holley G, et al. Comparative assessment of CT and sonographic techniques for appendiceal imaging. *Am J Roentgenol.* 2001;176:933–941.

227. Wall B, Hart D. Revised radiation doses for typical x-ray examinations. Report on a recent review of doses to patients from medical x-ray examinations in the UK by NRPB. National Radiological Protection Board. *Br J Radiol.* 1997;70:437–439.

228. Sharp H. The acute abdomen during pregnancy. *Clin Obstet Gynecol.* 2002;45:405–413.

229. Mourad J, Elliott J, Erickson L, Lisboa L. Appendicitis in pregnancy: New information that contradicts long held clinical beliefs. *Am J Obstet Gynecol.* 2000;182:1027–1029.

230. Ames Castro M, Shipp T, Castro E, Ouzounian J, Rao P. The use of helical computed tomography in pregnancy for the diagnosis of acute appendicitis. *Am J Obstet Gynecol.* 2001;184:954–957.

231. Stollman N, Raskin J. Diagnosis and management of diverticular disease of the colon in adults. *Am J Gastroenterol.* 1999;94:3110–3121.

232. Young-Fadok T, Roberts P, Spencer M, Wolff B. Colonic diverticular disease. *Curr Probl Surg.* 2000; 37:457–514.

233. Painter N, Burkitt D. Diverticular disease of the colon: A deficiency disease of Western civilization. *Br Med J*. 1971;2:450–454.

234. Place R, Simmang C. Diverticular disease. *Best Pract Res Clin Gastroenterol*. 2002;16:135–148.

235. Savides TJ, Jensen DM. Acute lower intestinal bleeding. In: Friedman SL, McQuaid KR, Kenneth R, Grendell JH, editors. *Current Diagnosis and Treatment in Gastroenterology*. 2nd ed. New York: McGraw-Hill; 2003. pp. 70–282.

236. Sherer D, Frager D, Eliakim R. An unusual case of diverticulitis complicating pregnancy at 33 weeks gestation. *Am J Perinatol*. 2001;18:107–111.

237. Longstreth GF. Epidemiology and outcome of patients hospitalized with acute lower gastrointestinal hemorrhage: A population based study. *Am J Gastroenterol*. 1997;92:419–424.

238. McGuire HH. Bleeding colonic diverticula. A reappraisal of natural history and management. *Ann Surg*. 1994;220:653–656.

239. Aldoori W, Ryan-Harshman M. Preventing diverticular disease: Review of recent evidence on high fiber diets. *Can Fam Physician*. 2002;48:1632–1637.

240. Aldoori W, Giovannucci E, Rimm F, Wing A, Trichopoulos D, Willett W. A prospective study of diet and the risk of symptomatic diverticular disease in men. *Am J Clin Nutr*. 1994;60:757–764.

241. Aldoori W, Giovannucci E, Rimm E, Ascherio A, Stampfer M, Colditz G, et al. Prospective study of physical activity and the risk of symptomatic diverticular disease in men. *Gut*. 1995;36:276–282.

242. Simpson J, Scholefield J, Spiller R. Origin of symptoms in diverticular disease. *Br J Surg*. 2003;90:899–908.

243. Halligan S, Saunders B. Imaging diverticular disease. *Best Pract Res Clin Gastroenterol*. 2002;16:595–610.

244. Buchanan G, Kenefick N, Cohen R. Diverticulitis. *Best Pract Res Clin Gastroenterol*. 2002;16:635–647.

245. Awasthi S, Bundy D, Savioli L. Helminthic infections. *BMJ*. 2003;327:431–433.

246. Colley D, LoVerde P, Savioli L. Medical helminthology in the 21st century. *Science*. 2001;293:1437–1438.

247. Muennig P, Pallin D, Sell R, Chan M. The cost effectiveness of strategies for the treatment of intestinal parasites in immigrants. *N Engl J Med*. 1999;340:773–779.

248. Fitzgerald J, Tronconi R, Sarigol S, Kay M, Wyllie R. Clinical quiz. *J Pediatr Gastroenterol Nutr*. 2000;30:556.

249. Clinch C, Stephens M. Case description of ascariasis. *Arch Fam Med*. 2000;9:1193–1194.

250. Gilman R. Intestinal nematodes that migrate through skin and lung. In: Strickland GT. *Hunter's Tropical Medicine and Emerging Infectious Disease*. 8th ed. Philadelphia: WB Saunders Company; 2000. pp. 730–736.

251. Mandell GL, Bennett JE, Dolin R. *Mandell, Douglas and Bennett's Principles and Practice of Infectious Disease*. 5th ed. Philadelphia: Churchill Livingstone; pp. 2941–2942.

252. Schuster H, Chiodini P. Parasitic infections of the intestine. *Curr Opin Infect Dis*. 2001;14:587–591.

253. Kato T, Kamoi R, Iida M, Kihara T. Endoscopic diagnosis of hookworm disease of the duodenum. *J Clin Gastroenterol*. 1997;24:100–102.

254. Chandra B, Long JD. Diagnosis of trichoris trichiura (whipworm) by colonoscopic extraction. *J Clin Gastroenterol*. 1998;27:152–153.

255. Epstein A, Isselbacher KJ. Gastrointestinal bleeding. In: Fauci AS, Braunwald E, Isselbacher KJ, Wilson JD, Martin JB, Kasper DL, et al., editors. *Harrison's Principles of Internal Medicine*. 14th ed. New York: McGraw Hill; 1998. pp. 246–249.

256. Zuckerman GR, Prakash C, Askin MP, Lewis BS. AGA technical review on the evaluation and management of occult and obscure gastrointestinal bleeding. *Gastroenterology*. 2000;118:201–221.

257. Elta G. Approach to the patient with gross GI bleeding. In: Yamada T, editor. *Texbook of Gastroenterology*. 4th ed. Philadelphia: Lippincott, Williams & Wilkins; 2003. pp. 698–715.

258. Lanas A, Sekar MC, Hirschowitz BI. Objective evidence of aspirin use in both ulcer and non-ulcer upper and lower gastrointestinal bleeding. *Gastroenterology*. 1992;103:862–869.

259. Wilcox CM, Alexander LN, Cotsonis GA, Clark WS. Nonsteroidal anti-inflammatory drugs are associated with both upper and lower gastrointestinal bleeding. *Dig Dis Sci*. 1997;42:990–997.

260. Pahor M, Guralnik JM, Furberg CD, Carbonin P, Havik R. Risk of gastrointestinal haemorrhage with calcium antagonists in hypertensive persons over 67 years old. *Lancet*. 1996;347:1061–1065.

261. Kaplan RC, Heckbert SR, Koepsell TD, Rosendaal FR, Psaty BM. Use of calcium channel blockers and risk of hospitalized gastrointestinal tract bleeding. *Arch Intern Med*. 2000;165:1849–1855.

262. Boley SJ, DiBiase A, Brandt LJ, Sammartano RJ. Lower intestinal bleeding in the elderly. *Am J Surg.* 1979;137:57–64.

263. Rogers BH. Endoscopic diagnosis and therapy of mucosal vascular abnormalities of the gastrointestinal tract occurring in elderly patients and associated with cardiac, vascular and pulmonary disease. *Gastrointest Endosc.* 1980;26:134–138.

264. Cello JP, Grendell JH. Endoscopic laser treatment for gastrointestinal vascular ectasias. *Ann Intern Med.* 1986;104:352–354.

265. Peura DA, Lanza FL, Gostout CJ, Foutch PG. The American College of Gastroenterology Bleeding Registry: Preliminary findings. *Am J Gastroenterol.* 1997;92:924–928.

266. Sorbi D, Norton I, Conio M, Balm R, Zinsmeister A, Gostout CJ. Post polypectomy lower GI bleeding: Descriptive analysis. *Gastrointest Endosc.* 2000;51: 690–696.

267. Bleday R, Breen E. Clinical features of hemorrhoids [monograph on the Internet]. 2004 [cited October 29]; Version 12.3. In: UpToDate [online subscriber service]. Available from: http://www.uptodate.com.

268. Gopal DV. Diseases of the rectum and anus: A clinical approach to common disorders. *Clin Cornerstone.* 2002;4:34–48.

269. MacRae HM, McLeod RS. Comparison of hemorrhoidal treatments: A meta-analysis. *Can J Surg.* 1997;40:14–17.

270. Breen E, Bleday R. Anal fissures [monograph on the Internet]. 2004 [cited October 29]; Version 12.3. In: UpToDate [subscription service online]. Available from: http://www.uptodate.com.

271. Pitt J, Williams S, Dawson PM. Reasons for failure of glyceryl trinitrate treatment of chronic fissure in ano: Multivariate analysis. *Dis Colon Rectum.* 2001; 44:864–867.

272. Scholefield JH, Bock JU, Marla B, Richter HJ, Athanasiadis S, Prols M, Herold A. A dose finding study with 0.1%, 0.2% and 0.4% gylceryl trinitrate ointment in patients with chronic anal fissures. *Gut.* 2003;52:264–269.

273. Minguez M, Herreros B, Espi A, Garcia-Granero E, Sanchez V, Mora F, et al. Long term follow-up (42 months) of chronic anal fissure after healing with botulinium toxin. *Gastroenterology.* 2002;123:112–117.

274. Brisinda G, Maria G, Bentivoglio AR, Cassetta E, Gui D, Albanese A. A comparison of injections of botulinum toxin and topical nitroglycerin ointment for the treatment of chronic anal fissure. *N Engl J Med.* 1999;341:65–69.

275. Nelson R. Nonsurgical therapy for anal fissure. *Cochrane Database of Systematic Reviews.* (4): CD003431,2003.

276. Nyam DC, Pemberton JH. Long-term results of lateral internal sphincterotomy for chronic anal fissure with particular reference to incidence of fecal incontinence. *Dis Colon Rectum.* 1999;42:1306–1310.

277. U.S. Cancer Statistics Working Group. *United States Cancer Statistics: 1999-2002 Incidence and Mortality Web–based Report Version.* Atlanta: Department of Health and Human Services, Centers for Disease Control and Prevention, *and* National Cancer Institute; 2005. Available at: www.cdc.gov/cancer/npcr/uscs.

278. Zuckerman GR, Prakash C. Acute lower intestinal bleeding. Part II: etiology, therapy, and outcomes. *Gastrointest Endosc.* 1999;49:228–238.

279. Macrae FA, St John DJ. Relationship between patterns of bleeding and hemoccult sensitivity in patients with colorectal cancers or adenomas. *Gastroenterology.* 1982;82:891–898.

280. Lawrence SP, Ahnen DJ. Clinical manifestations, diagnoses, and staging of colorectal cancer [monograph on the Internet]. 2004 [cited October 29] Version 12.3. In: UpToDate [online subscriber service]. Available from: http//www.uptodate.com.

281. Carraro PG, Segala M, Cesana BM, Tiberio G. Obstructing colonic cancer: Failure and survival patterns over a ten-year follow-up after one-stage curative surgery. *Dis Colon Rectum.* 2001;44:243–250.

282. Crucitti F, Sofo L, Doglietto GB, Bellantone R, Ratto C. Bossoal M, et al. Prognostic factors in colorectal cancer: Current status and new trends. *J Surg Oncol Suppl.* 1991;2:76–82.

283. Imperiale TF, Wagner DR, Lin CY, Larkin GN, Rogge JD, Ransohoff DF. Results of screening colonoscopy among persons 40–49 years of age. *N Engl J Med.* 2002;346:1781–1785.

284. Rex DK, Johnson DA, Lieberman DA, et al. Colorectal cancer prevention 2000: Screening recommendations of the American College of Gastroenterology. American College of Gastroenterology. *Am J Gastroenterol.* 2000;95:868–877.

285. Winawer SJ, Fletcher RH, Miller L, Codlee F, Stsolar MH, Mulrow DC, et al. Colorectal cancer screening:

Clinical guidelines and rationale. *Gastroenterology*. 1997;112:594–642.

286. Fletcher RH. Family history of colorectal cancer: Risks, pathogenesis and screening [monograph on the Internet]. 2004 [cited October 29]; Version 12.3. In: UpToDate [subscription service online] Available from: http//www.uptodate.com.

287. Woods JB, Martin JN Jr, Ingram FH, Odom CD, Scott-Conner CE, Rhodes RS. Pregnancy complicated by carcinoma of the colon above the rectum. *Am J Perinatol*. 1992;9:102–110.

288. Nesbitt JC, Moise KJ, Sawyers JL. Colorectal carcinoma in pregnancy. *Arch Surg*. 1985;120:636–640.

289. Ransohoff DF, Lang CA. Screening for colorectal cancer. *N Engl J Med*. 1991;325:37–41.

290. Cappell MS. Colon cancer during pregnancy. *Gastroenterol Clin North Am*. 2003;32:341–383.

291. Sugerbaker PH. Clinical evaluation of symptomatic patients. In: Steele G Jr, Osteen RT, editors. *Colorectal Cancer: Current Concepts in Diagnosis and Treatment*. New York: Marcel Dekker; 1986. pp. 57–70.

Chapter 18

The Abdomen: Kidney, Bladder, and Reproductive Problems

Diane Hodgman
Edie McConaughey
Diane Angelini

In addition to the many gastrointestinal problems that produce abdominal symptoms, specific conditions related to the urinary tract and reproductive organs may have a similar initial presentation. This chapter discusses infections of the upper and lower urinary tract, renal stones, and interstitial cystitis. Gynecologic problems including endometriosis, ectopic pregnancy, ovarian masses, and ovarian torsion are also presented. While this is by no means a complete survey of reproductive issues presenting as an abdominal complaint, it addresses those most likely to be seen by a midwife or women's health provider. The reader should refer to the history and physical examination sections in Chapter 17 to supplement the material presented here.

Urinary Tract Infections

Symptoms of urinary tract infections (UTIs) are common complaints both in emergency care facilities and nonurgent medical care settings. Close to 50% of women will experience at least one UTI in their lifetime, and more than 25% will have recurrent UTIs.[1] The incidence of UTIs is exceeded only by that of respiratory in-

fections.[2] Direct costs of screening, treatment, and follow-up care generate health care expenditures that exceed $1.6 billion annually in the United States.[3] The accurate diagnosis of UTIs is predicated on the knowledge of the etiology, anatomical considerations, medical and family history, and contraceptive and gynecologic history. This knowledge is used to determine the risk factors for infection, recurrence, and re-infection. Appropriate screening, treatment, and re-assessment can contribute to the management of this clinical problem in an efficient and cost-effective manner.

UTI refers to an infection in any part of the renal system. It can be delineated by location—upper or lower tract—as well as by level of severity or involvement of the infection (uncomplicated or complicated). Uncomplicated UTIs refer to those infections occurring in patients who have normal renal anatomy without obstruction or a history of instrumentation. A UTI is complicated if structural or functional abnormalities exist. Examples of these abnormalities include polycystic kidney disease, neurogenic bladder, diabetes, pregnancy, nephrolithiasis, immunosuppression, or indwelling urinary catheter.[4] Lower UTI consists of infections involving the urethra and bladder. Upper UTI refers to infections that occur in the kidney such as acute pyelonephritis or intrarenal and perinephric abscesses. Nephrolithiasis and interstitial cystitis are also discussed in this chapter. Management of renal problems during pregnancy is considered separately.

Lower Urinary Tract Infections

Lower UTIs include acute cystitis or UTI, and asymptomatic bacteriuria. Acute cystitis can refer to infection of the bladder (cystitis), or of the urethra (urethritis). Signs and symptoms of acute cystitis may include bacteriuria, frequency, urgency, suprapubic pain, and/or hematuria. A positive urine culture is defined as 100,000 colony forming units/milliliter (cfu/mL). However, 30% to 50% of women who have clinical symptoms will have less than 100,000 cfu. The criterion for diagnosing this entity is therefore lowered to 10^2 to 10^3 organisms/mL of urine in symptomatic women.[5] Asymptomatic bacteriuria is the presence of significant bacteriuria (>100,000 cfu/mL) of one to two bacterial species without symptoms. The criterion of 100,000 cfu/mL is applicable to specimens that were obtained from a clean catch, midstream voided sample. When the urine sample is obtained from a catheterized specimen or suprapubic aspirate, the criterion for infection is any amount of an organism.

A prospective study evaluated the incidence of asymptomatic bacteriuria in a young, sexually active female population and concluded that the prevalence was 5% to 6%. A symptomatic infection subsequently developed within one week in 8% of this population, demon-

strating the association of the two disease entities.[6] Asymptomatic bacteriuria has been shown to have a higher prevalence in women with both type I and type II diabetes, increasing from an incidence of 6% in controls to 21% in type I diabetics to 29% in type II diabetic women.[7] Elderly patients and those with long-standing indwelling bladder catheters also have an increased incidence of asymptomatic bacteriuria. A prospective study evaluating the incidence of asymptomatic bacteriuria in the elderly found that the incidence was higher in women than men in assisted living locations.[8]

It has been estimated that seven million episodes of acute cystitis are diagnosed in the United States annually.[4] A large prospective study to assess the independent risk factors for UTI found that risk for infection in sexually active young women included the following: recent sexual intercourse; recent use of a diaphragm with spermicide; and a history of recurrent UTIs.[4] This study was conducted in a setting of university students and women receiving care at a health maintenance organization. Although the results are not necessarily generalizable to all populations, it is one of the few prospective studies of independent risks. Other less significant risks include: blood group secretor status (a determinant of immunologic susceptibility to various diseases); ethnicity; parity; new sexual partner; sexual hygiene; and time interval to voiding after intercourse. Additional risk factors for UTI include a maternal history of UTI,[9] a history of childhood onset of UTI,[9] the presence of bacterial vaginosis,[10] and estrogen deficiency in postmenopausal women. A study that evaluated the relative influence of spermicide-coated or plain condoms found a higher incidence of UTIs in users of spermicide-coated condoms.[11] When women present for care with at least one symptom of a

UTI, the probability that such a diagnosis will be made has been found to be at least 50%.[12]

Etiology

The mechanism for colonization of the lower urinary tract is through adhesion to the uroepithelium, mediated by the papillae on the bacterial cell wall.[13] Bacteria commonly reach the urethra as a result of contamination from the rectum. The ascent of bacteria from the urethra may be facilitated by sexual intercourse, use of diaphragms, and spermicidal jelly. *E. coli* growth in the vagina is enhanced by the use of spermicides and diaphragms.[14] A normally functioning urinary system will prevent infection through several mechanisms. Fluid intake dilutes any bacteria that are present, and frequent voiding flushes the system. Bacterial growth is inhibited by the high urea content and osmolality of urine. Organic acids from mucosal cells and local antibody responses along with polymorphonuclear leukocytes in the bladder wall also destroy bacteria.[13] Urothelial mucosal cells secrete the tissue factors responsible for prohibiting or actively preventing attachment of bacteria to the mucosal surface. These cells have been found to be deficient in women who experience UTIs, especially recurrent infections.[13] A failure of some or all of these protective mechanisms, in addition to bacterial load and virulence, allows UTIs to develop.

E. coli, by far the most common pathogen, is seen in 80% to 85% of uncomplicated infections. The second most frequently seen organism is *Staphylococcus saprophyticus*; it has an incidence of 5% to 15%. Three other less commonly found organisms are *Klebsiella, Proteus*, and *Enterobacter*; their combined incidence varies from 5% to 10%.[15] Fungal infections are seen more frequently in hospitalized patients, diabetics, and patients who are immunocompromised. Group B streptococcal infections are seen more frequently in diabetics. *Enterobacter, Klebsiella* species, *Proteus mirabilis*, and *Staphylococcus saprophyticus* are gram negative organisms seen more commonly in complicated UTIs and in hospitalized patients.[16] Staphylococcus epidermidis, diptheroids, lactobacilli, and anaerobes are organisms commonly found on the skin and in the distal portion of the urethra and, therefore, represent probable contamination when seen in culture. The presence of trichomonas and yeast may also indicate vaginal contamination.

Signs and Symptoms

Signs of uncomplicated UTI include suprapubic and possibly low back pain. Symptoms include dysuria, frequency, urgency, voiding in small amounts, nocturia, incontinence, cloudiness of the urine, and hematuria as well as headache and malaise.

Essential History

Information obtained from the history dictates the extensiveness of the physical examination and the laboratory and imaging tests to be performed. Therefore, a complete and thorough history should screen for common symptoms of infection as well as determine whether any risk factors are present that increase the chances of infection. These include a prior history of recurrent infections or pyelonephritis and a history of childhood renal illnesses. Examples of these latter conditions include vesicoureteral reflux and unilateral kidney agenesis, which are thought to increase the chances of infection due to underlying anatomical and or functional abnormalities of the urinary tract.

Current symptoms, including the onset, severity, and duration of dysuria, and urgency should be investigated. Occasionally patients will describe symptoms of nocturia, low back pain, and loss of appetite. Systemic symptoms such as fever, malaise, chills, flank pain, or vomiting point to the possibility of an upper tract infection. Details of any attempt at self-treatment should be elicited, especially the use of herbal or homeopathic substances. Relevant medical conditions include diabetes, an immunocompromised state, a history of relapsing UTIs, recent urologic evaluations that included instrumentation, or a history of recent catheterization. When inquiring about a past history of UTIs, a recent infection (i.e., in the last 2 weeks) indicates the possibility of a relapsing infection. When taking a sexual history, noting the type of contraceptive (specifically, the type of condoms, use of spermicidal jelly, foam, or diaphragm) and whether anal-vaginal intercourse is practiced can identify an increased risk for UTI. Pregnancy, a peri- or postmenopausal state, and new environmental exposures may also increase risk. Other conditions that can have symptoms similar to UTIs include prior radiation exposure, chemotherapy for pelvic or bladder cancer, endometriosis, and interstitial cystitis.[17] A history of frequent or recurrent UTIs ideally should be corroborated by information from the culture prior to treatment.

Physical Examination

Information from the history dictates the components of the physical examination. Besides palpation of the abdomen, especially in the lower aspect, assessment of the back and costovertebral areas should be included if an upper UTI is suspected. A bimanual exam should be included as well as screening for vaginitis and for sexually transmitted diseases if the patient is sexually active. In menopausal women, inspection of the external genitalia and vagina for evidence of atrophic changes is appropriate.

Laboratory Examination

Urinalysis, including screening for the presence of leukocyte esterase and nitrites, is often the first step in assessment. The quality of the urine sample is influenced both by technique of collection and how the sample is handled. A first voided morning sample is desirable because the urine will have been in the bladder long enough to provide a more consistently accurate bacterial count. False negative tests can result from urine that has been too diluted by a large fluid intake[18] or urine that has spent a short time in the bladder. If an initial urine sample is contaminated, the subsequent urine should be collected after a sufficient time has elapsed for bacterial levels in the urinary tract to rise to detectable levels. Use of a tampon may reduce contamination by vaginal secretions during collection of the urine sample. Use of soap can result in a false positive result for the presence of protein.[19] Cleaning the urethral area with warm water is preferable. The urine sample needs to be transported and plated in a timely manner. If stored at room temperature for longer than one hour, bacteria numbers will increase, leading to an inaccurately high bacterial count.[2] If the sample remains at room temperature for greater than five hours, the alkalinity increases, and the sample will not provide an accurate culture.[20] Samples may be refrigerated for up to 48 hours without adversely affecting the accuracy of the analysis.[2]

Reagent strip (dipstick) analysis of a sample of urine from a midstream clean catch may be a more cost-effective and efficient approach to evaluating UTI symptoms than a urine culture is. Interpretation of the reagent strip from an uncontaminated sample is based on the following premises:

- Proteinuria may be an indicator of kidney damage
- Hematuria can be from either the upper or lower urinary tract
- Ketonuria is representative of the oxidation of fat (and is not reflective of a dehydrated state)
- Leukocyte esterase indicates the presence of white blood cells (WBCs)
- Nitrites are formed when nitrates are converted by the presence of bacteria[17]

Of these, the most useful measures of infection are the leukocyte esterase and nitrate tests. The sensitivity of the leukocyte esterase test has been found to have a range of 75% to 96% and a specificity of from 94% to 98% when compared to culture findings of at least 100,000 organisms, or greater than 10 leukocytes per high-powered field (HPF).[5]

Positive results from the urinalysis will distinguish a subset of samples that need to be examined microscopically for the presence of WBCs, epithelial cells, red blood cells (RBCs), casts, crystals, and bacteria. On a microscopic exam, five or more WBCs per HPF from a centrifuged, uncontaminated sample reflects true pyuria.[2] RBCs may indicate the presence of other diseases such as calculi, tumors, tuberculosis, vasculitis, or glomerulonephritis.[13] The presence of greater than four to six epithelial cells most likely reflects contamination. **Table 18-1** describes the common differential diagnoses that should be considered when evaluating abnormal findings found on urinalysis.

The decision to proceed with culture and sensitivity identification depends on risk status. Pregnant women, those with recurrent UTIs or failure of short course therapies, women unable to accurately identify their symptoms as being bladder-related, women with suspected renal involvement, and patients with recent urologic instrumentation require a urine culture. Culture is also indicated if the patient will be undergoing urologic surgery.[13] In general, those with uncomplicated UTIs can be treated based on history and urinalysis findings and do not require a culture, whereas those suspected of having a complicated UTI or underlying conditions that make eradication of infection more difficult should have a culture performed.

Controversy also exists about what cutoff values are important. Different authors cite varying criteria for the definition of pyuria, hematuria, and significant colony counts levels. Cutoff values reported to be significant for hematuria and pyuria range from two RBCs or WBCs per HPF to five RBCs or WBCs per HPF to as high as eight to ten RBCs or WBCs per HPF. In general, the higher the cutoff value deemed to be significant, the higher the positive predictive value of the test. **Table 18-2** lists predictive values of laboratory findings in infection. Using levels in the mid-range is prudent given that many samples in ambulatory practices are obtained via clean-catch technique. Reproductive-aged women, particularly those who are pregnant, are more likely to obtain samples that are contaminated by vaginal fluids, making the laboratory results less accurate and more difficult to interpret. Contamination cannot be determined by dipstick evaluation of a urine sample; however, microscopic findings of moderate to large numbers of epithelial cells indicate contamination. In this case, repeating

Table 18-1 DIFFERENTIAL DIAGNOSIS OF VARIOUS URINALYSIS AND MICROSCOPIC FINDINGS[21–23]

Dipstick Test	Dipstick Findings	Corresponding Microscopic Finding	Possible Causes
Leukocyte Esterase	Positive	6–10 WBCs/HPF [21,22]	Contamination with normal or infected vaginal fluids; cystitis, pyelonephritis.
Blood	Positive	3–5 RBCs/HPF or higher[23]	Coagulopathy; vaginal contamination; kidney damage or disease; cystitis; pyelonephritis; kidney stones, malignancy in older individuals; hemolytic anemias such as sickle cell; lesions in the bladder; excessive exercise.
Glucose	0–trace = normal 1/4 = 250 mg/dL 1/2 = 500 mg/dL 1 = 1000 mg/dL 2 ≥2000 mg/dL	NA	Positive with high sugar intake and/or diabetes. Spilled in urine when serum glucose level is 180mg/dL or higher
Proteint	0–trace = normal 1+ = 30 mg/dL 2+ = 100 mg/dL 3+ = 300 mg/dL 4+ ≥2000 mg/dL	NA	Positive in the presence of blood, vaginal contamination, amniotic fluid or bacteria and in conditions that increase filtration in the kidney (e.g., pregnancy, kidney damage). Transient increase with fever or excessive exercise.
Nitrate	Positive	Bacteria (may not be present in infections with lower colony counts of 10^2 or10^4)	Contamination with normal or infected vaginal fluids that contain nitrate reductase bacteria or in UTIs such as cystitis and pyelonephritis caused by these bacteria.

Abbreviations: WBC, white blood cells; HPF, high-powered field; RBCs, red blood cells; NA, not applicable; UTIs, urinary tract infections.

the sample via better clean-catch technique or catherization may result in more accurate findings. However, a high ratio of WBCs to epithelial cells in a contaminated sample suggests infection. In this case, the sample should be repeated and treatment individualized. **Table 18-3** describes the findings associated with common conditions affecting the urinary tract. **Figure 18-1** proposes an algorithm for evaluating UTIs in women.

Table 18-2 PREDICTIVE VALUE OF LABORATORY FINDINGS FOR URINARY TRACT INFECTION

Test	Sensitivity (%)	Specificity (%)	Positive Predictive Value (%)	Negative Predictive Value (%)
>5 WBC/HPF	80[21]	83[21]	46[21]	96[21]
>10 WBC/HPF	63[21]	90[21]	53[21]	93[21]
Nitrate	69[21]	90[21]	57[21]	94[21]
Leukocyte esterase	71–96[21,24]	85–94[21,24]	47[21]	94[21]
Nitrate and leukocyte esterase (either one positive)	75–86[21,25]	82–86[21,25]	54[21]	97[21]
Nitrate and leukocyte esterase (both positive)	75–96[5]	94–98[5]	75–93[26]	41–95[26]

Interpretation of the colony count found on culture is influenced by the presumed diagnosis based on prior history and current symptomatology. Historically, a colony count of 100,000 colony counts per milliliter (or 10^5) was considered indicative of infection. However, this older definition has been found to miss up to 50% of lower tract infections and up to 15% of cases of pyelonephritis.[5] Most authorities now agree that a diagnosis of infection can be based on cultures with a colony count of 10^2 to 10^3 bacteria/mL of urine in association with dysuria.[27] The colony count required to make the diagnosis of asymptomatic bacteriuria is still 10^5. Urine cultures that report three or more species with none being predominant are indicative of contamination and need repeating.

Treatment of Uncomplicated Urinary Tract Infections

Management of uncomplicated cystitis begins with obtaining a urinalysis. In the presence of pyuria or a positive leukocyte esterase test accompanied by symptoms, an empiric course of an antibiotic is given. Cultures do not need to be obtained from patients suspected of having an uncomplicated UTI who have clear symptoms of UTI and positive urinalysis results because the incidence of infection in this circumstance is 80% to 90%.[13] Women who meet the criteria for having a complicated UTI need a culture because these individuals are at higher risk of being infected with less common or antibiotic-resistant bacteria.

The patient's age, diabetes status, history of recurrent infections, kidney involvement, immune competence, and presumed severity of infection dictate the length of antibiotic treatment. Young women with new onset symptoms can safely receive a single dose therapy, although this is somewhat less effective than three- or five-day courses. For example, a one-day regimen of trimethoprim-sulfamethoxazole is estimated to eradicate infection in 87% of cases compared to 94% for three-day regimens.[25] There is no particular benefit in healthy women with uncomplicated UTIs receiving medication for more than three days. Longer courses do not

Table 18-3 DIPSTICK AND MICROSCOPIC FINDINGS SEEN IN COMMON URINARY TRACT CONDITIONS

Conditions	Laboratory Findings on Dipstick					Laboratory Findings on Microscopic Examination				
	Blood	Protein	Leukocytes	Esterace	Nitrates	WBC	RBC	Bacteria	Epithelial	Comments
Vaginal contam- ination	+/−	+/−	+/−	+/−	+/−	+/−	+/−	+/−	+++	Need to repeat the sample.
Urinary tract infection	+/−	+/−	++	++	++/−	++	++/−	+/−	0 to few	Pyuria is common in both cystitis and urethritis; however, hematuria differs according to what site is infected. Hematuria is common in cystitis but not urethritis.[24]
Acute pyleo- nephritis	+/−	+/−	++	++	++/−	+++/−	++/−	++	0 to few	Pyuria is common WBC. Casts may be present.
Kidney disease	++	++	−	−	−	+/−	++/−	−/−	0 to few	RBC casts are indicative of upper tract disease.

Figure 18-1 Evaluation of suspected urinary tract infection (UTI) symptoms using a proposed algorithm.

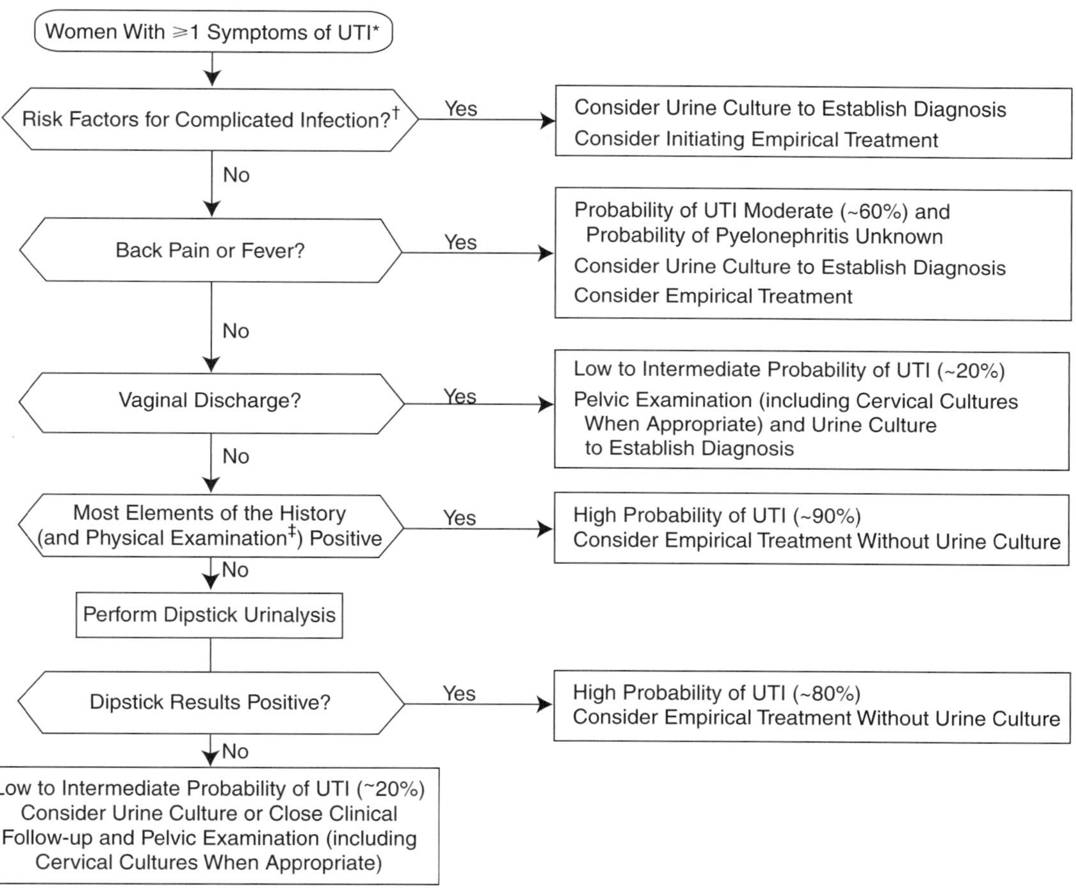

*In women who have risk factors for sexually transmitted diseases, consider testing for *Chlamydia*. The U.S. Preventive Task Force recommends screening for *Chlamydia* for all women age 25 or younger, and women of any age with more than one sexual partner, a history of sexually transmitted disease, or inconsistent use of condoms. † Complicated UTI is detailed in this chapter. ‡The only physical examination finding that increases the likelihood of UTI is costovertebral angle tenderness; clinicians may consider not performing this test in patients with typical symptoms of acute uncomplicated UTI (i.e., telephone management). *Source:* Reprinted with permission from the American Medical Association, ©2006.[12]

seem to be more effective in eradicating infection or preventing recurrences than a three-day course for acute uncomplicated cystitis and are associated with higher rates of adverse effects.[25] Older women generally require longer therapy as do those with complicated urinary tract infections. **Tables 18-4** and **18-5** list appropriate treatment regimens.

Empiric therapy is based on the knowledge of which bacteria are common causative agents as well as an understanding of local susceptibility patterns.[15] The optimal antibiotic exhibits the following characteristics:

- Able to achieve a high urine concentration
- Exhibits both Gram-negative and Gram-positive antimicrobial activity
- Has a minimal tendency to promote bacterial resistance
- Has a minimal effect on aerobic flora
- Eradicates aerobic Gram-negative rods from fecal and vaginal flora
- Has a long half-life
- Exhibits reasonable patient tolerance and minimal side effects
- Is inexpensive[13]

Cost, side effects profile, and risk of resistance all influence drug choice. Most urinary infections are sensitive to trimethoprim-sulfamethoxazole (TMP-SMX) or amoxicillin. TMP-SMX, trimethoprim, and the fluoroquinolones are the most frequently used antibiotics for treating UTIs. They all exhibit high rates of efficacy, are relatively well tolerated, and have a reasonable resistance rate.[28] The fluoroquinolones are the most expensive in this list and, depending on local antibiotic resistant patterns, could be reserved for UTI recurrences, treatment failures, or when allergies

Table 18-4 Treatment of Acute Uncomplicated Cystitis Using Single Dose Therapy[28]

Drug	Dose
Trimethoprim-sulfamethoxazole	4 single strength tablets PO
Trimethoprim	400 mg PO
Ciprofloxacin	500 mg PO
Fleroxacin	400 mg PO
Ofloxacin	400 mg PO
Pefloxacin	800 mg PO
Rufloxacin	400 mg PO
Amoxicillin	3 g PO
Fosfomycin trometamol	3 g PO

preclude the use of less expensive medications. There also is a greater risk of adverse events associated with their use. Other less efficacious

Table 18-5 Three- to Seven-Day Treatment of Urinary Tract Infections[3,13]

Antibiotic	Dose
Trimethoprim-sulfamethoxazole	160/800 mg bid for three days
Norfloxacin	400 mg bid for three days
Ofloxacin	200 mg bid for three days
Ciprofloxacin	250 mg bid for three days
Ciprofloxacin extended release	500 mg qd for three days
Levofloxacin	250 mg qd for three days
Lomefloxacin	400 mg qd for three days
Gatifloxacin	400 mg qd for three days
Nitrofurantoin	100 mg bid for seven days
Amoxacillin	500 mg tid for seven days
Sulfisoxasole	500 mg qid for seven days

choices for three-day therapy include amoxicillin, cefadroxil, or nitrofurantoin.[30,31]

Ampicillin, amoxicillin, and most of the cephalosporins rapidly achieve therapeutic levels in urine. The beta lactams are less frequently recommended for empiric treatment of acute cystitis because of their high frequency of resistance. Rates of resistance have shown regional variation. For example, resistance to TMP-SMX is 32% in the Western United States and 11% to 12% in the Northeast.[13] Some studies evaluating the susceptibility patterns of uropathogens have shown resistance rates for ampicillin as upwards of 25%.[13] As many as 33% of bacterial strains associated with uncomplicated cystitis and pyelonephritis in the United States exhibit resistance to amoxicillin and sulfonamides.[32] Therefore, it is imperative that health care providers have current knowledge of the resistance rates for the more frequently occurring pathogens in their local community. Resistance to TMP-SMX in outpatient settings is now estimated to be about 22% nationally, prompting some authorities to recommend extended release ciprofloxacin (Cipro XR) as the initial agent of choice for the outpatient treatment of uncomplicated UTIs and pyelonephritis.[24] However, increasing resistance to ciprofloxacin has also been documented, particularly in hospital-acquired infections. Consequently, different pharmacologic options may be recommended as first-line agents in the future.[24]

Recurrent Infections

Bacterial persistence refers to infection that recurs after successful eradication of the original organism. These infections result from a persistent focus within the urinary tract. In clinical practice, a UTI that occurs within two weeks of the original infection and is caused by the same organism is a relapse. A *recurrent infection*, by definition, is one that occurs more than two weeks after the prior one, regardless of whether the organism is the same or different. However, if the organism is the same as the original one and no cultures were obtained within two weeks of completion of antibiotics, then it is unclear whether the infection is due to a relapse or a re-infection. The majority of recurrences are re-infections.

Once a woman has had one UTI, the risk of recurrent infection has been estimated at between 20% and 40%.[33] A shorter than average anatomic distance from the urethra to the anus also increases the risk of recurrent UTIs. In postmenopausal women, three factors were found to have the most significant influence on the recurrence rate: urinary incontinence; presence of a history of UTI before menopause; and nonsecretor status.[34] The incidence of nonsecretor status of ABO blood group antigens is 3 to 4 times greater than in women who do not have recurrent UTIs.[34] Reduced bladder tone, post-void residual urine, bladder or uterine prolapse, or changes in the vaginal flora caused by a deficiency of estrogen (which makes uropathogens more prevalent) all increase the susceptibility of older women to recurrent UTIs. It has been hypothesized that administration of antibiotics that are active against the normal vaginal flora, such as the beta lactams, can alter the flora in such a way that bacterial colonization is facilitated.[35]

Management strategies for recurrent UTIs start with attempts at prevention. Decreasing or avoiding the use of spermicidal cream or jelly either alone or with diaphragms may help. Prompt postcoital voiding and adequate fluid intake to promote frequent voiding may be helpful in preventing some recurrences. Several small studies that investigated whether ingestion of cranberry juice could help reduce the risk of UTI had equivocal results.[36–38] One of these randomized 150 women with a history of UTI into three treatment groups: daily consumption of cranberry-lingonberry juice; consumption of a drink containing 100 mL of *Lactobaccilus* five days a week; or nothing. Women in the cranberry-consuming group had a 20% reduction in the absolute risk of having a recurrent infection.[38] A recent Cochrane review concluded that there was evidence that cranberry juice may decrease the number of symptomatic UTIs over a 12-month period in women, but that the optimum dose and route of administration (juice or pills) is unclear.[39]

Table 18-6 describes antibiotics to use post-intercourse to prevent UTIs.

Antimicrobial treatment for recurrent infections can be provided in a variety of ways. Prophylaxis is recommended for those women who have had either two infections in the prior six months or three infections in the prior 12 months. Patient preference as well as the frequency and severity of the infections will dictate the choice of postcoital medication, either three times weekly therapy or daily treatment. Intermittent self-treatment, in which the pa-

tient self-diagnoses the infection, can also be used effectively.[32,40] A short course of TMP-SMX or a fluoroquinolone is used for this purpose. Although the net number of recurrences may be slightly greater than with other treatment regimens, symptoms resolve quickly and the total amount of medication used is less.[32,40,41] Continuous prophylaxis is usually administered for six months. During this time one can expect to be free of symptomatic infection 95% of the time.[29] Some women will revert to recurrent infections; studies have shown a 60% recurrence rate after discontinuation of the prophylactic medication.[42] Long-term prophylaxis with TMP-SMX for up to two to five years has been used with success[43,44] and nitrofurantoin has also been used for long-term prophylaxis (**Table 18-7**).

TMP-SMX has the potential to reduce the effectiveness of estrogens by interrupting the enterohepatic recycling of estrogen.[45] It is possible that broad spectrum antibiotics may reduce the bioavailability of estrogen, but probably only in the first two weeks of use. At the present, the World Health Organization considers that the use of most broad spectrum antibiotics does not significantly affect the efficacy of combined hormonal contraceptives.[46]

Women who experience three or more infections in one year with the same organism may be candidates for further urologic evaluation including an intravenous pyelogram (IVP) or renal ultrasound and cystoscopy. While young women rarely have anatomic defects that require further evaluation, older women may need referral to a physician or practitioner competent in urogynecology.

Supportive therapy in the treatment of UTIs includes intake of adequate amounts of fluids

Table 18-6 POST-INTERCOURSE PROPHYLAXIS AGAINST URINARY TRACT INFECTION[29]

Medication	Dose
TMP/SMX	80 (tmp)/400 (smx) mg
TMP	100 mg
Nitrofurantoin	50–100 mg
Cephalexin	250 mg
Norfloxacin	200–400 mg
Ciprofloxacin	250 mg

Table 18-7 LONG-TERM LOW DOSE ANTIBIOTIC SUPPRESSION[29]

Medication	Dose
TMP/SMX	80 mg TMP/400 mg SMX mg daily at bedtime
	OR
	3 ×/week
TMP	100 mg daily at bedtime
Nitrofurantoin	50 mg daily at bedtime
Norfloxacin	200 mg 3 ×/week

to help flush the bacteria out of the urinary tract and also during administration of sulfonamides. Phenazopyridine, a urinary tract analgesic, may be used for a short (less than two-day) course in patients who have normal renal function. Two hundred milligrams may be administered by mouth three times per day as needed.

Several small studies indicate that the use of vaginal estrogen preparations may reduce the incidence of recurrent UTI in postmenopausal women.[34,47] The presumed mechanism of the estrogen replacement is the resultant increase of lactobacilli and lowering of vaginal pH.

Complicated Urinary Tract Infections

Complicated urinary tract infections are infections occurring in patients with functional or structural abnormalities. Infections occurring in pregnant women, diabetics, and elderly women, those who have structural or neurologic abnormalities, obstruction or stones, and persons with other immune or metabolic complications are all considered complicated UTIs.[17] Risks for the development of compli-

cated UTIs are a history of polycystic renal disease, nephrolithiasis, neurogenic bladder, and recent urinary instrumentation. A history of childhood renal illnesses will help to identify those patients who potentially have underlying anatomical and or functional abnormalities of the urinary tract, which require more aggressive screening and treatment.

A greater variety of organisms cause complicated UTIs, and an increased rate of antimicrobial resistance can be seen in these infections.[43,48] Some of the organisms involved are: *Escherichia coli (E. coli)*, *Klebsiella*, *Proteus*, *Serratia*, *Pseudomonas*, enterococci, and staphylococci.[8] Fungal infections are seen more frequently in hospitalized patients, diabetics, and patients who are immunocompromised. Group B streptococcal infections are seen more frequently in diabetics and pregnant patients.

Both a urinalysis and culture and sensitivity should be obtained when screening for a complicated UTI. Cultures should also be performed if the patient will be undergoing urologic surgery or has had recent instrumentation, including catheterization.[13] Empiric therapy can be started while waiting for culture results. A minimum of seven days is recommended for antibiotic treatment. If symptoms are mild, an oral fluoroquinolone can be used. Hospitalization is indicated in more severe infections, with administration of intravenous (IV) antibiotics such as imipenem, penicillin, a cephalosporin with an aminoglycoside, ceftriaxone or ceftrazidime.[8] Antibiotics should be continued for one to three weeks, depending on the severity of the infection and the individual rate of clinical improvement. A culture should be repeated two to four weeks after finishing the medication to confirm a cure.

Upper Urinary Tract Infections

Uncomplicated Pyelonephritis

Acute pyelonephritis is an upper tract infection that may or may not be associated with asymptomatic bacteriuria or cystitis. Commonly, it is an ascending infection arising from the urethra, moving to the bladder, and then to the kidneys. Other uncommon routes of infection are hematogenous, for example: in the case of debilitated or immunocompromised patients; or as a result of bacteremia or fungemia;[8] or lymphatic in origin.

Not all cases of pyelonephritis are accurately diagnosed. Although evidence of pyelonephritis has been found in 12% to 20% of autopsies, the diagnosis of that infection existed in only 20% of the cases.[49] The annual incidence of pyelonephritis in the United States is estimated to be 250,000.[50] Nicolle et al. studied hospitalization rates for pyelonephritis in Manitoba, Canada. Mean rates for hospitalization of women were 10.86 per 10,000 and included pregnant and/or diabetic women. Hospitalization rates were similar among young women (aged 20–29) and the elderly ($\geq$70).[51]

Signs and symptoms of pyelonephritis include complaints of cystitis and back pain, or more significant findings such as nausea and vomiting, flank pain, fever greater than 38°C (100.4°F), and costovertebral angle tenderness (CVAT). A study of women presenting to an emergency department for symptoms of pyelonephritis found that the presence of fever >38.7°C was strongly correlated with the diagnosis.[52] Symptoms of pyelonephritis can develop rapidly. The duration of symptoms prior to presentation for care is frequently less than four days. Symptoms of cystitis may or may not be present in patients with pyelonephritis. They may precede, be coincident with, or follow the development of pyelonephritis. Acute disease may be accompanied by systemic symptoms such as malaise, chills and shaking, flank pain, or vomiting associated with a high fever.[8]

The causative uropathogen in up to 80% of cases is *E. coli*. Uropathogenic strains constitute a unique subgroup of *E. coli*. They usually secrete hemolysin and/or aerobactin, factors that possess pyelonephritis-associated pili. In this instance, *pili* are specialized fine, keratinized filamentous growths that mediate bacterial conjugation;[5] they assist in the attachment of bacteria to uroepithelial cells.[8]

Certain laboratory findings are more suggestive of pyleonephritis. The standard criterion of $\geq$100,000 cfu/mL of pathogen is seen in 80% to 90% of cases.[53] Results suggestive of pyelonephritis on urine dipstick include protein, blood, nitrates, and leukocyte esterase. Microscopic results from the urinalysis usually show significant levels of leukocytes and bacteria. White cell casts can be seen in association with pyelonephritis and are generally considered pathognomonic; however, their absence does not rule out the diagnosis.[13]

All women in whom the diagnosis of pyelonephritis is suspected should have urine cultures obtained prior to the initiation of antibiotic therapy. Blood cultures should be considered in women who have a high fever and/or require hospitalization. Fifteen to 20% of these patients will have positive blood cultures.[8]

Management of uncomplicated pyelonephritis is straightforward. A urine culture is sent, and a 10- to 14-day course of antibiotic treatment is started immediately; treatment is not delayed pending results. TMP-SMX has been shown in several studies to have only a 1% failure rate.[5] However, resistance to TMP-SMX is rapidly increasing, so knowledge of local resistance patterns is essential in making appropriate treatment choices. Patients who have mild symptoms without high fever, nausea, or vomiting may be treated on an outpatient basis with a 10- to 14-day course of TMP-SMX, norfloxacin, ciprofloxacin, or ofloxacin. An alternative approach is parenteral gentamycin in the urgent care setting followed by a course of oral medication. Gentamycin plus ampicillin is a standard choice, because the combination provides a broad spectrum of coverage and is low in cost.

If the rate of resistance in the community is high, a quinolone may be a better choice. Follow-up culture should be done two to four days after finishing the antibiotic in order to identify those patients who may experience relapses. If the infection recurs, antibiotics may need to be taken for six weeks.

Complicated Pyelonephritis

The following conditions constitute complicated pyelonephritis and mandate hospitalization for treatment:

- Age ≥55 years
- Recurrence of pyelonephritis
- Presence of diabetes
- Presence of an immunocompromised state
- Presence of severe symptoms

Chronic pyelonephritis may have the same symptoms as acute pyelonephritis, and also include nonspecific symptoms such as malaise, fatigue, or abdominal pain. One type of complicated pyelonephritis, Xanthogrulomatous pyelonephritis, is caused by an obstructing stone that on radiologic exam may appear to be a mass-

like lesion. The advantage of treatment with ciprofloxacin in the case of complicated or chronic pyelonephritis is its ability to provide broad spectrum coverage of many Gram-negative and Gram-positive organisms with minimal toxicity.[54] The duration of antibiotic therapy is at least 10 to 14 days. If the follow-up culture is positive or the patient is still symptomatic after initiation of treatment, the duration of antibiotic administration should be extended to 21 days.[54] Subsequent antibiotic suppression may be considered (Table 18-7). Patients who experience recurrent pyelonephritis are also candidates for further urologic evaluation.

Subclinical Pyelonephritis

Not all women who have upper urinary tract infections present with the expected symptoms of high fever and flank pain.[55] Women may have symptoms of cystitis but fail to respond to the usual short course therapy. The factors increasing risk of a silent kidney infection are similar to those for complicated UTIs. Rapid relapse after short course therapy also suggests subclinical pyelonephritis. The diagnosis is often made with difficulty and in retrospect. Culture and sensitivity for persistent symptoms, and in those at risk, will help to support an effective choice of antibiotic. Two to six weeks of therapy may be required to eradicate the infection.

Nephrolithiasis

Kidney stones are formed by the crystals of salt precipitates that have grown by aggregation into large masses. Retention of these crystals in the renal collecting system leads to the development of nephrolithiasis. The most common stones in the United States are composed of calcium oxalate. Calcium stones evolve from a crystallization process that probably begins in the loop of Henle[56] or in the distal part of the distal tubule.[57] Any calcium phosphate crystals present in the urine may be dissolved as they reach the collecting ducts. At this point, the urine is usually supersaturated with calcium salts. Women who form calcium stones will experience the development of large crystals that then move slowly down the nephron and can adhere to the tubular cells.[58]

Knowledge of stone composition informs the diagnosis and management of kidney stones. Calcium-containing stones can be composed of pure calcium oxalate (either dehydrate or monohydrate), or be mixed with calcium phosphate. **Table 18-8** lists the common types of kidney stones.

Nephrolithiasis has a frequency of up to 12% of the general population, more commonly in Caucasians, and more frequently in an age range of 20 to 50 years. Recurrence rates are almost 50%,[61] and men are three times more likely than women to develop kidney stones.[59] Certain diseases are known to be associated with stone formation. Some examples include: hyperuricosuria, which is seen in patients with neoplastic states where cell turnover is very high; conditions such as sarcoidosis; and autoimmune diseases such as Sjögren syndrome.[62] Other associated conditions seen with nephrolithiasis are myeloma, use of certain drugs such as lithium, medulary sponge kidney, and gout.[62] Hyperthyroidism, hyperparathyroidism, Cushing's syndrome, immobilization, rapidly progressive bone disease, and Paget's disease also cause hypercalciurea and are associated with an increased incidence of nephrolithiasis.[63]

The primary symptom of urinary stones is acute flank pain radiating to the groin area. The pain may localize to the lower abdominal area in

Table 18-8 TYPES OF CALCULI[59,60]

Type	Incidence	Comments
Calcium oxalate	80%	60% increased incidence of urinary calcium; serum level can be normal. Seen in hypercalcemia, hyperparathyroidism, hyperthyroidism sarcoidosis, increased bone demineralization.
Struvite	2%–20%	Responsible for the majority of staghorn calculi. Caused by urease producing bacteria in UTIs.
Uric acid	6% (seen in 20% of patients with gout)	Formed by supersaturation of excess uric acid, low urine . volume
Cystine	1%	Autosomal recessive inherited disorder
Miscellaneous: Xanthine Silicate Indinavir	Less than 1%	

the vicinity of the stone and radiate to the pelvis. As the stone travels down the tubule, it may cause lower quadrant pain that radiates to the urethra or labia. Symptoms of urinary frequency, urgency, dysuria, and CVAT are often present. Findings on urinalysis include hematuria in 90% of cases.[64,65] Concurrent hydronephrosis and distention of the renal capsule may cause nausea and vomiting.[59] Radiologic examination of the kidneys and collecting system is used to evaluate the function and presence of anatomical abnormality. It also serves to confirm the diagnosis, helps to rule out other diagnoses with similar symptoms, has the potential to determine obstruction or infarction, and can identify the location of the stone.[59] The preferred imaging study for confirmation of the diagnosis of kidney stone is an unenhanced helical computed tomography (CT) of the abdomen and pelvis.[66] Unfortunately, CT cannot differentiate between severe and mild obstruction.[67] A study performed to compare the sensitivities of CT with IVP reported a higher sensitivity (96% vs. 87%) with the CT.[68] Follow-up with a plain abdominal x-ray will determine if the stone is radiopaque and aids in the diagnosis of the type of stone. Stones composed of calcium, magnesium salts, and uric acid are radiolucent.[20] Ultrasound can also be used to diagnose stones directly. In a prospective study done to compare the use of ultrasound with IVP, it was found that an experienced sonographer could identify stones with a 64% sensitivity and 100% specificity.[69]

Stone size and location in the renal system will influence the natural progression of the disease. Those stones that are less than 6 mm in diameter and located in the distal ureter have the highest rate of spontaneous passage.[70] Stones that are less than 5 mm will pass spontaneously 75% of the time.[62] Sixty-six percent of stones that pass spontaneously will do so within the first four weeks after onset of symptoms.[65] Complications such as renal function deterioration, sepsis, and ureteral stricture are seen at a rate of 20%.[71]

The medical management of nephrolithiasis in nonpregnant females consists primarily of increasing fluid intake as well as dietary modifications. Several studies have shown a reduced incidence of kidney stones in the general population with increased fluids.[72,73] Increased fluid intake also has been shown to reduce the incidence of stone recurrence.[74,75]

When women are prone to stone formation, dietary counseling may help to reduce recurrences. Dietary changes are thought to affect the excretion of calcium, oxalate, and uric acid, all of which are substances thought to promote stone development.[76] Counseling must take into account the type of stone, because dietary restrictions vary with stone type. For example, diets that contain large amounts of refined carbohydrates, animal proteins, and salt and a low intake of vegetables and fruit increase the risk of hypercalciuria and the development of calcium oxalate stones.[76] Diets low in calcium traditionally have been recommended for the treatment of calcium oxalate stones, but other dietary changes are now thought to be more effective and safer. Low calcium diets are believed to provoke hyperoxaluria, which can promote the development of stones and also may lead to a negative calcium balance and subsequent bone loss.[76] High oxalate-containing foods include walnuts, hazelnuts, peanuts, almonds, beets, spinach, rhubarb, parsley, chives, chocolate, cocoa, wheat germ, brown rice, and tea.[76] Hyperoxaluria is treated with avoidance of these foods, a reduction in the intake of carbohydrates, and animal protein, and encouragement of normal intake of calcium.[76] An observational study was able to show an association between the dietary intake of at least 40 mg pyridoxine (vitamin B_6) per day and the reduction of oxalate.[77] Uric acid stone disease is treated with limitation of meats and other foods high in purine.[76] A potassium-enriched diet derived from fruit, fruit juices, and vegetables can improve hypocitraturia.[76] Higher levels of citrate are thought to protect against calcium stones. Cystinuria treatment includes reduction of the intake of cystine and methionine amino acids and common salt.[76]

Drug therapy is reserved for more complicated cases. Medications are used when nephrolithiasis is accompanied by urinary abnormalities that diets have failed to ameliorate. Thiazides and indipamide have been shown to be effective in the reduction of stone recurrence.[76] Unfortunately, there are a number of side effects with these medications, such as hypotension, muscular cramps, asthenia, hypokalemia, hyponatremia, hypomagnesemia, hyperuricemia, hyperglycemia, and hypercholesterolemia.[76]

Uric acid stones can be treated by alkalinizing the urine because an alkaline state dissolves pure uric acid stones. Alkali, in the form of sodium bicarbonate or acetazolamide, can be used to elevate the urinary pH. If the daily uric acid level is greater than 1000 mg despite dietary reduction of purine and increased fluid intake, allopurinal may be administered to reduce uric acid production.[62,76] Side effects seen with the use of this drug include pruritis, urticaria, maculopapular and exfoliative skin eruptions, dyspepsia, and abdominal pain.[76] If this treatment fails, the approach to therapy should be the same as for radiopaque stones.[65]

Cystinuria is treated with alkalinizing salts (potassium citrate) as well as with drugs that bind the urinary cystine and form more soluble complexes. These drugs include tioprin and penicillamine.[76] Struvite stones are treated with the surgical removal of the stone and then long-term antibiotic administration. Acetohydroxamic acid inhibits the production of urease. It has the potential to reduce the formation of struvite calculi; however, it has a large number of side effects, such as phlebothrombosis, tremulousness, hemolytic anemia, and alopecia.[76]

Surgical Management of Stones

Obstruction is an indication for hospitalization. Open renal and ureteral surgery is the gold standard for definitive treatment of large stones. Three modalities are available for the treatment of stones that are too large to pass through the renal system: percutaneous nephrostolithotomy; rigid and flexible ureterorenoscopy; and shock wave lithotripsy. *Percutaneous nephrostolithotomy* is a technique in which an incision is made in the flank, a nephroscope is inserted into the kidney, and the stone is broken up and removed using a laser, ultrasound probe, or pneumatic device. *Ureterorenoscopy* is a procedure used to access middle and distal ureteral stones.[70] *Shock wave lithotripsy* uses high energy shock waves, delivered through a water medium, with the guidance of biplanar fluoroscopy. The stones are fragmented by the energy delivered to the surface of the stone. Open surgery is used for the management of complicated renal and ureteral calculi that cannot be resolved with the use of the prior techniques.[78] Morbidly obese patients may need open surgery because their body habitus may preclude localization by fluoroscopy or ultrasonography. Shock wave lithotripsy may fail because of wave attenuation by the excess tissue.[79]

Pregnancy Considerations

UTIs are frequently encountered in pregnancy. Pregnant women with asymptomatic bacteriuria have an increased incidence of pyelonephritis, leading to an increase in preterm birth and low birth weight.[80] Asymptomatic bacteriuria occurs in 2% to 10% of women, similar to the rate seen in a nonpregnant population. Cystitis and pyelonephritis combined have an incidence of approximately 3%.[81]

Anatomical and physiologic changes of pregnancy influence the frequency of infections. Pregnancy causes an increase in the volume, weight, and size of the kidney. The ureters, calyces, and renal pelvises undergo dilation. Because of the slight dextro-rotation of the uterus during pregnancy, and the more acute angle of the right ureter as it passes over the pelvic brim, dilation is usually seen more on the right. The dilated collecting system is responsible for up to an additional 200 cc volume of urine in the bladder. Both the glomerulofiltration rate and blood flow are increased, but simultaneously, higher progesterone levels seen in pregnancy contribute to decreased ureteral peristalsis and prolonged transit time of urine from the kidneys to the bladder. Incomplete bladder emptying and subsequent stasis of urine helps to increase the risk for UTIs. The higher renal threshold for glucosuria seen in pregnancy somewhat mimics a diabetic state with its concomitant increase in UTIs. Late in pregnancy, the distended uterus may contribute to a syndrome in which the patient experiences abdominal discomfort, hydronephrosis, and possibly, hypertension and an increase in serum creatinine levels.[82]

Routine screening for and treatment of asymptomatic bacteriuria in pregnancy has not changed the incidence of cystitis, but it has decreased the incidence of pyelonephritis approximately five-fold.[83,84] Asymptomatic bacteriuria, if untreated, will progress to pyelonephritis in 20% to 40% of pregnant women. Treating the bacteriuria will reduce the rate of pyelonephritis later in the pregnancy from 30% to 1% to 2%.[29]

The incidence of cystitis in pregnant women has been found to be 0.3% to 2%.[85] Women who have sickle cell trait or disease have an increased incidence of UTIs and should be screened each trimester in pregnancy. A colony count of 1000 or greater is considered positive for UTI in pregnancy if the patient is symptomatic and pyuria is seen in the urinalysis. Treatment of UTIs in pregnancy consists of a seven- to ten-day course of antibiotics (**Table 18-9**). Treatment suggestions by different authorities vary slightly, both in which specific antibiotic should be considered the best first-line agent as well as how long treatment should last. Based on their analysis of antibiotic resistance trends and the safety of antibiotics in pregnancy, the ACUTE Consensus Panel recommends various agents depending on the type of infection found in pregnancy: a beta-lactam, cephalexin, or nitrofurantoin for the treatment of asymptomatic bacteriuria; a five- to seven-day course of cephalexin for the treatment of cystitis; and a 7- to 14-day course of IV antibiotics for complicated UTIs such as pyelonephritis in pregnancy.[24] Repeat urine cultures should be obtained one to two weeks after completion of the drug therapy. Urinalysis and culture are then repeated at least once in each subsequent trimester of the pregnancy.

The incidence of pyelonephritis in pregnancy is estimated to be between 1% and 2.5% and is

Table 18-9 TREATMENT OF URINARY TRACT INFECTIONS IN PREGNANCY[24,81,86]

Medication	Dose	Category
Amoxicillin	500 mg tid × 7 d	B
Nitrofurantoin	100 mg PO bid × 7 d	C
		Folate antagonist
Cephalexin	500 mg qid × 7 d	B
Sulfisoxazole	Initial 2 g, then 1 g	C
	qid x 7 d	Avoid near term (hyperbilirubinemia)
Trimethoprim/	160/800 mg bid × 7 d	C
sulfamethoxazole		Folate antagonist
Cefixime	400 mg q 24 h × 7 d	B
Cefpodoxime proxetil	100 mg q 12 h × 7 d	B

highest toward the end of the second and beginning of the third trimester.[39] The recurrence rate during the same pregnancy is anywhere from 10% to 18%.[80] The most common organisms seen, in order of frequency, are *E. coli*, *Klebsiella*, *Enterobacter*, and *Proteus*.[80] The signs and symptoms of pyelonephritis in pregnant women are similar to those found in nonpregnant women, but the management is quite different. CVAT may be more pronounced on the right than the left. As with nonpregnant women, symptoms of cystitis may be present. Hospitalization is required to promptly correct dehydration and electrolyte imbalance and to initiate parenteral antibiotic therapy. Blood cultures may be obtained if high fevers are present because up to 10% of women will have bacteremia. Endotoxic shock is seen in approximately 3% of cases.[24,87]

Hospitalization for IV antibiotics is the preferred approach for the treatment of pyelonephritis in pregnancy.[24] The usual intravenous antibiotic choice is ceftriaxone, although ampicillin with gentamycin, extended-spectrum penicillins, or aztreonam are other choices.[24] Daily dosing of ceftriaxone has been found to be just as effective as multiple dosing of cefazolin.[88] Other antibiotic choices include TMP-SFX or ampicillin.[80] The cephalosporins are used more commonly now than the aminoglicosides unless *Enterobacter* is suspected or the patient appears at risk of septic shock.[80] In this circumstance, ampicillin or a cephalosporin and gentamycin would be appropriate.

During the initial stages of infection and early in the antibiotic treatment of pyelonephritis, the frequency of uterine contractions is often increased. Prompt antibiotic treatment and a course of tocolysis may help prevent preterm labor and delivery. One of the most concerning complications of pyelonephritis in pregnancy is the development of acute respiratory distress syndrome (ARDS), especially in the first 48 hours after initiating antibiotic therapy.[81,89] The following are factors that may increase the risk of developing ARDS or indicate its presence:

- Maternal heart rate ≥110 beats/min
- Fever ≥103°F in the first 24 hours
- Use of ampicillin as a single agent
- Fluid overload[90]

Once the patient is no longer febrile and is not exhibiting signs of preterm labor, she may be discharged home to finish a 10-day course of oral medication.

After one episode of pyelonephritis in pregnancy or any recurrent infection, patients should receive antibiotic suppression for the remainder of the pregnancy. Choices for antibiotic suppression include nightly dosing of nitrofurantoin (50–100 mg), amoxicillin (250 mg), cephalexin (250 mg)[91], or TMP-SFX (160/800 mg).[80] This treatment should be continued for six weeks postpartum. The effects of pregnancy on the renal system will not have resolved until that time (Table 18-7). An alternative approach is to follow patients closely with urinalysis and culture screening every two weeks until 36 weeks gestation. Lenke et al. found no significant difference in outcomes with this approach when compared to antibiotic suppression.[92] Yet another management scheme is the use of postcoital prophylaxis in the form of single oral doses of cephalexin (250 mg) or nitrofurantoin macrocrystals (50 mg).[92] Those patients who were catheterized during their hospitalization for delivery or who experienced periurethral or anterior vaginal trauma will be at slightly increased risk for UTIs during the early postpartum period.

The incidence of urolithiasis in pregnancy is 0.03% to 0.35%.[93] The most common type of stone seen in pregnancy is calcium oxalate. Staghorn stones, uric acid, and cystine stones are seen less commonly. Pregnant women with urolithiasis usually present with abdominal and flank pain. The symptoms of urolithiasis can be mistaken for appendicitis, diverticulitis, or placental abruption.[94] Also included in the differential diagnosis of urolithiasis are UTI, pyelonephritis, pelvic inflammatory disease, abdominal aortic aneurysm, and bladder cancer. Hematuria is seen in up to 90% of cases of urolithiasis.[60] Ultrasound of the renal collecting system is the preferred method of imaging in pregnancy because it provides adequate imaging of the calculi and avoids radiation exposure from abdominal x-rays. One study found the sensitivity and specificity of ultrasound in diagnosing calculi to be approximately 34% and 86%, respectively.[94] Newer techniques such as resistive index calculation, ureteral jet identification, and vaginal ultrasound improve the accuracy of the diagnoses.[95] If necessary, a limited IVP is acceptable to provide a definitive diagnosis of calculi in pregnancy.[60] Internal ureteral stents can be placed if the patient is unable to pass a ureteral calculus. Because of the associated risk of asymptomatic UTI, patients should be screened for infection at appropriate intervals during the pregnancy. Adequate pain relief and hydration is necessary for the treatment of urolithiasis in pregnancy. Fortunately, 70% to 80% of women will pass their stones spontaneously. Symptomatic obstructive hydronephrosis can be treated with sonographically guided percutaneous nephrostomy[96] or the placement of ureteral stents. Definitive stone treatment can then be deferred until the postpartum period.[97] When necessary, ureteroscopy can be safely used during the intrapartum period.[95]

Interstitial Cystitis

Interstitial cystitis is a painful bladder disease that is chronic in nature and characterized by discomfort in the bladder and pelvic areas; some motor and or sensory functions of the bladder may be affected as well. Frequently, the diagnosis is delayed because the symptoms—pressure, urgency, frequency, and bladder pain—are nonspecific. These symptoms are present with cystitis, but tend to be more pronounced, persistent, and severe in interstitial cystitis. Many women with interstitial cystitis also report nocturia and severe dyspareunia. It should be suspected if the patient reports multiple treatment failures for cystitis and whose testing fails to demonstrate infection.

The etiology of interstitial cystitis is unclear but may include an autoimmune reaction against bladder antigens and a deficiency in the glycosaminoglycan layer of the bladder surface that presumably allows toxins to penetrate the mucosa. Subsequent mast cell infiltration and activation lead to histamine release and local bladder wall damage from bacteria.[98] Other theories have proposed that interstitial cystitis results from damage due to occult infection, toxin exposure, or inflammatory changes in the smooth muscle of the bladder.[99] The National Institutes of Health have established a set of criteria for the clinical definition of interstitial cystitis. The diagnosis is derived from the inclusion and exclusion of particular symptoms, cystoscopic findings of bladder wall inflammation, and the absence of other diseases that can cause similar symptoms.

Submucosal hemorrhages or ulcers are commonly seen on cystoscopy. Histopathology from biopsy confirms the diagnosis.[98]

The prevalence of interstitial cystitis has been estimated at 30 cases per 100,000 in the United States.[98] About 9 out of 10 patients are female.[100] Symptoms include frequency, nocturia, and suprapubic pain. A study designed to investigate the natural history of interstitial cystitis reported that in a group of 374 women, the symptoms of interstitial cystitis progressed rapidly and then seemed to plateau within five years of onset of disease.[101]

After obtaining a detailed history of the symptoms experienced by the patient and information about any prior attempts at diagnosis, a thorough exam is done to rule out gynecologic or neurologic pathology. If the patient keeps a voiding diary, quantitative information about the frequency, amount of voided urine, and specific information about the ingestion of substances known to be bladder irritants can be obtained. Bladder irritants include caffeine, chocolate, citrus fruits, alcoholic beverages (especially red wine), spicy foods, tomatoes, aspartame, saccharine, monosodium glutamate, nuts, vinegar, onions, and soy sauce.[99] By eliminating all potential irritants from the diet and then gradually re-introducing them one at a time, it may be possible to identify those dietary changes that will reduce symptoms.

A urinalysis and culture should be obtained to evaluate for the presence of infection or hematuria. If hematuria is present, urine cytology should be done to look for cancerous or precancerous cells because hematuria can be a symptom of bladder cancer.

Measures that reduce the acidity of the urine may make voiding more comfortable. Increasing fluid intake can dilute urine, making it less acidic. Medications such as Prelief (which is an over-the-counter product sprinkled over food and ingested) and baking soda ($1/_2$ teaspoon with a glass of water three times per day) can also reduce the acidity of the urine.[99]

Initial attempts at medication therapy take an empiric approach, with the use of narcotic pain relievers as well as antidepressants and antihistamines. The latter are believed to decrease the stress associated with chronic pain, as well as reduce pain. Dimethyl sulfoxide has been approved by the Food and Drug Administration for instillation into the bladder. While the mechanism of action is unclear, its ability to permeate the bladder wall may make it reduce pain and inflammation more effectively. Initial instillations are performed in the urologist's office. Some women learn to perform the procedure at home. Pentosan polysulfate sodium (Elmiron) is an oral medication that provides relief from pain and frequency for some patients. Relief may take several months to develop, so long-term trials are necessary for the woman wishing to use this medication. The mechanism of action is unknown.

Women can use their voiding diary and autodilation to increase the time span between voidings. *Autodilation* refers to the process by which the patient gradually increases the time interval between voiding. In this way, the bladder is very gradually distended in small increments over a prolonged period of time. Patients should be seen frequently in order to monitor whether they are adhering to the voiding schedule and to receive support and encouragement.

Women suspected of having interstitial cystitis require a complete workup and should be referred to a specialist. A voiding cystogram is commonly ordered to evaluate for the presence of urethral defects. Urodynamic testing is done to screen for a neurogenic bladder, bladder instability, outlet obstruction, and the presence of sensory instability. The diagnosis is often made based on the clinical findings and the results of a cystoscopic evaluation. The most accurate information is obtained if biopsies are performed at the time of the cystocopy and if the cystoscopy is done using hydrodistension.[98] Because chronic inflammation may cause a contracted bladder with reduced capacity, evaluating the bladder capacity may help in the diagnosis. Hydrodistension ameliorates the symptoms in 20% to 30% of patients for as long as six months.[99] Refractory interstitial cystitis may be treated with percutaneous sacral nerve root neuromodulation. An electrode is placed in the S3 foramen and attached to a portable stim-

ulator unit. If this intervention improves symptoms, a permanent electrode lead and stimulator are implanted. Success rates as high as 73% have been seen with this technology.[99]

In rare instances, a surgical approach is utilized. Cystectomy, urethrectomy, and continent diversion have been the most successful treatments.[99] Ablation of the bladder lining has also been used with varying success rates.[99] Quality of life issues are a major component of the treatment of patients with this chronic disease.

Midwifery Management

The role of the midwife in the management of various urinary conditions will depend on the condition in question as well as the system in which the midwife practices. Certainly, independent management of UTIs is within the scope of midwifery practice in all practice settings. Asymptomatic bacteriuria and recurrent lower tract infections occurring in the nonpregnant population can be managed independently, as can uncomplicated pyleonephritis that responds appropriately to outpatient treatment. Complicated lower UTIs in the nonpregnant or pregnant women that do not respond to appropriate treatment may warrant further consultation or referral. Complicated cases of pyleonephritis in the nonpregnant woman and all cases of pyleonephritis in pregnancy should be co-managed or referred to the consulting physician. Knowledge of the risk factors for each type of UTI supports the delivery of health care to affected women in a safe, efficient, and cost-effective manner.

Given the chronicity and disability associated with interstitial cystitis for many women, those suspected of having this condition should have a thorough evaluation by a urogynecologist.

Follow-up care should be individualized and may be best managed using a team approach. Comprehensive care of patients with interstitial cystitis should include psychosocial assessments and multidisciplinary interventions, including behavioral and chronic pain counseling.

Pelvic Pain

While urinary-related conditions may account for a significant percentage of cases of lower abdominal pain, they are not the only cause. Infections of the vagina, the uterus, and ovaries as well as ovarian cysts, ectopic pregnancies, and uterine tumors can also cause pain. Women presenting with lower abdominal pain require a thorough evaluation of all potential urinary and pelvic problems. The differential should also include gastrointestinal conditions. Chapter 17 describes the general approach used to assess abdominal complaints; a more thorough discussion of the history and physical examination needed to evaluate women presenting with abdominal pain can be found there.

Essential History

Questioning includes the timing and normalcy of the last menstrual period, the regularity of the cycle, the presence of any cyclic pain, the amount of menstrual flow, and bleeding patterns. The cyclic or persistent nature of any pain provides clues to potential diagnoses. Responses to these questions can help to identify intrauterine or ectopic pregnancies, ovarian cysts, fibroids, and endometriosis. A sexual history can help determine whether sexually transmitted infections or pregnancy may be contributing to the problem. A medication history should be obtained because the use of certain medications, such as oral contraceptives, or birth control devices, such as in-trauterine devices (IUDs), may affect the likelihood that certain conditions will occur.

Essential Physical Examination

The pelvic examination, in combination with the general abdominal examination, provides essential information needed to determine the most likely diagnostic possibilities. Both speculum and bimanual examinations are required. Speculum examination provides not only an opportunity to collect specimens but an observation of cervical changes, any lesions or masses in the vagina or at the cervix, and bleeding sources. The bimanual examination allows an assessment of changes in the cervix; the size, shape, regularity, and position of the uterus and ovaries; localization of pain; and any associated masses. When appropriate, rectal examination is done to identify masses, nodularity, the size and shape of a retroverted uterus, and any bowel abnormalities.

Laboratory and other tests appropriate to diagnose the various conditions discussed below are included in the following sections.

Endometriosis

Endometriosis is defined as functioning endometrial tissue consisting of endometrial glands and stroma, growing outside of the uterine cavity, usually on the surface of abdominal organs, pelvic structures, and/or ligaments in the peritoneal cavity.[102–104] Little is known about the true prevalence or predisposing factors for the disease, because endometriosis can be definitely diagnosed only by surgery.[104] There is no definitive cure for endometriosis; women present with varying degrees of pain and altered fertility that do not necessarily correlate with the extent of the disease.[105] Women can experience mild symptoms or be asymptomatic. Diagnosis is often made incidentally when the woman undergoes laparoscopy for an unrelated reason such as tubal ligation or investigation of infertility. Conversely, other women may experience severe dysmenorrhea and dyspareunia. Because a cure is not available, the aim in management is symptom control.

Endometriosis occurs frequently, with an incidence in women of reproductive age approximating 45% when assessed via laparoscopy.[106] The average age of presentation is 27 years old. Most of these women have been symptomatic for two to five years prior to diagnosis. Because of its high prevalence and associated symptoms of pelvic pain and infertility, endometriosis is recognized as a leading cause of hospitalization and hysterectomy.[107]

Common sites for endometriosis include the peritoneum, posterior uterine surface, rectovaginal cul-de-sac, and uterosacral ligament.[102,104] Ovarian endometriosis can present as ovarian non-neoplastic cysts called *endometriomas*. These cysts can rupture and spill their contents into the peritoneum, producing tissue adhesions.[104,108]

Etiology

While the underlying cause of endometriosis is unknown, two different theories have been proposed: the retrograde menstruation theory and the coelomic metaplasia theory. The *retrograde menstruation theory* hypotheses that endometrial cells reach the intraperitoneal cavity through the open fimbrial endings of the fallopian tubes, as well as through lymphatic or vascular channels, during menstruation.[102,104,105] Retrograde menstruation occurs in approximately 90% of all women and is thought to seed the peritoneal cavity with endometrial cells.[105] These endometrial cells are stimulated by estrogen, causing a cascade of cytokines that can cause pain and infertility. They also produce inflammatory mediators (macrophages) that result in an inflammatory response.[105] The *coelomic metaplasia theory*, which is less widely held, proposes that the epithelium lining the peritoneum is influenced by increasing amounts of estrogen, causing it to undergo metaplastic transformation into endometrial cells.[102,104] Regardless of etiology, women are less at risk of developing endometriosis during episodes of physiologically induced (pregnancy) or artificially induced (hormonal) amenorrhea.

Diagnosis

The classic symptoms for which women present with endometriosis include: progressive pelvic pain associated with or occurring just prior to menses; dyspareunia; infertility; painful defecation; premenstrual staining; suprapubic pain; dysuria; and hematuria.[104] Pain is usually bilateral and varies in severity. Radiating back or leg pain is common. The active endometrial lesions release prostaglandins associated with inflammation, and the presence of prostaglandins is closely coupled with pain.[102]

Signs of endometriosis may include unusual tenderness during bimanual pelvic examination, nodularity along the uterosacral ligaments or the posterior cul-de-sac, decreased uterine mobility with or without pain, and adnexal mass or tenderness.[104,105] Deep lesions may be easily palpable during menses. In women with endometriomas, fixed adnexal masses may be appreciated.[104] The diagnosis of endometriosis can be assumed based upon clinical history and physical examination, but only surgery by laparoscopy or laparotomy with tissue histology is truly diagnostic.

Management

The goal of all endometriosis therapy is control of symptoms and enhancement of quality of life. Treatment options are aimed at controlling symptoms; only total hysterectomy and bilateral oophorectomy prevent recurrences.[102,105] Clinical diagnosis is predictive of laparoscopic findings. Medication therapy, if successful, will verify the diagnosis and diagnostic laparoscopy can be avoided.[105] Surgical treatment is warranted if treatment fails.

Medical treatment is based on the understanding that endometriosis is a disease that is hormonally responsive, and that the severity of endometriosis is decreased during pregnancy and after menopause. Treatment aims to simulate these conditions through the use of progestins or combined hormonal contraceptives and gonadotropin-releasing hormone (GnRH) analogs.[105]

Continuous, noncyclic oral contraceptives are the first line medical regimen for mild endometriosis in women who do not desire to become pregnant. The action of progestins can result in atrophy of the endometriotic lesions. Progestin compounds such as medroxyprogesterone acetate (20 to 30 mg/d) and depot medroxyprogesterone acetate (150 mg intramuscularly every 12 weeks) are alternatives to oral contraceptives. However, the side effect profile of weight gain and abnormal bleeding makes these drugs less attractive to women. Nonsteroidal anti-inflammatory drugs are the first choice for relief of dysmenorrhea. Danocrine (Danazol), an androgen, suppresses secretion of gonadotropins and inhibits ovulation.[105] It is highly efficacious for pain relief but is not commonly used because of the high incidence of side effects (including weight gain, edema, acne, decreased breast size, and other androgenic tendencies) associated with its use.

GnRH analogs such as leuprolide acaetate (Lupron), nafarelin acetate (Synarel), and goserelin acetate (Zoladex) are administered to induce a hypo-estrogenic state.[105] The GnRH analogs have become the medication of choice for moderate-to-severe symptoms of endometriosis. Side effects from these medications are related to hypoestrogenism (e.g., vasomotor symptoms, vaginal dryness, bone loss, and irritability) and can be mediated by "adding back" small amounts of estrogen, progesterone, or both in a fashion similar to the management of menopause. Therapy consists of monthly injections for 6 to 12 months concurrent with "add back" therapy. Approximately 90% of women experience symptom relief with fewer side effects than with danocrine alone. Treatment may not improve fertility, and recurrence is related to the severity of the disease.[105]

Surgical treatment via laparoscopy or laparotomy can be considered for women seeking to conceive, or for whom medical therapy is not effective. Areas of endometriosis can be removed or treated with laser or electrocautery. Conservative surgeries have the goal of restoring normal anatomy while removing visible lesions. In more severe disease, women who do not plan to have more children can opt for definitive therapies such as total hysterectomy and oophorectomy, or more limited surgeries combined with presacral neurectomy.

Ectopic Pregnancy

An *ectopic pregnancy* is defined as the implantation of any pregnancy outside the uterine cavity. Ninety-seven percent of these occur in the fallopian tubes, and the remaining 3% occur in the ovary, cervix, abdomen, or interstitial sites.[109,110] The rare occurrence of a heterotrophic pregnancy is a coexistent intrauterine pregnancy (IUP) and ectopic pregnancy. Ectopic pregnancy is a potential medical emergency with most morbidity and mortality occurring from ruptured ectopic. The goal of management is to identify and treat the ectopic before rupture occurs.

Epidemiology

Ectopic pregnancy appears in approximately 2% of all pregnancies in the United States. This rate has increased from 0.5% in 1970 to 1.97% in 1992.[109] Complications are the leading cause of maternal mortality in the first trimester, accounting for 9% to 13% of maternal deaths.[109–112] Ectopic pregnancy occurs more often in non-white women, mediated by less available access to health care and a higher reported rate of sexually transmitted infections.[113]

Risk factors include prior ectopic pregnancy or tubal surgery. Women with a history of sexually transmitted infections causing endothelial tubal damage are at higher risk. The current use of an IUD or failed tubal ligation also increase the relative risk of developing an ectopic pregnancy (although the overall incidence associated with these contraceptive options remains low given their high contraceptive effectiveness). Finally, women who are receiving infertility treatments by ovulation induction or who have had assisted reproductive techniques, such as in vitro fertilization, may be more at risk.[110–114]

The death rate from ectopic pregnancy has decreased even though the incidence has increased. This is a result of early diagnosis and treatment prior to the occurrence of rupture.[114] Testing now employs highly sensitive beta human chorionic gonadotropin (bHCG) sampling along with transvaginal ultrasound (TVUS). Additionally, the use of laparoscopic surgery, rather than open laparotomy, and con-

servative medical management with methotrexate are successful management options.[114]

Diagnosis

Early diagnosis of ectopic pregnancy is critical because it can reduce the risk of rupture, decrease tubal damage, and may prevent surgery.[112,115] A high index of suspicion should occur if a woman presents with the classic triad of amenorrhea, abdominal or pelvic pain, and abnormal vaginal bleeding.[109] Symptoms often occur between 6 and 11 weeks of gestation.[113] Pain and bleeding are the most common symptoms for which women seek care. At presentation, the woman may mistake irregular bleeding or spotting for menses. Pain can range from mild to severe cramping or colicky pain that can be located either midline, laterally, or both.[109] The cause of pain is degeneration of the pregnancy and breakdown in the uterine lining.[113] Other symptoms are shown in **Table 18-10**.

Management

Many women who seek care for symptoms of irregular bleeding or abdominal pain have a

---

Table 18-10 **SIGNS AND SYMPTOMS OF ECTOPIC PREGNANCY**[110–114]

Abdominal pain/tenderness

Adnexal pain/tenderness

Abnormal vaginal bleeding and/or amenorrhea

Nausea

Diarrhea

Right shoulder pain

Adnexal mass

Enlarged uterus (possibly)

Tissue passage (possibly)

Hypotension/peritoneal signs if ruptured ectopic

normally developing IUP.[112] A complete history and physical examination can differentiate the individual who needs immediate surgical evaluation from one who can be managed expectantly. Women with an ectopic pregnancy often do not experience common early pregnancy symptoms such as breast tenderness or nausea.[116] On physical examination, the abdomen is tender, the pelvic exam is painful, and cervical motion tenderness is present. A unilateral mass may be palpable in the adnexal area but is present in fewer than 10% of women.[109,116] The differential diagnosis of ectopic pregnancy includes, but is not limited to: IUP; corpus luteum cyst; ovarian torsion; threatened/incomplete abortion; pelvic inflammatory disease; appendicitis; and endometriosis.[108,111]

Laboratory testing consists of a complete blood count (CBC), blood type, and serum quantitative bHCG. Urine and blood pregnancy tests are used interchangeably to diagnose pregnancy. Depending on the specific test used, pregnancy can be detected at levels between 10 mIU and 25 mIU on urine samples, while blood tests are positive between 5 and 15 mIU.[117] While either test can reliably detect pregnancy, serial serum bHCG are used to determine whether the pregnancy is developing normally. Hormone levels typically double every 48 hours in the first 10 weeks of a healthy pregnancy. Abnormally low or high levels or hormone levels that fail to increase as expected may be indicative of complications such as ectopic pregnancy, spontaneous abortion, or molar pregnancy. A serum progesterone level has limited usefulness because an abnormal result might not differentiate a spontaneous abortion from an ectopic pregnancy.[111] However, serum progesterone levels less than 10 ng/mL suggest an abnormal gestation.

While serum HCG levels are very helpful in the diagnosis and management, a spot urine HCG is extremely helpful during the initial steps of a work-up for a suspected ectopic pregnancy because the results are immediately available and generally accurate. Due to the sensitivity of currently available urine HCG tests, it is highly unlikely that a woman with an ectopic pregnancy would have a false negative urine pregnancy test. It is estimated that only 1% of ectopic pregnancies would be missed using a urine pregnancy test sensitive enough to detect 50 mIU.[117]

A transvaginal ultrasound can confirm pregnancy status. At a bHCG level of 1000 to 1500 mIU/mL, a gestational sac may be seen in the uterus (which correlates with a post-conception age of 24 days/gestational age of 38 days). In all healthy pregnancies, the sac should be visible when the level has risen to 2000 mIU/mL. Transvaginal ultrasound findings indicative of an ectopic pregnancy include the absence of an intrauterine sac and a complex adnexal mass, possibly with a visible fetal sac or fetal heart beat in the tube[111] at a bHCG level of 1500 mIU/mL. A fluid collection may be seen in the cul-de-sac if rupture has occurred. Because transabdominal scanning cannot accurately detect uterine contents until the bHCG level is about 6500 mIU/mL, this mode is of less use to diagnose ectopic pregnancy. Few ectopic pregnancies have levels this high.[118]

Delays in diagnosis can result in rupture. Ruptured ectopic pregnancy presents with faintness, hypotension, complaints of acute pelvic pain and of referred pain secondary to diaphragmatic irritation from intraperitoneal blood, and severe anemia. The posterior fornix may be swollen due to bleeding into the cul-de-sac. The woman presenting with these symptoms and a positive pregnancy test needs immediate care.

When the midwife makes a presumptive diagnosis of ectopic pregnancy, immediate referral to a physician is mandatory. Early diagnosis and treatment can prevent tubal rupture and future infertility as well as maternal intra-abdominal hemorrhage.

Treatment

Treatment of an unruptured ectopic pregnancy is either by medical expectant management, surgical management, or a combination of both with the goal of preserving the woman's reproductive organs.[110] If the woman presents with acute peritoneal signs or hemorrhage, and laboratory testing and ultrasound suggest a ruptured ectopic, then immediate surgery is indicated.[111] Conservative/expectant treatment consists of either medical management with methotrexate or laparoscopic salpingostomy (surgical evacuation of the ectopic pregnancy from the tube).

Medical treatment maintains the integrity of the fallopian tubes.[110] Methotrexate, a folic acid antagonist, is the primary drug used for the woman who is hemodynamically stable with no evidence of hemoperitoneum on TVUS. The tubal mass should measure <3.5 cm and the bHCG should be $<15{,}000$ mIU/mL.[110,111,115] The dosage is 50 mg/m^2 body surface area given in a single intramuscular injection.[119] A repeat dose may be given after seven days. The success rate for methotrexate in unruptured ectopic pregnancies is 85% to 95% as a single dose and 98% with multiple doses and has the advantage of preserving the tube.[119] Contraindications for use include hepatic or renal disease, thrombocytopenia, leukopenia, and anemia.[111,115]

Following either medical or surgical treatment, quantitative bHCGs will need to be followed weekly until they are negative. In subsequent pregnancies, IUP can be diagnosed with quantitative bHCGs and early TVUS. There is a 12% recurrence rate of ectopic pregnancy in successive pregnancies.[112] Education about this risk will enable the woman to seek care early in pregnancy, which can prevent morbidity if ectopic pregnancy recurs.

Ovarian Mass

Evaluation of an ovarian mass is required when an asymptomatic mass is palpable during a pelvic exam or when imaging for symptomatic pain reveals a mass. Ultrasounds (transvaginal and possibly transabdominal) are the initial step whenever masses are suspected. The priorities are to determine the need for emergent intervention, which is required if an ectopic pregnancy, large ovarian cyst thought to be at risk of torsion, or malignancy is suspected.[120]

Types of Benign Ovarian Masses

FUNCTIONAL OVARIAN CYSTS

Nonmalignant follicular or corpus luteum cysts are common during the reproductive years. Dominant follicular cysts occur prior to ovulation, do not shrink after ovulation, and are characterized by anechoic fluid within the cavity and thin walls.[120–122] They often measure 20 to 25 mm.[103] With the lutenizing hormone surge at ovulation, the follicle can rupture and may cause temporary pain that quickly resolves.[123]

Corpus luteum cysts may have thickened or irregular walls and a more complex component that may be blood or clot filled.[103,120,122] If rupture occurs, acute lower abdominal pain can ensue due to intraperitoneal bleeding.[123] Most simple functional cysts will regress on their own over one or two menstrual cycles. However, repeat examination is indicated as part of expectant management to document regression.[122] If masses persist for more than two cycles, consideration should be given to possible surgical evaluation. The frequency of developing functional ovarian cysts can be decreased with the use of monophasic oral contraceptives.[124]

Endometriomas may occur in the premenopausal woman who complains of dysmenorrhea and pelvic pain.[120,124] They arise as cystic masses from endometrial implants on the ovaries. *Endometriomas* ("chocolate cysts") appear as complex masses on ultrasound with thin walls and contain thick, clotted blood. If rupture occurs, the contents produce a local tissue reaction in the peritoneum resulting in lower abdominal pain, dyspareunia, and irregular bleeding.[103,123] They may be associated with elevated serum cancer antigen 125 (CA-125) levels in premenopausal women.[120]

BENIGN NEOPLASTIC CYSTS

Benign neoplastic cysts, including serous cystadenomas and mucinous tumors, occur in all age groups. *Serous cystadenomas*, which occur in 30% of all epithelial ovarian neoplasms, are benign lesions that are often unilateral and large, have a smooth surface, and contain thin, clear yellow fluid.[125] Proliferation may produce firm projections within the cyst that form a serous cystadenofibroma.[23,125] *Mucinous tumors* are typical in women aged 30 to 50 with 75% to 85% presenting as benign. These mucinous tumors are the largest found in women, with several reported to weigh over 70 kg (154 pounds). They may cause nonspecific abdominal pain and, if present in the postmenopausal woman, may be associated with endometrial hyperplasia, with resulting vaginal bleeding.[125] Surgical investigation is necessary to rule out malignancy.

BENIGN NEOPLASTIC CYSTS OF GERM CELL ORIGIN

Complex cysts, including benign cystic teratoma or dermoid cysts, are the most common type of benign germ cell tumor found in reproductive age women.[103,124,125] They comprise 40% to 50% of all benign ovarian neoplasms and are usually asymptomatic unless accompanied by torsion or rupture.[125] Their ultrasound appearance ranges from cystic mass to solid, well defined mass with highly echogenic components, and they are often found on a pedicle.[103] Pain may occur as a result of enlargement or torsion; they are rarely malignant.

Ovarian Cancer

Epidemiology

Ovarian cancer, the leading cause of death from gynecologic malignancies, is diagnosed in 25,000 women annually with approximately 14,500 deaths each year. The incidence is 1.4% in the general population; one in 70 women will develop this disease during her lifetime mostly between the ages of 55 and 74. Known risk factors include advanced age, family history, nulliparity, late menopause, Caucasian, higher socioeconomic status, residence in North America or northern Europe, or women with genetic mutations where the incidence of ovarian cancer is estimated at 16% to 65%. Early detection is critical to increased survival rates, yet most women with ovarian cancer (80%) do not present until advanced stage disease.[122,124,126]

Diagnosis

Complete history, physical examination, and diagnostic testing, including imaging, are the cornerstones of diagnosis. It is critical to consider a woman's age and reproductive status because masses may be benign in women of reproductive age but abnormal in the postmenopausal woman. The history should focus on reproductive evaluation and symptoms including associated gastrointestinal and urinary factors. Clinical findings include abdominal pain with associated alterations in gastrointestinal function, urination, and possibly dysfunctional uterine bleeding.[122,124] Careful attention to the relationship of pain to the menstrual cycle may assist in narrowing the differential diagnosis.[120,127] **Table 18-11** lists the differential diagnosis for the woman presenting with pelvic pain.

The physical examination includes a thorough assessment of the abdomen as well as a

pelvic exam including bimanual. The bimanual examination evaluates the size, shape, and consistency of the uterus, the presence of tenderness or masses, and any cervical motion tenderness. A rectal exam allows for an examination of the cul-de-sac and posterior structures and is especially important to assess for occult blood.[127]

Diagnostic testing includes CBC, urinalysis and culture, pregnancy test, and cervical cultures in the sexually active woman. CA-125 is a diagnostic marker for ovarian cancer, but it is not sensitive for detection of early disease especially in the premenopausal woman.[120,124,126] A normal level is less than 35 U/mL; elevated levels occur in approximately 80% of ovarian cancers.[124] Elevations occur with conditions such as endometriosis, early pregnancy, and benign ovarian cysts. However, in postmenopausal women, it is crucial to obtain testing early in the evaluation process because the risk of ovarian cancer in this age group is greater. With abnormal CA-125 results and a documented mass, the risk of malignancy in this age group increases to over 80%.[120] **Figure 18-2** is an algorithm for the clinical approach for a patient presenting with a pelvic mass.

Ultrasound testing is vital in the evaluation of a pelvic mass and detects more early ovarian cancers than CA-125 alone.[120,124,126,127] Sixty to 97% of ovarian masses are visualized by sonography. Sonography and doppler imaging also can help distinguish benign from malignant ovarian masses in 93% to 97% of cases.[126] TVUS is useful for identifying the location of the mass (uterine versus ovarian), the presence of a pregnancy (intrauterine versus ectopic), abnormalities in pelvic structure, and the presence of fluid in the cul-de-sac (suggestive of a

---

Table 18-11 DIFFERENTIAL DIAGNOSIS OF ACUTE PELVIC PAIN[120,122–124]

Pelvic inflammatory disease
Tubo-ovarian abscess
Endometriosis
Ectopic pregnancy
Dysmenorrhea
Leiomyoma
Simple ovarian cysts
Hemorrhagic ovarian cyst
Ruptured ovarian cyst
Adnexal torsion
Ovarian neoplasms
Appendicitis
Diverticulitis
Irritable bowel syndrome
Constipation
Urinary tract disease (including renal stones)
Musculoskeletal

Figure 18-2 Algorithm for a patient presenting with a pelvic mass.

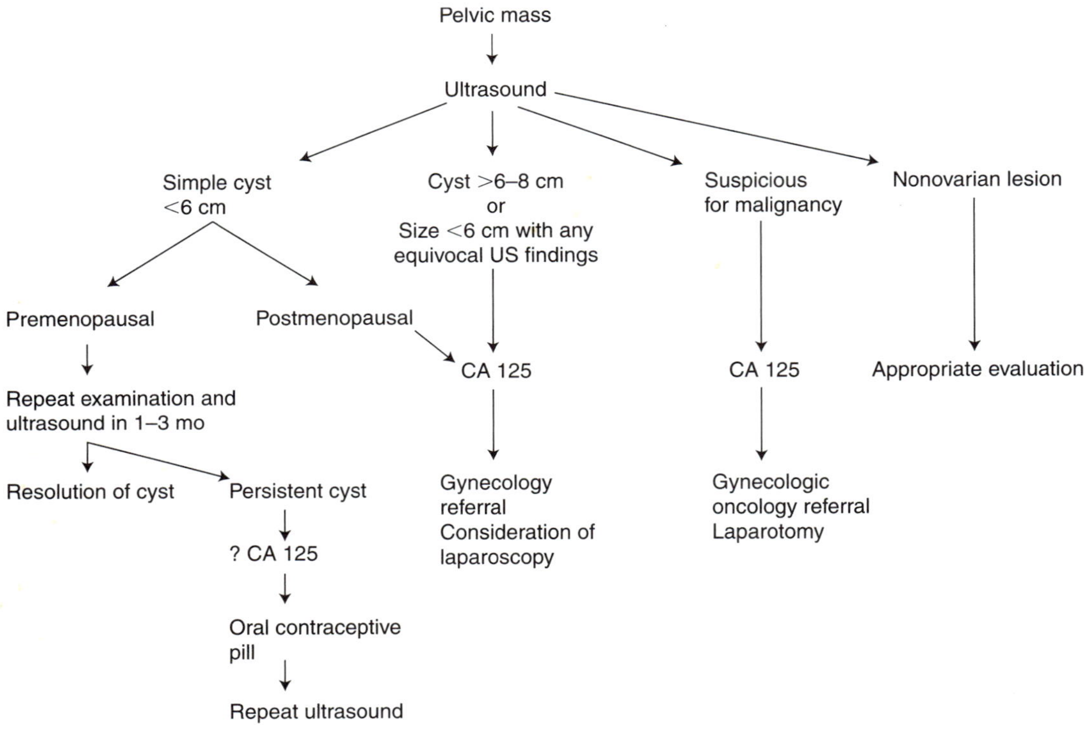

Source: Used with permission from Mosby Yearbook, Inc., ©2006.[120]

ruptured ovarian cyst).[120,124,127] Cysts with septations or other internal structures or those with combined cystic and solid masses warrant tissue diagnosis to exclude malignancy.[122] Furthermore, TVUS provides a preliminary assessment of the complexity of the mass and the likelihood of malignancy.[120,122,124] Because high frequency transducers can provide a high resolution of the mass, TVUS can detect solid components, mural nodules, thick internal septations, and wall irregularities that are associated with malignancy.[122] The addition of color-flow Doppler techniques can improve ultrasound results. Abdominal ultrasound is also useful in identifying intestinal and other abdominal structures. CT and magnetic resonance imaging (MRI), in addition to surgical intervention by laparoscopy or laparotomy, may be needed to clarify the diagnosis.

Prompt referral to a gynecologist or gynecologic oncologist is indicated to differentiate between benign and malignant ovarian masses. Benign cysts are typically unilateral, mobile, smooth, and cystic on palpation, whereas a malignancy is often bilateral, solid, irregular, and fixed on palpation. Malignant tumors are often associated with ascites and demonstrate rapid growth.[124] Because there are no effective screening tests for ovarian cancer, an accurate medical history, detailed physical exam, and appropriate use of diagnostic tests including ultrasound are essential.

Ovarian Torsion

In *ovarian torsion*, the ovary, the fallopian tube, or both twist on the vascular pedicle resulting in vascular compromise.[128] Ovarian torsion usually occurs with an adnexal mass that rotates around the pedicle, resulting in arterial, venous, or lymphatic obstruction, ischemia and ovarian infarction, and massive ovarian edema.[129–131] It is a rare gynecologic cause of lower abdominal pain. The lack of clinical findings on physical examination and specific laboratory and ultrasound findings make this difficult to diagnose without surgery.[131] Surgical intervention may be delayed because ovarian torsion presents with similar symtoms often seen with many other conditions.

Adnexal torsion is the fifth most common gynecologic emergency, with an incidence of approximately 3% of acute gynecological complaints.[129–131] Ovarian torsion primarily occurs in reproductive-aged women during adolescence and early adulthood.[131] Any woman of childbearing age who presents with complaints of abrupt onset lower abdominal pain needs to have adnexal torsion ruled out. The exact cause of ovarian torsion is unknown, but it is most often associated with an ovarian cyst or tumor.[131] Other associated findings include an enlarged ovary; excess length of fallopian tube and utero-ovarian ligaments; history of cyst or mass; ovarian hyperstimulation; and a history of pelvic surgery such as a tubal ligation.[130,132–134]

The most common symptom of ovarian torsion is the abrupt onset of colicky pain in the lower quadrant radiating to the side of the affected tube.[130,131,133] Women present most commonly with right-sided symptoms. They may also report that the pain radiates to the flank, back, or groin. Pain often increases in severity over time. Nausea and vomiting may occur along with urinary frequency and urgency. Physical examination reveals rigidity of the abdomen and rebound tenderness. A tender, palpable mass and cervical motion tenderness may be noted on vaginal exam.[130–137] Laboratory findings may reveal leukocytosis.[123,137] Other laboratory and imaging studies are not specific for ovarian torsion but can rule out abnormalities with similar clinical characteristics such as appendicitis, pelvic inflammatory disease, pyelonephritis, ruptured ovarian cyst, diverticulitis, gastroenteritis, ectopic pregnancy, and tubo-ovarian abscess.[131,132]

Doppler transvaginal sonography along with CT and MRI are useful diagnostic tools. Findings of ovarian enlargement and an absence of blood flow to the torsed ovary [120,133,135,136] are indicative of ovarian torsion. The absence of blood flow is 100% predictive. However, normal Doppler flow cannot rule out ovarian torsion, especially if the torsion is intermittent.[135] Confirmation by laparoscopy is the most specific diagnostic tool.

Early laparoscopy is the gold standard used to establish the diagnosis and, if possible, untwist the adnexa in an effort to preserve fertility when no malignancy is suspected.[131,133] Viability of the untorsed ovary is determined by the absence of ischemia. A resection is performed when the tissue is necrotic or if it contains a tubal or ovarian neoplasm.

In summary, clinical suspicion, knowledge of predisposing factors, and adjunct Doppler ultrasound will lead to a diagnosis by immediate laparoscopic surgery. Diagnosis is critical for salvaging the ovary, maintaining fertility, and lessening the morbidity related to adnexal torsion.

Conclusion

In all of the reproductive conditions discussed in this chapter, it is important that the midwife or nurse practitioner recognize the necessity of prompt evaluation. Initiating a work-up can be appropriate, but whenever there is a question of serious disease, consultation and referral should be employed.

References

1. Brown P. Antibiotic selection for urinary tract infection: New microbiologic considerations. *Curr Infect Dis Rep*. 1999;1(4):384–388.

2. Kass E, Finland M. Asymptomatic infections of the urinary tract. *J Urol*. 2002;168(2):420–424.

3. Foxman B, Barlow R, D'Arcy H, Gillespie B, Sobel J. Urinary tract infection: Self reported incidence and associated costs. *Ann Epidemiol*. 2000;10(8):509–515.

4. Hooton T, Scholes D, Stapleton A, Roberts P, Winter C, Gupta K, et al. A prospective study of asymptomatic bacteruria in sexually active young women. *N Engl J Med*. 2000;343(14):992–997.

5. Komaroff A. Acute dysuria and urinary tract infections. In: Carlson K, Eisenstat S, editors. *Primary Care of Women*. 2nd ed. St Louis: Mosby; 2002. pp. 176–182.

6. Schaeffer A. Infection and inflammation of the genitourinary tract. *J Urol*. 2001;165(4):1374–1381.

7. Geerlings S, Stolk R, Camps M, Netten P, Hoekstra J, Bouter K, et al. Asymptomatic bacteriuria may be considered a complication in women with diabetes. Diabetes Mellitus Women Asymptomatic Bacteriuria Utrecht Study Group. *Diabetes Care*. 2000;23(6): 744–749.

8. Stamm W, Hooton T. Current concepts: Management of urinary tract infections in adults. *N Engl J Med*. 1993;329(18):1328–1334.

9. Scholes D, Hooton T, Roberts P, Stapleton A, Gupta K, Stamm W. Risk factors for recurrent urinary tract infection in young women. *J Infect Dis*. 2000;182(4): 1177–1182.

10. Harmanli O, Cheng G, Nyirjesy P, Chatwani A, Gaughan J. Urinary tract infections in women with bacterial vaginosis. *Obstet Gynecol*. 2000;95(5):710–712.

11. Fihn S, Boyko E, Normand E, Chen C Jr, Hunt M, Yarbro P, et al. Association between use of spermicide coated condoms and *Escherichia coli* urinary tract infection in young women. *Am J Epidemiol*. 1996; 144(5):512–520.

12. Bent S, Nallamothu B, Simel D, Fihn S, Saint S. Does this woman have an acute uncomplicated urinary tract infection? *JAMA*. 2002;287(20):2701–2710.

13. Jackson N. Urinary tract problems. In: Leppert P, Peipert J, editors. *Primary Care for Women*. 2nd ed. Philadelphia: Lippincott; 2004. pp. 495–502.

14. Hooton T, Roberts P, Stamm W. Effects of recent sexual activity and use of a diaphragm on the vaginal microflora. *Clin Infect Dis*. 1994;19(2):274–278.

15. Hooton T, Stamm W. Diagnosis and treatment of uncomplicated urinary tract infection. *Infect Dis Clin North Am*. 1997;11(3):551–581.

16. Offerdahl T, Umland E. Urinary tract infection. (Chapter 35). In: Singleton J, Sandowski S, Green-Hernandez C, Horvath T, DiGregorio R, Holzemer S, editors. *Primary Care*. Philadelphia: Lippincott; 1999. pp. 379–389.

17. Dembry L-M, Andriole V. Urinary tract infections. In: Faro S, editor. *Infectious Diseases in Women*. Philadelphia: WB Saunders and Company; 2001. pp. 354–367.

18. Anonymous. Urine studies. In: Fischbach F., editor. *Manual of Laboratory and Diagnostic Tests*. 7th ed. Philadelphia: Lippincott Williams & Wilkins; 2003. pp. 164–263.

19. U.S. Public Health Service. Urinalysis. *Am Fam Physician*. 1994;50(2):351–353.

20. Bakerman S. *Bakerman's ABCs of Interpretive Laboratory Data*. 4th ed. Scottsdale, AZ: Interpretive Laboratory Data, Inc; 2002.

21. Wallach J. Pyleonephritis. In: *Interpretation of Diagnostic Tests*. 7th ed. Philadelphia: Lippincott Williams & Wilkins; 2000. p. 736.

22. O'Connell L, Siroky M. The abnormal urinalysis. In: Siroky M, Oates R, Babayan R, editors. *Handbook of Urology: Diagnosis and Therapy*. Philadelphia: Lippincott Williams & Wilkins; 2004. pp. 1–15.

23. Rose B, Fletcher R. Evaluation of hematuria in adults. [monograph on the Internet; subscription service]. 2005 Up to Date. Available from http://www.uptodate.com. Accessed 5/11/2005.

24. Anonymous. Optimizing Antibiotic Selection for CAP and cUTI in the Emergency Department and Hospital Setting: A Systematic Review and Evidence-based Treatment Recommendations—Year 2005 Update. In: Hospital Medicine Consensus Reports; 2005. Available at http://www.clinicalconsensusreports.com/.

25. Fihn S. Acute uncomplicated urinary tract infection in women. *N Engl J Med*. 2003;349:259–266.

26. Orenstein R, Wong E. Urinary tract infections in adults. *Am Fam Physician*. 1999;59(5):1225–1234.

27. Stamm W, Hooten T. Management of urinary tract infections in adult. *N Engl J Med*. 1993;329(18):1328–1334.

28. Warren J, Abrutyn E, Hebel J, Johnson J, Schaeffer A, Stamm W. Guidelines for antimicrobial treatment of uncomplicated acute bacterial cystitis and acute pyelonephritis in women. Infectious Diseases Society of America (IDSA). *Clin Infect Dis*. 1999;29(4):745–758.

29. Nicolle L. Urinary tract infection: Traditional pharmacologic therapies. *Dis Mon*. 2003;49(2):111–128.

30. Norby S. Short term treatment of uncomplicated lower urinary tract infections in women. *Rev Infect Dis*. 1990;12(3):458–467.

31. Hooton T, Winter C, Kuwamura L, Roberts P, Stamm W. A comparison of amoxicillin (a), cefadroxil (c), nitrofurantoin (n), and trimethopirn/sulfamethoxazole (T/S) in 3 day regimens for the treatment of uncomplicated UTI in women [abstract]. In: Program and Abstracts of the 31st Interscience Conference on Antimicrobial Agents and Chemotherapy. Chicago. Sept 29–Oct 2, 1991. Washington, DC: American Society for Microbiology; 1991. p. 260.

32. Gupta K, Hooton T, Roberts P, Stamm W. Patient initiated treatment of uncomplicated recurrent urinary tract infections in young women. *Ann Intern Med*. 2001;135(1):9–16.

33. Mabeck C. Treatment of uncomplicated urinary tract infection in non-pregnant women. *Post Med J*. 1972;48:69–75.

34. Raz R, Gennesin Y, Wasser J, Stoler Z, Rosenfeld S, Rottensterich E, et al. Recurrent urinary tract infections in post menopausal women. *Clin Infect Dis*. 2000;30:152–156.

35. Stapleton A, Stamm W. Prevention of urinary tract infection. *Infect Dis Clin North Am*. 1997;11(3):719–733.

36. Avorn J, Monane M, Gurwitz J, Glynn R, Choodnovskiy I, Lipsitz L. Reduction of bacteriuria and pyuria after ingestion of cranberry juice. *JAMA*. 1994;271(10):751–754.

37. Walker E, Barney D, Mickelson J, Walton R, Mickelsen R. Cranberry concentrate: UTI prophylaxis (letter). *J Fam Pract*. 1997;45(2):167–168.

38. Kontiokari T, Sundqvist K, Nuutinen M, Pokka T, Koskela M, Uhari M. Randomized trial of cranberry-lingonberry juice and lactobacillus GG drink for the prevention of urinary tract infections in women. *BMJ*. 2001;322(7302):1571–1573.

39. Jepson R, Mihaljevic L, Craig J. Cranberries for preventing urinary tract infections. *Cochrane Database Syst Rev*. 2004:CD001321.

40. Schaeffer A, Stuppy B. Efficacy and safety of self start therapy in women with recurrent urinary tract infections. *J Urol*. 1999;161(1):207–211.

41. Fang LS-T. Approach to dysuria and urinary tract infections in women. In: Goroll A, Mulley AJ, editors. *Primary Care Medicine*. 4th ed. Philadelphia: Lippincott Williams & Wilkins; 2000. pp. 770–775.

42. Nicolle L. Prophylaxis: Recurrent urinary tract infection in women. *Infection*. 1992;20(suppl 3):S203–S205.

43. Stamm W, McKevitt M, Roberts P, White N. Natural history of recurrent urinary tract infections in women. *Rev Infect Dis*. 1991;13:77–84.

44. Nicolle L, Harding G, Thompson M, Kennedy J, Urias B, Ronald A. Efficacy of five years of continuous, low dose trimethoprim-sulfamethoxazole prophylaxis for urinary tract infections. *J Infect Dis*. 1988;157(1):1239–1242.

45. *The Medical Letter's Handbook of Adverse Drug Interaction*. Marlborough, MA: The Medical Letter, Inc., Skyscape; 2000. p. 196.

46. Department of Reproductive Health and Research (RHR). Medical Eligibility Criteria for Contraceptive Use. 3 ed. [monograph on the Internet] World Health Organization; 2004. [retrieved 4/30/05]. Available

from: http://www.who.int/reproductive-health/publi cations/RHR_00_2_medical_eligibility_criteria_3rd/.

47. Parsons C, Schmidt J. Control of recurrent lower urinary tract infections in the postmenopausal woman. *J Urol.* 1982;128(6):1224–1226.

48. Nicolle L. A practical guide to antimicrobial management of complicated urinary tract infection. *Drugs Aging.* 2001;18(4):243–254.

49. Mansfield J, Mallory G, Ellis L. The differential diagnosis of Bright's disease: Clinicopathological correlation. *N Engl J Med.* 1943;220:387.

50. Stamm W, Hooton T, Johnson J, Johnson C, Stapleton A, Roberts P, et al. Urinary tract infections: From pathogenesis to treatment. *J Infect Dis.* 1989;159(3): 400–406.

51. Nicolle L, Friesen D, Harding G, Roos L. Hospitalization for acute pyelonephritis in Manitoba Canada during the period from 1989 to 1992; impact of diabetes, pregnancy and aboriginal origin. *Clin Infect Dis.* 1996;22(6):1051–1056.

52. Pinson A, Philbreak J, Lindbeck G, Schorling J. Fever in the clinical diagnosis of acute pyelonephritis. *Am J Emerg Med.* 1997;1(2):148–151.

53. Levi M, Redington J, Reller L. The patient with urinary tract infection. In: Schrier R., editor. *Manual of Nephrology.* Philadelphia: Lippincott Williams & Wilkins; 2005. pp. 91–114.

54. McLaughlin S. Urinary tract infections in women. *Med Clin North Am.* 2004;88(2):417–429.

55. Kurowski K. The woman with dysuria. *Am Fam Physician.* 1998;57(9):2155.

56. Kok D. Intratubular crystallization events. *World J Urol.* 1997;15(4):219–228.

57. Höjgaard I, Tiselius H. Crystallization in the nephron. *Urol Res.* 1999;27(6):397–403.

58. Tiselius H. Medical evaluation of nephrolithiasis. *Endocrinol Metab Clin North Am.* 2002;31(4): 1031–1050.

59. Manthey D, Teichman J. Nephrolithiasis. *Emerg Med Clin North Am.* 2001;19(3):633–654.

60. Coe F, Parks J, Asplin J. The pathogenesis and treatment of kidney stones. *N Engl J Med.* 1992;327(16): 1141–1152.

61. Sierakowski R, Finlayson B, Landes R, Finlayson C, Sierakowski N. The frequency of urolithiasis in hospital discharge diagnoses in the United States. *Invest Urol.* 1978;15(6):438–441.

62. Agarwal S, Caeser R. Nephrolithiasis. In: Leppert P, Peipert J, editors. *Primary Care for Women.* 2nd ed. Philadelphia: Lippincott; 2004. pp. 507–513.

63. Asplin J, Coe F, Favus M. Nephrolithiasis. In: AS F, Braunwald E, Isselbacher K, Wilson J, Martin J, Kasper D, et al., editors. *Harrison's Principles of Internal Medicine.* 14th ed. New York: McGraw Hill, Health Professions Division; 1998. pp. 1569–1574.

64. Bove P, Kaplan D, Dalrymple N, Rosenfield A, Verga M, Anderson K, et al. Reexamining the value of hematuria testing in patients with acute flank pain. *J Urol.* 1999;162(3 Pt 2):685–687.

65. Teichman J. Clinical practice. Acute renal colic from ureteral calculus. *N Engl J Med.* 2004;350(7):684–693.

66. Vieweg J, Teh C, Freed K, Leder R, Smith R, Nelson R, et al. Unenhanced helical computerized tomography for the evaluation of patients with acute flank pain. *J Urol.* 1998;160(3 Pt 1):679–684.

67. Bird V, Gomez-Marin O, Leveillee R, Sfakianakis G, Rivas L, Amendola M. A comparison of unenhanced helical computerized tomography findings and renal obstruction determined by furosemide (99m) technetium mercaptoacetyltriglycine diuretic scintirenography for patients with acute renal colic. *J Urol.* 2002;167(4):1597–1603.

68. Miller O, Rineer S, Reichard S, Buckley R, Donovan M, Graham I, et al. Prospective comparisons of unenhanced spiral computed tomography and intravenous urogram in the evaluation of acute flank pain. *Urology.* 1998;52(6):982–987.

69. Sinclair D, Wilson S, Toi A, Greenspan L. The evaluation of suspected renal colic: Ultrasound scan versus excretory urography. *Ann Emerg Med.* 1989;18(5): 556–559.

70. Segura J, Preminger G, Assimos D, Dretler S, Kahn R, Lingeman J, et al. Ureteral Stones Clinical Guidelines Panel summary report on the management of ureteral calculi. *J Urol.* 1997;158(5):1915–1921.

71. Ueno A, Kawasmura T, Ogawa A, Takayasu H. Relation of spontaneous passage of ureteral calculi to size. *Urology.* 1977;10(6):544–546.

72. Curhan G, Willett W, Rimm E, Stampfer M. A prospective study of dietary calcium and other nutrients and the use of symptomatic kidney stones. *N Engl J Med.* 1993;328(12):833–838.

73. Frank M, DeVries A, Tikva P. Prevention of urolithiasis. *Arch Environ Health.* 1996;13(5):625–630.

74. Hosking D, Erickson S, Van Den Berg C, Wilson D, Smith L. The stone clinic effect in patients with idiopathic calcium urolithiasis. *J Urol.* 1983;130(6): 1115–1118.

75. Strauss A, Coe F, Deutsch L, Parks J. Factors that predict relapse of calcium nephrolithiasis during treatment. *Am J Med.* 1982;72(1):17–24.

76. Borghi L, Meschi T, Schianchi T, Allegri F, Guerra A, Maggiore U, et al. Medical treatment of nephrolithiasis. *Endocrinol Metab Clin North Am.* 2002; 31(4):1051–1064.

77. Goldenberg R, Girone J. Oral pyridoxine in the prevention of oxalate kidney stones. *Am J Nephrol.* 1996; 16(6):552–553.

78. Metlaga B, Assimos D. Changing indications of open stone surgery. *Urology.* 2002;59(4):490–493.

79. American Urological Association. Ureteral Stones Clinical Guidelines Panel. *Report on the Management of Ureteral Calculi.* Linthicum, MD: American Urological Association, Inc.; 1997.

80. Gibbs R, Sweet R, Duff W. Maternal and fetal infectious disorders. In: Creasy R, Resnick R, Iams J, editors. *Maternal-Fetal Medicine Principles and Practice.* 5th ed. Philadelphia: Saunders; 2004. pp. 741–801.

81. Cunningham F, Lucas M. Urinary tract infections complicating pregnancy. *Baillières Clin Obstet Gynaecol.* 1994;8(2):353–373.

82. Thorsen M, Poole J. Renal disease in pregnancy. *J Perinat Neonat Nurs.* 2002;15(4):13–26.

83. Harris R. The significance of eradication of bacteriuria during pregnancy. *Obstet Gynecol.* 1979;53(1): 71–73.

84. Swenson K, Chisholm C. Renal, hepatic, and gastrointestinal disorders and systemic lupus erythemataosus in pregnancy. In: Bankowski B, Hearne A, Lambrou N, Fox H, Wallach E, editors. *John Hopkins Manual of Gynecology and Obstetrics.* Philadelphia: Lippincott Williams & Wilkins; 2002. pp. 204–212.

85. Bales G, Gerber G. Urologic complications. In: Cohen, W, editor. *Cherry and Merkatz's Complications of Pregnancy.* Philadelphia: Lippincott Williams and Wilkins; 2000. pp. 295–302.

86. Briggs G, Freeman R, Yaffee S. *Drugs in Pregnancy and Lactation.* Philadelphia: Lippincott; 2002.

87. Anonymous. Infection of the urinary tract. In: Gabbe S, Niebyl J, Simpson J, editors. *Obstetrics - Normal and Problem Pregnancies.* 4th ed. New York: Churchill Livingstone, Inc., 2002. On line text accessed January 21, 2006, at http://home.mdconsult.com/das/book/54272898-2/view/1007/1.html/top.

88. Sanchez-Ramos L, McAlpine K, Adair C, Kaunitz A, Delke I, Briones D. Obstetrics: Pyelonephritis in pregnancy. Once-a-day ceftriaxone versus multiple doses of cefazolin: A randomized, double-blind trial. *Am J Obstet Gynecol.* 1995;172(1 Pt 1):129–133.

89. Ovalle A, Levancini M. Urinary tract infections in pregnancy. *Curr Opin Urol.* 2001;11:55–59.

90. Towers C, Kaminskas C, Garite T, Nageotte M, Dorchester W. Pulmonary injury associated with antepartal pyelonephritis: Can patients at risk be identified? *Am J Obstet Gynecol.* 1991;164:974–978.

91. Plattner M. Pyelonephritis in pregnancy. *J Perinat Neonat Nurs.* 1994;8(1):20–27.

92. Lenke R, Van Dorsten J, Schifrin B. Pyelonephritis in pregnancy: A prospective randomized trial to prevent recurrent disease evaluating suppressive therapy with nitrofurantoin and close surveillance. *Am J Obstet Gynecol.* 1983;146(8):953–957.

93. Butler E, Cox S, Eberts E, Cunningham F. Symptomatic nephrolithiasis complicating pregnancy. *Obstet Gynecol.* 2000;96(5 Pt 1):753–756.

94. Stothers L, Lee L. Renal colic in pregnancy. *J Urol.* 1992;148(5):1383–1387.

95. McAleer S, Loughlin K. Nephrolithiasis and pregnancy. *Curr Opin Urol.* 2004;14(2):123–127.

96. Davison J, Lindheimer M. Renal disorders. In: Creasy R, Resnick R, Iams J, editors. *Maternal-Fetal Medicine Principles and Practice.* 5th ed. Philadelphia: Saunders; 2004. pp. 901–923.

97. Denstedt J, Razvi H. Management of urinary calculi during pregnancy. *J Urology.* 1992;148(3 Pt 2): 1072–1075.

98. Bouchelouche K, Nordling J. Recent developments in the management of interstitial cystitis. *Curr Opin Urol.* 2003;13(4):309–313.

99. Aguilar V. Interstitial cystitis. In: Leppert P, Peipert J, editors. *Primary Care for Women.* 2nd ed. Philadelphia: Lippincott; 2004. pp. 536–541.

100. Metts J. Interstitial cystitis: Urgency and frequency syndrome. *Am Fam Physician.* 2001;64 (7): 1199–1206.

101. Koziol J, Clark D, Gittes R, Tan E. The natural history of interstitial cystitis: A survey of 374 patients. *J Urol.* 1993;149(3):465–469.

102. Gould D. Endometriosis. *Nurs Stand.* 2003;17(27): 47–55.

103. Hopkins C. Sonographic evaluation of gynecologic pain and dysfunctional uterine bleeding: The basic scan. In: Menihan C, editor. *Limited Sonography in Obstetric and Gynecologic Triage.* Philadelphia: Lippincott Williams & Wilkins; 1998. pp. 97–116.

104. Hornstein M, Barbieri R. Endometriosis. In: Ryan K, Berkowitz R, Barbieri R, Dunaif A, editors.

Kistner's Gynecology and Women's Health. 7th ed. St. Louis: Mosby, Inc; 1999. pp. 492–518.

105. Winkel C. Evaluation and management of women with endometriosis. *Obstet Gynecol*. 2003;102(2): 397–408.

106. Sangi-Haghpeykar H, Poindexter A. Epidemiology of endometriosis among parous women. *Obstet Gynecol*. 1995;85(6):983–992.

107. Eskenazi B, Warner M. Epidemiology of endometriosis. *Obstet Gynecol Clin North Am*. 1997;24: 235–258.

108. Holdredge A. Clinical assessment of gynecologic vaginal bleeding. In: Menihan C, editor. *Limited Sonography in Obstetric and Gynecologic Triage*. Philadelphia: Lippincott Williams & Wilkins; 1998. pp. 73–86.

109. Della-Giustina D, Denny M. Ectopic pregnancy. *Emerg Med Clin North Am*. 2003;21(3):565–584.

110. Lemus J. Ectopic pregnancy: An update. *Curr Opin Obstet Gynecol*. 2000;12(5):369–375.

111. Danakas G. Ectopic pregnancy. In: Ferri F, editor. *Ferri's Clinical Advisor: Instant Diagnosis and Treatment*. St. Louis: Mosby, Inc; 2004. pp. 297–298.

112. Gracia C, Barnhart K. Diagnostic ectopic pregnancy: Decision analysis comparing six strategies. *Obstet Gynecol*. 2001;97(3):464–470.

113. Shima T. Ectopic pregnancy. *Top Emerg Med*. 2002; 24(4):12–20.

114. Lipscomb G, Stovall T, Ling F. Primary care: Nonsurgical treatment of ectopic pregnancy. *N Engl J Med*. 2000;343(18):1325–1329.

115. Buster J, Heard M. Current issues in medical management of ectopic pregnancy. *Curr Opin Obstet Gynecol*. 2002;12(6):525–527.

116. Closson S. Clinical assessment of first trimester bleeding in pregnancy. In: Menihan C, editor. *Limited Sonography in Obstetrics and Gynecologic Triage*. Philadelphia: Lippincott Williams & Wilkins; 1998. pp. 119–127.

117. Stewart S. Pregnancy testing and management of early pregnancy. In: Hatcher R, Trussell J, Stewart F, Nelson A, Cates W, Guest F, et al., editors. *Contraceptive Technology*. 18th ed. New York: Ardent Media Inc.; 2004. pp. 629–649.

118. Anonymous. Ectopic pregnancy. In: Stenchever M, Droegemueller W, Herbst A, Mishell D, editors. *Comprehensive Gynecology*. 4th ed. St. Louis: Mosby; 2001. pp. 443–478.

119. Miller J, Griffin E. Methotrexate administration for ectopic pregnancy in the emergency department— one hospital's protocol/ competencies. *J Emerg Nurs*. 2003;29(3):240–244.

120. Carlson K, Schiff I. Pelvic masses. In: Carlson K, Eisenstat S, Frigoletto F, Schiff I, editors. *Primary Care of Women*. 2nd ed. St. Louis: Mosby, Inc; 2002. pp. 366–369.

121. Persutte W. Ultrasonography in the first trimester of pregnancy: The basic examination. In: Menihan C, editor. *Limited Sonography in Obstetric and Gynecologic Triage*. Philadelphia: Lippincott Williams & Wilkins; 1998. pp. 129–154.

122. Morgan A. Adnexal mass evaluation in the emergency department. *Emerg Med Clin North Am*. 2001; 19(3):799–816.

123. Holdredge A. Clinical assessment of pelvic pain. In: Menihan C, editor. *Limited Sonography in Obstetrics and Gynecologic Triage*. Philadelphia: Lippincott Williams & Wilkins; 1998. pp. 73–86.

124. Schrecengost A. Ovarian mass - benign or malignant? *AORN J*. 2002;76(5):792–810.

125. Purcell K, Wheeler J. Benign disorders of the ovaries and oviducts. In: DeCherney A, Nathan L, editors. *Current Obstetrics and Gynecologic Diagnosis and Treatment*. 9th ed. New York: McGraw Hill Companies, Inc; 2003. Accessed January 21, 2006, at http://www.accessmedicine.com/resourceTOC.aspx? resourceID=9.

126. Funt S, Hann L. Detection and characterization of adnexal masses. *Radiol Clin North Am*. 2002;40(3): 591–608.

127. Quint E. Acute pelvic pain in adolescents. *J Pediatr Adolesc Gynecol*. 2003;16(4):254–257.

128. Rha S, Byun J, Jung S, Jung J, Choi B, Kim B, et al. CT and MR imaging features of adnexal torsion. *Radiographics*. 2002;22(2):283–294.

129. Helvie M, Silver T. Ovarian torsion: Sonographic evaluation. *J Clin Ultrasound*. 1989;17(5):327–332.

130. Houry D, Abbott J. Ovarian torsion: A fifteen year review. *Ann Emerg Med*. 2001;38(2):156–159.

131. Krissi H, Shalev J, Bar-Hava I, Langer R, Herman A, Kaplan B. Fallopian tube torsion: Laparoscopic evaluation and treatment of a rare gynecological entity. *J Am Board Fam Pract*. 2001;14(4):274–277.

132. Bayer A, Wiskind A. Adnexal torsion: Can the adnexa be saved? *Am J Obstet Gynecol*. 1994;171(6): 1506–1511.

133. Kruger E, Heller D. Adnexal torsion: A clinicopathologic review of 31 cases. *J Reprod Med.* 1999;44(2): 71–75.

134. Germain M, Rarick T, Robins E. Management of intermittent ovarian torsion by laparoscopic oophoropexy. *Obstet Gynecol.* 1996;88(suppl 4 Pt 2): 715–717.

135. Pena J, Ufberg D, Cooney N, Denis A. Usefulness of Doppler sonography in the diagnosis of ovarian torsion. *Fertil Steril.* 2000;73(5):1047–1050.

136. Chen C, Wang W, Wang T. Adnexal torsion during late pregnancy. *Am J Emerg Med.* 1999;17(7):738–739.

137. Dart R. Acute pelvic pain. In: Marx J, editor. *Rosen's Emergency Medicine: Concepts and Clinical Practice.* 5th ed. St. Louis: Mosby; 2002. pp. 219–226.

Mary Ellen Rousseau

Breast Health and Disease

Chapter 19

Women often present with breast concerns in the ambulatory setting, and most of these concerns are related to normal hormone fluctuations in the menstrual cycle. However, some presentations are more serious and may in fact be breast cancer. Awareness of breast cancer by professionals, the media, and the public has increased the use of mammograms and other diagnostic tests in the United States. The quality of the data regarding risks and benefits of various screening and treatment choices must be considered when making management decisions about breast problems. Best practice requires that clinicians be current with the latest management protocols and care guidelines. Midwives must also be mindful of their fiscal responsibility and order tests only when needed. As primary care providers, midwives are called upon to screen, evaluate, and manage breast symptoms, and to manage general breast health including recommendations for clinical breast exam (CBE), self breast exam (SBE), mammogram and other diagnostic tools as appropriate. These include such procedures as fine needle aspiration (FNA), ultrasound, and excisional biopsy. As the primary care provider, midwives are responsible for ordering these tests, explaining their results, and for coordinating care between women and specialists as appropriate.

Clinical Presentation

Women themselves usually discover a breast lump or other breast problem. In a study of women under the age of 40, 80% of the masses were self-identified, while the other 20% were found on clinical exam and not known to the patient until that time.[1] Women also commonly seek care for other changes such as nipple discharge and breast discomfort. A thorough evaluation of these problems is dependent on understanding the normal physiologic changes that occur over time, characteristics of breast-related problems that are more worrisome, and particular patient profiles that raise concern. This chapter discusses how to evaluate breast problems, provide a description of various breast conditions, and describe appropriate screening approaches for both healthy and at-risk women.

Essential History, Physical, and Laboratory Evaluation

Thorough, yet focused, history, physical, and laboratory evaluations are essential when evaluating breast problems. **Table 19-1** lists screening recommendations from three nationally recognized authorities.

History

The initial questions asked when a woman presents with a breast problem will depend on whether she is seeking care for concerns about a mass, nipple discharge, or breast tenderness. Questions to ask the woman who presents to your care with a mass include, first, information about the mass: when she first noted the lesion; whether or not she has pain with the mass; and whether the mass is stable in size. Further questions include: where she is in her menstrual cycle or her menopause status; her history of previous breast biopsies and results; history of cyst aspiration; whether she has had a mammogram or breast ultrasound as well as the results; and her personal history of breast cancer as well as that of her first- or second-degree relatives. A complete history also includes: parity; age of first pregnancy; history of nursing her children and for how long; history of colon or ovarian cancer in a first-degree relative; and a personal history of proliferative breast diseases (i.e., fibroadenoma, sclerosing adenosis, florid ductal hyperplasia, and intraductal papilloma).

If a woman reports breast tenderness, inquiries should be made regarding onset, frequency, and area of concern. Whether there is an association to the menstrual cycle is important because some physiologic tenderness is experienced by women in the luteal phase of their cycle from the effects of the gonadotropins on the mammary lobules, stroma, and ducts. While pregnancy and lactation also can cause physiologic breast tenderness, the woman should be screened for signs of mastitis including: temperature; malaise; a wedge-shaped reddened area of the breast; warmth in the affected area; and pain with nursing.

If, for example, a woman reports nipple discharge, several differential diagnoses direct your history taking because nipple discharge can be either physiologic or pathologic. The provider should include questions concerning onset, color, and characteristics of the nipple discharge; whether both breasts are affected; or if a mass is present. The provider should also determine if the discharge is spontaneous or if it must be expressed (the former being more serious), as well as if only one or many ducts are affected.

The most common physiologic reasons for *galactorrhea* (milky discharge) are pregnancy, birth, or nursing within the last year. With continued nipple stimulation, women may experience galactorrhea for many months after a spontaneous or therapeutic abortion, childbirth, and lactation. Some women nurse for a number of years, so that milk may be found upon physical exam and be a surprise for the examiner who has not considered this possibility.

Physical

Women seeking care for a breast problem require a thorough CBE. Examination includes observation of her sitting erect and with arms at her waist. The breasts are then observed while the patient is still sitting and leaning forward to see if there is any area that is attached to the wall of the chest. Upon inspection whether sitting or

Table 19-1 SCREENING RECOMMENDATIONS

American Cancer Society (ACS)[2]	U.S. Preventive Services Task Force (USPSTF)[3]	National Cancer Institute (NCI)[4]
Begin mammography at age 40	Mammography every 1–2 years for women beginning at age 40	Women in their 40s should be screened every 1–2 years with mammography
CBE every 3 years from ages 20–40; annually age 40 on	Insufficient evidence to recommend for or against CBE alone	Women aged 50 and older should be screened every 1–2 years
Benefits and limitations of SBE explained to women age 20 on, including prompt reporting of new findings	Insufficient evidence to recommend for or against teaching or performing SBE	Women who are at higher than average risk of breast cancer should seek expert medical advice about whether they should begin screening before age 40 and the frequency of screening
Women who choose to do SBE should be taught correct technique	It is *cost effective* to screen older women (>65 y) for breast cancer every 2 years[5]	
High-risk women need earlier screening, shorter intervals, or *consider* addition of screening modalities other than mammogram and physical exam (MRI not a recommendation)		
Older women should consider risks and benefits in light of current health status and estimated life expectancy		
Women should be informed of both benefits and limitations of screening and the possibility of harm from false-positive findings		

Abbreviations: CBE, clinical breast exam; SBE, self breast exam.

supine, the following should be noted: size and symmetry of the breasts; contour (masses, dimpling, retraction); edema; venous pattern; and the shape and size of the nipples as well as any lesions or discharge on the nipples.

Next, examination requires flattening the breast tissue against the woman's chest while she is in a supine position. This is of particular importance for the woman with larger breasts. To palpate the lateral portion of the large-breasted woman, having her roll onto her contralateral hip and rotate her shoulder back while placing her hand on her forehead allows for the best flattening of the tissue. To examine the medial portion of the breast, the woman should rest flat on her back so that the breast falls laterally in the larger breasted woman. The entire breast should be palpated from the area bordered by the clavicle, to the midsternum, the midaxillary line, and the bra line inferiorly. Pennypacker and Pilgrim[6] and Baines and colleagues[7] have done much of the work in standardizing the CBE. They recommend beginning in the axilla, proceeding to the bra line along the midaxillary line, and continuing between the clavicle and the bra line with overlapping rows. Pads of three middle fingers (excluding the pinkie) are used to examine the breast. Then each area is palpated by making small circles using different pressures (light, medium, and deep) to examine all levels of tissue. Upon finding an area that is clearly suspicious or even mildly suspicious, careful documentation is necessary; it should describe the characteristics of the area of concern and whether similar findings are present in the opposite breast. It is often helpful to draw the lesion on a schematic of the breast, including descriptors such as size, shape, and other qualities (i.e., cystic or solid, solitary, discrete, firm, hard, sensitive or not).

Evaluation of Breast Masses in Pregnancy

Breast masses are more difficult to discern during pregnancy and lactation because of the normal physiologic changes. There is increased glandular and areolar development and an overall increase in the parenchymal-to-adipose tissue ratio, and an increase in vascular flow. A lactating woman presenting with a mass is more likely to have a lactating adenoma, a fibroadenoma, or a galactocele than cancer.[8]

Ultrasound and mammography are used in pregnant and lactating women with varying success. It has been suggested that mammograms are less sensitive than usual because of increased breast density and other physiologic changes, although one small study by Swinford et al. showed no increased mammographic density in half the pregnant women studied.[9] Regardless of whether a woman is pregnant or lactating, an ultrasound can tell the difference between a solid or cystic mass.[8] If the results are indeterminate or suspicious, a biopsy is performed to rule out malignancy.

Midwives must recognize that breast cancer, while uncommon in a pregnant or lactating woman, is a real phenomenon that requires a full diagnostic work-up when symptoms are present. Delay in the diagnosis must be minimized by evaluating and referring pregnant and lactating women to a surgeon in a timely manner.

Tests and Laboratory Evaluations

Tests that help in diagnosing breast problems include a variety of media. Foremost is mammography for women age 40 and older. In a *screening mammogram*, each breast is compressed for two films: craniocaudal and lateral. The cost is between $50 and $200. Because there is no provider evaluation included, the screening mammogram should always follow the clinical exam done by the provider so that the data from the clinical exam can be used to choose the type of mammogram ordered and how the radiologist will examine the patient.

If there is a clinical concern other than breast tenderness, a *diagnostic mammogram* is required in which the area of concern is magnified and films taken to identify any problems. The diagnostic mammogram answers the question, "does this mass require a biopsy or is a follow-up diagnostic film sufficient?" A diagnostic film may be recommended in a certain period of time to show resolution, stability, or heightened concern that may require a biopsy.

If there is a strong likelihood that a mass is cystic (fluid filled), it is necessary to determine whether it is solid or fluid filled. This can be done by FNA or ultrasound. FNA is done with a 22-gauge needle and is an inexpensive means of obtaining an immediate answer to the question of whether the mass is a cyst. If solid material is withdrawn (i.e., in the case of a solid mass from which no fluid could be obtained), then it can be sent for a biopsy. For a premenopausal woman, if the fluid is not bloody and the cyst disappears with aspiration, no further diagnostic steps are necessary. Because the fluid is rarely malignant (<1%), there is no need to send it to cytology.[10] If the fluid is bloody, does not disappear completely upon aspiration, or recurs within a short period of time, a biopsy to rule out intracystic carcinoma is needed.

Ultrasound is another option to determine if the mass is cystic. Fluid-filled cysts are easily identified on sonogram; if they have the classic features of a simple cyst, no further work-up is needed. Cystic masses that look like simple cysts on ultrasound may be aspirated if the diagnosis is in doubt or to relieve pain, but cysts containing solid components should not be aspirated because they may then become difficult to palpate and find for biopsy. If no fluid is aspirated,

then the lesion is considered solid and further evaluation is required.

To aspirate a palpable cyst, raise a wheal with 1% lidocaine. With a 19-gauge needle on a 5-cc syringe, enter the cyst (upon entering the cyst, there is a "popping" feeling). The color and consistency of the fluid should be noted. Often, a simple cyst will have greenish black fluid that is similar in consistency to motor oil. As the cyst is aspirated, most of the mass should disappear. If the fluid appears bloody or the woman is postmenopausal, it should be sent to cytology for evaluation.

If a breast mass is found in a woman who is postmenopausal, then referral to a surgeon is required immediately without an aspiration. Expediency requires that a diagnostic mammogram be ordered concurrently so that the surgeon has the results when seeing the patient. The radiologist will determine at the time of the diagnostic mammogram whether an ultrasound of the breast will be useful. An ultrasound may be ordered for evaluation of a probable cyst to suggest problems such as irregular borders or increased blood flow, but it is not a substitute for a mammogram; in a woman over the age of 40, an ultrasound is strictly a secondary test.

Several tests should be considered for use when evaluating nipple discharge. Prolactin levels should be obtained as part of a work-up for pituitary adenoma, because it may cause a milky discharge. However, this should not be ordered if a breast exam has been done in which the nipple has been manipulated, because that in and of itself can raise the elevated prolactin level. The patient should be counseled to return for the prolactin level on another day when she has not been examined or sexually stimulated. *Nipple aspiration* is another method for early diagnosis and risk assessment for breast cancer.[11] Obtaining the aspirate, however, may be difficult and some training is involved. Additionally, cytological examination of nipple discharge is a specific but insensitive method to find a malignancy.[12] For this reason it is not usually part of a work-up for nipple discharge. Nipple discharge is discussed later in this chapter; the qualities of the discharge determine other laboratory tests that may be ordered.

MAMMOGRAPHY

All centers must meet the Mammography Quality Standards Act of 1994. Sensitivity depends on quality of the equipment, the experience of the technician, and the density of the breast tissue.

Findings on mammogram include the presence of a variety of findings: significant masses; calcifications; fibrocystic changes; focal asymmetric densities; the particular view where abnormalities are seen, and at what depth. The radiologist will also compare films and comment on any interval changes noted from previous films. The final report will include an impression, an indication as to whether further work-up is needed to make a diagnosis (such as obtaining additional films or views and/or biopsy), and a recommendation regarding when and how the patient should be followed in the future (i.e., return for routine annual or biannual mammogram or ultrasound). The woman needs to obtain a copy of any previous mammograms if done at a different facility, because comparison of films over time by the radiologist is an essential component of the mammographic evaluation.

Findings on mammogram may include *macrocalcifications*, which are associated with benign conditions, and most likely the result of degenerative changes such as aging arteries, old injuries, or inflammations. They are found in up to 50% of women over the age of 50. *Microcalcifications* are tiny mineral deposits that appear as small white spots in film. They are less than $\frac{1}{50}$ inch and appear singly or in clusters. Shape and arrangement help to determine the significance of the findings on mammogram. They do not always indicate a malignancy. The radiologist will recommend a biopsy or follow-up diagnostic mammogram, depending on the degree of concern associated with the finding.

Screening mammography is recommended for women who meet the criteria of increased risk for breast cancer. For most women, age is the only risk factor and mammographic screening usually begins at age 40. Table 19-1 provides guidelines for screening. For a woman who has a family history of premenopausal breast cancer in first-degree relatives, a yearly screening mammogram should begin at approximately five years before the age of the relative's diagnosis.[13] Screening for women younger than age 40 and over age 65 may prove to be efficacious but has not yet been validated.

Diagnostic mammogram is recommended for women with a solid dominant mass if age appropriate. Diagnosis may also include ultrasonography or aspiration. The purpose of the diagnostic mammogram is to screen the normal surrounding breast tissue and the opposite breast for nonpalpable cancers, rather than to make a diagnosis.[13] It is not generally done on women younger than age 40 because increased breast density makes it more difficult to interpret the findings and to identify microcalcifications. A normal mammogram still requires further evaluation of a suspicious mass. During a diagnostic mammogram the area involved is magnified. It attempts to answer the question, "does this mass require a biopsy or is another follow-up diagnostic mammogram indicated and, if so, when should this occur?"

Ultrasound is most useful in distinguishing between solid and cystic masses. It is especially useful when a palpable mass is not well defined on the mammogram. Ultrasound is the first option for screening in a woman younger than 40 years when breast density precludes mammogram use as a first-line screening. Simple cysts are diagnosed if four criteria are met: round or oval in shape; sharply defined margins; lack of internal echoes; and posterior acoustic enhancement.[13] Ultrasound is not used as first-line screening after the age of 40 because of its inability to identify microcalcifications.

Magnetic resonance imaging (MRI) is more sensitive for detecting breast cancers than mammography, ultrasound, or CBE alone,[14] and while it may be found efficacious for women at highest risk for breast cancer (i.e., those with a family history of BRCA 1 or BRCA 2), whether surveillance regimens that include MRI will reduce mortality from breast cancer in high-risk women requires further investigation. MRI, with its poor specificity, high cost, and complexity, is currently precluded from a major role in breast cancer diagnosis.[13]

FNA is used to diagnose and eliminate fluid-filled cysts or for aspiration of tissue to send to cytology or histology for evaluation of solid masses such as fibroadenoma. FNA provides single cells only and offers no appreciation of the architectural qualities of the mass. Although the false positive rates are low, the false negative rates may be as high as 15% to 20%.[13] Consequently, if a mass remains after aspiration of a cyst or a suspicious mass remains after a negative finding, then a biopsy is recommended.

Excisional biopsy (lumpectomy) provides a complete pathological assessment. This is done on a palpable mass and on nonpalpable masses with stereotactic or ultrasound-guided biopsy or mammographic localization. Lesions suspicious for malignancy are removed with at least a 1 cm margin while nonsuspicious lesions such as a fibroadenoma need only minimal margins. The whole lesion is removed intact. Stereotactic biopsy uses x, y, and z coordinates on the mammogram to find a nonpalpable mass.

Classifications of Benign Breast Lesions

Understanding how to interpret the findings of tests commonly ordered during the evaluation of breast problems is dependent on understanding how various breast disorders are classified, their particular characteristics, and their potential for developing cancer in the future. The main classifications for benign disorders include: 1) nonproliferative; 2) proliferative without atypia; 3) and proliferative with atypia. These classifications and various specific disorders are listed in **Table 19-2**.

NONPROLIFERATIVE LESIONS

Nonproliferative lesions include approximately 70% of the lesions of the breast and carry no increased risk for the development of carcinoma.[13] They can occur anywhere in the breast, including the ducts, lobes, and stroma. A *cyst*, which is a fluid-filled pocket, is the most common finding. Cysts large enough to palpate are termed gross cysts. Other lesions include papillary (nipple) apocrine (sweat gland) change, which is characterized by a growth of ductal epithelial cells in which all of the cells show apocrine features. Epithelial-related calcifications are frequently observed in breast tissue and can be found in normal ducts, lobules, or in almost any pathologic condition.

Table 19-2 CLASSIFICATIONS OF BENIGN AND ATYPICAL BREAST DISORDERS

Classifications	Lesions	Characteristics	Clinical Significance	Refer if:
Nonproliferative	Cyst	Fluid-filled sac	None	Solid structures within cyst
	Papillary apocrine change	Nipple and sweat gland features	Incidental finding	
Proliferative without atypia	Fibroadenomas	Firm, rubbery, unilateral, age usually <30	Small association with increased risk of breast cancer	Patient requests lumpectomy; if age >40
	Ductal hyperplasia or (moderate or florid) hyperplasia	Increased number of cells relative to normal above basement membrane; moderate is 3 cells above membrane; florid is 70% of lumen occluded	Increased risk of breast cancer 0.5–2 times normal	Found on biopsy, therefore a surgeon is involved
	Intraductal papillomas	Tumor of major lactiferous ducts; 3–4 mm usually; rarely 4–5 cm	Seen in women ages 30–40; bloody nipple discharge	Present
	Sclerosing adenosis	Proliferation of glandular and stromal structures	Enlarges and distorts lobes; associated with diffuse calcifications	Seen on mammogram or in biopsy
Proliferative with atypia	Atypical lobular hyperplasia (ALH)	Possess some but not all characteristics of cancer in situ	Composed of cells identical to those found in LCIS	Risk greater than that associated with ADH; (RR 4.3)[15]
	Lobular Carcinoma in situ (LCIS): Distinguishing hyperplasia from neoplasia is based on identification of a clonal cell	Noninvasive disease but morphologic similarities between wells of LCIS and frankly invasive lobular carcinoma; no	Usually diagnosed between ages of 40 and 50; difficult to manage because it is multifocal and clinically undetectable	If found on mammogram, refer

Table 19-2 CLASSIFICATIONS OF BENIGN AND ATYPICAL BREAST DISORDERS
(continued)

Classifications	Lesions	Characteristics	Clinical Significance	Refer if:
Proliferative with atypia (cont'd)	process. Clonality means uniformity of morphology and phenotype (i.e., cytokeratin expression or hormone receptor expression)	palpable lump; often invisible on mammogram; usually an incidental finding on biopsy; often multifocal and bilateral		
	Atypical ductal hyperplasia (ADH)	Identified by micro-calcifications on mammogram	Has some architectural and cytologic features of low-grade DCIS	Increased risk for development of breast cancer, approximately 3.5 to 5.0 times that of the reference population

Abbreviations: DCIS, ductal carcinoma in situ; RR, relative risk.

The conditions described below may be found on biopsy but are of little clinical relevance to the provider who screens for breast cancer.

- *Apocrine metaplasia* describes changes in the epithelial lining the wall of the cyst and is composed of columnar cells. Although not a typical constituent of the microscopic anatomy of the mammary gland, any benign proliferative lesion of the breast may contain metaplastic cells with apocrine cytologic features.
- *Ductal ectasia* occurs when the ductules of the breast are filled with desquamated ductal epithelium and secretory proteinaceous contents. It is a condition that involves the periareolar tissues in the nonlactating breast and is a conse-

quence of disruption of the epithelial interface, with subsequent entry of normal skin flora.
- *Calcifications*, which are calcium deposits, are often seen in ductal, lobular, and stromal tissues of the breast, are macroscopic or microscopic, and can be seen in blood vessels or lobules, free in the stroma, or associated with the epithelium.

PROLIFERATIVE LESIONS WITHOUT ATYPIA

Proliferative lesions, on the other hand, are those that have grown beyond what is considered normal and are characterized by a tendency to bridge and distend the involved tissue. Such lesions have the potential for the development of invasive breast cancer $1\frac{1}{2}$ to 2 times normal.[13] This type of lesion includes:

- Fibroadenoma
- Usual ductal hyperplasia (moderate or florid hyperplasia)
- Intraductal papilloma
- Sclerosing adenosis (an incidental finding for the most part)
- Radial and complex sclerosing lesions
- Lactating adenoma

Fibroadenomas are now included in the proliferative lesion category.[16] Whereas adenomas are well-circumscribed tumors made up of benign epithelial cells with sparse, inconspicuous stroma,[17] in fibroadenomas the stroma is an integral part of the tumor. *Fibroadenomas* are hyperplastic breast lobules considered to be an aberration of normal development and involution. Because fibroadenomas most often are found in young women, it was long thought to have no association with breast cancer. However, women with a diagnosis of complex fibroadenoma (containing cysts >3 mm in diameter, sclerosing adenosis, epithelial calcifications, or papillary apocrine changes) have a two to three times increased risk of breast cancer.[18] These masses are the most common benign tumors of the female breast and are the most common breast tumor in women under the age of 25. Although they most often do not change with the menstrual cycle, they may contain estrogen receptors and can change in size with cycling. In general, they are firm, rubbery, and usually are well delineated and not tender.

Florid ductal epithelial hyperplasia has an increased risk of invasive breast cancer of between 0.5 and 2 times normal. This is a variant of proliferative lesions in which there are an increased number of cells relative to what is normally seen above the basement membrane. Moderate hyperplasia is when there are three more than expected number of cells above the basement membrane; with florid hyperplasia, 70% of the duct lumen is involved.

Sclerosing adenosis is a proliferation of glandular and stromal elements that enlarges and distorts the lobular units and is associated with diffuse calcifications. Intraductal papillomas are tumors of the major lactiferous ducts and are usually between 3 and 4 mm but occasionally as large as 4 to 5 cm. They are usually seen in women between the ages of 30 and 50. Women often present with bloody nipple discharge.

Intraductal papillomas (benign tumors of the epithelium) are found in the major lactiferous ducts and usually are attached to the wall of the duct by a stalk. When they are multiple, they are more peripheral, more bilateral and appear to be more susceptible to malignant transformation.

Lactating adenomas are mobile masses during pregnancy or the postpartum period. Such masses are uncommon, well-differentiated benign tumors of secretory mammary epithelium. The origin of a lactating adenoma, though controversial, is believed to be de novo or a variant of pre-existing tubular adenoma or fibroadenoma that reflects the morphologic changes resulting from the physiologic state of pregnancy.[19]

PROLIFERATIVE LESIONS WITH ATYPIA

This type of lesion is also called *atypical hyperplasia*. Such lesions possess some but not all of the features of carcinoma in situ,[20] which include:

- Atypical ductal hyperplasia (ADH) — has some features of LCIS
- Atypical lobular hyperplasia (ALH) — identical cells to those found in LCIS
- Lobular carcinoma in situ (LCIS)
- Ductal carcinoma in situ (DCIS)

Women with a diagnosis of DCIS are at 3.5 to 5.0 times increased risk for developing breast cancer. Women with ALH involving both the ducts and lobules have a 6.8 times risk of developing breast cancer.[21] Findings suggest that the risk of breast cancer in patients with atypical hyperplasia is approximately equal in both breasts, which suggests that atypical hyperplasia (ductal or lobular) is a marker of generalized increased risk.[16] If a woman has atypical hyperplasia prior to menopause, it puts her at greater risk for breast cancer than when it is diagnosed in a postmenopausal woman.[16]

Management of Specific Conditions

Clinical management strategies for some of the more common breast conditions and diseases are discussed here. **Table 19-3** summarizes the findings suggestive of a specific problem and suggestions for management.

Benign Breast Diseases

Love et al.[22] divide benign breast disorders into six general categories: physiologic swelling and tenderness; nodularity; mastalgia; dominant lumps; nipple discharge; and breast infection.[22] Most women experience some swelling and tenderness in the luteal half of the menstrual cycle because of the increase in gonadotropins on the mammary lobules, stroma, and ducts. After the engorgement, the epithelial cells lining the ducts desquamate with menses. As cycles continue throughout a woman's reproductive lifespan, changes occur in the breast that are not abnormal and represent breast parenchymal responsiveness to hormonal stimulation.[13] These changes include nodularity with or without tenderness, which involves the whole breast or just a portion and can be either unilateral or bilateral.

Fibrocystic changes include symptoms and physical findings such as pain, nodularity, and cysts. The common features of fibrocystic breasts are likely to have an endocrine etiology and persist over the span of a woman's reproductive life.[13] Fibrocystic disease/changes have been called mammary dysplasia, cystic disease, cystic mastopathy, and cystic hyperplasia. These can be characterized as cystic change, ductal epithelial hyperplastic change, or fibrotic change. Microcysts are <1 mm in size, while macrocysts are >3 mm in size. Hyperplastic ductal alterations can occur where the ductal epithelium has undergone benign proliferation of the superficial cells. Fibrosis is a palpable, nonmobile, flat, button-like, firm, irregular mass.[13] Fibrotic change is when the breast parenchyma is reacting to an irritative factor, probably ductal inflammation.[13]

In general, most attempts at treatment of discomforts associated with fibrocystic changes have been of little help. Autopsy reports show that most women have such changes and that the incidence increases throughout life even though there is some regression after menopause. Love et al. were the first to recommend the name change from disease to "fibrocystic changes"[22]; Europeans call such changes *aberrations of normal development and involution.*[23]

Cysts are thought to be the result of cystic lobular involution. Acini within the lobule distend to become microcysts that may develop into macrocysts. Clinical occurrence is reported to be approximately 7% of women, with as many as 23% incidence of cysts >1 cm found on autopsy.[24,25] Cysts often fluctuate in size and discomfort with the menstrual cycle. Although they can occur at any age, they are most frequently

Table 19-3 BENIGN BREAST CONDITIONS

Signs and Symptoms	Physiology	Presentation	Screening/ follow-up	Treatment
Physiologic swelling and tenderness	Physiologic; hormonal influence; resolved by menopause	Sometimes increases in perimenopause	CBE Writing breast journal; return to office in 3 months for evaluation	Avoid salt and caffeine. Take vitamin E, Evening primrose oil
Mastalgia	Cyclic	Pain in luteal phase	CBE Writing breast journal; return to office in 3 months for evaluation	Avoid salt, caffeine. Take Vitamin E, Evening primrose oil, NSAIDs
Nodularity	Noncyclic	Ropiness	CBE Mammogram* and/or US	NSAIDs none
Fibrocystic changes	Reaction to irritation or inflammation; endocrine response	Palpable nonmobile, flat, firm, irregular areas of denser breast tissue	CBE, mammogram*	None age <39; mammogram age 40 or greater
Gross cysts (i.e., fluid-filled sac that is either silent or painful)	Cystic lobular involution	Ages 35–50; solitary or multiple; breast discharge or not	FNA, US, mammography*	Avoid salt, caffeine. Take Vitamin E, Evening primrose oil, NSAIDs
Galactocele	Milk-filled cyst from over-distention of lactiferous duct	Mobile, non-tender mass in lactating woman	FNA; occasionally must be repeated	Surgical resection rarely needed
Fibroadenoma	Abnormal development of lobes; most common mass in women 20–40	Not painful; discrete mass; usually solitary and in upper outer quadrant; cyclic response sometimes	FNA; CBE, mammogram*	Leave in place with follow-up clinical exam or refer for excision
Intraductal papilloma	Lactiferous ducts tumors	Solitary or multiple; occur in large ducts; 3–4 mm but occasionally as	Mammogram Refer to surgeon	Surgical resection

Table 19-3 BENIGN BREAST CONDITIONS *(continued)*

Signs and Symptoms	Physiology	Presentation	Screening/ follow-up	Treatment
		large as 4–5 cm; appears during ages of 30–50; bloody nipple discharge		
Nipple discharge	Physiologic: post-childbirth; lactating; fibrocystic changes	Clear, milky, multicolored, sticky, or watery	CBE, expression of discharge; possibly send to cytology?	If suspicious, refer to surgeon: one nipple, one pore, spontaneous post-menopause, associated with mass
	Drug related: with use of phenothiazines triclic anti-depressants, rauwolfia alkaloids, methyldopa or OCPs[13]			
	Pathologic: pituitary adenoma; thyroid disease; intra-ductal papilloma	Sanguinous, serosanguinous	Prolactin, thyroid function studies	Pituitary adenoma: Bromocryptine
	Purulent - mastitis	*S. aureus*		Dicloxicillin 250–500 mg qid for 10 days
	Cancer: yellow, serous, serosan-guinous and sanguinous	3%–4% incidence; risk increases when spontaneous, one breast, one duct, persistent, associated with a lump	Mammogram*, referral to surgeon	Biopsy and histology
Infection (mastitis)	Intrinsic: related to breast architecture or function; e.g., postpartum engorgement, lactational mastitis	Sore, inflamed breast, fever, flu-like symptoms, leukocytosis	CBE, continue nursing; refer to surgeon if not responsive to antibiotics	Dicloxacillin 250–500 mg qid for 10 days

(continues)

Table 19-3 BENIGN BREAST CONDITIONS *(continued)*

Signs and Symptoms	Physiology	Presentation	Screening/ follow-up	Treatment
Infection (mastitis) *(cont'd)*	(retrograde infection), or breast abscess; extrinsic infection in an adjacent organ or structure			
Duct ectasia	Involves the periare-olar tissues and results from disruption of the epithelial interface with subsequent entry of normal skin flora such as *S. aureus* and streptococcal bacteria	Noncyclic mastalgia, nipple retraction or discharge	Refer to surgeon	Simple drainage is usually all that is needed, but the condition may recur.
Mondor's disease	Caused by a super-ficial thrombo-phlebitis of the lateral thoracic veins.	Local acute pain in lateral half of breast or anterior chest wall with tender, palpable subcutane-ous cord or linear skin dimpling; followed by a tender, firm cord "string phlebitis" that follows the superficial veins.	May occur after local trauma or surgery but no follow-up needed	Resolves spontaneously; NSAIDs for pain. No inter-vention required
Unconfirmed mass	Unknown	Variable	CBE. Mammogram if >40 years; return after next menses if <40 for repeat CBE	None, unless problem is found on other diagnostic exams

* If age appropriate.

Abbreviations: CBE, complete breast exam; FNA, fine needle aspiration; NSAIDs, nonsteroidal anti-inflammatory drugs; US, ultrasound; OCPs, oral contraceptive pills; mg, milligram; qid, four times a day.

found in women in their 40s and are rare in the postmenopausal woman, so any mass in this group should be viewed with a high degree of suspicion. All cysts need to be evaluated to determine if they are fluid filled or solid, using sonograms and/or FNA. For premenopausal women, this evaluation may be sufficient. However, women over 40 years and younger women with high-risk profiles or suspicious findings on sonogram require further evaluation. At a minimum, they will require a mammogram and, in certain situations, a follow-up biopsy. The Laboratory Evaluation section above has further details.

Efficacy of therapies to help with cyclic breast pain associated with breast cysts, such as avoidance of caffeine and salt as well as the use of B and E vitamins, has not yet been proven.

Fibroadenomas are usually solitary, round or oval, nontender, and mobile rubbery lesions. Such lesions may present as multiple lesions 10% to 15% of the time. The most frequent location is the upper outer quadrant. If there is a reoccurrence, it is usually in the same quadrant as before.[26] On ultrasound, fibroadenomas appear round or oval, circumscribed, homogenous, solid masses with low-level internal echoes in a uniform distribution and intermediate acoustic attenuation.[27] If a fibroadenoma looks like cancer with irregular margins and acoustic shadowing on ultrasound, a biopsy with FNA is required for diagnosis. It was believed that these lesions grew to 2 to 3 cm in size and remained unchanged[28]; however, newer studies have demonstrated that between 16% and 59% of fibroadenomas resolve spontaneously.[29,30] Although fibroadenomas are associated with a slightly increased risk of breast cancer, this evidence does not change the clinical management strategy.

Fibroadenomas may be managed by excision of the whole lesion. This provides a definitive diagnosis and relieves the woman of anxiety about the mass; continued follow-up is not needed. On the other hand, doing nothing has no negative impact on the woman's health, while surgery has the risk of scarring and added expense. Alternatively, the mass may be managed by combining physical examinations, ultrasonography, and/or FNA. For women younger than age 35 who have clinically benign masses, if all three modalities are consistent with fibroadenoma, then they may be followed for clinical physical exam every six months until age 40.[1]

Palpable mass, vague thickening, or nodularity can be managed using various approaches depending upon age, cycle status, menopause status, and whether the woman has breast pain. Other factors include whether it is a bilateral finding, and whether it is a solitary mass or multiple masses. If fibrocystic changes are suspected, then reassurance is usually all that is needed. Analgesics such as ibuprofen and elimination of caffeine in coffee, tea, and chocolate may help, although efficacy of these suggestions is not proven. Reducing salt intake may help some women. It is appropriate to re-examine the patient in one to two cycles, or refer to a gynecologist or surgeon if the problem is persistent. A mammogram is recommended if the woman is age 40 or older. The section above on Benign Breast Diseases contains a more in-depth discussion of various breast findings.

Unconfirmed mass is a problem of clinical significance. In this case, the patient presents with a breast mass that is not palpable on CBE. Should the provider convince the patient that the findings of the CBE are correct? What should be done if she has breast pain? The provider should always take this concern seriously, documenting a careful history with regard to onset, duration, and exacerbating circumstances. If the woman feels a lump and it is not discernible on palpation, the location of the mass should be documented with a diagram or descriptive narrative. A standard CBE technique should be conducted with particular emphasis on the area the woman best feels the lump. This area should be compared to the same area in the other breast. If the patient is still concerned, then a follow-up appointment should be made. If she still is cycling, then an examination should be repeated in the follicular phase of her cycle. A consult with a collaborative physician should be obtained if there is still concern. If the woman is over 40 years of age, then a screening mammogram is appropriate.

Mastalgia may be physiologic breast fullness or tenderness often occurring in the luteal phase of the menstrual cycle; true cyclic mastalgia is a more extreme form of this occurrence. For most women, reassurance is the only measure needed. For women 40 years or older, a screening mammogram is recommended as part of the work-up. For younger women, a mammogram is not needed for mastalgia alone because of the difficulty in interpreting the findings.

The primary care provider needs to distinguish whether the woman is more worried that the pain might indicate a malignancy or whether the pain itself is the problem. Based on the history and physical examination, breast pain can be categorized into cyclic, noncyclic, or extramammary pain.

There are many theories regarding the etiology of extreme breast pain, including endocrine abnormalities, particularly estrogen, progesterone, and prolactin, but none of them has been proven beyond doubt. It has also been proposed

that women who suffer with mastalgia are at a higher risk for anxiety and depression.[31] Because no consistent histologic, endocrine, or behavioral assessments are available, breast pain often is not thought to be a clinical condition.[22]

Evaluation of breast pain begins with history and should include the type of pain, relationship to menses, duration, location, and relationship to other medical problems. The provider should establish if the woman wants specific treatment or if reassurance that the pain does not represent a more serious problem is acceptable.

While the patient is sitting and lying supine, the physical exam should start with a general exam of the breast and then proceed to the affected area. If the woman is then turned half on her side so that the breast tissue can fall away from the chest wall, it is possible to discern whether the pain is located in the breast tissue, chest wall, or rib area. Some women have nodularity at the site of the pain and yet the extent of the nodularity bears no relationship to the intensity of the pain.[32] Some women have no physical findings whatsoever.

No other treatment than reassurance should be instituted unless the symptoms are present for at least six months. When appropriate, a pain diary along with a pain analogue chart and a menstrual diary should be recommended for a few months, so that the woman can note any association of the pain with the menstrual cycle or other precipitating factors.

Treatment, after excluding disease and offering reassurance, should include the use of nonsteroidal anti-inflammatory drugs (NSAIDs), which have been shown to be successful.[33] Other options include drugs such as Danazol, an antigonadotropin that may relieve pain in up to 93% of cases.[34,35] However, Danazol has a high side effect profile that includes irregular menses, nausea, headache, and depression. Tamoxifen, a partial anti-estrogen/partial estrogen agonist has been shown effective for breast pain but is off label for breast pain and may cause hot flashes. Efficacy of gamma-linolenic acid (evening primrose oil) is still in dispute for breast pain but might be effective for cyclical pain. Vitamin E and caffeine reduction may play a role in treatment for breast pain. Progestins have been used for breast pain, but efficacy has not been shown.

Mastitis most often occurs as lactational mastitis, which usually involves the interlobular connective tissue of the breast parenchyma along a peripheral wedge of the breast and stems from nipple fissuring or milk stasis. A secondary retrograde bacterial infection occurs, with *Staphylococcus aureus*, *Escherichia coli*, or *Streptococcus* species usually being the offending agents, the source of which is the baby's flora. One or more of the ducts may drain poorly or become blocked, resulting in bacterial growth in the retained milk. It may occur in up to 24% of women, according to a study including a large cohort of women in Finland who were between 5 and 12 weeks postpartum.[36] When women have sore or cracked nipples, they are at a higher risk for mastitis because such breaks in the skin allow the bacteria to enter. Women present with a very sore, inflamed breast and often feel like they have the flu. The breast symptoms often occur in a wedge-shaped section in the upper outer quadrant, where the area will be erythematous, edematous, tender, and warm. Axillary lymphadenopathy may be present. An abscess may develop, presenting as a palpable, tender, inflamed, and fluctuant mass. Breast engorgement may develop as well. Diagnosis is based on history and physical findings, and culture and sensitivity may be performed. Women are encouraged to continue to nurse while taking antibiotics. The usual first-line antibiotic is di-

cloxacillin 250 mg or 500 mg, depending on severity, four times daily for 10 days.

The differential diagnosis includes simple breast engorgement, which generally presents with generalized breast swelling and is often noted during the first days of breast feeding. It is relieved with the use of the following techniques: frequent nursing; milk expression between feedings; and the use of hot showers or massage. Mastitis is not relieved after using those techniques. When a blocked duct-lump area is noted in one area of a lactating breast and it remains unrelieved by breast feeding with massage, then early treatment with antibiotics often prevents progression or the need for incision and drainage when the condition is well advanced.

Other measures that help to resolve lactational mastitis, and should be encouraged, include: application of warm, moist compresses to the area affected prior to breast feeding; frequent nursing with the unaffected breast until let down occurs in the affected breast; and then nursing from the affected breast until it has emptied completely.[37] Fluid intake should be increased to two to three liters a day. Bed rest may be required for very symptomatic women. Acetaminophen or NSAIDs are recommended for pain, inflammation, and fever. Cold compresses may help with pain.

Ten percent of all cases will develop into an abscess that will require aspiration or incision and drainage[38]; these women should be referred to a physician.

Patient teaching to avoid mastitis should include: adequate instruction in proper breast-feeding techniques; early and frequent nursing to prevent engorgement; adequate rest and fluid intake; and, after nursing, leaving a small amount of milk on each nipple to prevent cracking and allowing nipples to air dry. Early identification of signs and symptoms of abscess formation and need for prompt notification of the midwife should also be emphasized.

Nonlactational mastitis may be from many possible causes including abscess, inflammatory breast cancer, duct ectasia, and granulomatous lesions.[39] Women with sporadic infectious mastitis or noninfectious inflammation of the breast should have mammography followed by prompt drainage of the abscess and biopsy of any viable tissue near or within the abscess cavity.[13]

Nonlactational mastitis may present as subareolar abscess, with tenderness, redness, swelling; a palpable mass usually is not accompanied by fever or malaise. Subareolar abscess is often associated with nipple inversion or retraction. A peripheral abscess occurs anywhere in the breast with pain, tenderness, and swelling. Women with a mass other than in the periareolar area should be assessed for systemic diseases that predispose them to abscess development, including diabetes and immunosuppression.

Galactocele is an uncommon milk-filled breast cyst caused by a duct that is usually clogged by protein. It is formed by an over-distention of a lactiferous duct and presents as a firm nontender lesion. It usually occurs in lactating females and is generally unilateral. *Galactostasis* is milk retention, while galactocele represents a further stage of retention, including local cystic extension of ducts with thickened milk and chronic inflammatory infiltrate in the ductal wall. The lesions are known to occur singly or in multiples. Diagnostic aspiration is often curative. Although rarely needed, needle aspiration, followed by excision should the cyst recur, is the standard method of diagnosing and treating galactocele.

Mondor's disease is a rare condition that presents clinically as local pain with tender, palpable subcutaneous cord, or linear skin dimpling caused by a superficial thrombophlebitis of the lateral thoracic vein. It nearly always resolves spontaneously and NSAIDs may offer relief. Often no underlying pathology is found; it may occur after local trauma or surgery to the breast. The patient presents with acute pain in the lateral half of the breast or anterior chest wall followed by a tender, firm cord "string phlebitis" that follows the superficial veins. No intervention is usually required because it resolves on its own.

Duct ectasia usually involves the periareolar tissues and results from disruption of the epithelial interface with subsequent entry of normal skin flora such as *S. aureus* and streptococcal bacteria. It presents with noncyclic mastalgia, nipple retraction, or discharge. It is a superficial condition that is associated with cellulitis and may be the result of sebaceous gland involvement. Simple drainage is usually all that is needed, but the condition may recur.

Nipple discharge can be either physiologic or pathologic. Spontaneous nipple discharge in nonlactating and nonpregnant women is considered abnormal and requires further evaluation.[40] While breast cancer can be associated with nipple discharge, most pathologic breast lesions associated with such a discharge are benign.[12] To be significant, a discharge should be true, spontaneous, persistent, and nonlactational. It can be milky, multicolored and sticky, purulent, clear (watery), yellow (serous), pink (serosanguinous), or bloody (sanguineous). Watery, serous, serosanguinous, and sanguineous discharges are often caused by intraductal papillomas (unilateral and hemorrhagic), fibrocystic disease, or other physiologic disturbances, but they also could be cancerous (13%).[40] Referral to a surgeon is recommended if the discharge is unilateral, found in a postmenopausal woman, or is confined to one duct with clear, serous, bloody, black, or serosanguinous characteristics. Suspicion increases if there is an associated lump, if the woman is older, and if it is associated with mammographic findings. If the discharge is green in color, it is usually not suspicious but rather hormonally induced by, for example, a hormonal contraceptive or hormone therapy use.

When the discharge is bilateral or includes multiple ducts, usually the condition is benign. If milk is expressed, a work-up for galactorrhea is necessary that includes at a minimum thyroid stimulating hormone and prolactin (drawn on a day when there has been no breast exam or sexual contact that might elevate the prolactin level). Galactorrhea may be the result of phenothiazines, tricyclic antidepressants, rauwolfia alkaloids, methyldopa, or oral contraceptives. Multicolored sticky discharge is usually the result of duct ectasia (see above).

Breast Cancer

Invasive breast cancers are generally divided into ductal and lobular types, but either type can arise in either location.[41] These are further divided into the following classifications:

- Special types
  - Tubular
  - Mucoid
  - Cribiform
  - Papillary
  - Medullary
  - Classical lobular
- No special type
  - Commonly known as NOS (not otherwise specified)
  - Useful prognostic information is obtained by grading such cancers (degree of differentiation of the tumor)[41]

Staging

Staging of invasive cancer is an attempt to communicate systematically the status of the tumor through measurements and clinical evaluation by a pathologist. There are two generally accepted systems of staging: the Tumor Node Metastasis and the International Union Against Cancer System. Both use clinical measurements of tumor size and location and assessment of lymph node status (**Table 19-4**).

Table 19-4 TUMOR NODE METASTASIS CLASSIFICATION OF BREAST TUMORS

Classification	Definition
T_{is}	Cancer in situ
T_1	2 cm (T_{1a} 0.5 cm; T_{1b} >0.5–1; T_{1c} >1–2 cm)
T_2	>2 cm–5 cm
T_3	>5 cm
T_{4a}	Involvement of chest wall
T_{4b}	Involvement of skin (includes ulceration, direct infiltration, peau d'orange, and satellite nodules)
T_{4c}	T_{4a} and T_{4b} together
T_{4d}	Inflammatory cancer
N_0	No regional node metastases
N_1	Palpable mobile involved ipsilateral axillary nodes
N_2	Fixed involved ipsilateral axillary nodes
N_3	Ipsilateral internal mammary node involvement (rarely clinically detectable)
M_0	No evidence of metastasis
M_1	Distant metastasis (includes ipsilateral supraclavicular nodes)

Neither system is particularly accurate,[41] yet prognosis and treatment recommendations are linked to staging because no other better data system is yet available.

Breast Cancer in Perspective

Because of the possibility of breast cancer, finding a breast lump is one of the most upsetting experiences a woman can experience. While biomedical science has made progress in screening and treatment of breast cancer (**Figure 19-1**), our knowledge is still relatively primitive and reflects our imperfect understanding of the biological world. Technologies such as mammograms and fetal heart monitoring are often difficult to interpret and sometimes lead to unnecessary interventions or produce insufficient data to interpret with enough sophistication to make much more than marginal gains in quality of life or survival. Mastectomies, radiation, and chemotherapy can produce toxic physiologic and psychologic side effects. In contrast, other better technologies have cost-effective, nontoxic, and widely applicable uses that either prevent or cure disease. Examples of these include the polio and smallpox vaccines, and iodization of salt. Although Phase II trials have begun for more sophisticated technologies for breast cancer (i.e., anti-angiogenesis, which may offer nontoxic therapy to block a vital component of progressive breast cancer), the mainstays of care at the current time are aimed at early detection. These techniques include: regular SBE, CBE, mammograms, and providing education and support to women.

Breast cancer can be a frightening disease. What makes it more tragic is that it often occurs when women have maximal social re-sponsibility.[15] In addition, midwives often care for underserved women who statistically bear an excess burden with regard to breast cancer morbidity and mortality. Although white women have an increased overall incidence of breast cancer, African-American women have a higher mortality rate (Figure 19-1).[42] Breast cancer is the leading cause of cancer death among African-American women, and while the breast cancer death rate for white women fell in the United States from 1992 to 1995, the death rate for African-American women rose 2.6% during that same time period.[42]

The National Cancer Institute estimates that 13.4% of women (often expressed as "1 in 7") born today will be diagnosed with breast cancer at some time in their lives,[43] and the mortality rate of those with breast cancer is 1 in 30.[15] Because rates of breast cancer increase with age, estimates of risk at specific ages are more meaningful than estimates of lifetime risk. With each passing decade, women are more likely to develop breast cancer, making age the most important risk factor for women. Although progress has been made in identifying other risk factors for breast cancer, 50% of women who have the disease have no known major predictors. Both the incidence and mortality rate increase with age: 94% of new cases and 96% of deaths due to breast cancer during the years 1996 to 2000 occurred in women aged 40 and older.[42] In 2003, it was estimated that 211,300 new cases of invasive breast cancer were diagnosed with an additional estimated 55,700 cases of in situ disease.[42] Rapid advances in detection and treatment have led to increases in disease-free survival of women diagnosed with breast cancer.[42] However, age-based estimates of risk are not particularly helpful for a specific woman because individual risk is modified by age, family history, repro-

---

Figure 19-1 Mortality trends for groups 1990–2000.[42]

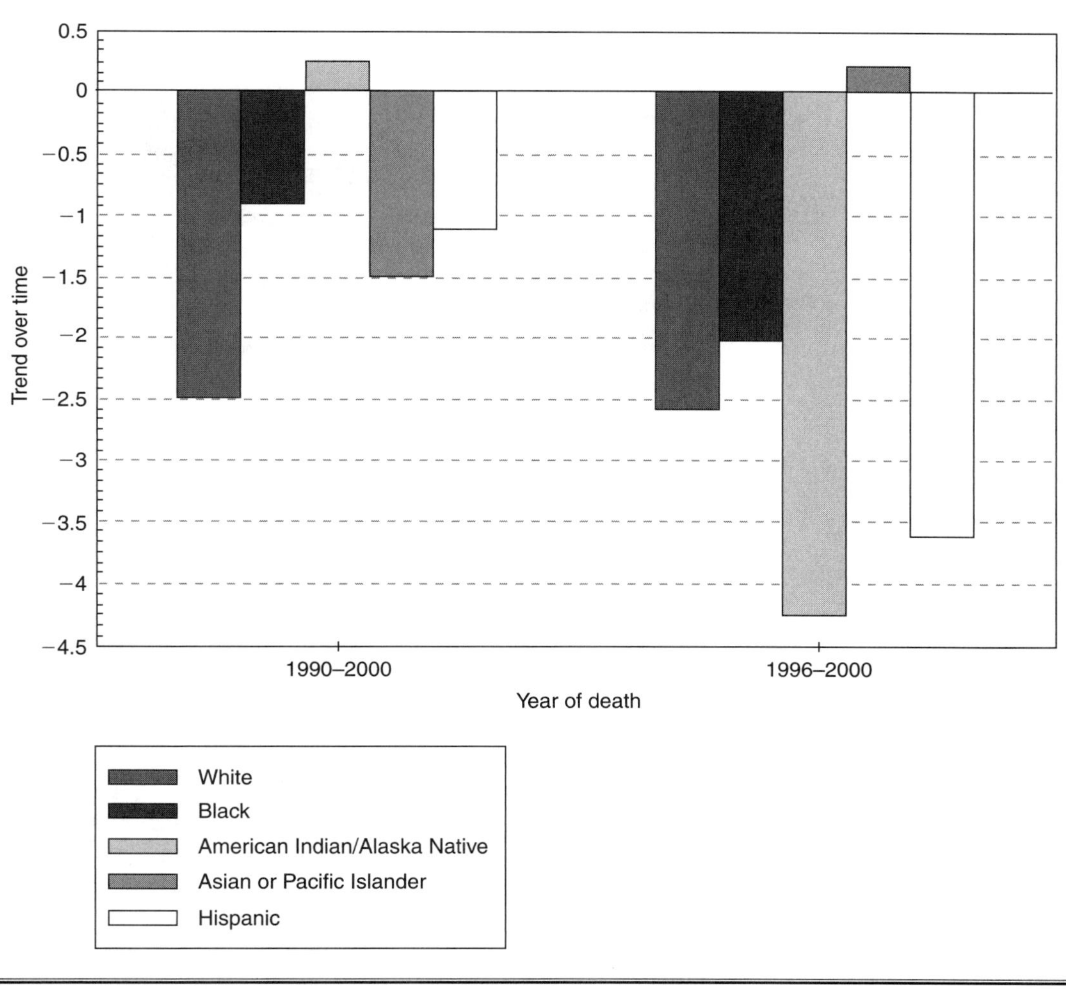

Source: Statistics are provided by the *SEER Program* for research purposes only. {(www.seer.cancer.gov) released, April 2004 #90}

---

ductive history, race/ethnicity, and other factors. Estimated lifetime risk of breast cancer has gone up gradually over the past several decades (**Figures 19-2** and **19-3**).

The etiology of breast cancer, while not well understood, is thought to result from a complex interaction between environment, genetic, and hormonal factors.[44] Other determinants include growth factors, dysfunction of cell growth, cell death (*apoptosis*), and tissue remodeling.[45] The cancer genes (called *oncogenes*) encode defective proteins that would otherwise serve in the normal regulation of these functions. Breast cancer is a progressive rather than a systemic disease,[46]

Figure 19-2 SEER Incidence—Age adjusted rates for white/black/other, 1973–2001.[42]

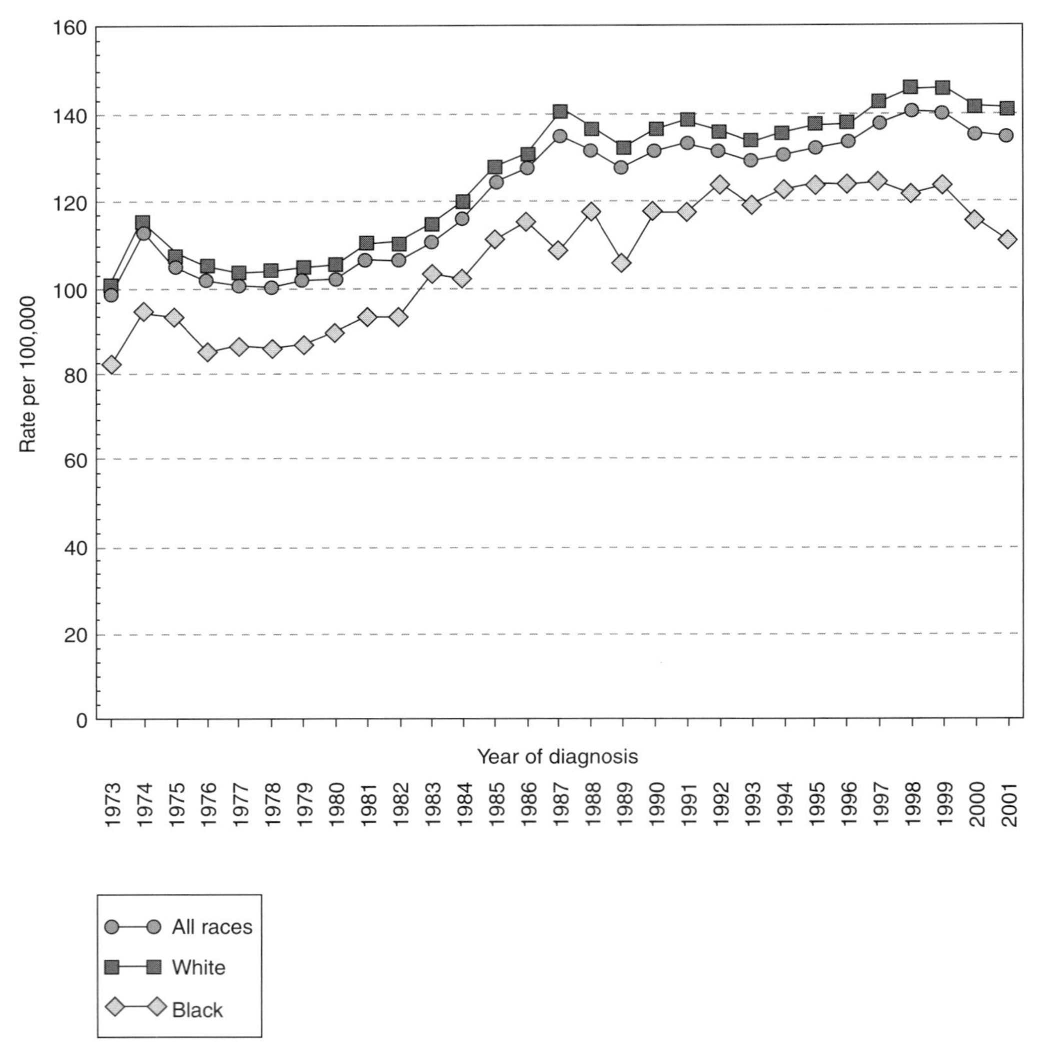

Notes: • Statistics were generated from malignant cases only.
  • Rates are expressed as cases per 100,000.
  • Statistics are provided by the *SEER Program* for research purposes only. {(www.seer.cancer.gov) released, April 2004 #90}

Figure 19-3 SEER incidence—crude rates for additional races/registries, 1992–2001.[42]

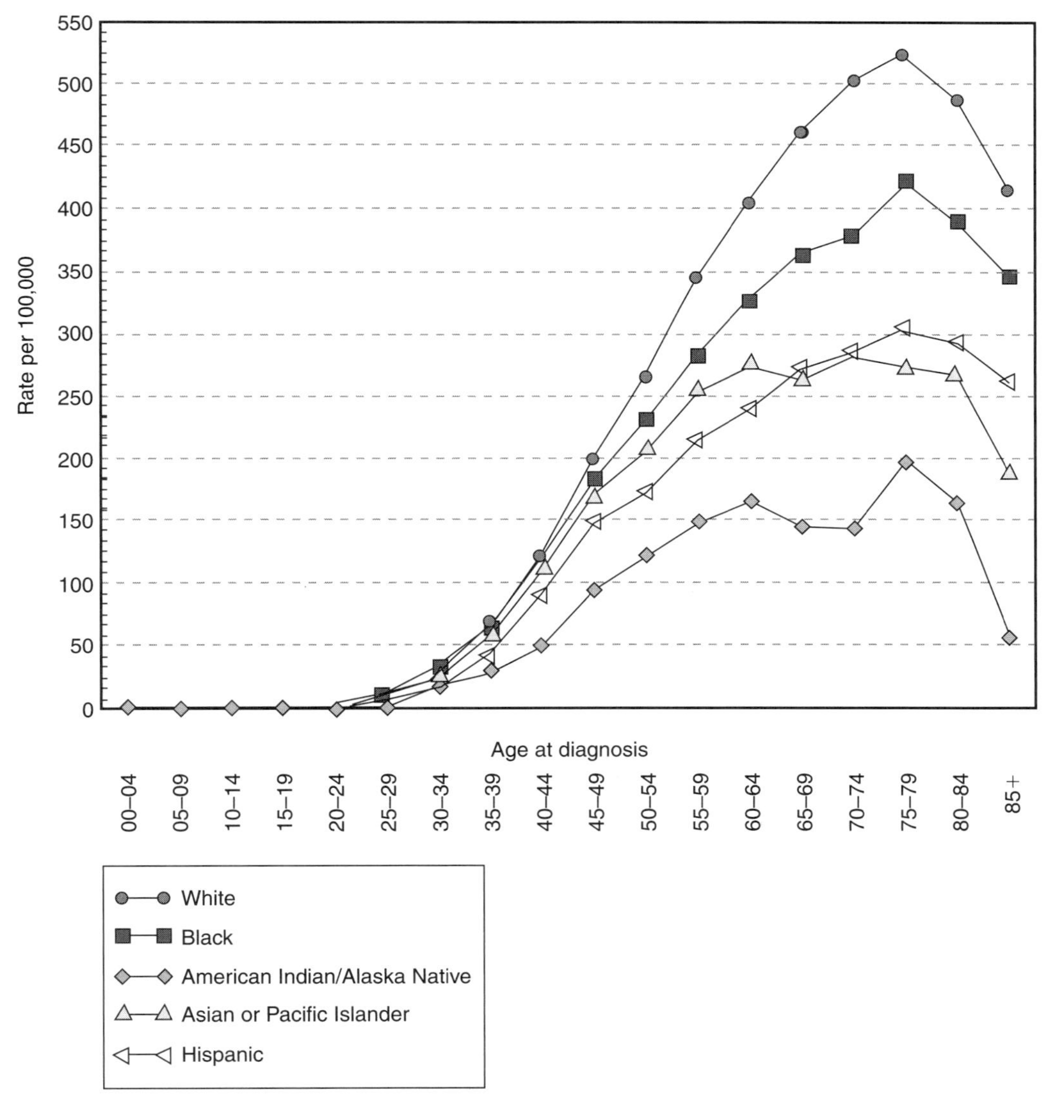

Notes: • Statistics were generated from malignant cases only.

• Rates are expressed as cases per 100,000.

• Statistics are provided by the *SEER Program* for research purposes only. {(www.seer.cancer.gov) released, April 2004 #90} meaning that most cancers grow from small size of low-grade histology and low metastatic potential to larger size and greater metastatic potential. Some of these events initiate tumor growth while others promote its growth.[47]

Breast Cancer Risks

Most women who develop breast cancer have no risk factors other than female gender and age. Some of the more commonly accepted factors include: first-degree relative with breast cancer; age at first live birth (earlier provides increased protection); age at menarche and menopause (earlier menarche increased risk, later menopause increased risk); number of breast biopsies; history of atypical hyperplasia; personal history of breast cancer; and incidence of ovarian and colon cancer. Ten percent of women who have breast cancer will develop a second primary cancer in their lifetime (**Table 19-5**).

When working in primary care, providers need tools to reliably estimate a woman's susceptibility to breast cancer in order to identify individuals at risk. Such risk assessment has potential implications for medical decision making; women might benefit from preventive measures or genetic counseling.[48] However, current risk assessment systems do not permit combining multiple risk factors or allow a calculation of a woman's lifetime probability of breast cancer. The Gail model is the most widely used and accepted tool for calculating risk of breast cancer.[49] Other statistical models include those by Claus et al.[50] and the BRCAPRO,[51] but none are comprehensive or could be used as a stand-alone tool. **Table 19-6** compares the advantages and disadvantages of each model. For women without a strong family history of breast cancer, the Gail model is usually the most helpful (National Cancer Institute Web site: http://bcra.nci.nih.gov/brc/). The genetic models by Claus et al. and the BRCAPRO are available on the Cancergene Web site (http://caroll.vjf.cnrs.fr/cancergene/HOME.html).

Non-Mass Type Breast Cancers Found on Physical Exam

Inflammatory breast cancer is an aggressive form with high rates of morbidity and mortality; it occurs most often in women between the ages of 50 and 55 years, and constitutes only 2% of all breast cancers.[52] The differential diagnosis of an inflamed breast includes: acute mastitis; abscess; tuberculosis (rare); duct ectasia; lymphoma; generalized dermatitis (insect bites, allergic reactions); and cancer. Women with mastitis often present with a localized painful lump and often have systemic symptoms including fever and leukocytosis.[52] Inflammatory cancer, on the other hand, is rarely associated with either fever or leukocytosis. Inflammatory cancer often involves at least one-third of the breast tissue and is not well demarcated, whereas duct ectasia is often well demarcated and affects less than one-

Table 19-5 BREAST CANCER RISK FACTORS

Female
Age
First-degree relative with breast cancer
Later age at birth of first child
Early menarche
Late menopause
Number of breast biopsies
History of atypical hyperplasia
History of fibroadenoma
Personal history of breast cancer
Personal history of ovarian or colon cancer

Table 19-6 STATISTICAL MODELS TO ASSESS INDIVIDUAL ABSOLUTE RISKS FOR BREAST CANCER

Gail Model[49]	Claus Model[50]	BRCAPRO Model[51]
First-degree relatives with diagnosis of breast cancer	First- and second-degree relatives diagnosed with breast cancer	Age-specific and cumulative breast and ovarian cancer incidence curves for *BRCA* gene mutation
Age at menarche	Ages of relatives at diagnosis	Age of first- and second-degree relatives with breast cancer
Age combined with number of breast biopsies	Whether inheritance pattern of breast cancer is present	Whether unilateral or bilateral breast cancer with age
Age at first live birth combined with number of first-degree relatives with breast cancer	Includes only genetic susceptibility, overlooks personal history of breast conditions	Relatives with ovarian cancer with age
Lifetime risk to age 90	Lifetime risk to age 79	Lifetime risk to age 85
Personal history of atypical hyperplasia		No calculation for births or a typical hyperplasia/lobular neoplasia
Overlooks bilateral disease		
Overlooks second-degree relatives		
Overlooks ovarian cancer in relatives		
Overlooks personal history of LCIS		
Age at diagnosis not considered		

third of the breast.[52] With inflammatory breast cancer, the patient often has pain, tenderness, and firmness in the breast with an increase in breast size. Within four weeks of onset of symptoms, the skin becomes warm, red, raised, hard, and painful. The typical peau d'orange appearance of the breast is sometimes evident.

Diagnosis and treatment must not be delayed in the case of inflammatory breast disease by providing prolonged use of antibiotics, thinking that the treatment is for mastitis. If the problem is not resolved with 10 days of antibiotic treatment, then a mammogram and ultrasound should be ordered, and a referral to a breast surgeon should be expedited.

Paget's disease is an erythematous scaling eruption involving the nipple that most often represents a cutaneous extension from an underlying carcinoma. Paget's disease of the nipple presents as unilateral erythema and scaling. Although usually not painful, it can be pruritic and can be exudative or ulcerative. Induration and infiltration may be present, and an underlying nodule may be palpated in later stages. Lymph node involvement occurs later and carries a poorer prognosis. Clinical outcomes for this cancer depend mainly on early referral by the midwife, which leads to early diagnosis and treatment.

Paget's disease of the breast is insidious and slow-growing. The peak ages of occurrence are between 50 and 60 years. Women will often present with erythema, mild eczematous-like scaling or flaking of the nipple skin that advances to crusting, skin erosion, and ulceration, with exudation or frank discharge. Some women experience tingling, pruritus, hypersensitivity, burning, or pain. Fu et al.[53] studied the symptoms of 41 patients diagnosed with Paget's; women presented with eczema (39%); bleeding (37%); ulcer (32%); and mass (22%). Women's symptoms lasted more than four months before definitive therapy began in 29.3% (12/41) of patients in this study. The diagnosis is made by biopsy, so a referral to a breast surgeon is indicated if the lesion does not respond to treatment for eczema or dermatitis. Paget's disease is most often associated with underlying DCIS and/or invasive ductal cancer. The prognosis of patients who have the disease is determined by the extent of the associated carcinoma.[53]

Treatment for Paget's disease is similar to surgical options for patients with invasive breast cancer. Women with Paget's disease confined to the nipple-areolar complex are now being considered as potential candidates for breast preservation. Physical examination and mammography are used in efforts to identify multicentric disease that would require mastectomy.

High-Risk Women

Between 5% and 10% of breast cancer involves aberrant genes. Women in such families have to face the question of whether to get genetic testing, and midwives can be a source of information. Only women at high risk are suitable for testing, including those with a high incidence of premenopausal breast cancer in their families. Most women who get tested have negative re-

sults. Seven percent of breast cancers are attributed to an autosomal pattern of inheritance of a genetic alteration in either the *BRCA1* or *BRCA2* gene.[54] Estimates for women with *BRCA1* or *BRCA2* gene mutation run a lifetime breast cancer risk of between 40% and 90%, depending on the population sampled and the risk factors involved. Women in a high-risk family also have an increased risk of ovarian cancer, colon cancer, and an increased chance of cancer in the contralateral breast. The primary care provider may refer a high-risk woman to a genetic counselor (costs range from $600–$2000). Some women choose not to be tested for fear that they will be denied insurance coverage in the future. At a minimum, however, every woman should be screened to identify those whose family history places them at higher risk and offered testing.

Close surveillance is the best defense, including more frequent breast exams (SBE monthly beginning at age 18–25; CBE annually or semi-annually beginning at age 18–25; mammogram annually beginning at age 25).[54] Some sources recommend that mammography should be ordered five years earlier than the diagnosis was made for the first-degree family member with breast cancer. Options for women in high-risk families include bilateral mastectomy, medications such as Tamoxifen, and early mammography (which may not be helpful because of dense breasts found in younger women).

Breast Cancer Screening and Controversies

The use of various screening modalities for breast cancer varies among different populations of women. Compliance is poor among women over the age of 60, women in lower socioeconomic groups, and in ethnic minority women. Access to care, in particular financial barriers, certainly contributes to this problem. Midwives should be aware that another significant factor affecting compliance is that too few providers recommend screening to their patients. (Several models mentioned above are used to predict the risk of breast cancer.)

Mammography

Mammogram screening has allowed breast cancer to be identified at earlier stages, which correlates positively with better cure rates and easier treatment management.[46] However, recent reviews have called into question the efficacy of mammograms. In a 2001 review of mammography screening trials, Olsen and Gotzsche[55] claimed that there was no survival benefit from mammography screening and that screening leads to more aggressive treatment. When this article was published, the media raised major concerns that screening was doing no good and may be doing harm.[55] Because breast cancer trials show a significant reduction in breast cancer mortality with the invitation to participate in screening, there has been little change in thinking about the benefit of mammography in the United States, the United Kingdom, The Netherlands, or Sweden.[56] While controversy endures, particularly regarding the cost-effectiveness of screening in certain age groups, the evidence that screening reduces deaths from breast cancer has grown and there is still a consensus for its use.[56] The U.S. Preventive Services Task Force (USPSTF) concluded in 2002 that mammography could be recommended as a Category B intervention on the grounds that the

quality of evidence was fair and the net gain was moderate.[15] According to the USPSTF, the reduction in mortality among women invited to be screened appeared to be 23%. Consequently, the task force recommends screening mammography, with or without CBE, every one to two years for women over the age of 40. It also concludes that the evidence is insufficient to recommend for or against routine clinical screening alone or for or against teaching or performing routine BSE.

Following these controversies, several expert panels concluded to re-evaluate the evidence. One in Sweden concluded that the advantageous effect of breast screening for breast cancer mortality persists after long-term follow-up.[57] The International Agency for Cancer Research met in 1992 with experts from 11 countries who assessed the quality of seven trials; they concluded that criticisms such as those raised by Gotzsche and Olsen were unsubstantiated. The working group concluded that trials have provided sufficient evidence of efficacy for mammograms between ages 50 and 69 but only limited evidence of reduction in mortality in women between the ages of 40 and 49.[58] The USPSTF looked at seven trials of women over the age of 50 and found that the odds ratio was 0.77 (95% CI, 0.67–0.89) for mortality.

For women in the youngest and oldest age groups, recommendations for mammogram screening should be personalized to take into account the woman's risk factors, because of the ongoing debate over the efficacy of screening. In the group of women between the ages of 40 and 49, the number needed to screen with mammography to prevent one death from breast cancer (after 14 years of observation) was

838 women.[15] In 2002, USPSTF looked at seven trials with women between the ages of 40 and 49 at entry. Two trials showed no benefit; five trials suggested a benefit (risk reduction 13%–43%), and one trial (the Gothenburg trial) showed a statistically significant risk reduction. The odds ratio as presented by the USPSTF overall was 0.83 (95% CI, 0.64–1.04).

There is only limited direct evidence of efficacy of mammographic screening for women age 65 and older. The USPSTF found only two trials that included women over the age of 65; they showed relative risk reductions among women between the ages of 65 and 74 to be 0.68 (95% CI, 0.51–0.89) and 0.79 (95% CI, 0.51–1.24) among women 70 to 74 years.[59] In a review of Swedish trials, the summary relative risk for women between 65 and 74 years of age was 0.78.[57]

Common convention in most parts of the United States includes participation in mammographic screening with the understanding that it can reduce breast cancer mortality. Table 19-1 shows the recommendations for screening. When quality assurance programs are in place, mammography is beneficial to women[56]; thus, midwives should encourage all women between the ages of 50 and 69 to have screening. After childbearing is finished, women from lower socioeconomic strata often do not seek out medical care for themselves. Outreach to women ages 50 and older should be included for midlife health care, including recommendations for screening mammograms.

Clinical Breast Exam

What are the contributions of CBE and SBE? While there have been no trials to look at CBE without mammography, the examination is commonly used either for screening in asymptomatic women or diagnosis when a woman presents with a problem such as pain or a mass. Because CBE is used to find cancer, there are legal reasons to performing it well. Failure to diagnose breast cancer is a leading reason for malpractice claims, and primary care providers do most of the CBEs for both screening and diagnosis.[60] CBE has not been standardized and techniques can differ widely. Furthermore, the sensitivity of CBE is far from perfect, and providers vary considerably in the prevalence of abnormalities they find on CBE. Barton et al.[60] reported that the sensitivity of CBE is approximately 54% and the specificity of the exam is about 94%. Duration of the exam may correlate with accuracy of lump detection.[60] A careful examination of an average size breast (B cup) should take three minutes per breast[60] whereas the average actual time spent was closer to 1.8 minutes.[61] The CBE should be performed in a systematic search pattern, with thoroughness, varying palpation pressure, and with three fingers, using the finger pads in a circular motion.

The accuracy of CBE varies according to the expertise of the person performing the exam and specific qualities of the breast(s) being examined. Practitioners with previous experience with an abnormal breast lump may be more accurate in their findings. Younger women have denser breasts that make it more difficult to discern an abnormal finding. Breasts of older women become more fatty, which makes the detection of an abnormality easier.[62] Clinical breast exam sensitivity is slightly lower in women with larger breasts. It is more difficult to distinguish a suspicious mass in women with fibrocystic changes.[22] Since disease prognosis generally follows cancer size at the time of diagnosis, it is important to find and act on small cancers (i.e., ≤2 cm).[60]

In menstruating women the physical exam is best done in the follicular phase of the menstrual cycle. In the pregnant or lactating woman, hormone levels continue to increase and the breast becomes increasingly firmer, larger, and often contains increased nodularity. If a breast lump is found in a cycling, lactating, or pregnant woman, a follow-up exam in two to four weeks is recommended for evaluation. If there is still a suspicious area, a referral to a breast surgeon is advised. Concurrently, an ultrasound and/or mammography may be ordered to allow the radiologist to make the decision about which test is more appropriate. Generally, however, mammograms are not usually ordered in women younger than 40 because of the increased density in breast tissue of younger women and also because of the increased density during pregnancy and lactation.

The importance of breast inspection as part of the CBE is unproven.[60] Whereas many authorities recommend inspection to look for nipple abnormalities, dimpling, and retraction of the skin with the woman in varying positions, in a series of 296 breast cancers found on examination, 96% were found on palpation, only 1% by retraction alone, and another 3% were visible nipple abnormalities.[63] This series did not report the women's position when the inspection yielded a positive result. It is best to use inspection while performing palpation when pressed for time.

Should CBE be done on women of all ages? No screening trial has examined the benefits of CBE alone (without accompanying mammography) compared to no screening, and in addition, design characteristics limit the generalizability of the studies that have examined CBE. Therefore, the USPSTF could not determine the benefits of using CBE alone as a screening tool or the incremental benefit of adding CBE to mammography. Therefore, the available data were judged to be insufficient to determine whether the potential benefits of routine CBE outweigh the potential harms. The USPSTF gave CBE a rating of I (insufficient evidence).[3] Currently, CBEs should be done for women with symptoms as well as for those who are at risk for breast cancer and for whom screening has been found to be effective (i.e., women over the age of 40).[60] Because breast cancer is a concern for providers and their clients, CBE is usually done routinely at an annual gynecology exam despite the lack of evidence. Spending the time to perform a complete exam may detect up to 50% of asymptomatic breast cancers.[60]

Self Breast Examination

Systematic SBE has been recommended for the past 70 years; however, studies report conflicting results. Rates of monthly SBE are low; one study showed that only 21% of American female physicians reported doing this exam.[64] A study of African-American women found that only 13% of the women in the study practiced monthly SBE during the 12-month period before enrollment.[65] While only some women will do SBE at regular intervals, the use of SBE may increase breast awareness and prompt women to come to care.[66] If women are conscious of changes in their breasts or notice a lump, it is likely that they will present in a timely fashion with these breast symptoms; palpation of a lump is the most common reason for presentation. Therefore, clinicians should think of SBE as an entry to care strategy.[67]

There are both false positive and false negative costs associated with SBE. However, many women might still opt for the potential costs associated with finding a lump on their own and the diagnostic evaluation that likely will follow. While it has been reported that SBE has not detectably improved survival,[68] other studies have reported a reduction in primary tumor size dependent on SBE.[69] Smaller tumor size at detection may improve outcomes because tumor size has been found to be inversely related to survival.

The USPSTF concludes that there is insufficient evidence to recommend for or against teaching or performing routine SBE, particularly because of design limitations of published and ongoing studies of SBE. They found poor evidence to determine whether SBE reduces breast cancer mortality and found fair evidence that SBE is associated with an increased risk for false-positive results and biopsies.

For providers who want to teach SBE, the prime opportunity to teach is during the CBE using the method described in the above section on physical exam. The MammaCare method, a standardized approach to teaching the detection of breast lumps using silicone breast models, is another way that women can learn breast exam. By practicing with the silicone models, women have the opportunity to find masses of different sizes and at various depths.[70,71] Several studies showed that the MammaCare Method doubled detection abilities in patients and medical and nursing students.[70,71] SBE frequency and proficiency may improve by participating in an education class.[65] However, some women may be reluctant to learn about SBE whether individually or in a group because of fears of exposing their bodies, or they may have suffered from past sexual abuse and are reluctant to be touched, particularly by clinicians.[65] Taylor and Jones[65] recommend that educational activities for BSE be developed that are culturally sensitive. Culturally sensitive SBE programs, which can foster behavior change in populations at risk, should present information in a way that decreases a woman's fears, using language and images that women are familiar with.

Missed Diagnosis

Breast cancer holds intense media attention. On the positive side, this has led to increased surveillance and detection, but it also has increased anxiety on the part of women regarding the disease and providers who may be fearful of missing significant breast disease. First and foremost, every midwife needs to know the standard of practice in the clinical setting and in the community in which she works. Second, every provider should always assume that the medical record will be read by another.

Screening for breast cancer is not synonymous with mammographic screening.[72] Despite the earlier discussion, the physical examination is likely to be considered the standard of care for clinical practice. Because most specialty boards recommend regular mammographic screening for women who are between the ages of 50 and 69, midwives should recommend it to all women in that age range. Although there is no consensus for women younger than 50 and older than 69 years, screening mammography can still serve as a risk management tool.

Delay in diagnosis is the leading cause of malpractice litigation.[72] Medical malpractice cases are governed by civil law, specifically tort law, the primary claim of which is negligence.[72] Reasons for lawsuits include: dissatisfaction with rapport (the hurried provider); lack of ability to administer care and treatment consistent with expectations; suspicion of cover-up; need for information;

desire to protect others; and inability to effectively communicate with the provider.[73,74] Lawsuits are likely to be the result of an adverse outcome, but the litigation is concerned not with outcome but with conduct of providers.[72]

Another important aspect of litigation is standard of care, which means care that is reasonable and prudent and that another provider would exercise under similar circumstances. The benchmark for conduct is "reasonableness." It is the duty of the clinician to obtain a reasonable history, perform a reasonable exam, and arrive at a reasonable management plan. The management plan should be developed with the patient, ensuring that she understands the goals and rationale. A patient should never be advised to "return as needed" because the midwife will be considered to have "superior knowledge" that a patient might not comprehend. Abandonment may be found if a clinical condition exists and appropriate transfer of care is not successfully completed.

The acronym FACT (<u>f</u>actual, <u>a</u>ccurate, <u>c</u>omplete, and <u>t</u>imely) should be used when charting about breast findings. The chart should be legible; each entry should include the time and date and be signed. The midwife should record all efforts to contact the patient and any follow-up that is done. Entries should include significant changes in condition for the better or worse. The patient's emotional response should be recorded if it is significant. Any contact made with other professionals about the breast condition should be recorded; this includes supervisory or consultative conversations. The woman should be informed of diagnostic and treatment risks and alternative therapies when appropriate. Document limiting factors (such as "patient declines mammogram, biopsy" "interview terminated prior to obtaining complete history;"

"patient distracted due to children in exam room with her—plan finish interview/exam in 1 hour/2 days.") Charting the characteristics of a breast mass may include such modifiers as "cystic or solid, solitary, discrete, firm/hard."

The main reasons for failure to diagnose or correctly manage a breast pathology include the following: no pathology is identified when pathology is present; pathology is misidentified; severity of problem not recognized; failure to advise patients of findings; improper reporting; failure to advise of limited scope of assessment; failure to advise of follow-up care needed; failure to advise of alternatives or appropriateness of requested care or evaluation; and failure to timely communicate assessments or recommendations.

The midwife as a primary care provider will be judged on the written record. Midwives carry major responsibility for recording the problem, getting the woman to the proper care, and providing appropriate communication with all of the team members—including the woman—throughout the entire process. Specific plans for follow-up should always be documented whether it be a return appointment in a certain time period, a consultation, or a referral. Postmenopausal women with any breast mass require a referral to a surgeon whenever a breast mass is identified.

Conclusion

Midwives and nurse practitioners, as primary care providers, have a major responsibility for breast health, screening, and referral. The evaluation of benign lesions and management of problems such as mastitis are well within the scope of practice. All at-risk women benefit from early detection and treatment of cancer, and midwives are ideally positioned to help women to access the best care. This requires being knowledgeable about the signs of disease, the best risk reduction strategies, the latest referral guidelines, and the best resources available in the community to maximize the best prognosis possible. Communication between health professionals is another important role that midwives can play. Communicating with women about clinical assessment, test results, associated risks, and management options is essential to the role and will serve to optimize the flow of care and follow-up evaluation, and to minimize error, confusion, and delay in the quality of care.

References

1. Marrow M, Wong S, Venta L. The evaluation of breast masses in women younger than forty years of age. *Surgery.* 1998;124:634.

2. Smith RA, Saslow D, Sawyer KA, Burke W, Costanza ME, Evans WPR, et al. American Cancer Society Breast Cancer Advisory Group. American Cancer Society guidelines for breast cancer screening: Update 2003. *CA Cancer J Clin.* 2003;53(3):141–169.

3. USPSTF. Screening for Breast Cancer: Recommendations and Rationale. February 2002. Agency for Healthcare Research and Quality, Rockville, MD. Available at: http://www.ahrq.gov/clinic/3rduspstf/breastcancer/brcanrr.htm.

4. National Cancer Institute (NCI). NCI Statement on Mammography Screening, February 21, 2002 update. Available on the Internet at: http://www.cancer.gov/newscenter/mammstatement31jan02.

5. Mandelblatt J, Saha S, Teutsch S, Hoerger T, Siu AL, Atkins D, et al. Cost Work Group of the U.S. Preventive Services Task Force. The cost-effectiveness of screening mammography beyond age 65 years: A systematic review for the U.S. Preventive Services Task Force. *Ann Intern Med.* 2003;139(10):835–842.

6. Pennypacker HS, Pilgrim CA. Achieving competence in clinical breast examination. *Nurse Pract Forum.* 1993;4(2):85–90.

7. Baines CJ, Miller AB, Bassett AA. Physical examination. Its role as a single screening modality in the Canadian National Breast Screening Study. *Cancer.* 1989;63(9):1816–1822.

8. Talele AC, Slanetz PJ, Edmister WB, Yeh ED, Kopans DB. The lactating breast: MRI findings and literature review. *Breast J.* 2003;9(3):237–240.

9. Swinford AE, Adler DD, Garver KA. Mammographic appearance of the breasts during pregnancy and lactation: False assumptions. *Acad Radiol.* 1998;5(7):467–472.

10. Brenin DR. Management of the palpable breast mass. In: Harris JR, Lippman ME, Morrow M, Osborne CK, editors. *Diseases of the Breast.* 3rd ed. Philadelphia: Lippincott Williams & Wilkins; 2004.

11. Klein P, Glaser E, Grogan L, Keane M, Lipkowitz S, Soballe P, et al. Biomarker assays in nipple aspirate fluid. *Breast J.* 2001;7(6):378–387.

12. Johnson TL, Kini SR. Cytologic and clinicopathologic features of abnormal nipple secretions: 225 cases. *Diagnostic Cytopathology.* 1991;7(1):17–22.

13. Zylstra S. Office management of benign breast disease. *Clin Obstet Gynecol.* 1999;42(2):234–248.

14. Warner E, Plewes DB, Hill KA, Causer PA, Zubovits JT, Jong RA, et al. Surveillance of BRCA1 and BRCA2 mutation carriers with magnetic resonance imaging, ultrasound, mammography, and clinical breast examination. *JAMA.* 2004;292(11):1317–1325.

15. Humphrey LL, Helfand M, Benjamin KS, Chan MS, Woolf SH. Breast cancer screening: A summary of the evidence for the U.S. Preventive Services Task Force. *Ann Intern Med.* 2002;137(5 (Part 1)):347–360.

16. Schnitt SJ, Connolly JL. Pathology of benign breast disorders. In: Harris JR, editor. *Diseases of the Breast.* 2nd ed. Philadelphia: Lippincott Williams & Wilkins; 2000.

17. Hertel BF, Zaloudek C, Kempson RL. Breast adenomas. *Cancer.* 1976;37(6):2891–2905.

18. Dupont WD, Page DL, Parl FF, Vnencak-Jones CL, Plummer WDJ, Rados MS, et al. Long-term risk of breast cancer in women with fibroadenoma. *N Engl J Med.* 1994;331(1):10–15.

19. Choudhury M, Singal MK. Lactating adenoma—cytomorphologic study with review of literature. *Can J Pathol Microbiol.* 2001;44(4):445–448.

20. Page DL, Rogers LW. Combined histologic and cytologic criteria for the diagnosis of mammary atypical ductal hyperplasia. *Hum Pathol.* 1992;23(10):1095–1097.

21. Page DL, Kidd TEJ, Dupont WD, Simpson JF, Rogers LW. Lobular neoplasia of the breast: Higher risk for subsequent invasive cancer predicted by more extensive disease. *Hum Pathol.* 1991;22(11):1232–1239.

22. Love SM, Gelman RS, Silen W. Sounding board. Fibrocystic "disease" of the breast—a nondisease. *N Engl J Med.* 1982;307(16):1010–1014.

23. Hughes LE, Mansel RE, Webster DJ. Aberrations of normal development and involution (ANDI): A new perspective on pathogenesis and nomenclature of benign breast disorders. *Lancet.* 1987;2(8571):1316–1319.

24. Sterns EE. The natural history of macroscopic cysts in the breast. *Surg Gynecol Obstet.* 1992;174:36–40.

25. Haagensen CD. *Diseases of the Breast.* 3rd ed. Philadelphia: WB Saunders; 1986.

26. Foster ME, Garrahan N, Williams S. Fibroadenoma of the breast: A clinical and pathological study. *J R Coll Surg Edinb.* 1988;33:16–19.

27. Cole-Beugler C, Soriano RZ, Kurtz AB, Goldberg BB. Fibroadenoma of the breast: Sonomammography correlated with pathology in 122 patients. *Am J Roentgenol.* 1983;140:369–375.

28. Haagensen CD. Chapter 12. *Diseases of the Breast.* 2nd ed. Philadelphia: WB Saunders; 1971. p. 191.

29. Wilkinson S, Anderson TJ, Rifkind E, Chetty U, Forrest AP. Fibroadenoma of the breast: A follow-up of conservative management. *British Journal of Surgery.* 1989;76(4):390–391.

30. Sainsbury JRC, Nicholson S, Needham GK, Wadehra A, Farndon FR. Natural history of the benign breast lump. *Br J Surg.* 1988;75:1080–1082.

31. Ramirez AJ, Jarrett SR, Hammed H, Smith P, Fentiman IS. Psychological adjustment of women with mastalgia. *Breast.* 1995;4:48.

32. Fentiman IS. Management of breast pain. In: Harris JR, Lippman ME, Morrow M, Osborne CK, editors. *Diseases of the Breast.* 3rd ed. Philadelphia: Lippincott Williams & Wilkins; 2004.

33. Colak T, Turgut I, Kanik A, Ogetman Z, Aydin S. Efficacy of topical nonsteroidal antiinflammatory drugs in mastalgia treatment. *JACS.* 2003;196(4):525–530.

34. Doberl A, Tobiassen T, Rasmussen T. Treatment of recurrent cyclical mastodynia in patients with fibrocystic breast disease. *Acta Obstet Gynecol Scand Suppl.* Supplement 1984;123:177–184.

35. Mansel RE, Wisbey JR, Hughes LE. Controlled trial of the antigonadotrophin danazol in painful nodular benign breast disease. *Lancet.* 1982;1:928–930.

36. Jonsson S, Pulkkinen MO. Mastitis today: Incidence, prevention and treatment. *Ann Chirurg Gynaecol Suppl.* 1994;208:84–87.

37. Inch S, Fisher C. Mastitis: Infection or inflammation? *Practitioner.* 1995;239(1553):472–476.

38. Love SM. *Dr. Susan Love's Breast Book.* 2nd ed. Reading, MA: Addison-Wesley; 1995.

39. Appling SE. Mastitis. *Lippincott's Prim Care Pract.* 1998;2(2):184–188.

40. Leis HPJ, Greene FL, Cammarata A, Hilfer SE. Nipple discharge: Surgical significance. *South Med J.* 1988;81(1):20–26.

41. Sainsbury JRC, Anderson TJ, Morgan DAL. ABC of breast diseases: Breast cancer. *BMJ.* 2000;321(7263):745–750.

42. National Cancer Institute. SEER Cancer Statistics Review. Incidence Breast Cancer. In: National Cancer Institute; 2004. At http://seer.cancer.gov accessed January 8, 2006.

43. National Cancer Institute. Surveillance, Epidemiology, and End Results Program, 1975–2000; at http://seer.cancer.gov accessed January 8, 2006.

44. Russo J, Russo IH. Development of the human mammary gland. In: Neville M and Daniel CW, editors. *Mammary Gland Development Regulation and Function.* New York: Plenum Press; 1987. pp. 67–93.

45. Dickson RB, Russo J. Biochemical control of breast development. In: Harris JR, editor. *Diseases of the Breast.* 3rd ed. Philadelphia: Lippincott Williams & Wilkins; 2004.

46. Tabar L, Duffy S, Vitak B, Chen H, Prevost TC. The natural history of breast carcinoma. What have we learned from screening? *Cancer.* 1999;86(3):449–462.

47. Benson J, Baum M. Breast cancer, desmoid tumours, and familial adenomatous polyposis—a unifying hypothesis. *Lancet.* 1993;342(8875):848–850.

48. Claus EB. Risk models used to counsel women for breast and ovarian cancer: A guide for clinicians. *Fam Cancer.* 2001;1(3-4):197–206.

49. Gail MH, Brinton LA, Byar DP, Corle DK, Green SB, Schairer C, et al. Projecting individualized probabilities of developing breast cancer for white females who are being examined annually. *JNCI.* 1989;81(24):1879–1886.

50. Claus EB, Risch NJ, Thompson WD. Age at onset as an indicator of familial risk of breast cancer. *Am J Epidemiol.* 1990;131(6):961–972.

51. Berry DA, Parmigiani G, Sanchez J, Schildkraut J, Winer E. Probability of carrying a mutation of breast-

ovarian cancer gene BRCA1 based on family history. *JNCI*. 1997;89(3):227–238.

52. Dahlbeck SW, Donnelly JF, Theriault RL. Differentiating inflammatory breast cancer from acute mastitis. *Am Fam Phys*. 1995;52(3):929–934.

53. Fu W, Mittel VK, Young SC. Paget disease of the breast: Analysis of 41 patients. *Am J Clin Oncol*. 2001; 24(4):397–400.

54. de Carvalho M, Jenkins J, Nehrebecky M, Lah lLT. The role of estrogens in BRCA1/2 mutation carriers: Reflections on the past, issues for the future. *Cancer Nurs*. 2003;26(6):421–430.

55. Olsen O, Gotzsche PC. Cochrane review on screening for breast cancer with mammography. *Lancet*. 2001; 358(9290):1340–1342.

56. Boyle P. Mammographic breast cancer screening: After the dust has settled. *Breast*. 2003;12(6):349–356.

57. Nystrom L, Andersson I, Bjurstam N, Frisell J, Nordenskjold B, Rutqvist LE. Long-term effects of mammography screening: Updated overview of the Swedish randomised trials. *Lancet*. 2002;359(9310): 909–919.

58. International Agency for Research on Cancer (IARC) Working Group (WG). Mammographic Screening: World Health Organization; 3/19/2002. Press release. Contact www@iarc.fr for press releases issued prior to 1998.

59. Andersson I, Aspegren K, Janzon L, Landberg T, Lindholm K, Linell F, et al. Mammographic screening and mortality from breast cancer: The Malmo mammographic screening trial. *BMJ*. 1988;297(6654): 943–948.

60. Barton MB, Harris R, Fletcher SW. The rational clinical examination. Does this patient have breast cancer? The screening clinical breast examination: Should it be done? How? *JAMA*. 1999;282(13):1270–1280.

61. Kahn KL, Goldberg RJ. Screening for breast cancer in the ambulatory setting [abstract]. *Clin Res*. 1984. p. 649A.

62. Stomper PC, D'Souza DJ, DiNitto PA, Arredondo MA. Analysis of parenchymal density on mammograms in 1353 women 25–79 years old. *Am J Roentgenol*. 1996;167(5):1261–1265.

63. Mahoney L, Csima A. Efficiency of palpation in clinical detection of breast cancer. *CMAJ*. 1982;127(8): 729–730.

64. Frank E, Rimer BK, Brogan D, Elon L. U.S. Women physicians' personal and clinical breast cancer screening practices. *J Women's Health Gender Based Med*. 2000;9(7):791–801.

65. Taylor G, Jones A. Effects of a culturally sensitive breast self-examination intervention. *Outcomes Manag*. 2002;6(2):73–78.

66. Austoker J. Breast self examination [editorial]. *BMJ*. 2003;326(7379):1–2.

67. Epstein RJ. Breast self examination. Breast self examination provides entry strategy [letter]. *BMJ*. 2003;326(7391):710–711.

68. Thomas DB, Gao DL, Ray RM, Wang WW, Allison CJ, Chen FL, et al. Randomized trial of breast self-examination in Shanghai: Final results. *JNCI*. 2002; 94(19):1445–1457.

69. Koibuchi Y, Iino Y, Takei H, Maemura M, Horiguchi J, Yokoe T, et al. The effect of mass screening by physical examination combined with regular breast self-examination on clinical stage and course of Japanese women with breast cancer. *Oncol Rep*. 1998;5: 151–155.

70. Campbell HS, Fletcher SW, Pilgrim CA, Morgan TM, Lin S. Improving physicians' and nurses' clinical breast examination: A randomized controlled trial. *Am J Prevent Med*. 1991;7(1):1–8.

71. Fletcher SW, O'Malley MS, Earp JL, Morgan TM, Lin S, Degnan D. How best to teach women breast self-examination. A randomized controlled trial. *Ann Intern Med*. 1990;112(10):772–779.

72. Brenner RJ. Breast cancer evaluation: Medical legal issues. *Breast J*. 2004;10(1):6–9.

73. Hickson GB, Clayton EW, Githens PB, Sloan FA. Factors that prompted families to file medical malpractice claims following perinatal injuries. *JAMA*. 1992;267(10):1359–1363.

74. Hickson GB, Federspiel CF, Pichert JW, Miller CS, Gauld-Jaeger J, Bost P. Patient complaints and malpractice risk. *JAMA*. 2002;287(22):2951–2957.

Chapter 20

Cervical and Ovarian Cancer Screening

Molly Fey Persinger
Margaret W. Beal

Cancer is estimated to be the cause of one out of every four American deaths, second only to heart disease. For women in the United States of all races, breast cancer is the leading malignancy, followed by lung and colorectal cancers (**Figure 20-1**).[1,2] Genital tract cancers account for nearly 13% of invasive cancers in women. Of these, approximately 13% to 17% are cervical malignancies and 29% to 30% are ovarian malignancies.[1] Regular screening is crucial to prevent or detect the early stage of many cancers, including those of the cervix and ovaries.

Cervical Cancer Screening

In the United States, more than 12,000 cases of cervical cancer are diagnosed annually, and approximately 4000 women die from the disease.[3] Invasive cervical cancer was once a leading cause of cancer death in the United States but is now relatively uncommon (**Figure 20-2**). Over the past 50 years, the incidence of cervical cancer in the United States has declined to approximately eight cases per 100,000 women.[4] This decrease is attributable to implementation of nationwide cervical cytology screening programs.[5] In developed countries, the incidence of and mortality from cervical cancer have declined more than 70% since the introduction of Papanicolaou (Pap) testing as a widespread screening approach in the 1950s. Cervical cancer is still a leading cause of cancer death in women in many developing countries due to the lack of screening programs. Eighty percent of cervical cancer deaths occur in underdeveloped nations.

Cervical cancer incidence and mortality increase with age and are rare among women under 30 (**Figures 20-3** and **20-4**). Mortality is 40% higher in African-American women younger than 65 when compared to white women of the same age. Despite an overall decline in incidence secondary to screening programs, African-American women still have 72% greater incidence of cervical cancer and 13% lower survival rate when compared to Caucasians, largely because of socioeconomic factors influencing access to and utilization of health care services.[5,6]

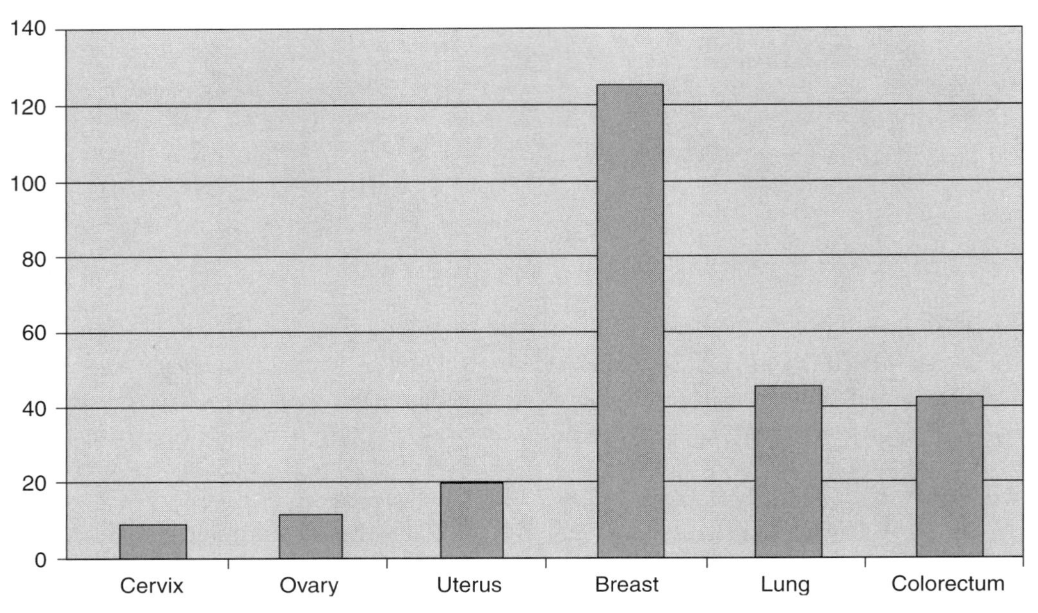

Figure 20-1 Cancer incidence per 100,000 American women, 1998–2000.

Source: Surveillance, Epidemiology, and End Results (SEER) Program (www.seer.cancer.gov). SEER*Stat Databases: Incidence—SEER 13 Regs Public-Use, Nov 2004 Sub for Expanded Races (1992–2002) and Incidence - SEER 13 Regs excluding AK Public-Use, Nov 2004 Sub for Hispanics (1992–2002), National Cancer Institute, DCCPS, Surveillance Research Program, Cancer Statistics Branch, released April 2005, based on the November 2004 submission.

Signs and Symptoms

Early cervical cancer produces no signs or symptoms, and early lesions are rarely visible to the naked eye. Abnormal vaginal bleeding and discharge are the most common presenting complaints of advanced disease. Symptoms include postcoital bleeding and bloody discharge between periods or after menopause. The discharge may be watery, heavy, or have a foul odor. As the cancer progresses, the cervix may appear red, friable, ulcerated, or enlarged. Symptoms resulting from impingement of the surrounding anatomic structures occur as the tumor grows larger. More often, cervical cancer is diagnosed by screening methods prior to onset of clinical symptoms.

Human Papillomavirus Infection

Cervical cancer is caused by the sexually transmitted human papillomavirus (HPV), a non-enveloped, double-stranded DNA virus. Over 100 types of HPV have been identified, and those that infect the anogenital tract have been divided into two groups based on the associated level of risk for cervical cancer (**Table 20-1**).[4,7] Low-risk viral strains are associated with condyloma (genital warts) and low-grade cervical lesions that usually spontaneously regress. These strains are of low or no oncogenic risk, and the resulting lesions rarely progress to cancer. High-risk HPV strains have the highest oncogenic potential. HPV 16 and

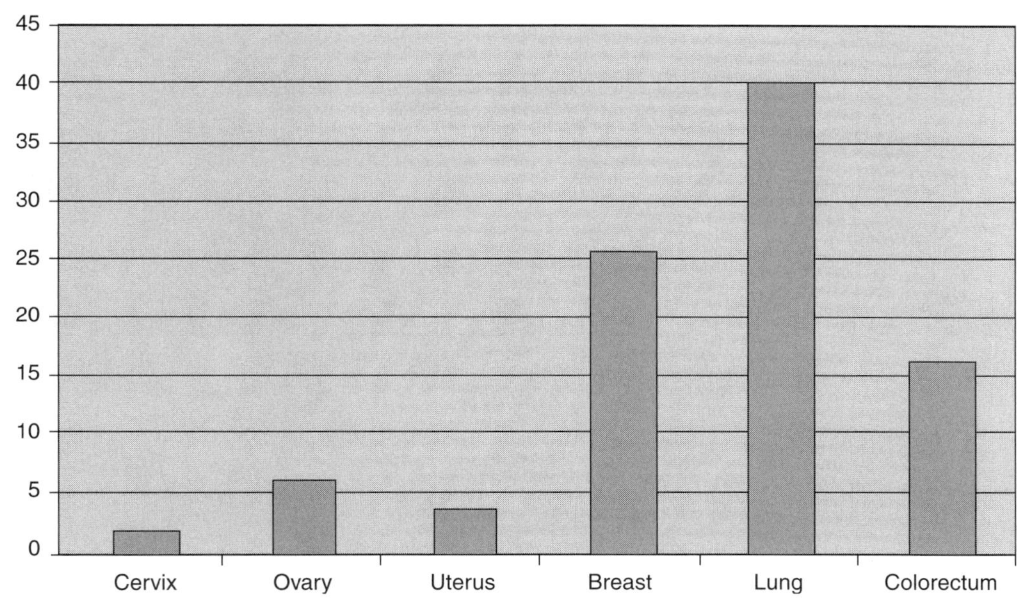

Figure 20-2 Cancer mortality per 100,000 American women, 1998–2000.

Source: Surveillance, Epidemiology, and End Results (SEER) Program (www.seer.cancer.gov) SEER*Stat Database: Mortality—All COD, Public-Use with State, Total U.S. (1969–2002), National Cancer Institute, DCCPS, Surveillance Research Program, Cancer Statistics Branch, released April 2005. Underlying mortality data provided by NCHS (www.cdc.gov/nchs).

18 are the most prevalent high-risk strains worldwide, with HPV 16 accounting for more than 50% of high-risk infections.[4,7,8] HPV causes cervical cancer by incorporating itself into the host cell genome, then activating oncogenes and suppressing immune response. HPV protein products impede host cell DNA repair and programmed cell death, leading to instability and unchecked cell growth.

HPV is spread by skin-to-skin contact. Condoms reduce but do not eliminate the risk of transmission because only a portion of the genitals is covered, and infection may occur via contact with or without intercourse.[9] While limited data exist to confirm avenues of HPV transmission, initial studies suggest that infection also occurs from hand-genital contact, oral sex, and genital contact with infected objects such as sex toys. As a result, women who have sex with women are equally at risk for infection with HPV and need to be adequately screened for cervical cancer. Nonsexual human to human transmission has also been postulated.[10–13]

NATURAL HISTORY OF HPV INFECTION

HPV is the most common sexually transmitted disease worldwide, yet only a small number of women with HPV will go on to develop cervical cancer (**Figure 20-5**). Eighty percent of high-risk HPV infections are transient, asymptomatic, and are cleared from the cervix without treatment. As a result, most carriers are unknowingly infected and unaware that they may pass the virus to others.[14]

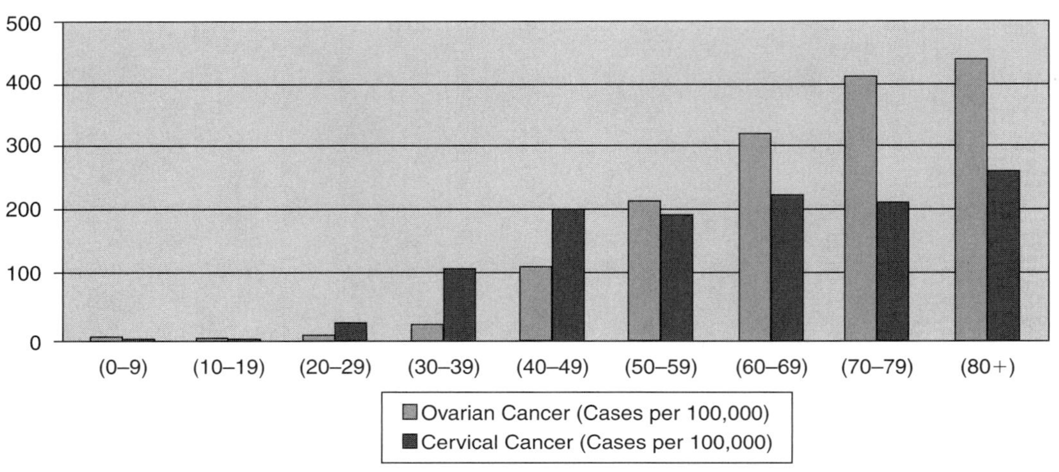

Figure 20-3 Incidence of cervical and ovarian cancers by age.[2]

Most high-risk HPV infections lead only to minor cervical lesions and low-grade dysplasia, and then spontaneously clear. However, persistent high-risk HPV infection is the key etiologic factor leading to high-grade dysplasia and then cervical cancer. For HPV that persists, ultimately causing advanced lesions, the average time from initial infection to invasive cervical cancer is 15 years.[15]

The regression of HPV-related irregularities and local clearance of HPV from the cervix are mediated by host immunologic factors and oncogenic risk potential of the viral strain. The more advanced the lesion, the less likely it is to spontaneously resolve. Only 15% to 25% of low-grade cervical dysplasia will advance to high-grade severity. Median duration of detectable HPV in the cervix ranges from 6 to 14 months. Patient age is also a key factor influencing persistent HPV infection, yet the nature of this correlation is not well understood. In adolescents, HPV is most often temporary and regressive. In older women, infection is more likely to persist, perhaps mediated by hormonal or immune changes that occur with age.[14,16,17]

Systemic response to genital HPV infection is under intense study. Preliminary evidence indicates that many women clear HPV from the cervix with only local immune response. In such cases, there is no systemic antibody response or recognition of the virus. Other women mount a systemic antibody response and acquire protective immunity to specific HPV strains. Further research is needed to understand the mechanisms of lesion regression and HPV clearance.[18,19]

HPV PREVALENCE AND RISK FACTORS

Lifetime risk of HPV infection is estimated to be as high as 80% in sexually active individu-

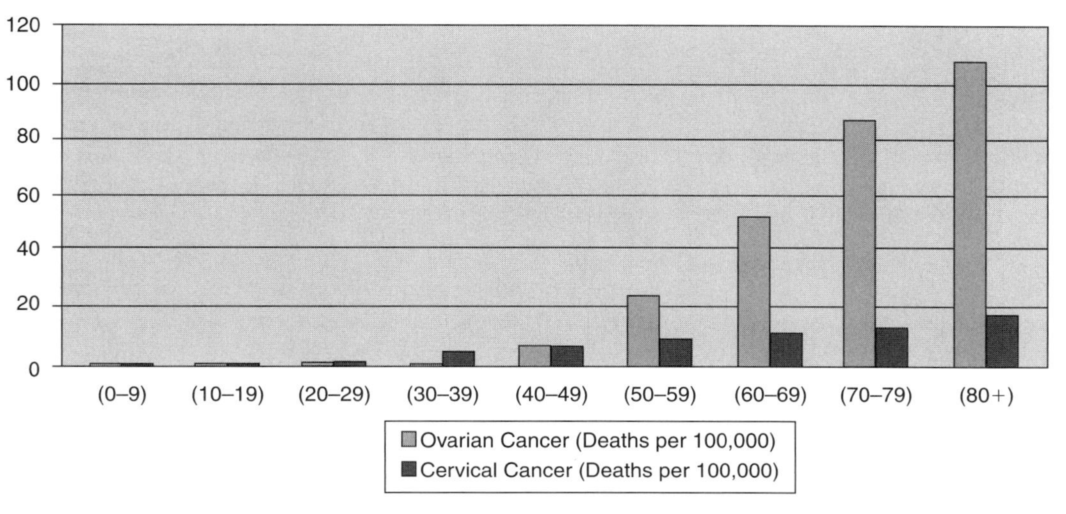

Figure 20-4 Age at death due to cervical and ovarian cancers.[2]

als. Five and half million Americans become infected annually.[20] The most significant risk factor associated with HPV infection is the total number of lifetime sexual partners. Earlier age at onset of sexual activity is also a factor. This risk is further augmented by the following: an increase in the total number of sexual partners in the last six months; history of sexually transmitted infections; alcohol and drug use related to sexual behaviors; and an increase in the number of partner's sexual partners.[21]

HPV is most prevalent in young women. It is highest, nearing 50%, among women age 20- to 24-years-old, followed closely by the 15- to 19-year-old age group. Prevalence decreases beginning at age 24, dropping sharply in women over 30. This drop may be explained by a decrease in the number of sexual partners and thus decreased risk of exposure to HPV, or by age-related maturation of the cervix as ectopy decreases and the vulnerable transformation zone regresses.[7,16]

Cofactors for Cervical Cancer Risk

Persistent high-risk HPV infection is the major cause of cervical cancer, yet many women are infected for years with minimal sequelae. Only a small minority develop rapidly progressive cervical dysplasia, suggesting that the malignant transformation is modulated by additional cofactors that contribute to cervical cancer risk (**Table 20-2**).

SMOKING

Active and passive tobacco smoke exposure increases cervical cancer risk up to twice that of non-smokers. The mechanism by which this exposure influences cervical cancer has yet to be clearly defined. Nicotine metabolites are found in the cervical mucus of women who smoke and probably play a direct role. Indirect effects of tobacco-induced antioxidant depletion or immunosuppression are also under investigation.[4,22]

Table 20-1 HUMAN PAPILLOMAVIRUS (HPV) STRAINS AND ASSOCIATED LEVEL OF CERVICAL CANCER RISK[4,7,8]

Classification	Viral Strains	Associated Risk
High-risk HPV	16, 18, 31, 33, 35, 39, 45, 51, 52, 56, 58, 59, 68	Confers highest risk for high-grade cervical lesions and progression to cervical cancer.
Low-risk HPV	6, 11, 42, 43, 44	Confers low to no oncogenic risk and is associated with condyloma/genital warts.

PARITY

High parity is also associated with an increased risk for cervical cancer. A direct relationship exists between the number of full-term pregnancies and increased risk of cervical malignancy. Women with seven or more full-term pregnancies have three- to sixfold increased risk when compared to nulliparous women who are also infected with high-risk HPV. It is hypothesized that the increased ectopy found in parous women facilitates

Figure 20-5 Natural history of HPV infection.

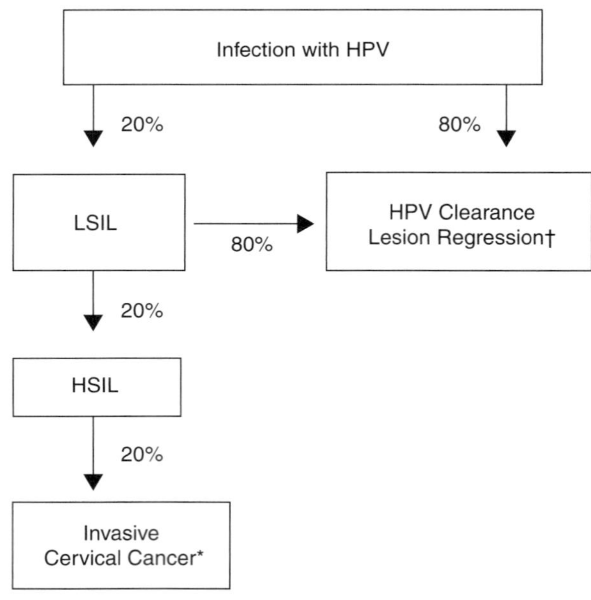

*The average time from infection to invasive cervical cancer is 15 years.
†HPV clearance is mediated by the woman's immune status and infection cofactors.
Source: Reprinted with permission from The American College of Nurse-Midwives.[3]

Table 20-2 RISK FACTORS FOR CERVICAL CANCER[16–24]

Primary

Persistent infection with high-risk HPV

Cofactors

Cigarette smoking
High parity (>7)
Immunocompromise
Vitamin and nutrient deficiency

the malignant progression induced by HPV. Parity does not influence risk of initial acquisition of HPV infection or duration of HPV infection.[23]

ORAL CONTRACEPTION

The effects of oral contraceptive pill use on cervical cancer risk are controversial. The preliminary evidence is inconsistent but indicates possible increased risk, particularly with oral contraceptive pill use for longer than five years. Risk for cervical cancer is more strongly associated with duration of use than age at first use. Like parity, the neoplastic progression caused by HPV may be enhanced by oral contraceptive pills, while risk for initial infection or persistence is unchanged.[24,25] Current research does not warrant discontinuing oral contraceptive pills in the case of an abnormal Pap test or HPV infection. The newer combined hormonal contraceptives (i.e., the patch and vaginal ring) may carry similar risks, although they have not been accessible long enough for data to be available.

NUTRIENT DEFICIENCY

Evidence exists that a diet high in vitamins A, B_6, B_{12}, C, and E may reduce the risk for cervical cancer. Increased dietary intake of folate and beta carotene may also decrease HPV persistence or lesion progression. The extent and nature of nutrient effects, whether they are independent of other cofactors for cervical cancer, and benefits of supplementation have yet to be determined.[26,27]

IMMUNOSUPPRESSION

Compromised immune status contributes significantly to cervical cancer risk and is associated with greater risk for rapidly advancing neoplastic changes due to persistent HPV infection. Women with human immunodeficiency virus are four times more likely to be infected with HPV, and even those with a relatively intact immune function based on CD4 lymphocyte count are at greater risk than uninfected women for development of cervical dysplasia. Incidence and severity of preneoplastic cervical lesions increase with progressive immune compromise.[28–31]

Screening Techniques

The Pap smear is the mainstay of cervical cancer screening and has resulted in greater success than any other screening approach for malignancy. A direct relationship exists between the proportion of a population screened and the resulting decline in incidence and mortality attributable to cervical cancer.[6]

A Pap test entails the removal of a sample of epithelial cells from the cervix. The *transformation zone*, or *squamocolumnar junction*, of the cervix is the most vulnerable to neoplastic changes and formation of abnormal lesions. Screening is directed at obtaining a sample of cells from this dynamic area where endocervical and ectocervical cells meet. The os of the cervix must be visible in order to obtain an accurate cytologic specimen. Historically, Pap test samples have been obtained using both a spatula for the exocervix and a cotton applicator or cytobrush for the endocervix. Newer liquid-based tests require the use of a cervical broom. Cells should be collected prior to testing for sexually transmitted infections or performing the bimanual exam.

In premenopausal women, mid-cycle is the ideal time to perform Pap testing, because estrogen levels are highest. Thus, the epithelial cells of the cervix are most mature and easiest to examine microscopically. Ideally, women should be advised not to douche, use vaginal creams, tampons, or have intercourse for 24 to 48 hours prior to the Pap test. While these factors or bleeding may detract from ideal testing conditions, they are not a contraindication to screening. Sampling is not advised during menses because red blood cells may obscure the epithelial cell sample.

Screening Inefficiencies

The traditional Pap smear is performed by manual transfer of sampled cervical cells to a glass slide. Fixative spray must be applied within seconds to avoid air drying of the cells. The slide is then sent to a laboratory for microscopic examination. Despite the huge success of cervical cancer screening with Pap testing, cervical cancer has not been eradicated, and the rate of reduction has reached a plateau. About half of all cervical cancers occur in women who were adequately screened. Research suggests that Pap screening is unlikely to prevent more than 60% of cervical cancers in any given population.[32]

Several factors account for these inefficiencies. Sensitivity for detection of cytologic abnormalities is reduced by interpretation errors made by laboratory technicians. Slide analysis is a subjective process that is poorly reproducible even among expert technicians. Sensitivity of traditional Pap testing decreases further with inadequate sampling and errors in slide preparation. In 5% to 10% of conventional Pap tests, fewer than 20% of cells sampled are successfully transferred to the slide.[6,33] The rate of false negative results for a single conventional slide Pap is estimated at 25% to 50%, thus emphasizing the need for serial testing to adequately detect those women who are at risk.[34]

Decreased specificity is also a concern with traditional Pap screening. Misclassification of abnormal slides is common, and false positive rates reach as high as 15%.[33] Equivocal and mildly irregular slides have a low yield for underlying high-grade cancer precursor lesions, which results in great costs for referral and follow-up. As a result of these inadequacies, several new technologies have been developed to improve the sensitivity and specificity of Pap testing.

Pap Test Technology

The liquid-based or thin-layer Pap test technique was developed to improve slide quality in cervical screening. In this method, cells are transferred to a liquid preservative instead of a slide. After cervical sampling, the spatula and brush are swished vigorously in a small amount of liquid preservative to obtain as many cells as possible, transferring them from the collection device to the media.

The liquid is spun through a microfilter at the lab, removing excess cells from blood, mucus, and vaginal secretions contaminating the sample. The slide is mechanically plated and fixed. This process allows a greater number of cervical epithelial cells to be transferred to the slide for interpretation, and production of a clearer slide for interpretation.

When compared to conventional slide preparation, liquid-based cytology is more sensitive but less specific than traditional Pap smear sampling for the detection of cervical cancer precursors, particularly in populations with higher disease prevalence.[35] Liquid-based cytology is also more costly, although residual liquid samples can be tested for sexually transmitted infections such as HPV, chlamydia, and gonorrhea. Neither test is currently recommended over the other. The gains and drawbacks of liquid-based cytology versus conventional testing must be weighed individually for each practice setting.

Computer-assisted slide interpretation is another technique used to improve Pap test screening. A high-speed camera scans Pap slides and a computer interprets the slide images, indicating to cytologists those slides that are normal and those that contain irregularities requiring human review. Approximately 25% of all slides are deemed normal, thus reducing manual screening loads by one quarter. Long-term costs and benefits of automated slide scanning and liquid-based cytology have yet to be determined.[3,6,35,36]

TESTING FOR HIGH-RISK HPV

The role of HPV testing in screening and prevention has been under intense study following confirmation of the etiologic link between high-risk HPV infection and cervical cancer. Samples are obtained via reflex testing of residual cell suspension leftover from a liquid-based Pap sample, or by direct collection with a cytobrush or spatula. A modified enzyme-linked immunosuppression assay with non-radioactive RNA probes is used to identify the presence or absence of 13 strains of high-risk HPV. One drawback of the test is that it does not test for individual viral strains. A positive or negative result is given based on the finding of any one or more high-risk HPV strains.[32,37,38] Low-risk HPV strains may be still present in the case of a negative test result.

SCREENING GUIDELINES

No consensus exists among different authoritative bodies, but several well recognized groups have published recommendations on the onset, duration, and frequency of Pap testing (**Table 20-3**). The objective of screening is to detect severe cervical dysplasia or high-grade squamous intraepithelial lesions (HSIL), which is an indicator of persistent, nontransient, high-risk HPV infection and an identified precursor lesion of cervical cancer.

Initiation of Screening Cervical cancer screening is unlikely to be beneficial prior to onset of sexual activity and thus, any potential exposure to HPV. As a result, most U.S. organizations, including the American Cancer Society (ACS), the American College of Obstetricians and Gynecologists (ACOG), and the U.S. Preventive Services Task Force (USPSTF), recommend starting Pap test screening within three years of initiation of sexual activity and no later than the age of 21 (**Table 20-4**). Nondisclosure in women's reporting of sexual activity, the high prevalence of sexual activity by age 21, and concern that providers may fail to take a sexual history have prompted these and other groups to include the additional age-based criterion for screening. The window of three years after first intercourse is provided based on current knowledge of the natural history of HPV. Evidence suggests there is very low risk of missing a clinically significant cervical lesion due to persistent HPV until three to five years after initial exposure to the virus.[39–41,44]

Frequency of Screening: Women under 30 For women under 30, the ACS recommends annual Pap screening by conventional cervical smear or biannual screening using liquid-based cytology. ACOG recommends annual screening regardless of testing methods. The USPSTF supports

Table 20-3 PUBLISHED GUIDELINES FOR CERVICAL CANCER SCREENING, FOLLOW-UP, AND TREATMENT

Organization and Title	Publication Year
American Cancer Society (Saslow et al.)[39]	2002
Guideline for the Early Detection of Cervical Neoplasia and Cancer	
United States Preventive Services Task Force[40]	2003
Recommendations and Rationale, Screening for Cervical Cancer	
American College of Obstetricians and Gynecologists[41]	2003
Clincial Management Guidelines for Obstetrician Gynecologists: Cervical Cytology Screening	
The 2001 Bethesda Workshop, National Cancer Institute (Solomon et al.)[42]	2002
The 2001 Bethesda System: Terminology for Reporting Results of Cervical Cytology	
The American Society for Colposcopy and Cervical Pathology Consensus Conference (Wright et al.)[43]	2002
2001 Consensus Guidelines for the Management of Women with Cervical Cytological Abnormalities	
The American Society for Colposcopy and Cervical Pathology Consensus Conference (Wright et al.)[29]	2003
2001 Consensus Guidelines for the Management of Women with Cervical Intraepithelial Neoplasia	

recommendations of most U.S. organizations to screen annually based on the known low sensitivity of Pap testing (60%–80%) to detect high-grade cervical lesions, but reports no direct evidence supporting optimal screening intervals or improved outcomes for screening more frequently than every three years.[39–41,44]

Frequency of Screening: Women over 30 For women over 30 who have had at least three consecutive negative and satisfactory cytology results, a majority of U.S. organizations recommend a prolonged screening interval of every two to three years.[39–41,44] Women over 30 have a lower likelihood than younger women of acquiring high-risk HPV infection of the cervix, possibly due to decreased cervical ectopy. Ad-

ditionally, the rate of disease progression is slow, and high-grade dysplasia is unlikely to develop in less than three years in an immunocompetent woman who has had multiple normal smears. More frequent screening may slightly increase sensitivity, but does not outweigh the increases in patient harm due to cost, anxiety, and inconvenience.[39–41,44,45]

Since the Food and Drug Administration approval of HPV testing for primary screening of women over 30, clinicians have a second option and may screen this age group using combined HPV testing and cervical cytology. Women over 30 with a negative result for both tests should be screened no more frequently than every three years. This lengthened screening interval is not recommended for younger women, because of the

Table 20-4 **CERVICAL CANCER SCREENING GUIDELINES**[29,40,41]

Onset	Within three years of initiation of sexual activity No later than age 21 (whichever comes first)
Frequency **Age <30 years** **Age ≥30 years**	Annual cervical cytology screening by Pap test. If three consecutive negative and satisfactory Pap test results, choose to continue using one of two approaches: 1. Cervical cytology alone. Screen every two to three years. 2. Combined cervical cytology and HPV testing. Screen no more frequently than every three years if both results negative. *Note:* More frequent screening is required for women who are immunocompromised or were previously diagnosed with cervical cancer.
Duration	Discontinue screening in any of the following cases: 1. For women aged 65 to 70 if they have a 10 year history of negative and satisfactory Pap test results. 2. After complete hysterectomy for benign disease. 3. For women with severe comorbid or life-threatening illness. Continue screening in the following cases: 1. Older women if no previous screening or if past screening results are unavailable. 2. Older women who are immunocompromised and in good health. 3. Older women with a history of cervical cancer who are in good health. 4. After subtotal hysterectomy with a retained cervix. 5. After total hysterectomy for women with a history of invasive cervical cancer. Continue screening vaginal samples.

increased prevalence and decreased persistence of HPV infection in women under 30.[39–41,44]

Screening Women with HIV Infection Women who are infected with HIV should be screened via a Pap test twice in the first year following diagnosis, and if results are normal, annually thereafter. Screening frequency does not increase based upon a changing immune status.[30,31]

Discontinuation of Screening The USPSTF recommends that clinicians discontinue cervical cancer screening for women over 65 years of age if they have had adequate recent screening, normal Pap results, and are not at high risk for cervical cancer. The ACS recommends that screening continue through age 70 if a woman has had a 10-year period of normal cytology results. Because of a lack of studies on the impact of continuing screening in older women, ACOG does not set an upper age limit; instead, it suggests that the decision on when to stop screening be made based on a woman's medical history and anticipated future health status.[39–41,44]

Discontinuation of screening for older women is not appropriate when a woman has not been screened previously or if previous screening results are unavailable. Although most cases of cervical cancer and deaths from cervical cancer occur in women over age 50, these are women who have not adequately been screened throughout their reproductive years. The incidence of new cases of cervical disease in older women is very low for those who have been properly screened on a regular basis. Ongoing screening in older women is associated with low screening yield and potential harm such as frequent false-positives and needless invasive procedures. These drawbacks offset screening benefits.

Screening may be discontinued for women who suffer from severe comorbid or life-threatening disease. Women who have a history of cervical cancer or are immunocompromised should continue screening as long as they are in good health.[39–41,44]

After Hysterectomy Women without a cervix following hysterectomy for benign disease do not need to be screened for cervical cancer because of the low yield of detectable abnormalities.[39–41] For women with a history of invasive cervical cancer, vaginal screening should be continued, although limited data on screening yield exist.[39] Vaginal screening recommendations range from annually[41] to every four months[39] until three consecutive negative results are obtained, at which point screening is discontinued.[39,41] Women who have had a subtotal hysterectomy and retain their cervix should continue cervical cancer screening.[39–41,44]

Reporting of Cervical Cytology: 2001 Bethesda Classification Guidelines

The Bethesda System for reporting cervical cytology was first developed in 1988 to provide a clear and standardized presentation of results as well as to facilitate simplified guidelines for clinical management. The Bethesda Guidelines and terminology were updated most recently in 2001 to keep up with advances in the understanding of the natural history of HPV and evidence that most mild, low-grade cervical lesions resolve spontaneously (Table 20-3). Identification of women with high-grade cervical lesions is the screening focus of the current Bethesda classification system.

BETHESDA CATEGORIZATION

Normal Result Pap test results with normal or non-neoplastic epithelial cell findings are reported as "Negative for Intraepithelial Lesion or Malignancy" (**Figure 20-6A**). The presence of organisms or other changes may be reported as ancillary findings despite normal epithelium. These include *Trichomonas vaginalis*, *Candida* species, shifts in flora secondary to bacterial vaginosis (BV), or cellular changes due to herpes simplex virus.[42]

Women with ancillary Pap findings who have symptomatic vaginitis should be re-evaluated. Recommendations for further evaluation of asymptomatic women vary. Detection of *Trichomonas vaginalis* with the liquid-based Pap is reliable and warrants treatment without further testing.[46] Detection of *Trichomonas vaginalis* by conventional slide Pap is less reliable, so follow-up of asymptomatic women with suspected infection is necessary to confirm diagnosis by wet mount or culture.[47] Asymptomatic *Candida* does not require follow-up or treatment. Non-pregnant asymptomatic women with floral changes indicative of BV do not require treatment. Pregnant asymptomatic women with suspected BV based on Pap findings should be re-evaluated because BV during pregnancy is associated with adverse outcomes.[48]

Figure 20-6 Examples of cervical cytology slides.

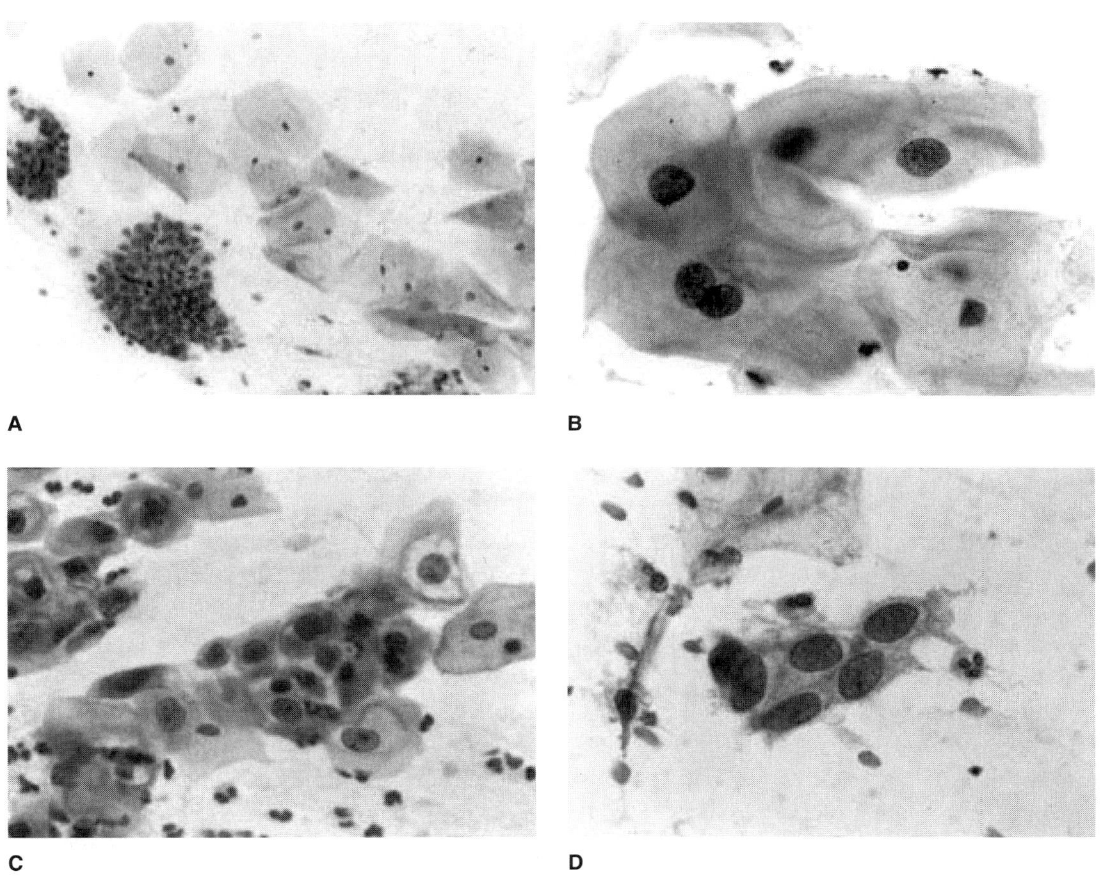

(A) Normal squamous cells. Squamous cells have a small blue nuclei and abundant pink/green cytoplasm. A group of endocervical glandular cells can be seen in the lower left corner with a "honeycomb" arrangement. (B) Atypical squamous cells of undetermined significance (ASCUS). Squamous cells show some nuclear enlargement but still abundant cytoplasm. (C) Low-grade squamous intra-epithelial lesion (LSIL). Squamous cells show enlarged dark blue nuclei and occasionally a clear ring of cytoplasm. (D) High-grade squamous intra-epithelial lesion (HSIL). Very enlarged blue nuclei with less abundant cytoplasm can be seen, resulting in a high nuclear-to-cytoplasmic ratio.

Source for slides: Diane Solomon, M.D. at the National Cancer Institute (http://www.cancer.gov).[42]

Atypical Squamous Cells *Atypical squamous cells* (ASC) are a nonspecific categorization of epithelial cell abnormality (**Table 20-5**). An equivocal result, ASC generally represent mild or transient cervical dysplasia and are the most common abnormal Pap test results in the United States (**Figure 20-6B**). Each year, approximately two million American women

Table 20-5 CLASSIFICATION OF CYTOLOGIC EPITHELIAL CELL ABNORMALITIES[3,9]

Pap Test Result	Cytology Interpretation
ASC-US	Atypical squamous cells, undetermined significance
ASC-H	Atypical squamous cells, cannot exclude HSIL
LSIL	Low-grade squamous intraepithelial lesion
	Includes mild dysplasia
	Associated with CIN 1 histology
HSIL	High-grade squamous intraepithelial lesion
	Includes moderate-to-severe dysplasia
	Associated with CIN 2, CIN 3, and CIS histology
AGC	Atypical glandular cells
	Endocervical, endometrial, or not otherwise specified
	May indicate favor neoplastic cells

receive this mildly atypical report and require some form of follow-up. Despite the category's ambiguity, participants of the 2001 Bethesda Forum support that maintaining an equivocal classification is essential to sensitive screening, as 10% to 20% of women who receive an ASC result have underlying moderate-to-severe dysplasia upon colposcopy.[42]

The Bethesda System further divides the ASC category into "atypical squamous cells, undetermined significance" (ASC-US) and "atypical squamous cells, cannot rule out HSIL" (ASC-H). The ASC-H category is thought to represent 5% to 10% of all ASC cases. Both ASC-US and ASC-H are equivocal findings but are kept as separate classifications. ASC-H has demonstrated an even higher positive predictive value for underlying moderate to high-grade dysplasia than ASC-US. As a result, the category of ASC-H was retained to further improve the system's ability to identify underlying high-grade cervical lesions, despite the fact that it is not highly reproducible among pathologists.[42]

Squamous Intraepithelial Lesion *Low-grade squamous intraepithelial lesion (LSIL)* and *high-grade squamous intraepithelial lesion (HSIL)* are the two tiers of Bethesda classifications representing noninvasive squamous cell abnormalities. LSIL is usually associated with transient HPV infection, HPV cytopathic effect (*koilocytosis*), and low-grade dysplasia (CIN I; **Figure 20-6C**). It is thought to represent 2% to 8% of all Pap test results. HSIL is usually associated with persistent HPV infection, moderate-to-severe dysplasia (CIN 2 and 3), and higher risk of progression to cervical cancer (**Figure 20-6D**). HSIL represents less than 1% of Pap results.[29,42] A Pap report may indicate simply SIL if the cytologist has been unable to categorize the irregularity more specifically.

LSIL and HSIL are diagnosed by cytologic (cell) interpretation of a Pap test sample. *Cervical intraepithelial neoplasia (CIN)* is a histologic (tissue) interpretation that must be diagnosed by biopsy done via colposcopy. CIN is often associated with SIL, but cannot be diagnosed from a cytologic Pap sample.

Atypical Glandular Cells The cytologic interpretation of *atypical glandular cells (AGC)* is an uncommon finding, detected in less than 1% of all Pap test results in the United States. This classification is indicative of abnormalities of the glandular cells that line the endocervix and uterus. An AGC result is often attributable to benign conditions such as polyps or reactive changes; however, it may also be associated with underlying high-grade squamous dysplasia or glandular cell neoplasia.[49] The rate of underlying high-grade squamous or glandular disease for AGC is 10% to 39%, which is even higher than the risk of serious abnormality with ASC-US.[42] Depending upon the cytologic interpretation, AGC may be identified as endocervical, endometrial, or not otherwise specified. Furthermore, the result may or may not be classified as "favor neoplastic."[42]

Endometrial Cells   The 2001 Bethesda System classifies normal endometrial cells under the category of "Other." This finding is only reported for women age 40 and older, regardless of the date of the last menstrual period, because endometrial cancer is rare under the age of 40. A Pap test result with endometrial cells may indicate endometrial hyperplasia or carcinoma, particularly if it is not associated with the secretory phase of menses or if it occurs in a post-menopausal woman.[42,50]

Follow-Up of Abnormal Pap Test Results

In response to the updated Bethesda Classification parameters and new insights into the role of HPV testing, the American Society for Colposcopy and Cervical Pathology (ASCCP) hosted a consensus conference in 2001 to revise evidence-based guidelines for management of women with cervical cytological abnormalities (Table 20-3).

ASC-US

The ASCCP offers three choices for follow-up of women with an ASC-US Pap result (**Figure 20-7**). The preferred approach in most cases is HPV testing for high-risk strains by reflex testing with liquid-based cytology, or HPV testing of a separate sample collected at the time of the initial Pap. If the HPV test is positive, referral for colposcopy is indicated. If the HPV test is negative, the recommendation is to repeat the cytology screening after one year. The second option for ASC-US follow-up is serial cytology, which repeats the Pap test at four- to six-month intervals until two consecutive negative results are achieved. After two normal Pap results, routine annual screening may be resumed. If a second result of ASC-US or more severe abnormality is reported, referral for colposcopy is indicated. The last option for ASC-US follow-up is immediate referral for colposcopy without prior HPV testing or repeat cytology. If negative for abnormal histologic findings, the woman may return to a routine screening schedule.[29]

When comparing options for management of ASC-US results, several factors must be considered. The goal of screening and follow-up is to identify and treat those women who are at true risk for cervical cancer with a high-grade precursor lesion. Women with ASC-US Pap results have a 10% to 20% percent chance of underlying high-grade cervical lesion. The chosen method must be adequately aggressive to achieve this goal, while also preventing unnecessary procedures, expenditures, and undue patient anxiety and discomfort. Over 80% of women with ASC-US have either no lesion or a low-grade HPV related lesion that is likely to regress without intervention.[29,42,51]

HPV testing is the most cost-effective choice because it can eliminate the need for a repeat

Figure 20-7 Triage for women with ASC-US pap test results.*

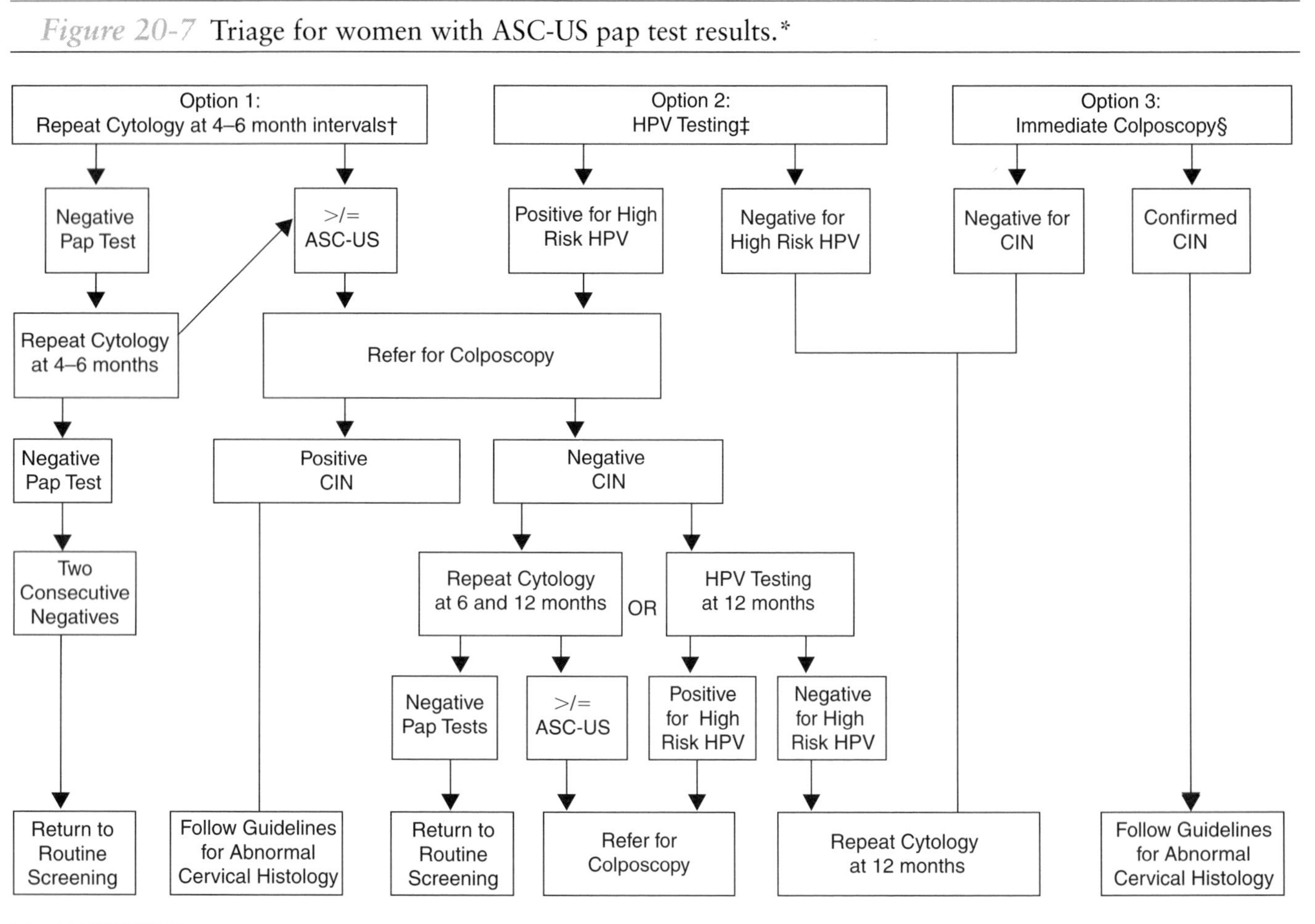

*Management of pregnant women and non-pregnant women is the same. †For postmenopausal women, cytology may be repeated approximately one week after a course of intravaginal estrogen. ‡HPV testing is the preferred approach when liquid-based cytology or co-collection of HPV sample is performed. §Recommended for immunosuppressed women.

Source: Reprinted with permission from The American College of Nurse-Midwives.[3]

office visit in many cases. Data from two landmark clinical trials support this recommendation. The first, a multisite trial conducted by Kaiser Permanente included nearly 1000 women with ASC-US Pap results. Each woman was followed up with liquid-based cytology, HPV testing, and colposcopy with histologic evaluation.[52] The ASCUS/LSIL Triage Study randomized approximately 3500 women to ASC-US follow-up with immediate colposcopy, HPV testing, or repeat cytology.[53] Both trials illustrate the increased sensitivity of HPV testing over repeat cytology for detection of high-grade cervical lesions.[52–54] Furthermore, a negative HPV test result carries a negative predictive value of greater than 98% for high-grade cervical lesions. As a result, the ASCCP recommends HPV testing as the preferred approach to ASC-US management. Using this approach, 30% to 60% of women will test positive for high-risk HPV, especially those in the younger age groups, but HPV testing still refers no more women for colposcopy than do serial cytologies. HPV testing is a less expensive, more objective method than Pap slide interpretation and requires a much shorter timeline than the serial cytology approach.

Universal referral for colposcopy continues to be an option following an ASC-US result, but is the least cost-effective method. While it is the most highly sensitive approach for identification of underlying high-grade lesions, universal colposcopy subjects many women with no or low grade lesions to unnecessary overtreatment.[29,53]

ASC-H

Women with an ASC-H Pap test result should be referred for colposcopy, as this result is much more likely to be indicative of an underlying high-grade lesion than ASC-US (**Figure 20-8**).

For those with ASC-H, estimates for biopsy confirmed high-grade lesion range greatly, from 24% to 94%.[29,42] The specific management plan for an individual woman will depend on the physical findings noted on colposcopy, the results of the biopsy, HPV status, and other factors outlined below. Follow-up with serial cytology or HPV testing is indicated only if histologic findings are negative for CIN.[29]

LSIL

Most women with LSIL should be referred for colposcopy. HPV testing is not an option for follow-up of LSIL because the HPV prevalence in this group is greater than 80%, and 15% to 30% will have an underlying high-grade lesion. HPV testing has proven to be less specific for identifying underlying high-grade lesion in women with LSIL than with ASC-US Pap test results.[29,54]

Adolescent and postmenopausal women are an exception to the rule of universal colposcopy for LSIL follow-up. Instead, it is acceptable in these groups to forgo colposcopy and manage LSIL with repeat cytology at 6 and 12 months, or HPV testing 12 months after the initial LSIL Pap test result. Adolescents have a higher likelihood of spontaneous regression of LSIL, and of those that progress to HSIL, only a small percentage will evolve into *carcinoma in situ* (CIS), a process that usually takes years. Because of the high prevalence of HPV, high rates of viral clearance, and low rates of HSIL in younger women, a more conservative approach is acceptable. Referral of all adolescents for colposcopy following LSIL would result in the overtreatment of many low-grade lesions and HPV infections that might otherwise spontaneously regress if given time.[29]

For low-risk postmenopausal women with a negative screening history, it is also acceptable

Figure 20-8 Algorithm for triage of women with positive ASC-H and LSIL pap test results.

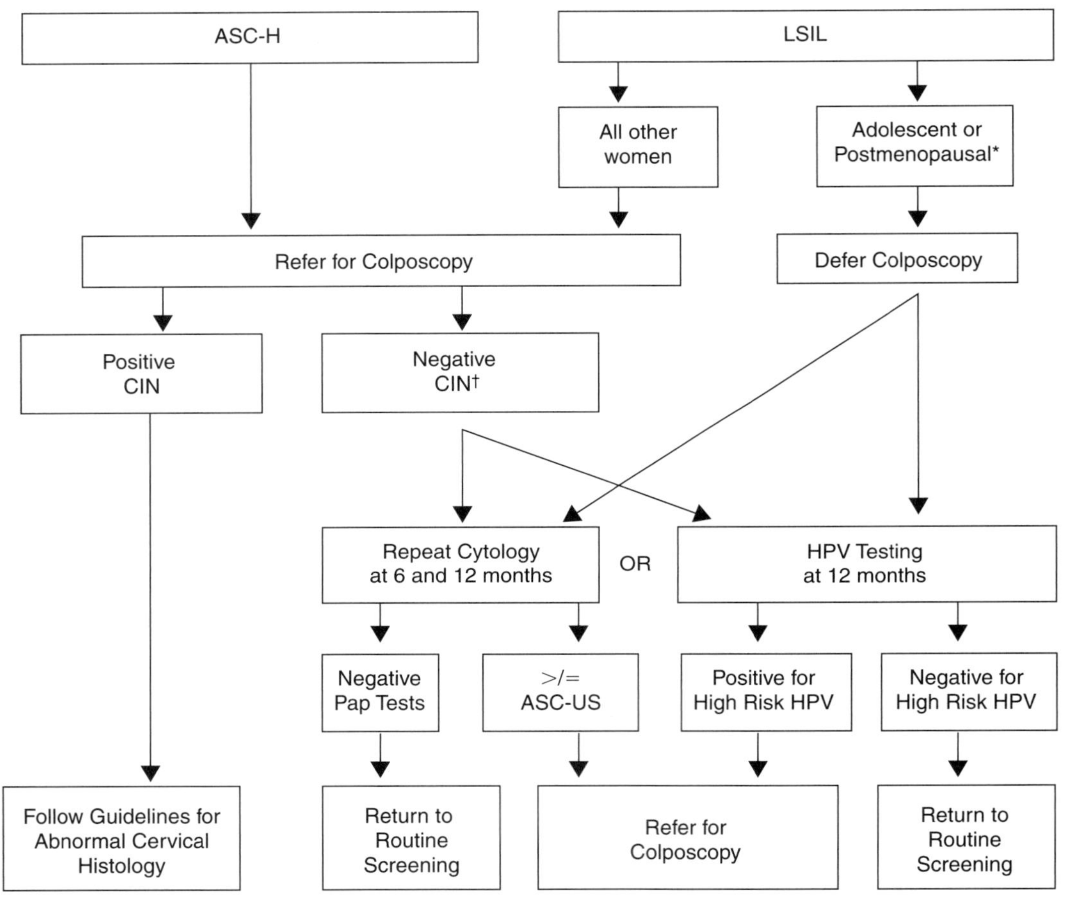

*Colposcopy deferral is only for postmenopausal women who are at low risk with a negative screening history; cytology may be repeated approximately one week after a course of intravaginal estrogen. †Following a result of ASC-H, if negative for biopsy confirmed CIN: re-review of all samples is recommended; diagnosis is subject to change.

Source: Reprinted with permission from The American College of Nurse-Midwives.[3]

to defer colposcopy for follow-up of LSIL. While few concrete data exist to support this advice, the more conservative approach is recommended by the ASCCP based on clinical experience. Postmenopausal women are less likely to be pos-itive for HPV, and more likely to have false-pos-itive Pap test results. Cervical epithelial cells of a postmenopausal woman are more likely to ap-pear atypical secondary to the age-related de-crease in hormone stimulus. Cytology may be repeated approximately one week after a course of intravaginal estrogen.[29]

HSIL

Following an HSIL Pap result, women should be referred immediately for colposcopy. This result, while uncommon, is indicative of a 70% to 75% chance of underlying high-grade lesion, and 1% to 2% chance of invasive cervical cancer. No other triage approach is acceptable in this scenario.[29]

AGC

This category of cytologic interpretation is associated with a higher risk for cervical neoplasia than ASC-US and LSIL. It is recommended that all women, regardless of subclassification, be referred for colposcopy. Younger women with abnormal bleeding and older women over the age of 35 also require an endometrial biopsy. AGC in younger women is associated with higher risk of CIN 2, 3, and adenocarcinoma in situ and with endometrial hyperplasia or cancer in older women. Women of any age who receive a result of "AGC, endometrial" should have endometrial sampling in conjunction with colposcopy.[29]

ENDOMETRIAL CELLS

The follow-up needed if normal endometrial cells are reported will depend on age and risk status. Normal endometrial cells are unlikely to be pathologic in reproductive-aged women, particularly if they occur within 10 days of the onset of menses. Normal endometrial cells have been thought to indicate a higher risk of pathology if found on the Pap smears in postmenopausal women, although recent research is conflicting on whether their presence is an accurate marker of risk.[55,56] Therefore the management of these findings will need to be individualized but may warrant follow-up with an endometrial biopsy to screen for endometrial hyperplasia or carcinoma.[29,42,50,55,57]

PREGNANT WOMEN

The management of an abnormal Pap result for pregnant women is generally the same as for nonpregnant women. While a biopsy is often obtained during a colposcopy for nonpregnant women, it is usually avoided in pregnancy. Due to risks of preterm labor, infection, and blood loss, biopsy during pregnancy is indicated only if there is strong suspicion that lesions are indicative of high-grade precursors or invasive disease. Biopsy may be deferred until the second trimester to minimize the risk of spontaneous abortion.[57] Pregnant women who require colposcopy should be followed by a provider familiar with the colposcopic changes induced by pregnancy.[29]

IMMUNOSUPPRESSED WOMEN

All women who have HIV or are immunosuppressed should be referred for colposcopy following any abnormal Pap test result, regardless of immune status or antiretroviral therapy.[29] Management of ancillary findings is the same as for immunocompetent women.[48]

Patient Education

Many women have only a vague understanding of the purpose of Pap smears. Most are unfamiliar with the relationship between HPV and cervical cancer. The news that an abnormal Pap is due to an asymptomatic, sexually transmitted viral disease can be quite stressful. Midwives and other primary care providers need to address the psychological impact of an abnormal Pap or

HPV test result, reassuring women that HPV is very common and associated with low risk for cervical cancer, yet emphasizing the importance of appropriate follow-up.

Diagnosis of Cervical Cancer

The Pap test is a screening tool, one that examines a cytological or cell sample. It does not provide a formal diagnosis of cervical epithelial abnormality. Colposcopy and direct biopsy of the cervix are necessary in order to make a diagnosis. This diagnosis is based upon abnormal histological (tissue) findings obtained via biopsy during a colposcopy or other surgical procedure. The colposcope utilizes illuminated 5 to 15× magnification to examine the cervix, vagina, and external genitalia, allowing identification of cervical lesions not seen by the naked eye. Application of 3% to 5% acetic acid aids in the identification of these otherwise invisible irregularities by staining them white. Tissue biopsies are obtained from the identified areas.

Histologic abnormalities are reported as CIN. CIN represents disordered tissue growth of the cervical epithelial lining that is a precursor to cancer. Most patients with CIN have lesions that are identifiable with the colposcope.[58] CIN 1 is characterized by abnormal growth of the outer one-third of basal epithelial lining.[9] CIN 2 indicates irregular cell growth in two-thirds thickness of the epithelium, and CIN 3 indicates irregular growth in greater than two-thirds thickness of the epithelium. CIS is a localized, full thickness epithelial malignancy.[9]

Histologic abnormalities categorized as CIN 1 are generally associated with the level of squamous cell abnormalities represented by LSIL Pap test results. CIN 2 and 3 are generally associated with the level of cellular change represented by HSIL Pap test results. In some situations, Pap test and colposcopic biopsy results do not correlate in this way. If histologic results obtained from biopsy during colposcopy are of greater severity than Pap results, they should be considered more significant than Pap results in clinical decision making and are used to direct the management plan. However, if the converse occurs (i.e., the Pap smear reports cytological abnormalities but no CIN is found on biopsy), the guidelines illustrated in Figures 20-7 and 20-8 should be followed. In the case of HSIL followed by colposcopy that is negative for CIN, a re-review of all samples is recommended because it is possible that the lesion was missed on colposcopy but sampled by the Pap smear. If the cytologic evaluation of HSIL is upheld, a diagnostic excisional procedure should be performed.[29]

Treatment for Cervical Cancer and Precursor Lesions

In 2001, the ASCCP published guidelines for management of women with CIN (summarized in **Figures 20-9, 20-10, and 20-11** and Table 20-3).[29] Recommendations are based on whether the colposcopy is considered to be satisfactory or unsatisfactory. In a satisfactory colposcopy, the entire squamocolumnar junction and the margins of any lesion have been visualized. The ASCCP guidelines also take into consideration special circumstances such as adolescence, pregnancy, and immunosuppression.

PROCEDURES

Several localized treatments for pre-invasive CIN exist. Laser surgery and cryocauterization are treatment options that ablate the affected tissue. *Loop electrosurgical excision procedure* (LEEP) excises cancerous cells using a wire loop that passes an electrical current. Cervical conization entails removal of a cone-shaped piece of cervix with a scalpel. One of the advantages of using a conization or LEEP procedure for treatment is that it can provide additional tissue samples. Because these tissue samples have been incised, they will have "clean edges" as opposed to obscured edges as is seen with destructive procedures. Therefore, they can be used to determine the likelihood that the entire lesion was excised; in this case, normal tissue will be seen at the edges and abnormal tissue will be seen only in the interior of the sample. These tissue samples are typically sent to pathology to confirm that the original histological classification seen on colposcopy is correct.[9]

CIN 1
The ASCCP offers several options for follow-up of biopsy-confirmed CIN 1 depending on the quality of the colposcopic exam (Figure 20-9). Women whose colposcopies were considered adequate may be managed in any of the following ways. Women may be treated immediately with a locally ablative or excisional procedure. However, because most cases of CIN 1 regress without intervention, the ASCCP states that the preferred approach is to follow up with repeat Pap testing at 6 and 12 months, or HPV testing at 12 months. This less aggressive approach carries a 9% to 16% risk of lesion progression, but the majority of resulting invasive cancers in this group are in women who are lost to follow-up. If consistent follow-up cannot be ensured, immediate treatment is suggested. Several topical agents are currently being evaluated for treatment of CIN 1, but adequate published data to provide guidelines on efficacy or appropriate use are not yet available.[43]

Follow-up should be more aggressive in a woman with biopsy-confirmed CIN 1 whose colposcopy is unsatisfactory, because there is a significant risk of missing occult invasive cancer. The preferred treatment is a diagnostic excisional procedure (Figure 20-10). The ASCCP makes an exception to this rule for women at lower risk of having higher grade lesions or invasive cancer. For adolescent women, CIN 2 and CIN 3 are rare following unsatisfactory colposcopy and biopsy-confirmed CIN 1. Thus, follow-up without treatment is acceptable (Figure 20-9).[29]

CIN 2 and CIN 3
Biopsy-confirmed CIN 2 and CIN 3 have a higher likelihood of progression to CIS. Thus, all patients with CIN 2 and CIN 3 should be referred for cervical ablation or exision (Figure 20-11). Either technique is generally accepted for treatment because no differences in outcomes have been demonstrated. Excisional techniques are preferred and chosen by some, particularly in the case of recurrent CIN, because they produce an excised tissue specimen that can be further reviewed for pathology.[29]

Adolescents with satisfactory colposcopy and CIN 2 who are reliable for follow-up may receive colposcopy and cytology at four- to six-month intervals. This is because of the higher rates of regression and lower rates of cervical cancer in the younger age group. Adolescents with CIN 3 require ablation or excision of the cervix.[29]

For women with biopsy-confirmed CIN 2 or CIN 3 and an unsatisfactory colposcopy, there is up to a 7% chance of underlying invasive cervical carcinoma. As a result, a diagnostic exisional procedure is the recommended approach (Figure 20-11).[29]

Figure 20-9 Algorithm for managing women with biopsy-confirmed cervical intraepithelial neoplasia grade 1 (CIN 1) and satisfactory colposcopy.

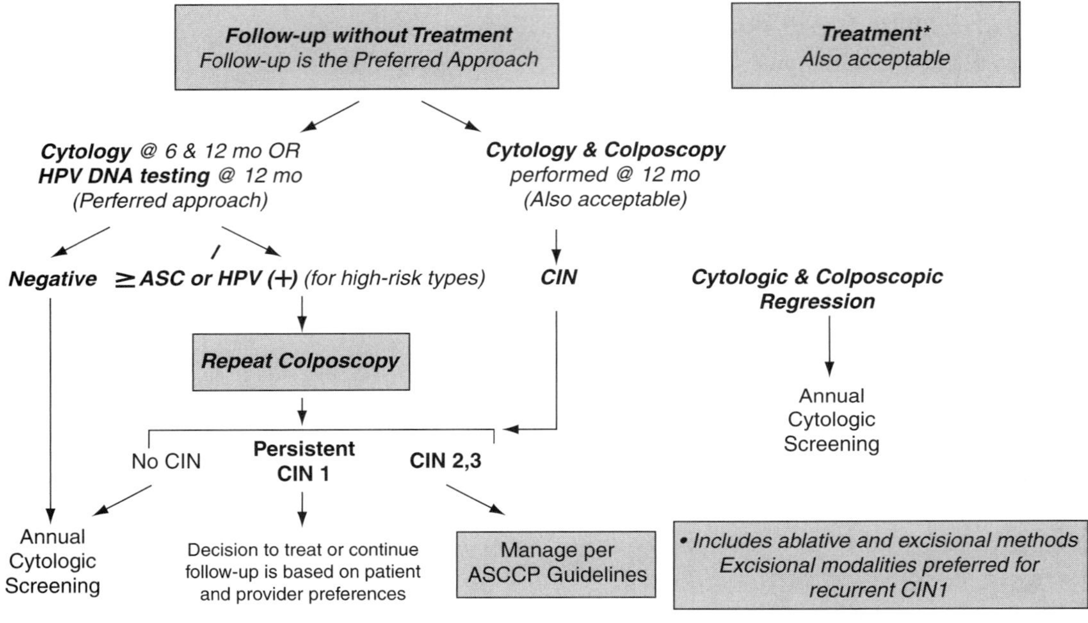

Source: Reprinted with permission from the American Society for Colposcopy and Cervical Pathology, ©2002.

Pregnancy The goal of management for pregnant women with CIN is to identify invasive cancer. Progression of CIN 1, 2, and 3 to invasive cancer during pregnancy is rare, so follow-up without treatment for pregnant women with CIN is acceptable (Figure 20-10).[29] Excisional procedures during pregnancy can cause complications such as miscarriage, hemorrhage, incompetent cervix, and infection, so conservative management is preferred. Biopsies and other excisional procedures should be reserved for use in situations only when invasive cancer cannot be ruled out.[43,57,58]

Immunosuppression In women with HIV, the risk of recurrence of CIN 2 and CIN 3 is 40% to 60%.[59] Level of risk correlates with degree of immunosuppression. Standard treatments have low efficacy for eliminating persistent or recurrent CIN 2 and CIN 3 in HIV-infected women, but appear to successfully prevent progression to invasive cervical cancer and thus are indicated.[43,59] One preliminary study indicates that application of 5% topical vaginal 5-fluorouracil biweekly for six months significantly reduces recurrence or persistence of CIN 2 and CIN 3 after treatment.[60] Since CIN 1 may regress sponta-

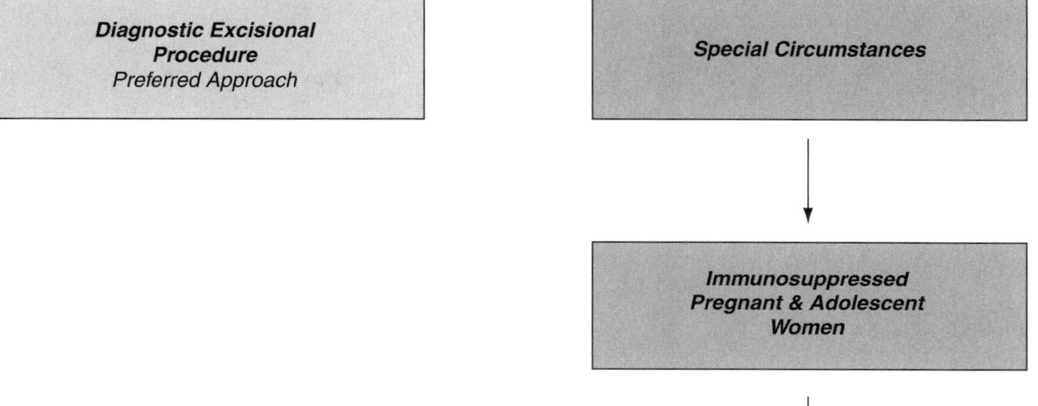

Figure 20-10 Algorithm for managing women with biopsy-confirmed cervical-intraepithelial neoplasia grade 1 (CIN 1) and unsatisfactory colposcopy.

Source: Reprinted with permission from the American Society for Colposcopy and Cervical Pathology. ©2002.

neously, no specific therapy is required for women with CIN 1 and a satisfactory colposcopy except close follow-up (Figures 20-9 and 20-10).[43,59]

Follow-Up

After treatment for CIN, the recommended follow-up is serial Pap screening at four- to six-month intervals. HPV testing at least six months after treatment is also an alternative. Repeat colposcopy is recommended if greater than or equal to ASC-US cytology or if high-risk HPV is identified. If three negative Pap test results are obtained or the woman is negative for high-risk HPV, returning to annual screening is acceptable follow-up.[43]

CIS CIS or invasive cervical malignancy warrants referral to a gynecologic oncologist. Treatment requires simple or radical hysterectomy, radiation, and/or chemotherapy.

Treatment Outcomes

With appropriate intervention, survival rates for women with pre-invasive cervical malignancy approaches 100%. Localized invasive cervical cancer detected at an early stage has a five-year survival rate of greater than 90% and is one of the most successfully treated cancers.[1]

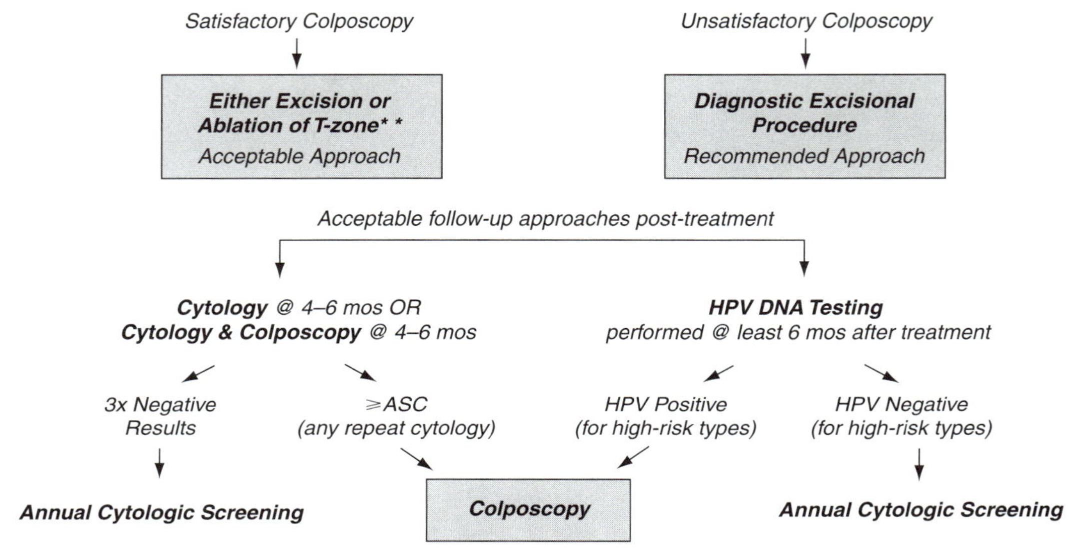

Figure 20-11 Algorithm for managing women with biopsy-confirmed cervical intraepithelial neoplasia grades 2 and 3 (CIN 2 and CIN 3).

*Management options may vary if the woman is pregnant, immunosuppressed, or an adolescent—(see text).
**Excisional modalities preferred for recurrent CIN 2, 3.
Source: Reprinted with permission from the American Society for Colposcopy and Cervical Pathology. ©2002.

Future of Cervical Cancer Prevention: HPV Vaccines

Vaccines targeted at HPV prophylaxis are under development and in the future may become the primary approach to cervical cancer prevention. Current vaccine studies focus upon HPV 16, 18, 31, and 45, the most prevalent high-risk strains. Preliminary results for an HPV 16 vaccine appear promising and have demonstrated nearly 100% efficacy thus far. The duration of protection afforded by this vaccine, as well as its impact on long-term outcomes, is not yet known. Multivalent vaccines that offer protection against several strains of HPV are also under investigation. If outcomes are shown to improve with vaccine use, identification of an optimal vaccine schedule, as well as determining the best way to integrate this vaccine into current screening programs, will become top research priorities.[61,62]

Ovarian Cancer Screening

Ovarian cancer is the leading cause of death due to cancer of the female reproductive system although it is only the fifth most prevalent cancer diagnosed in the United States. The incidence of ovarian cancer in the United States is 17 per 100,000. Nearly 80% of ovarian cancer occurs in postmenopausal women, although it can occur at any age, including in prepubescent girls. About 75% of ovarian cancers are ovarian in origin, while about 25% have metastasized from other sites, including the breast, stomach, colon, and endometrium. The majority of cases of premenopausal onset are associated with genetic risk factors.

Barnholtz-Sloan et al.[63] recently published an analysis of patterns of diagnosis and survival of women in the United States diagnosed with primary invasive epithelial ovarian cancer. Two-, five-, and 10-year survival rates during the 1970s, 1980s, and 1990s were compared using data from the Surveillance, Epidemiology, and End Results (SEER) Program. While many confounding factors complicate comparisons across the three decades, the two- and five-year survival rates have improved significantly, whereas the proportion of those surviving at 10 years post-diagnosis remains stable at about 34%. Long-term survival has not improved because many cancers continue to be diagnosed at an advanced stage. The following factors are associated with poorer outcomes: older age, more advanced staged disease at diagnosis, receiving no surgery, and African-American race.[2,62] Women who present with more advanced metastatic illness, as is true in the majority of cases of ovarian cancer, are less likely to have surgery.

Risk Factors

Ovarian cancer is a disease of the industrialized world, with the highest rates being found in countries with lower birth rates.[64] As early as 1978, Beral et al. hypothesized that parity accounted for the international differences in rates of ovarian cancer.[65] More recently the risk of ovarian cancer has been seen to decrease with multiparity, breastfeeding, and use of oral contraceptives and increase with polycystic ovarian syndrome (PCOS) and unopposed estrogen treatment (**Table 20-6**).[66] Multiparity confers

Table 20-6 RISK FACTORS FOR OVARIAN CANCER[47,48]
Nulliparous
Polycystic ovarian syndrome
Unopposed estrogen treatment
Genetic factors
Family history of breast or ovarian cancer
BRCA1, BRCA2 mutation (increased in families of Ashkenazi Jewish and Icelandic descent)
MSH2, MLH1 mutation (increased in families with a history of colorectal cancer)

significant protection against ovarian cancer, with a 13% to 19% decrease in risk per pregnancy, while the use of oral contraceptives for greater than five years has been associated with a 50% decrease in risk. Rates of ovarian cancer are higher in married nulliparous women than in those who are not married, perhaps because of an association with PCOS and infertility.

Women at genetic risk account for only 10% of cases of ovarian cancer. However, the lifetime risk of developing ovarian cancer is as high as 50% in women with two first-degree relatives diagnosed with ovarian cancer.[66] The most commonly discussed genetic factors are the *BRCA1* and *BRCA2* mutations, which are mutations to the tumor suppression genes on chromosomes 17 and 13. A second kind of genetic risk is conferred from mutations in the *MSH2* and *MLH1* genes on chromosomes 2 and 3. These genes are involved in correction of errors in cell replication.

Screening Challenges

The essential problems of diagnosis and treatment of ovarian cancer are threefold: 1) symptoms do not present until the disease is fairly advanced; 2) advanced disease is unlikely to be cured; and 3) no screening modality currently exists that is sensitive, specific, and cost-effective enough to be used for mass population-based screening. Clinical trials of ovarian cancer screening in low-risk groups similar to the general population have detected both nonmalignant and malignant masses in study participants, and resulted in an increased number of surgeries with a low yield of malignant tumors.[67] In 1983, an assay was developed that allowed for serum measurement of the glycoprotein antigen now known as CA 125. CA 125 is a tumor marker that is often elevated in early cases of epithelial ovarian cancer, but unfortunately CA 125 testing is neither sensitive nor specific enough to be used in mass screening. Serum levels may be normal in as many as 50% of women with stage I/II ovarian cancer, and false positives may be obtained with conditions such as pregnancy, benign ovarian and uterine conditions, and pelvic inflammatory disease.[64,68] The ACS, ACOG, and USPSTF all recommend against routine screening of the general population for ovarian cancer.[69]

Because of the low incidence of the disease, successful mass screening programs will require the development of highly specific tests and multiple approaches such as combining CA 125 blood tests with high-tech transvaginal ultrasonography, perhaps including color Doppler and three-dimensional (3-D) technology to evaluate ovarian morphology as well as volume. Large, multi-armed, randomized studies of such protocols are ongoing in both the United States and the United Kingdom. Outcome measurements will include rates of ovarian cancer morbidity and mortality, quality of life, and compliance with annual screening, but the results of these studies will not be available for several years.[67,70] Researchers in another large, multisite study have recently identified three new promising markers for ovarian malignancy, which when used in combination were found to perform with a greater sensitivity and specificity than CA 125. These biomarkers need to be evaluated in larger populations before such testing is applied beyond the basis of clinical trials.[71]

Ovarian cancer screening services today focus their efforts on women at known risk, such as those with a family history of ovarian and/or breast cancer. Increased rates of the *BRCA1* genetic mutation have been found in women who are of Icelandic and Ashkenazi Jewish background, and the *MSH* and *MLH* mutations may occur in families with a history of colorectal cancer.[66] Women with such family history should be advised to obtain as much information as they can on the age of onset and type of cancer that occurred in their family members, including male relatives, and should be referred for genetic counseling.

The age of onset of disease is an important factor, because malignancies that develop early in life are more likely to be the result of genetic risk. A family history that includes two or more first-degree relatives with early age onset of breast, ovarian, colon, or endometrial cancer is more likely to be followed by positive results on genetic screening than a history of second-degree relatives with older age onset of disease.[72] In geographical areas where genetic counseling services are limited, it is important for primary providers to collaborate with their consultants in oncology and genetics in order to develop referral policies that reflect individual and community-related trends in risk.

Monitoring of Women at Increased Risk

Ideally, women who are at increased risk for ovarian cancer should be offered a face-to-face consultation with a gynecological oncologist.[73] Women at increased risk include those with positive results on genetic testing as well as those with a history of PCOS or infertility. Established approaches for monitoring women at increased risk include annual screening with vaginal ultrasound and serum testing for the tumor marker CA 125. As mentioned above, CA 125 testing is not highly sensitive or specific in either premenopausal or postmenopausal women, although high levels in postmenopausal women accompanied by pelvic mass are often associated with malignancy. However, women with any stage of ovarian cancer may have normal levels of CA 125, and a number of benign gynecological conditions in premenopausal women are commonly associated with elevated levels of CA 125.

Newer screening approaches under investigation include the use of 3-D ultrasound, the tumor marker lysophosphaticid acid, and mass spectroscopy.[74] Prevention approaches include oral contraception to suppress ovarian activity and prophylactic oophorectomy. Oral contraceptive use has been shown to decrease the risk of ovarian cancer, but evidence is lacking on the efficacy of other hormonal contraceptive approaches. Recent reports of fallopian tube malignancy and dysplasia found in high-risk women undergoing prophylactic oophorectomy raise the question of the possibility of tubal involvement in the elaboration of ovarian epithelial cancer.[75,76] Prophlactic oophorectomy has been reported to reduce the risk of ovarian cancer for high-risk women carrying the BRCA 1 and BRCA 2 mutations by 90%.[77]

Signs and Symptoms

Ovarian cancer can present with a variety of abdominal symptoms such as fullness or bloating, vague pain, indigestion, and changes in gastrointestinal functioning such as smaller stool size.[74,78,79] Some women report change in urinary function. By the time a woman presents with secondary shortness of breath, fluid in the abdomen, and weight gain, she is likely to have advanced stage illness. Given this nonspecific clinical picture, many women with ovarian cancer are not diagnosed early in the course of disease. Research has shown that women may experience abdominal symptoms for up to a year prior to diagnosis. The possibility of ovarian cancer must be considered in women presenting with such complaints. Screening for gastrointestinal symptoms is an essential component of the history and is a particularly important component in the evaluation of any woman with an adnexal mass.

Appropriate Referral for Women with Clinical Findings

Clinical findings indicative of possible ovarian cancer include the symptoms listed above, nodular or fixed pelvic mass associated with elevated CA 125, and ascites. The current ACOG Committee Opinion entitled, "The Role of the Generalist Obstetrician-Gynecologist in the Early Detection of Ovarian Cancer," recommends a two-part approach for streamlining diagnosis and correct staging of ovarian cancer.[73] The first is for generalists to have a high index of suspicion for ovarian cancer in women exhibiting symptoms. Physical and pelvic examination and vaginal ultrasound should be performed, and CA 125 may be helpful in the evaluation of postmenopausal women. The second recommendation is to refer women with a suspicious or complex mass to a gynecological oncologist or other surgeon trained in comprehensive surgical staging. It is important that, whenever possible, the appropriate staging procedures be conducted with the initial surgery. Thus, primary care providers will need to carefully consider their patterns of referral and consultation for women who present at risk for or with clinical findings indicative of possible ovarian cancer.[73]

Prevention of Ovarian Cancer

Providers of primary and contraceptive care should consider how what is known about ovarian cancer can be used in prevention. The underlying pathologic mechanisms are thought to relate to repetitive cyclical ovarian stimulation and ovulation. Most women are unaware that low parity in the absence of ovulatory suppression is a risk factor for ovarian cancer. It is possible that some women might choose hormonal contraception or, if contraception is not needed, hormonal suppression for the purpose of decreasing their cancer risk

if this benefit were explicitly addressed. Women being seen for annual gynecologic or primary care evaluation who are nulliparous and who have not used hormonal contraception may benefit from a discussion on their personal risks and the benefits that may accrue from the use of hormonal contraceptive methods.

Conclusions

Population-based cervical cancer cytology screening is one of the success stories of the twentieth century. Current efforts to include HPV testing as an integral part of cervical cancer screening has the potential to improve the efficacy and specificity of established programs for early detection of cervical cancer. In contrast, early detection of ovarian cancer has proven to be much more difficult. Perhaps the development of ovarian cancer screening programs will be a hallmark achievement of oncology researchers of the 21st century. In the meantime, primary care providers need to attend to careful use of their skills in history-taking and physical examination, and build referral networks that allow for appropriate collaboration with generalist and specialist consultants in gynecology, oncology, and genetics testing services.

References

1. American Cancer Society. Cancer Facts and Figures. [monograph on the Internet] 2004 [cited 2004 May 29]. Available from: http://www.cancer.org/docroot/pro/content/pro_1_1_Cancer_Statistics_2004_presentation.asp.

2. National Cancer Institute. Surveillance, Epidemiology, and End Results (SEER) Cancer Statistics Review, 1975–2001 [monograph on the Internet]. 2003 [cited 2004 May 04]; Available from: http://SEER.cancer.gov/csr/1975-2001/sections.html.

3. Fey MC, Beal MW. Role of human papillomavirus testing in cervical cancer prevention. *J Midwifery Women's Health*. 2004;49:4–13.

4. Franco EL, Duarte-Franco E, Ferenczy A. Cervical cancer: Epidemiology, prevention and the role of human papillomavirus infection. *CMAJ*. 2001;164(7):1017–1025.

5. National Cancer Institute. Cervical Cancer: Screening [Online]. 2004 [cited 2004 Feb 6]; Available

from: http://www.cancer.gov/cancerinfo/pdq/screen ing/cervical/health professional.

6. Janicek MF, Averette HE. Cervical cancer: Prevention, diagnosis, and therapeutics. *CA Cancer J Clin.* 2001; 51(2):92–114.

7. Jastreboff AM, Cymet T. Role of the human papilloma virus in the development of cervical intraepithelial neoplasia and malignancy. *Postgrad Med J.* 2002;78(918):225–228.

8. Bosch FX, Manos MM, Munoz N, Sherman M, Jansen AM, Peto J, et al. Prevalence of human papillomavirus in cervical cancer: A worldwide perspective. *J Natl Cancer Inst.* 1995;87(11):796–802.

9. Holschneider CH. Premalignant and malignant disorders of the uterine cervix. In: *Current Obstetric and Gynecologic Diagnosis and Treatment.* 9th ed. New York: McGraw Hill [online]. 2002 [cited 2004 Feb 23]. Available from: http://pco.ma.ovid.com/lrpbooks/ decherney/textbook/chapters/ch0047.htm.

10. Marrazzo JM, Stine K, Koutsky LA. Genital human papillomavirus infection in women who have sex with women: A review. *Am J Obstet Gynecol.* 2000;183(3): 770–774.

11. Sonnex C, Strauss S, Gray JJ. Detection of human papillomavirus DNA on the fingers of patients with genital warts. *Sex Transm Infect.* 1999;75(5):317–319.

12. Pao CC, Tsai PL, Chang YL, Hsieh TT, Jin JY. Possible non-sexual transmission of genital human papillomavirus infections in young women. *Eur J Clin Microbiol Infect Dis.* 1993;12(3):221–222.

13. Tay SK, Ho TH, Lim-Tan SK. Is genital human papillomavirus infection always sexually transmitted? *Aust N Z J Obstet Gynaecol.* 1990;30(3):240–242.

14. Helmerhorst TJ, Meijer CJ. Cervical cancer should be considered as a rare complication of oncogenic HPV infection rather than a STD. *Int J Gynecol Cancer.* 2002;12(3):235–236.

15. Meijer CJ, Snijders PJ, van den Brule AJ. Screening for cervical cancer: Should we test for infection with high-risk HPV? *CMAJ.* 2000;163(5):535–538.

16. McFadden SE, Schumann L. The role of human papillomavirus in screening for cervical cancer. *J Am Acad Nurse Pract.* 2001;13(3):116–125.

17. Ho GY, Bierman R, Beardsley L, Chang CJ, Burk RD. Natural history of cervicovaginal papillomavirus infection in young women. *N Engl J Med.* 1998;338(7): 423–428.

18. Konya J, Dillner J. Immunity to oncogenic human papillomaviruses. *Adv Cancer Res.* 2001;82:205–238.

19. Vinther J, Norrild B. Clearance of cervical human papillomavirus infections. *Int J Cancer.* 2003;104(2): 255–256.

20. Centers for Disease Control and Prevention. Tracking the Hidden Epidemics 2000. Trends in STDs in the United States: A Closer Look at HPV Infection [monograph on the Internet]. 2001 [cited 2002 Apr 28]. Available from: http://www.cdc.gov/nchstp/od/ news/RevBrochure1pdfcloselookhpv.htm.

21. Kahn JA, Rosenthal SL, Succop PA, Ho GY, Burk RD. Mediators of the association between age of first sexual intercourse and subsequent human papillomavirus infection. *Pediatrics.* 2002;109(1):E5.

22. Coker AL, Bond SM, Williams A, Gerasimova T, Pirisi L. Active and passive smoking, high-risk human papillomaviruses and cervical neoplasia. *Cancer Detect Prev.* 2002;26(2):121–128.

23. Munoz N, Franceschi S, Bosetti C, Moreno V, Herrero R, Smith JS, et al. Role of parity and human papillomavirus in cervical cancer: The IARC multicentric case-control study. *Lancet.* 2002;359:1093–1101.

24. Moreno V, Bosch FX, Munoz N, Meijer CJ, Shah KV, Walboomers JM, et al. Effect of oral contraceptives on risk of cervical cancer in women with human papillomavirus infection: The IARC multicentric case-control study. *Lancet.* 2002;359:1085–1092.

25. Skegg DC. Oral contraceptives, parity, and cervical cancer. *Lancet.* 2002;359:1080–1081.

26. Castellsague X, Bosch FX, Munoz N. Environmental co-factors in HPV carcinogenesis. *Virus Res.* 2002;89: 191–199.

27. Massion CT. Nutrients and cervical cancer prevention. *Alt Ther Women's Health.* 2000;2(8):57–62.

28. Kuhn L, Sun XW, Wright TC Jr. Human immunodeficiency virus infection and female lower genital tract malignancy. *Curr Opin Obstet Gynecol.* 1999;11(1): 35–39.

29. Wright TC Jr., Cox JT, Massad LS, Twiggs LB, Wilkinson EJ. 2001 consensus guidelines for the management of women with cervical cytological abnormalities. *JAMA.* 2002;287(16):2120–2129.

30. U.S. Public Health Service/Infectious Diseases Society of America. 2001 Guidelines for the Prevention of Opportunistic Infections in Persons Infected with Human Immunodeficiency Virus [monograph on the Internet]. 2001 [cited 2004 May 30]. Available from: http://aidsinfo.nih.gov.

31. Bartlett JG. *Medical Management of HIV Infection.* 2003 ed. Baltimore: Johns Hopkins University; 2003.

32. Sasieni PD. Human papillomavirus screening and cervical cancer prevention. *J Am Med Women's Assoc.* 2000;55(4):216–219.

33. Bovicelli A, Bristow RE, Montz FJ. HPV testing: Where are we now? *Anticancer Res.* 2000;20(6C):4673–4680.

34. Mandelblatt JS, Lawrence WF, Womack SM, Jacobson D, Yi B, Hwang YT, et al. Benefits and costs of using HPV testing to screen for cervical cancer. *JAMA.* 2002;287(18):2372–2381.

35. Cohn DE, Herzog TJ. New innovations in cervical cancer screening. *Clin Obstet Gynecol.* 2001;44(3):538–549.

36. Nuovo J, Melnikow J, Howell LP. New tests for cervical cancer screening. *Am Fam Physician.* 2001;64(5):780–786.

37. Jin XW, Xu H. Cervical cancer screening from Pap smear to human papillomavirus DNA testing. *Compr Ther.* 2001;27(3):202–208.

38. Cuzick J, Sasieni P, Davies P, Adams J, Normand C, Frater A, et al. A systematic review of the role of human papilloma virus (HPV) testing within a cervical screening programme: Summary and conclusions. *Br J Cancer.* 2000;83(5):561–565.

39. Saslow D, Runowicz CD, Solomon D, Mosicki AB, Smith RA, Eyre HL, et al. American Cancer Society guideline for the early detection of cervical neoplasia and cancer. *Cancer J Clin.* 2002;52(6):342–376.

40. United States Preventive Services Task Force. Recommendations and Rationale, Screening for Cervical Cancer [monograph on the Internet]. 2003 [cited 2004 Jan 20]. Available from: http://www.ahrq.gov/clinic/3rduspstf/cervcan/cervcanrr.htm.

41. American College of Obstetricians and Gynecologists. ACOG News Release. Cervical Cancer Screening: Testing Can Start Later and Occur Less Often Under New ACOG Recommendations [monograph on the Internet]. 2003 [cited 2004 Feb 6]. Available from: http://www.acog.org/from_home/publications/press_releases/nr07-31-03.cfm.

42. Solomon D, Davey D, Kurman R, Moriarty A, O'Connor D, Prey M, et al. The 2001 Bethesda system: Terminology for reporting results of cervical cytology. *JAMA.* 2002;287(16):2114–2119.

43. Wright TC Jr, Cox JT, Massad LS, Carlson DO, Twiggs LB, Wilkinson EJ. 2001 Consensus Guidelines for the Management of Women with Cervical Intraepithelial Neoplasia. *Am J Obstet Gynecol.* 2003;189(1):295–304.

44. American College of Obstetricians and Gynecologists. ACOG Practice Bulletin Number 45. Clinical Management Guidelines for Obstetrician-Gynecologists: Cervical Cytology Screening. *Obstet Gynecol.* 2003;102(2):417–427.

45. Frame PS, Frame JS. Determinants of cancer screening frequency: The example of screening for cervical cancer. *J Am Board Fam Pract.* 1998;11(2):87–95.

46. Lara-Torre E, Pinkerton JS. Accuracy of detection of trichomonas vaginalis organisms on a liquid-based papanicolaou smear. *Am J Obstet Gynecol.* 2003;188(2):354–356.

47. Krieger JN, Tam MR, Stevens CE, Nielsen IO, Hale J, Kiviat NB, et al. Diagnosis of trichomoniasis. Comparison of conventional wet-mount examination with cytologic studies, cultures, and monoclonal antibody staining of direct specimens. *JAMA.* 1988;259(8):1223–1227.

48. Centers for Disease Control and Prevention. Sexually transmitted diseases treatment guidelines 2002. *MMWR Recomm Rep.* 2002;51(RR-6):1–78.

49. Krane JF, Lee KR, Sun D, Yuan L, Crum CP. Atypical glandular cells of undetermined significance. *Am J Clin Pathol.* 2004;121(1):87–92.

50. Wu HH, Schuetz MJ 3rd, Cramer H. Significance of benign endometrial cells in Pap smears from postmenopausal women. *J Reprod Med.* 2001;46(9):795–798.

51. Ferris DG, Wright TC Jr., Litaker MS, Richart RM, Lorincz AT, Sun XW, et al. Comparison of two tests for detecting carcinogenic HPV in women with Papanicolaou smear reports of ASCUS and LSIL. *J Fam Pract.* 1998;46(2):136–141.

52. Manos MM, Kinney WK, Hurley LB, Sherman ME, Shieh-Ngai J, Kurman RJ, et al. Identifying women with cervical neoplasia: Using human papillomavirus DNA testing for equivocal Papanicolaou results. *JAMA.* 1999;281(17):1605–1610.

53. Solomon D, Schiffman M, Tarone R. Comparison of three management strategies for patients with atypical squamous cells of undetermined significance: Baseline results from a randomized trial. *J Natl Cancer Inst.* 2001;93(4):293–299.

54. Sherman ME, Schiffman M, Cox JT. The Atypical Squamous Cells of Undetermined Significance/Low-Grade Squamous Intraepithelial Lesion Triage Study Group. Effects of age and human papilloma viral load on colposcopy triage: Data from the randomized Atypical Squamous Cells of Undetermined Significance/

Low-Grade Squamous Intraepithelial Lesion Triage Study (ALTS). *J Natl Cancer Inst.* 2002; 94(2):102–107.

55. Cherkis RC, Patten SF Jr, Andrews TJ, Dickinson JC, Patten FW. Significance of normal endometrial cells detected by cervical cytology. *Obstet Gynecol.* 1988; 71(2):242–244.

56. Gomez-Fernandez C, Ganjei-Azar P, Averette H, Nadji M. Normal endometrial cells in Papanicolaou Smears: Prevalence in women with and without endometrial disease. *Obstet Gynecol.* 2000, 96:874–878.

57. Ward RM, Bristow RE. Cancer and pregnancy: Recent developments. *Curr Opin Obstet Gynecol.* 2002; 14(6): 613–617.

58. Holschneider C. Premalignant and malignant disorders of the uterine cervix. In: De Cherney AH, Nathan L, editors. *Obstetric & Gynecologic Treatment.* 9th ed. New York: Lange Medical/McGraw-Hill; 2003. pp. 894–915.

59. Levine AM. Evaluation and management of HIV-infected women. *Ann Intern Med.* 2002;136(3):228–242.

60. Maiman M, Watts DH, Andersen J, Clax P, Merino M, Kendall MA. Vaginal 5-fluorouracil for high-grade cervical dysplasia in human immunodeficiency virus infection: A randomized trial. *Obstet Gynecol.* 1999; 94(6):954–961.

61. Koutsky LA, Ault KA, Wheeler CM, Brown DR, Barr E, Alvarez FB, et al. A controlled trial of a human papillomavirus type 16 vaccine. *N Engl J Med.* 2002; 347(21):1645–1651.

62. Kulasingam SL, Myers ER. Potential health and economic impact of adding a human papillomavirus vaccine to screening programs. *JAMA.* 2003;290(6): 781–789.

63. Barnholtz-Sloan JS, Schwartz AG, Qureshi F, Jacques S, Malone J, Munkarah AR. Ovarian cancer: Changes in patterns at diagnosis and relative survival over the last three decades. *Am J Obstet Gynecol.* 2003;189(4): 1120–1127.

64. Look KY. Epidemilogy, etiology and screening of ovarian cancer. In: Rubin SC, Sutton GP, editors. *Ovarian Cancer.* 2nd ed. Philadelphia: Lippincott, Williams & Wilkins; 2001. pp. 167–180.

65. Beral V, Fraser P, Chilvers C. Does pregnancy protect against ovarian cancer? *Lancet.* 1978;1(8073): 1083–1087.

66. Dorigo O, Baker VV. Premalignant and malignant disorders of the ovaries and oviducts. In: *Current Obstetric and Gynecologic Diagnosis and Treatment.* 9th ed. New York: McGraw Hill; 2003.

67. Menon U, Jacobs IJ. Ovarian cancer screening in the general population. *Curr Opin Obstet Gynecol.* 2001; 13(1):61–64.

68. Jacobs I, Bast RC Jr. The CA 125 tumour-associated antigen: A review of the literature. *Hum Reprod.* 1989; 4(1):1–12.

69. Screening for ovarian cancer: Recommendation statement. *Ann Fam Med.* 2004;2(3):260–262.

70. Alexander-Sefre F, Menon U, Jacobs IJ. Ovarian cancer screening. *Hosp Med.* 2002;63(4):210–213.

71. Zhang Z, Bast RC Jr, Yu Y, Li J, Sokoll LJ, Rai AJ, et al. Three biomarkers identified from serum proteomic analysis for the detection of early stage ovarian cancer. *Cancer Res.* 2004;64(16):5882–5890.

72. Murff HJ, Spigel DR, Syngal S. Does this patient have a family history of cancer? An evidence-based analysis of the accuracy of family cancer history. *JAMA.* 2004;292(12):1480–1489.

73. American College of Obstetricians and Gynecologists. ACOG Committee Opinion: Number 280, December 2002. The role of the generalist obstetrician-gynecologist in the early detection of ovarian cancer. *Obstet Gynecol.* 2002;100:1413.

74. Schwartz PE. Diagnosis and treatment of epithelial ovarian cancer. *Minerva Ginecol.* 2003;55(4):315–326.

75. Piek JM, Verheijen RH, Kenemans P, Massuger LF, Bulten H, van Diest PJ. BRCA1/2-related ovarian cancers are of tubal origin: A hypothesis. *Gynecol Oncol.* 2003;90(2):491.

76. Leeper K, Garcia R, Swisher E, Goff B, Greer B, Paley P. Pathologic findings in prophylactic oophorectomy specimens in high-risk women. *Gynecol Oncol.* 2002; 87(1):52–56.

77. Newman L. Prophylactic oophorectomy in the genome age: Balancing new data against uncertainties. *JNCI.* 93(3):173–175.

78. Koldjeski D, Kirkpatrick MK, Swanson M, Everett L, Brown S. Ovarian cancer: Early symptom patterns. *Oncol Nurs Forum.* 2003;30(6):927–933.

79. Goff BA, Mandel LS, Melancon CH, Muntz HG. Frequency of symptoms of ovarian cancer in women presenting to primary care clinics. *JAMA.* 2004; 291(22):2705–2712.

Todd Ambrosia

Jan M. Kriebs

Chapter 21

Musculoskeletal Conditions

Musculoskeletal complaints are common in primary care women's health practice. Orthopedic conditions cannot be diagnosed or managed without knowledge of skeletal and muscular anatomy and the nervous system. It is essential that women's health clinicians who take responsibility for managing these conditions review and update their knowledge. Clinicians should be able to assess whether care is within their competence, or whether referral to an orthopedist or physical medicine specialist is required.

Structures of the Musculoskeletal System

Bones, muscles, joints, tendons, ligaments, cartilage, and bursae compose the musculoskeletal system (MS), which functions to permit support and movement of the body. If any component of the system is compromised due to injury or trauma, quality of life can be impacted. Disability from pain and immobility affects proper functioning of the organs in this system and can decrease the woman's ability to perform her daily routine.

The framework of the MS is composed of the 206 bones that provide skeletal support to the associated soft tissue structures of the body. The bones are classified into four types: *long bones*, such as the humerus and femur; *short bones*, such as the metacarpals and phalanges; *irregular bones*, such as the carpal bones of the hand; and *flat bones*, such as the ribs.

Joints, the functional units of the MS, permit mobility. Joints connect all elements of the MS and are classified into two distinct types: non-synovial joints, which are composed of fibrous tissue or cartilage that are immovable or slightly movable, like that of intervertebral joints; and synovial joints, which are freely movable joints enclosed in a joint cavity that is filled with a lubricant. The synovial fluid reduces friction between the component parts of the joint. *Bursae* are sacs surrounding the synovial joints to contain this fluid.

Cartilage is the fibrous tissue that covers the surface of opposing bones, such as in the knee or shoulder joints. *Ligaments* are fibrous bands running directly from one bone to another to strengthen the joint. They help prevent movement in undesirable directions.

Lastly, *tendons* are strong fibrous cords that attach skeletal muscle to bone. Skeletal muscles are functionally attached to joints in order for their contraction to produce movement.

Assessment

History

When a woman mentions problems related to the MS as the chief complaint, most women's health providers will need to re-focus their history and physical examination to include the appropriate questions. A detailed assessment of the MS includes the following history items. First, it must be determined whether the complaint is due to an injury or to a chronic problem with an acute exacerbation. The clinician must elicit: the time and mechanism of injury or onset of chronic problem; the length of time the complaint has been present; and the area(s) of the body affected by the problem. It is important to ascertain any aggravating and alleviating factors (i.e., activity or rest) as well as any additional symptoms that accompany the complaint, such as skin breakdown, spasm, or immobility. The examiner must ask the woman questions regarding the location, duration, and quality of any pain; any weakness, stiffness, or difficulty with balance or coordination.

The examiner also needs a current list of any medications or allergies the client may have as well as any previous illness or surgery. Questions regarding the client's family, occupational, and social history provide information about any genetic predisposition, living or work conditions that may cause or exacerbate the condition, and the woman's ability to access resources to assist with daily needs.

Physical Examination

The physical examination of the MS begins with an assessment of the client's gait, balance, and posture. The clinician can begin this assessment as the woman enters the exam room and while she is seated during the initial history, noting any gait abnormalities, movement difficulties, or abnormal posturing. Gait should be assessed by noting the base of support, stride, and stance. Posture is assessed by the woman's ability to sit or stand erect, with the head midline, and the midwife noting any deviation. Grimacing or guarding of particular areas of the body are noted as are the woman's overall appearance and demeanor.

A full musculoskeletal assessment incorporates an evaluation of the spinal column, thorough palpation of all muscles and joints, active and passive range of motion and determination of muscle strength of all joints, comparing each side of the body bilaterally. Size, symmetry, and alignment of bilateral structures are assessed. If the woman presents with a unilateral complaint, care should be taken to evaluate the unaffected side prior to the affected side. The clinician must note any swelling, deformity, increased curvature, crepitus, laxity, or immobility, tremors or muscle spasm, muscle weakness, or complaint of pain. It is important to assess the level of pain; however, the examination of a particular area is not continued past the point where motion or pressure becomes painful.

A neurovascular assessment rules out any compromise of the nerves and vascular structures related to the affected areas. This is accomplished by assessing peripheral pulses and noting the color, turgor, and sensation of the overlying skin and associated soft tissues.

Laboratory testing and diagnostic procedures are specific to the diagnoses being considered and are discussed in the appropriate sections below.

Low Back Pain

The most common musculoskeletal complaint seen in primary care is low back pain, with close to 90% of adults having one or more episodes of back pain at some point during their lifetime. About 85% of adults with low back pain have a musculo-ligamentous injury, another 5% have injury to the vertebral disc, and 4% have compression fractures.[1] Description of various symptoms can be used to help identify the cause of pain, such as areas of local tenderness, loss of lower extremity sensation, and loss of motor control. The evaluation of a low back complaint includes ruling out underlying medical disorders including infection, metastatic cancers, pyelonephritis, and referred pain from an abdominal or pelvic disorder. Psychogenic pain secondary to depression must also be considered. Other conditions affecting the back include scoliosis and osteoporosis, which may or may not be associated with pain; these are discussed later in this chapter.

The common musculoskeletal causes of low back pain are shown in **Table 21-1**.

Low back pain can occur as a result of injury to the spinal muscles or lumbar strain, compression of a nerve root that arises from the vertebral column due to degenerative disc disease, herniated nucleus pulposa, inflammation, or vertebral fracture. In the most common presentation, the patient presents with a complaint of pain in the low back, buttock, and posterior thigh, which is described as aching or having a "spasm" like quality. There is often local tenderness and decreased spinal motion. Loss of sensation secondary to nerve damage can cause weakness or numbness in the buttocks and lower extremity, along the affected dermatome (area of spinal nerve distribution).[2]

Diagnosis of Low Back Pain

A thorough medical history, inclusive of any previous injury or trauma, medications, surgeries, and chronic illnesses provides a basis for the examination and eventual diagnosis of low back pain. Psychosocial factors must also be considered, including employment, hobbies, sports, and potential stressors in the home or work environment. Specific history questions related to the back pain must include time of onset, duration, location, and type of pain (shooting, burning, etc.). The presence or absence of sciatica should be determined, as this is a major contributor to the differential diagnosis. It is also important for the clinician to establish any potential aggravating or alleviating factors, such as lifting, movement, heat, or massage. The presence of fever, worsening neurologic deficits, loss of bladder control, or bilateral pain (as opposed to unilateral or central) may signal more significant problems.

A thorough examination of a patient presenting with back pain includes gait evaluation, assessment of active and passive range of motion, and a neurologic examination that assesses sensation, peripheral motor function, and deep tendon reflexes. The symmetry of the spine and muscle tone and mass are evaluated. An abdominal, pelvic, and rectal examination may be necessary to rule out gastrointestinal (GI) involvement, uterine and ovarian causes, and cauda equina syndrome, respectively. Finally, clues to possible systemic causes of pain such as malignancy should be sought.

Straight leg raises (SLR) should be performed as part of the musculoskeletal exam for low back pain. During SLR, reported pain in the low back or buttock is considered a positive and indicates nerve root involvement. The examiner checks to

Table 21-1 COMMON CAUSES OF LOW BACK PAIN

Disorder	Type of Pain	Location	Clinical Signs	Average Age of Onset
Lumbosacral strain	Spasmodic Aching Worsens with movement	Low back area Buttocks	Point tenderness Decreased ROM	20–45
Herniated nucleus pulposa	Shooting pain Lower extremity numbness Increases with bending	Buttocks Lower extremity Calf	Lower extremity weakness Decreased lower extremity reflexes Straight leg raises – positive	30–55
Osteoarthritis	Aching/shooting pain Pinching quality Increases with activity	Low back Lower extremity	Asymmetric LE reflexes Weakness of LE	≥ 50

Abbreviations: ROM, range of motion; LE, lower extremity.

be sure that the pain is reproducible when the patient is distracted from the exercise. Sciatic pain is differentiated from tightness on the posterior leg.[3]

If a clear diagnosis of muscle and ligament strain exists, further diagnostic studies are not warranted. Plain film x-rays are not indicated in the initial management of patients with acute back pain. Certain factors shown in **Table 21-2** increase the risk of serious disease. If these are present, or if the patient does not improve after four to six weeks, further evaluation is warranted. The patient should be referred to a clinician skilled in managing musculoskeletal problems.

A trial in the United Kingdom found no benefit to ordering x-rays even with chronic pain, so long as the symptoms continued to be those of low back strain.[4] **Table 21-3** indicates reasons to consider radiography. Magnetic resonance imaging (MRI) and computed tomography scans may be ordered for prolonged cases and those in which increased soft tissue and nerve root involvement is suspected.

LUMBOSACRAL STRAIN

Low back pain that presents with a sharp pain in the low back region as *lumbosacral strain* prevents the woman from walking or enjoying her normal activities. Lumbosacral strain is common in women aged 16 to 40. Immediate pain may be associated with the movement that initiates the strain, but pain often develops or worsens 12 to 36 hours after an injury, as associated soft tissues become swollen. Symptoms are usually confined to the low back, buttocks,

Table 21-2 RED FLAGS FOR PATIENTS PRESENTING WITH LOW BACK PAIN

Age over 50 years
Temperature >100.4°F/38°C
Loss of bowel or bladder function
Weight loss

and thighs. Common descriptors are spasm, burning or "twinging." Standing and bending are aggravating factors for pain caused by lumbosacral strain; lumbosacral strain also may worsen on inspiration or with sudden movement. Rest and reclining tend to provide relief.

For pain relief, nonsteroidal anti-inflammatory drugs (NSAIDs) such as diclofenac, naproxen, and ibuprofen are commonly used. Common NSAID used in musculoskeletal injury are shown in **Table 21-4**. Muscle relaxants have not been shown to be more effective than NSAIDs and need not be used as adjunctive therapy for this condition. Narcotics may be beneficial for relief of acute pain for a short period of time, not greater than 72 hours duration. However, caution should be taken when using narcotics for acute lumbar strain, as pro-

Table 21-3 INDICATIONS FOR RADIOGRAPHS IN PATIENTS WITH ACUTE LOW BACK PAIN

History of trauma
Neurologic deficit
Symptoms of systemic illness
Temperature >100.4°F/38°C
History of:
    Cancer
    Glucocorticoid use
    Substance abuse (drugs or alcohol)

longed use may lead to dependence. Additionally, intermittent application of ice packs during the first 48 to 72 hours may be beneficial, with heat application if necessary after 72 hours. The cold reduces swelling and bleeding into the tissues, while heat relaxes the muscles and promotes blood flow.

Activity should not be restricted, as prolonged bed rest may worsen lumbosacral strain. Stretching and strengthening exercises have been demonstrated to be most effective, regardless of whether the pain is an acute incident or a chronic condition. Programs should be individualized to encourage patient adherence.[5,6] Low impact aerobic exercise is a good adjunct to therapy after two weeks, including activities such as walking, swimming, and light biking. Participation in structured exercise programs appears to have long-term benefits, including decreased work absence and decreased pain scores.[7] Physical therapy and chiropractic may offer small incremental advantages and in one study significantly improved patient satisfaction with care.[8] Massage therapy has been demonstrated to be beneficial for chronic subacute pain, but data regarding acupuncture for this purpose are unclear.[9] Consideration also should be given to patient lifestyle, because maintaining normal weight and increasing regular exercise activities may assist in limiting recurrence.

Lumbosacral strain usually resolves without further treatment; however, follow-up to assess recovery is recommended one month following the initial visit.

OTHER CONDITIONS PRESENTING AS LOW BACK PAIN

In those clients presenting with a herniated disc (herniated nucleus pulposus), pain is felt in the buttock or radiating down into the lower

Table 21-4 NONSTEROIDAL ANTI-INFLAMMATORY DRUGS FOR MANAGEMENT OF MUSCULOSKELETAL INJURY

Ibuprofen (Motrin, Advil)	Rx 600–800 mg po every 6–8 hours
	OTC 200–400 mg po every 4–6 hours, package labeling specifies not more than 6 tablets/day
Celecoxib (Celebrex)	400 mg po, then 200 mg po every 12 hours
Diclofenac potassium (Cataflam)*	50 mg po tid
Diflunisal (Dolobid)	1000 mg po then 500 mg po every 8–12 hours
Naproxen sodium** (Anaprox 275 mg)	550 mg po then 275 mg po every 6–8 hours or 550 mg every 12 hours
(Anaprox DS)	550 mg po every 12 hours
(Aleve) OTC	220 mg po every 6-8 hours

*Diclofenac sodium (Voltaren, Voltaren XR) is used primarily for symptoms of arthritis, rather than musculoskeletal injury.
**Naproxen (Naprosen, EC-Naprosen) has a slower onset of action and is not generally used for this purpose.
Comment: Use of nonsteroidal anti-inflammatory drugs increases the incidence of gastrointestinal disorders and may also increase the risk of cardiovascular events. Medications used for long-term therapy should be carefully monitored for adverse effects.
Abbreviations: OTC, over the counter; DS, double strength.

extremity as opposed to localizing in the low back area. This condition is related to compression of the nerve root as it emanates from the spinal column, most often at the L4-L5 level, with the possibility of the L5-S1 level being affected either alone or with other vertebrae.

Sciatica is the term used for this irritation of the nerve root. The pain is sharp and radiates down the posterior or lateral portion of the leg to the foot. Numbness and tingling are common. If the compression is progressive weakness, decreased muscle tone and diminished reflexes of the affected lower extremity will develop.[1] Clients with these symptoms should be referred to orthopedics or physical medicine for further evaluation and treatment. Herniation at the thoracic level is rare; however, it should be considered as part of the differential diagnosis of chest and upper extremity complaints. When suspected, a referral for care should be obtained promptly.[10]

Compression fractures are most commonly seen in association with osteoporosis, glucocorticoid use, and metastatic cancer. The pain has a sharp onset. Typically, the distribution of the pain is lateral, rather than extending into the lower extremities. As with herniation of a lumbar disc, patients in whom compression fracture is suspected should be promptly referred to an orthopedic specialist. Any condition that presents with loss of bowel and bladder function (cauda equina syndrome) and those involving paralysis or suspected aneurysm should be considered emergent and be referred to a surgeon immediately.

Some patients suffering from depression will present with somatic symptoms as their primary complaint. In general, these patients will have symptoms that are more severe than the history and examination suggest.

Thorough evaluation is still required to ensure that the medical diagnosis is not obscured by the psychologic one.

Malingering must be considered as a possibility in patients presenting with low back pain. Maneuvers such as axial loading, where the examiner places downward pressure on the top of the head, that elicit pain, and inappropriate complaints of pain on palpation to the areas of the low back that are not involved should clue the examiner to consider malingering as a potential diagnosis.

Clinicians also must be aware that patients with drug-seeking behavior will feign back pain to garner narcotic medication. In the absence of a secure diagnosis, it is not advisable for the midwife or women's health practitioner to provide controlled substances for pain relief. In addition, if the patient has a clinician who is managing a chronic condition such as low back pain, all prescriptions for controlled substances are deferred to that clinician.

Sprain Injuries

Unlike a *strain*, in which there is injury to a segment of a muscle related to excessive forcible stretch such as lumbosacral strain, a *sprain* is an injury to the ligamentous structures of the body. Sprains occur near a joint whereas strains present within the muscle body, which often helps to differentiate between the two forms of injury. Common sites of sprain injury are the wrist, elbow, knee, and ankle.

Loss of continuity when the ligaments are overstretched may result in one of three types of sprains:

- First degree: mildly stretched
- Second degree: moderate stretch with some tearing of the ligament
- Third degree: severe stretch with complete tear (avulsion) of the ligament

The most common sprain is that of the ankle, and these injuries typically occur when someone is walking or running on an uneven surface. Inversion injury to the lateral area of the ankle is the most common presentation. Cardinal signs of ankle sprain include immediate pain, immediate inability to bear weight, the sensation of a "pop" or "snap" and locking of the ankle, and joint swelling within one hour of injury.

Diagnosis of sprain requires a thorough examination of both ankles, beginning with the unaffected side. All structures of the ankle joint are observed and palpated, looking for inflammation, swelling, deformity, hematoma or pallor, intact pulses, crepitation, and decreased active and/or passive range of motion. The inability to bear weight and joint instability are also assessed. **Figure 21-1** illustrates the different parts of the ankle.[11]

Ankle sprains do not require radiography unless criteria suggestive of fracture are met. The Ottawa criteria recommend radiologic studies if there is pain at either the lateral or medial malleolus with bone tenderness at the posterior edge or tip, or an inability to bear weight both immediately after the injury and in the emergency department.[12,13]

Management of sprain is a two-step process. The therapeutic plan for the first 48 hours includes avoidance of weight-bearing activity, using crutches or splints as necessary, NSAIDs for pain relief, and RICE therapy (**Table 21-5**).[11]

After the first two days, soaking the affected joint alternately in warm and cold water, dorsiflexion/plantarflexion exercises, and isometric resistance exercises can be started. Use of compression bandages can be continued to reduce swelling and stabilize the joint. Plastic braces also may be used to stabilize the ankle during recovery. For first and second degree sprains,

Figure 21-1 Lateral view of the ankle.[11]

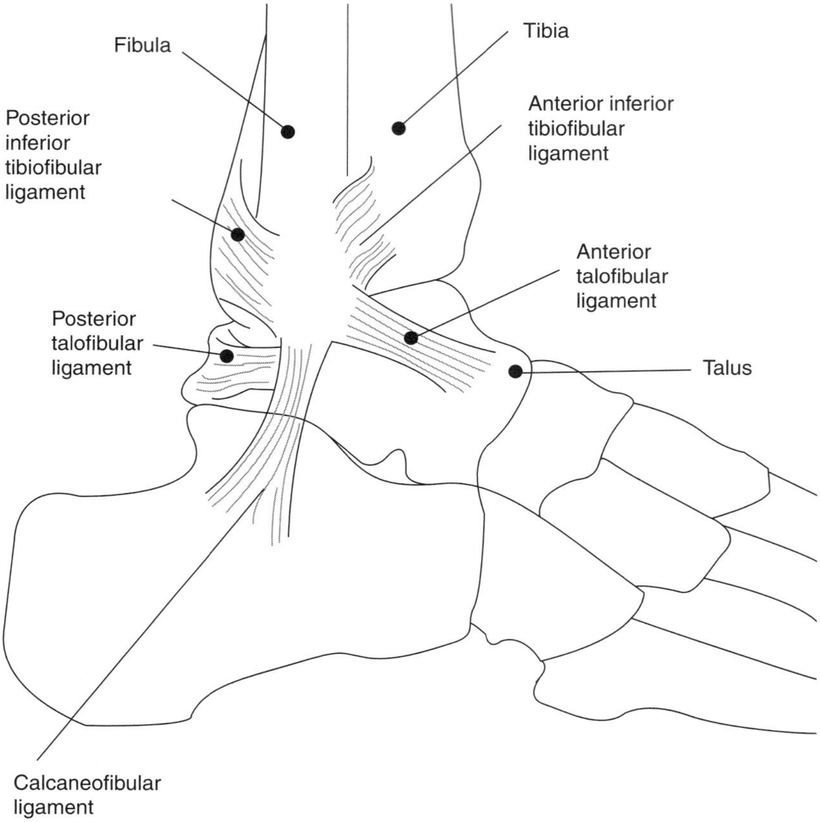

these measures will usually suffice. However, third degree sprains with complete ligament tear often require surgery.[14]

Four to six weeks is an average time for complete recovery. During that time, the clinician should monitor for a possible fracture and for neurovascular compromise. Ankle fractures are rare and involve the malleoli either unilaterally or bilaterally.

Although sprains often are regarded as minor injuries, severe sprains require orthopedic evaluation and joint immobilization during healing. If the degree of injury is unclear or the examination suggests the need for radiology, referral to an orthopedic provider is indicated. Finally, patients need to understand that resolution of pain does not indicate complete recovery of ligament strength, which may take several months, depending on the severity of the injury.

Costochondritis

Costochondritis is an inflammation in the interface between the bony and cartilaginous area of

Table 21-5 MANAGEMENT OF PAIN FROM A SPRAIN USING THE RICE MNEMONIC[11]

- **Rest** – Use a cane on the opposite side from the injury, crutches as necessary, and reduce activity to the minimum necessary.
- **Ice** – Applied for 20 minutes 4 to 8 times a day.
- **Compression** – Elastic bandages, an air cast, or splints may be applied for support.
- **Elevation** – Above the level of the heart if possible.

the thoracic cage, the costochondral junction, which causes chest pain. Often, more than one area may be involved; edema may be associated with the affected joints. The woman with costochondritis usually presents with unilateral pain and can point to the location of maximum discomfort. The pain may be sharp or dull, and the duration varies. The pain is increased on movement and with deep inspiration and expiration, and is usually relieved with rest, change of position, and quiet breathing.

The patient may report trauma due to repetitive movements or moving heavy objects. However, in some cases, women may not be aware of the condition until the affected area is palpated, such as during breast exam or chest percussion. On examination, pain is elicited by palpating the involved costochondral joint(s).

A chest x-ray may be ordered to rule out more serious conditions such as pneumonia, and to assess the possibility of any rib fractures. Anyone presenting with chest pain should be evaluated for a potential cardiac or respiratory condition such as myocardial infarction, pericarditis, or pleurisy before a diagnosis of costochondritis is finalized (see Chapters 13 and 14).

Management of costochondritis includes NSAIDs, cold and heat applications, and light exercise to stretch the chest wall muscles. Narcotic analgesics are not indicated. The course of the condition is self-limiting, with complete resolution in four to six weeks.

Carpal Tunnel Syndrome

Carpal tunnel syndrome is a frequent cause of pain and numbness in the hands and a major contributor to work absences. Estimates of lifetime risk are as high as 10%.[15] Atroshi et al.'s survey reported that close to 15% of their sample had symptoms of pain, numbness, or tingling along the median nerve; after clinical examination and electrophysiological testing, about 20% of those who were symptomatic met the criteria for diagnosis of carpal tunnel syndrome.[16] Women have an increased incidence relative to men, but the magnitude of the reported difference varies. Work-related carpal tunnel syndrome is most common in women between 20 and 40 years of age, and nonwork related incidence peaks after age 50.

Clients who engage in occupations that involve repetitive wrist movements, whether in an office or manual labor settings, are most likely to be affected. Hobbies that require frequent repetitive movements, such as knitting, can also increase risk, and medical conditions such as hypothyroidism, diabetes mellitus, and rheumatoid arthritis may play a role. Excessive computer use is frequently cited as likely to increase risk of carpal tunnel syndrome. At least one large survey found a minimal effect other than with use of a computer mouse for more than 30 hours a week.[17]

Women are also prone to injury when their estrogen levels are lower than usual, including pregnancy, lactation, and menopause. Most commonly, the syndrome presents late in pregnancy as a transient problem.[16,18–19] Pregnancy-associated carpal tunnel syndrome is associated with edema of the hands and wrists.[20]

Carpal tunnel syndrome is an entrapment neuropathy caused by compression of the median nerve and hand tendons as they pass through the carpal tunnel, a narrow ligamentous passage between the small bones of the wrists. The pressure results in inflammation and swelling of the soft tissue structures. Carpal tunnel syndrome presents with a complaint of pain in the wrists and numbness in the hands and fingers. Occasionally, the pain will radiate up the affected arm. The pain is related to ischemia of the median nerve more often than actual nerve damage. Discomfort is often first noticed at night.

Numbness of the hand occurs mainly in the thumb, index, and middle fingers, with the most significant loss of sensation centrally. A protracted course of carpal tunnel pain can involve the fourth digit and the distal portion of the fifth digit. Grip may be decreased as nerve innervation of the hand muscles is impaired.

Examination of the patient reveals decreased sensation of the palm in the distribution of the median nerve as well as the fingers. **Figure 21-2** shows the area of the hand innervated by the median nerve. In persistent conditions, thumb weakness and thenar atrophy (decreased muscle mass at the base of the thumb) can be found. Attention should be given to other conditions that may produce similar symptoms, testing for diabetes or arthritis, and looking for indication of strains or fractures.[19] Assessment of other possible neurologic causes is also necessary. While carpal tunnel syndrome and related symptoms are the most common cause of hand pain, cervical spine injury and other nerve entrapments can exist.

Two easy tests for in-office screening involve Phalen and Tinel signs. A positive *Phalen sign*

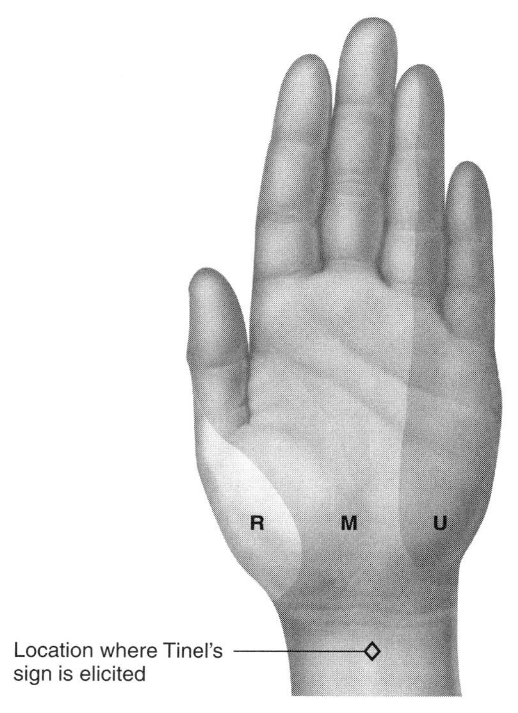

Figure 21-2 Distribution of sensation by the radial (R), median (M), and ulnar (U) nerves.

results in numbness and paresthesia in the affected area after 60 seconds of hyperflexion of the wrist. *Tinel sign* is positive when tapping over the median nerve on the volar aspect of the wrist elicits paresthesia. Both are standard parts of the evaluation when carpal tunnel is suspected. Positive results indicate the need for further evaluation.

Electromyelogram (EMG; nerve conduction) studies are necessary for a definitive diagnosis; the EMG also provides information about the severity of median nerve compromise. X-rays and MRI have little value in making a diagnosis; ultrasound is not regularly used but is being studied.[21]

Mild carpal tunnel syndrome is managed with NSAIDs, wrist rests, and assistive devices that prevent the injured area from being subjected to the repetitive trauma of certain activities. The use of wrist splints when at rest can maintain the wrist and hand in a neutral position to promote relief. Inexpensive wrist splints are available at medical supply houses. For most effective use, splints should be fitted by a physical therapist or orthopedic clinician. Corticosteroid injections may be necessary and should be considered based on the severity of nerve involvement. Surgery is the definitive treatment for severe carpal tunnel syndrome, although it does not lead to complete resolution in all cases.

Except for the transient syndrome of late pregnancy, midwives should refer women with carpal tunnel syndrome to an orthopedist if the relief measures above do not provide prompt relief. Options for treatment are limited during the course of pregnancy. Early onset in pregnancy is associated with poorer outcomes.[22]

Scoliosis

Scoliosis is a progressive disorder usually identified in childhood that affects young women twice as often as young men. Most commonly it is an idiopathic disease, although other conditions may underlie its development, such as cerebral palsy or polio. It also appears as part of some congenital syndromes. There is lateral curvature of the spinal column with vertebral rotation. Pain rarely accompanies this condition; however, pain may be present in clients with adjunct clinical conditions of the spine such as *spondylolisthesis* (forward subluxation of a vertebrae) or spinal tumor. **Figure 21-3** depicts the spine curvatures attributable to scoliosis.[23]

Idiopathic scoliosis usually develops after age 10. The overall incidence is about 3 to 5 per 1000 children. The plan of management is based on degree of spinal deformity and bone maturity.[23]

Idiopathic scoliosis has been studied over a 50-year period by Weinstein and colleagues. Their findings included a generally high standard of function and productive adult life. The incidence of back pain and shortness of breath were higher than in the comparison group. No other significant difficulties were reported.[24] Increased risk of osteoporosis related to bracing for treatment of scoliosis has been posited. Snyder and colleagues studied adolescent females and found increases in spinal bone density appropriate for age and menstrual status.[25]

Unlevel shoulders and protruding scapulae are commonly seen clinically and are cues for the examiner to evaluate the client for scoliosis. A right thoracic curvature is most common, and presents with the right shoulder deviating in a forward rotation and the medial border of the scapula deviating posteriorly. Physical examination to evaluate for scoliosis includes a baseline assessment of client posture and body contour. An abnormal rib cage shape or an asymmetric waist also should trigger consideration of scoliosis. A forward-bend test is used to assess the potential extent of spinal curvature. The patient is asked to bend forward from the waist, presenting the spine to identify any curvature. Whenever a forward bend test (one where the spine is not aligned normally) is positive, the patient should be referred for orthopedic care.[23]

Scoliosis is best managed by an orthopedic physician. Common treatments for milder forms of scoliosis include observation with follow-up

---

Figure 21-3 Curve patterns of the spine.[23]

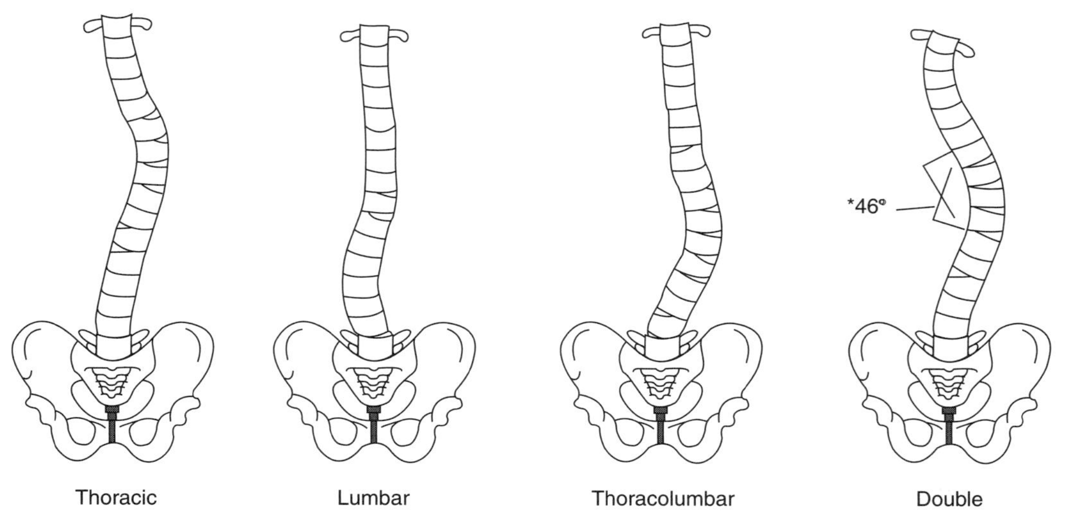

---

x-rays at regular intervals. More severe forms are treated with mechanical bracing and surgery. Exercise, chiropractic, transcutaneous electrical stimulation, or nutritional interventions have not been shown to help.[23] Based on the progressive nature of scoliosis, aggressive follow-up is necessary. The midwife's participation in management is limited to encouraging the patient to follow through with orthopedic visits.

During pregnancy, uncorrected scoliosis may be problematic for the mother because of the increased stress placed on the spine by the enlarging uterus. At delivery, women who have had surgery to repair the spinal curve may be unable to have regional anesthesia. When the midwife is aware of a history of scoliosis repair or, indeed, any spinal surgery, an anesthesia consult should be scheduled prior to the onset of labor. This holds true even when the management plan for labor does not include regional anesthesia. In the event of an emergency, the mother and her fetus will be best served by a well-informed anesthesia team.

Arthritic Conditions

There are more than 100 causes of arthritic pain. The etiologies are diverse, and management of arthropathies is beyond the scope of this text or of women's health care. Including the rheumatoid diseases, they range from infections such as Lyme disease to lupus to fibromyalgia. Four of the most common conditions are presented here, because all primary care clinicians should be able to recognize and refer appropriately women with these joint diseases. *Osteoarthritis* is the most common of these, affecting as many as 20% of those over 65 years of age. It is a degenerative disease of the cartilage with associated bone overgrowth.[26] In contrast, *rheumatoid arthritis* is a chronic inflammatory process with an immunologic basis. Three percent of women and 1% of men have a sure or probable diagnosis.[27] *Gout*, the cause of about 5% of arthritis diagnoses, is the result of uric acid deposits in tendons and joints.[28] *Fibromyalgia*, a syndrome classed with the rheumatic diseases, is a condition found predominantly in women.

Symptoms common to many of the arthritic and rheumatoid diseases are shown in **Table 21-6**.

Relevant history for arthritic and rheumatoid conditions includes the onset, persistence, and quality of pain; effect of activity and rest; number of joints affected; recent illnesses or injuries; current medications; and whether family members have a history of these conditions. Often patients are asked to maintain a daily journal of symptoms. The examination includes assessment of the joints for erythema, warmth, pain, and range of motion. A number of different laboratory tests and procedures may be ordered, depending on the differential diagnosis for each patient.[29]

Table 21-6 COMMON SYMPTOMS OF ARTHRITIS[29]

- Swelling in one or more joints
- Stiffness around the joints that lasts for at least one hour in the early morning
- Constant or recurring pain or tenderness in a joint
- Difficulty using or moving a joint normally
- Warmth and redness in a joint

As with other health problems considered in this chapter, NSAIDs are often considered as a treatment option for arthritic conditions. All NSAIDs share an increased risk of gastric toxicity, which can limit their utility. The adverse effects can range from stomach discomfort to bleeding or perforation.[30] The cyclooxygenase-2 (COX-2) specific inhibitors were developed to offer similar pain relief with reduced GI effects. However, at least two of the drugs in this class (valdecoxib [Bextra] and rofecoxib [Vioxx]) have been withdrawn from the market, based on inceased risk of cardiovascular events such as myocardial infarction and ischemic stroke, and other drugs in this class also have a demonstrated increase in cardiovascular risk.[31,32] Providers using these medications should be aware of these and other risks associated with NSAID and COX-2 use and advise patients carefully. There is some evidence[33,34] that patients may neither receive adequate information regarding medication options, or be followed with appropriate monitoring to reduce risks of medication use.

Osteoarthritis

Osteoarthritis is primarily a chronic hypertrophic arthropathy in which there is degeneration of the articular cartilage and reactive osteophyte formation in a joint space, leading to degenerative joint disease. Osteoarthritis has a peak incidence at age 65, with women being affected more than men at a rate of 2:1. The joints most commonly involved are the knees, hips, hands, cervical spine, and lumbar spine. Osteoarthritis usually affects joints unilaterally and asymmetrically.[26]

Development of osteoarthritis is associated with overuse, physical stressors, obesity, and joint laxity. Secondary forms of osteoarthritis also may develop following autoimmune diseases, avascular necrosis, chronic illness, and infection.

There is a strong genetic component for hand and hip osteoarthritis, but less so for knee problems. The role of estrogen in the prevention or development of osteoarthritis is unclear, but it may have a mild protective benefit related to increased bone mass.[29,35] Maintaining a normal weight throughout life can be important in reducing the risk of osteoarthritis.[36] Particularly for older women, obesity is strongly linked to osteoarthritis in the knees, and weight reduction programs can reduce the risk by more than 50%.[37,38]

Bony sclerosis, loss of cartilage, and osteophyte formation all lead to joint space narrowing. The narrowed joint space causes symptoms that include pain that is aggravated by weight-bearing pressure and morning stiffness. Acute inflammatory flares due to overuse and environmental temperature change are common to osteoarthritis. Over time, progressive deformation of the joints leads to increasing disability, pain, limitation in range of motion, and joint instability.

Diagnosis is made with a combination of history, examination, and radiography. When suspected in a women's health setting, osteoarthritis should be referred to a clinician with skills in orthopedic diagnosis and management.

Treatment options for osteoarthritis include acetaminophen and ibuprofen, tramadol (a synthetic opioid agonist), rest, weight reduction; intra-articular corticosteroid injection; and physiotherapy. End-stage osteoarthritis may require surgery. Capsaicin creams have demonstrated some benefit. Although a number of complementary therapies have been suggested, none have demonstrated long-term benefits. In several cases, a strong placebo effect has been noted.[26,39]

Rheumatoid Arthritis

Rheumatoid arthritis is a chronic inflammatory arthropathy that occurs bilaterally in joints of the hands, hips, and knees. The condition usually begins in one to two joints and often will progress to 20 or more, initially affecting the proximal interphalangeal, metacarpophalangeal, and metatarsophalangeal joints. It affects small joints primarily, but any peripheral joint may be affected. There is often synovial proliferation (pannus), inflammation synovitis, and erosion of the articular surfaces of the bones in affected joints.

Rheumatoid arthritis is characterized clinically by inflammation of a joint, tenderness to palpation of the affected joints, limited joint function, and morning stiffness that lasts longer than an hour. There may also be associated fever, fatigue, and inflammatory vascular conditions accompanying this autoimmune disorder.[40] The disease exists in both remitting-relapsing and progressive forms.

Young age at onset and female sex have been identified in some studies as being related to poorer outcomes. Level of joint erosion at diagnosis may also provide clues as to eventual disability, although clinical markers are most predictive of the likelihood of remissions (**Table 21-7**).[41]

Because of the possibility of multisystem involvement, rheumatoid arthritis is best evaluated and managed by a specialist such as a rheumatologist or physiatrist. Diagnostic laboratory testing includes rheumatoid arthritis factor and erythrocyte sedimentation rate. A positive rheumatoid arthritis factor result and increased erythrocyte sedimentation rate support the diagnosis of rheumatoid arthritis.

Table 21-7 Features of
Rheumatoid Arthritis[29]

- Tender, warm, swollen joints
- Symmetrical pattern of affected joints
- Joint inflammation often affecting the wrist and finger joints closest to the hand
- Joint inflammation sometimes affecting other joints, including the neck, shoulders, elbows, hips, knees, ankles, and feet
- Fatigue, occasional fevers, a general sense of not feeling well
- Pain and stiffness lasting for more than 30 minutes in the morning or after a long rest
- Symptoms that last for many years
- Variability of symptoms among people with the disease

Women in whom rheumatoid arthritis is suspected should be told that early diagnosis and management improve the likelihood of maintaining functional capacity. Management can include pain control with NSAIDs, corticosteroids for symptomatic relief on a short-term basis, medications to delay or prevent disease progression, and regular monitoring of symptoms. Surgery can be used to replace destroyed joints. Prevention of osteoporosis, to which rheumatoid arthritis patients are prone secondary to inactivity and steroid treatment, is an additional concern.[27]

Gout

Gout is an erosive arthritis that results from the deposition of sodium urate crystals in connective tissue or in one or more joints, with the first occurrence often being in the big toes. About 5% of all arthritis diagnoses are gout. Gout is most common in males over 40.[42] The incidence range is 5.0 to 6.6 per 1000 in men and 1.0 to 3.0 per thousand in women, although self-reported cases are approximately twice those levels.[43] A condi-

tion that resembles gout in clinical findings is called pseudogout, or chostrocalcinosis; it is caused by calcium phosphate deposits.

The pathologic basis of gout is either overproduction or under-excretion of uric acid. Many cases are idiopathic. Among the associated factors for increased risk are genetic predisposition, obesity, excessive alcohol intake, high purine diet (e.g., liver, dried beans), lead exposure, medications including diuretics, salicylates, and niacin.[42]

Prevention of gout includes dietary changes, specifically the avoidance of dietary fats and purine-rich foods such as organ meats and aged cheeses. Rapid weight loss diets can stimulate new attacks and should be avoided. Avoidance of alcohol, particularly of excessive drinking, is essential to prevent recurrences.[28]

The classic presentation of gout is unilateral pain in the first metatarsophalangeal joint (podagra). In the first episode, sudden onset of pain, worsening over several hours, is followed by complete recovery within days or weeks. On examination there is pain to palpation, swelling, decreased mobility, and inflammation of the affected joint. Intermittent periods without any symptoms occur, although these become shorter over time. As the disease advances, multiple joints can be involved and healing is slowed.[43]

Intermittent hyperuricemia is found in gout but is not pathognomonic. Diagnosis is made by aspiration of synovial fluid for evaluation.[43] Initial plain films of joints affected by gout are negative, as involvement is confined to the soft tissues and involves asymmetric inflammation in affected joints. Later stages of chronic gout show notable changes, and "punched-out" lesions appear in the bony structures on x-ray. After several years of chronic gout, large *tophi* (collections of sodium urate crystals imbedded in an inflammatory response) are a hallmark sign and can be seen on x-ray along with joint space narrowing.

Treatment of acute gout is accomplished with NSAIDs, particularly indomethacin (Indocin), and rest of the affected joint. Injectable corticosteroids may also be used to provide local pain relief. Long-term treatment of gout includes allopurinal, probenecid, and colchicine. Allopurinol is not used during an acute attack, because it may aggravate symptoms. As with the other arthritic conditions, referral for physician management is most appropriate.

Fibromyalgia

Fibromyalgia is a chronic disorder that is characterized by diffuse muscle pain, fatigue, and multiple tender points on various areas of the body. It affects as many as one in 50 Americans and approximately 80% to 90% of diagnoses are in women. Persons with other rheumatic diseases (i.e., lupus and rheumatoid arthritis) are also prone to fibromyalgia.[44]

Fibromyalgia is considered a rheumatic disorder; however, it is not a true arthritis. There is no inflammation of the joints, nor is there any destruction of the associated tissues such as cartilage or muscle. Pain and fatigue, headache, sleep disturbances, morning stiffness, increased sensitivity to heat or cold, and extremity numbness and tingling are common symptoms. By virtue of the potential myriad of possible symptoms, it is considered a syndrome rather than a disease. The actual cause of fibromyalgia is unknown. There may be musculoskeletal, neurologic, genetic, and psychologic factors that contribute to the development of this disorder. Recent research suggests that fibromyalgia demonstrates a familial pattern, and it may be linked to strong family history of mood disorders.[45,46]

For a diagnosis of fibromyalgia to be considered, the examiner must elicit 11 of 18 tender points on various areas of the body (**Figure 21-4**), while applying at least 4 kg of pressure to the site. Complaints of widespread pain lasting three months or longer and affecting all four quadrants of the body (above and below the waist and bilaterally) are other criteria that must be met for a diagnosis.

A team treatment approach has been proven to be most effective, with primary care, physi-

Figure 21-4 Tender points of the body.[44]

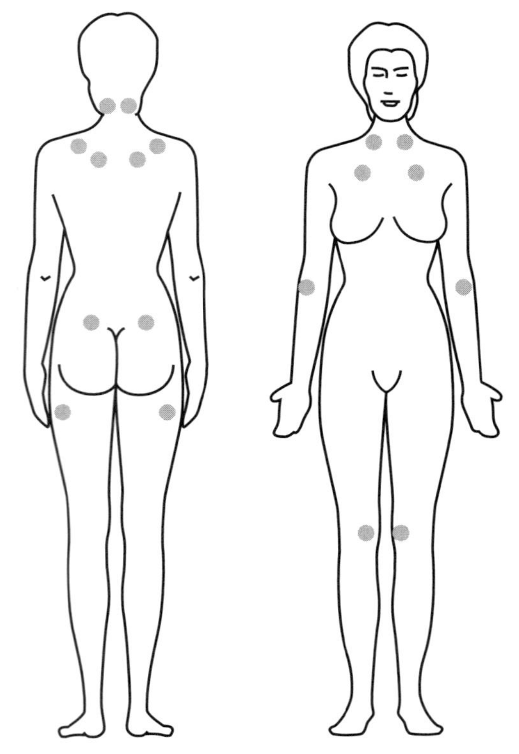

Note: Location of the nine paired tender points that comprise the 1990 American College of Rheumatology Criteria for Fibromyalgia.

cal medicine, and psychotherapy professionals lending clinical expertise to provide a well-rounded treatment plan. Women's health practitioners need to be aware of the diagnosis and management for fibromyalgia, but should not offer primary care for women with a suspected diagnosis outside of such a team setting.

Ample data demonstrate that structured exercise programs are a major contributor to improved health and quality of life.[47–49] Counseling or other interventions to deal with comorbid mood disorders can benefit women for whom these are affecting fibromyalgia management.[50,51] Combinations of exercise, patient education, provision of behavioral therapy, and medication are most frequently effective.[48,52]

The U.S. Food and Drug Administration has not approved any drugs specifically for the treatment of fibromyalgia. Clinicians often incorporate analgesics such as acetaminophen and NSAIDs, to provide pain relief, antidepressants to deal with depressive symptoms, pain and fatigue, benzodiazepines to relax muscles and promote rest, and other drugs such as gabapentin (Neurontin).[44]

Complementary therapies that have been explored include massage, chiropractic, acupuncture, and a variety of dietary supplements, but no solid evidence supports their effectiveness at this time.[44] However, given the interrelationship of mental status and pain in fibromyalgia, patients should discuss these therapies with their primary provider.

Osteoporosis

Osteoporosis affects more than 10 million Americans, more than half of all persons over 50; an additional 34 million have osteopenia. Eighty percent of cases are in women.[53] As many as 40% of Caucasian women over 50 will have an osteoporosis-related fracture during the remainder of their lives.[54] Rates are also rising among Hispanic women.[55] As the population ages, dramatic increases are predicted for rates of fracture and the resultant morbidity.

The 2004 Surgeon General's Report on Bone Health and Osteoporosis[56] cited a yearly rate of 1.5 million osteoporotic fractures, with more than 0.5 million hospitalizations and placement of almost 200,000 persons in nursing homes.

Osteoporosis is a diffuse skeletal disease with increased bone fragility and fracture risk.[57] The condition is characterized by the deterioration of bone mass, with *osteoclast* (bone resorbing) activity exceeding *osteoblast* (bone forming) cell activity. Primary osteoporosis is seen in both males and females at all ages. Secondary osteoporosis can be the result of medications, disease states, or genetic predisposition. Medications can induce osteoporosis by causing hypogonadism or interfering with vitamin D metabolism. **Table 21-8** lists risk factors for both primary and secondary osteoporosis.

Peak bone mass is attained in 95% of women by age 16, although further small increases are possible before age 30.[60,61] Genetic factors account for about 75% of the variation in peak bone mass.[62] Until menopause, there is little further alteration in a woman's bone mass and structure. Following the decrease in circulating estrogens that accompanies the cessation of menses, bone density drops dramatically over several years. Women using hormonal therapy delay but do not prevent this change.

Screening

Clinically, osteoporosis is defined as decreased bone mineral density (BMD) that is more than 2.5 standard deviations below that of a healthy 25 year-old individual of the same sex, as

Table 21-8 RISK FACTORS FOR PRIMARY AND SECONDARY OSTEOPOROSIS[57–59]

Primary
  Older age
  Low body weight
  Low BMI
  Sedentary lifestyle
  Fair skin
  Female gender
  Postmenopausal status (without current HRT)
  Hypogonadic states
  Low calcium intake
  Family history
  Tobacco use
  Excess alcohol use
Secondary
  Medications include:
    Medroxyprogesterone
    Corticosteroids
    Antiepileptics
    SSRI antidepressants
    Excess thyroid hormone
    Chronic heparin, coumadin treatment
    Methotrexate
    Cholestyramine
  Diseases include:
    Malnutrition (e.g., anorexia nervosa)
    Vitamin B_{12} deficiency
    Diabetes mellitus
    Hyperthyroidism
    Hyperparathyroidism
    Hyperprolactinemia
    Cushing's disease
    Rheumatoid arthritis
    Organ transplant survivors
    Gastrectomy patients
    Inflammatory Bowel disease
  Genetic risks include:
    Marfan syndrome
    Thalassemia
    Celiac disease
    Hemochromatosis
    Osteogenesis imperfecta
    Homocystinuria
    Ehlers Danlos syndrome

evaluated by Dual Energy X-ray (DEXA) Absorption scan of the lumbar vertebrae and hip. Osteopenia is the term used when bone density is decreased to 1 to 2.5 standard deviations below the mean. The term used to describe these scores is "T score." The "Z score" is a measurement of BMD in relation to age and sex adjusted norms; a normal Z score does not rule out osteoporotic changes in adults because bone loss is common in older individuals. Therefore while a "Z-score" provides a comparative assessment of age-matched bone density levels, it is not used to indicate whether treatment is needed. Treatment is based on the "T score." The complete World Health Organization criteria for diagnosis are shown in **Table 21-9**.

Both the United States Preventive Services Task Force[64] and the National Osteoporosis Foundation (NOF)[65] recommend BMD screening in all women age 65 and older, regardless of risk factors. Each also recommends screening for women with risk factors, although the age cutoff varies. See Chapter 3 for details on recommendations made by other organizations.

Other methods of screening for osteoporosis include peripheral dual x-ray absorptiometry (pDXA) and single-energy x-ray absorptiometry (SXA), which measure bone density in the

Table 21-9 WHO CRITERIA FOR DIAGNOSIS OF OSTEOPOROSIS[63]

DEXA score for women after menopause	T score
Normal	-1.0 to $0+$
Osteopenia	-2.5 to -1.0
Osteoporosis	<-2.5
Severe Osteoporosis	$<-2.5 + \geq$ fragility fracture

forearm, finger, or heel; quantitative computed tomography, which measures trabecular and cortical bone density at various sites; and ultrasound densitometry. Ultrasound measurements are generally not as precise as pDXA or SXA, but appear to predict fracture risk as well as other measures of bone density. Serum or urine biochemical markers can identify changes in bone turnover, but are not used in lieu of BMD evaluation.[65] Plain radiographs will not reveal changes unless bone loss is greater than 30%.[58] Because this reflects a significant increase in risk, x-ray is not an acceptable method of screening for osteoporosis.

Several screening tools are available for provider use; none are specific enough to use instead of BMD, although they can be used to screen for additional women who are at risk and require evaluation. Two of these tools, the Simple Calculated Osteoporosis Risk Estimation and the Osteoporosis Risk Assessment Instrument, had similar sensitivity to the NOF recommendations. None of these three methods was specific; between 60 and 90 percent of in the group identified for screening were without osteoporosis.[66,67]

Osteoporosis Prevention

The most effective preventive measures for osteoporosis are those that increase peak bone mass in the young adult years and promote adequate calcium and vitamin D intake. Thus, counseling to increase exercise, promote healthy dietary habits, and decrease tobacco and alcohol use are core parts of health maintenance visits for all women of reproductive age, beginning in adolescence. Assessments of dietary intake of calcium and sun exposure for stimulation of vitamin D production are also valuable. All women whose diets are deficient should be encouraged to supplement appropri-

ately. Recommendations for calcium and vitamin D intake are shown in **Table 21-10**. At least one author has identified the necessary vitamin D intake for those without sun exposure to be 1000 IU/day.[69] Many women who are postmenopausal, even those on osteoporosis therapy, remain vitamin D deficient, which directly impacts the body's ability to maintain bone mass.[70]

Following menopause, consideration should be given to beginning a preventive regimen of bisphosphonates or a selective estrogen receptor modulator. Continued exercise and appropriate dietary supplements are also recommended. Although the use of hormonal therapy has decreased in the wake of evidence that risks of cardiovascular disease and cancer are increased, they remain available and can be considered in the context of individual risks and benefits; however, they are not the first choice to consider.

Because medroxprogesterone acetate (Depoprovera) has been shown to have at least a short-term effect on BMD in young women,[71] discussion of risks of bone loss should be part of contraceptive counseling for this product. Additionally, in recommending Depoprovera,

---

Table 21-10 RECOMMENDATIONS FOR CALCIUM AND VITAMIN D INTAKE IN WOMEN[68]

Calcium	
Age	Milligrams/day
9–18	1300
19–50	1000
51 and older	1200
Vitamin D	
Age	IU/day
9–50	200
51–70	400
71 and older	600

the midwife should consider whether additional risk factors for decreased bone mass exist, remembering that young women can also develop osteoporosis. Studies indicate that bone density increases to normal levels following discontinuation of depoprovera.[72] Combined hormonal contraception, in contrast, does not have a significant effect on bone density.[73]

Pregnancy and lactation have been shown to produce a short-term decrease in BMD in some women, but this effect does not increase osteporosis risk in later life.[74–77]

Presentation

Osteoporosis can present silently or with minimal symptoms, reinforcing the importance of screening and attention to risk factors presented in the history. Loss of height and changes in spinal curvature suggest its presence. A decrease in height is an indicator of loss of height of the vertebrae. For this reason, it is necessary to monitor a woman's height at each preventive visit. On examination, an increased thoracic kyphosis or decreased curvature of the lumbar lordosis is commonly seen when the woman is in a standing position.

Localized spinal tenderness may be present, with spinal flexion increasing pain more than extension. When the vertebrae are involved in osteoporosis, the woman may present with neck or back pain. Osteoporosis of the spinal column causes weakening and pathologic wedge-fracture of the vertebrae, which, in turn may sublux and exert pressure on spinal peripheral nerve roots.

Fracture is a late presentation in osteoporosis. Most commonly, the wrist, lumbar vertebrae, and hip at are risk. Relative risk of fracture increases two to three times with each 1.0 decrease in T score. However, there is significant overlap between T scores of those with and without fracture.[78] Increasing age also inde-

Table 21-11 MEDICATIONS USED IN THE PREVENTION OR TREATMENT OF OSTEOPOROSIS

Bisphosphonates
  Alendronate (Fosamax)
    Prevention: 5 mg daily or 35 mg once per week.
    Treatment: 10 mg daily or 70 mg once per week.
  Risendronate (Actonel)
    Prevention/ Treatment: 5 mg daily or 35 mg once per week
Selective Estrogen Receptor Modulators
  Raloxifene (Evista)
    Prevention/Treatment: 60 mg daily
Hormone Therapies
  Estrogens (such as Climara, Estrace, Estraderm, Estratab, Menostar, Ogen, Ortho-Est, Premarin, Vivelle)
    Prevention: dosage varies
  Estrogens and Progestins (such as Activella, FemHrt, Premphase, Prempro)
    Prevention: dosage varies
  Calcitonin (Miacalcin)
  Treatment: 100 Units IM or SC, every other day, or three times a week
Calcium Supplements
  1200–1500 mg elemental calcium daily
Vitamin D Supplements
  800 IU daily

Abbreviations: IM, intramuscular; SC, subcutaneous; IU, international units.

pendently increases fracture risk due to factors including bone changes such as decreased flexibility and increased brittleness, decreasing weight with age, decreased visual acuity, mental confusion, and loss of stability.

Hip fracture has been demonstrated to be the most likely injury to reduce survival, resulting in a 10% to 20% excess mortality. A quarter of women with hip fracture as a result of osteoporosis will require nursing home care; only 40% will recover full function.[65]

Management of Osteoporosis

Management of osteoporosis is best accomplished using a combination of medications; nonpharmacologic therapy including calcium supplementation and vitamin D supplements; and weight-bearing exercise. The NOF recommends beginning therapy to reduce fracture risk in postmenopausal women with BMD T-scores below −2 in the absence of risk factors and in women with T-scores below −1.5 if one or more risk factors are present.[65] Currently approved therapies for prevention and treatment of osteoporosis are listed in **Table 21-11**.

Current pharmacologic options for osteoporosis treatment are bisphosphonates (alendronate and risedronate), calcitonin, parathyroid hormone (PTH 1-34), and raloxifene. Other bisphosphonates are also available, but are not indicated for osteoporosis treatment. Potential treatments include tamoxifen, which exerts an estrogen-like effect on bone cells, and teriparatide (Forteo) a recombinant parathyroid hormone.

Counseling includes the importance of adequate calcium and vitamin D supplementation, increasing activity by adding weight bearing and muscle strengthening exercises, and fall prevention. A 30-minute walk at least three times a week is effective exercise.

Conclusion

This chapter has presented a range of conditions that primary care providers, including midwives and other women's health practitioners, can expect to see in practice. Not all are appropriate for management in the women's health setting. Others, such as osteoporosis, are central to the care of older women. In making decisions about when to treat and when to refer, the clinician should always be aware of both her own skill set and the resources available.

References

1. Goroll AH, Mulley AG. Evaluation of low back pain. In: Goroll AH, Mulley AG, editors. *Primary Care Medicine*. 4th ed. Philadelphia, Lippincott Williams & Wilkins; 2000.

2. National Institute of Arthritis, Musculoskeletal and Skin Diseases. Health Topics. Spinal stenosis [database on the Internet; accessed 7/05, 12/05]. Available from http://ww.niams.nih.gov/hi.

3. National Institute of Arthritis, Musculoskeletal and Skin Diseases. Health Topics. Back pain [Database on the Internet; accessed 7/05, 12/05]. Available from http://ww.niams.nih.gov/hi.

4. Kendrick D, Fielding K, Bentley E, Miller P, Kerslake R, Pringle M. The role of radiography in primary care patients with low back pain of at least 6 weeks duration: A randomized (unblended) controlled trial. *Health Technol Assess*. 2001;5:1–69.

5. Hayden JA, van Tulder MW, Tomlinson G. Systematic review: Strategies for using exercise therapy to improve outcomes in chronic low back pain. *Ann Intern Med*. 2005;142:776–785.

6. Hayden JA, van Tulder MW, Malmivaara AV, Koes BW. Meta-analysis: Exercise therapy for nonspecific low back pain. *Ann Intern Med*. 2005;142:765–775.

7. Moffett JK, Torgerson D, Bell-Syer S, Jackson D, Llewelyn-Phillips H, Farrin A, Barber J. Randomised controlled trial of exercise for low back pain: Clinical outcomes, costs, and preferences. *BMJ*. 1999;319:279–283.

8. Cherkin DC, Deyo RA, Battie M, Street J, Barlow W. A comparison of physical therapy, chiropractic manipulation, and provision of an exercise booklet for the treatment of low back pain. *N Engl J Med*. 1998;339:1021–1029.

9. Cherkin DC, Sherman KJ, Deya RA, Shelleke PG. A review of the evidence for the effectiveness, safety and cost of acupuncture, massage therapy, and spinal manipulation for back pain. *Ann Intern Med*. 2003;138: 898–906.

10. National Institute of Arthritis, Musculoskeletal and Skin Diseases. Health Topics. Back pain [Database on the Internet; accessed 7/05, 12/05]. Available from http://www.niams.nih.gov/hi.

11. National Institute of Arthritis, Musculoskeletal and Skin Diseases. Health Topics. Sprains and strains [Database on the Internet; accessed 7/05, 12/05]. Available from http://www.niams.nih.gov/hi.

12. Stiell I, Greenberg GH, McKnight RD, Nair RC, McDowell I, Worthington JR. A study to develop clinical decision rules for the use of radiography in acute ankle injuries. *Ann Emerg Med*. 1992;21: 384–390.

13. Stiell IG, McKnight RD, Greenberg GH. Implementation of the Ottawa ankle rules. *JAMA*. 1994; 271:827–832.

14. Wolfe MW, Uhl TL, Mattacola CG, McCluskey LC. Management of ankle sprains. *Am Fam Physician*. 2001;63:93–104.

15. Franzblau A, Werner RA. What is carpal tunnel syndrome? *JAMA*. 1999;282:186–187.

16. Atroshi I, Gummesson C, Johnsson R, Omstein E, Ranstam J, Rosen I. Prevalence of carpal tunnel syndrome in a general population. *JAMA*. 1999;282: 153–158.

17. Andersen JR. Computer use and the carpal tunnel syndrome. *JAMA*. 2003;289:2963–2969.

18. Jupiter JB, Ring D. Approach to minor orthopedic problems of the elbow, wrist, and hand. In: Goroll AH, Mulley AG, editors. *Primary Care Medicine*. 4th ed. Philadelphia: Lippincott Williams & Wilkins; 2000.

19. National Institute of Neurological Disorders and Stroke. National Institutes of Health. [Information on the Internet; accessed 7/05, 12/05] Carpal tunnel syndrome fact sheet. Available from: http://ninds.nih. gov/disorders/carpal_tunnel/detail_carpal_tunnel_pr. htm.

20. Padua L, Aprile I, Caliandro P, Carboni T, Meloni A, Massi S, et al. Symptoms and neurophysiological picture of carpal tunnel syndrome in pregnancy. *Clin Neurophysiol*. 2001;112:1946–1951.

21. Keles, I, Karagulle Kendi AT, Aydin G, Zog SG, Orkun S. Diagnostic precision of ultrasonography in patients with carpal tunnel syndrome. *Am J Phys Med Rehabil*. 2005;84:443–450.

22. Padua L, Aprile I, Caliandro P, Mondelli M, Pasqualetti P, Tonali PA; for the Italian Carpal Tunnel Syndrome Study Group. Carpal tunnel syndrome in pregnancy: Multiperspective follow-up of untreated cases. *Neurology*. 2002;59:1643–1646.

23. National Institute of Arthritis, Musculoskeletal and Skin Diseases. National Institutes of Health. Health Topics. Scoliosis. [Database on the Internet; accessed 12/05]. Available from http://niams.nih.gov/hi/ topics/scoliosis/scochild.htm.

24. Weinstein SL, Dolan LA, Spratt KF, Peterson KK, Spoonamore MJ, Ponsetti IV. Health and function of patients with untreated idiopathic scoliosis: A 50-year natural history study. *JAMA*. 2003;289:559–567.

25. Snyder BD, Katz DA, Myers ER, Breitenbach MA, Emans JB. Bone density accumulation is not affected by brace treatment of idiopathic scoliosis in adolescent girls. *J Pediatr Orthop*. 2005;25:423–428.

26. Goroll AH, Mulley AG. Management of osteoarthritis. In: Goroll AH, Mulley AG, editors. *Primary Care Medicine*. 4th ed. Philadelphia: Lippincott Williams & Wilkins; 2000.

27. Goroll AH, Mulley AG. Management of rheumatoid arthritis. In: Goroll AH, Mulley AG, editors. *Primary Care Medicine*. 4th ed. Philadelphia: Lippincott Williams & Wilkins; 2000.

28. Goroll AH, Mulley AG. Management of gout. In: Goroll AH, Mulley AG, editors. *Primary Care Medicine*. 4th ed. Philadelphia: Lippincott Williams & Wilkins; 2000.

29. National Institute of Arthritis, Musculoskeletal and Skin Diseases. National Institutes of Health. Health Topics. Arthritis and rheumatic diseases. [Database on the Internet; accessed 7/05, 12/05]. Available from: http://www.niams.nih.gov/hi/topics/arthritis/artrheu. htm.

30. Laine L. The gastrointestinal side effects of nonselective NSAIDs and COX-2-selective inhibitors. *Semin Arthritis Rheum*. 2002;32 (3Suppl 1):25–32.

31. Mukherjee D, Nissen SE, Topol EJ. Risk of cardiovascular events associated with selective COX-2 inhibitors. *JAMA*. 2001;286:954–959.

32. Solomon SD, McMurray JJV, Pfeffer MA, Wittes J, Fowler R, Finn P, et al. Cardiovascular risk associated with celecoxib in a clinical trial for colorectal adenoma prevention. *N Engl J Med*. 2005;352:1071–1080.

33. Fraenkel L, Wittink DR, Concato J, Fried T. Informed choice and the widespread use of antiinflammatory drugs. *Arthritis Rheum*. 2004;51:210–214.

34. Patino FG, Olivieri J, Allison JJ, Mikuls TR, Moreland L, Kovac SH, et al. Nonsteroidal antiinflammatory drug toxicity monitoring and safety practices. *J Rheumatol*. 2003;30:2680–2688.

35. Felson DT. Osteoarthritis: New insights. Part 1: The disease and its risk factors. *Ann Int Med*. 2000;133:635–646.

36. Gelber AC, Hochberg MC, Mead LA, Wang NY, Wigley FM, Klag MJ. Body mass index in young men and the risk of subsequent knee and hip osteoarthritis. *Am J Med*. 1999;107:542–548.

37. Felson DT, Anderson JJ, Naimark A, Walker AM, Meenan RF. Obesity and knee osteoarthritis: The Framingham Study. *Ann Intern Med*. 1988;109:18–24.

38. Felson DT, Shang Y, Anthony JM, Naimark A, Anderson JJ. Weight loss reduces the risk for symptomatic knee arthritis in women: The Framingham study. *Ann Intern Med*. 1992;116:535–539.

39. Felson DT. Osteoarthritis: New insights. Part 2: Treatment approaches. *Ann Intern Med*. 2000;133:726–737.

40. National Institute of Arthritis, Musculoskeletal and Skin Diseases. National Institutes of Health. Health Topics. Rheumatoid arthritis. [Database on the Internet; accessed 7/05, 12/05]. Available from http://www.niams.nih.gov/hi/topics/arthritis/rahandout/htm.

41. Gossec L, Dougados M, Goupille P, Cantarel A, Sibilia J, Meyer O, et al. Prognostic factors for remission in early rheumatoid arthritis: A multiparameter prospective study. *Ann Rheum Dis*. 2004;63:675–680.

42. National Institutes of Arthritis and Musculoskeletal Diseases. National Institutes of Health. Health Topics. Questions and answers about gout. [Database on the Internet; accessed 7/05, 12/05]. Accessed from http:/www.naims.nih.gov/hi/topics/gout/gout.htm.

43. Harris MD, Siegel LB, Alloway JA. Gout and hyperuricemia. *Am Fam Physician*. 1999;59:925–934.

44. National Institute of Arthritis, Musculoskeletal and Skin Diseases. Health Topics. Fibromyalgia. [Database on the Internet; accessed 7/05, 12/05]. Available from http://www.nih.gov/hi/topics/fibromyalgia/fibrofs.htm.

45. Arnold LM. A controlled family study in patients with fibromyalgia. [monograph on the Internet] National Institutes of Arthritis and Musculoskeletal Diseases. National Institutes of Health. Spotlight on Research. Highlights 2004. [accessed 7/05; 12/05]. Available from http://www.niams,nih.gov/ne/highlights/spotlight/2004/fibro_sum.htm.

46. Raphael KG. Fibromyalgia, depression, and myofascial TMD. [accessed 7/7/05]. Preliminary report at www.niams.nih.gov/ne/highlights/spotlight/2004/fibro_sum.htm.

47. Gowans SE, Dehueck A, Voss S, Silaj A, Abbey SE. Six-month and one-year followup of 23 weeks of aerobic exercise for individuals with fibromyalgia. *Arthritis Rheum*. 2004;51:890–898.

48. Lemstra M, Olszynski WP. The effectiveness of multidisciplinary rehabilitation in the treatment of fibromyalgia. *Clin J Pain*. 2005;21:166–174.

49. Mannerkorpi K. Exercise in fibromyalgia. *Curr Opin Rheumatol*. 2005;17:190–194.

50. Thieme K, Turk DC, Flor H. Comorbid depression and anxiety in fibromyalgia syndrome: Relationship to somatic and psychosocial variables. *Psychosom Med*. 2004;66:837–844.

51. Turk DC, Robinson JP, Burwinkle T. Prevalence of fear of pain and activity in patients with fibromyalgia syndrome. *J Pain*. 2004;5:483–490.

52. Goldenberg DL, Burckhardt C, Crofford L. Management of fibromyalgia syndrome. *JAMA*. 2004;292:2388–2395.

53. National Osteoporosis Foundation. Fast Facts. [Database in the internet, accessed 7/23/2005]. Available at www.nof.org/osteoporosis/diseasefacts.htm.

54. Cummings SR, Melton LJ, III. Epidemiology and outcomes of osteoporotic fractures. *Lancet*. 2002;359(9319):1761–1767.

55. Zingmond DS, Melton LJ, III , Silverman SL. Increasing hip fracture incidence in California Hispanics, 1983–2000. *Osteoporos Int*. 2004; 15:603–610.

56. U.S. Department of Health and Human Services. Bone Health and Osteoporosis: A Report of the Surgeon General. Rockville, MD: Public Health Service, Office of the Surgeon General; Washington, DC, 2004.

57. Osteoporosis Prevention, Diagnosis, and Therapy. *NIH Consens Statement*. 2000 March 27–29;17(1):1–36.

58. Up to Date. Epidemiology and causes of osteoporosis. [Monograph on the Internet, accessed 7/18/2005.] Available at www.utdol.com/application/topic.

59. Tannirandorn P, Epstein S. Drug induced bone loss. *Osteoporos Int.* 2000;11:637–659.

60. Theintz B, Ruchs R, Rizzoli R, Slosman D, Clavien H, Sizonenko C, Bonjour J. Longitudinal monitoring of bone mass accumulation in healthy adolescents: Evidence for a marked reduction after 16 years of age at the levels of lumbar spine and femoral neck in female subjects. *J Clin Endo Metab.* 1992;75: 1060–1065.

61. Recker RR, Davies KM, Hinders SM, Heaney RP, Stegman MR, Kimmel DB. Bone gain in young adult women. *JAMA.* 1992;268:2403–2408.

62. Matcovic V, Fontana D, Tominac C, Goel P, Chestnut CH, III. Factors that influence peak bone mass formation: A study of calcium balance and the inheritance of bone mass adolescent females. *Am J Clin Nutr.* 1990;52: 878–888.

63. World Health Organization. Assessment of fracture risk and its application to screening for postmenopausal osteoporosis: Report of a WHO Study Group. (Technical report series 843.) Geneva Switzerland: World Health Organization; 1994.

64. U.S. Preventive Services Task Force. *Guide to Clinical Preventive Services.* 3rd ed. Available at www.arhq.gov/clinic/uspstfix.htm.

65. National Osteoporosis Foundation. Physician's Guide to Prevention and Treatment of Osteoporosis. Available at www.nof.org/_vti_bin/shtml.dll/physguide/index/htm.

66. Cadarette SM, Jaglal SB, Murray TM, McIsaac WJ, Joseph L, Brown P, Canadian Multicentre Osteoporosis Study. Evaluation of decision rules for referring women for bone densitometry by dual-energy x-ray absorptiometry. *JAMA.* 2001;286:57–63.

67. Mauck KF, Cuddihy MT, Atkinson EJ, Melton LJ. Use of clinical prediction rules in detecting osteoporosis in a population-based sample of postmenopausal women. *Arch Intern Med.* 2005;165:530–536.

68. United States Department of Health and Human Services. National Women's Health Information Center. *Osteoporosis.* [Monograph on the Internet, Accessed 7/23/2005.] Available from www.4woman.gov/faq/osteopor.

69. Holick MF. Vitamin D: Importance in the prevention of cancers, type 1 diabetes, heart disease and osteoporosis. *Am J Clin Nutr.* 2004;79:362–371.

70. Holick MF, Siris ES, Binkley N, Beard MK, Khan A, Katzer JT, et al. Prevalence of vitamin D inadequacy among postmenopausal North American women receiving osteoporosis therapy. *J Clin Endocrinol Metab.* 2005 Jun;90(6):3215–3224.

71. Clark MK, Sowers MR, Nichols S, Levy B. Bone mineral density changes over two years in first time users of depot medroxyprogesterone acetate. *Fertil Steril.* 2004;82:1580–1586.

72. Scholes D, La Croix AZ, Ichiwara LE, Barlow WE, Ott SM. Change in bone mineral density among adolescent women using and discontinuing depot medroxyprogesterone acetate contraception. *Arch Pediatr Adolesc Med.* 2005 Feb;159:139–144.

73. Berenson AB, Breitkopf CR, Grady JJ, Rickert VI, Thomas A. Effects of hormonal contraception on bone mineral density after 24 months of use. *Obstet Gynecol.* 2004;103(5 Pt 1):899–906.

74. Kalkwarf HJ, Specker BL. Bone mineral changes during pregnancy and lactation. *Endocrine.* 2002;17: 49–53.

75. Ritchie LD, Fung EB, Halloran BP, Turnlund JR, Van Loan MD, Cann CE, King JC. A longitudinal study of calcium homeostasis during human pregnancy and lactation and after resumption of menses. *Am J Clin Nutr.* 1998;67:693–701.

76. Kalkwarf HJ. Lactation and maternal bone health. *Adv Exp Med Biol.* 2004;554:101–114.

77. Kalkwarf HJ, Specker BL, Ho M. Effects of calcium supplementation on calcium homeostasis and bone turnover in lactating women. *J Clin Endocrinol Metab.* 1999;84:464–470.

78. Wainwright SA, Marshall LM, Ensrud KE, Cauley JA, Black DM, Hillier T, et al. Study of Osteoporotic Fractures Research Group. Hip fracture in women without osteoporosis. *J Clin Endocrinol Metab.* 2005; 90:2787–2793.

Chapter 22

Dermatology

Mary Ellen Rousseau

In the course of women's health care, knowledge of skin conditions is an integral part of care. Many disorders such as pruritic urticarial papules and plaques of pregnancy (PUPPP), candidiasis, and herpes simplex II are commonly seen in obstetrics/gynecology practice. However, other conditions should not be overlooked. The skin is the easiest organ in which to identify problems and can be easily evaluated when the woman is undressed during annual examinations. Midwives and women's health providers can play an important role in the early identification of serious problems such as skin cancer and the treatment of more common conditions such as acne and eczema.

The Skin

The skin is a two-layered membrane. The *epidermis* is a continually renewing, stratified, squamous epithelium that keratinizes and gives rise to derivative structures (pilosebaceous units, nails, and sweat glands) called appendages. This layer is approximately 0.4 to 1.5 mm in thickness.

The lower thick, spongy *dermis* is one to two millimeters thick. It is an integrated system of fibrous, filamentous, and amorphous connective tissue that accommodates nerve and vascular networks. The dermis makes up the bulk of the skin and provides its pliability, elasticity, and tensile strength. It protects the body from mechanical injury, binds water, aids in thermal regulation, and includes receptors of sensory stimuli, and interacts in repairing and remodeling the skin as wounds are healed.[1] Collagen is the major dermal constituent; it accounts for approximately 75% of the dry weight of the skin and provides both tensile strength and elasticity.

Burden of Skin Diseases

The skin receives messages from the environment, responding to both tactile and emotional stimuli.[2] Tactile stimuli are felt by the person through the skin and cause a reaction in the skin, whether it be to temperature, ultraviolet light, or other conditions. Blushing and blanching are two examples of emotional responses. Beginning in infancy, tactile and emotional messages are filed away in memory and are eventually incorporated into the individual's personality.[2] Thus, the skin is an organ that responds to life's events whether good or bad and can lead to psychogenic skin disease.

Humans, beginning in infancy, depend on touching, stroking, and positive support for a strong healthy body image. When a skin disease causes disfigurement, there can be a profound negative effect on the individual's psyche.[2] Psychologic factors that can also bring about dermatologic conditions include: stress, mood, and anxiety disorders; lack of social support; and specific psychological or personality disorders (perfectionism, hostility).[3] Up to 30% of dermatologic conditions are considered to be related to psychiatric or psychologic factors.[4]

Some dermatologic disorders involving sensitive areas of the body such as the face, hands, and genitals can cause significant distress for women. However, the distress experienced is not always in concert with the seriousness or extent of the disease. For example, teens who are dealing with core developmental issues related to body image and sexuality can have a significant psychosocial reaction to even mild disfigurement from acne. Depression, suicidal ideation, and sexual dysfunction can coexist with skin diseases that affect sensitive areas or those that involve disfigurement, so consideration of psychiatric and psychosocial factors must be addressed when assessing patients with dermatologic problems. It is important to recognize the patient who may be at high risk of developing psychosocial and psychiatric comorbidity.[4]

Comorbidity is seen between dermatologic diseases and some major psychiatric syndromes such as depressive illness. Major life events have been reported to exacerbate some skin disorders and, conversely, psychosocial stress may result from the impact of the skin disorder upon the quality of life of the patient.[4] When a woman presents with severe pruritus, in addition to asking questions about exposure to environmental factors, inquiries should be made about depression and recent life events that might influence skin complaints. Acne, for example, has been associated with disorders related to body image such as bulimia.[5] Management of the distressed patient with skin conditions requires aggressive treatment; this patient is likely to be best served by immediate referral to a dermatologist. The patient may also benefit from referral to a psychiatric provider for assessment and treatment of any mental health comorbidity.

Racial Differences

Racial differences in skin have been minimally studied by objective measures, and results have been contradictory.[6] The current model for skin is based on physical properties of what is known about Caucasian skin; differences may exist in the properties of the skin in non-Caucasian peoples. Furthermore, race and ethnicity are ill defined. While anthropologists divide race into Caucasoid, Mongoloid, Australoid, and Congoid/Negroid, ethnicity is often defined as how individuals see themselves, taking into account ancestry, skin color, religion, language, and so on.[7] It is plausible that differences exist in the skin of individuals depending on genetic variations or subjective labels such as race/ethnicity. These differences may affect the presentation of various skin conditions and how they respond to treatment.

For the purposes of this chapter, *skin photo types (SPTs)* will be used when there are different responses seen in groups. The SPT is based on a person's own estimate of sunburning and tanning. **Table 22-1** defines the SPT categories and descriptions. The SPT of some groups has not been determined. However, some Asians

Table 22-1 SKIN PHOTO TYPE (SPT)

SPT Class	Tanning	Descriptors	Constitutive Color	Other Factors
I	Never	Melanocompromised	White	Regardless of hair and eye color, always burns within 30 minutes of exposure
II	Rarely	Melanocompromised	White	Sunburns easily; tans with difficulty
III	Over time	Melanocompetent	White	Some sunburn with short exposures, but over time develop deep tanning
IV	Easily	Melanocompetent	White	Tans easily and never sunburns with short exposures
V	Always-rare burn	Melanocompetent	Brown	Can sunburn with long exposures
VI	Always tans	Melanocompetent	Black	Can sunburn with long exposures

and Latinas have SPT I and II. Certain conditions that relate to skin color will be discussed below in the section on pigment disorders.

Clinical Presentation

History

History taking includes all the essential components of any medical history including menstrual, gynecologic, obstetric, sexual, medical, surgical, and family histories. In collecting the complete history, hormonal changes, potential exposures, and other risk factors may appear. The general condition of the woman's health is assessed; family history of atopy is determined. Atopy is an immune response to common naturally occurring allergens with the continual production of IgE antibodies. It commonly presents as atopic dermatitis, although allergic rhinitis and allergic asthma, which are related disorders, occur even more frequently. These conditions likely have a shared genetic basis because they are often clustered in families. A family history of any of these conditions increases the chance that a woman may present with an atopy-related condition.

Further details of the condition in question should be ascertained; in particular, its relationship to chemical exposures, travel, temperature extremes such as heat or cold, and drug ingestion. Other questions should elicit information about timing (onset and duration), initial appearance and change over time, whether this is an isolated or recurrent problem, and if recurrent, a description of prior episodes. Inquiries should also be made regarding previous treatments including the use of over-the-counter (OTC) medications, prescription drugs, or complementary therapies.

Physical Examination

While it has been reported that dermatologists provide greater accuracy in diagnosis and more appropriate treatment of skin disorders than primary care providers,[8] looking is the most important skill in diagnosing and treating skin diseases and is one that can be learned by primary care providers. Because diseases have locations of predilection, the midwife must know where to look as well as how to look. Not to look is more serious than not knowing exactly what is observed (**Figure 22-1**).

What is seen may be the result of secondary irritation such as excoriation with severe moniliasis. Scratching or previous treatment with OTC preparations may alter the look of the lesion. When observing a skin lesion, more than looking

Figure 22-1 Differential diagnosis by body region.

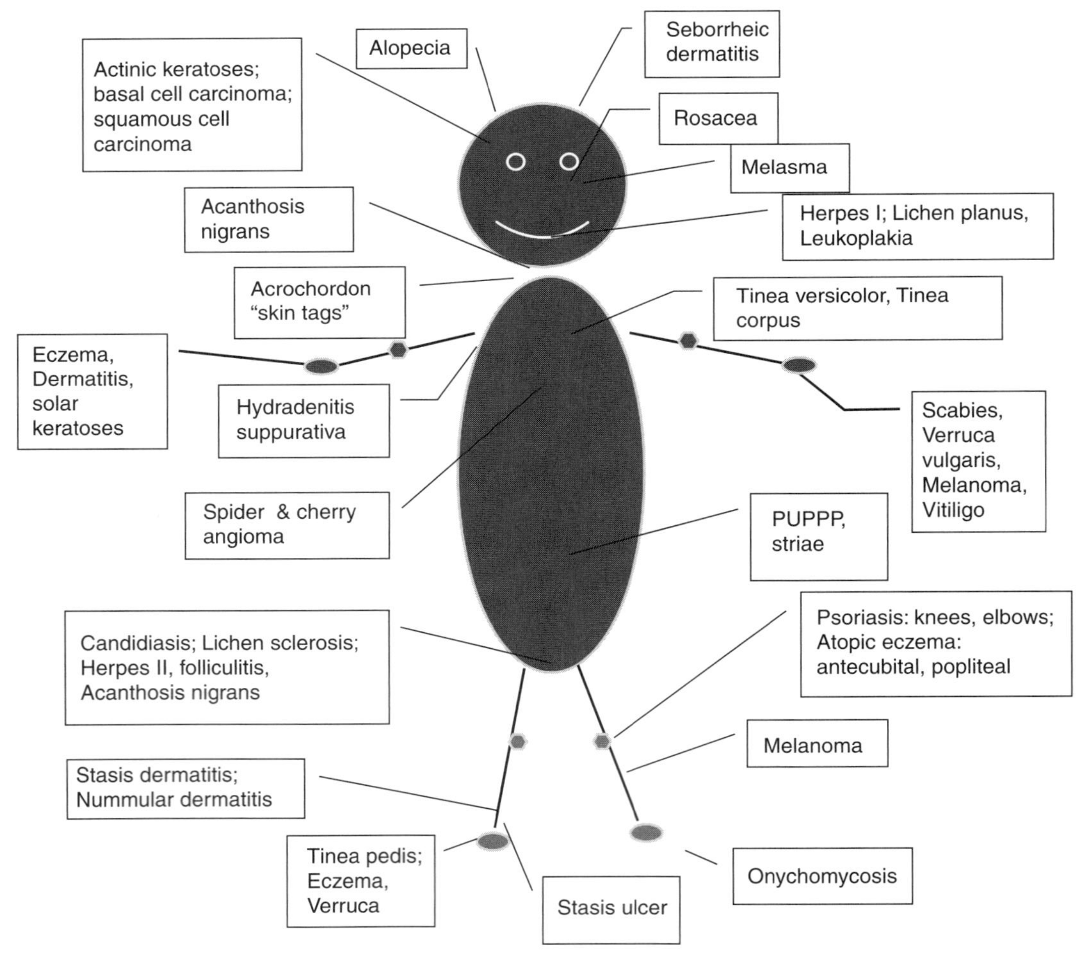

is required. The lesion must be viewed with good lighting from various angles but may need to be touched, stretched, pinched, or moistened in order to appreciate the characteristics of the lesion.

Full body examination provides the opportunity for identifying serious skin problems. It has been estimated that 85% of the U.S. population sees a health provider at least once in a two-year period.[9] Annual gynecologic examinations can be used to both examine and educate women regarding skin health. Melanomas are six times more likely to be detected on screening if all, rather than part of, the skin is visible.[10] Because women are fully undressed at the annual gynecology visit, it is the perfect opportunity for detection. This is an opportunity to observe for atypical nevi, in particular. Hair, nails, and mucous membranes are all ectodermal structures closely related to skin and so should be included in the examination. **Table 22-2** contains a mnemonic useful for detecting melanoma.

Examination of the lesion or rash is the first step in evaluation of the skin. This allows the provider to focus the history in a productive

---

Table 22-2 MNEMONIC FOR MALIGNANT MELANOMA

A	Asymmetry
B	Border is irregular with irregularly scalloped edges
C	Color is mottled, haphazard colors in various shades of brown, black, blue, gray, red, and white
D	Diameter is large, greater than the tip of a pencil eraser. Enlargement in size may be the most important sign.
E	Elevation is almost always present with surface distortion; in situ and acral (foot) lesions may be flat

manner. The history of this occurrence should be obtained while doing the physical examination. Knowledge about various dermatologic conditions allows the midwife to focus on suspected areas of probable involvement. For example, psoriasis is often found on elbows and knees but can also involve the nails. Mucous membranes of the genital area and the oral cavity are often affected by the same lesions; lichen planus (LP) is such a lesion.

Inspection should be done with good lighting. Dim lighting reduces color and increases shadows, but too much light interferes with observation of skin surfaces. Daylight is the optimal light source for viewing lesions. The next choice is a blue incandescent light. Skin diseases assume unusual hues when observed under white fluorescent lighting; such lighting is too strong.[11] Evaluation of skin lesions should be done from not more than 20 cm away; a 5 to 10x magnifying glass is also helpful. Application of water or oil to the surface of a lesion allows better observation of its shape, color, and margins, in the way that oil immersion does in microscopic exams.[11]

To define the differential diagnoses, a description of the lesion is essential. The four main descriptors of skin lesions include type (macules, nodules, and cysts), shape, arrangement, and distribution. Terms for various colors of the skin or lesion are described:

- White – leukoderma, hypomelanosis
- Red – erythema, pink, violaceous
- Brown – hypermelanosis, hemosiderin
- Black, blue, gray, orange, yellow
- Purpuric – red or purple lesions that do not blanch with pressure

Shape can be variously described as round, oval, annular, serpiginous (snakelike), or umbilicated.

The margins can be well defined or not. Grouped arrangements are described as linear, annular (circular), arciform (arc), herpetiform (blisters in clusters), zosteriform (similar to herpes zoster), reticulated (weblike). Disseminated lesions can be described as scattered or diffuse. Distribution includes the extent of the involvement: isolated, localized, and regional. Patterns can be described as characteristic such as those seen in Lyme disease, candidiasis, or acne; or described using more general terms such as symmetrical; or by location such as present in exposed or intertriginous areas.

Skin lesions are described as papule, plaque, wheal, nodule, pustule, vesicle, bulla, crust, desquamation (scaling), ulcer, erosion, excoriation, exudation, and lichenification (see Glossary for descriptions of lesions).

Simple office-based tests can be done to help determine the diagnosis. One is to stroke the flexor surface of the forearm or upper back with a wooden tongue depressor. In certain conditions, a red linear wheal called *dermographism* will occur. However, in women with atopic dermatitis, stroking will cause a white line without urtication to form where the skin was stroked. *Diascopy* is the use of a glass slide to dehematize a lesion by applying pressure. If pressure on the glass slide causes a red lesion to blanch, the lesion is caused by vascular dilation. Extravascular lesions such as hemorrhages, pigmentations, and cellular infiltrates will not blanch under pressure. In trying to determine if a lesion is a vesicle or a solid papule, puncture with a fine sterile needle will demonstrate the difference. When trying to distinguish between a verruca (wart) and a molluscum contagiosum lesion, light application of liquid nitrogen will show the characteristic central umbilication of the molluscum. Dermatologists use a Wood's light (ultraviolet light at 360 nm) to diagnose certain types of fungal infections.

Potassium hydroxide (KOH) preparation of scales is diagnostic for fungal organisms of the skin and can be done in the office setting of the primary care provider (Table 22-3).

Tests and Laboratory Evaluations

Although visualization of the skin is the most important component of diagnosis for most lesions in a gynecology practice, at times, laboratory examination may contribute to the diagnosis. Examples of tests to consider include cultures for bacteria and virology, microscopy for wet mounts including yeast, laboratory evaluation of blood for signs of diabetes, polycystic ovarian syndrome, and serology for syphilis.

Table 22-3 **KOH WET MOUNT FOR CUTANEOUS FUNGAL INFECTIONS**

1. Hold a # 15 surgical blade perpendicular to the skin surface and smoothly but firmly draw the blade against the scale of the lesion with several short strokes. If a border is present, the blade should be held at right angles to the fringe of the scale.
2. The scale is separated and placed on the slide and covered with the cover slip. KOH 10–20% is applied by a toothpick or eyedropper to the edge of cover slip and allowed to seep beneath the cover slip by capillary action.
3. The slide is gently heated under a low flame and pressed to separate the epithelial cells from the fungal hyphae.
4. Lower the condenser of the microscope and dim the light to enhance the contrast, making identification of the hyphae easier.

Biopsies of the skin, especially of the vulva, are commonly done in a gynecology practice.

Classifications of Dermatologic Conditions

General Dermatoses

URTICARIA

Urticaria is a common, distinctive, and variably pruritic reaction to a variety of stimuli. The transient wheals (hives) are edematous papules and plaques, and larger edematous areas that involve the dermis. When the subcutaneous tissue is involved, it is called *angioedema*.[12] In either case it can be acute or chronic. The various types include:

1) Immunologic (IgE-mediated)
   a. Associated with atopic background
   b. Antigens include: food (eggs, milk, wheat, shellfish, nuts), therapeutic agents (penicillin), and parasites
2) Physical urticaria
   a. Dermographism (urticaria appears after stroking with a tongue depressor; 4.2% incidence in the general population; most have no untoward effects and fading occurs within 30 minutes)
   b. Cold urticaria seen in children and young adults (ice cube test establishes diagnosis)
   c. Solar urticaria (histamine is one of the mediators)
   d. Cholinergic urticaria (brought on by exercise to the point of sweating; provokes typical, small papular lesions, which establish the diagnosis)
   e. Vibratory or pressure urticaria (swelling of the buttocks when seated)
3) Mast cell releasing agents found in radiocontrast media as a consequence of intolerance to salicylates, dyes, and benzoates
4) Vascular/connective tissue autoimmune disease
5) Hereditary angioedema (a serious autosomal dominant disorder)

Midwives and other women's health providers would not manage any of the serious forms of urticaria but may see transient urticaria in which the plaques change size and shape by peripheral extension and regression. Differential diagnoses include drug eruption, viral exanthema, and insect bites. All suspected triggers should be stopped (e.g., food, aspirin) and antihistamines such as hydroxyzine 10 to 25 mg should be administered every four to six hours. Non-drowsy H1 blockers, including loratidine (Claritin), cetirizine (Zyrtec), and fexofenadine (Allegra), do not work as well but are useful during the daytime. Prednisone (e.g., 60 mg for 2 days, 40 mg for 5 days, and 20 mg for 7 days) can be used if the antihistamines are ineffective. Epinephrine is administered in extensive cases. Children and adults with serious known allergies in which urticaria occurs carry epinephrine (administered intramuscularly using an Epipen) for emergency response to contact with allergens. If there is an urticarial allergic response making it difficult for the woman to breathe, or she experiences swelling in the throat or tongue, 9-1-1 should be called immediately. The individual who is having a mild-to-moderate response should be kept cool physically and removed from stressors if possible. Cool baths are soothing but hot showers must be avoided or the pruritus and urticaria can worsen. Topical steroids are not effective in this case.[13]

PRURITIS

Itching affects everyone to a greater or lesser extent at various times. However, itching is the major symptom of many skin diseases, especially inflammatory skin diseases. Whatever the underlying cause, itch evokes the behavior of scratching, which increases inflammation and stimulates nerve fibers, leading to a vicious cycle called the "Itch-Scratch Cycle."[14] This cycle can alter the integrity of the skin, leading to barrier damage.[15] Another negative effect of the itch-scratch cycle is disrupted sleep.

Clinical features seen as a response to scratching include the following. *Lichenification* is a well-developed plaque with marked accentuation of the skin creases, which develops over time from incessant rubbing and scratching. The common sites for lichenification are those the person can easily scratch, such as the nape of the neck, below the elbow, the ankle, the buttock, and the genitals. Postinflammatory hyperpigmentation or hypopigmentation is common in skin types 4 to 6. The butterfly sign is found on the back, which may show a hypopigmented area in the pattern of a butterfly, where it is impossible to scratch.

Dry skin, *xerosis*, which is characterized by a rough, scaly, and flaky skin surface, has long been associated with sensations of itching. Types of xerosis include seasonal/winter xerosis, atopic dermatitis, and senile xerosis. It has also been found to be associated with anorexia nervosa; in one study, 58% of 19 hospitalized women with anorexia also had severe generalized itch.[16] Although the clinical association between dry skin and itching is well established, the data to support skin hydration and barrier impairment

do not support an association between skin hydration and water loss and itch.[17]

Pruritis is a common symptom of some systemic diseases, including renal failure, cholestatic jaundice, primary biliary cirrhosis, hepatitis C, cholestasis of pregnancy, polycythemia vera, iron deficiency anemia, multiple myeloma, Hodgkin's disease, non-Hodgkin's lymphoma, hyperthyroidism, and hypothyroidism.[18] Individuals can also suffer significant pruritis under certain circumstances such as with keloids or scarring, after a burn, and with infectious diseases such as fungal and parasitic infestations. Pruritis is the most common dermatologic symptom in patients with human immunodeficiency virus (HIV).[18] Pruritis of the lower legs often accompanies venous insufficiency. Some emotional and psychiatric states such as depression can cause itching or lower the itch threshold for itching sensation.[19]

Exogenous and endogenous factors are known to aggravate pruritis by lowering the threshold for itch or prolonging the itch duration. A short list includes wool fiber, extreme cold, warm temperature, soaps, disinfectants, oral medications such as aspirin, antimalarials and opiates, dust mites, molds, furry animals, alcoholic beverages, spicy food (chili pepper), and nuts. Endogenous factors include emotional stress, depression, obsessive-compulsive disorder, xerosis, and perspiration.[18] When obtaining a history from an individual with a complaint of itch, questions should be asked about all of the above categories.

Management of pruritis depends on the etiology. Categories include pruritoceptive itch, neuropathic and neurogenic itch, and psychogenic itch. These will be described below in the section on management of skin diseases.

INTERTRIGO

Intertrigo is a clinical description of an inflammatory dermatosis involving body folds and results from chafing and moisture. Because many diseases can affect the skin folds, it is difficult to predict the prevalence of this condition. Mistiaen et al. concluded that there is little evidence on which to base recommendations for the prevention and treatment of intertrigo.[20] Research articles on the subject are scarce and most of the empirical evidence focuses on the effectiveness of treating this condition with antifungal agents. However, several studies have found that very few patients had a positive fungal culture before treatment, raising doubt about what role fungal infections play in the etiology of intertrigo.[21,22]

Obese sedentary individuals as well as athletes are thought to be prone to intertrigo. Hypothetically, in the obese patient, there is little chance for perspiration to dry so the individual is at risk for developing a secondary bacterial (erythrasma) or fungal infection (*Candida*). Common sites for intertrigo include: beneath the breasts; in the axillae; antecubital fossae; inguinal folds; and in abdominal folds above the symphysis pubis. Red plaques seen with intertrigo oppose each other on either side of the skin fold, creating almost a mirror image. Heat is thought to aggravate the condition. It is hypothesized that poor hygiene may contribute to the incidence but the condition has been little studied. Chronic intertrigo can develop after inflammatory hypopigmentation or hyperpigmentation.

There is general agreement in the literature that the best prevention is to keep the affected areas clean and dry by minimizing skin-on-skin friction, heat, and moisture in and around skin folds.[20] Experience and expert opinion suggest that these goals can be achieved by the following interventions: 1) using various techniques to promote dryness (such as the use of cotton, talcum powder, or disrobing and exposing affected areas to the heat of a hair dryer or electric light bulb for 30 minutes twice a day) and 2) using treatments that encourage healing (such as the application of wet tea bags, Domeboro soaks, hydrocolloid dressings, Burrow's solution, diluted vinegar, or witch hazel compresses).[20] Women with intertrigo should be advised to wear light, nonconstrictive, absorbent clothing. Biotextiles are now available, which are cotton or polyester gauze fabric in which antiseptic molecules such as zeolite or triclosane are fixed.[23]

In an early study by McMahon and Buckeldee, little consensus was found among nurses who were asked about what treatment(s) they recommended for their patients with intertrigo.[24] The nurses recommended 12 different creams and a variety of other substances such as rose oil and yogurt. There was disagreement as to whether absorbing powders should be used and no consensus as to which antibacterial and antifungal products should be used. Also, the respondents disagreed on whether to treat with or without a culture. Clearly, this is a topic about which little is known, including what preventive measures will be effective, what fabrics should be worn, and what therapy should be pursued. Further research is needed to determine the most effective treatment approach.

Conditions of Pregnancy

Physiologic Changes of Pregnancy

Skin changes are common in pregnancy. Women's skin is affected by hormonal influences throughout life, and pregnancy is no exception. Localized or generalized hyperpigmentation occurs to some extent in 90% of pregnant women.[25] Such lesions are apt to be more pronounced in darker skinned individuals but are noticeable in light-skinned women as well. The most commonly seen change is darkening of the line between the umbilicus and the symphysis pubis, the *linea nigra*. It often occurs several months into the first pregnancy and earlier in subsequent pregnancies. Darkening of the nipples, areola, the external genitalia, and the axillae are usual. Melasma, formerly called chloasma, or mask of pregnancy, occurs on the face in some women and can also occur with use of hormonal contraception. *Striae distensae* (stretch marks) occur in nearly all women by the end of the pregnancy. They are commonly seen on the abdomen but may be observed on the breasts, hips, and thighs. They are pink to purple atrophic lines that develop at right angles to the skin tension lines. After the birth of the baby, they typically become more flesh colored or pale and thinner, but they never disappear completely.

Hair and nails also undergo changes in pregnancy. Hair growth is seen, particularly in dark skinned women or women who already have abundant hair. *Telogen effluvium* is a condition that results in the loss of terminal scalp hairs about one to five months postpartum. This can cause great distress in some women. It is hypothesized that pregnancy interrupts the normal hair shedding cycle, allowing hair to continue growing.[25] After birth, the hair follicles resume the normal pattern of growth and loss. Women often need reassurance that it is a self-limiting process and that baldness will not occur.

Nails can become brittle and soft in the early months of pregnancy. In some women nails grow faster during the pregnancy.

Mucous membranes become more vascularized in pregnancy. Gingivitis, nosebleeds, and postcoital spotting are common as a result of these changes. A dental checkup and use of a soft toothbrush that massages the gums is recommended.

Varicosities of the vulva and legs can occur for the first time in pregnancy and are often exacerbated by the pressure exerted on venous return by the growing uterus. Spider angiomas often occur for the first time in pregnancy, especially in light-skinned women. They are recognized by a central redness with radiating branches.

Polymorphic Eruption of Pregnancy

Polymorphic eruption of pregnancy (PEP), also called PUPPP, is the most common dermatosis of pregnancy.[26] It has also been called prurigo of late pregnancy and toxemic erythema of pregnancy. The term PUPPP is still widely used, but PEP includes the full range of clinical morphologic lesions including papules, plaques, target lesions, polycyclic erythematous wheals, vesicles, and occasional bullae. It is an inflammatory process associated only with pregnancy and no associations have been found with pre-eclampsia, atopy, or autoimmune disease.[27] It is most often characterized by itching and papules that occur on the abdomen (90% of the time) in the third trimester. The incidence is approximately 1 in 160 pregnancies and is most common in first pregnancies.[13] The mean duration is six weeks; however, the rash is usually not severe for more than a week.

Itching typically occurs on the abdomen, sometimes in the striae distensae (stretch marks) with 1- to 3-mm erythematous papules quickly coalescing into urticarial plaques with polycyclic shape and arrangement. The lesions may extend to the thighs, back, and buttocks. Women often suffer with the itching, but excoriation is not frequently seen. PEP may be confused with other disorders, particularly *Pemphigoid (herpes) gestationis (PG)*. Lesions overlying striae are common in PEP but seldom seen in PG. In PEP, vesicles are rarely larger than 2 to 3 mm, but with PG vesicles usually evolve into larger tense bullae. PEP usually does not involve the periumbilical area, whereas PG does. Direct immunofluorescence can be used to differentiate between the two diseases (**Figure 22-2**).[28]

Because PEP is self-limiting and without serious sequelae, reassurance and symptomatic treatment is usually all that is necessary. The mother should be told that the itching will end either before or at the time of birth. Cool wet compresses, oatmeal baths, antipruritic lotions, and topical steroids can be used. Medium potency steroids such as clobetasone butyrate 0.05% (Class V) are generally needed to control itch, but milder presentations may respond to lower potency steroids such as hydrocortisone 0.01%. Prednisone in a tapering dose of 30 to 40 mg may be used daily for seven to ten days in extreme cases. Antihistamines are not as effective as topical corticosteroids in controlling itch, but may be a helpful adjunctive measure. Since the itchiness associated with PEP can be especially bothersome at night, antihistamines may be particularly useful if taken in the evening. Not only can they help control itch, but they may also promote sleep. Antihistamines can cause drowsiness; therefore they are often used as a sleep aid in pregnancy.

Pemphigoid (Herpes) Gestationis

PG is a rare (1:10,000 births) autoimmune bullous disease that occurs during pregnancy and the postpartum period. It may occur from nine weeks gestation through the postpartum period but is usually seen in the latter part of pregnancy. Its etiology and effects on the fetus are unknown. Circulating complement-fixing IgG antibodies are present in the serum. PG is not

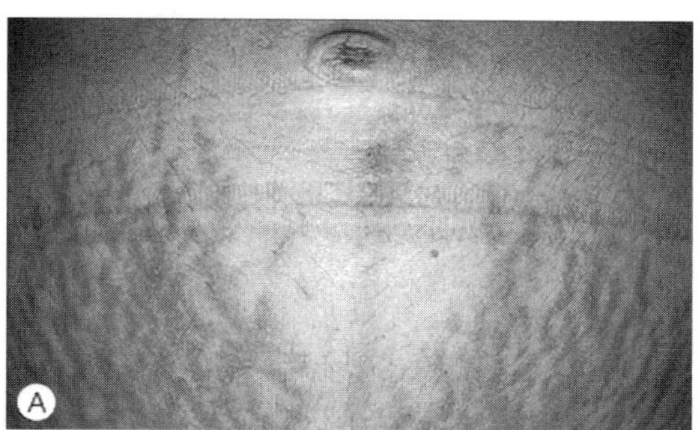

Figure 22-2 Example of polymorphic eruption of pregnancy (PEP).

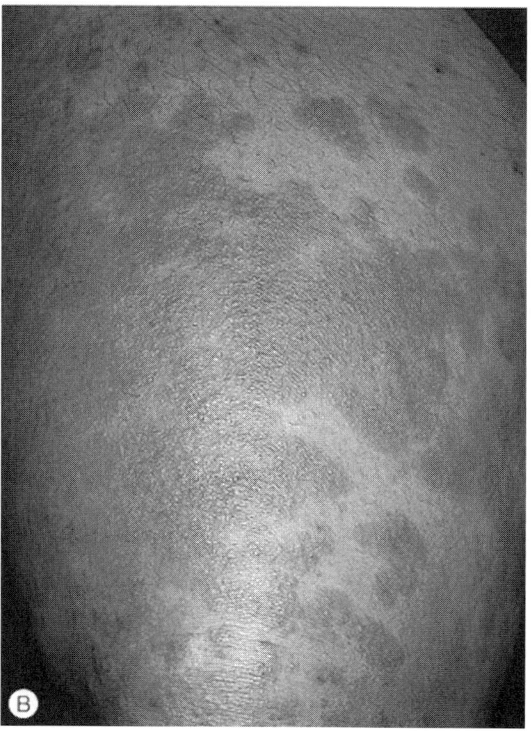

Source: Reprinted with permission from Elsevier, © 2003. Dermatology Online. Bolognia JL, Jorizzo JL, Rapini RP, editors. [subscriber site on the Internet]. Available from: http://www.dermtext.com.

known to be related to any viral infection. Lesions vary from papulovesicular eruptions to large bullae, erosions, and crusts. Grouping of the lesions (thus the name herpes) is pronounced; they frequently occur on the abdomen and lateral sides of the trunk but may extend to palms, soles, chest, face, and neck. The name herpes is a description of the arrangement of the vesicles, not to be confused with the viral infection. Consequently, the name pemphigoid gestationis is preferred.

PG may occasionally be related to other autoimmune diseases such as Crohn's disease and alopecia areata. It may be associated with trophoblastic tumors, hydatidiform mole, and choriocarcinoma.[29]

Therapy includes relief of pruritis, suppression of blister formation, and prevention of erosions.[30] Aggressive use of topical corticosteroids combined with emollients and systemic antihistamines are usual. Once bullae have developed, however, it is necessary to use systemic steroids. The patient with PG should be referred to a maternal fetal medicine specialist.

Prurigo Gestationis (Besnier) of Pregnancy

Prurigo of pregnancy occurs in one in 300 pregnancies with onset between 25 and 30 weeks gestation, and may persist for up to three months postpartum. The lesions are discrete erythematous or skin-color papules (**Figure 22-3**). Lesions are extremely pruritic with excoriation soon following. Most often the lesions are found on the extensor surfaces of the extremities and the trunk and do not proceed to vesicle formation.[31] The entity has been little studied but it is hypothesized that prurigo of pregnancy might be pruritis gravidarum occurring in atopic women.[32] Symptomatic relief in-

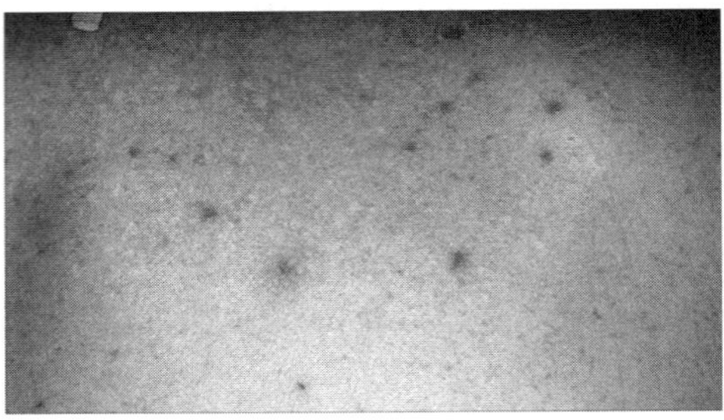

Figure 22-3 Prurigo of pregnancy.

Source: Reprinted with permission from Elsevier, © 2003. Dermatology Online. Bolognia JL, Jorizzo JL, Rapini RP, editors. [subscriber site on the Internet]. Available from: http://www.dermtext.com.

cludes moderately potent topical corticosteroids such as Class IV or V-clobetasone butyrate 0.05% cream. Cordran tape (translucent polythene adhesive film impregnated with flurandrenolone) can be helpful in the management of smaller number of papules.

Other lesions that can be found in or exacerbated by pregnancy include vascular and hematologic changes such as hemorrhoids, varicosities, spider angiomas, and palmar erythema of pregnancy to name a few (**Figure 22-4**).

Genital Lesions

Condyloma accuminata

Human papilloma viruses (HPV) commonly infect the mucosa (genital warts, venereal warts, verruca acuminata) and are extremely contagious. Warts are probably more contagious than subclinical infections.[12] Women are usually asymptomatic, although pruritis is occasionally

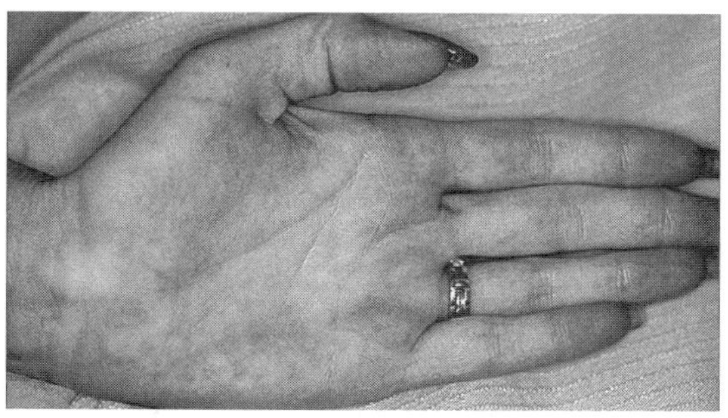

Figure 22-4 Palmar erythema of pregnancy.

Source: Reprinted with permission from Elsevier, © 2003. Dermatology Online. Bolognia JL, Jorizzo JL, Rapini RP, editors. [subscriber site on the Internet]. Available from: http://www.dermtext.com.

reported. Women are concerned over the cosmetic appearance of the warts.

The skin appears pale pink with numerous, discrete projections on a broad base with a cauliflower appearance (**Figure 22-5**). Subclinical lesions can be seen with the application of acetic acid (white vinegar) and appear as white patches. The color may be pink, skin colored, or gray. They may be solitary or in clusters. Lesions start as pin-size papules that grow into filliform papules or plaques that are often found symmetrically on opposing surfaces. Condyloma acuminata spread rapidly over moist areas such as under the foreskin and the vulva. Management of genital warts is discussed in Chapter 23.

Herpes Type I and II

Two different virus types cause *herpes simplex virus* (HSV) infections: HSV-1 and HSV-2. The former is usually associated with oral infections and the latter with genital infections, but both types can be found in either location, perhaps

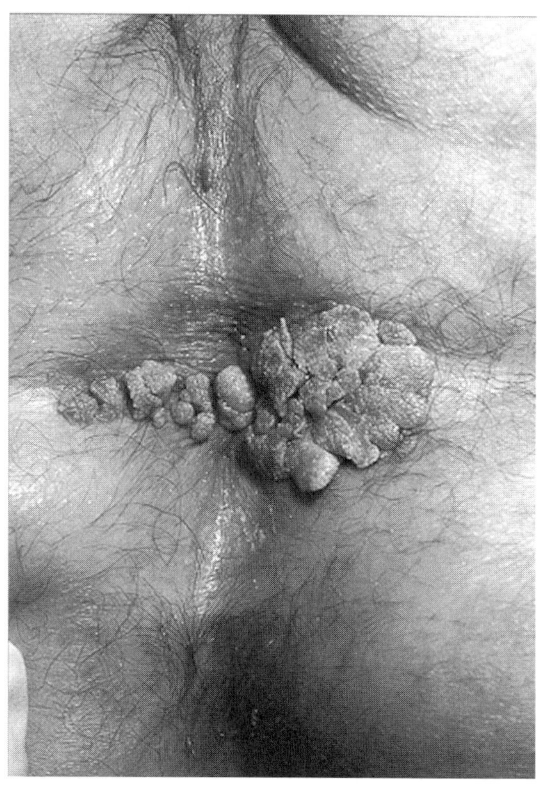

Figure 22-5 Condyloma acuminata.

Source: Reprinted with permission from Elsevier, © 2003. Dermatology Online. Bolognia JL, Jorizzo JL, Rapini RP, editors. [subscriber site on the Internet]. Available from: http://www.dermtext.com.

because of oral genital sexual activity. It is estimated that up to 30% of genital herpes are type 1.[12] HSV has two phases of infection: 1) the primary infection, after which the virus becomes established in a nerve ganglion, and 2) the secondary phase, characterized by recurrent outbreaks at the same site.[12] Both types produce identical patterns of infection and can occur anywhere on the skin as well as the mucous membranes. Lesions last for two to six weeks and heal without scarring. Recurrences occur with local skin trauma including ultraviolet light exposure. Prodromal symptoms last from 2 to 24 hours and include tenderness, pain, mild paresthesias, or burning. Within 12 hours, a group of lesions evolves from an erythematous base to form papules and then vesicles. The dome-shaped tense vesicles rapidly umbilicate and rupture in two to four days to form erosions covered by crusts (**Figure 22-6**). The crusts are

---

Figure 22-6 Herpes type II.

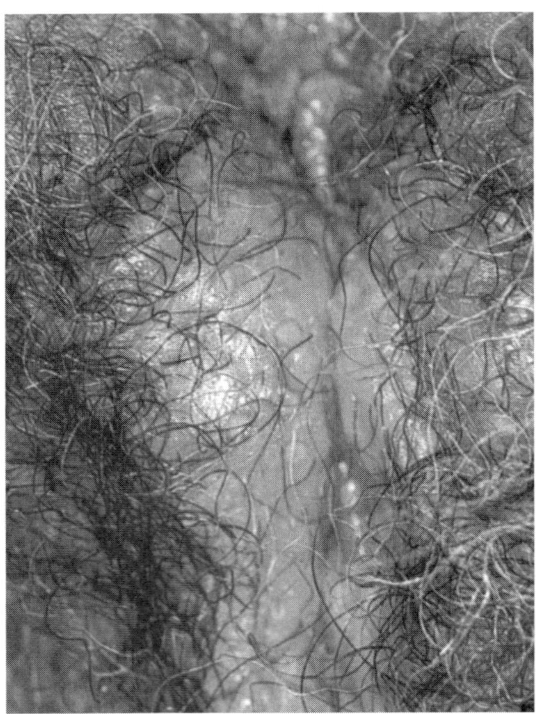

Source: Reprinted with permission from Mosby, © 2001. *Skin Disease: Diagnosis and Treatment.* Habif TP, Campbell JL Jr, Quitadamo M, Zug KA, editors. Chicago: Mosby; 2001. p. 140.

shed in eight or so days with a pink re-epithelialized surface exposed. Management and treatments issues are discussed in Chapter 23.

Molluscum Contagiosum

Molluscum contagiosum is caused by a poxvirus and transmitted by skin-to-skin contact. Usually found in the pubic and genital area, the papules are between 2 and 5 mm, with a keratotic plug, which gives the lesion a central dimple or umbilication (**Figure 22-7**). The infection is spread through autoinoculation after scratching or touching a lesion. Papules can be difficult to see because of pubic hair, and since most women have only a few lesions, they can be easily overlooked. In healthy individuals the lesions resolve spontaneously. Molluscum in the genital area can be removed to avoid sexual transmission by mechanically disrupting the surface with a small curette and extruding the white material containing the molluscum bodies.[33]

Lichen Dermatoses

Lichen simplex chronicus (LSC), *lichen planus* (LP), and *lichen sclerosis* (LS) are each histologically distinctive diseases. The name "lichen" is intended to evoke the image of a rough-surfaced lichen heaped on a smooth-surfaced rock.[34] A dermatologist would have little problem distinguishing one from another, but for the primary care provider a biopsy is definitive.

A pathology report noting "hyperkeratosis and parakeratosis" usually refers to LSC. This is the result of persistent rubbing or scratching of the skin that produces leathery secondary changes called *lichenification.*

LP has a classic description of five Ps: purple polygonal papules and plaques that are pruritic. These are found on the inner wrists and anterior shins. A second or erosive form of LP occurs

Figure 22-7 Molluscum contagiosum.

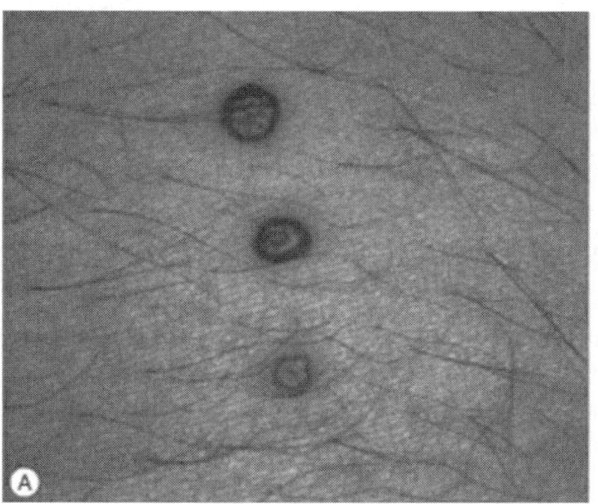 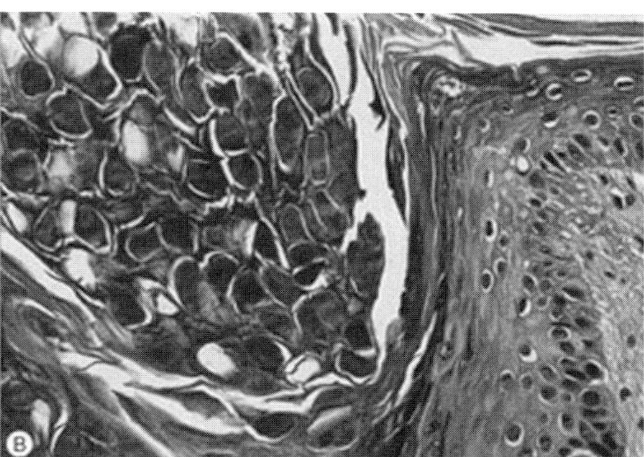

Source: Reprinted with permission from Elsevier, © 2003. Dermatology Online. Bolognia JL, Jorizzo JL, Rapini RP, editors. [subscriber site on the Internet]. Available from: http://www.dermtext.com

both in the mouth and on the vulva. Forty to sixty percent of individuals with LP have oropharyngeal involvement.[12]

LS is one of the major vulvar dermatoses and is estimated to occur in between 1 in 300 to 1 in 1000 people.[35] The skin is white and wrinkly, but the dermis beneath is thickened and sclerotic (**Figure 22-8**). LS often involves the vulva and the anus in a "keyhole" pattern. It is most commonly observed in the prepubertal, perimenopausal, and postmenopausal periods. It has not been determined whether there is an association with autoimmune disease.[36] There is a 6% incidence of development of squamous cell carcinoma from LS, but LS has been found in about 60% of vulvectomy specimens with squamous cell carcinoma.[35,37]

Women with LS experience intense pruritis so serious that it may interfere with sleep. The initial signs are pallor, thickening, and excoriations followed by edema and shrinkage of the labia minora. Eventually, the skin loses its pigmentation and acquires a thinned texture of parchment paper. Atrophy and scarring can result. The disfigurement can be extreme with almost total closure of the introital opening.

Potent topical corticosteroids such as clobetasol propionate 0.05% should be applied to the area once daily at night.[38,39] Because of the small surface area affected by LS, a 30 gm tube should last for three months. This class of steroids should be used only for two weeks at a time followed by a week of rest. It may be resumed if treatment is still needed after the first two weeks. Estrogen creams are not effective for treatment of LS,[36] and although once widely used, topical testosterone is no longer an acceptable treatment option.[40]

Because several conditions result in the formation of white plaques, a biopsy is recommended to establish a definite diagnosis. The differential diagnoses for leukoplakia (white

Figure 22-8 Lichen sclerosis.

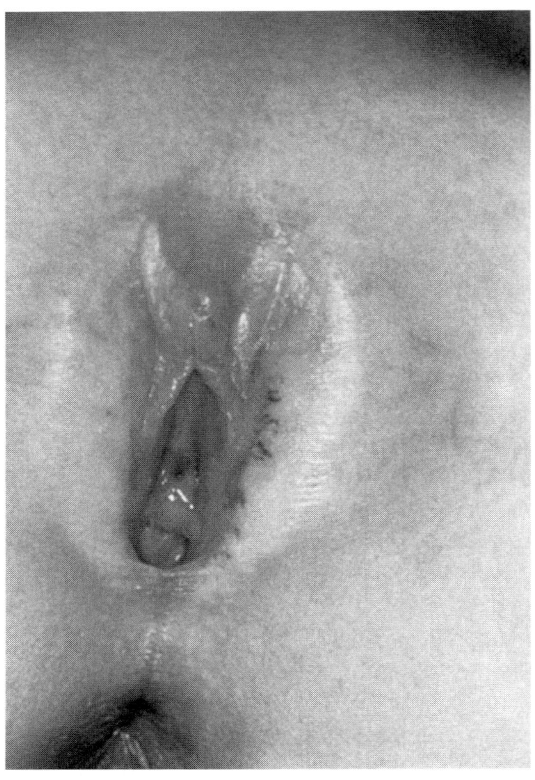

Source: Reprinted with permission from Elsevier, © 2003. Dermatology Online. Bolognia JL, Jorizzo JL, Rapini RP, editors. [subscriber site on the Internet]. Available from: http://www.dermtext.com.

plaques) includes HPV, LP, and vulvar intra-epithelial neoplasia.

Eczematous Disorders

Eczema is from the Greek word meaning to erupt, ferment, or boil. *Acute eczema* is an inflammation of the skin characterized by erythema, edema, and vesiculation with weeping of acute lesions. Pruritis is severe. *Subacute eczema* is more organized and often associated with excoriation, scaling, and erythematous papules or plaques, grouped or scattered over erythematous skin.[41] In chronic eczema, thickened, lichenified skin is seen. Some authors complain that the definition has become a catch-all label that is devoid of meaning,[42,43] and others believe the name should be replaced with the term *"spongiotic dermatitis."*[44] Spongiosis refers to the histopathologic changes that underlie most of the so-called eczemas: edema between the keratinocytes of the stratum that result in a spongy appearance.

The mainstay of treatment is avoidance of irritants and keeping the skin moisturized. In acute flares, cool wet compresses and topical steroid creams allow vasoconstriction and suppress inflammation and itching. Oral corticosteroids are used only for severe or generalized or acute eczema.

Atopic Eczema

Atopy (*atopic dermatitis*, AD) is now thought to be a result of interactions between genetics and environmental factors.[45] The term is used to describe individuals with an inherited tendency toward hypersensitivity, such as asthma and allergic rhinitis, and has come to include the cutaneous manifestation of this condition.[46] Half of children with AD develop asthma or allergic rhinitis by the age of 7.[47] Women with atopy tend to have inherently dry skin that makes them vulnerable to environmental irritants. They also have a lower itch threshold that is triggered by seasonal changes or contact with substances such as sweat, occlusive clothing, or wool.[48] Emotional stress may also be a trigger.[13] The role of dust mites and food allergies is controversial. Most children outgrow AD.

Adult manifestations include flexural involvement, hand manifestations, and upper eyelid dermatitis (**Figure 22-9**).

Treatment includes topical corticosteroids for inflammation and oral antibiotics if lesions become secondarily infected. The skin barrier should be restored and preserved with emollients such as petroleum jelly, Aquaphor, or Unibase applied at least once daily after bathing. Aggravating factors should be avoided. Clothing should be soft and light; cotton is an excellent choice. Stress reduction techniques may be helpful. Pruritus can be controlled with oral antihistamines with a sedating effect such as diphenhydramine (Benadryl) or hydroxyzine (Atarax).

Contact Dermatitis

Contact dermatitis is a generic term applied to acute or chronic inflammatory reactions to substances that come in contact with the skin. The disease is closely linked to occupation because of irritants encountered on the job. The response may be immediate or delayed, and symptoms include pruritis and inflammation (**Figure 22-10**). Common contact allergens include: neomycin; procaine (benzocaine); sulfonamides; turpentine; formalin; mercury; nickel; cobalt sulfate (cement, galvanization, industrial oils, cooking agents); fragrances; frequent wet work (health care providers); latex; and many more.

Allergic contact dermatitis is a delayed hypersensitivity resulting in eczematous dermati-

Figure 22-9 **Atopic eczema.**

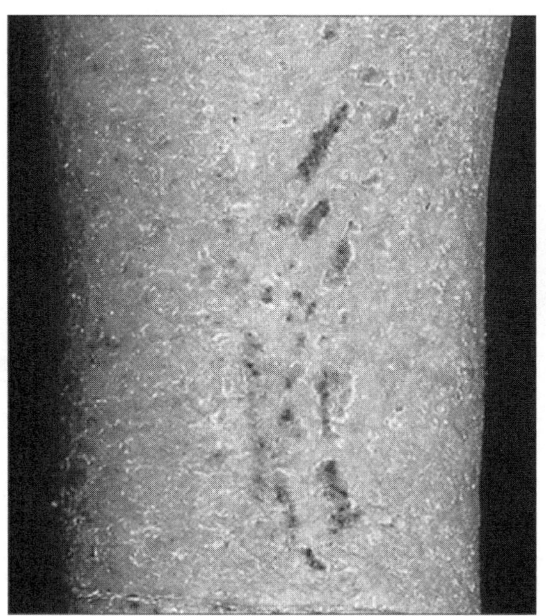

Figure 22-10 **Contact dermatitis.**

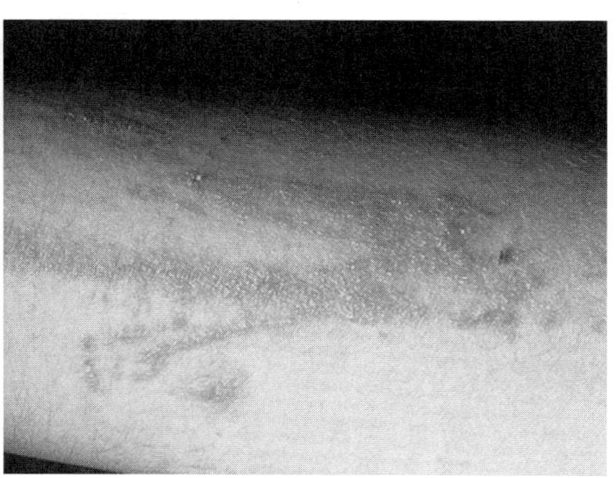

tis. Poison ivy is such a condition. Subacute allergic contact dermatitis to nickel may be seen when a woman develops an inflammation where her watch comes in contact with her skin. Avoidance of the offending irritant is the recommended action.

Other varieties of dermatitis that are frequently seen in a primary care or gynecologic practice include: nummular dermatitis; stasis dermatitis; seborrheic dermatitis (dandruff); and cradle cap in infants.

NUMMULAR ECZEMA

Nummular eczema is a chronic, pruritic, round, coin-shaped plaque composed of grouped small papules and vesicles on an erythematous base, scale, and crust (**Figure 22-11**). The margins are often more pronounced than the central portion. This condition is often seen in atopic individuals. It is commonly seen on the lower legs in men and on the trunk, hands, and fingers in

Figure 22-11 **Nummular eczema.**

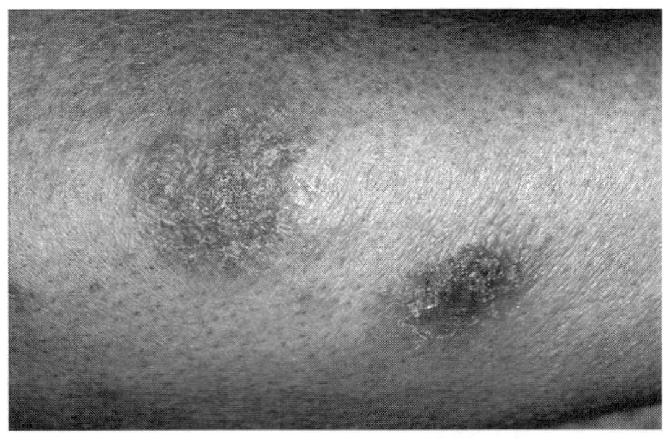

young women. Lesions usually respond to treatment with Class III to IV corticosteroids, but severe presentations may require more potent steroids. Coal tar preparations are useful in resistant cases.

STASIS DERMATITIS

Stasis dermatitis, the result of chronic venous insufficiency, may be seen in older women. It is associated with varicosed and dilated veins, edema, hyperpigmentation, and thickening of the skin. It must be distinguished from contact dermatitis. The lesion may appear pink, red, or brown (hemosiderosis), and ulceration or erosion may occur (**Figure 22-12**). Excoriation may be evident from incessant scratching. Differential diagnoses include contact dermatitis and cellulitis.[13]

Cool water compresses applied for 20 minutes twice a day for acute exudative inflammation will help relieve pruritis. Class II to IV topical steroids can be applied twice daily for two weeks; the cream is used if the dermatitis is acute and ointment if chronic.[13] Lubrication with creams, which are more effective than lotions, will help the dryness. Support hose or socks will provide compression to the ankle. Referral to a dermatologist or podiatrist should be made.

SEBORRHEIC DERMATITIS

Dandruff and cradle cap are forms of eczema known as *seborrheic dermatitis*. Both genetic and environmental factors are thought to be involved.

In infants there is a yellow, greasy adherent scale that develops on the vertex of the scalp that may accumulate and thicken. It might be accompanied by diaper rash or inflammation in the axillae. Milder cases require no attention because cradle cap is often self-limited. Use of

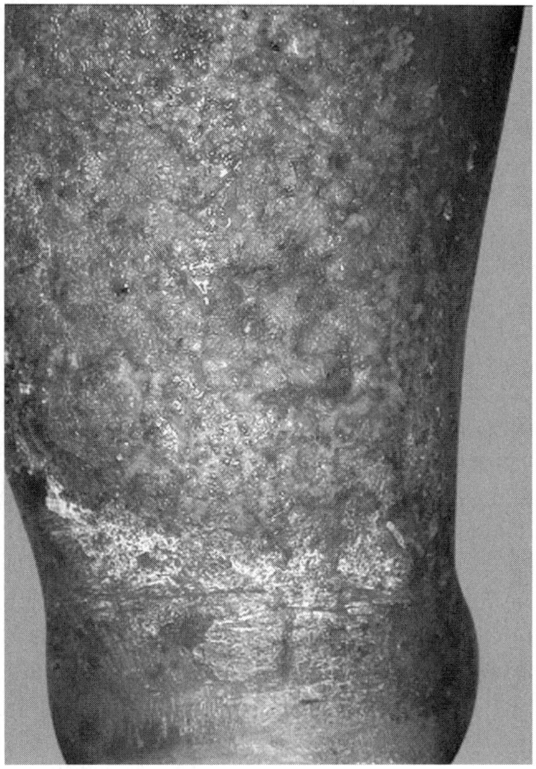

Source: Reprinted with permission from Elsevier, © 2003. Dermatology Online. Bolognia JL, Jorizzo JL, Rapini RP, editors. [subscriber site on the Internet]. Available from: http://www.dermtext.com.

shampoos containing sulfur or salicylic acid may facilitate faster resolution. The differential diagnosis includes atopic dermatitis, zinc deficiency, and Langerhans cell histiocytosis.

In adults, greasy scales and yellow–red coalescing macules, patches, and papules may be diffuse in location and are commonly found on the scalp, scalp margins, eyebrows, base of the lashes, nasolabial folds, external ear canals, posterior auricular fold, presternal skin, and upper back.[13] White scales adherent to eyelashes and lid margins with variable amounts of erythema can be seen in *seborrheic blepharitis*. Seborrheic dermatitis in adults tends to be chronic with periods of remission and exacerbation. Treatment includes oral, anti-staphylococcal antibiotics (dicloxacillin, cephalexin) if heavy exudate and crust are present. Ketoconazole (Nizoral cream) can be applied daily. For the scalp, mild scale is removed by frequent shampooing with products containing sulfur, salicylic acid, or both.[13] For ongoing remissions products containing salicylic acid, sulfur, zinc pyrithrione (Head and Shoulders, ANP Bar soap), selenium (Selsun lotion, Selsun Blue), or tar shampoo (T-Gel, Reme-T, Pentrax) are useful.

Psoriasis

Psoriasis is a papulosquamous disease; that is, it is manifested as scale, with papules, and plaques (**Figure 22-13**). Most frequently, it affects the elbows, knees, and scalp but can affect any portion of the skin, nails, and joints. The lesions are sharply marginated with a silvery white scale. It is a hereditary disorder; if one parent has the disease, the offspring have an 8% chance of having the disease, but if both parents have psoriasis, the child has a 41% chance.[12]

Most patients will already have a diagnosis of psoriasis when they present to a gynecologic visit. The expression "the heartbreak of psoriasis" is not a joke. The name literally means "humiliation."[12] It can be disfiguring and very difficult to treat. It is lifelong and characterized by recurrent exacerbations and remissions. Psoriasis may be worsened by stress and is often worse in the winter months. Drugs that may precipitate or exacerbate

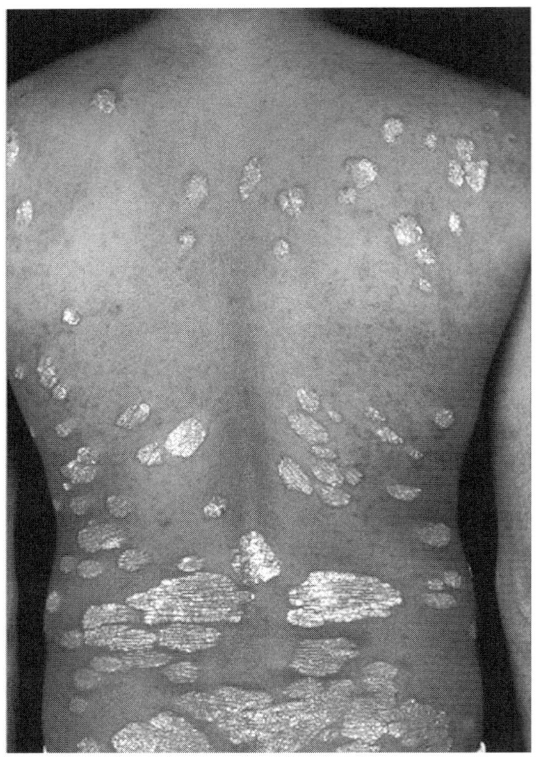

Figure 22-13 Psoriasis.

Source: Reprinted with permission from Elsevier, © 2003. Dermatology Online. Bolognia JL, Jorizzo JL, Rapini RP, editors. [subscriber site on the Internet]. Available from: http://www.dermtext.com.

the condition include lithium, beta-blockers, antimalarials, and systemic steroids.[13]

Smallpox Vaccine

The Centers for Disease Control and Prevention (CDC) issued a statement in 2003 on the contraindications for use of the smallpox vaccine. Individuals with certain skin conditions should not receive this vaccine.[49] The smallpox vaccine is made from a live virus related to smallpox called vaccinia, which stimulates the immune system to react against the virus in order to develop immunity. Immunity to vaccinia also provides immunity to smallpox. While live virus vaccines are safe and effective, individuals with eczema and atopic dermatitis should *not* get the vaccine because such individuals are more likely to have a rare but serious reaction (eczema vaccinatum). This results when virus from the vaccine penetrates broken skin and causes a rash, which can lead to serious scarring or death.

Individuals who have *ever* been diagnosed with eczema, even if the condition was mild, not presently active, or if only present as a child, should not receive smallpox vaccine. Persons with *Darier sign* (where stroking a lesion produces a wheal surrounded by intense erythema) also should not be vaccinated. Persons closely associated with someone who has ever been diagnosed with eczema should not get the vaccine because of the risk it poses to that contact. Close contacts include anyone living in the household or persons with whom there is a sexual contact.

Conditions that warrant waiting before being vaccinated include: impetigo, varicella, pityriasis rosea, acute contact dermatitis (e.g., poison ivy), recent significant burns greater than 2 cm diameter, moderate or extensive psoriasis, severe acne, and pemphigus vulgaris. The skin must be completely healed prior to immunization.

The caveat here is that an individual who has been directly exposed to smallpox should be vaccinated, because the disease poses greater risk than the vaccine. Public health authorities will make vaccine recommendations if there is a smallpox outbreak. For more information, contact the CDC [http://www.cdc.gov/smallpox; hotline, 888-246-2675 (English) or 888-246-2857 (Español)].

Diseases of the Sebaceous and Apocrine Glands

Acne

Acne is an inflammation of the pilosebaceous unit (pustular eruption) of the face and trunk that occurs in adolescence and may persist into adulthood. It may manifest itself as comedones, papulopustules, or nodules plus cysts. Pitted, depressed, or hypertrophic scarring may occur with all types, but this happens more frequently with nodulocystic acne. Women may have premenstrual flares. Controversy remains about whether diet influences acne.[50] Most authorities have concluded that restricting certain foods, like chocolate or fried foods, has little or no impact on the course of acne. However others feel that low-glycemic diets high in fruits and vegetables may minimize outbreaks.

Comedones result from abnormalities in the proliferation and differentiation of ductal keratinocytes in the skin. With acne there is retention of hyperproliferating ductal keratinocytes and corneocytes in the duct. It may be that abnormalities in the sebaceous lipid composition, androgens, local cytokine production, and colonization by particular bacteria encourage comedone formation.[51] It is hypothesized that comedone formation may be primarily an inflammatory process. This would explain why antibacterial agents (benzoyl peroxide) and antimicrobial therapy (oral and topical antibiotics) work so well. *P. acnes* has been implicated in the pathogenesis of acne for more than 100 years.[52] Topical retinoids, which are a mainstay of therapy for many patients, are thought to normalize keratinization and reduce follicular plugging.

Ongoing use prevents formation of microcomodones, which are precursor lesions to all forms of acne.[50]

Acne lesions are divided into noninflammatory and inflammatory lesions. The former consist of open comedones (whiteheads) and closed comedones (blackheads). The latter are characterized by the presence of papules, pustules, and nodules (cysts).[13] The pustules have a visible central core of purulent exudates. *Nodules* are larger than 5 mm, and they become suppurative (cysts) or hemorrhagic. Recurring rupture and re-epithelialization of cysts lead to epithelial-lined tracts, often accompanied by severe scarring.

Recommendations to patients with acne should include washing—not scrubbing—the face no more than two or three times daily. For blocked pores, agents that induce drying and peeling are used. Examples include benzoyl peroxide, azelaic acid (Azelex cream), tretinoin (Retin-A), and other related drugs. The newer drugs in the class of tretinoins are less irritating.

Treatment approaches vary according to the severity of the presentation. Tretinoins are often prescribed as initial therapy in mild to moderate cases. If no response is seen in four to eight weeks, topical antibiotics or benzoyl peroxide agents are added. It takes up to two months for most topical regimens to show their full effect.

Oral antibiotics may be prescribed initially if inflammatory lesions are present or as adjunctive therapy if milder presentations do not improve with topical agents. Options include clindamycin (Cleocin), erythromycin, and some sulfa drugs. Usually the dosage is started at the high end and tapered when control is achieved.[13] Oral contraceptives with a low androgen profile, such as drospirenone/ethinyl estradiol (Yasmin) or norgestimate/ethinyl estradiol (Ortho Tri-Cylen Lo) can also be used as adjunctive therapy. Isotretinoin (Accutane) is reserved for use with severe cystic acne, with acne that causes scarring, and for persistent cases unresponsive to less aggressive therapy. It also has been suggested for the treatment of very oily skin. Isotretinoin is a class X drug (not to be used in pregnancy). Exposure to isotretinoin during pregnancy can cause severe cardiofacial, cardiac, and central nervous system anomalies. Women taking it should have monthly pregnancy tests and use two forms of contraception. Dermatologists register any women taking the drug, and the patient must sign a consent form.

Acne is a chronic condition. Therapy is usually continuous and prolonged so referral to a dermatologist is indicated for moderate to severe cases. Women with milder presentations who respond well to topical agents or hormonal contraception do not require a referral.

Women over the age of 25 with acne usually have long-term low-grade acne. A workup for polycystic ovarian syndrome (PCOS) is indicated if the woman has any of the following: irregular cycles, hirsutism, or obesity. The diagnosis can be made on clinical evidence alone. If irregular cycles are present, the woman can have complications of unopposed estrogen effect on the lining of her uterus and so should be cycled with oral contraception, the contraceptive patch, or with a progestin. She may also need help conceiving a pregnancy and have an increased rate of spontaneous abortion compared to women who do not have PCOS. PCOS is associated with increased insulin resistance and increased unbound androgen levels. Such women are likely to be prediabetic. They should have a glucose tolerance test and be counseled to make changes to improve lifestyle such as diet, exercise, and maintaining optimal weight to avoid health problems later in life related to diabetes and heart disease.

Rosacea (Rosacea Acne)

Rosacea is a common, chronic facial disorder of the pilosebaceous unit. Increased activity of the capillaries leads to flushing and eventually to telangiectasia (**Figure 22-14**). Individuals with rosacea are usually over age 30 and are likely to be of Celtic origin with skin phototypes I and II. It is rare in dark skinned persons, although it is seen in some individuals from southern Italy.[12] With rosacea, there is often a long history of

Figure 22-14 Rosacea.

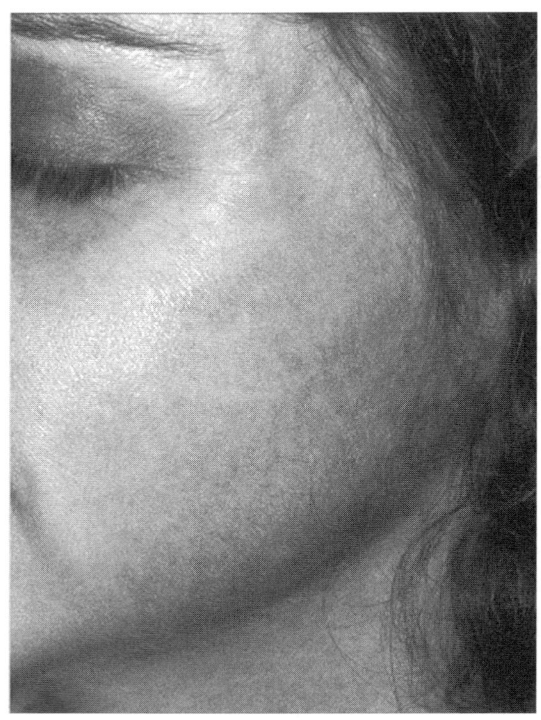

Source: Reprinted with permission from Elsevier, © 2003. Dermatology Online. Bolognia JL, Jorizzo JL, Rapini RP, editors. [subscriber site on the Internet]. Available from: http://www.dermtext.com.

flushing with hot fluids, spicy foods, or alcohol. It may follow acne but usually arises de novo.

Treatment includes avoidance of triggers through lifestyle modifications. Hot beverages, not necessarily caffeine, and alcohol should be eliminated. Emotional stressors may contribute to the flares.

Dermatologists usually prescribe oral antibiotics and topical therapy to bring the inflammation under control, followed by long-term treatment with topical medication to maintain remission. Metronidazole (pregnancy Class B) gel or cream 0.75% twice daily is usually the first antibiotic used. Topical antibiotics such as erythromycin may also be used. If both of these fail or the disease is severe, then oral tetracycline, minocycline, or doxycycline (all pregnancy Class D) can be used. Once the inflammation is controlled, the underlying telangiectasia may become more visible. Surgical techniques such as using a laser or intense pulsed light source may erase the vessels.

Hidradenitis Suppurativa

Hidradenitis suppurativa is another chronic disease of apocrine gland–bearing skin in the axillae and the groin. It is commonly seen in gynecology practice.

Families may give a history of nodulocystic acne and hidradenitis suppurativa occurring separately or together in blood relatives.[12] Predisposing factors include acne, obesity, and apocrine duct obstruction. Symptoms include pain and tenderness related to abscess formation.

The initial lesion is an inflammatory nodule or abscess that may either resolve or point to the surface and drain purulent or seropurulent material (**Figure 22-15**). A relationship to a hair follicle is not apparent. Eventually, sinus tracts form with fibrosis and scarring; hypertrophic and keloidal

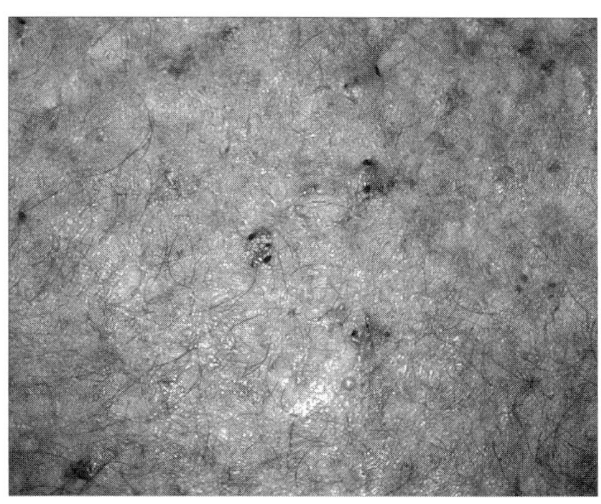

Figure 22-15 Hidradenitis suppurativa.

Source: Reprinted with permission from Elsevier, © 2003. Dermatology Online. Bolognia JL, Jorizzo JL, Rapini RP, editors. [subscriber site on the Internet]. Available from: http://www.dermtext.com.

scars and contractures may ensue. Comedones or double comedones may be present.

Treatment is complicated because this condition is not just an infection. A combination of intralesional corticosteroids, surgery, oral antibiotics, and isotretinoin are used.

Disorders of Hair Follicles

Alopecia

Hair loss in women is often very disturbing to the individual. As previously discussed in the section on pregnancy, most women experience self-limited loss in the postpartum period; reassurance is usually all that is needed.

Androgenic alopecia, male pattern hair loss, is another disease that is most distressing to affected women. It is a physiologic reaction to androgens in genetically predisposed individuals of both sexes. In women, there is central, diffuse hair thinning that begins at an early age (20s or 30s), in contrast to the hair loss that occurs as part of aging that begins in the 50s or 60s. Hair loss is gradual. Menstrual cycles are normal, as are pregnancies. There is no association with infertility or galactorrhea.[13] Contrary to the common belief that baldness is inherited from the maternal grandfather, alopecia can be inherited from either side of the family.[53] It may be beneficial to avoid the term "male pattern baldness" and replace it with hereditary hair thinning or female pattern hair loss to avoid the stigma inferred from the more commonly used term.

Most women with alopecia do not require laboratory hormonal evaluation. If however, the woman has irregular menstrual cycles, acne, hirsutism, infertility, or galactorrhea, then DHEAS, serum-free or total testosterone, and prolactin levels may help to point to a diagnosis of PCOS, pituitary adenoma (galactorrhea), or other constitutional disease. A thyroid stimulating hormone level should be obtained to rule out thyroid disease, which may affect the menstrual cycle.

Treatment includes use of 2% topical minoxidil solution (Rogaine), applied twice a day; a 5% solution is used on men. Use of the stronger solution by women may result in increased hair growth on the forehead and face. There are no restrictions on hair washing, combing, or coloring the hair. Estrogen is not prescribed for thinning hair. If hormonal contraception is desired, a product low in androgenic activity (i.e., Yazmin or Ortho Tri-Cyclen Lo) should be considered.

Hirsutism

Hirsutism is excessive hair growth in androgen-dependent hair patterns: the face, chest, areola, linea nigra, inner thighs, and external genitalia. Defining this condition is difficult because there is considerable individual and ethnic variation in the degree and pattern of body hair.[54] The development of body hair growth in women is not a disease; rather, it is along the spectrum of biological variation. In the extreme on this spectrum, however, there may be an association with endocrinopathy that produces a state of hyperandrogenism. This is the case with PCOS (discussed above), where decreased insulin sensitivity drives the pancreas to produce more insulin, which in turn drives the ovary to produce more testosterone. This results in increased hirsutism. Because PCOS puts the affected women at increased risk of infertility, endometrial pathology, diabetes, and heart disease, intervention is necessary.

Other rare causes of hirsutism that must be considered include: congenital adrenal hyperplasia, androgen secreting tumors, Cushing syndrome, hyperprolactinemia, HAIR-AN syndrome (often seen with PCOS: hyperandrogenism, insulin resistance, and acanthosis nigricans), pregnancy, and postmenopausal hirsutism. The latter is the result not of increased testosterone in the postmenopause but a decrease in the estrogen/androgen ratio when the ovaries no longer produce the strongest estrogen, estradiol. Consequently, the androgen effect is greater since there is less circulating estrogen; this results in increased hair growth in some women.

For most women, reassurance that they have no masculinizing or other serious disease is all that is needed. Some women will ask about cosmetic treatments, but others will want to be referred to a dermatologist for additional remedies. Oral contraceptives with a low androgenic profile should be chosen for women who require contraception, but hormonal contraception does nothing to decrease established hirsutism.

Infectious Folliculitis

Infectious folliculitis is an inflammatory reaction, usually in the superficial aspect of the follicle. The inflammation may be the result of bacterial, fungal, or viral infections. Folliculitis in the axillae or the groin/genital region that proceeds to the boil stage is a common presentation in a gynecologic practice.

Predisposing factors include shaving hairy regions such as the axillae and the pubic area. Removing hair, such as by bikini waxing, can also lead to folliculitis. Investigation of causative factors should include use of hot tubs, swimming pools, exposure to chemicals, and the possibility of other associated dermatitis.

Dome-shaped pustules with small erythematous halos arise in the center of a follicle. *Furuncles* (boils) develop as a result of the spread of the bacterial infection into the tissues of the follicle. The furuncle begins as a small, painful, inflammatory follicular nodule that becomes pustular, develops central necrosis within a few days, and heals after a discharge of necrotic material, often leaving a scar. Predisposing conditions for development of furuncles include chronic staphylococcal carrier state, diabetes mellitus, malnutrition, and HIV infection.[55] Culture is not usually necessary because *Staphylococcus aureus* is the most common infecting organism. Inspection of scrapings from the lesion under the microscope with KOH should be done to rule out fungal organisms.

Folliculitis is responsive to antibiotic and hygienic measures. Heat and friction should be minimized. Antibacterial soaps are useful in this instance although not beneficial for daily use in the genital region. Warm or cold compresses offer some relief for the pain and itching. Mupirocin (Bactroban) is an effective topical treatment for limited, superficial involvement. Oral antibiotics are indicated for extensive or spreading disease. If a boil is present, oral anti-staphylococcal antibiotics such as oxacillin, dicloxacillin, or cefuroxime (all Pregnancy Class B) should be used.

Fungal Infections

Candidiasis

Candidiasis is a common condition that affects the vulvovaginal region and is often the result of a disturbance in the normal flora (**Figure 22-16**). Women are prone to *Candida* in pregnancy, with hormonal contraceptive use, diabetes, topical steroid therapy, and antibiotic therapy. *Candida vulvovaginitis* appears as a bright erythema with edema. The primary lesion is a pustule that peels away the stratum corneum, leaving a denuded, glistening surface. Yeast grows best in a warm, moist environment, so it usually is confined to the mucous membranes and intertriginous areas. See Chapter 23 for management of vaginal candida infections. In addition to the vulva, women who are obese and have pendulous breasts or overhanging abdominal folds are at risk for *Candida* in these areas.

Tinea Corpus

Tinea corpus can be easily recognized in the annular form, ringworm. It can be contacted from animals, contaminated soil, or autoinoculation from

Figure 22-16 Candida.

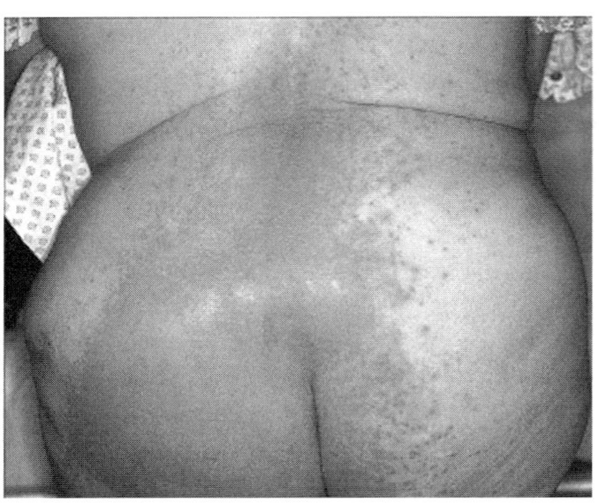

Source: Reprinted with permission from Elsevier, © 2003. Dermatology Online. Bolognia JL, Jorizzo JL, Rapini RP, editors. [subscriber site on the Internet]. Available from: http://www.dermtext.com.

other parts of the body, that is, from tinea pedis or tinea capitis. The most likely organisms are *E. floccosum* and *T. rubrum*. The incubation period can be from days to months. Lesions range widely in size as sharply marginated plaques with or without pustules or vesicles at margins (**Figure 22-17**). Central clearing follows peripheral enlargement of the lesion. Examination of scrapings with KOH preparation usually shows abundant hyphae. Mild itching is the most common complaint. It can be confused with pityriasis rosea, but the scaling ring of pityriasis does not reach the edge of the border as it does in tinea.

Tinea corpus may be found in the intertriginous folds beneath the breasts and the abdominal fold over the symphysis in obese women. The arcuate raised borders and clear areas of the rash help to distinguish it from intertrigo or seborrhea.[33] A KOH smear will clarify the diagnosis.

Superficial lesions respond to antifungal creams applied twice daily for a minimum of two weeks. Treatment should be continued for one week after the lesions have resolved. Extensive lesions or those with red papules require oral therapy including griseofulvin and should be treated by a dermatologist.

Pityriasis (Tinea) versicolor

Pityriasis versicolor (PV) is a chronic asymptomatic scaling dermatosis caused by the lipophilic yeast, *Pityrosporum orbiculare*. Excess heat, perspiration, and oily skin can be predisposing factors. It is often seen in adolescence or young adulthood, a time with high sebaceous activity. The organism is part of the normal skin flora but is opportunistic in the right circumstances. It is particularly common in individuals exposed to high humidity, such as those residing in subtropical or tropical zones. Self-care practices that increase local humidity of the skin can also facilitate the growth of *Pityrosporum orbiculare*. For example, applications of grease or cocoa butter in children will predispose them to PV. Certain circumstances may also lower the skin's resistance to this organism and allow for its overgrowth including pregnancy, malnutrition, corticosteroid therapy, immunosuppression, and hormonal contraception.[13]

The lesions present as small, circular, white scaling patches on the upper trunk (**Figure 22-18**). Lesions are white in tanned individuals, and pink or brown in untanned fair women; they are hyperpigmented in black women. Clinical findings can be confirmed by positive KOH preparation. The scale is scraped off onto a slide with a #15 surgical blade, covered with a slip, and gently heated. Hyphae can be observed.

The greatest concern for women who have PV is cosmetic, because of the blotchy pigmen-

Figure 22-17 Tinea corpus.

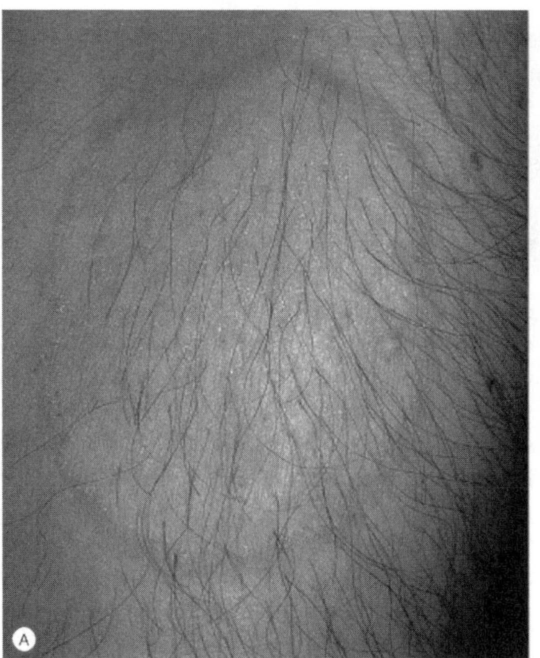

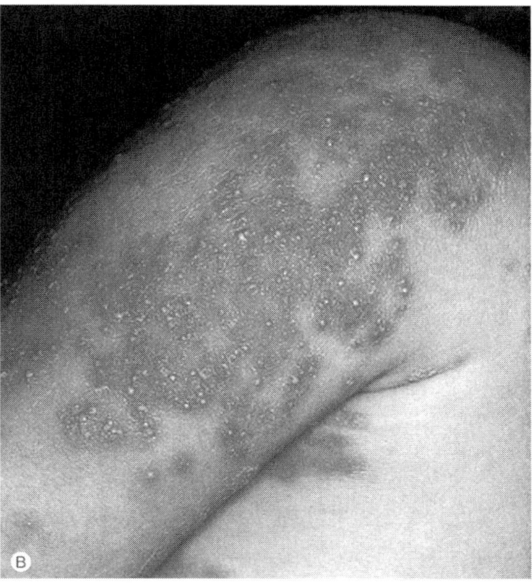

Source: Reprinted with permission from Elsevier, © 2003. Dermatology Online. Bolognia JL, Jorizzo JL, Rapini RP, editors. [subscriber site on the Internet]. Available from: http://www.dermtext.com.

tation. Topical agents used in treatment include selenium sulfide (2.5%) lotion or shampoo applied daily for 10 to 15 minutes, followed by a shower, for one week. Alternately, azole creams (ketoconazole, econazole, miconazole, clotrimazole) can be applied twice a day for two weeks. Systemic agents such as oral ketoconazole are off label for use for PV, so if topical agents are not successful, referral to a dermatologist is recommended. **Table 22-4** is a list of antifungal agents.

Bacterial Infections

Impetigo

Impetigo in adults is often a secondary bacterial infection (usually *Staphylococcus aureus*). Predisposing factors include: warm ambient temperature; humidity; presence of another skin disease, especially atopic dermatitis; prior antibiotic therapy; poor hygiene; crowded living conditions; and neglected minor skin trauma. Transient superficial small

Figure 22-18 **Pityriasis versicolor.**

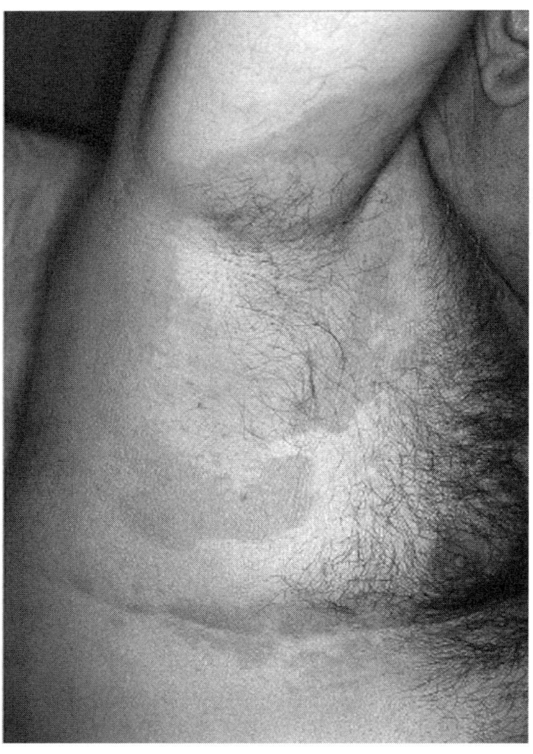

Source: Reprinted with permission from Elsevier, © 2003. Dermatology Online. Bolognia JL, Jorizzo JL, Rapini RP, editors. [subscriber site on the Internet]. Available from: http://www.dermtext.com.

vesicles or pustules rupture and result in erosions, which in turn become crusted.

The disease is self-limiting, but if not treated may be of long duration. Sometimes severe systemic sequelae occur that include glomerulonephritis and serious secondary infections such as osteomyelitis, septic arthritis, and pneumonia.[13] Treatment for localized infections is usually with mupirocin ointment or cream (Bactroban). Oral antibiotics are administered for widespread infection. A penicillinase-resistant antibiotic such as dicloxacillin or cephalexin (Keflex) four times a day for 5 to 10 days is recommended.[13] The development of antibiotic-resistant staphylococci is a concern when oral erythromycin is used.

Cellulitis

Cellulitis involves the skin down to subcutaneous tissues and is characterized by erythema, edema, and pain. It typically occurs in patients with serious systemic disease such as diabetes, cirrhosis, and kidney failure. Cellulitis also develops frequently near surgical wounds or trauma sites. The lower extremities are most at risk. Other dermatoses, such as athlete's foot or stasis dermatitis, may provide the entry for infection. If cellulitis is suspected, then referral is required for evaluation and treatment.

If the leg is affected, elevation improves circulation to the area. Pain can be alleviated somewhat with Burrow's solution compresses. The patient should be treated empirically with oral antibiotics aimed at staphylococcal and streptococcal organisms. Dicloxacillin 500 to 1000 mg orally every six hours, amoxicillin 250 to 500 mg, or erythromycin 250 to 500 mg every six hours is used for 10 to 14 days. Severe infections require hospitalization.

Erythrasma Intertrigo

Erythrasma intertrigo is a chronic bacterial infection caused by *Corynebacterium minutissimum* that affects the intertriginous areas of the toes, axillae, and the groin (**Figure 22-19**). It is often mistaken for a widespread fungal infection, but the KOH prep will be negative. This microbe is normal skin flora that can cause superficial infection under circumstances such as diabetes, increased humidity, and prolonged periods of occlusion or maceration. Obese women often

Table 22-4 ANTIFUNGAL AGENTS

Generic Name	Brand Name	Uses
Miconazole	Monistat, Monistat-Derm	*Candida*
Clotrimazole	Lotrimin, Mycelex	*Candida*
Fluconazole	Diflucan	*Candida*
Griseofulvin	Grisfulvin V; Gris-PEG	Tinea
Ketoconazole	Nizoral	Tinea, *Candida*; drink citrus or cranberry juice for better absorption
Terbinafine	Lamisil	Onychomycosis
Nystatin	Nilstat	*Candida*
Itraconazole	Sporanox	Onychomycosis
Clotrimazole and betamethasone dipropionate	Lotrisone	Antifungal with potent topical steroid for inflamed fungal infections (short duration only)
Nystatin and Triamcinolone topical	Mycolog II	Antifungal with medium potency steroid (short duration only)

have chronic chafing and inflammation in intertriginous areas. Deep body folds are less able to dry out with perspiration, which can lead to erythrasma, tinea, or candidiasis. Once a yeast infection is ruled out, Benzoyl peroxide 2.5% gel for seven days or topical erythromycin solution twice a day for seven days will treat the bacterial infection. Alternately, oral erythromycin 250 mg four times a day for 14 days may be used. Regular use of a benzoyl peroxide bar or wash is usually all that is needed to prevent further episodes.

Viral Infections

Verruca Vulgaris

Verruca vulgaris (warts) are classified by clinical morphology and location. They are caused by HPV. As with other viral infections, there is no definitive cure but there are medical and destructive options available.

Common warts make up about 70% of cutaneous warts.[56] They may occur anywhere on the skin but have an affinity for the backs of hands, fingers, palmar, and plantar surfaces. Flat warts (*verrucae planae*) are found in 4% of the patients with warts (**Figure 22-20**).[57] They are frequently multiple and involve the face, back of the hand, and legs when women shave. Plantar warts occur more commonly in adolescents and young adults.

In general, warts have no symptoms, but in some areas such as the palmar aspects of the fingers, they may be tender. Periungual and subungual warts may interfere with nail growth. Most warts regress spontaneously unless the patient is immunocompromised. The goal of therapy is to alleviate the discomfort, both physical and psychological, and also to prevent the spread of infection to other parts of the body and to other individuals.

Aggressive therapies against warts can be painful and may be followed by scarring. Because most warts resolve on their own, such

Figure 22-19 Erythrasma.

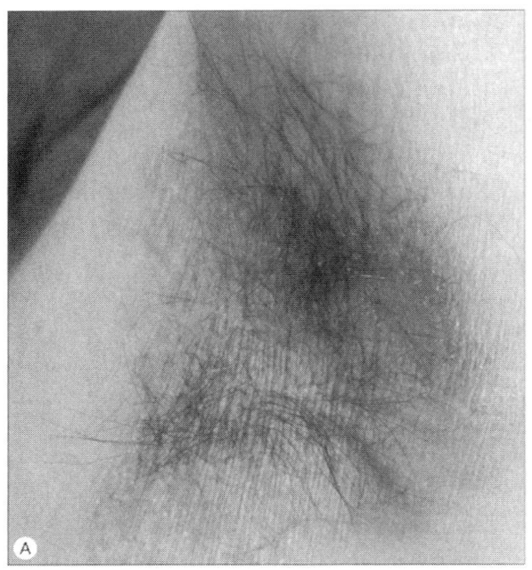
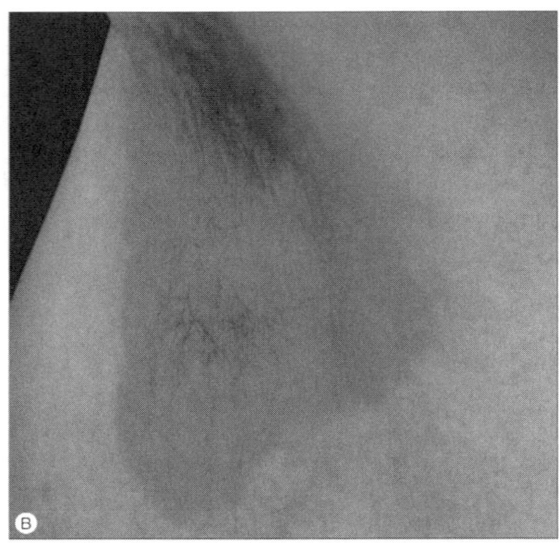

Source: Reprinted with permission from Elsevier, © 2003. Dermatology Online. Bolognia JL, Jorizzo JL, Rapini RP, editors. [subscriber site on the Internet]. Available from: http://www.dermtext.com.

therapies are usually avoided. Patients may initiate therapy on their own with OTC preparations such as salicylic acid and lactic acid in a colloidal solution. This must be repeated daily for long periods of time. Occlusion of the wart with impregnated bandages provides for better penetration. These are available OTC at pharmacies. Persistent warts unresponsive to topical treatment should be referred to a dermatologist. Liquid nitrogen cryotherapy for 15 seconds is an option. A follow-up visit in two weeks for re-treatment may be necessary.

Herpes Zoster

Herpes zoster (shingles) is caused by the reactivation of latent varicella zoster virus and occurs in 10% to 20% of all persons. It usually occurs in the elderly or in the immunocompromised but can occur in any age group. Herpes zoster may be the first clinical manifestation of the development of HIV.

It appears as small grouped vesicles on a pink/red base that occur unilaterally, usually without crossing the midline of the body. The rash usually appears along a single dermatome. Although shingles are thought to be most common on the trunk, they may appear on any dermatome throughout the body. Pre-eruptive tenderness, hyperesthesia, pain, itching, or burning in only one dermatome is usually a predictive sign of the disease. The patient may also have constitutional symptoms including fever, malaise, and headache prior to the rash. An episode of zoster does not confer immunity, so an individual may have more than one attack over the course of her life.

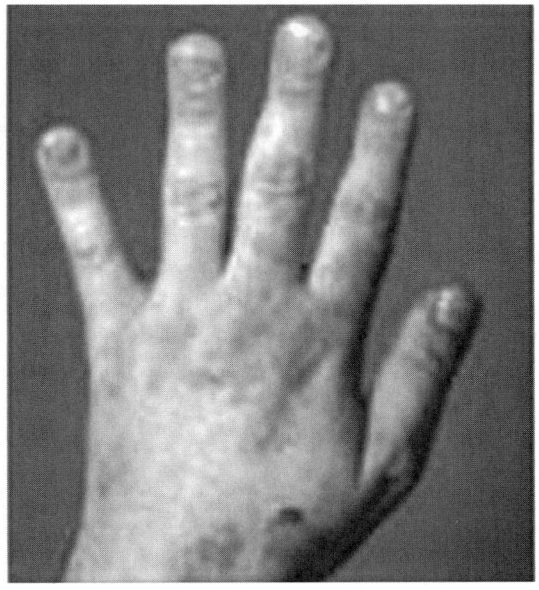

Figure 22-20 Flat warts.

Source: Reprinted with permission from Elsevier, © 2003. Dermatology Online. Bolognia JL, Jorizzo JL, Rapini RP, editors. [subscriber site on the Internet]. Available from: http://www.dermtext.com.

Pain is the major cause of morbidity with this disease; the incidence and duration of pain increase with age. It can be intractable and exhausting. Treatment includes cool tap water compresses when the vesicles are present. Oral steroids can reduce acute pain and help resolve the rash more quickly. Sympathetic blocks (stellate ganglion or epidural with bupivacaine 0.25%) may help with the pain and may alleviate or prevent post-herpetic neuralgia.[13] While oral antiviral drugs may help to decrease acute pain, viral shedding, and the duration and severity of post-herpetic neuralgia, the efficacy for severe post-herpetic neuralgia is doubtful. Many therapeutics have been tried, including tricyclic antidepressants, steroids, narcotics, and topical capsaicin cream (Zostrix; a product made from hot peppers). Capsaicin should not be applied to unhealed skin.

Pityriasis Rosea

Pityriasis rosea is a self-limited exanthematous disease of unknown etiology that has long been suspected to be viral in origin.[58] The diagnosis of pityriasis is primarily a clinical one, only rarely requiring a skin biopsy for diagnosis. However, it may be confused with tinea corporis or nummular eczema, especially when only the herald patch is present. The possibility of secondary syphilis should also be considered. Pityriasis can occur in multiple individuals in group residences such as fraternity houses and military bases.[13]

It has a distinctive morphology and runs a characteristic course. Some patients have a mild prodrome of fever, malaise, headache, or arthralgias. The first clinical manifestation is a herald patch, present in 40% to 60% of all patients (**Figure 22-21**).[59] This is a solitary round or oval lesion from 2 to 10 cm across that appears anywhere on the body, but usually on the trunk or upper arms. This patch is annular with a raised border of fine adherent scales. Within 10 to 14 days, small lesions appear and reach their maximum number in one to two weeks. Apart from the herald patch, the eruption is symmetrically oriented along lines of skin cleavage. On the back the rash looks like drooping pine tree branches. While the rash lasts for 2 to 12 weeks, the post-inflammatory hyper- or hypopigmentation may last for many months. Relapse is rare. The diagnosis of pityriasis rosea is made clinically. The treatment is symptomatic: patients who are pruritic may benefit from emollients,

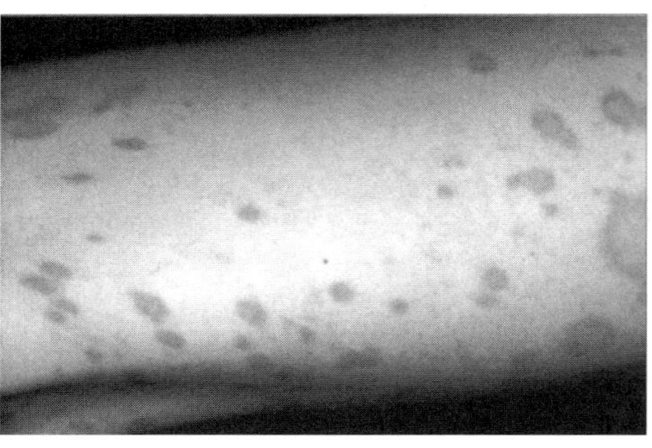

Figure 22-21 Pityriasis rosea.

Source: Reprinted with permission from Elsevier, © 2003. Dermatology Online. Bolognia JL, Jorizzo JL, Rapini RP, editors. [subscriber site on the Internet]. Available from: http://www.dermtext.com.

mild topical corticosteroids, and antipruritic medications. There are no data on the effect on a fetus, but no clinical reports have lent credence to adverse outcomes if the mother contracts the rash.

Infestations

Pediculosis Pubis

Pediculosis pubis (crab lice) is an infestation of hair bearing-regions. It is the most contagious sexually transmitted problem known, with the chance of acquiring the infestation from one's infected partner being 90%.[12,13] Lice all have three sets of legs, but the crab louse has enlarged posterior claws that grasp large diameter body hairs (hence the name). The life cycle from egg (nit) to adult is 22 to 27 days, and the incubation period is seven to eight days.[12] Transmission can occur from adults to children (eyelashes) and from inanimate objects such as hats or earphones.

On physical examination, the nits are firmly attached to the hair in the pubic or anal regions. All agents used for treatment attack the louse's nervous system. The treatment should be repeated one week after the first. Nix, an OTC 1% permethrin rinse, is usually the first line drug of choice. OTC synergized pyrethrin shampoos (RID, A-200) are also used. They are applied and washed off after 10 minutes. Permethrin 5% (Elimite cream) is prescribed when OTC preparations have not proven efficacious. Other options include lindane (Kwell) shampoo and Malathion lotion (Ovide).

Nits are not affected by the treatments above, so they must be physically removed. Shaving the pubic and abdominal hair is an option. Fomite control (household decontamination) is essential.

Scabies

Scabies is an infestation by the mite, *Sarcoptes scabiei*, that is usually spread by close, prolonged skin-to-skin contact. The symptoms are the result of an allergic response to the mites. It is manifested by severe, intractable pruritis with few dermatologic findings. The itching is worse at night. Scabies should be considered whenever any generalized pruritic eruption does not respond to topical corticosteroids or oral prednisone.

The burrow is the classic lesion, linear, curved, or S-shaped. It is 1 to 2 mm wide and up to 15 mm long. The lesion looks pink-white and is slightly elevated. Commonly found in the webbing between the fingers, on the wrists, sides of hands or feet, it can also be found in skin folds, the genital area, and in warm intertriginous regions. In secondary lesions (resulting from infection or from scratching) there is a honey-colored crust like that seen with impetigo. Mites can be identified with a wet prep with KOH after scraping the burrow with a #15 blade, which is then applied to a slide.

Scabies is usually treated topically with permethrin cream 5% (Elimite, Acticin) applied overnight for 8 to 14 hours. It is applied to the entire skin surface below the neck, including under the fingernails, toenails, and in the umbilicus. Treatment should be repeated in one week.

Other choices are available. Lindane 1% lotion (gamma benzene hexachloride; Kwell) is less expensive than permethrin cream but associated with more significant (although rare) side effects. It also may be less effective. Seizures have been reported with lindane use after a bath or with severe dermatitis. Aplastic anemia has also been reported.[12] Lindane should never be used on infants, young children, or pregnant or lactating women; neither should it be used after a shower or with open lesions. Because of these potential reactions, permethrin is also preferred if the mites have infested the head and neck. The only oral treatment is single dose ivermectin, given in a single oral dose. However, it is not approved for scabies in the United States. Regardless of the treatment used, itching may continue for a week after treatment is completed because of the continued reaction to the dead mites and mite excrement. Severe cases of pruritis may be treated with a 14-day tapered steroid course, beginning with prednisone 70 mg on the first day.

The home and the examining room need to be cleaned thoroughly and all clothing and bedding washed and dried by machine. Stuffed animals or other unwashable material should be kept away from contact with humans for 72 hours; storage in a sealed black garbage bag is suitable. Insecticides, fumigation, and extermination are not necessary.[60]

Lyme Disease

Lyme disease is a three-stage tick-borne disease caused by the spirochete *Borrelia burgdorferi*. It is a disease that is often overdiagnosed; as many as 80% of individuals originally diagnosed with Lyme disease are re-diagnosed with another disorder.[13] Like syphilis, it affects many systems, occurs in stages, and mimics other diseases. Three to 21 days after the tick bite, a skin lesion appears that is accompanied by influenza-like symptoms. In stage 2, there are cardiac and neurologic effects; stage 3 is characterized by arthritis and chronic neurologic syndromes.

The original bite has a local reaction with pain, erythema, and a papule that may proceed to a slowly enlarging ring. The central erythema gradually fades, leaving a normal to light blue surface. The ring remains flat, blanches with pressure, and does not desquamate, vesiculate, or have a scale at the periphery. The erythema migrans border may enlarge to form a broad round to oval area of erythema up to 10 cm. This border may advance for days or weeks. Some patients will have multiple concentric rings. Diagnosis without the appearance of erythema migrans is difficult. Laboratory testing is not useful except for serology. Poor sensitivity and inter-laboratory variability are problematic.[13]

Adults with Lyme disease should be treated with 21 days of doxycycline 100 mg twice a day, amoxicillin 500 mg three times a day, or cefuroxime axetil (Ceftin) 500 mg twice a day. Erythromycin, penicillin V, and azithromycin are less effective. A physician experienced in infectious disease should manage the treatment of Lyme disease.

Benign Skin Tumors and Conditions

Acrochordon

Skin tags are common, benign findings, variously called soft fibroma or cutaneous papillomas. They may vary in size from <1 mm to 10 mm. Skin tags occur most often in middle and old age, and are more prevalent in women than in men. Skin tags are frequently found in intertriginous areas including the axilla, inframammary, and the groin, and are associated with obesity. These lesions often first appear or grow in pregnancy. Undisturbed tags are usually asymptomatic. If they are tender as a result of torsion, management is accomplished by excision with a scissors, or with cautery or cryosurgery. Histologic testing is not usually performed.

Dermatofibroma

Dermatofibromas are button-like nodules usually found on the legs. Commonly found in women, they are important only because of cosmetic concerns or by being mistaken for another lesion. They appear as dome shaped, but some can be depressed beneath the skin surface; dermatofibromas are usually smaller than 0.7 cm, although they can rarely grow as large as 3 cm in diameter (**Figure 22-22**). Dermatofibromas are fixed in the skin but can be moved over the underlying subcutaneous fat. On palpation, they feel like a button or a pea. When the skin on either side is squeezed together, a dimple will be evident. The lesions may remain stable for many years, and some regress. There is no intervention indicated.

Figure 22-22 Dermatofibroma.

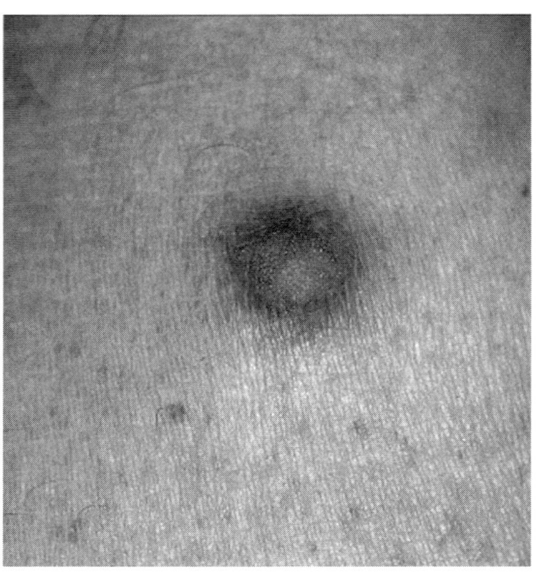

Source: Reprinted with permission from Elsevier, © 2003. Dermatology Online. Bolognia JL, Jorizzo JL, Rapini RP, editors. [subscriber site on the Internet]. Available from: http://www.dermtext.com.

Keloids

Keloids are hypertrophic scars gone wild, resulting from fibrous tissue repair. Hypertrophic scars remain confined to the site of the original injury but keloids extend beyond. They appear much more commonly on blacks than lighter complexioned individuals. There are usually no symptoms associated with keloids, although they can cause great concern cosmetically. Moreover, they may continue to progress in size for decades. Individuals prone to keloids should be advised to avoid unnecessary trauma to the skin such as piercings. Prior to surgery, keloids may be pretreated with Triamcinolone acetate 5 mg/mL injected into the site. Intralesional corticosteroids may be used to reduce pruritis and sensitivity and to reduce volume and flatten the keloid. Surgical excision is avoided because it may result in the development of a larger keloid than the original one.

Syringoma

Syringomas are benign adenomas (a benign epithelial structure usually arranged like a gland) of the intra-epidermal eccrine ducts. There may be a familial tendency. Syringomas occur most frequently in women beginning at puberty. They are 1 to 2 mm, firm, skin-colored or yellow papules; most often they appear as multiple papules around the eyes but are also found on the labia (**Figure 22-23**). The papules are asymptomatic, stable in size, and persistent. If the lesions are considered disfiguring, they can be removed with electrosurgery.

Seborrheic Keratosis

Seborrheic keratoses are very common, benign persistent lesions of variable appearance, usually occurring after age 30. These lesions affect both sexes and all races equally. Most are between 0.2 and 2.0 cm in size, and may appear flat or raised (**Figure 22-24**). Their surface may be smooth, velvety, or verrucous (wart-like). The color of the lesions varies from white to pink to jet-black and may vary within a single lesion.[13] Most appear as "stuck on." *Dermatosis papulosa nigra* describes seborrheic dermatoses more commonly found in SPTs 5 and 6. These lesions are 1 to 2 mm, dark brown keratotic papules concentrated around the eyes and on the cheeks.

Seborrheic keratoses may be found anywhere on the body, especially in the presternal area. Lesions may be localized to the areola. Keratoses tend to persist and grow slowly; with time, the lesions may become very large. Most individuals have fewer than 20, but some women have

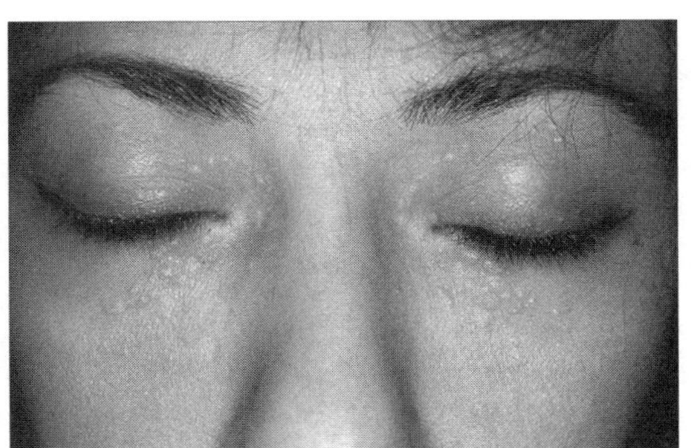

Figure 22-23 **Syringoma.**

Source: Reprinted with permission from Elsevier, © 2003. Dermatology Online. Bolognia JL, Jorizzo JL, Rapini RP, editors. [subscriber site on the Internet]. Available from: http://www.dermtext.com.

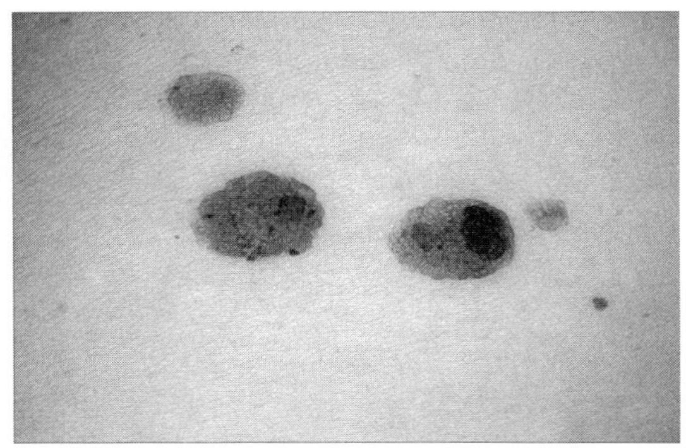

Figure 22-24 **Seborrheic keratosis.**

Source: Reprinted with permission from Elsevier, © 2003. Dermatology Online. BoloJgnia JL, Jorizzo L, Rapini RP, editors. [subscriber site on the Internet]. Available from: http://www.dermtext.com.

untold numbers. Treatment is usually done only for cosmetic reasons. Because seborrheic keratoses may resemble melanoma, any concerning lesion is an indication for immediate referral to a dermatologist.

Epidermal Cyst: Inclusion Cyst

An *epidermal cyst* is a firm, mobile, subcutaneous cyst originating from true epidermis, most often from a hair follicle (**Figure 22-25**). These lesions are formed by a cystic enclosure of epithelium within the dermis that becomes filled with keratin and lipid-rich debris. They grow slowly and may persist indefinitely; they may be subject to external trauma and rupture because of their thin walls. These cysts can occur on the labia where sebaceous glands are large and numerous. Inflammation after rupture of an epidermal cyst can be misdiagnosed as an infection.[13] Symptomatic or recurrent cysts can be removed. Asymptomatic cysts occurring anywhere other than the face need no attention.

Disorders of Blood Vessels

Cherry Angioma

These are common, asymptomatic, bright-red to violaceous, domed vascular lesions usually found on the trunk in individuals over the age of 30 (**Figure 22-26**). Angiomas are less easily blanched than telangiectases. They may first appear in pregnancy and in patients with elevated prolactin levels.[13] Sudden occurrence of these lesions may be associated with occult malignancy; in this situation, the woman should be referred to dermatology.

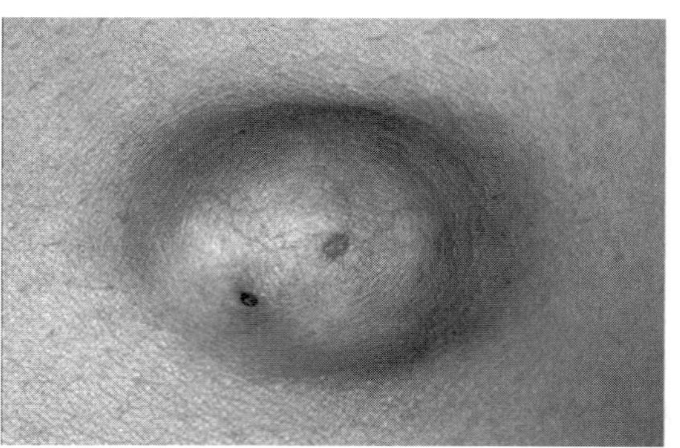

Figure 22-25 Epidermal cyst.

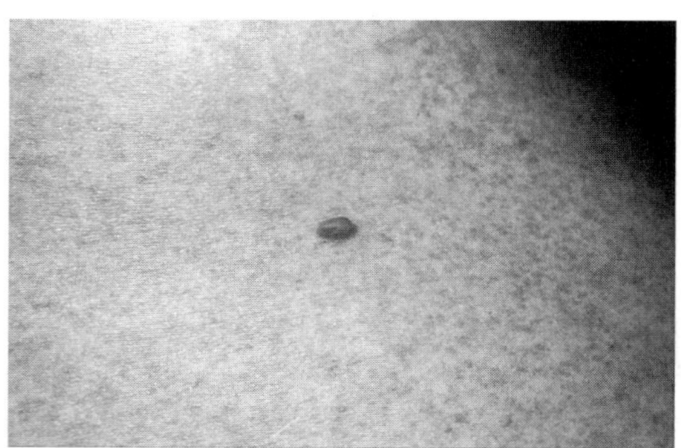

Figure 22-26 Cherry angioma.

Source: Reprinted with permission from Elsevier, © 2003. Dermatology Online. Bolognia JL, Jorizzo JL, Rapini RP, editors. [subscriber site on the Internet]. Available from: http://www.dermtext.com.

Source: Reprinted with permission from Elsevier, © 2003. Dermatology Online. Bolognia JL, Jorizzo JL, Rapini RP, editors. [subscriber site on the Internet]. Available from: http://www.dermtext.com.

Angiokeratoma

Asymptomatic multiple lesions occur on the vulva in middle and later life and persist indefinitely. *Angiokeratomas* appear as deep red to maroon or blue to black sharply defined, 0.5 to 1.0 cm papules. They may occur in younger women on oral contraceptives or during pregnancy, possibly because of increased venous pressure.

Spider Angioma

These lesions are common, asymptomatic vascular papules with a distinct clinical appearance. They are found in 10% to 15% of adults and are also common in young children. They result from dilation of a previously existing blood vessel, and most commonly are found on the face, neck, and upper trunk. They often increase in number in pregnancy and with chronic liver disease. It has been suggested that spider angiomas occur in a state of estrogen excess.[13] Some lesions arising in pregnancy will resolve after the birth. Most spider angiomas in children also tend to resolve spontaneously.

Nail Disorders

Brittle Nails

The most common cause of *brittle nails* is dehydration of the nail plate, usually from exposure to damaging agents. Common causes include acetone, alkaline liquids, organic solvents, and frequent hand washing.[61] Direct trauma to the nail plate, nail biting, typing, playing a musical instrument, or using the nail as a tool to pry or scrape can lead to trauma, which can lead to dehydration. Frequent hand washing causes the nail plate to expand and contract repeatedly as the nail absorbs and loses water, which places a strain on the protein structures and onychocyte bridges, and results in weakening and destruction of the protein links between the cells that comprise the nail.[61] As a consequence, the nail loses its ability to retain water and becomes brittle and susceptible to splitting, cracking, and peeling. Brittleness occurs because of a loss of flexibility.

Brittle nails are also associated with aging. Atherosclerosis of small arteries will decrease blood flow to the nail matrix and can reduce growth and flexibility.[62] Longitudinal ridges that also contribute to brittleness can occur in humans by the late 20s. Thickening of the nails also occurs with aging.

Poor nutrition can also cause brittle nails, so eating disorders should be considered as well as deficiencies in vitamins A, B_6, and C when evaluating this condition.[63]

Suggestions to help with brittle nails include regular trimming to avoid direct trauma. This should be done after bathing when the nails are soft. Filing after trimming keeps the edges smooth, and buffing gently keeps the surfaces smooth. Wearing gloves to avoid precipitating factors such as exposure to chemicals and soaps will help. Avoiding all contact with water is impossible, but the nails and the periungal skin should be moisturized several times a day and after each hand washing. For extreme problems, a nightly routine may be suggested. Soaking the hands (or feet) for 20 minutes in lukewarm water, followed by application of a moisturizer and covering with white cotton gloves is very effective in treating brittle and splitting nails.[61] Applying nail enamel that does not contain formaldehyde and toluene may improve nails but the polish should not be removed more frequently than once weekly. Studies have shown that gelatin, iron, zinc [61] or calcium supplementation do not improve nail strength.[64]

Onychomycosis

Dermatophytes are a unique group of fungi that are capable of infecting nonviable keratinized cutaneous tissues including nails and hair. *Tinea unguium* is a fungal infection of the nail that accounts for up to 50% of nail dystrophy.[61] It occurs more commonly on the feet and is acquired in locker rooms, swimming pools, or from soil. The appearance of the nail can vary depending on the specific infecting organism. Separation of the nail from the underlying nail bed, debris from under the nail, thickening, flaking, and changes in color of the nail are red flags for *onychomycosis*.

Fungal infections of the nail do not resolve spontaneously, so treatment is always necessary. Topical agents are of little value.[13] Terbinafine (Lamisil) may provide the highest cure rates and longest remission, but it may not be effective for some candidal species.[13] Length of treatment varies according to the site of infection: 6 weeks for infections of the fingernail and 3 months for those affecting toenails. Other options include itraconazole (Sporanox) and fluconazole. Griseofulvin is only active against dermatophytes; it may interact with other medicines and has serious side effects. It also may decrease the efficacy of hormonal contraception and some antibiotics.

Pigment Disorders

Vitiligo

Vitiligo is a disease in which the melanocytes are destroyed, resulting in pigment loss. The disease may begin at any age but occurs most fre-quently between the ages of 10 and 30 years. It affects 1% of all races and occurs with equal frequency in both men and women. Macules are chalk white and range in size from 5 mm to 5 cm. Common sites include the dorsa of the hands, face, body folds, the axillae, and the genitalia. There is no increased risk of malignancy in the white skin, but photoaging may occur in the vitiligo macules. There is an association between vitiligo and thyroid disease, especially in women.

Management includes use of sunscreens, cosmetic cover-up, and repigmentation. The latter is done with topical corticosteroids, as well as with topical and systemic photochemotherapy; these treatments are beyond the scope of this chapter. Sunscreens are used to protect the macules and to prevent tanning of the normal skin. This limits the contrast between normal skin and depigmented skin. Sunscreens with a protection factor of 30 are recommended.

Lentigo

Lentigo is a benign condition that occurs as brown macules, most commonly in Caucasians. Freckles are included in this category; they occur in childhood as an autosomal dominant trait. Lentigines are nearly universal in Caucasian skin. These lesions do not darken in response to sun exposure as freckles do. Juvenile lentigines are round to oval macules 2 to 10 mm in size that are darker than freckles; prepubertal children have a mean number of 20 such macules.[13] Solar lentigines occur on sun-exposed skin. They develop in response to actinic damage and increase in number with age (**Figure 22-27**).

Sunscreens may help to prevent new freckles and darkening in the summer. Juvenile lentigines need no intervention. Solar lentigines are best

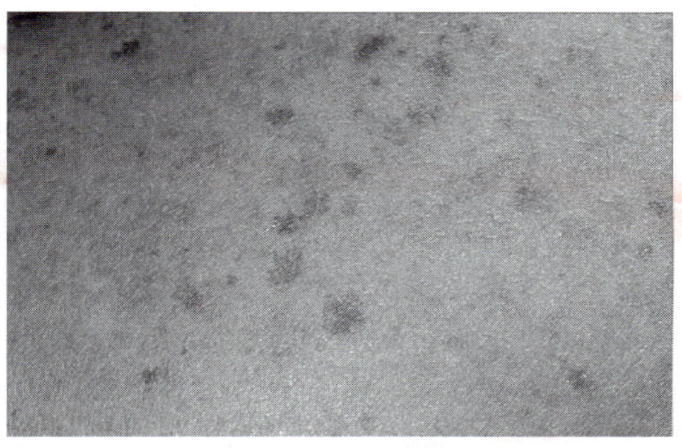

Figure 22-27 Solar lentigine.

Source: Reprinted with permission from Elsevier, © 2003. Dermatology Online. Bolognia JL, Jorizzo JL, Rapini RP, editors. [subscriber site on the Internet]. Available from: http://www.dermtext.com.

prevented by protection from sun exposure in the first place. When lesions occur, they should be monitored because although they are not premalignant lesions, the lentigines are apt to look like actinic keratoses, which do have malignancy potential. Any lentigo that develops a localized area of hypopigmentation, an irregular outline, or localized thickening should be biopsied.

Acanthosis Nigricans

Acanthosis nigricans is thickened, velvety, hyperpigmented skin. The margins blend imperceptibly into surrounding skin edges. Lesions usually develop in the flexures such as the axillae and the groin and on the neck. Between the ages of 12 and 30, the most common association is with obesity.[65] Skin tags are frequently seen with acanthosis nigrans. Many times these conditions will disappear with weight loss. Women with these lesions are apt to have an underlying organic disease such as diabetes, pituitary dysfunction or tumors (ir-

regular menses, pituitary adenoma), or hypothyroidism. Individuals with other serious diseases such as Addison's disease, neurofibromatosis, epilepsy, achondroplasia, and Turner's syndrome may also have acanthosis nigricans.

In gynecologic practice, acanthosis nigricans is important because it can be a marker for PCOS, hyperinsulinemia, and insulin resistance in women with obesity.[65] Treatment may be necessary for diabetes or prediabetes, infertility, and protection of the endometrial lining of the uterus from unopposed estrogen effect. Weight reduction and exercise are the most important interventions.[66] Losing as little as 10% of body weight may help the woman resume ovulatory menstrual cycles. This in turn protects the endometrium from overgrowth, which can occur with irregular menstrual cycling. Fertility also improves with weight loss, as does hyperinsulinemia and insulin resistance. Without intervention young women with obesity and acanthosis nigricans have higher risk from the effects of long-term diseases like diabetes and heart disease.

The Skin and Aging

Damage done to the skin over a lifetime is seen as aging. Signs of photoaging are apparent by the age of 40 and include: fine wrinkles; deep furrows on the forehead and at angles of the mouth; uneven and blotchy skin pigmentation; distinct solar lentigines; skin dryness; and loose inelastic skin. Pilosebaceous units are prominent and dilated (solar comedones). Sometimes the blood vessels in exposed areas become telegiectatic. Bruising occurs more easily on the hands and arms. *Poikiloderma* describes the combination of epidermal atrophy, hyperpigmentation and hypopigmentation, and telegiectasia. This is often seen on sun-exposed surfaces of the face and neck. Progressive damage occurs even when further sun exposure is avoided. Some lesions such as actinic keratoses may regress with protection from the sun.

Treatment with topical tretinoin reverses some photoaging, causing the pigmentation to become lighter and more uniform. New collagen and new blood vessels form within the papillary dermis. However, treatment must be continued for effects to remain. Peeling agents can also improve skin texture and appearance. Alpha-hydroxy acids reduce hyperkeratosis and promote epidermal hyperplasia. Laser resurfacing damages the papillary dermis, which causes a thin zone of scar formation (new collagen), effectively reducing wrinkles.

Premalignant and Malignant Skin Tumors

Skin cancer accounts for one-third of all new cancers in the United States, making it the most common malignancy.[67,68] *Non-melanoma skin cancers (NMSC)* include basal cell carcinoma (BCC) and squamous cell carcinoma (SCC), which account for 90% of the cutaneous cancers.[69] NMSC affect one million Americans annually. They are estimated to cause 2300 deaths per year.[10] BCC is four times as common as SCC[70] and is the most common tumor in white individuals.[71]

As with most diseases, the etiology of skin cancer is a combination of inherent individual characteristics and exogenous environmental factors. Ultraviolet radiation (UVR) has long been established as an important etiologic factor for all forms of skin cancers. Skin types I and II (fair skin, blue eyes, red hair, and the tendency to burn) have long been associated with higher risk of skin cancer, but an even stronger association

is seen with hair color and a tendency to freckle for both NMSC and melanoma.[69] Pigmented nevi are another important risk factor for melanoma: the greater the number of nevi, the greater the risk. Such lesions are both markers of increased risk and direct precursors of melanoma, because 30% of melanomas arise in pre-existing moles.[72,73]

Finally, heredity plays a role in the development of skin cancers. Family history significantly increases the risk for melanoma, especially if there is also a history of atypical moles.[69] A first-degree relative with melanoma increases the personal risk of an individual eight times.[10]

Actinic Keratoses

Actinic keratosis (AK) is the most common in situ cancerous skin lesion. The word actinic means "pertaining to radiation (sunlight)" but does not address the malignant nature of these lesions.[74] *Keratosis* is a horny growth. Hyperkeratosis is an overgrowth of the horny layer of the skin. AK appears as rough, scaly, often hyperkeratotic flesh-colored macules or papules with discrete or diffuse borders (**Figure 22-28**). The key to clinical diagnosis is the gritty, sand paper–like sensation felt when palpating these lesions.[74] These lesions are considered to have undergone invasive malignant transformation when they become palpable, indurated, and ulcerated or bleed.[75] Moreover, substantial evidence suggests that AKs may develop into invasive SCC.[74] The bottom line is that primary care practitioners need to have a clear understanding of the aggressiveness of the disease. Referral to a dermatologist is obligatory.

Basal Cell Carcinoma

BCC is the most common type of skin cancer.[76] BCCs are usually slow growing tumors

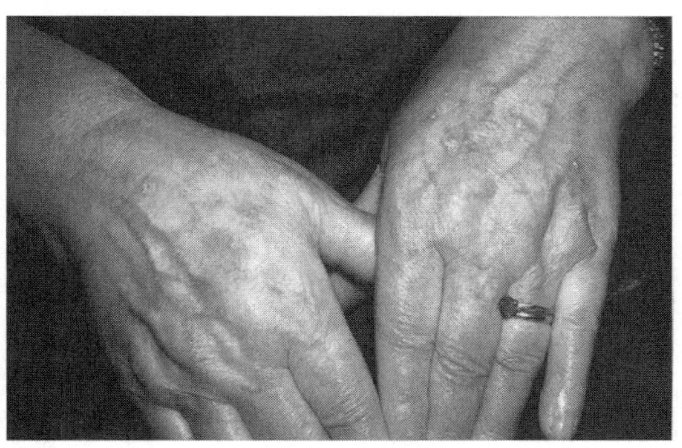

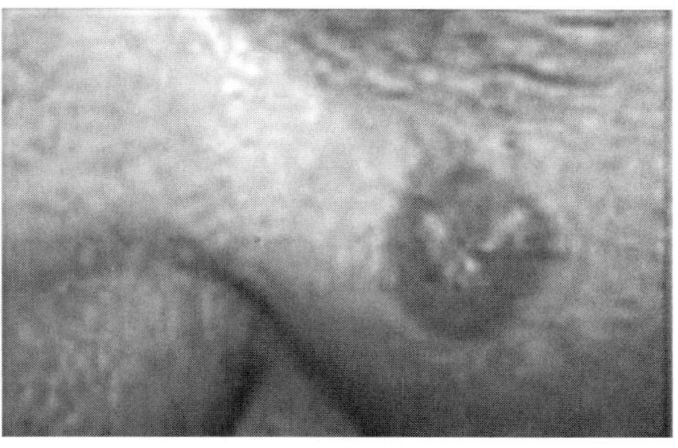

that rarely spread to distant parts of the body but have diverse clinical appearances and morphology. The clinical course of BCC is unpredictable; the lesion may remain small for years, or it may grow rapidly or proceed by successive spurts of extension. Approximately 80% occur on the head and neck, with the rest mainly on the trunk and lower limbs, particularly in women. BCC on the backs of the hands is rare. The classic presentation of the nodular-ulcerative form is a smooth skin-colored indurated (hardened) nodule with a rolled edge (**Figure 22-29**). There is often an ulcerated center. Early BCCs are commonly small, translucent or pearly, with raised areas through which dilated vessels may show telangiectasia. Pinching or stretching a BCC to blanch it may highlight the pearly quality. A pigmented BCC may be confused with melanoma, but the BCC usually has a pink or reddish component with a suggestion of waxiness (**Figure 22-30**).

The tumor may occur at any age, but the incidence of BCC increases markedly after the age of 40.[76] The incidence in younger people is increasing, however, possibly as a result of increased childhood and adolescent sun exposure. Risk factors are fair skin, tendency to freckle, high degree of sun exposure, excessive use of sun beds, previous radiotherapy, phototherapy, male sex, and genetic predisposition.[77] The first-line treatment of BCC is surgical excision.[76] Many alternatives are available, including curettage, cryosurgery, and laser treatment.

A novel approach to treatment of BCC includes the use of Imiquimod, the first member of a new class of topically applied therapeutic agents that have indirect antiviral effects, resulting largely from induction of interferon-alpha.[78] This produces an immunological cascade of events that stimulates innate immunity and cytolytic antiviral activity. Immune

Figure 22-30 Basal cell carcinoma (BCC), superficial spreading.

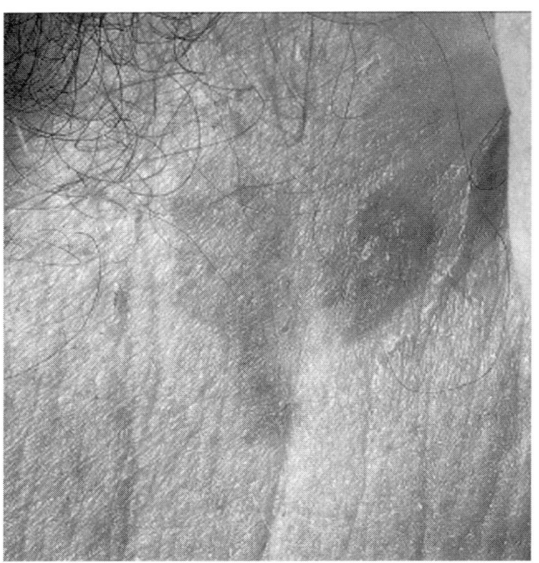

Source: Reprinted with permission from Elsevier, © 2003. Dermatology Online. Bolognia JL, Jorizzo JL, Rapini RP, editors. [subscriber site on the Internet]. Available from: http://www.dermtext.com.

Figure 22-31 Squamous cell carcinoma (SCC).

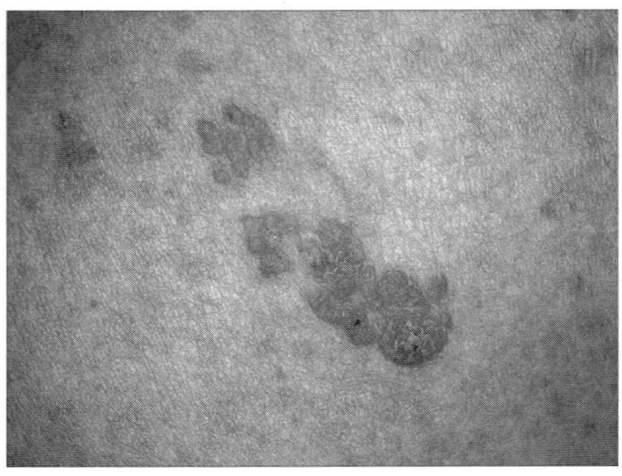

Source: Reprinted with permission from Elsevier, © 2003. Dermatology Online. Bolognia JL, Jorizzo JL, Rapini RP, editors. [subscriber site on the Internet]. Available from: http://www.dermtext.com.

modulation also has indirect antiproliferative and antitumor activity; preliminary data suggest a role in the management of localized skin cancers such as BCC, intraepithelial neoplasias, and SCC in situ.[78]

Squamous Cell Carcinoma

SCC lesions are often tender, with an elevated pink base peripheral to an overlying crust, and may feel indurated (**Figure 22-31**).[69] They may appear as a discrete pink to red patch or plaque without the threadlike, waxy border of BCC. SCC is also more likely to be scaly than BCC, with pinpoint erosions or hyperkerato-sis. These sometimes occur as an indurated keratotic nodule or scale within long-standing scars.

Malignant Melanoma

Most dermatologists have an 89% to 97% sensitivity of visual assessment of melanomas,[10] but for the primary care provider, clinical assessment and suspicion are not so easy. While the ABCDE guidelines for recognizing melanoma (Table 22-2) are a useful reminder for identifying potential dangerous lesions, there is no single criterion that is absolutely indicative of whether a lesion is benign or malignant.[69] A high index of suspicion should be maintained for any pigmented lesion, particularly those that are new or have changed.

Atypical moles are sometimes a precursor to melanoma. They are the strongest predictor of risk.[9,72,79,80] Melanocytic nevi originate in childhood and are the result of sun exposure.[81] These nevi increase the risk of melanoma. There is an inverse relationship in case control studies between children who used broad-spectrum sunscreens and the development of new melanocytic nevi.[81] Normal moles are characterized by symmetry, the presence of a single color, discrete borders, and size less than 6 mm.[69] Atypical nevi are often seen in an abnormal distribution in patients with a great number of moles or large sized moles. Atypical moles have irregular scalloped borders and irregular pebbly surfaces as opposed to ordinary moles[69] and appear in multiple shades of brown that are sized greater than 6 mm.

The typical nodular form of melanoma is an elevated brown-black papule or nodule. The superficial spreading form, which has a higher incidence in younger individuals, is a flat, irregularly pigmented macule, patch, or plaque. The acral-lentiginous melanoma is a flat spreading lesion found on the soles, palm, or fingers/ toes as a variably pigmented tan to brown to black patch or plaques. The acral-lentiginous is the only type that occurs equally in all races.[69]

The relationship between sun exposure and melanoma is complicated. Most studies do not show an association between chronic, cumulative sun exposure and melanoma, and exposure may offer protection[69]; however, intense intermittent exposure, as in sunburn, does seem to be associated. Sunburns in children younger than age 15 appear to be a strong predisposing factor.[68,79,80] Because melanomas frequently occur on areas that are normally clothed, intermittent sunburn that occurs in those areas is especially risky.

Tumor thickness is the single most important prognostic indicator used to predict mor-

bidity and mortality in patients with all types of melanoma.[82] While most melanomas are found by individuals, screening by providers may be beneficial. 99% of melanomas detected through a screening program were found to be less than 1.5-mm thick, suggesting the importance of regular screening (**Figures 22–32** and **22–33**).[9,10,80]

Inflammatory Breast Cancer

Inflammatory breast cancer is the most aggressive manifestation of primary breast cancer[83] but is relatively rare (1%–6% of the breast cancers in the United States).[84] Women present with a rapid onset of swelling, diffuse erythema, edema involving more than two-thirds of the breast, peau d'orange skin, tenderness, induration, warmth, and diffuseness of the tumor on palpation (**Figure 22-34**). Referral to a breast surgeon is necessary if a woman presents with these skin symptoms.

Figure 22-32 **Melanoma in situ.**

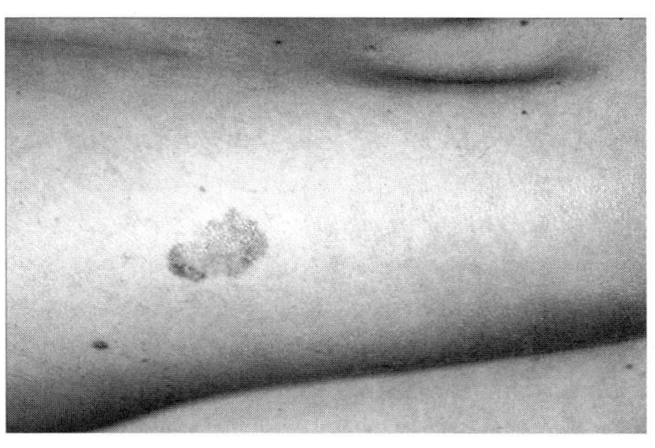

Source: Reprinted with permission from Elsevier, © 2003. Dermatology Online. Bolognia JL, Jorizzo JL, Rapini RP, editors. [subscriber site on the Internet]. Available from: http://www.dermtext.com.

Figure 22-33 Malignant melanoma.

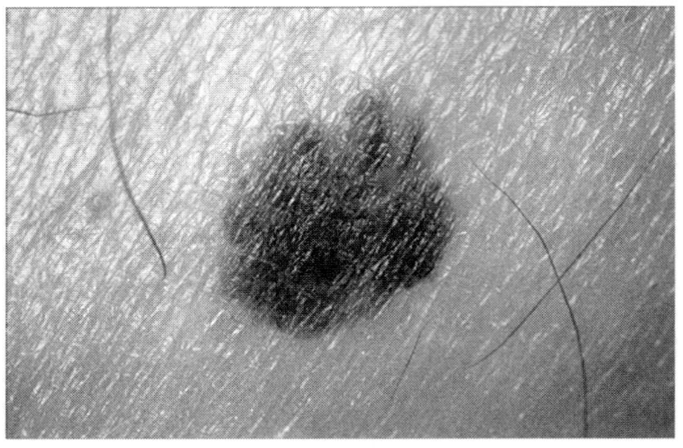

Source: Reprinted with permission from Elsevier, © 2003. Dermatology Online. Bolognia JL, Jorizzo JL, Rapini RP, editors. [subscriber site on the Internet]. Available from: http://www.dermtext.com.

Paget's Disease

Paget's disease of the breast presents as a skin lesion. It is a rare intraepithelial adenocarcinoma resulting from intraductal mammary carcinoma that extends from the epidermis of the nipple and the areola through a lactiferous duct; it may also arise from invasive breast cancer that reaches the epidermis via direct extension from the dermis (**Figure 22-35**). Clinical features mimic inflammatory and infectious diseases such as eczema. Paget's disease is confined to the nipple and areola complex from where it may spread onto surrounding skin. The appearance is usually a demarcated, thickened, eczematous, erythematous weeping of a crusted lesion with irregular borders. Nipple discharge or ulceration may be present, and a breast tumor may be palpable. Differential diagnoses include eczema and psoriasis. Paget's disease is slow growing, but if a lesion does not respond to a course of corticocosteroids, then cancer must be sus-

Figure 22-34 Inflammatory breast cancer.

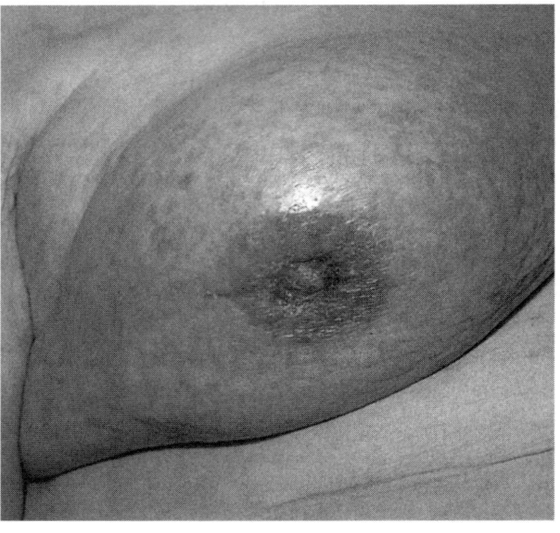

Source: Reprinted with permission from Mosby, © 2001. *Skin Disease: Diagnosis and Treatment.* Habif TP, Campbell JI Jr, Quitadamo M, Zug KA, editors. Chicago: Mosby; 2001. p. 395.

pected. Ultrasound and mammography are necessary once other inflammatory diseases are ruled out.

Prevention and Education

Prevention is the most important aspect of primary care for melanoma and NMSC. The annual gynecology exam and the antepartum visit are opportunities for teaching women ways to minimize their, as well as their families, risks. Simple measures such as avoiding UVR, especially in childhood and adolescence, and between the hours of 10 AM and 4 PM at any age, and wearing tightly woven clothing and hats can be protective. Such points should be made to young women in their childbearing years and

---

Figure 22-35 Paget's disease of the breast.

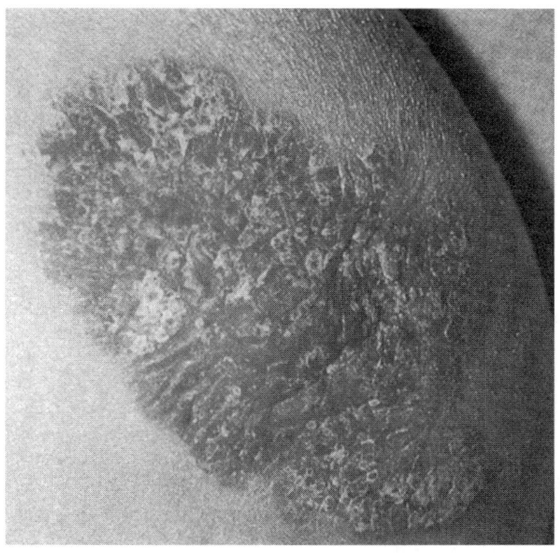

Source: Reprinted with permission from Mosby, © 2001.
Skin Disease: Diagnosis and Treatment. Habif TP, Campbell JL Jr, Quitadamo M, Zug KA, editors. Chicago: Mosby; 2001. p. 395.

are just as important as other health messages, such as the benefit of avoiding exposure to smoke for young children, the need for all children to use car seats and seat belts, and similar topics. Parents should be taught to require the use of sunscreens for their children. When children use sunscreens, they are more apt to continue to use them as adults. Use of sunscreens during the first 18 years of life may produce as much as a 78% reduction in lifetime incidence of BCC and SCC.[10] Use of sunscreens can also reduce development of new actinic keratoses and increase remission of existing lesions.[69] This is important to stress to individuals because some may not use sunscreens if they think that the damage is already done. Recent sun exposure, as opposed to childhood exposure, is important risk factor for the development of nonmelanoma skin cancers.

Management of Common Symptoms

Management of specific skin diseases has been discussed in previous sections of this chapter. However, there are a number of overriding issues in treatment that pertain to many types of lesions. Inflammation, infection, pruritis, moisture, and dryness are common to many diseases. Each of these qualities, regardless of their cause, can respond to similar treatments that include both nonpharmacologic as well as pharmacologic therapeutics (**Table 22-5**).

Preserving the integrity of normal skin is the first and foremost requirement for healthy skin. This is done with a variety of products that restore water and lipids to the epidermis. These products include lotions, creams, and ointment that should be applied after bathing and then patted dry. Repeated applications are important, especially for women who wash frequently. There is no need for expensive preparations because ingredients are very similar despite wide differences in price. Because creams are thicker than lotions, they are generally more lubricating. Vaseline, petroleum jelly, and mineral oil are all inexpensive and effective choices. Products containing urea 5% to 10% (Aquacare, Carmol) or lactic acid 5% to 12% (Lac Hydrin) are particularly useful in helping hydrate skin that has a thick epidermal layer.

Mild soaps are available for women with dry or inflamed skin. Examples include Cetaphil, Dove, Keri, Basis, Oil of Olay, and many others. Ivory is probably the most drying product available.

Table 22-5 TREATMENT FOR DERMATOLOGIC LESIONS

Category	Condition	Nonpharmacologic Measures	Pharmacologic Measures
Inflammatory	Intertrigo	Use of hair dryer; loose, cotton clothing	Anti-yeast or antibacterial Rx
	PUPP	Cool, wet compresses Burrow's solution	Oral antihistamines, topical corticosteroids
	Lichen sclerosis		Class I-2 corticosteroid
	Eczema/dermatitis	Avoidance of irritants Keeping the skin moisturized Cool, wet compresses	Topical corticosteroids Oral corticosteroids for acute flares
	Psoriasis	Cool, wet compresses; loose, cotton clothing PUVA (psoralen plus ultraviolet A) required therapy 3 × a week	Oral and topical corticosteroids
	Acne	Non-comedone forming moisturizers to combat over-drying induced by some of the medications used for treatment of acne. Scrubbing and over washing should be avoided.	Agents to induce drying and peeling are used. Benzoyl peroxide, Azelaic acid (Azelex cream), and Tretinoin (Retin-A). Oral and topical antibiotics Isotretinoin (Accutane) – Class X
Infection	Tinea	Topical application of selenium or selenium-containing shampoos (Head and Shoulders Intensive Treatment) can be used for the treatment of tinea versicolor. Leave on skin for 24 hours and then wash off. Repeat at weekly intervals for four weeks.	Antifungal creams
	Impetigo	Hygiene measures	Dicloxacillin, Cephalexin (Keflex)
	Erythrasma	Benzoyl peroxide bar or wash	Benzoyl peroxide 2.5% gel Topical erythromycin solution Oral erythromycin
	Warts	Use of occlusive dressing after application of topical OTC	Imiquimod

Table 22-5 TREATMENT FOR DERMATOLOGIC LESIONS *(continued)*

Category	Condition	Nonpharmacologic Measures	Pharmacologic Measures
		salicylic acid preparations may enhance effectiveness.	
	Condylomata		Imiquimod Trichloroacetic acid Podophyllin
	Molluscum		None needed unless multiple and persistent lesions are present
	Folliculitis	Hygienic measures Avoidance of heat & friction Antibacterial soaps Warm & cold compresses	Mupirocin topical Oxacillin Dicloxacillin Cefuroxime
	Candida	Compresses for itch and pain Cotton underwear Sleep nude	Clotrimazole Fluconazole Nystatin Miconazole
	Herpes	NSAIDs for pain	Acyclovir Famcyclovir Zanamivir
	Scabies	Wash clothes and bedding in hot water	Lindane (not in pregnancy) Kwell Prednisone PO may be necessary for severe itch
	Lyme disease	Inspect for ticks after being outdoors Wear long sleeves and pants tucked into socks outdoors	21 days Doxycycline 100 mg bid, Amoxicillin 500 mg tid Cefuroxime axetil 500 mg bid
Dryness	General dryness, winter itch	Moisturizers to restore barrier function Substitution of cetyl alcohol preparations (Cetaphil) for soaps Avoidance of excessive bathing, harsh detergents Humidification of home. Use of urea 5% to 10% or alpha hydroxyl acid (lactic acid) 5% to 12% containing	

(continues)

Table 22-5 TREATMENT FOR DERMATOLOGIC LESIONS *(continued)*

Category	Condition	Nonpharmacologic Measures	Pharmacologic Measures
		products are especially effective in more pronounced cases.	
Itch	Eczema or atopy	Emollients are first-line therapy to restore altered barrier function; put on immediately after bath	Topical corticosteroids Oral prednisone in severe cases
		Low pH cleansers to maintain acidic surface to reduce irritation	
		Cooling agents with menthol, phenol, or camphor	
		Topical anesthetics	
		Topical antihistamines	
		Capsaicin	
		Avoid spicy foods & alcohol, which release histamines	
		Keep nails short	
		Use detergents free of enzymes, dyes, & perfumes	
		Avoid fabric softeners	

Exudative lesions respond well to wet compresses. A wet compress is created by soaking a dressing in a solution (such as plain water or Burrows solution), wringing it out so that it remains sopping wet but is not dripping, and placing it on the affected area for 30 minutes. Repeated use of compresses promotes healing, debrides accumulated crust, and will eventually dry the lesion.

Topical corticosteroids are most effective for treating inflammatory problems whether eczema, poison ivy, or other pruritic condition. It is questionable whether generic products are equivalent to brand-name products, particularly with regard to vasoconstrictor assays.[13]

Topical corticosteroids are grouped by strength from I to VII (strongest to weakest; **Table 22-6**).

When choosing a product, the group to which it belongs is the indicator of the strength, not the percent as noted on the package. Percent noted on the package refers to the concentration of the active ingredient in the vehicle (cream, ointment, etc.).

It is essential that the product chosen be the correct strength for the specific condition being treated and be used for an appropriate amount of time. It is of little value to prescribe a product from the weaker categories when it is not of sufficient strength to be therapeutic. Weaker, supposedly "safer" strengths can fail to provide adequate activity and control.

The super potent topical steroids from Class I are the strongest agents available; they are used for difficult-to-treat conditions such as psoriasis

Table 22-6 TOPICAL CORTICOSTEROIDS BY CLASS

I Super	II High	III Medium	IV Medium	V Medium Low	VI Low	VII Very Low
Augmented betamethasone dipropionate 0.05% (Diprolene lotion or cream)	Augmented betamethasone dipropionate 0.05% (Diprolene AF cream)**	Betamethasone dipropionate cream 0.05% (Diprosone cream)	Triamcinolone acetonide 0.1% (Kenalog ointment)	Triamcinolone acetonide (Kenalog cream 0.1%, ointment 0.025%)	Triamcinolone acetonide 0.025% (Kenalog cream)	Topicals with hydrocortisone, dexamethasone, flumethasone, prednisolone
Clobetasol propionate 0.05% (Temovate)	Amcinonide 0.1% (Cyclocort ointment)	Amcinonide 0.1% (Cyclocort lotion)	Amcinonide 0.1% (Cyclocort cream)**			
Flurandrenolide (Cordran tape)	Desoximetasone 0.25% (Topicort cream, ointment)	Diflorasone diacetate 0.05% (Florone)	Flurandrenolide 0.05% (Cordran ointment)	Flurandrenolide 0.05% (Cordran cream, lotion)	Desonide 0.05% (DesOwen cream, ointment, lotion)	
	Fluocinonide 0.05% (Lidex cream, gel, ointment, solution)	Fluocinonide 0.05% E-cream**	Fluocinonide acetonide 0.025% (Synelar ointment)	Fluocinonide acetonide 0.025% (Synelar cream)	Prednicarbate 0.05% (Aclovate cream, ointment)	
			Hydrocortisone valerate (Westcort ointment 0.2%)	Hydrocortisone valerate (Westcort cream 0.2%)		

** Some sources differ in their potency rating for this corticosteroid

and hand eczema. They are reserved for use in only the most serious conditions because they have the potential to cause serious side effects. Hypothalamic-pituitary-adrenal axis suppression, hyperglycemia, and glucosuria occur rarely with the use of topical corticosteroids, but have been reported if the area being treated is large, occlusive dressings are used, or treatment is prolonged. Adverse dermatological reactions are more common. These include thinning of the epidermis, striae, purpura, and maceration. To lessen these risks, no more than 45 to 60 grams of a Class I steroid should be used in a week's time. Side effects are minimized and efficacy increased when the medication is used twice daily for only two weeks followed by a week of rest.[13]

In general Class I and II corticosteroids should be used sparingly in the primary care setting and are best prescribed under the direction of a dermatologist. Class III through VII are prescribed more commonly in primary care practice. While adverse reactions are less common with use of mid- to low-potency steroids, following certain guidelines will minimize the risk. They should be applied no more than twice a day and be limited to two to six weeks' duration. If no improvement is seen, then a referral to a dermatologist is necessary. Steroid atrophy and other dermatologic reactions can develop in the areas being treated if an individual is treated for too long a time or with too strong a product.

Particular care should be used in treating skin conditions found on the face or in intertriginous areas such as the groin and axilla. Use of lower potency corticosteroids in these areas is more likely to result in side effects than if same-strength products are used on other parts of the body. Therefore, using the lowest potency products available (Class VI or VII) for the shortest period of time is recommended for treating skin conditions in more vulnerable areas. Referral to a dermatologist is warranted if prompt improvement is not seen.

Using occlusive dressings can also increase the potency of corticosteroids. While they can markedly improve the response to treatment in more severe presentations, they also increase the risk of developing serious side effects related to corticosteroid use. Generally, lesions requiring this level of intervention are best managed by a dermatologist.

Topical corticosteroids are mixed in various bases: creams, lotions, gels, or ointments. Ointments are usually petroleum based, which allows greater penetration than creams or lotions and, therefore, are more potent. The type of vehicle can affect potency to such an extent that it can change the classification of a corticosteroid. For example, hydrocortisone valerate (Westcort) ointment 0.2% is classified as a Class IV steroid; however, it is categorized as a Class V corticosteroid if prescribed as a cream. Ointments are also usually preservative-free, whereas creams are more likely to contain preservatives that may cause irritation. However, many patients prefer the feel of a cream or lotion to gels or ointments and may discontinue use of products that feel "greasy." Therefore, careful attention to the choice of a vehicle is just as important as the strength of corticosteroid in ensuring treatment success.

Steroid mixtures include lotrisone cream, which contains an antifungal agent as well as the corticosteroid betamethasone diproprioate, a Class II or III steroid. It is expensive and not usually indicated because most inflammatory skin diseases do not have a fungal origin. Another combined product is Mycolog II, which is an antifungal agent with triamcinalone (Class VI).

Conclusion

As primary care providers, midwives and women's health providers have innumerable opportunities to observe skin lesions, become familiar with characteristics of various diseases, treat simpler and more straightforward problems, and refer in a timely matter to the dermatologist for management of more persistent or severe presentations.

Glossary

Annular—ring shaped.

Antihistamine—substance that is capable of reducing inflammation, swelling, and general allergic reactions.

Atopic, atopy—genetic tendency to experience immediate allergic reactions because of the presence of an antibody in the skin; atopic dermatitis.

Atrophy—a depression in the skin resulting from thinning of the epidermis and dermis.

B cells—lymphocytes that make and carry surface immunoglobulins.

Bulla—blister; greater than 0.5 cm (pea size); circumscribed, elevated superficial cavity filled with fluid; derived from cleavage at various levels of the skin.

Bullous diseases—autoimmune blistering.

Comedone—a plug of sebaceous and keratinous material lodged in the opening of a hair follicle; when dilated it is a blackhead, and when narrowed it is a whitehead or closed comedo.

Crusts—from crusta, a Latin word meaning bark, rind, shell; develops when serum, blood, or purulent exudates dries on the skin.

Dermatoheliosis—photoaging.

Dermis—the layer of the skin below the epidermis and above the subcutaneous tissue, composed of connective tissue in which is embedded hair follicles, sweat glands, superficial and deeper blood vessels, and nerve fibers.

Desquamation—scaling.

Dyschromia—abnormal color of skin, hair, nails, or mucosa.

Elastosis—fine nodularity and inelasticity.

Emollient—making soft or supple; soothing to skin or mucous membranes.

Epidermis—the outermost layer of the skin; contains several active zones of skin cells, including cells that participate in immune reactions (e.g., eczematous reactions).

Erosion—defect of only of the epidermis; heals without a scar.

Erythema—a reaction in the skin characterized by an active or passive redness of the skin more or less sharply defined, usually temporary, that disappears upon finger pressure.

Erythroderma—a persistent inflammatory reddening of all the skin with lichenification and scaling.

Exanthema—erythematous macules and/or papules; less frequently, vesicles, petechiae; usually central (i.e., head, neck, trunk, proximal extremities); diffuse erythema of cheeks (i.e., "slapped cheek") with erythema infectiosum.

Excoriation—erosions caused by scratching.

Fissure—linear loss of epidermis and dermis with sharp vertical walls.

Folliculitis—suppurativa, acneform, and keratotic eruptions that primarily involve the pilosebaceous unit.

Granulomatous—heaped up.

Hidroses—functional or organic disturbance of the apocrine or eccrine sweat glands.

Hypertrophy—persistent localized extensive thickening of all or many layers of skin.

Immunoglobulin—an antibody that is an antigen-binding protein secreted by specific white cells of the immune system.

Intertriginous—areas of the body where the skin is in contact with other skin surfaces such as in the axillae and the groin.

Intertrigo—skin changes that occur in intertriginous areas because of chafing and chronic inflammation.

Keratosis—a localized moderate thickening of the horny layer.

Leukoderma—secondary postinflammatory decrease in melanin.

Leukoplakia—a clinical term that describes a sharply defined, white, macular or slightly raised area that cannot be rubbed off.

Lichenification—thickening upper layers of the skin in response to trauma.

Macule—Latin for "spot"; a non-palpable, circumscribed change in skin color without elevation or depression of surrounding skin.

Melanoderma—secondary postinflammatory increase in melanin.

Melanosis—endogenous or primary melanin hyperpigmentation without preceding disease.

Moisturizer—often used interchangeably with emollient but implies the addition of water to the skin.

Nodule—Latin meaning, "nodulus, small knot"; a palpable, solid round lesion that involves dermis, epidermis, or subcutaneous tissue. Depth and size of mass differentiate it from a papule.

Onychosis—disease that affects the nail plate and surrounding structures.

Papule—Latin for "pimple"; superficial solid mass less than 0.5 cm, mostly located on the skin's surface.

Parakeratosis—nuclei are retained in the outmost layers of the skin with increased proliferation of epithelial cells as in psoriasis.

Pemphigus—loss of a fragile blister roof.

Petechia—a circumscribed deposit of blood less than 0.5 cm in diameter.

Pruritus—itch.

Purpura—extravasation of red blood cells; a circumscribed deposit of blood greater than 0.5 cm;

minute: petechia; extensive: ecchymosis; massive: hematoma.

Pustule—a circumscribed, superficial cavity that contains a purulent exudate that may be white, yellow, greenish yellow, or hemorrhagic.

Scar—abnormal formation of connective tissue from dermal damage.

Sclerosis—a condensation and or overproduction of connective tissue with or without other morphologic changes such as atrophy or telangiectasia.

Subcutaneous tissue—the deepest layer of skin composed of fat, tissue that separates the fat in lobules, nerves and blood vessels; the fatty tissue is biologically active and subject to inflammatory responses.

Suppurative—producing or associated with generation of pus or an agent producing pus formation.

T cell—a white blood cell of the immune system that participates in a number of immune responses.

Telangiectasia—permanent dilation of superficial blood vessels.

Trichosis—condition where the abnormality is primarily of the hair itself.

Ulcer—Latin meaning, "sore"; loss of epidermis and partial layer of dermis; heals with scar formation.

Urticaria—hives.

Verrucosities—wave-like projections of the Malpighian layer and the papillae with or without a thickened stratum corneum.

Vesicle—Latin meaning, "little bladder"; A collection of free fluid causing a ballooning of epidermal cells; less than 0.5 cm in size.

Wheal—hive.

Xeroxis—dryness.

References

1. Chu DH, Haake AR, Holbrook K, Loomis CA. The structure and development of skin. In: Freedberg IM, Eisen AZ, Wolff K, Austen K, Goldsmith LA, Katz SI, editors. *Fitzpatrick's Dermatology in General Medicine*. 6th ed. New York: McGraw-Hill; 2003. pp. 58–87.

2. Sands G. Three monosymptomatic hypochondriacal syndromes in dermatology. *Dermatol Nurs*. 1996;8(6): 421–425.

3. Folks DG, Kinney FC. The role of psychological factors in dermatologic conditions. *Psychosom Med*. 1992; 33(1):45–53.

4. Gupta MA, Gupta AK. Psychiatric and psychological co-morbidity in patients with dermatologic disorders. *Am J Clin Dermatol*. 2003;4(12):833–842.

5. Gupta MA, Gupta AK. The psychological comorbidity in acne. *Clin Dermatol*. 2001;19(3):360–363.

6. Wesley NO, Maibach HI. Racial (ethnic) differences in skin properties: The objective data. *Am J Clin Dermatol.* 2003;4(12):843–860.

7. Oppenheimer GM. Paradigm lost: Race, ethnicity, and the search for a new population taxonomy. *Am J Public Health.* 2001;91(7):1049–1055.

8. Federman DG, Reid MC, Feldman SR, Greenhoe J, Kirsner RS. The primary care provider and the care of skin disease. *Arch Dermatol.* 2001;137(1):25–29.

9. Koh HD, Geller AC, Miller DR, Lew RA. The early detection of and screening for melanoma: International status. *Cancer.* 1995;75(2 suppl):674–683.

10. Rhodes AR. Public education and cancer of the skin: What do people need to know about melanoma and nonmelanoma skin cancer? *Cancer.* 1995;75(suppl): 613–636.

11. Jackson R, Alghareeb M, Alaradi I, Tomi Z. The diagnosis of skin disease. *Dermatol Nurs.* 1999;11(4): 275, 278–283.

12. Fitzpatrick TB, Johnson RA, Wolff K, Polano MK, Suurmond D. *Color Atlas and Synopsis of Clinical Dermatology: Common and Serious Diseases.* 3rd ed. New York: McGraw-Hill; 1997.

13. Habif TP, Quitadamo MJ, Campbell JL, Zug KA. *Skin Disease: Diagnosis and Treatment.* St. Louis: Mosby; 2001.

14. Hagermark O, Wahlgren C. Treatment of itch. *Semin Dermatol.* 1995;14(4):320–325.

15. Yosipovitch GH, Jennifer L. Practical guidelines for relief of itch. *Dermatol Nurs.* 2004;16(4):325–328.

16. Morgan JF, Lacey JH. Scratching and fasting: A study of pruritus and anorexia nervosa. *Br J Dermatol.* 1999;140(3):453–456.

17. Kato A, Hamada M, Maruyama T, Maruyama Y, Hishida A. Pruritis and hydration state of stratum corneum in hemodialysis patients. *Am J Nephrol.* 2000;20(6):437–442.

18. Yosipovitch G. Pruritis. *Curr Prob Dermatol.* 2003;15: 135–164.

19. Arnold LM, Auchenbach MB, Mcelroy SL. Psychogenic excoriation. Clinical features, proposed diagnostic criteria, epidemiology and approaches to treatment. *CNS Drugs.* 2001;15(5):351–359.

20. Mistiaen P, Poot E, Hickox S, Jochems C, Wagner C. Preventing and treating intertrigo in the large skin folds of adults: A literature overview. *Dermatol Nurs.* 2004;16(1):43–46, 49–52, 54–57.

21. McMahon R. An evaluation of topical nursing interventions in the treatment of submammary lesions. *J Wound Care.* 1994;3(2):365–366.

22. Hedley K, Tooley P, Williams H. Problems with clinical trials in general practice—a double-blind comparison of cream containing miconazole and hydrocortisone with hydrocortisone alone in the treatment of intertrigo. *Br J Clin Pract.* 1990;44(4): 131–135.

23. Benigni JP, Casaubon M, Dijian B. Les biotextiles antiseptiques: Leru interet dans la contention medicale [Antiseptic biotextiles and their role in medical support]. *Angeiologie.* 2000;52(3):43–45.

24. McMahon R, Buckeldee J. Skin problems beneath the breasts of inpatients: The knowledge, opinions and practice of nurses. *J Adv Nurs.* 1992;17(10): 1243–1250.

25. McKay M. Physiologic skin changes of pregnancy. In: Black MM, McKay M, Braude PR, Vaughan-Jones SA, Margesson LJ, editors. *Obstetric and Gynecologic Dermatology.* 2nd ed. New York: Mosby; 2002. pp. 17–22.

26. Black MM. Polymorphic eruption of pregnancy. In: Black MM, McKay M, Braude PR, Vaughan-Jones SA, Margesson LJ, editors. *Obstetric and Gynecologic Dermatology.* 2nd ed. New York: Mosby; 2002. pp. 39–44.

27. Charles-Holmes R. Polymorphic eruption of pregnancy. *Semin Dermatol.* 1989;8(1):18–22.

28. Saurat JH. Immunofluorescence biopsy for pruritic urticarial papules and plaques of pregnancy. *J Am Acad Dermatol.* 1989;20(4):711.

29. Jenkins RE, Shornick JK, Black MM. Pemphigoid gestationis. *J Eur Acad Dermatol Venereol.* 1993;2(2): 163–173.

30. Jenkins RE, Shornick J. Pemphigoid (herpes) gestationis. In: Black MM, McKay M, Braude PR, Vaughan-Jones SA, Margesson LJ, editors. *Obstetric and Gynecologic Dermatology.* 2nd ed. New York: Mosby; 2002. pp. 29–37.

31. Hayashi RH. Bullous dermatoses and prurigo of pregnancy. *Clin Obstet Gynecol.* 1990;33(4):746–753.

32. Black MM, Jones SV. The papular and pruritic dermatoses of pregnancy. In: Black MM, McKay M, Braude PR, Vaughan-Jones SA, Margesson LJ, editors. *Obstetric and Gynecologic Dermatology.* 2nd ed. New York; Mosby; 2002. pp. 45–49.

33. McKay M. Differential diagnosis of the vulvar ulcer. In: Black MM, McKay M, Braude PR, Vaughan-Jones SA, Margesson LJ, editors. *Obstetric and Gynecologic Dermatology.* 2nd ed. New York: Mosby; 2002. pp. 187–207.

34. McKay M. Vulvar manifestations of skin disorders. In: Black MM, McKay M, Braude PR, Vaughan-Jones SA, Margesson LJ, editors. *Obstetric and Gynecologic Dermatology*. 2nd ed. New York: Mosby; 2002. pp. 109–135.

35. Wallace HJ. Lichen sclerosus et atrophicus. *Trans St Johns Hosp Dermatol Soc*. 1971;57(1):9–30.

36. Neill SM. Vulvar lichen sclerosis. In: Black MM, McKay M, Braude PR, Vaughan-Jones SA, Margesson LJ, editors. *Obstetric and Gynecologic Dermatology*. 2nd ed. New York: Mosby; 2002. pp. 137–142.

37. Leibowitch M, Neill S, Pelisse M, Moyal-Baracco M, Neill SM. The epithelial changes associated with squamous cell carcinoma of the vulva: A review of the clinical, histologic and viral findings in 78 women. *Br J Obstet Gynecol*. 1990;97(12):1135–1139.

38. Garzon MC, Paller AS. Ultrapotent topical corticosteroid treatment of childhood lichen sclerosus. *Arch Dermatol*. 1999;135(5):525–528.

39. Dalziel K, Millard PR, Wojnarowska F. The treatment of vulvar lichen sclerosus with a very potent topical corticosteroid (clobetaasol propionate 0.05%) cream. *Br J Dermatol*. 1991;124(5):461–464.

40. Sideri M, Origoni M, Spinaci L, Gerrari A. Topical testosterone in the treatment of lichen sclerosus. *Int J Obstet Gynecol*. 1994;46(1):53–56.

41. Jones SV. Eczema and pregnancy. In: Black MM, McKay M, Braude PR, Vaughan-Jones SA, Margesson LJ, editors. *Obstetric and Gynecologic Dermatology*. 2nd ed. New York: Mosby; 2002. pp. 73–77.

42. Altekrueger I, Ackerman AB. "Eczema" revisited. A status report based upon current textbooks of dermatology. *Am J Dermatopathol*. 1994;16(5):517–522.

43. Ackerman AB, Ragaz A. A plea to expunge the word "eczema" from the lexicon of dermatology and dermatopathology. *Am J Dermatopathol*. 1982;272(3–4):407–420.

44. Phelps RG, Miller MK, Singh F. The varieties of "eczema": Clinicopathologic correlation. *Clin Dermatol*. 2003;21(2):95–100.

45. Marsh DG, Meyers DA, Bias WB. The epidemiology and genetics of atopic allergy. *N Engl J Med*. 1981;305(26):1551–1559.

46. Borirakchanyavat K, Kurban AK. Atopic dermatitis. *Clin Dermatol*. 2001;18(6):649–655.

47. Berth-Jones J, Graham-Brown RA, Marks R, Camp RD, English JS, Freeman K, et al. Long term efficacy and safety of cyclosporine in severe adult atopic dermatitis. *Br J Dermatol*. 1997;136(1):76–81.

48. Morren MA, Przybilla B, Bamelis M, Heykants B, Reynaers A, Degreef H. Atopic dermatitis: Triggering factors. *J Am Acad Dermatol*. 1994;31(3 pt1):467–473.

49. Anonymous. Recommendations for using smallpox vaccine in a pre-event Vaccination Program Supplemental Recommendations of the Advisory Committee on Immunization Practices (ACIP) and the Healthcare Infection Control Practices Advisory Committee (HICPAC). *MMWR Recommendations and Report*. 2003;52(RR07);1–16.

50. Katsambas AD, Cunliffe WJ. Commentary: Acne and its treatment. *Clin Dermatol*. 2004;22(5):367–374.

51. Cunliffe WJ, Holland DB, Jeremy A. Comedone formation: Etiology, clinical presentation, and treatment. *Clin Dermatol*. 2004;22:367–374.

52. Farrar MD, Inghan E. Acne: Inflammation. *Clin Dermatol*. 2004;22(5):380–384.

53. Ellis JA, Harrap SB. The genetics of androgenetic alopecia. *Clin Dermatol*. 2001;19(2):149–154.

54. Dawber RP, Sinclair RD. Hirsuties. *Clin Dermatol*. 2001;19(2):189–199.

55. Lulemo-Aguilar J, Sabat-Santandreu M. Folliculitis: Recognition and management. *Am J Clin Dermatol*. 2004;5(5):301–310.

56. Plasencia JM. Cutaneous warts. *Dermatology*. 2000;27(2):423–434.

57. Micali G, Dall'Oglio F, Nasca MR, Tedeschi A. Management of cutaneous warts: An evidence-based approach. *Am J Clin Dermatol*. 2004;5(5):311–317.

58. Nelson JS, Stone MS. Update on selected viral exanthems. *Curr Opin Pediatr*. 2000;12(4):359–364.

59. Chuh AA. Pityriasis rosea: Roles of the dermatology nurse. *Dermatol Nurs*. 2004;16(2):130–134.

60. Scheinfeld N. Controlling scabies in institutional settings. *Am J Clin Dermatol*. 2004;5(1):31–37.

61. Scher RK, Fleckman P, Tulumbas B, McCollam L, Enfanto P. Brittle nail syndrome: Treatment options and the role of the nurse. *Dermatol Nurs*. 2003;15(1):15–23.

62. Kechijian P. Brittle fingernails. *Dermatol Clin*. 1985;3(3):421–429.

63. Scher RK, Bodian AB. Brittle nails. *Semin Dermatol*. 1991;10(1):21–25.

64. Reid IR. Calcium supplements and nail quality. *N Engl J Med*. 2000;343(24):1817.

65. Hermanns-Le T, Scheen A, Pierard GE. Acanthosis nigricans associated with insulin resistance. *Am J Clin Dermatol*. 2004;5(3):199–203.

66. Hermanns-Le T, Hermanns JF, Pierard. GE. Juvenile acanthosis nigricans and insulin resistance. *Pediatr Dermatol*. 2002;19(1):12–14.

67. Kopf AW, Salopek TG, Slade J, Marghoob AA, Bart RS. Techniques of cutaneous examination for the detection of skin cancer. *Cancer*. 1995;75(suppl):684–690.

68. Marks R. An overview of skin cancers: Incidence and causation. *Cancer*. 1995;75(suppl):607–612.

69. Bruce AJ, Brodland DG. Overview of skin cancer detection and prevention for the primary care physician. *Mayo Clin Proc*. 2000;75(5):491–500.

70. Pariser DM, Phillips PK. Basal cell carcinoma: When to treat it yourself, and when to refer. *Geriatrics*. 1994;49:39–44.

71. Scotto J, Fears TR, Fraumeni JFJ. Incidence of Nonmelanoma Skin Cancer in the United States. Bethesda, MD: U.S. Department of Health and Human Services, National Institutes of Health; 1983.

72. Marks R, Dorevitch AP, Mason G. Do all melanomas come from "moles"? A study of the histological association between melanocytic naevi and melanoma. *Aust J Dermatol*. 1990;31(2):77–80.

73. Ross PM. Apparent absence of benign precursor lesion: Implications of malignant melanoma. *J Am Acad Dermatol*. 1989;21(3 pt 1):529–538.

74. Anwar J, Wrone D, Kimyai-Asadi A, Alam M. The development of actinic keratosis into invasive squamous cell carcinoma: Evidence and evolving classification schemes. *Clin Dermatol*. 2004;22(3):189–196.

75. Marks VJ. Actinic keratosis. A premalignant skin lesion. *Otolaryngol Clin N Am*. 1993;26(1):23–35.

76. Bath-Hextall F, Bong J, Perkins W, Williams H. Interventions for basal cell carcinoma of the skin: Systematic review. *BMJ*. 2004;329(7468):705.

77. Gilbody J, Aitken J, Green A. What causes basal cell carcinoma to be the commonest cancer? *Aust J Public Health*. 1994;18:218–221.

78. Garland SM. Imiquimod. *Curr Opin Infect Dis*. 2003;16(2):85–89.

79. Osterlind A. Etiology and epidemiology of melanoma and skin neoplasm. *Curr Opin Oncol*. 1991;2:355–359.

80. Goldstein AM, Tucker MA. Etiology, epidemiology, risk factors, and public health issues of melanoma. *Curr Opin Oncol*. 1993;5(2):358–363.

81. Scarlett WL. Ultraviolet radiation: Sun exposure, tanning beds, and vitamin D levels. What you need to know and how to decrease the risk of skin cancer. *J Am Osteopath Assoc*. 2003;103(8):371–374.

82. Ridgeway CA, Hieken TJ, Ronan SG, Kim DK, das Gupta TK. Acral lentiginous melanoma. *Arch Surg*. 1995;130(1):88–92.

83. Cristofanilli M, Buzdar AU, Hortobagyi GN. Update on the management of inflammatory breast cancer. *Oncologist*. 2003;8(2):141–148.

84. Levine PH, Steinhorn SC, Reis LG. Inflammatory breast cancer. The experience of the Surveillance, Epidemiology and End Results (SEER) program. *J Natl Cancer Inst*. 1985;74:291–297.

Chapter 23

Infectious Diseases in Women

Jan M. Kriebs

Previous chapters have addressed a variety of infectious complaints, ranging from colds and flu to *H. pylori*. In this chapter, infections of the female genital tract and some other serious chronic infections are discussed. Every woman's health care provider is—or should be—familiar with these topics. A comprehensive survey of infectious diseases would fill its own text; here, those most likely to be addressed in a gynecologic setting are reviewed.

Vaginal Ecology

The female lower genital tract is a complex environment. A balanced mix of vaginal flora help to maintain the normal pH, prevent adherence of infectious organisms to the epithelial cells, prevent overgrowth of bacteria and yeasts, and contribute to the normal vaginal discharge. The dominant organisms in the healthy vagina are usually *Lactobacillus spp.*, including *L. crispatus*, *L. jensenii*, *L. acidophilus*, and others. Glycogen stores in the mucosal tissue are metabolized into lactic acid by these bacteria, helping to maintain an acidic environment. Most healthy women have hydrogen peroxide (H_2O_2)-producing strains of lactobacilli that play an active role in supporting normal flora; the release of H_2O_2 acts to decrease bacterial adherence to epithelial cells.[1,2] Diphtheroids, *Staphylococcus* and *Streptococcus* species, *Gardnerella vaginalis*, *Mycoplasma hominis*, *Escherichia coli*, *Klebsiella*, *Bacteroides*, other bacteria, and *Candida* can also be found in healthy asymptomatic women.[3–6] The relative quantity of various microorganisms as well as their efficiency in producing antibacterial substances or utilizing their environment acts to control the constituents of the microflora.[4] A normal vaginal wet mount can be seen in **Figure 23-1**.

Events that affect the hormonal balance of the vagina or disrupt the growth of normal flora are associated with increased risk of infection. During pregnancy, the presence of H_2O_2-producing lactobacilli has been demonstrated to decrease the likelihood of bacterial vaginosis and *Chlamydia* infections.[7] After menopause, women who do not take hormone therapy have a decrease in lactobacilli, elevated vaginal pH, and increased *E. coli*.[8] Race or ethnicity also may play a role. Newton et al.[9] found that African-American women consistently had more abnormal flora than Mexican-American women. In another study,[10] black women were found to have a greater likelihood than whites

Figure 23-1 Normal vaginal wet mount.

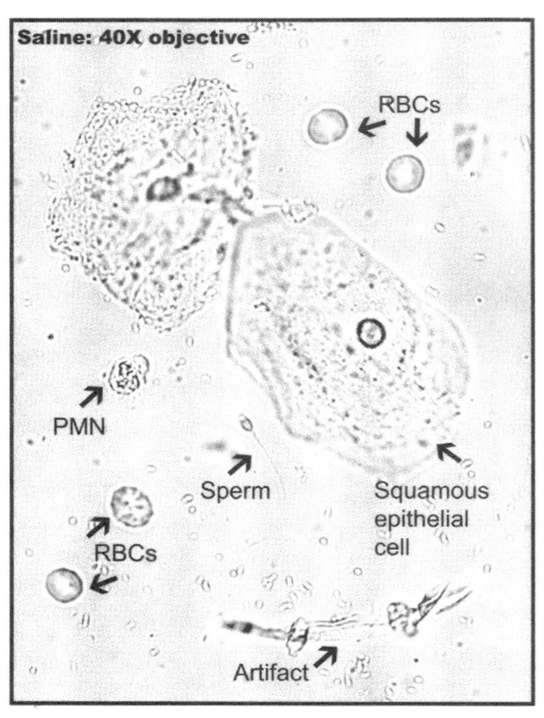

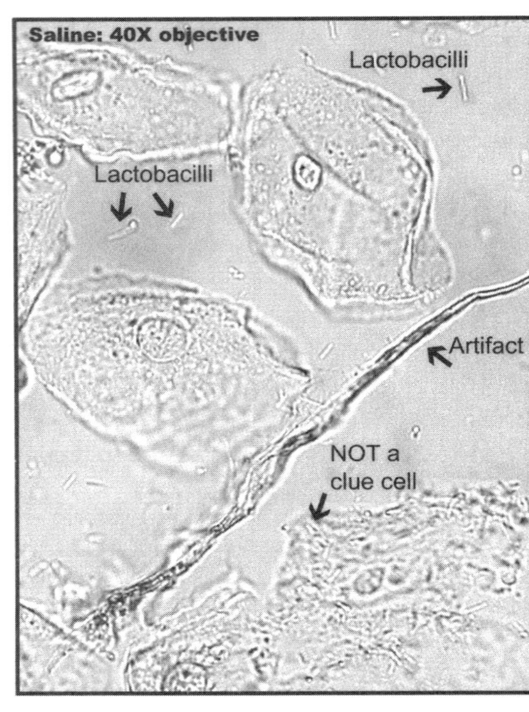

Source: Seattle STD/HIV Prevention/Training Center at the University of Washington. 11/99. Used by permission.

of decreased lactobacilli and increased Gram negative rods and *Mobiluncus* during pregnancy.

Vaginal pH changes with age. During the reproductive years, vaginal pH hovers between 3.8 and 4.2. After menopause, declining serum estradiol is associated with a shift in the vaginal pH to between 5.0 and 6.5.[11]

Other aspects of vaginal anatomy and physiology also play a role in disease transmission risk. These include: the exposed columnar epithelium found in adolescent women; increased ectropion with combined hormonal contraception and in pregnancy; and the thin epithelium of postmenopausal women and anyone with decreased estrogen status (e.g., breastfeeding women).

Counseling and Testing for Infectious Diseases

When women present to the clinical setting with complaints such as vaginal irritation or odor, pelvic pain, or an abnormal discharge, the physical examination and laboratory testing frequently can be driven by symptomatology and the woman's history. Other women present requesting testing for "everything" based on suspicion of partner infidelity or fear of a prior exposure. In the absence of specific patient concerns, counseling to address risks of serious infection is frequently omitted, based on provider assumptions about which women are at risk for infection and for which infections the woman is at risk. No group of sexually active women can be presumed to be risk-free. However, in one study, both obstetrician-gynecologists and general medical practitioners frequently omitted questions that would lead them to offer sexually transmitted disease (STD) prevention messages.[12]

Further, many women may not recognize their own risks or seek out information. Whiteside et al.[13] surveyed 103 women at several urban clinic sites. Although this population was known to be at risk for sexually transmitted infections (STIs), one-third had not heard of pelvic inflammatory disease (PID) and almost 80% were unaware of any adverse sequelae to STDs. More than half could not identify any method to prevent infection; only 18% mentioned use of a barrier contraceptive for this purpose.

Many clinicians associate the phrase "counseling and testing" with human immunodeficiency virus (HIV), but the general population's risk of HIV is statistically small. Concerns regarding possible sexual transmission of infections should be addressed by counseling prior to the examination and laboratory testing as well as in the management phase of the visit. The function of such counseling is to educate the woman about her own health, help her understand why certain tests are performed or recommended, and reduce the risk of future STDs. Introducing these topics before the examination allows the woman to participate in the decision-making process regarding testing. It also offers the opportunity to

explain which STD tests are performed, because many women expect testing to include more infections than are part of a standard evaluation. For example, human papilloma virus (HPV) or herpes simplex virus (HSV) testing is not routine in an asymptomatic woman.

History/Review of Systems

When screening for infections is done as part of an annual examination, a complete health history is taken or reviewed, and additional questions incorporated as needed to obtain a complete picture. Often, visits relating to genital infections occur as isolated problem visits. At that time, focusing on aspects of health history that affect the gastrointestinal and genitourinary systems is appropriate. This medical history should emphasize prior urinary infections, hepatitis or jaundice, and a history of unexplained pelvic or lower abdominal pain. When recurrent candidal infections are the complaint, additional questions might include diabetes, chronic antibiotic use, immune suppressive drugs, and HIV status. The social history should include questions about substances of abuse that provide direct risks (such as risk of HIV or hepatitis C transmission with intravenous drug use) as well as indirect risks associated with decreased inhibitions when using substances that reduce self-control (e.g., alcohol).

It is important to assess prior obstetric and gynecologic history whenever infection is a consideration; equally, one should anticipate the possibility of prior genital infections in any history taken in the gynecologic setting. Many of the questions asked to completely assess risk of STIs are quite personal. These questions need to be asked after other aspects of the history have been explored, when the woman is aware of her provider's interest in her general health. They can be introduced with a comment about asking all women questions that can help identify risks. The woman should be reassured that asking these questions is not a reflection on her as an individual. As with any sensitive topic, the clinician works from the most general question to the most specific, and from the least invasive to those that are more intimate. The woman's behaviors should be observed for signs of distress or withdrawal, and her emotional concerns addressed before further questions are asked.

The obstetric history is useful to identify whether infection may have played a role in any adverse reproductive outcome. Gynecologic history questions include any history of vaginal infections, PID, STD or abnormal Papanicolau (Pap) smears. The sexual history links to these questions and includes age at onset of sexual activity, number and gender of partners, number of current partners, and use of a protective barrier for sexual activity. At least among adolescents, underreporting of both STDs and pregnancies has been documented.[14]

Asking about partner behaviors can assess risk associated with sexual activity. Women who self-identify as lesbian or report having a female partner also need to be asked these questions, because many of these women have had previous experience in heterosexual relationships.[15] Further, transmission of infections between partners of the same sex is well documented.[16] **Table 23-1** lists questions that are asked to assess sexual risk factors.

The review of systems serves as a bridge between prior history and the physical examination. Gastrointestinal or genitourinary complaints need to be elicited and explored for the following:

onset; duration; quality; factors that improve or worsen the symptom; recurrence; and related symptoms or activities. With regard to STDs, this offers an additional time to incorporate questions about symptoms the current partner may be experiencing. For example, if the woman complains of an open sore, it is prudent to ask whether she has noticed similar lesions on her partner.

Physical Examination

Physical examination for possible STDs goes well beyond an examination of the genitalia because symptoms of various diseases appear in a variety of organ systems. Thus, the skin is inspected for jaundice, rashes, open sores, vesicles, solid lesions, or scarring from prior lesions. The presence or absence of lymphadenopathy is noted. Abdominal examination specifically includes assessment of hepatomegaly, any tenderness to shallow or deep palpation, and the location of any palpable masses.

Table 23-1 **SEXUAL RISK ASSESSMENT**[17,18]

Are you sexually active at this time?
How long ago were you last sexually active?
Are your sex partners male, female, or both?
Do you have vaginal sex? Oral sex? Anal sex?
Do you have sex with people you don't know well, or with someone you just met?
Do you and your partner talk about preventing infections?
What do you use to protect yourself during sex?
Do you use condoms? Always? How often?
When was the last time you had unprotected sex?
Do you or your partner have any symptoms you don't recognize?

During the genital examination, the first step in assessing for disease is to inspect the appearance of the external genitalia. Excoriation, lesions, visible discharge, changes in skin color, and any alteration in anatomy need to be noted. Edematous or swollen areas should be palpated; the Bartholin and Skene glands and the urethra should be checked for discharge.

As the speculum is inserted, attention should be paid to the tone and appearance of the vaginal walls. During the speculum examination, the speculum can be gently rotated to view all aspects of the vaginal wall and search for lesions or masses. Abnormalities of the cervix are noted, as are as the presence or absence or any discharge. Characteristics of the discharge such as appearance, color, texture, quantity, adherence to tissue, and odor are noted. The amount of ectropion present should be observed. Friability, erosion, and lesions are all recorded.

Samples for microscopic analysis or laboratory testing are collected from the appropriate location within the vagina and cervix (**Figure 23-2**). Wet mount specimens are collected from the lateral vaginal wall or pooled discharge in the posterior fornix. Samples for STD cultures or DNA testing are collected at the endocervix. Cultures for HSV are taken from visible lesions; when checking for asymptomatic shedding, both the vulva and cervix are swabbed. When testing for *group B Streptococcus*, the sample is taken from the outer third of the vagina and the rectum.

Vaginal pH can be collected at the same time. Samples for pH are taken in the posterior fornix or along the vaginal wall. The pH of the cervix is approximately 7.0 while the normal vaginal pH of reproductive age women is 3.8 to 4.2. The material obtained is applied directly to the nitrazine paper or other testing material.

The bimanual examination that follows allows the examiner to assess for cervical motion tenderness, uterine size and shape, and adnexal pain or masses.

In Office Laboratory Testing

Use of light microscopy to identify vaginal pathogens (and for fern tests) is considered a moderately complex test by the Centers for Medicare and Medicaid Services under the Clinical Laboratory Improvement Amendments (CLIA) regulations. There are specific requirements for maintaining an on-site microscope that can be reviewed at the Centers for Disease Control and Prevention (CDC) Web site.[20] Most gynecologic offices will need to maintain CLIA approval to expedite treatment of common infections.

The saline wet mount is used to identify the presence or absence of normal epithelial cells, lactobacilli, red or white blood cells, clue cells, and *Trichomonas vaginalis*. *Candida* species may also be seen on wet mount, although use of a potassium hydroxide (KOH) preparation is preferred for accuracy. The slide is prepared by placing the vaginal sample into a test tube with a small amount of saline, and plating that specimen within 15 minutes. Delay in proceeding to visualization of the slide can cause a loss of cellular integrity. A slide can be plated at the same time with a drop of KOH solution added to the specimen. The slide should be allowed to stand while the saline specimen is examined to allow for lysis of cells. Both slides are examined under 10x and 40x power.[21]

This specimen can also be used to perform the "whiff" test for bacterial vaginosis (BV). A positive whiff test is recognized by the release of amines from the lysed anaerobic bacteria when

Figure 23-2 Specimen collection.[19]

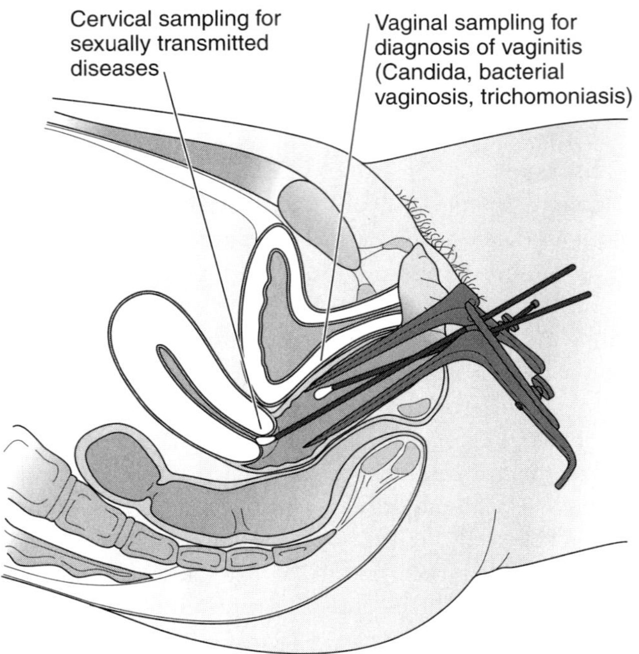

an alkaline solution is added, causing a potent fishy odor.

Laboratory tests used to diagnose specific diseases are discussed further under each heading below. **Table 23-2** compares symptoms of the common vaginal infections.

Infections Characterized by Discharge

Changes in vaginal discharge are among the first symptoms noticed by women concerned that they may have acquired an infection. Odor, irritation, changes in texture, color, or amount of fluid may be introduced as the reason for a visit. The woman's description of vaginal discharge can contribute to the plan of evaluation and be a foundation of the differential diagnosis. The astute clinician will remember that menarche, hormonal contraception, topical irritation by chemicals or latex, foreign objects left in the vagina, pregnancy, and menopause all produce changes in vaginal discharge that must be distinguished from infection. Some of these changes may precipitate infection; others are benign variations.

Candida Albicans and Other Yeasts

More than three quarters of vaginal yeast infections are the result of *C. albicans* overgrowth when lactobacilli are reduced. *C. glabrata* and

Table 23-2 SIGNS AND SYMPTOMS OF COMMON VAGINAL INFECTIONS[6,21]

	Candida albicans	Bacterial vaginosis	Trichomoniasis
Primary complaint	Itching, pain	Odor, burning	Irritation, some odor
Discharge	Internal only	Visible at introitus	Visible at introitus
Mucosal irritation	Significant erythema common	Absent	Variable
Color	White or cream	Gray	Yellow-gray, Green-gray
Viscosity	Thick	Thin	Thin
Consistency	Clumps	Homogeneous	Homogeneous, sometimes frothy
pH	~4.0	>4.5	>4.5
"Whiff" test	Absent	Present	Present ±
Wet mount	Pseudohyphae, spores, best seen with KOH *C. glabrata* – spores only	Clue cells, *Mobiluncus*, decreased white cells	Mobile trichomonads, increased white cells
Other diagnostic techniques	Culture for severe, resistant infection	Gram stain Culture less useful than PCR	Pap smear

Abbreviations: KOH, postassium hydroxide; PCR, polymerase chain reaction

C. tropicalis are other species known to cause vaginal infections. The incidence of non-*albicans* infections has been increasing, possibly as a result of selective resistance to antifungal medications and immune suppression with HIV.[22–24]

Candida spp. are considered normal in small amounts in the vagina, although colonization is heavier in women prone to recurrent infection. Giraldo et al.[25] found that polymerase chain reaction (PCR) testing identified *Candida* in about 30% of women, regardless of prior history. Both culture and wet mount were less accurate in identifying colonized women. Beigi et al.[26] identified a 70% colonization rate in young women over the course of a year, although less than 5% were colonized at every study visit.

While *Candida* infections (vulvovaginal candidiasis, VVC) are commonly reported to be about 40% of all benign vaginal infections, this cannot be easily confirmed, because many cases are self-diagnosed or diagnosed by clinicians without laboratory confirmation.[22,27,28] Self-diagnosis and inadequate triage leading to misdiagnosis contribute to unclear data regarding both frequency and treatment effectiveness.[29,30]

A clear etiology for uncomplicated VVC is frequently not seen. *Candida* is frequently present asymptomatically in the normal vagina. Onset of sexual activity, hormonal contraception, diaphragm use, and antibiotic use all have been associated with infection; the role of douching, tight clothing, feminine hygiene products, and diet have not been confirmed as contributors.[23,31,32] At least one study found an association with current or recent infection with gonorrhea and current BV.[33]

Presenting symptoms among women with VVC include painful itching and a thick clumpy (sometimes called curdy or cottage cheesy), white vaginal discharge. Other symptoms include dyspareunia, dysuria, swelling, and inflammation. The history may not provide specific clues to the diagnosis; uncontrolled diabetes and immune suppression are both associated with increased risk and with persistent recurrences.

On examination, localized edema, fissures, and excoriation of the vulva may be noted. The characteristic discharge is thickened, clumped, white or cream colored. It is frequently adherent to the vaginal walls or cervix. Wet mount findings include yeast hyphae and spores. These are best seen on KOH preparation, when other structures have been dissolved. Vaginal pH is in the normal range.

Microscopy is the most accurate diagnostic technique in the clinical setting (**Figure 23-3 A&B**). Culture is useful when frequent recurrences or failure to heal with first-line therapy indicate a more complicated infection.

The use of over-the-counter (OTC) antifungals has been widely promoted by the pharmaceutical industry and by clinicians for the treatment of uncomplicated yeast infections. There is evidence that women are frequently mistaken in their self-diagnosis, even when they read the package information and have had prior infections.[27] For this reason, initial prescriptions for new patients should never be provided without office examination, and multiple recurrent infections or inadequate response should be re-evaluated clinically, not by symptoms alone.

The standard topical azoles, whether prescriptive or OTC, have similar effectiveness rates. Short course therapies should be reserved for uncomplicated infections in healthy nonpregnant women. Oral single dose fluconazole is popular with women who can then avoid "messy" creams or suppositories. A review of oral and intravaginal methods found similar effectiveness rates in the treatment of uncomplicated VVC. Both oral and intravaginal products cure about 80% of infections in the short term.[34] However, neither short course, narrow spectrum topical products, or oral fluconazole treat non-*albicans* infections as effectively. Any factor associated with increased risk of infection or persistent recurrences should be treated initially with a seven-day course of therapy. Sequential doses of fluconazole (one 150-mg tablet orally with a second dose 3 days later) has improved outcome relative to a single oral dose.[35] Terconazole is preferable for use with recurrent infection because it has a broader antifungal spectrum. During pregnancy, standard remedies for VVC can be used safely. **Table 23-3** lists the currently available therapies for vaginal yeast infections.

Boric acid has been used as a remedy for women with persistent VVC, and has good efficacy against *Torulopsis glabrata* (also known as *C. glabrata*).[37] It requires access to a compounding pharmacy to obtain the vaginal preparation, which is a gelatin capsule with 600-mg boric acid. These are inserted vaginally at bedtime for 14 days. Vaginal irritation is an uncommon side effect. Boric acid is poisonous if taken by mouth.

Lactobacilli recolonization through ingestion of active culture yogurt has been studied with inconsistent results. However, with the exception of gastrointestinal upset in the lactose intolerant, it is a benign therapy. The evidence regarding vaginal application of yogurt is minimal and inconclusive. Tea tree oil and garlic, applied vaginally, have each been suggested to have benefit, but the data are weak.[38]

Women presenting with VVC often have symptoms they may be embarrassed to reveal, such as dyspareunia. They also may have concerns regarding the etiology of their infection. While yeast can be transmitted between partners, it is in no way a "sexually transmitted

Figure 23-3 Vulvovaginal candidiasis (VVC).

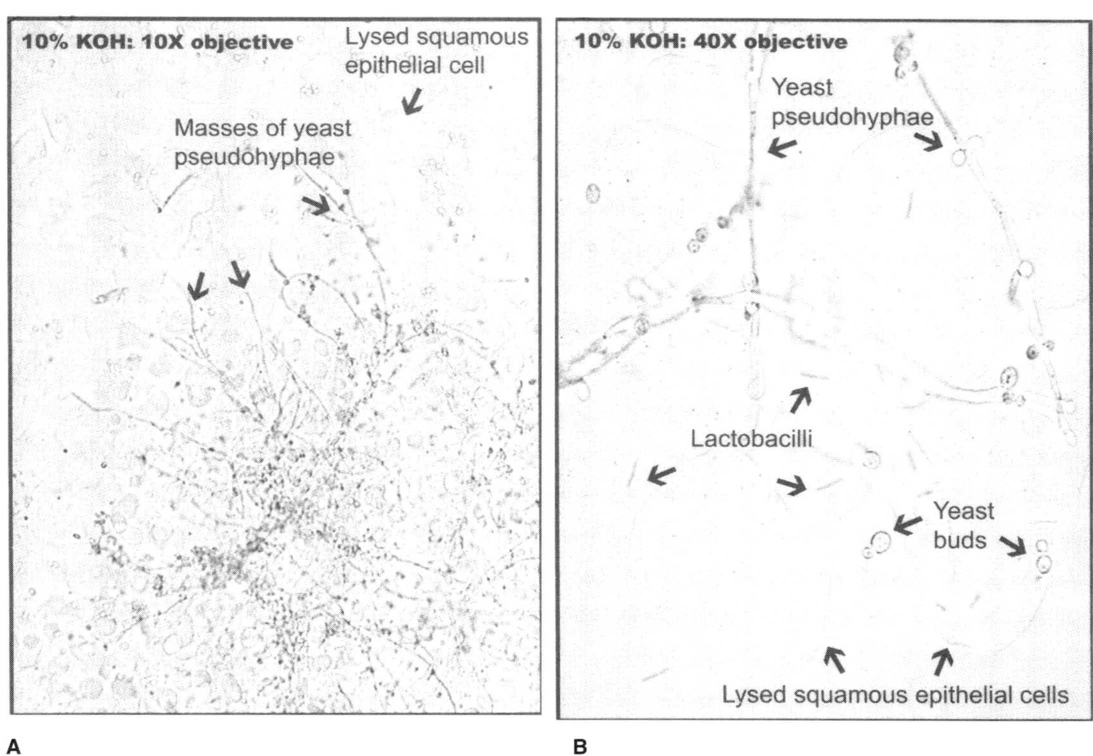

A. The 10x view shows masses of yeast pseudohyphae and a lysed squamous epithelial cell. **B.** The 40× view shows lactobacilli, yeast pseudohyphae and buds, and lysed squamous epithelial cells.
Source: Seattle STD/HIV Prevention/Training Center at the University of Washington. 11/99. Used by permission.

infection." Patient counseling includes: hygiene measures appropriate for all women; self-care during the infection; prevention of recurrent infection; consideration of changing contraceptive measures; testing for diabetes and HIV when appropriate; and reassurance that this is a common and essentially benign complaint.

Bacterial Vaginosis

BV is a noninflammatory vaginal condition characterized by overgrowth of any of several anaerobic and facultative bacteria and loss of lac-tobacilli. **Table 23-4** lists the organisms generally associated with BV, which constitutes about 40% of benign vaginal conditions. Prevalence estimates range from 5 to 37%, with the highest estimates found in STD clinics. Approximately 12% of all women have BV, although half of these women are asymptomatic.[39]

Commonly identified associations with BV include: sexual activity; early onset of sexual activity; multiple sexual partners and STIs; and African-American ethnicity. BV is found in virginal women, indicating that the infection is

Table 23-3 MEDICATIONS USED FOR VULVO-VAGINAL CANDIDIASIS[36, pp. 46–48]

Intravaginal Agents
Butoconazole (Gynazole) 2% cream
    5 g (Butaconazole1-sustained release)
       intravaginally in a single dose
    5 g intravaginally for 3 days
Clotrimazole (Gyne-Lotrimin)*
    1% cream, 5 g intravaginally for 7 to 14 days
    100 mg vaginal tablet for 7 days
    100 mg vaginal tablet, two tablets for 3 days
    500 mg vaginal tablet, one tablet in a single
       application
Miconazole (Monistat)*
    2% cream, 5 g intravaginally for 7 days
    100 mg vaginal suppository, one suppository
       for 7 days
    200 mg vaginal suppository, one suppository
       for 3 days
Tioconazole (Gyno-Troysd) 6.5% ointment
    5 g intravaginally in a single application
Terconazole (Terazol)
    0.4% cream, 5 g intravaginally for 7 days
    0.8% cream, 5 g intravaginally for 3 days
    80-mg vaginal suppository, one suppository
       for 3 days
Nystatin 100,000-unit vaginal tablet
    One tablet intravaginally for 14 days
Oral Agent
Fluconazole (Diflucan) 150-mg oral tablet
    One tablet in a single dose

*Over-the-counter (OTC) preparations.
The most current information on the CDC STD treatment guidelines can be accessed at http://www.cdc.gov/std.

Table 23-4 ORGANISMS ASSOCIATED WITH BACTERIAL VAGINOSIS

Gardnerella vaginalis
Mobiluncus sp.
Prevatella spp.
Mycoplasma hominis
Peptostreptococcus sp.
Ureaplasma urealyticum

In BV, the absence of lactobacilli, as opposed to a relative decrease, is associated with multiple sexual partners and douching more than two times per month. Beigi and colleagues have suggested that the presence or absence of H_2O_2-producing lactobacilli is a factor in co-infection with or increased risk of transmission of HIV and other STDs.[40]

In all diagnoses of infection where African-American ancestry or ethnic minority status is cited as a risk or associated factor, it is essential for the reader to recognize that these are often markers for other conditions, such as poor access to health care, poverty, over-crowding, and the like, which are more likely to be the true associations.

In turn, BV is a strong predictor of infections with *N. gonorrhoeae* and *Chlamydia* when the partner has symptoms of urethritis.[41]

Women with BV often complain of a foul "fishy" odor and associate it with sexual activity or onset of the menses. Burning or irritation is also noted. Some women may complain of feeling "wet." Just as with yeast, the symptoms are not pathognomonic. As indicated by the epidemiology, sexual activity is an essential piece of the history to collect.

On examination, a thin white discharge may be evident at the introitus. Inflammation or

not a strictly sexually transmitted condition. Recolonization after treatment is not uncommon; conversely, BV will resolve spontaneously without recurrence in some women.

erythema of the vaginal tissue is absent. The release of amines associated with a higher vaginal pH is often noticeable as the examiner approaches the perineum.

Clinically, BV is most accurately diagnosed by a combination of findings known as Amsel criteria (**Table 23-5**) or in the laboratory with the use of Gram staining. Culture is relatively less useful as many of the species found in BV are also found in normal flora. Collection of material for diagnosis with Amsel criteria is described in the section on examination of the patient; no additional procedures are necessary. Gram staining detects BV by comparing the frequency of lactobacillus morphotypes to those of *Gardnerella* and *Bacteroides*, and to curved Gram-variable rods.[42] Use of Gram staining eliminates the possibility of subjectivity in applying clinical criteria.[43] Pap smears may report the presence of a shift in microorganisms. Cervical smears that do not include vaginal sampling do not have good sensitivity. However, their specificity and positive predictive value is high, suggesting that the report of bacterial changes is a good predictor of BV.[44]

Gutman et al. recently suggested that if vaginal pH is obtained first, then a pH greater than 4.5 plus any other criterion (discharge, amines, clue cells) gives equivalent results.[45] Others

have reported that a positive whiff test plus the presence of clue cells offer an effective tool for rapid diagnosis.[46] In this study, the use of Gram staining to identify bacterial morphology to quantify relative numbers of lactobacilli versus others, or to identify clue cells, did not improve outcomes. Both of these studies described vaginal discharge as being the least useful criterion in making a diagnosis.

Wet mount findings associated with a diagnosis of BV include clue cells, decreased lactobacilli, possible *Mobiluncus*, and no increase in white blood cells (WBCs). When WBCs are seen on a slide that meets the criteria for BV, other vaginal or cervical infections should be suspected, including trichomonas, yeast, chlamydia, and gonorrhea.[47] In identifying clue cells, the clinician must recognize most visible cells as covered with adherent bacteria, causing loss of a regular cell outline and obscuring the nucleus. **Figure 23-4** illustrates clue cells.

Treatment of BV can be accomplished with any of several regimens, of which the traditional standard therapy has been a seven-day course of metronidazole. The single dose regimen is less effective in treating BV. For women with infrequent and uncomplicated infections, the use of a vaginal preparation is a reasonable option. Metronidazole and metronidazole gel have similar efficacy, while clindamycin cream is less effective.[38, p. 46] **Table 23-6** contains the CDC recommendations for the treatment of BV. Women taking oral metronidazole need to be reminded not to ingest any alcohol during and 24 hours after completing their treatment. A recent case report suggested that tinidazole, which like metronidazole is an imidazole, may be useful in treatment of refractory BV infections.[48] However, it is not currently recommended and there is little information available. Treatment

---

Table 23-5 **A**MSEL **C**RITERIA TO **D**IAGNOSE **B**ACTERIAL **V**AGINOSIS

Thin, white vaginal discharge
Amine release (positive "whiff" test)
Vaginal pH >4.5
Clue cells on wet mount

Three out of four indicators are required to diagnose BV.

Figure 23-4 Clue cells in bacterial vaginosis.

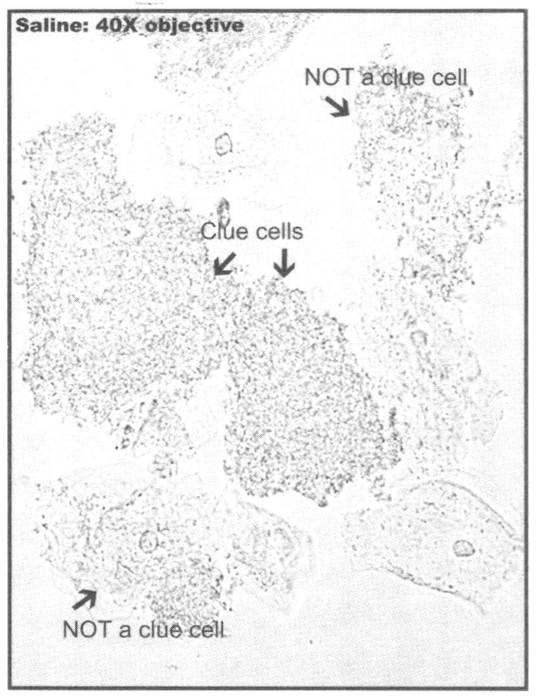

Source: Seattle STD/HIV Prevention/Training Center at the University of Washington. 11/99. Used by permission.

Table 23-6 TREATMENT REGIMENS FOR BACTERIAL VAGINOSIS[36, pp. 43,44]

Metronidazole (Flagyl)
   500 mg PO twice a day for 7 days
Metronidazole gel (Metrogel) 0.75%
   One applicator (5 g) intravaginally,
     once a day for 5 days
Clindamycin (Cleocin) cream 2%
   One applicator (5 g) intravaginally at
     bedtime for 7 days

Pregnancy regimens include:

   Metronidazole 250 mg PO tid for 7 days
   Clindamycin 300 mg PO bid for 7 days

Note: Metronidazole prescriptions should include a warning to avoid alcohol intake.

increased in women with BV and other abnormalities of genital flora. The clinician must decide whether the risks associated with asymptomatic, and probably transient, colonization outweigh the value of treatment on an individual basis.

The use of oral lactobacillus cultures in yogurt and vaginal lactobacillus capsules or suppositories has been shown to have some efficacy against BV. Tea tree oil as a suppository has been suggested to be beneficial, but there are no good data to support its use at this time.[38,49]

During pregnancy, a prior adverse pregnancy outcome associated with BV should increase the midwife's watchfulness for recurrent symptoms. Any woman who presents with symptoms should be evaluated and treated at the first prenatal visit if possible. Treatment early in pregnancy may be more effective than in the mid-trimester, when bacteria may already have colonized the cervix and lower uterine segment. However, the 2004 *Cochrane Review* found little benefit to global screening and treatment of BV

of male partners does not affect resolution or recurrence of symptoms and is not recommended.

The question of whether to treat asymptomatic colonization has been a matter of some debate. It is commonly accepted that BV is associated with a variety of both gynecologic and obstetric complications. These include: PID; post-abortal infections; post-surgical infections; endometritis; abnormal vaginal bleeding; spontaneous abortion; preterm birth; preterm premature rupture of membranes; and chorioamnionitis. Sexual acquisition of HIV is

during pregnancy.[50] The CDC recommendation is to treat with oral metronidazole or clindamycin during pregnancy.[36, p. 44] Many clinicians prefer to defer metronidazole until organogenesis is complete, although there is no evidence that first trimester use of metronidazole has risks for the fetus. Women treated in the first trimester should be evaluated for recolonization one month after treatment is complete.

Patient counseling includes information about sexual transmission of infections, use of barriers to decrease risks of infection, and the fact that BV is not an STD that requires partner treatment. Specific information about precautions for metronidazole use is essential, as is information about common side effects such as stomach upset and metallic taste. Recent information suggests that there may be an increase in preterm deliveries with metronidazole use. At this time, the recommendations have not changed; however, clinicians need to be aware of the potential risk and counsel women accordingly.[51,52]

Trichomonas Vaginalis

T. vaginalis is a flagellate protozoan that inhabits the vagina, urethra, and Bartholin and Skene glands. There are more than 7.4 million new cases in the United States each year, making it the most common non-viral STD.[53] Although it is considered an STD (in opposition to VVC and BV), there is some evidence that it can live in moist conditions for varying lengths of time. Transmission by this route has not been effectively documented.[54] Sexual transmission from male to female is more effective (67%–100%) than the reverse (14%–60%). Men are also more likely to clear *T. vaginalis* spontaneously.[55] Same sex couples can transmit *Trichomonas* during sexual activities.

Infection with *Trichomonas* is associated with: older age; African-American ethnicity; current or previous STD; and substance abuse. A variety of sequelae are reported for trichomoniasis, including: PID; preterm birth; preterm premature rupture of membranes; low birthweight babies; and increased likelihood of HIV transmission.

Presenting symptoms may include odor, irritation, dysuria, and a discolored vaginal discharge. This is a disease for which assessment of sexual relations is essential to eradicate the infection; without partner treatment, the woman will soon be re-infected.

On examination, the clinician may notice a malodorous, profuse, often frothy discharge that ranges in color from gray to yellow or green, and vulvar irritation. The vaginal pH will be >5.0. However, many women are asymptomatic, and findings on speculum examination will be the first suggestion of the presence of *Trichomonas*. These findings can include friable vaginal and cervical tissue, and occasionally, the presence of a "strawberry" cervix, the punctate surface of which is so damaged as to have visible petechiae. These are most commonly seen with colposcopy.

On microscopy, the clinician will see moving teardrop-shaped bodies, with four anterior flagella in motion (**Figure 23-5**). If the specimen has been left to sit for long, the death of the trichomonads will make diagnosis more difficult. Clinical diagnosis was only 60% accurate compared to culture results in one study.[56]

Culture is the most sensitive method of diagnosis generally available but is not typically performed at the time of the initial diagnosis. Urine cultures may be obtained when dysuria is present and a wet mount is inconclusive. Where PCR testing is available, it can be used when lack of a clear diagnosis is complicating patient management. Pap test reports of

---

Figure 23-5 Trichomonads.

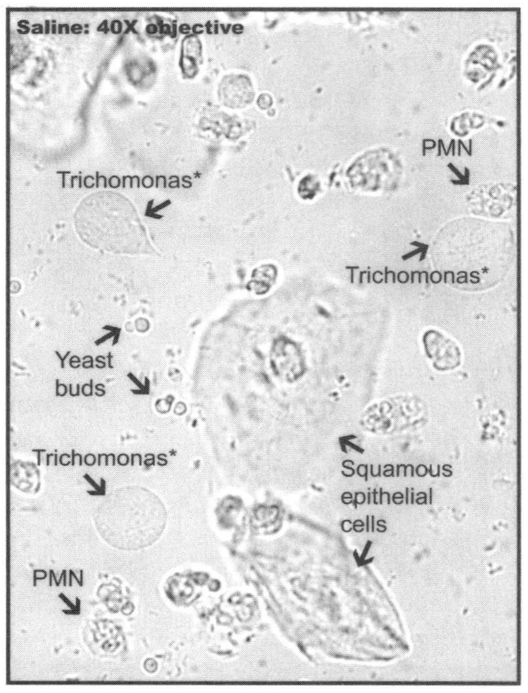

Source: Seattle STD/HIV Prevention/Training Center at the University of Washington. 11/99. Used by permission.

STD clinic is necessary. Because asymptomatic disease is common, a note stating the reason for recommended treatment should be provided. Recurrence rates are high, running 36% in one study of HIV infected women.[58] Because most re-infection involves an untreated partner, the issue of partner treatment cannot be overstated.

Metronidazole in a single 2-gram dose is the most effective therapy and will cure more than 90% of infections. Although a 1.5-gram dose has been tested and found to be efficacious in a small trial, it is not recommended.[59] A week-long course of twice daily 500 mg orally of metronidazole can be used as an alternative or for re-treatment. Persistent infection (not re-infection) requires three to five days of 2-gram daily dosing. Resistance is still rare but possible. At this time, an infectious disease consultation needs to be made when there is a question of metronidazole resistance.[36, p. 45] Potential therapies for resistant *Trichomonas* include tinidazole and paromomycin cream.[60] Paromomycin is associated with vaginal irritation and ulceration. Metronidazole gel is not an effective treatment for *T. vaginalis* infection.[61] **Table 23-7** identifies the current CDC recommended treatments for trichomoniasis.

All STDs require abstinence until treatment is complete and symptoms are resolved. After that time, use of condoms or another effective

trichomonads are not generally sensitive enough to be useful in making a diagnosis.[56] In high prevalence areas (>20%), treatment based on Pap testing can be recommended.[57] When a Pap smear result suggests the presence of *T. vaginalis*, the woman can be contacted and offered a screening visit as appropriate. The clinician must keep in mind that wet mounts have poor sensitivity as well.

Treatment of trichomoniasis involves both the woman and her partner(s). If the midwife does not prescribe for male partners, a referral for the woman's partner to another provider or the local

---

Table 23-7 TREATMENT REGIMEN FOR TRICHOMONAS[36, pp. 44–45]

Metronidazole 2 g orally in a single dose
Metronidazole 500 mg PO bid for 7 days

Single dose therapy is preferred. Note: Metronidazole prescriptions should include a warning to avoid alcohol intake. *Source:* The most current information on the CDC STD treatment guidelines can be accessed at http://www.cdc.gov/.std

barrier is advisable. When metronidazole is prescribed, a warning regarding avoidance of alcohol is required.

Vaginal trichomoniasis is associated with adverse pregnancy outcomes similar to those found in BV, particularly preterm premature rupture of the membranes, preterm birth, and low birth weight babies. Women who are symptomatic should be treated according to the CDC guidelines. The use of metronidazole in the absence of symptoms is debatable. The incidence of adverse outcomes, at least among asymptomatic women, is not lessened by treatment. It has been suggested that an inflammatory response or release of toxins from dying organisms is responsible for the failure to reduce preterm birth.[62]

Mucopurulent Cervicitis

The presence of purulent discharge from the cervix is a clear indicator of cervical infection. *N. gonorrhoeae*, *C. trachomatis*, and BV species are all associated with the presence of cervicitis. Mycoplasma was identified by one study of archived cervical specimens as being a factor associated with mucopurulent cervicitis in the absence of other identified causes.[63] Regardless of the cause, diagnosis and treatment are essential to prevent the ascending infections that can lead to chronic pain, infertility, and ectopic pregnancy. If BV species are identified along with any STD, treatment of BV will improve resolution of the cervicitis.[64]

Gonorrhea

Neisseria gonorrhoeae is the cause of about 330,000 new STDs per year in the United States.[65] It is most commonly diagnosed in young adults 15 to 24 years old. In addition to youth, belonging to an ethnic minority and concurrent infection with other STDs are risk factors. Male-to-female transmission is more common than female-to-male, with estimates of transmission as high as 50% per contact.[66] Gonorrhea is associated with increased risk of PID, co-infection with other STDs and HIV, preterm labor and birth, chronic pelvic pain, infertility, and ectopic pregnancy.

Infected men are usually symptomatic and complain of a discharge from the penis. Gonorrhea infections in women are found most commonly on routine screening; or because the woman has complaints or a history suggesting STD exposure; or because she has been told by her partner that he is infected.

On speculum examination, a mucopurulent cervical discharge is frequently seen, and indicates the presence of either gonorrhea or another cervicitis, most commonly chlamydia. The presence of BV with increased leukorrhea or increased WBCs on wet mount is also associated strongly with the presence of either gonorrhea or chlamydia.[41,67] The bimanual examination may identify mild cervical, uterine, or adnexal tenderness that does not meet the criteria for cervical motion tenderness. Women with these findings can and should be treated empirically.

Diagnosis with culture or DNA probe is the standard. Both can produce false negative findings with inadequate sampling or improper technique. Specimens are collected at the endocervix. If other body sites (i.e., rectum, throat) have been exposed, these sites should also be tested. In the symptomatic woman, treatment is not delayed while waiting for culture results. Where testing for *C. trachomatis* is not routine, treatment for both infections is accomplished simultaneously on the presumption that the two are frequently associated. If a test of cure is planned, use of DNA probes should be avoided for three to four weeks after treatment. A false positive result can be obtained if re-testing is done before bacterial DNA has been shed from the vagina.

Treatment regimens for *N. gonorrhoeae* are outlined in **Table 23-8**. An advantage of a single injection of ceftriaxone is the guarantee of observed therapy. When cefixime is available, it is a desirable regimen, with easy oral administration and minimal side effects. Cefixime manufacture was discontinued in 2002; although a generic product has been approved, it has not yet been released in tablet form. Other cephalosporins have been used, but their cure rate falls below the

---

Table 23-8 **Treatment for *N. gonorrheae*[36, pp. 37–38]**

Ceftriaxone 125 mg IM in a single dose‡
Ciprofloxacin 500 mg orally in a single dose*
Ofloxacin 400 mg orally in a single dose*
Levofloxacin 250 mg orally in a single dose*

Plus, if chlamydial infection is not ruled out:

Azithromycin 1 g orally in a single dose
Doxycycline 100 mg orally bid for 7 days

Alternatively, when other medications are contraindicated:

Spectinomycin 2 g IM†

---

* Quinolones should not be used in communities with increased gonococcal resistance to quinalones, or if the infection is believed to have been transmitted in the Pacific region. Information about quinolone resistance can be gathered from the local health department or CDC.

‡ Ceftriaxone is the preferred cephalosporin regimen. However, other single dose cephalosporins that are effective against uncomplicated gonorrhea include: cefixime 400 mg orally; ceftizoxime 500 mg IM; cefoxitin 2 g, administered IM with probenecid 1 g orally; and cefotaxime 500 mg, administered IM.

† Associated with much lower cure rates.

Source: The most current information on the CDC STD treatment guidelines can be accessed at http://www.cdc.gov/std.

95% the CDC considers acceptable, or they have not been adequately studied. Thus, substitution of another cephalosporin for cefixime is not recommended.[63] Other oral regimens are the fluoroquinolones, which cannot be used during pregnancy. The rise of fluoroquinolone-resistant strains of *N. gonorrhoeae* in Asia and on the west coast of the United States has led to a CDC recommendation that these drugs not be used in Hawaii and for any infection where exposure may have occurred in the Pacific basin. In addition, almost 20% of all cases in the United States are resistant to penicillin, tetracycline, or both. Treatment failure requires culture and sensitivity testing. When *N. gonorrhoeae* is identified at the pharynx, the CDC recommendation is to treat with ceftriaxone or with ciprofloxacin 500 mg orally, recognizing that this site is more difficult to treat and success rates are rarely above 90%.[36, p.37]

Azithromycin (2 g orally) in a single dose is effective against *N. gonorrhoeae*; however, severe gastrointestinal side effects make it less useful. If used, the 500-mg tablet form given with food should be administered.[68] The single gram dose used to treat *C. trachomatis* is not effective against *N. gonorrhoeae*.[69]

When one of the recommended regimens is used, test of cure is not necessary. Persistent symptoms are followed with culture and evaluation for other possible causes of the symptoms.

In pregnancy, fluoroquinolones are contraindicated. Women unable to take cephalosporins are treated with spectinomycin and are given a test of cure four weeks later. Exposure at birth to infectious cervical secretions can cause opthalmia neonatorum, which manifests within a few days after birth. The associated risk is infant blindness. When an infant is positive for gonococcal conjunctivitis, the risk of disseminated disease, including sepsis, meningitis, and joint inflammation should be considered.[36, pp. 38–39]

Patient teaching for gonococcal infections includes: safe sex practices; the need to have all partners treated to avoid re-infection; risks of untreated infection; and side effects of the medication prescribed. All partners within the last 60 days should be seen and evaluated. The importance of having a single, stable, faithful partner is also an essential message. Many young women define single partner and long-term relationship very differently than a clinician will.

Chlamydia

C. trachomatis is a obligate intracellular parasitic bacterium. It is the single most commonly diagnosed STD in women, with almost 930,000 new cases in the United States in 2004.[70] The primary associations are with young age and concurrent or prior STD, and the sequelae are essentially as those for gonorrhea. As many as two-thirds of tubal factor infertility cases and one-third of all ectopics can be attributed to prior chlamydia infection.[71]

Chlamydia is rarely symptomatic until ascending infection has damaged the upper genital tract. The prevalence of the infection in adolescents and women under 25 means that clinicians must be sensitive to any history suggesting unprotected sexual activity, and to any partner complaints of penile discharge or burning.

On examination, yellowish mucopurulent cervicitis may be seen. The cervix is particularly friable. One study suggested that opacity of the discharge is also a valid clinical indicator and can be used to assist in evaluation for empiric therapy.[71]

Treatment for chlamydial infection is either a single 1 g dose of azithromycin or a week

of a tetracycline. **Table 23-9** lists CDC recommended therapies. Despite its cost, the opportunity for directly observed therapy, particularly in an adolescent population, suggests the real utility of using azithromycin. During pregnancy the tetracycline antibiotics are contraindicated.

Pregnancy considerations include the very real risk of preterm birth, premature preterm

Table 23-9 **TREATMENT FOR** *T. CHLAMYDIA*[36, p. 34]

Azithromycin 1 g orally in a single dose*‡
Doxycycline 100-mg orally bid for 7 days‡
Erythromycin base 500-mg orally qid for 7 days†
Erythromycin ethylsuccinate 800-mg orally qid for 7 days†
Ofloxacin 300-mg orally bid for 7 days†
Levofloxacin 500-mg orally for 7 days†

Pregnancy

Azithromycin 1-g orally, single dose†
Erythromycin base 500-mg orally qid for 7 days†
Amoxicillin 500-mg PO orally for 7 days†

Alternative regimens in pregnancy

Erythromycin base 250-mg orally qid for 14 days†
Erythromycin ethylsuccinate 800 mg orally qid for 7 days†
Erythromycin ethylsuccinate 400 mg orally qid for 14 days†

* The CDC lists Azithromycin as an alternative regimen; however, the benefit of directly observed or single dose treatment suggests priority use.

‡ Women using these regimens do not need a test of cure except in pregnancy.

† Regimens requiring a test of cure.

Source: The most current information on the CDC STD treatment guidelines can be accessed at http://www.cdc.gov/std.

rupture of membranes, low birthweight, and decreased infant survival.[72] In addition, infants exposed to *C. trachomatis* at birth have a risk of opthalmia neonatorum that approaches 50%, and of neonatal pneumonia.

In addition to the patient counseling discussed for gonorrhea, women and girls with chlamydia need to know that not all partners may be symptomatic. Partner treatment, a mutually monogamous relationship, and condom use cannot be overemphasized in this situation.

Infections Characterized by Lesions

Just as some infections are most commonly described by the characteristics of the associated discharge, others are identified, at least in part, by the lesions produced. Visual inspection and laboratory evaluation combine to make the diagnosis. Women's health care providers should be prepared to diagnose, initiate treatment, and appreciate complications requiring referral for each of these diseases.

Syphilis

The bacterium *Treponema pallidum*, a spirochete, is responsible for syphilis. More than half of all new syphilis cases are in the southern states. Rates of syphilis in the United States are very low, with approximately 7980 new cases of primary and secondary syphilis reported in 2004,[73] but this number may underestimate total new cases. Latent phase syphilis can go undetected unless the infected person is tested in a screening program. Rates of syphilis are higher among men than women, reflecting the rise in syphilis among men who have sex with men (MSM). Rates among African Americans are 16 times

higher than in whites. The peak age at diagnosis is 20 to 29 years.

Syphilis is a moderately infectious disease, and the chance of infection from a single sexual act with an infected partner is 3% to 10%.[6] Syphilis transmission occurs when mucous membranes are exposed to the bacterium, or when abraded skin is exposed to infectious lesions. Mother-to-child transmission is possible during pregnancy and birth. Because the disease passes through stages of greater and less infectivity, and is frequently asymptomatic, diagnosis is often delayed, increasing risks of further transmission. While syphilis is curable, undiagnosed cases will persist and cause progressive damage.

After inoculation with *T. pallidum*, the time until the chancre of *primary syphilis* appears can be up to 90 days, and averages 3 weeks. The chancre is a flat, erythematous, circular open lesion with slightly raised edges. More than one may be present. It is not painful, and women often do not notice an extragenital or vaginal chancre. Spontaneous resolution occurs within a few weeks. Lymphadenopathy, with small rubbery nodes, is common during primary syphilis. Primary syphilis is the period of highest infectivity.

Secondary syphilis is the term given to the next symptomatic phase, which can occur weeks or months after the primary lesion resolves. At this point, syphilis has ceased being a localized disease and become systemic. During this second period of heightened infectivity, a reddish, painless, peeling rash appears, extending from the trunk to head, neck, and limbs, including the palms of the hands and soles of the feet. Other signs of secondary syphilis include condyloma lata (round, smooth surfaced, moist lesions arising in the genital area), patchy alopecia, and mucous lesions of the mouth, throat, and cervix.

The term used to describe the less infectious resting periods of syphilis is the *latent phase*. Early latent phase is an asymptomatic period of less than one year following exposure to syphilis. Late latent phase must be presumed when there is not a known time of exposure, and occurs at any time after the first year of untreated disease. Recurrent signs of secondary syphilis may appear during latency.

Although it is rare to see today, *tertiary syphilis* incorporates injury to liver, bones, heart, brain and skin; gummous tumors; and chronic central nervous system damage. The damage occurring during tertiary syphilis can be treated but not reversed.

Diagnosis of syphilis most commonly occurs for women during screening or as part of an STD evaluation. Since the primary lesion is painless, it is not always significant enough to bring women in for testing. In parts of the country where syphilis is more prevalent, screening during pregnancy is routine. Women presenting with STDs should also be screened as part of a complete evaluation. Both syphilis and HIV testing are often omitted from these evaluations because of their relatively low rates. Unfortunately, these are among the most damaging of all STDs. Another group who should be offered testing for syphilis is women diagnosed with pityriasis rosaea, which is a benign and self-limiting rash with an appearance similar to that of secondary syphilis.

Laboratory evaluation is a two-step process. A nonspecific treponemal antibody test (known as non-treponemal tests) is followed by an antigen-specific fluorescent antibody test (FTA) or particle agglutination test. False positive results on the antibody screen are common and can be caused by a number of bacterial and viral diseases, autoimmune diseases, pregnancy, or other medical conditions.[6,74]

The most commonly used nontreponemal antibody tests are VDRL (venereal disease research laboratory) and RPR (rapid plasma reagin) tests. Positive results on these tests must be confirmed by a positive result on a more specific test. The two most commonly used confirmation tests are the FTA and Mita-TP; these are both classified as treponemal tests. False-positive treponemal tests are very rare but can occur in individuals with lupus, other autoimmune disorders, and leprosy.[6,74]

In addition to serving as the initial test, the nontreponemal tests can be used to follow infectivity. Quantitative reporting should be done by the same lab whenever possible to reduce variation. A rise or fall of two dilutions (4-fold change) indicates a true change in disease progress. A rise from 1:32 to 1:128 would be significant, as would a fall from 1:16 to 1:4. Nontreponemal tests usually become negative over time, although some women will have persistent low titers for life, even after a cure has been effected. Treponemal tests usually remain positive for life.

Treatment with Penicillin G is always the preferred technique, so much so that the CDC recommends desensitizing allergic persons to the drug. Treatment guidelines can be found in **Table 23-10**. Partner identification and treatment should extend back for the presumed period of symptoms plus 90 days. Thus, if primary syphilis is diagnosed, partners for the prior 90 days plus the current duration of symptoms should be identified. For secondary cases, the reach back period is six months plus symptom duration, and for early latent syphilis it is one year.

Effectiveness of treatment is tracked with repeat testing every three months for one year, and every six months for the second year. A sustained reduction at that point indicates a true cure.

Table 23-10 TREATMENT OF SYPHILIS[36, pp. 19–26]

Stage	Regimen
Primary/secondary	Benzathine penicillin G 2.4 million units IM in a single dose.
Early latent syphilis Less than 12 months since documented negative test	Benzathine penicillin G 2.4 million units IM in a single dose.
Late latent syphilis or latent syphilis of unknown duration	Benzathine penicillin G 7.2 million units total, administered as three doses of 2.4 million units IM each at 1-week intervals.
Pregnancy	Seropositive pregnant women are considered infected unless an adequate treatment history is documented in the medical records and sequential serologic antibody titers have declined. Treatment during pregnancy is the same as for nonpregnant women based on stage of syphilis determined at diagnosis. Women allergic to penicillin should be desensitized and given the usual dose of penicillin. There is not good evidence regarding the effectiveness of the standard penicillin doses in preventing transmission. A second dose of penicillin can be given one week after the single dose regimen if desired.

Source: The most current information on the CDC STD treatment guidelines can be accessed at http://www.cdc.gov/std.
Abbreviation: IM, intramuscular.

During pregnancy, penicillin therapy is necessary, as it is the only agent proven to affect the fetus.[36, pp. 18–25] Treatment is the same as for nonpregnant women, although some experts will recommend an additional dose of penicillin. Untreated or inadequately treated syphilis can cause fetal syphilis (seen on ultrasound as hepatomegaly, ascites, and hydrops); preterm labor or stillbirth; and congenital syphilis. Signs of congenital syphilis include nonimmune hydrops, rhinitis (snuffles), rash, liver or splenic enlargement, and jaundice. The initial infant tests can be positive from maternal antibody, so testing of the asymptomatic infant continues every three months until a negative result is obtained. In 2004, there were 353 cases of congenital syphilis in the United States, reflecting the decline in rates among women.[73]

An uncommon but significant febrile reaction to therapy is called the Jarisch-Herxheimer reaction. Muscle aches and headache may accompany the fever. It may trigger preterm labor or fetal distress when it occurs during the second half of pregnancy.[36, pp. 18–25]

All patients who test positive for syphilis should also be tested for HIV.

Chancroid

Chancroid is a relatively rare disease in the United States, with only 30 diagnoses in 2004, the most recent reporting year.[75] Most cases are found in discrete outbreaks; cases occurred in 16 states or jurisdictions in 2004. Minority ethnicity, multiple sexual partners, prostitution, and drug use (primarily cocaine), are associated risk factors for chancroid. The disease is more common in the developing world.[76] It is included here to remind the reader that when evaluating a patient with open vulvo-vaginal lesions, herpes and syphilis are not the only possible diagnoses.

H. ducreyi is difficult to culture, and no other approved tests are available. For this reason, it is likely that the infection is underdiagnosed. The diagnosis is made by the presence of a painful genital ulcer, negative tests for syphilis and herpes, and bilateral inguinal lymphadenopathy. The ulcer is usually deeper, softer at the edges, and more irregular than a syphilitic chancre. It is always painful. One or more lesions may be present. If the adenopathy is *suppurative* (i.e., open and draining purulent discharge), the clinical presentation is classic.[36, p. 12]

Syphilis and HIV are both common co-infections with chancroid. As many as 10% of persons with chancroid will also have syphilis. Because the diagnosis of chancroid is made by exclusion, testing for *T. pallidum* should be automatic; HIV testing needs to be included as well.

Table 23-11 lists the approved regimens for treatment of chancroid. Following treatment, the woman should be re-examined within one week. If treatment is successful, marked improvement will already be apparent. Complete resolution, however, may take several weeks. All sex partners during a period of time extending back 10 days prior to the appearance of symptoms should be treated.[36, pp.11–12]

Herpes Simplex

Although herpes virus type 2 is thought of as "genital herpes," both serotypes are responsible for HSV infections on any part of the body. About two-thirds of genital infections are caused by HSV 2, the remaining third by HSV

Table 23-11 TREATMENT FOR CHANCROID[36, pp. 11–12]

Azithromycin 1 g orally, single dose
OR
Ceftriaxone 250 mg IM, single dose
OR
Ciprofloxacin 500 mg orally, twice daily for 3 days
OR
Erythromycin base 500 mg orally, 3 times daily for 7 days

Note: Ciprofloxacin is contraindicated in pregnancy.
Source: The most current information on the CDC STD treatment guidelines can be accessed at http://www.cdc.gov/std.

1. As many as 25% of Americans are positive for HSV 2 by serology, although most have had mild or subclinical infections and are not aware of their exposure.[77] HSV 1 is becoming more prevalent as a genital infection, particularly among adolescents.[78] The high prevalence of HSV 1 in the United States makes further increase in the number of genital infections likely.

Among risk factors for HSV 2 are: African-American ethnicity; female sex; older age; multiple lifetime sexual partners; young age at onset of sexual activity; less education; history of STD infections; an uncircumcised partner; smoking; douching; abnormal vaginal flora (e.g., group B streptococcus or BV); and lack of HSV 1 antibody.[79,80] The incidence is increased in women relative to men, possibly as a result of anatomic susceptibility or increased efficiency of transmission.

Transmission of HSV occurs through viral contact with mucous membranes or non-intact skin. Oral-genital transmission occurs, as can occupational transmission if abraded skin is inoculated with the virus. Subclinical shedding of

HSV can also be responsible for transmission. Wald and colleagues[81] found that overall, women with HSV experienced subclinical shedding as much as 2% of the time, or one-third of all days that the virus was reactivated. The duration of episodes of viral shedding was similar (1.5 vs. 1.8 days), whether or not symptoms were present. More recent infection and more frequent clinical recurrences were both associated with increased risk of shedding. In another study, the same team identified similar risks of viral shedding in seropositive persons without a history of clinical HSV.[82]

Prevention of all HSV transmission is not possible when couples are discordant. Prior HSV 1 infection may reduce a woman's chance of acquiring HSV 2 from a partner.[83] Condom use will reduce but not eliminate risk.[84] Subclinical shedding exposes partners who are relying on condoms to prevent infection. Suppression with valacyclovir has been demonstrated to reduce heterosexual transmission.[85] For this reason, the American College of Obstetricians and Gynecologists recommends that serodiscordant couples use suppressive therapy for the infected partner as an additional protective mechanism.[86]

The presentation of HSV is diverse, both at the time of infection and during recurrences of shedding. Approximately one-third of those with an initial HSV 2 infection will experience a primary outbreak with multiple lesions, severe pain, and systemic effects such as myalgia, lymphadenopathy, and malaise. Many others who have clinical symptoms present with the classic blisters but do not experience more severe symptoms.

Most women with clinical outbreaks notice a prodrome of burning, pain, paresthesias, or irritation along the nerve line where the virus lies dormant, lasting 12 to 24 hours prior to the onset of clinically apparent lesions. HSV lesions are typically multiple round vesicles that erode to form exquisitely tender ulcers. As the infection progresses, these develop a golden crust before resolving. In recurrent infection, the number of vesicles is fewer, and some women only have prodromal symptoms—stinging or irritation—along the nerve line, or reddened, irritated tissue. Single isolated, deep ulcers may also represent herpetic infection. Extragenital lesions are common.[87] An illustration of herpes is found in Figure 22-6.

Diagnosis of HSV should not be limited to observation of the lesions because this will miss many infected persons.[87] Culture will be most sensitive during the vesicular stage and decrease in sensitivity as the infection progresses. Type-specific serology should also be performed at this time. While one-third of initial episodes are caused by type 1 virus, the recurrence rate for these women will be much lower. Knowing the viral type influences counseling as well as the anticipated lifetime course of the infection.

Pharmacotherapy for management of HSV is shown in **Table 23-12**. Antiviral therapy is always indicated for initial outbreaks and can be prescribed empirically for women with a classic presentation. Severe disease (usually seen in primary infection and with immune suppression) requires intravenous therapy and physician management in a hospital.

Management of recurrent episodes can decrease the healing time. Suppressive therapy for those with frequent recurrences reduces the frequency and severity of outbreaks, and 70% to 80% of recurrences can be eliminated with suppression therapy. However, neither intermittent nor suppressive therapy will protect against recurrences when medication is stopped.

During pregnancy, the greatest risk of transmission of HSV to the newborn is at the time of birth. Transmission is most common among women who do not have a history of clinical

Table 23-12 AMBULATORY TREATMENT REGIMENS FOR HERPES SIMPLEX GENITALIS[36, pp. 12–17]

Primary*	
Acyclovir 400 mg	Orally 3 times a day for 7–10 days
Acyclovir 200 mg	Orally 5 times a day for 7–10 days
Famciclovir 250 mg	Orally 3 times a day for 7–10 days
Valacyclovir 1 g	Orally 2 times a day for 7–10 days
Recurrent‡	
Acyclovir 400 mg	Orally 3 times a day for 5 days
Acyclovir 200 mg	Orally 5 times a day for 5 days
Acyclovir 800 mg	Orally 3 times a day for 5 days
Famciclovir 125 mg	Orally 2 times a day for 5 days
Valacyclovir 500 mg	Orally 2 times a day for 3–5 days
Valacyclovir 1.0 g	Orally 1 time a day for 5 days
Suppression	
Acyclovir 400 mg	Orally 2 times a day,
Famciclovir 250 mg	Orally 2 times a day
Valacyclovir 500 mg	Orally 1 time a day
Valacyclovir 1.0 g	Orally 1 time a day

* Treatment of primary infection can be extended if healing is not complete.

‡ Short courses (2 days of acyclovir 800 mg PO tid or 3 days of valacyclovir 500 mg PO bid) have been studied and have similar efficacy to longer regimens.[88,89]

Source: The most current information on the CDC STD treatment guidelines can be accessed at http://www.cdc.gov/std.

outbreaks. Transmission risk is highest—up to 50%—when new infection occurs in the third trimester. Women with a history of recurrent herpes, or new infections in early pregnancy, rarely transmit. Suppressive therapy for women with frequent recurrences can be used in the late third trimester to decrease the risk of perinatal transmission. On admission in labor, all women should be evaluated for lesions or prodrome as part of the admission examination. Cesarean birth is recommended for those women who have evidence of active HSV.

Patient counseling and education for HSV includes the natural history and incurable nature of the infection, modes of transmission, and ways to decrease risks. The emotional nature of the diagnosis for many women also dictates that community resources be offered and supportive counseling provided. Many women have concerns about the safety of childbearing and about transmission to future sexual partners. An international study of patient satisfaction with care found that having educational materials easily available, taking the time for counseling at the initial visit, and effective diagnosis and treatment methods all improved patient perception of quality of care.[90]

Molluscum Contagiosum

Molluscum contagiosum is found most commonly in tropical areas, although the distribution is worldwide. A member of the pox viruses, it is frequently seen in children as a skin infection. Among adults, sexual transmission is more common. Overcrowding, poverty, and inadequate resources for good hygiene are all associated with higher rates of infection.[91]

The virus causes a benign infection of the skin. Firm raised flesh-colored nodules with a softly indented (umbilicated) center form from small papules. The average size is less than 0.5 cm. The central area is filled with a soft curd-like material that can be expressed. The nodules can appear on the genitals, buttocks and thighs, or chest. In immune-suppressed patients, large lesions may be seen on the face. See Figure 22-7 for an image of molluscum contageosum.

Transmission occurs through contact with infected skin. In addition to sexual transmission, it can be transferred from personal objects that have been in contact with lesions, and by skin-to-skin contact. The infection can be spread on the body by touching infected areas and then touching other body parts before washing. The incubation period averages two to three months after the initial exposure.[92]

A presumptive diagnosis can be made on clinical presentation. Staining of the material expressed from the nodules can identify typical "molluscum" bodies in the cytoplasm. The most accurate diagnosis is by biopsy and histopathology.[93]

Because molluscum is a benign disease with a limited course, it will resolve spontaneously after weeks or month. The potential for auto-inoculation and ease of spread through intact skin, and the appearance of the lesions, are reasons for treatment. Cryotherapy, scraping the core material out with a sharp object, curetting the lesions, application of podophyllin in the office or podopfilox at home, imiquimod cream, and other methods are equally successful.[91]

Lymphogranuloma Venereum

Lymphogranuloma venereum (LGV) is caused by some subgroups of *C. trachomatis* and is rarely seen in the United States. A genital ulcer may appear at the site of initial infection, but it quickly resolves. The more recognizable presentation is tender lymphadenopathy, most commonly in the inguinal/femoral area, but also perianally. Diagnosis is by exclusion of other causes of lymphadenopathy or by complement fixation testing.

LGV is treated with doxycycline 100 mg orally twice a day for 21 days or erythromycin base 500 mg orally four times a day for 21 days. The patient is seen regularly until all symptoms resolve. All partners counting back 30 days from onset of symptoms should be tested for *Chlamydia* and treated as above.[36, p. 18]

External Genital Warts (Human Papilloma Virus Infection)

HPV infections are found in as many as 50% of sexually active adults. More than 100 strains are known to exist; at least 30 of these strains are found predominantly in the anogenital area.[94] Their effects range from visible warts to cervical dysplasia. The association of HPV with cervical cancer is discussed in Chapter 20 and is not addressed here.

HPV types 6 and 11 are responsible for the visible warts found on the external genitalia and perianal region, vaginally, and at the cervix. Neither of these types is strongly associated with dysplasia. Many more women have subclinical infections without any obvious lesions. The viral types associated with cervical dysplasia are less commonly found in visible external lesions.[16,18,31,33,35] They are also associated with the development of vulvar neoplasia.

The appearance of visible warts is of a fleshy, exophytic mass that is easily friable and non-tender unless injured or secondarily infected. Warts found on mucous tissue are more moist in appearance, but have a similar pattern of growth. Other HPV types produce flat lesions best seen with application of acetic acid, or during colposcopy. These can occur both externally and inside the vagina. Internal HPV frequently has an associated dirty appearing vaginal discharge; this discharge is exaggerated by the presence of co-infections with vaginitis or STDs. Over time, HPV may improve spontaneously or may form progressively larger masses.

Diagnosis of HPV lesions is most commonly accomplished by visual inspection. HPV must be distinguished from condyloma lata of secondary syphilis and from neoplastic lesions. Biopsy and viral typing are not necessary to make an initial diagnosis, but they can be useful when lesions do not resolve with treatment, or when the appearance of the lesions is not clearly that of HPV.

Treatment plans for HPV focus on resolving symptomatic warts. Often treatment is followed by a period without new lesions. Most recurrences happen within the first 90 days after treatment. It is not clear whether treating warts will reduce infectivity.[36, p. 53]

Many women may prefer to use a home-based method such as imiquimod (Aldara) cream, rather than return to the office for repeated treatments. In that case, careful instructions as to use and the period of time after which the woman should return for re-evaluation should be documented. Imiquimod cream is an immune modulator that may work by stimulating alpha-interferon production. The most common side effect of imiquimod use is an erythematous "sunburn" rash over the area of application. Cure rates with this method are equivalent to office-applied therapies, and recurrence rates may be lower.[95]

Table 23-13 lists the standard treatment regimens for external warts. Use of cryotherapy, excision, or laser ablation can remove intravaginal lesions or large masses of external warts. Treatment of partners does not appear to change the natural history of infection.

Table 23-13 TREATMENT REGIMENS FOR EXTERNAL GENITAL WARTS[36, pp. 53–57]

Treatment	Comments
Imiquimod 5% cream*	Patient applies at bedtime every other day for up to 16 weeks
Podofilox 0.5% solution or gel*	Patient applies twice a day for three days, then no treatment for four days, repeated for up to four weeks.
Podophyllin resin 10%–25%* in a compound tincture of benzoin	Provider applies weekly in the office. Airdry before patient leaves the exam table. Can be washed off after 4 hours.
Trichloroacetic acid or Bichloroacetic acid 80%–90%	Provider applied weekly, only to warts and allowed to dry, at which time a white "frosting" develops. Sodium bicarbonate, talc, or liquid soap can be used to reduce discomfort after treatment.

*Not approved for treatment during pregnancy.

Source: The most current information on the CDC STD treatment guidelines can be accessed at http://www.cdc.gov/std.

During pregnancy, office-applied treatment is limited to trichloracetic acid. Use of cryotherapy, laser, or excision is not contraindicated. Cesarean section is not recommended unless the mass of warts is such as to block the birth canal or produce excessive bleeding.

Pelvic Inflammatory Disease

PID includes any infection of the upper genital tract that has ascended from the vagina and cervix, whether of the endometrium, fallopian tubes or peritoneum, and tubo-ovarian abscesses. PID is most common among women aged 15 to 24. **Table 23-14** lists organisms as-

---

Table 23-14 ORGANISMS ASSOCIATED WITH THE DEVELOPMENT OF PELVIC INFLAMMATORY DISEASE (PID)[36, p. 48,96]

N. gonorrhoeae
C. trachomatis
G. vaginalis
Prevotella sp.
H. influenzae
E. coli
S. agalactiae
S. pyogenes
S. pneumoniae
Cytomegalovirus
M. hominis
U. urealiticum
Other vaginal anaerobes associated with BV and enteric Gram negative rods

---

Source: The most current information on the CDC STD treatment guidelines can be accessed at http://www.cdc.gov/std.

sociated with the development of PID. The diversity of these organisms as well as the often vague symptoms can make acute PID difficult to diagnose when laboratory screening tests are negative or are omitted. In addition, subclinical PID can persist and cause damage. The etiologies of acute and subclinical PID are similar.[97]

While STDs are associated with most cases of PID, the risk factors for acquiring upper genital tract infection vary with the organisms involved. Studies have identified race, young age, early onset sexual activity, multiple sexual partners, sex during the menses, short duration for symptoms, and history of *N. gonorrheae* infection with prior PID as risk factors for a sexually transmitted bacterial infection causing PID.[98–100] Intrauterine device (IUD) use and recent pelvic surgery have been implicated in non-STD related PID.[100] The risk associated with IUD use appears restricted to the period immediately following insertion and is related to the introduction of vaginal flora into the uterine cavity.[101] Antibiotic prophylaxis does not appear to alter this risk.[102] Consistent use of a barrier contraceptive reduces risk of PID. However, no single characteristic, whether it be historical, physical, or laboratory based, is adequate to make the diagnosis of PID or to exclude it.[36, p. 48]

The presentation of acute PID can be vague enough that the diagnosis will be missed when clinicians are not alert to the possibility of upper genital tract disease. Vague lower abdominal pain or pain with intercourse may be the presenting symptom, as can an abnormal vaginal discharge (particularly when BV organisms are involved) or unexplained vaginal bleeding. In some women, acute lower abdominal pain, especially in the adnexa, may signal tubal disease.

On examination, vaginal discharge or mucopurulent cervicitis will suggest the need for appropriate testing. Uterine or adnexal tenderness or cervical motion tenderness on bimanual examination in sexually active women prompts empiric treatment for acute PID while laboratory results are pending; a pregnancy test should also be performed to exclude ectopic pregnancy from the differential diagnosis. Whenever the question of PID arises, cultures or DNA screens should be collected from the cervix, and a wet mount performed.

The CDC recommends the use of additional criteria to improve diagnostic accuracy.[36, pp. 48–49] These include:

- Oral temperature $>101°F$
- Mucopurulent discharge
- Increased WBCs on wet mount
- Elevated erythrocyte sedimentation rate
- Elevated C-reactive protein
- Positive test for gonorrhea or chlamydial infections

Laparoscopy, endometrial biopsy, or imaging can be used to obtain definitive diagnosis when indicated.

Alternative diagnoses need to be considered as explanations for pelvic pain, bleeding, and/or abnormal discharge. These include ectopic pregnancy, appendicitis, endometriosis, bladder infections or interstitial cystitis, and pelvic masses. Beckmann and colleagues[103] reported on data from the National Hospital Ambulatory Medical Care Survey related to emergency department care for adolescents with STDs. Among their findings was incomplete or incorrect treatment for PID in as many as 65% of all adolescent females with that diagnosis. In addition, less than half of these sexually active teens had a pregnancy test, and only 1% had HIV testing. These findings underscore the need for careful, thorough assessment of women presenting with symptoms suggestive of PID as well as the importance of considering other possible diagnoses (e.g., ectopic) and complete STD screening.

Treatment for PID incorporates broad spectrum antibiotics, with verification of efficacy not later than 72 hours after beginning medication. Patients should be asked to return for follow-up in that time frame. **Table 23-15** lists oral regimens recommended for acute uncomplicated PID. Midwives and other women's health practitioners should consult regarding PID management and refer women who need hospitalization or those for whom invasive procedures such as laparoscopy are required. Partner therapy is necessary, including all partners for two months prior to the diagnosis.

Table 23-15 ORAL MEDICATION REGIMENS FOR PELVIC INFLAMMATORY DISEASE (PID)[36, pp. 49–50]

Ofloxacin 400 mg orally, twice a day for 14 days
OR
Levofloxacin 500 mg orally, daily for 14 days
PLUS CONSIDER
Metronidazole 500 mg orally, twice a day for 14 days
Ceftriaxone 250 mg IM once
OR
Cefoxitin 2 g IM and Probenicid 1 g orally once
PLUS
Doxycycline 100 mg orally for 14 days
PLUS CONSIDER
Metronidazole 500 mg orally, twice a day for 14 days

Source: The most current information on the CDC STD treatment guidelines can be accessed at http://www.cdc.gov/std.

At times, hospitalization is required to effectively manage upper genital tract disease. During pregnancy, an initial period of hospital-based intravenous therapy is appropriate, because of the risks of chorioamnionitis and preterm birth from intrauterine infection. Women unable to accurately take medications at home, or who are too unwell to do so, need hospitalization. Tubo-ovarian abscess diagnosed with sonography or other imaging modalities, and an acute (surgical) abdomen also warrant hospitalization.

Sequelae of PID include tubal factor infertility, ectopic pregnancy, and chronic pelvic pain. Because this diagnosis represents an ascending infection that has already affected the uterus and fallopian tubes, even prompt treatment may not prevent these future problems. Prevention of STD transmission will greatly reduce the incidence of PID and is thus the best preventive for its sequelae.

Hepatitis and HIV as Sexually Transmitted Diseases

Both HIV and several forms of hepatitis are transmitted sexually. For convenience, Hepatitis A, which is transmitted through the oral-fecal route, has been grouped in this section with other forms of liver infections that are transmitted through blood and body fluids. The severity and chronic nature of many of these conditions means that midwives and nurse practitioners are unlikely to be the primary care provider. However, any person providing primary care for women needs to be familiar with the diagnosis, natural course, and general principles of management for hepatitis and HIV.

Hepatitis

The term *hepatitis* refers to any of a group of viral infections of the liver as well as to other inflammatory conditions that are not necessarily the result of infection. The discussion here is limited to the three most common viral hepatic infections: hepatitis A, B, and C (**Table 23-16**). While all health care providers should know the basics of hepatitis diagnosis and treatment, the responsibility for managing these diseases lies outside the scope of midwifery and most other women's health care providers.

HEPATITIS A

Hepatitis A virus (HAV) is transmitted by the oral-fecal route but can be an STD, as can most enteric infections; bloodborne transmission is rare. The incubation period averages one month. Virus is being shed in stool for two weeks prior to the onset of clinical disease.

Recent declines in the incidence of HAV in the United States have been attributed in large part to immunization practices.[104] A childhood vaccine is available and commonly administered. Adults who require vaccination are those at high risk, including: travelers to endemic areas; drug users; chronic liver disease patients; and MSM. Persons who are exposed to HAV can be given immune globulin to promote passive immunity. Close household and work contacts of infected persons are those most at risk.

Symptoms and signs of HAV include: flu-like syndrome; upper right quadrant abdominal pain; enlarged tender liver; splenomegaly; muscle or joint aches; itching and rash; and weight loss. Laboratory abnormalities include elevations of the aminotransferases and bilirubin.

Diagnosis is made through serology testing. A positive immunoglobulin M antibody is representative of acute infection. When a screening

Table 23-16 DIAGNOSIS OF HEPATITIS[19]

History

Blood transfusion or blood products/organs
    prior to June 1992
Previous incidence of hepatitis or jaundice
Exposure to someone who has hepatitis or is
    jaundiced
Multiple sex partners
MSM
Women having sex with MSM
Intravenous drug use—even one episode—
    even in the remote past
Immigration or travel from a country with
    endemic hepatitis
Occupation (health care worker or public
    safety worker, day care worker)
Hemophilia
History of dialysis

Clinical signs of hepatitis

Anorexia
Nausea
Vomiting
Upper-right quadrant abdominal pain
Epigastric pain
Malaise
Weakness
Fatigue
Arthralgia
Arthritis
Urticaria
Myalgia

Physical examination

Tender, enlarged liver
Enlarged spleen
Jaundice (of sclera or entire body)

Laboratory tests

Positive hepatitis screening test or
    identification of specific hepatitis antigens and
    antibodies
Elevated liver function tests AST (SGOT),
    ALT (SGPT), LDH, and bilirubin

serology is drawn, the total HAV antibody reported does not distinguish between current or past infections and prior vaccination.

Because HAV is an acute and not a chronic disease, care is palliative. The course is worse in those acquiring infection in the developing world, those with underlying liver damage, and in older adults. The elderly have an increased risk of hospitalization during the acute infection, severe complications (e.g., pancreatitis, ascites, and cholycystitis), and death.[105,106]

Pregnancy does not affect the course of HAV, nor does HAV affect the fetus. Vertical transmission has not been documented. Breastfeeding is not contraindicated.[107,108]

Patient instructions should include avoidance of exposure and the importance of vaccination for high-risk persons. Unfortunately, neither good general hygiene nor condom use will prevent transmission during sexual activity.

HEPATITIS B VIRUS

Unlike HAV, *hepatitis B virus (HBV)* is principally transmitted through exposure to blood and body fluids. About two-thirds of these transmissions are sexual. Also unlike HAV, HBV can persist as a chronic disease with risk of cirrhosis, hepatocellular carcinoma, and death. The CDC cites rates of 2% to 6% for chronic infection; up to 25% of those chronically infected will have progressive disease.[36, p. 61]

Risk factors for acquiring HBV include: any exposure to blood, semen, saliva, or vaginal secretions from an infected person, such as with unprotected sex; multiple sexual partners; intravenous drug users (IVDU); MSM; women who are intimate with MSM; infants born to infected mothers; hemodialysis patients; and residents in an endemic area (including emigrants from those areas). Both a vaccine and immune globulins are available for use in the prevention of HBV.

The incubation period for HBV averages two to three months, with a range that extends to six months. Symptoms and signs found in HBV include: nausea and vomiting; right upper quadrant abdominal pain; enlarged tender liver; jaundice; fever; chills; weakness; and headache. A rash, myalgia, arthritis, and fever may precede more classic signs. Seventy percent of those infected will have subclinical disease.

During the acute phase of the disease, palliative care is often all that is required. Fulminant liver disease is rare. Persistence of Hepatitis B surface antigen six months after the acute episode indicates a chronic infection. Most chronic HBV carriers are asymptomatic or have only vague complaints. The chronic state carries risks of chronic active liver disease, cirrhosis, and hepatocellular carcinoma. **Table 23-17** relates the various laboratory markers in HBV to the stage of disease.

The need to institute therapy is based on elevated alanine aminotransferase (ALT), presence of measurable HBV DNA, and possibly liver biopsy results. Treatment of chronic HBV can be accomplished with antiviral alpha interferon therapy. Nucleoside analogues (also used in treating HIV) appear to be effective. Combination therapies are becoming the standard of treatment. Interferon produces a number of side effects, including: fatigue and fever; various aches, weight loss, nausea, vomiting, and diarrhea; pancytopenia; neurologic and psychologic abnormalities; increased risks of infection; and autoimmune effects. Management of these medications requires an experienced infectious diseases team.[109,110]

The course of pregnancy is unchanged by HBV, unless liver damage already exists. The primary concern during pregnancy is transmission to the newborn. Ninety percent of infected infants will develop chronic disease. This risk can be reduced to about 3% by the administra-

Table 23-17 SEROLOGIC MARKERS OF HEPATITIS B STATUS[19]

Stage of HBV Infection	Hepatitis B Surface Antigen	Hepatitis B Surface Antibodies	Hepatitis B Core Antibodies	Total IGM (Anti-HBc Detects both IgM and IgG)
Late incubation	+	−	−	±
Acute	+	−	+	+
Chronic	+	− (Rarely +)	+	−
Recent (< 6 months window)	−	±	+	+
Distant (> 6 months; resolved)	−	+	+	−
Immunized	−	+ with titer >10 mIU/mL	−	−

tion of immune globulins immediately after the birth and initiation of a vaccination series. HBV infected mothers can safely breastfeed.

HEPATITIS C

Hepatitis C virus (HCV) is primarily a bloodborne disease. The highest risks are among those with repeated exposures to infected blood, whether through IVDU, transfusion with infected blood, or occupational injury. Poverty, risky sex, and lack of education are associated with increased risk. Sexual transmission is relatively uncommon and accounts for 5% to 20% of infections. Needlestick injury carries a transmission risk of 2%.

It is possible that 2.7 million Americans have active HCV with viremia.[111,112] Infected persons with high viral loads are more likely to transmit than those with low or negative RNA levels.

Incubation of HCV ranges up to six months, with an average of six to seven weeks. The acute phase is often asymptomatic. Fewer than 30% of those infected will present with jaundice, and less than half will exhibit the diagnostic signs and symptoms of hepatitis. However, progression to chronic disease occurs in 70% to 85% of those infected. Long-term risks of persistent viremia include cirrhosis, liver failure, and hepatocellular carcinoma.

The diagnosis is made with HCV antibody tests or HCV-RNA tests. Anti-HCV will be positive within three weeks after exposure, and ALT levels begin to rise within 12 weeks. Quantitative PCR testing is used to monitor the course of the disease. Screening is usually targeted to groups at risk because there is no effective preventive vaccine and no treatment for acute disease. Chronic disease is defined by persistent HCV RNA presence for six months after diagnosis.

Therapy is commonly reserved for those with viremia, abnormal ALT, and some degree of liver damage. Management of chronic disease can include treatment with ribaviron and alpha interferon. Slightly more than half of those treated have a sustained response without disease progression. Courses of medication run for several months. Ribavirin is teratogenic, so it cannot be used in pregnant women or partners of women trying to conceive.[111,112]

During pregnancy, infection in the last trimester, with the accompanying high viral loads of acute disease, may carry a risk of mother-to-child transmission as high as 33%, although 10% transmission is cited as a background rate in antibody-positive women.[113]

Patient education for both HBV and HCV deals with transmission risks to sexual partners, prevention of co-infections, signs of disease progression, and long-term sequelae.

Human Immunodeficiency Virus

HIV is an RNA retrovirus with a strong affinity for T-helper lymphocytes (CD4 cells). It has an insidious course and can remain silent for many years, thus promoting its spread by undiagnosed persons.

The natural history of HIV begins with a period of rapid viral replication; the body does not yet have an antibody response. CD4 counts drop and the viral load rises. During this period, the newly infected person may experience a flu-like syndrome with muscle aches, fever, malaise, sore throat, and lymphadenopathy. As the body mounts an immune response, viral replication is suppressed. Although rapid multiplication is still going on, the amount of circulating virus is decreased. Over time, as the immune system begins to decline, viral replication again becomes dominant and the CD4 count decreases. A normal CD4 count is above 500 cells/mm3. Levels lower than 200 cells/mm3 are one of the criteria that define acquired immune deficiency syndrome (AIDS).

Many factors play a role in determining the length of time spent in an asymptomatic state. Age, gender, race, and strain of HIV all play a role; in general, women with equivalent viral loads progress more rapidly toward AIDS than men.[114]

Although transmission was initially thought to be primarily among MSM and IVDU, the maturation of the HIV pandemic has identified heterosexual transmission as the dominant route worldwide. In the United States, men living with HIV infection still outnumber women. More than 27% of all new diagnoses are in women, and sexual transmission accounts for 80% of those new infections.[115] Fewer than 100 new perinatal infections were identified in 2003.

The wide availability of antiretroviral drugs in the developed world has created a "two-track" pandemic. For those able and willing to access antiretroviral therapy, HIV is a chronic disease whose course can be at least partially controlled. Without that access, HIV is still a progressive, invariably fatal disease. Lack of access to medications, available laboratory facilities needed to monitor for adverse events and disease progression, and well prepared clinicians are all restricting factors in the battle to control the spread of HIV.

HIV testing is accomplished as a two-step process. The initial screening test's positive predictive value is dependent on community prevalence. The enzyme-linked immunoabsorbent assay (ELISA) is a laboratory-based test detects the presence of antibodies. Several "rapid" tests have also become available, which provide a turnaround from test to results in hours rather than days. Regardless of whether a standard ELISA or one of the rapid diagnostic tests is used, confirmation with a Western blot is required before the test is reported as positive. When a single test is used to give results (as in the labor and delivery setting), the woman should always be told that the diagnosis is not assured until the confirmatory test is done. However, the high level of sensitivity for rapid tests offers an opportunity for one-visit screening, and for emergency treatment pending final results. The combination of ELISA and Western blot gives sensitivity between 99.3% and 99.7%, and a specificity of 99.7%.[116]

Risk factors for HIV infection have been well identified and include: heterosexual intercourse; African-American or Hispanic ethnicity; age <25; urban residence; intravenous drug abuse; and MSM. Infections with STDs and BV and loss of lactobacilli have been demonstrated to be associated with increased risk of HIV acquisition and viral shedding.[117–119] Among the societal factors that increase risk of transmission are lack of understanding regarding risks and sexual inequity. In addition, the CDC recommends offering testing universally in any setting where the prevalence of HIV exceeds 1%.[120]

Testing for HIV has shifted from an "opt-in" approach, in which the woman was counseled and offered testing that she had to affirmatively accept, to the "opt-out" approach, which provides testing unless specifically declined. Under this model, women still need to receive counseling about reducing risks of STD and HIV transmission, and information specific to their situation. The presence of a window after exposure during which the lack of an antibody response will cause the test to be falsely negative and the possibility of indeterminate or false positive results on the initial screening test should be mentioned. After the test is complete, women who test negative should have counseling that reinforces risk reduction. Women who test positive present greater challenges in post-test counseling. For many women, the emotional impact of being told that an HIV test is positive overshadows any other information they are given. A second encounter may be necessary to present basic information and make referrals for care. Among the topics to discuss are: interpretation of test results; monitoring health and disease progression; what treatment is available; where to find competent care; disclosure; partner notification; discrimination; and behavior changes to protect her health and prevent transmission. Observation for emotional distress or depression is essential.

Issues of disclosure are frequently difficult for newly diagnosed women. Indeed, some women will go for months or years without revealing their status to anyone. O'Brien et al. found that advancing disease was an incentive for disclosure, and that young age was linked with nondisclosure. In this study, immediate family members and primary sexual partners were most likely to be told, but less than one quarter of the patients told casual sexual partners.[121] Risky sex without disclosure has also been found to be the case for nonexclusive partners, with nondisclosure rates of 13% in serodiscordant couples.[122] Many women decrease sexual activity or increase their use of barriers after diagnosis, whether or not they have disclosed their status. Fear of violence or disruption of a stable relationship may influence some women's decisions not to share their diagnosis. Clinicians need to be aware of resources for supportive counseling and partner notification programs that women can use to inform partners of HIV exposure.

Primary care for women living with HIV includes regular assessment of disease progression, initiation of medications when the body's defenses weaken, monitoring for adverse events related to medication use, and observation for complications. Virtually all medications currently available are members of one of three classes. The nucleoside reverse transcriptase inhibitors and non-nucleoside reverse transcrip-

tase inhibitors interrupt the attempt of the virus to duplicate its genetic code, while protease inhibitors block the production of new virions through enzyme inactivation. Antiretroviral therapy is prescribed when the body's own defenses are suppressed.

Among the most common HIV complications in women are persistent, difficult to treat yeast infections, rapid progress of HPV infections and associated Pap smear abnormalities, and pneumonia.[119] Many women will still be asymptomatic when their CD4 count has dropped low enough to become an AIDS-defining condition. At that point, interventions to prevent the acquisition of opportunistic infections are necessary.

Co-infection with an STD indicates that the woman is engaging in high-risk sexual behaviors. In addition, the cumulative effect of multiple infections may worsen the course of both HIV and the STD. Close monitoring and aggressive follow-up are essential in sexually active women with risky behaviors.

Gynecologic care of the HIV seropositive woman requires particular attention to Pap smear abnormalities and aggressive management of cervical abnormalities, careful observation for lesions of the vulva and vagina, and choice of contraceptives selected with drug interactions in mind. **Table 23-18** lists common drug-drug interactions that might be seen in the gynecologic and obstetric settings.

Information about the diagnosis and management of HIV is available from many sources, including the CDC Web site.

Safer Sex and Prevention of STD Transmission

There is good evidence that consistent use of male condoms or another adequate barrier, such as the

Table 23-18 DRUG COMBINATIONS CONTRAINDICATED OR HAVING INCREASED RISK IN THE WOMEN'S HEALTH SETTING[*][123]

Drug(s)	Combination and Comments
Ergot alkaloids (methergine)	All protease inhibitors, delavirdine, efavirenz
St. John's wort	All protease inhibitors, delavirdine, efavirenz
Ketoconazole	Nevirapine
H2 blockers proton pump inhibitors	Delavirdine, atazanavir
Oral contraceptives	Additional method of contraception required with: nevirapine, efavirenz, ritonavir, amprenavir, nelfinavir, lopinavir/r, fosamprenavir
Methadone	Nevirapine, efavirenz, and some protease inhibitors will decrease methadone levels substantially and cause withdrawal

*This is not a comprehensive list. As with any medication, the prescribing provider should check for possible interactions as well as for side effects before prescribing or dispensing medications.

female condom, can reduce the transmission of STDs. For those infections that are easily transmitted, such as chlamydia or gonorrhea, consistent use with every sexual act is essential for effective prevention.[124–126] For some infections, such as genital herpes, the inability of condoms to cover all potentially infectious tissue decreases the benefit. It has been demonstrated that even intermittent use should lower the risk of transmission for HIV.[127] Although both male and female condoms are recommended as barriers to exposure to semen, and thus infection, the male condom is a more effective barrier. According to Galvao et al.,[128] patient education decreased the number of problems reported with use.

Condoms are not a perfect barrier. Breakage and slippage are both possible. Oil-based lubricants or medications (e.g., clindamycin cream) can degrade latex and cause it to tear.

For midwives and other women's health practitioners, teaching about safer sex is not the only route to prevention of genital infections. Primary prevention begins with education about delay-

ing the onset of sexual activity, limiting numbers of partners, and maintaining a monogamous relationship. Decreasing barriers to care—cost, accessibility, stigma—makes asking for information and obtaining treatment easier. The Institute of Medicine published *The Hidden Epidemic: Confronting Sexually Transmitted Diseases* in 1997.[129] Nearly a decade later the disease burden is still high, and millions of women are affected. Openly addressing these issues is an essential part of providing care to women.

After all is said and done, the other barrier to reduction of the STD burden in society may be the unwillingness of providers to adhere to CDC guidelines and standard diagnostic procedures. A number of studies have documented inadequate data collection for accurate diagnoses, failure to comply with CDC recommendations for screening and treatment, and follow-up such as management of partners.[130–132] Landers et al.[130] evaluated the predictive value of clinical diagnosis of lower genital tract disease and found that diagnosis by symptoms led to a significant number of misdiagnoses and underdiagnosis. Clinical testing improved the predictive value but still did not identify all cases correctly. Trichomoniasis and BV were more accurately diagnosed in the office than yeast. Accuracy in diagnosing gonorrhea and chlamydia required laboratory testing.[130] An evaluation of emergency department care found that fewer than 10% of cases reviewed complied with all aspects of the CDC recommendations for diagnosis and management of urethritis, cervicitis, and PID.[131] Nor is switching away from public health settings the route to improved quality of care. A quality review of the transitional period from health department to private office care in one county in Washington state found that significant variations in treatment for PID existed, Gram stains were not available, and medical records were incomplete.[132]

The message for women's health practitioners generally is clear. Self-diagnosis or symptomatic diagnosis is an inadequate technique. Where clinical testing can be provided in the office, it must be. When the result is unclear, or a laboratory test is demonstrated to be superior, then the best techniques available should be used. Before a diagnosis of refractory or recurrent disease is made, laboratory confirmation is required. The health and quality of life for women will be improved by staying with this level of evidence in making diagnoses, and knowing and following sound recommendations for care.

References

1. Hillier SL, Krohn MA, Rabe LK, Klebanoff SJ, Eschenbach DA. The normal flora, H_2O_2 producing lactobacilli, and bacterial vaginosis in pregnant women. *Clin Infect Dis*. 1993;16 Suppl 4:S273–S281.

2. Eschenbach DA, Davick PR, Williams BL, Klebanoff SJ, Young-Smith K, Critchlow CM, et al. Prevalence of hydrogen peroxide-producing *Lactobacillus* species in normal women and women with bacterial vaginosis. *J Clin Microbiol*. 1989;27:251–256.

3. Mardh P-A. The vaginal ecosystem. *Am J Obstet Gynecol*. 1991;165:1163–1168.

4. Larsen B, Monif GRG. Understanding the bacterial flora of the female genital tract. *Clin Infect Dis*. 2001; 32:e69–e77.

5. Zhou X, Bent SJ, Schneider MG, Davis CC, Islam MR, Forney LJ. Characterization of vaginal microbial communities in adult healthy women using cultivation independent methods. *Microbiology*. 2004;150: 2566–2573.

6. Droegemueller W. Infections of the lower genital tract. In: Stenchever MA, Droegemueller W, Herbst AL, Mishell DR, editors. *Comprehensive Gynecology*. 4th ed. St. Louis: Mosby; 2001. pp. 641–705.

7. Hillier SL, Krohn MA, Klebanoff SJ, Eschenbach DA. The relationship of hydrogen peroxide producing lactobacilli to bacterial vaginosis and genital microflora in pregnant women. *Obstet Gynecol*. 1992;79:369–373.

8. Pabich WL, Fihn SD, Stamm WE, Scholes D, Boyko EJ, Gupta K. Prevalence and determinants of vaginal flora in postmenopausal women. *J Infect Dis*. 2003; 188:1054–1058.

9. Newton ER, Piper JM, Shain RN, Perdue ST, Peairs W. Predictors of the vaginal microflora. *Am J Obstet Gynecol*. 2001;184:845–855.

10. Royce RA, Jackson TP, Thorp JM, Hillier SL, Rabe LK, Pastore LM, Savitz DA. Race/ethnicity, vaginal flora patterns, and pH during pregnancy. *Sex Transm Dis*. 1999;26:96–102.

11. Caillouette JC, Sharp CF, Zimmerman GJ, Roy S. Vaginal pH as a marker for bacterial pathogens and menopausal status. *Am J Obstet Gynecol*. 1997;176: 1270–1277.

12. Haley N, Maheux B, Rivard M, Andre Gervais. Sexual health risk assessment and counseling in primary care: How involved are general practitioners and obstetrician-gynecologists. *Am J Public Health*. 1999;89:899–902.

13. Whiteside JL, Katz T, Anthes T, Boardman L, Peipert JF. Risks and adverse outcomes of sexually transmitted diseases: Patients' attitudes and beliefs. *J Repro Med*. 2001;46:34–38.

14. Clark LR, Brasseux C, Richmond D, Getson P, D'Angelo LJ. Are adolescents accurate in self-report of frequencies of sexually transmitted diseases and pregnancies? *J Adolesc Health.* 1997;21:91–96.

15. Diamant AL, Schuster MA, McGuigan K, Lever J. Lesbians' sexual history with men: Implications for taking a sexual history. *Arch Internal Med.* 1999;159:2730–2736.

16. Marrazzo JM, Koutsky LA, Handsfield HH. Characteristics of female sexually transmitted disease clinic clients who report same sex behaviour. *Int J STD AIDS.* 2001;12:41–46.

17. STD/HIV Risk Assessment: A Quick Reference Guide. [Monograph on the Internet]; Accessed January 2005 Seattle STD/HIV Prevention Training Center. Seattle: University of Washington Center for Health Education and Research. Available from: http://www.seattlestdhivptc.org.

18. Anderson JR. *A Guide to the Clinical Care of Women with HIV.* Rockville, MD: United States Department of Health and Human Services, Health Resources and Services Administration; 2001.

19. Kriebs JM, Gegor CL. *Varney's Pocket Midwife.* 2nd ed. Sudbury, MA: Jones and Bartlett Publishers; 2005.

20. Centers for Disease Control. CLIA provider performed (PPM) procedures. [Monograph on the Internet; Accessed January 2005]. Atlanta: Department of Health and Human Services. Available from: http://www.phppo.cdc.gv/clia/ppm.aspx.

21. Lowe S, Saxe JM. *Microscopic Procedures for Primary Care Providers.* Philadelphia: Lippincott Williams & Wilkins; 1999.

22. Anderson MR, Klink K, Cohressen A. Evaluation of vaginal complaints. *JAMA.* 2004;291:1368–1379.

23. Spinillo A, Capuzzo E, Gulminetti R, Marone P, Colonna L, Piazzi G. Prevalence of and risk factors for fungal vaginitis caused by non-albicans species. *Am J Obstet Gynecol.* 1997;176:138–141.

24. Sobel JD, Faro S, Force RW, Foxman B, Ledger WJ, Nyirjesy PR, et al. Vulvovaginal candidiasis: Epidemiologic, diagnostic, and therapeutic considerations. *Am J Obstet Gynecol.* 1998;178:203–211.

25. Giraldo P, Von Nowaskonski A, Gomes FAM, Linhares I, Neves NA, Witkin SS. Vaginal colonization by Candida in asymptomatic women with and without a history of recurrent vulvovaginal candidiasis. *Obstet Gynecol.* 2000;95:413–416.

26. Beigi RH, Meyn LA, Moore DM, Krohn MA, Hillier SL. Vaginal yeast colonization in nonpregnant women: A longitudinal study. *Obstet Gynecol.* 2004;104:926–930.

27. Schaaf VM, Perez-Stable EJ, Borchardt K. The limited value of symptoms and signs in the diagnosis of vaginal infections. *Arch Intern Med.* 1990;150:1929–1933.

28. Wiesenfeld HC, Macio I. The infrequent use of office based diagnostic tests for vaginitis. *Am J Obstet Gynecol.* 1999;181:39–41.

29. Ferris DG, Dekle C, Litaker MS. Women's use of over-the-counter antifungal pharmaceutical products for gynecologic symptoms. *J Fam Pract.* 1996;42:595–600.

30. Allen-Davis JT, Beck A, Parker R, Ellis JL, Polley D. Assessment of vulvovaginal complaints: Accuracy of telephone triage and in-office diagnosis. *Obstet Gynecol.* 2002;99:18–22.

31. Foxman B. The epidemiology of vulvovaginal candidiasis: Risk factors. *Am J Public Health.* 1990;80:329–331.

32. Spinillo A, Capuzzo E, Acciano S, de Santolo A, Zara F. Effect of antibiotic use on the prevalence of symptomatic vulvovaginal candidiasis. *Am J Obstet Gynecol.* 1999;180:14–17.

33. Eckert LO, Hawes SE, Stevens CE, Koutsky LA, Eschenbach DA, Holmes KK. Vulvovaginal candidiasis: Clinical manifestations, risk factors, management algorithm. *Obstet Gynecol.* 1998;92:757–765.

34. Watson MC, Grimshaw JM, Bond CM, Mollison J, Ludbrook A. Oral versus intra-vaginal imidazole and triazole anti-fungal agents for the treatment of uncomplicated vulvovaginal candidiasis (thrush): A systematic review. *BJOG Int J Obstet Gynaecol.* 2002:109:85–95.

35. Sobel JD, Chaim W. Treatment of Torulopsis glabrata vaginitis: Retrospective review of boric acid therapy. *Clin Infect Dis.* 1997;24:649–652.

36. Centers for Disease Control and Prevention. Sexually transmitted diseases treatment guidelines 2002. *MMWR* 2002;51(no. RR-6). (The most current information on the CDC STD treatment guidelines including the STD treatment guidelines can be accessed at http://www.cdc.gov/std/.)

37. Sobel JD, Kapernick PS, Zervos M, Reed BD, Hooon T, Soper D, et al. Treatment of complicated Candida vaginitis: Comparison of single and sequential doses of fluconazole. *Am J Obstet Gynecol.* 2001;185:363–369.

38. Van Kessel K, Assefi N, Marrazzo J, Eckert L. Common complementary and alternative therapies for yeast vaginitis and vacterial vaginosis: A systematic review. *Obstet Gynecol Surv.* 2003;58:351–358.

39. French JI, McGregor JA. Bacterial vaginosis. In: Faro S, Soper D. *Infectious Diseases in Women*. Philadelphia: WB Saunders Company; 2001.

40. Beigi RH, Wiesenfeld HC, Hillier SL, Straw T, Krohn MA. Factors associated with absence of H_2O_2 producing *Lactobacillus* among women with bacterial vaginosis. *J Infect Dis*. 2005;191:924–929.

41. Wiesenfeld HC, Hillier SL, Krohn MA, Landers DV, Sweet RL. Bacterial vaginosis is a strong predictor of Neisseria gonorrhea and Chlamydia trachomatis infection. *Clin Infect Dis*. 2003;36:663–668. [Epub 2003].

42. Nugent RP, Krohn MA, Hillier SL. Reliability of diagnosing bacterial vaginosis is improved by a standardized method of Gram stain interpretation. *J Clin Microbiol*. 1991;29:297–301.

43. Schwebke JR, Hillier SL, Dobel JD, McGregor JA, Sweet RL. Validity of the vaginal Gram stain for the diagnosis of bacterial vaginosis. *Obstet Gynecol*. 1996; 88:573–576.

44. Davis JD, Connor EE, Clark P. Correlation between cervical cytological results and Gram stain as diagnostic tests for bacterial vaginosis. *Am J Obstet Gynecol*. 1997:177:532–535.

45. Gutman RE, Peipert JF, Weitzen S, Blume J. Evaluation of clinical methods for diagnosing bacterial vaginosis. *Obstet Gynecol*. 2005;105:551–556.

46. Thomason JL, Gelbart SM, Anderson RJ, Walt AK, Osypowski PJ, Broekhuizen FF. Statistical evaluation of diagnostic criteria for bacterial vaginosis. *Am J Obstet Gynecol*. 1990;162:155–160.

47. Geisler WM, Yu S, Venglarik M, Schwebke JR. Vaginal leukocyte counts in women with bacterial vaginosis: Relation to vaginal and cervical infections. *Sex Transm Infect*. 2004;80:401–405.

48. Baylson FA, Nyirjesy P, Weitz MV. Treatment of recurrent bacterial vaginosis with tinidazole. *Obstet Gynecol*. 2004;104:931–932.

49. Reid G, Bocking A. The potential for probiotics to prevent bacterial vaginosis and preterm labor. *Am J Obstet Gynecol*. 2003;189:1202–1208.

50. Shennan A, Crawshaw S, Briley A, Hawken J, Seed P, Jones G, et al. A randomised controlled trial of metronidazole for the prevention of preterm birth in women positive for cervicovaginal fetal fibronectin: The PREMET Study. *BJOG*. 2006;113:65–74.

51. Okun N, Gronau KA, Hannah ME. Antibiotics for bacterial vaginosis or Trichomonas vaginalis in pregnancy: A systematic review. *Obstet Gynecol*. 2005 Apr;105:857–868.

52. McDonald H, Brocklehurst P, Parsons J, Vigneswaran R. Antibiotics for treating bacterial vaginosis in pregnancy. *The Cochrane Database of Systematic Reviews*. 2003, Issue 1. Art No. CD000262. DOI:10.1002/ 1461858.CD000262.

53. Centers for Disease Control and Prevention. Trichomonas. Fact Sheet available on the Internet. Accessed July 2005. Available at: http://www.cdc. gov/std/trichomonas/stdfact-trichomoniasis.htm.

54. Mou S, Faro S. Trichomonas vaginalis. In Faro S, Soper DE. *Infectious Diseases in Women*. Philadelphia: WB Saunders Company; 2001.

55. Krieger JN. Trichomoniasis in men: Old issues and new data. *Sex Transm Dis*. 1995;22:83–96.

56. Krieger JN, Tam MR, Stevens CE, Nielsen IO, Hale J, Kiviat NB, et al. Diagnosis of trichomoniasis: Comparison of conventional wet mount examination with cytologic studies, cultures, and monoclonal antibody staining of direct specimens. *JAMA*. 1988;259: 1223–1227.

57. Wiese W, Patel SR, Patel SC, Ohl CA, Estrada CA. A meta-analysis of the Papanicolau smear and wet mount for the diagnosis of vaginal trichomoniasis. *Am J Med*. 2000;108:301–308.

58. Nicollai LM, Kopicko JJ, Kassie A, Petros H, Clark RA, Kissinger P. Incidence and predictors of reinfection with Trichomonas vaginalis in HIV infected women. *Sex Transm Dis*. 2000;27:284–288.

59. Spence MR, Harwell TS, Davies MC, Smith JL. The minimum single oral metronidazole dose for treating trichomoniasis: A randomized, blinded study. *Obstet Gynecol*. 1997;89:699–703.

60. Sobel JD, Nyirjesy P, Brown W. Tinidazole therapy for metronidazole-resistant vaginal trichomoniasis. *Clin Infect Dis*. 2001;33:1341–1346. [Epub 2001].

61. duBouchet L, McGregor JA, Ismail M, McCormack WM. A pilot study of mertonidazole vaginal gel versus oral metronidazole for the treatment of Trichomonas vaginalis vaginitis. *Sex Transm Dis*. 1998;25: 176–179.

62. Klebanoff MA, Carey JC, Hauth JC, Hillier SL, Nugent RP, Thom EA, et al. Failure of metronidazole to prevent preterm delivery among pregnant women with asymptomatic Trichomonas vaginalis infection. *N Engl J Med*. 2001;345:487–493.

63. Manhart LE, Critchlow CW, Holmes KK, Dutro SM, Eschenbach DA, Stevens CE, et al. Mucopurulent

cervicitis and Mycoplasma genitalium. *J Infect Dis.* 2003; 187:650–657.

64. Schwebke JR, Weiss HL. Interrelationships of bacterial vaginosis and cervical inflammation. *Sex Transm Dis.* 2002;29:59–64.

65. Centers for Disease Control and Prevention. STD Surveillance 2004 Gonorrhea. Database on the Internet, Accessed January 2006. http://www.cdc.gov/std/stats/gonorrhea.htm.

66. Ram S, Rice P. Gonococcal infections. In Faro S, Soper DE. *Infectious Diseases in Women.* Philadelphia: WB Saunders Company; 2001.

67. Steinhandler L, Peipert JF, Heber W, Montagno A, Cruikshank C. Combination of bacterial vaginosis and leucorrhea as a predictor of cervical chlamydial or gonococcal infection. *Obstet Gynecol.* 2002;99:603–607.

68. Centers for Disease Control and Prevention. Oral alternatives to cefixime for the treatment of uncomplicated Neisseria gonorrheae urogenital infections. *MMWR.* 2004;53:335–338.

69. Paavonen J, Eggert-Kruse W. Chlamydia trachomatis: Impact on human reproduction. *Hum Reprod Update.* 1999;5:433–447.

70. Centers for Disease Control and Prevention. STD Surveillance 2004 Chlamydia. Database on the Internet. Accessed January 2006. http://www.cec.gov/std/stats/chlamydia.htm.

71. Sellors JW, Walter SD, Howard M. A new visual indicator of chlamydial cervicitis? *Sex Transm Infect.* 2000;76:46–48.

72. Ryan GM Jr, Abdella TN, McNeeley SG, Baselski VS, Drummond DE. Chlamydia trachomatis infection in pregnancy and the effect of treatment on outcome. *Am J Obstet Gynecol.* 1990;162:34–39.

73. Centers for Disease Control and Prevention. STD Surveillance 2004. *Syphilis* [Database on the Internet; accessed January 2006.]. http://www.cdc.gov/std/stats/syph/htm.

74. Livengood CH. Syphilis. In: Faro S, Soper DE. *Infectious Diseases in Women.* Philadelphia: WB Saunders Company; 2001. pp. 403–429.

75. Centers for Disease Control and Prevention. *STD Surveillance 2004. Other Sexually Transmitted Diseases.* [database on the Internet; accessed January 2006]. Available from: http://www.cdc.gov/std/stats/other stds.htm.

76. Schmid GP. Genital Ulcer Disease. In: Faro S, Soper DE. *Infectious Diseases in Women.* Philadelphia: WB Saunders Company; 2001. pp. 504–522.

77. Stanberry L, Cunningham A, Mertz G, Mindel A, Peters B, Reitano M, et al. New developments in the epidemiology, natural history, and management of genital herpes. *Antiviral Res.* 1999;42:1–14.

78. Cowan FM, Copas A, Johnson AM, Ashley R, Corey L, Mindel A. Herpes simplex virus type 1 infection: A sexually transmitted infection of adolescence? *Sex Transm Infect.* 2002;78:346–348.

79. Cherpes TL, Meyn LA, Krohn MA, Hillier SL. Risk factors for infection with Herpes simplex virus type 2. *Sex Transm Dis.* 2003;30:405–410.

80. Gottlieb SL, Douglas JM, Schmid DS, Bolan G, Iatesta M, Malotte CK, et al. Seroprevalence and correlates of herpes simplex virus type 2 infection in five sexually transmitted disease clinics. *J Infect Dis.* 2002; 186:1381–1389.

81. Wald A, Zeh J, Selke S, Ashley RL, Corey L. Virologic characteristics of subclinical and symptomatic genital herpes infections. *N Engl J Med.* 1995;333:770–775.

82. Wald A, Zeh J, Selke S, Warren T, Ryncarz AJ, Ashley R, et al. Reactivation of genital herpes simplex virus type 2 infection in asymptomatic seropositive persons. *N Engl J Med.* 2000;342:844–850.

83. Mertz GJ, Benedetti J, Ashley R, Selke SA, Corey L. Risk factors for the sexual transmission of genital herpes. *Ann Internal Med.* 1992;116:197–202.

84. Wald A, Langenberg AG, Link K, Izu AE, Ashley R, Warren T, et al. Effect of condoms on reducing the transmission of herpes simplex virus type 2 from men to women. *JAMA.* 2001;285:3100–3106.

85. Corey L, Wald A, Patel R, Sacks S, Tyring SK, Warren T, et al. Once-daily valacyclovir to reduce the risk of transmission of genital herpes. *N Engl J Med.* 2004: 350:11–20.

86. American College of Obstetricians and Gynecologists. Gynecologic herpes simplex infections. ACOG Practice Bulletin No. 57. *Obstet Gynecol.* 2004;104: 1111–1117.

87. Lautenschlager S, Eichmsnn A. The heterogeneous clinical spectrum of genital herpes. *Dermatology.* 2001;202:211–219.

88. Wald A, Carrell D, Remington M, Kexel E, Zeh J, Corey L. Two-day regimen of acyclovir for treatment of recurrent genital herpes simplex virus type 2 infection. *Clin Infect Dis.* 2002;34:944–948.

89. Leone PA, Trottier S, Miller JM. Valacyclovir for episodic treatment of genital herpes: A shorter 3-day treatment course compared with 5-day treatment. *Clin Infect Dis.* 2002;34:958–962.

90. Patrick DM, Rosenthal SL, Stanberry LR, Hurst C, Ebel C. Patient satisfaction with care for genital herpes: Insights from a global survey. *Sex Transm Infect.* 2004;80:192–197.

91. Hanson D, Diven DG. Molluscum contageosum. [Monograph on the Internet, ©2003; accessed January 5, 2005]. Dermatology Online Journal 9(2): 2. Accessed from: http://dermatology.cdlib.org/92/reviews/molluscum/diven.html.

92. American Social Health Association. Facts and Answers about STDs: Molluscum Contagiosum. [Monograph on the Internet; January 5, 2005]. Accessed from: http://www.ashastd.org/stdfaqs/molcon.html.

93. Phillips-Smith L, Hall GS. Specimen collection and diagnostic procedures for the laboratory diagnosis of infections in females. In: Faro S, Soper DE. *Infectious Diseases in Women.* Philadelphia: WB Saunders Company; 2001.

94. Centers for Disease Control and Prevention. Human Papillomavirus (HPV) Infection. Internet site, accessed 7/1/2005 http://www.cdc.gov/HPV/default/htm.

95. Edwards L, Ferenczy A, Eron L, Baker D, Owens ML, Fox TL, et al. Self-administered topical 5% imiquimod cream for external anogenital warts. *Arch Dermatol.* 1998;134:25–30.

96. Soper DE. Pelvic inflammatory disease. In: Faro S, Soper DE. *Infectious Diseases in Women.* Philadelphia: WB Saunders Company; 2001.

97. Wiesenfeld HC, Sweet RL, Ness RB, Krohn MA, Amortegui AJ, Hillier SL. Comparison of acute and subclinical pelvic inflammatory disease. *Sex Transm Dis.* 2005;32:400–405.

98. Jossens MOR, Schachter J, Sweet RL. Risk factors associated with pelvic inflammatory disease of differing microbial etiologies. *Obstet Gynecol.* 1994;83: 989–997.

99. Jossens MOR, Eskenazi, Schachter J, Sweet RL. Risk factors for pelvic inflammatory disease: A case control study. *Sex Transm Dis.* 1996;23:239–247.

100. Miller HG, Cain VS, Rogers SM, Gribble JN, Turner CF. Correlates of sexually transmitted bacterial infections among U.S. women in 1995. *Fam Plan Perspect.* 1999;31:4–9, 23.

101. Grimes DA. Intrauterine devices and pelvic inflammatory disease: Recent developments. *Contraception.* 1987;36:97–109.

102. Walsh T, Grimes D, Frezieres R, Nelson A, Bernstein L, Coulson A, Bernstein G. Randomised

103. Beckmann KR, Melzer-Lang MD, Gorelick MH. Emergency department management of sexually transmitted infections in U.S. adolescents: Results from the National Hospital Ambulatory Medical Care Survey. *Ann Emerg Med.* 2004;43:333–338.

104. Samandari T, Bell BP, Armstrong GL. Quantifying the impact of hepatitis A immunization in the United States, 1995–2001. *Vaccine.* 2004;22:4342–4350.

105. Kyrlagkitis I, Cramp ME, Smith H, Portmann B, O'Grady J. Acute hepatitis A virus infection: A review of prognostic factors from 25 years experience in a tertiary referral center. *Hepatogastroenterology.* 2002;49:524–528.

106. Brown GR, Persley K. Hepatitis A epidemic in the elderly. *South Med J.* 2002;95:826–833.

107. Koff RS. Seroepidemiology of HAV in the United States. *J Infect Dis.* 1995;171 Suppl 1:s19–23.

108. Lawrence ML, Lawrence RA. The evidence for breastfeeding: Given the benefits of breastfeeding, what contraindications exist? *Pediatr Clin North Am.* 2001;48:1.

109. Belefer AS, Di Bisceglie AM. Hepatitis B. *Infect Dis Clin North Am.* 2000;14:617–632.

110. Lai CL, Ratziu V, Yuen M-F, Poynard T. Viral hepatitis B. *Lancet.* 2003;362:2089–2094.

111. National Institutes of Health. NIH Consensus Statement of Management of Hepatitis C: 2002. *NIH Consens State Sci Statements.* 2002;19:1–46.

112. Lauer GM, Walker BD. Hepatitis C virus infection. *N Engl J Med.* 2001;345:41–52.

113. Sabatino G, Ramenghi LA, di Marzio M, Pizzigallo E. Vertical transmission of hepatitis C virus: An epidemiological study on 2,980 pregnant women in Italy. *Eur J Epidemiol.* 1996;12:443–447.

114. Farzadegan H, Hoover DR, Astemborski J, Lyles CM, Margolick JB, Markham RB, et al. Sex differences in HIV-1 viral load and progression to AIDS. *Lancet.* 1998;352:510–514.

115. Centers for Disease Control and Prevention. HIV/AIDS among women. [Monograph on the Internet; accessed July 2005]. Accessed from: http://www.cdc.gov/hiv/pubs/facts/women.htm.

116. Iweala OI. HIV diagnostic tests: An overview. *Contraception.* 2004;70:141–147.

117. Beck EJ, Mandalia S, Leonard K, Griffith RJ, Harris JRW, Miller DL. Case-control study of sexually

transmitted diseases as cofactors for HIV-1 transmission. *Int J STD AIDS*. 1996;7:34–38.

118. Martin HL, Richardson BA, Nyange PM, Lavreys L, Hillier SL, Chohan B, et al. Vaginal lactobacilli, microbial flora, and risk of human immunodeficiency virus type 1 and sexually transmitted disease acquisition. *J Infect Dis*. 1999;180:1863–1868.

119. Rotchford K, Strum AW, Wilkinson D. Effect of co-infection with STDs and STD treatment on HIV shedding in genital-tract secretions. *Sex Transm Dis*. 2000;27:243–248.

120. Centers for Disease Control and Prevention. Advancing HIV prevention: New strategies for a changing epidemic—United States 2003. *MMWR*. 2003; 52:329–332.

121. O'Brien ME, Richardson-Alston G, Ayoub M, Magnus M, Peterman TA, Kissinger P. Prevalence and correlates of HIV serostatus disclosure. *Sex Transm Dis*. 2003;30:731–735.

122. Ciccarone DH, Kanouse DE, Collins RL, Miu A, Chen JL, Morton SC, Stall R. Sex without disclosure if positive HIV serostatus in a U.S. probability sample of persons receiving care for HIV infection. *Am J Public Health*. 2003;93:949–954.

123. Bartlett JG. *Pocket Guide to Adult HIV/AIDS Treatment*. Baltimore: The Johns Hopkins University AIDS Service; 2005.

124. Roper WL, Peterson HB, Curran JW. Commentary: Condoms and HIV/STD prevention—clarifying the message. *Am J Public Health*. 1993;83:501–503.

125. Cates W Jr, Stone KM. Family planning, sexually transmitted diseases, and contraceptive choice: A literature update. *Fam Plan Perspect*. 1992;24:75–84.

126. Weller SC. A meta-analysis of condom effectiveness in reducing sexually transmitted HIV. *Soc Sci Med*. 1993;36:1635–1644.

127. Pinkerton SD, Abramson PR. Occasional condom use and HIV risk reduction. *J AIDS Hum Retrovirol*. 1996;13:456–460.

128. Galvao LW, Oliviera LC, Diaz J, Kim D, Marchi N, van Dam J, et al. Effectiveness of female and male condoms in preventing exposure to semen during vaginal intercourse: A randomized trial. *Contraception*. 2005;71:130–136.

129. Committee on Prevention and Control of Sexually Transmitted Diseases. *The Hidden Epidemic: Confronting Sexually Transmitted Diseases*. Washington, DC: National Academy Press; 1997.

130. Landers, DV, Wiesenfeld HC, Heine RP, Krohn MA, Hillier SL. Predictive value of the clinical diagnosis of lower genital tract infection in women. *Am J Obstet Gynecol*. 2004;190:1004–1008.

131. Kane BG, Degutis LC, Sayward HK, D'Onofrio G. Compliance with the Centers for Disease Control and Prevention Recommendations for the diagnosis and treatment of sexually transmitted diseases. *Acad Emerg Med*. 2004;11:371–377.

132. Eubanks C, Lafferty WE, Kimball AM, MacCornack R, Kassler WJ. Privatization of STD services in Tacoma Washington: A quality review. *Sex Transm Dis*. 1999;26:537–542.

Index

T